# MYELIN BIOLOGY *and* DISORDERS

VOLUME 2

# MYELIN BIOLOGY *and* DISORDERS 2

Robert A. Lazzarini

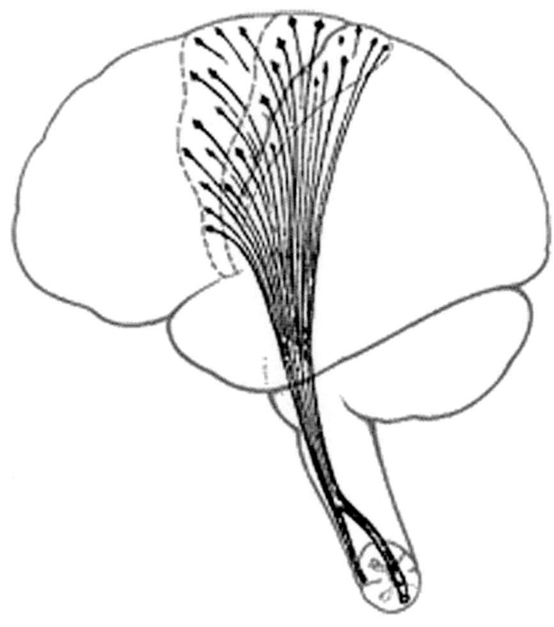

*Section Editors:*

**Robert A. Lazzarini John W. Griffin Hans Lassman Klaus-Armin Nave**

**Robert H. Miller Bruce D. Trapp**


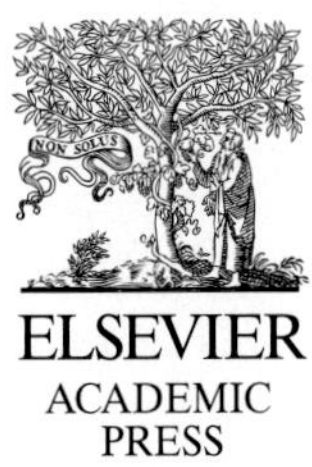

ELSEVIER
ACADEMIC
PRESS

Amsterdam • Boston • Heidelberg • London • New York • Oxford • Paris • San Diego • San Francisco • Singapore • Sydney • Tokyo

Elsevier Academic Press
525 B Street, Suite 1900, San Diego, California 92101-4495, USA
84 Theobald's Road, London WC1X 8RR, UK

This book is printed on acid-free paper. ♾



**Library of Congress Cataloging-in-Publication Data**

Lazzarini, Robert A.
Myelin biology and disorders / Robert A. Lazzarini
p. cm.
Includes index.
ISBN 0-12-439510-4 (alk. paper)
1. Myelin sheath. 2. Myelin sheath–Pathophysiology. 3. Myelin sheath–Diseases–Animal models. 4. Demyelination. I. Title

QP752.M9L39 2003
612.8′1–dc22

2003062808

**British Library Cataloguing in Publication Data**
A catalogue record for this book is available from the British Library

International Standard Book Number: 0-12-439510-4 (set)
International Standard Book Number: 0-12-439511-2 (vol. 1)
International Standard Book Number: 0-12-439512-0 (vol. 2)

For all information on all Academic Press publications
visit our website at www.academicpress.com

Printed in China
03 04 05 06 07 08 9 7 6 5 4 3 2 1

# Contents

## VOLUME 2

## 25. Integrins

*Charles ffrench-Constant*



## 26. The Periaxin Gene

*Diane L. Sherman and Peter J. Brophy*



## 27. The QKI Gene

*Rebecca J. Hardy*

# Contributors

**Mihaela Anitei** Department of Neuroscience, University of Connecticut Medical School, Farmington, Connecticut 06030-3401

**Jack Antel** Department of Neurology and Neurosurgery, McGill University, Montreal, Quebec, Canada H3A 2B4

**D. L. Arnold** Magnetic Resonance Spectroscopy Laboratory, Brain Imaging Center, Montreal Neurological Institute, Montreal, Quebec, Canada H3A 2B4

**Edgardo J. Arroyo** Department of Neurology, The University of Pennsylvania Medical Center, Philadelphia, Pennsylvania 19104

**Lakshmi Bangalore** Department of Neurology and PVA/EPVA Center for Neuroscience Research, Yale University School of Medicine, New Haven, Connecticut 06510

**Rashmi Bansal** Department of Neuroscience, University of Connecticut Medical School, Farmington, Connecticut 06030-3401

**Susan C. Barnett** Division of Clinical Neuroscience, University of Glasgow, G61 1BD Glasgow, United Kingdom

**A. Baron-Van Evercooren** The French Institute of Health and Medical Research (INSERM), CHU Pitié Salpêtrière, 75634 Paris, France

**Amit Bar-Or** Neuroimmunology Unit, Montreal Neurological Institute, Montreal, Quebec, Canada H3A 2B4

**Hugo J. Bellen** Howard Hughes Medical Institute, Department of Molecular and Human Genetics, Division of Neuroscience, Department of Molecular and Cell Biology, Program in Developmental Biology, Baylor College of Medicine, Houston, Texas 77030

**Manzoor A. Bhat** Cardiovascular Research Institute, Department of Medicine, Mount Sinai School of Medicine, New York, New York 10029

**A. J. Bieber** Department of Neurology and Program in Molecular Neuroscience, Mayo Medical and Graduate Schools, Rochester, Minnesota 55905

**W. F. Blakemore** Department of Clinical Veterinary Medicine, University of Cambridge, Cambridge, United Kingdom

**Peter E. Braun** Department of Biochemistry, McGill University, Montreal, Quebec, Canada H3G 1Y6

**Michael Brenner** Department of Neurobiology, University of Alabama at Birmingham, Birmingham, Alabama 35294-0021

**Peter J. Brophy** Department of Preclinical Veterinary Sciences, University of Edinburgh, EH9 1QH Edinburgh, Scotland

**Anthony T. Campagnoni** Neuropsychiatric Institute, University of California Medical School, Los Angeles, California 90024

**Celia W. Campagnoni** Neuropsychiatric Institute, University of California Medical School, Los Angeles, California 90024

**Alberto Cifelli** Center for Functional Magnetic Resonance Imaging of the Brain, Department of Clinical Neurology, University of Oxford, John Radcliffe Hospital, OX3 9DU Oxford, United Kingdom

**Alastair Compston** Department of Neurology, University of Cambridge Clinical School, Addenbrooke's Hospital, CB2 2QQ Cambridge, United Kingdom

**Andre Dautigny** Laboratory of Neurogenetics, National Center for Scientific Research (CNRS), UMR 7624, 75252 Paris, France

**Maria Laura Feltri** Department of Biological and Technological Research (DIBIT), San Raffaele Scientific Institute, 20132 Milan, Italy

**Robin J. M. Franklin** Department of Clinical Veterinary Medicine and Brain Repair Center, University of Cambridge, CB3 OE5 Cambridge, United Kingdom

**Charles ffrench-Constant** Cambridge Center for Brain Repair, University of Cambridge, CB2 2PY Cambridge, United Kingdom

**James Y. Garbern** Department of Neurology, Wayne State University School of Medicine, Detroit, Michigan 48201

**John Georgiou** Samuel Lunenfeld Research Institute, Mount Sinai Hospital, Toronto, Ontario, Canada M5G 1X5

**James E. Goldman** Department of Pathology and the Center for Neurobiology and Behavior, Columbia University College of Physicians and Surgeons, New York, New York 10032

**Steven A. Goldman** Department of Neurology and Neuroscience, Cornell University Medical College, New York, New York 10021

**Alexander Gow** Center for Molecular Medicine and Genetics, Departments of Pediatrics and Neurology, Wayne State University School of Medicine, Detroit, Michigan 48301

**John W. Griffin** Department of Neurology, The John Hopkins University School of Medicine, Baltimore, Maryland 21287-7608

**Ian R. Griffiths** Institute of Comparative Medicine, Glasgow, United Kingdom

**Michel Gravel** Department of Biochemistry, McGill University, Montreal Quebec, Canada H3G 1Y6

**Rebecca J. Hardy** MRC National Survey of Health and Development, Department of Epidemiology and Public Health, University College London Medical School, WC1E 6BT London, United Kingdom

**Lynn D. Hudson** National Institute of Neurological Disorders and Stroke, National Institutes of Health, Bethesda, Maryland 20892-4160

**K. R. Jessen** Department of Anatomy and Developmental Biology, University College London, WC1E 6BT London, United Kingdom

**Richard T. Johnson** Department of Neurology, John Hopkins School of Medicine, Baltimore, Maryland 21287

**John A. Kamholz** Department of Neurology, Wayne State University, Detroit, Michigan 48201

**Grahame J. Kidd** Department of Neuroscience, Lerner Research Institute, Cleveland Clinic Foundation, Cleveland, Ohio 44195

**Daniel A. Kirschner** Biology Department, Boston College, Chestnut Hill, Massachusetts 02467-3811

**Kleopas A. Kleopa** The Cyprus Institute of Neurology and Genetics, 1683 Nicosia, Cyprus

**Hans Lassmann** Division of Neuroimmunology, Brain Research Institute, University of Vienna, A 1090 Wien, Austria

**Christopher Linington** Neuroimmunology Department, Max Planck Institute, Martinsried, Germany

**Fred D. Lublin** Corinne Goldsmith Dickinson Center for Multiple Sclerosis, Mount Sinai Medical Center, New York, New York 10032

**Eugene O. Major** Laboratory of Molecular Medicine and Neuroscience, National Institute of Neurological Disorders and Stroke, National Institutes of Health, Bethesda, Maryland 20892

**Cecilia B. Marta** Department of Neuroscience, University of Connecticut Medical School, Farmington, Connecticut 06030-3401

**P. M. Matthews** Magnetic Resonance Spectroscopy Laboratory, Brain Imaging Center, Montreal Neurological Institute, Montreal, Quebec, Canada H3A 2B4

**Albee Messing** Department of Pathobiological Sciences, University of Wisconsin School of Veterinary Medicine, Madison, Wisconsin 53706

**Robert Miller** Department of Neuroscience, Case Western Reserve University, School of Medicine, Cleveland, Ohio 44106

**R. Mirsky** Department of Anatomy and Developmental Biology, University College London, WC1E 6BT London, United Kingdom

**Hugo W. Moser** Neurogenetics Research, Kennedy Krieger Institute, Baltimore, Maryland 21205

**Klaus-Armin Nave** Max Planck Institute of Experimental Medicine, Göttingen, Germany

**Pedro Pasik** Department of Neurology, Mount Sinai School of Medicine, New York, New York 10029

**Tauba Pasik** Department of Neurology, Mount Sinai School of Medicine, New York, New York 10029

**David L. Paul** Department of Molecular Cell Biology, Weizmann Institute of Science, 76100 Rehovot, Israel

**Elior Peles** Department of Molecular Cell Biology, Weizmann Institute of Science, 76100 Rehovot, Israel

**Steven E. Pfeiffer** Department of Neuroscience, University of Connecticut Medical School, Farmington, Connecticut 06030-3401

**Danielle Pham-Dinh** The French Institute of Health and Medical Research (INSERM), U 546, University of Paris, 75013 Paris, France

**James M. Powers** Department of Pathology and Laboratory Medicine, University of Rochester School of Medicine, Rochester, New York 14627

**Mahendra Rao** Laboratory of Neurosciences, Gerontology Research Center, National Institute on Aging, National Institutes of Health, Baltimore, Maryland 21224

**Richard Reynolds** Department of Neuroinflammation, Division of Neuroscience, Imperial College Faculty of Medicine, Charing Cross Campus, W68 RF London, United Kingdom

**John C. Roder** Samuel Lunenfeld Research Institute, Mount Sinai Hospital, Toronto, Ontario, Canada M5G 1X5

**M. Rodriguez** Departments of Neurology, Immunology, and Program in Molecular Neuroscience, Mayo Medical and Graduate Schools, Rochester, Minnesota 55905

**Neeta S. Roy** Department of Neurology and Neuroscience, Cornell University Medical College, New York, New York 10021

**Steven S. Scherer** Department of Neurology, The University of Pennsylvania Medical Center, Philadelphia, Pennsylvania 19104

**Karen L. Schulze** Howard Hughes Medical Institute, Department of Molecular and Human Genetics, Division of Neuroscience, Department of Molecular and Cell Biology, Program in Developmental Biology, Baylor College of Medicine, Houston, Texas 77030

**Kazim Sheikh** Department of Neurology, Johns Hopkins University School of Medicine, Baltimore, Maryland 21287

**Diane L. Sherman** Department of Preclinical Veterinary Sciences, University of Edinburgh, EH9 1 QH Edinburgh, Scotland

**Ueli Suter** Institute for Cell Biology, Eth Zurich, 8093 Zurich, Switzerland

**Kunihiko Suzuki** Brain and Developmental Research Center, University of North Carolina, Chapel Hill, North Carolina 27599

**Peter K. Stys** Department of Medicine, Division of Neuroscience, University of Ottowa, Ottowa, Canada K1Y 4E9

**Christopher M. Taylor** Department of Neuroscience, University of Connecticut Medical School, Farmington, Connecticut 06030-3401

**Bruce D. Trapp** Department of Neuroscience, Lerner Research Institute, Cleveland Clinic Foundation, Cleveland, Ohio 44195

**Michael B. Tropak** Samuel Lunenfeld Research Institute, Mount Sinai Hospital, Toronto, Ontario, Canada M5G 1X5

**Stephen G. Waxman** Department of Neurology and PVA/EPVA Center for Neuroscience Research, Yale University School of Medicine, New Haven, Connecticut 06510, and Rehabilitation Research Center, VA Connecticut Healthcare System, Westhaven, Connecticut 06516

**Martha S. Windrem** Department of Neurology and Neuroscience, Cornell University Medical College, New York, New York 10021

**Lawrence Wrabetz** Department of Biological and Technological Research (DIBIT), San Raffaele Scientific Institute, 20132 Milan, Italy

## SECTION IV

# HUMAN DISEASES OF MYELIN

CHAPTER

# 28

# The Leukodystrophies: Overview and Classification

*James M. Powers*

## DISORDERS OF CENTRAL WHITE MATTER: LEUKOENCEPHALOPATHIES, LEUKODYSTROPHIES DEMYELINATION, DYSMYELINATION

"When I use a word," Humpty Dumpty said
in a rather scornful tone, "It means just what
I choose it to mean. Neither more nor less."
*Through the Looking Glass*
Lewis Carroll

Myelin, the lipid-protein insulating coat of axons, is largely restricted to white matter of the central nervous system (CNS) and to larger axons of the peripheral nervous system (PNS). Therefore, diseases that specifically affect myelin, often referred to as primary diseases of myelin (Figures 28.1A, B), by necessity affect either CNS white matter, myelinated axons in the PNS, or both. The converse is not always true. That is, there are several disease processes that affect CNS white matter, or less commonly myelinated PNS fibers, but do not specifically or primarily affect myelin or myelinating cells. These latter entities are in reality secondary or coincidental disorders of myelin, and their etiologies are diverse. One of the clearest examples of this secondary type of myelin loss, usually referred to as secondary demyelination, is due to a primary loss of axons from the death of its distant parent neuron (Wallerian or Wallerian-like degeneration) (Fig. 28.1C). Another is vascular disease, such as subcortical arteriosclerotic leukoencephalopathy (often referred to as "Binswanger disease"), which is attributed to the small vessel lesions of chronic hypertension (Fig. 28.1D) (Babikian and Ropper, 1987). In "Binswanger disease," there is a predominant destruction of cerebral white matter (Fig. 28.2) that varies from lacunar (small cystic) infarcts to concomitant and equivalent losses of myelin and axons to a preferential loss of myelin, in association with markedly hyalinized regional blood vessels (De Reuck *et al.*, 1980). Another cerebral leukoencephalopathy presumed to be due to ischemia is its rare occurrence in amyloid angiopathy (Gray *et al.*, 1985); here, however, the vascular lesions reside in amyloidotic leptomeningeal arteries/arterioles. Vascular lesions displaying the preferential loss of myelin share the major neuropathologic characteristic of primary diseases of myelin: loss of myelin and oligodendrocytes with relative sparing of axons; but the primary cause of this myelin loss is ischemia (vascular insufficiency) in which oligodendrocytes and their myelin sheaths are more affected than their neighbors. The vulnerability of oligodendrocytes to oxygen deprivation, particularly in the human post-natal period when they are heavily involved in myelination, and their destruction by

 

## White Matter Lesions

A Normal

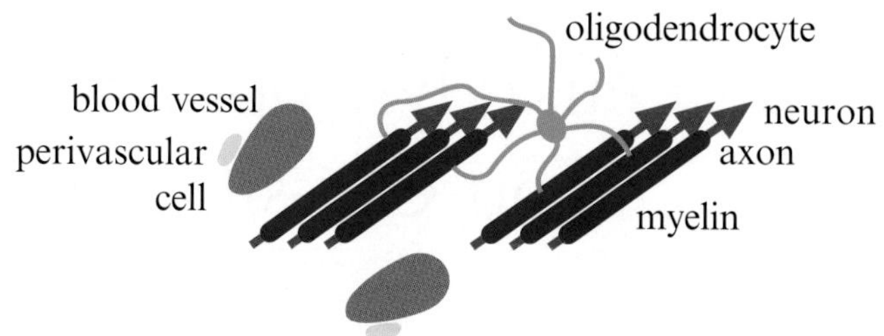


B Primary demyelination

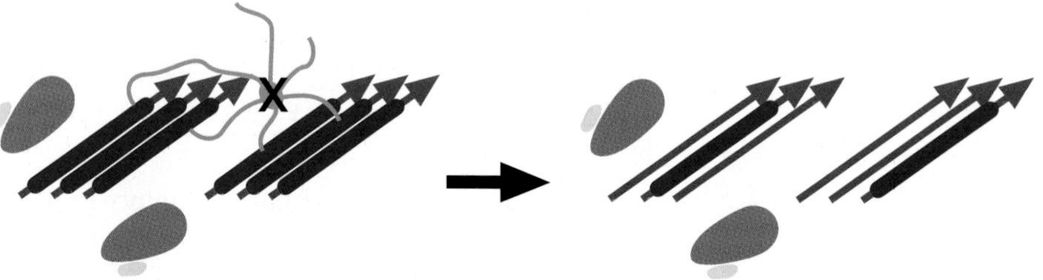

C Secondary demyelination

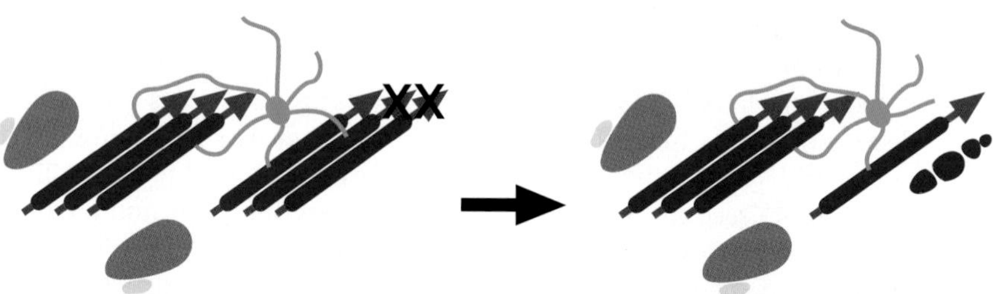

D Leukoencephalopathy

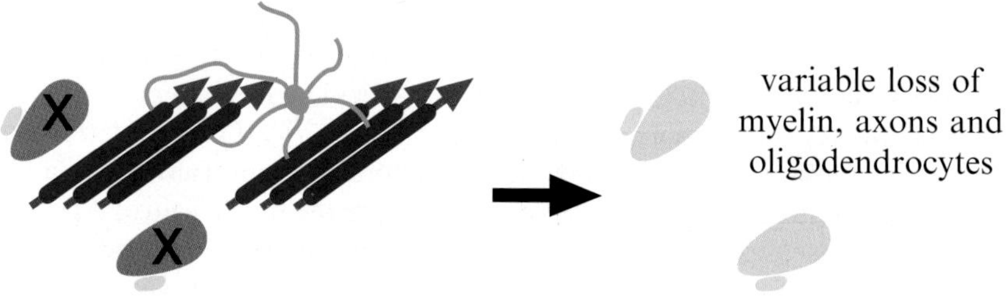


FIGURE 28.1
Schematic diagrams of primary and secondary lesions of myelin. X identifies the initial or primary lesion in B, C, and D.

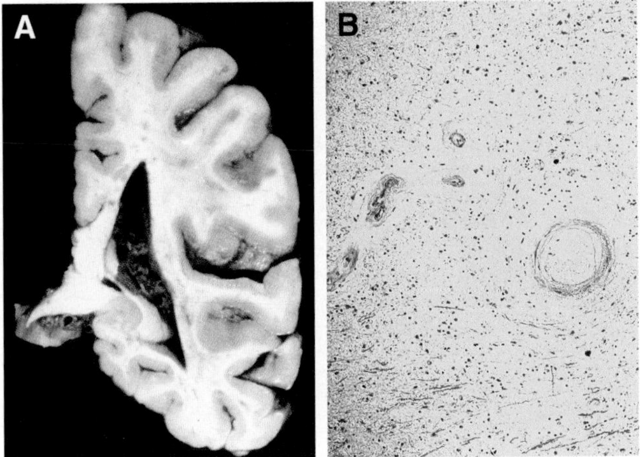


FIGURE 28.2
Diffuse atrophy with focal gray discoloration and cavitation of parietal white matter in "Binswanger disease." (B) Hyalinized blood vessels within myelin-depleted white matter of "Binswanger disease." Hematoxylin-eosin.

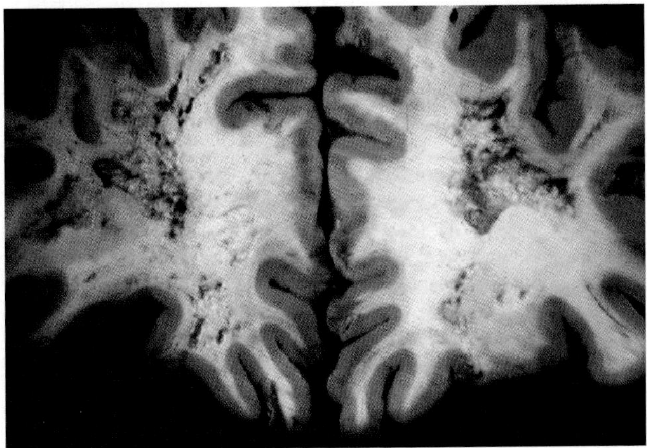

FIGURE 28.3
Bilateral symmetrical necrosis of frontal white matter with sparing of cortical gray in severe hypoxia-ischemia, such as CO poisoning.

hypoxic-ischemic insults are well documented (reviewed in Ludwin, 1997). The clinical presentation of such an hypoxic or ischemic destruction of white matter may occur cataclysmically, as in the delayed leukoencephalopathy of carbon monoxide (CO) poisoning (Fig. 28.3) (Grinker's myelinopathy) (Plum *et al.*, 1962), or more surreptitiously as in "Binswanger disease." The latter's chronic and progressive clinical course mimics that of primary diseases of myelin, in particular the major focus of this chapter: the leukodystrophies. CADASIL (cerebral autosomal dominant arteriopathy with subcortical infarcts and leukoencephalopathy) also may exhibit a chronic and progressive clinical course, often dementing, due primarily to the destruction of cerebral white matter; it is familial and is associated with a defect in the Notch 3 gene (Joutel *et al.*, 1996; Tournier-Lasserve *et al.*, 1993). In view of its genetic causation, its progressive clinical course, and its predominant white matter lesion, CADASIL has been included by some under the rubric of "leukodystrophies." In my opinion, this is inappropriate because CADASIL lacks the most important pathogenetic criterion of the leukodystrophies: the primary involvement of myelin sheaths/myelinating cells. Available evidence for the destruction of cerebral white matter in CADASIL indicates that it too is fundamentally ischemic and due to arterial abnormalities (Fig. 28.4) obvious at both light (granular medial myocytic degeneration) and electron (granular osmiophilic material, GOM) microscopic levels (Baudrimont *et al.*, 1993). Cer-

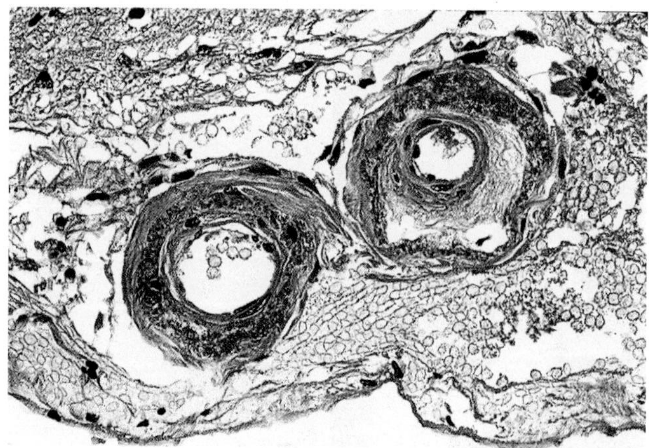

FIGURE 28.4
Granular degeneration of medial myocytes in small arteries of CADASIL. Hematoxylin-eosin.

tain chemotherapeutic agents and illicit drugs or toxins, such as solvent vapor exposure, also can lead to confluent losses of cerebral myelin (Kornfeld *et al.*, 1994).

"It was the best of times, it was the worst of times . . . it was the season of Light, it was the season of Darkness," wrote Charles Dickens concerning England and France in 1775 (Dickens, 1894). In respect to our molecular understanding of genetic diseases, including those of myelin, the present is the best of times and a season of Light; one only has to witness the transformation of the single volume of Stanbury *et al.*'s *The Metabolic Basis of Inherited Disease* of 1983 to its four-volume heir, Scriver *et al.*'s *The Metabolic and Molecular Bases of Inherited Disease* of 2001. Many of the pathogenetic advances that have expanded this tome were derived from mouse mutants, both natural and genetically engineered, and by other powerful molecular methodologies. At the same time, it would profit us to interpret these modern data within the context of a large repository of clinical and basic neuroscience, such as classical neuropathologic studies of the leukodystrophies (reviewed in Powers, 1996). While darkness no longer prevails, there still are many persistent glimmers in our current scientific world that are aggravated by the imprecise use of language. Sometimes a linguistic imprecision reflects a limited understanding of a scientific process, such as the difficulty in determining neuropathologically whether a developmental delay or a complete arrest in myelination is responsible for some cases of "hypomyelination," but too often it is due to an ignorance of, or unwillingness to acknowledge, well-documented scientific precedent. Enlightened scientific discourse can be facilitated by the persistent use of traditional terms and concepts, rather than their distortion or the fabrication of neologisms. As cases in point, consider the current designation of Alzheimer's disease by some as an inflammatory disease, the same historical etiologic category as bacterial meningitis; or the term "intracellular amyloid" for a substance (amyloid) defined in part for over a century by its extracellular localization; or the inclusion of CADASIL within the leukodystrophies. The latter decision ignores both the pathologic data mentioned above and its neuropathologic appellation: *leukoencephalopathy*.

A more relevant, and pervasive, linguistic impropriety has occurred with the terms "demyelination" and "dysmyelination, which has led to much confusion. Some use "demyelination" to describe any loss of myelin staining in CNS white matter. Such linguistic promiscuity has been rightly condemned by Raine, one of the world's experts in myelin diseases (discussed in Raine, 1997, p. 627, and the earlier editions 1991 and 1985); he also objects to the term "secondary demyelination" as used earlier. Moreover, both he and Prineas (Prineas *et al.*, 2002, and the previous edition 1997), another leader in this field, equate "demyelinating" diseases with acquired autoimmune and suspected autoimmune diseases usually accompanied by perivascular demyelination/inflammation, in keeping with the historical precedents set by Adams and Kubik (1952) for demyelinating diseases and Poser (1962, 1968). Poser divided the primary diseases of myelin into two major types: myelinoclastic (currently referred to as demyelinating or demyelinative) and dysmyelinating (Poser, 1968). These two major types were established primarily on the basis of their differing pathogeneses: acquired immune and inflammatory for demyelinating disorders versus an heredofamilial metabolic abnormality in myelin without inflammation for dysmyelinating disorders. To quote Poser: "The first, the 'myelinoclastic' type, constitutes the true demyelinating diseases.... The other type, exemplified by the leukodystrophies...groups together the 'dysmyelinating' diseases." While Adams's and Poser's classifications were not universally accepted and had some flaws (as do all classification schemes), most found their concepts of demyelinating and dysmyelinating diseases to be rational and useful. To quote Raine: "'Demyelination' is a term carefully avoided by most authors in reference to the hereditary dysmyelinating diseases (metachromatic leukodystrophy, Krabbe's disease, adrenoleukodystrophy, etc.).... Thus, there is currently consensus among neuropathologists that 'demyelination' should be a term reserved for the multiple sclerosis group of conditions." (Raine, 1997, 1991, 1985). Would that life were that simple! Recently, two other good friends and colleagues, as preeminent in the neuroradiological elucidation of pediatric myelin disorders as Adams and Poser were in the neuropathologic elucidation of adult and pediatric myelin disorders, respectively, re-examined these concepts through a semantic eye; this approach led to dramatically different definitions.

> Demyelinating disorders are...metachromatic leukodystrophy, multiple sclerosis.... Dysmyelination is, as the literal translation of the name implies, reserved for conditions in which the process of myelination is disturbed, leading to abnormal, patchy, irregular myelination, sometimes but not necessarily combined with signs of myelin breakdown. Examples: some amino acidopathies, damaged structure of unmyelinated white matter after perinatal hypoxia or encephalitis" (van der Knaap and Valk, 1995).

These latter definitions fly in the face of the neuropathologic precedents mentioned previously and in particular those concepts proposed by Poser, whom they quote: "The dysmyelinating disorders comprise those disorders in which 'myelin is not formed properly, or in which myelin formation is delayed or arrested, or in which the maintenance of already formed myelin is disturbed.' Examples are metachromatic leukodystrophy and adrenoleukodystrophy."

Semantic considerations do have some merit, particularly when a conceptual framework is being established or fine tuned. When they threaten or disassemble an established framework, however, they cause confusion and distract us from more important issues. For example, a reviewer of this chapter argued similarly that "dysmyelination is defined as a process of defective myelin formation during development, while demyelination describes a process where myelin is formed correctly during development but is destroyed later. In this sense, ALD and MLD, for instance, should be demyelinating diseases." The easiest way to respond to this latter criticism is again to cite the historical scientific precedents described earlier and perhaps specifically foreseen by Poser when he defined dysmyelinating diseases: "or in which the maintenance of already formed myelin is disturbed." Note that he does not say "attacked" or "destroyed," hallmarks of the acquired immune "demyelinating" diseases. The words "maintenance" and "disturbed" reflect the metabolic imbalance in myelin that he believed was operative in these diseases (Poser, 1962, 1968). One could also play the semantic card and define "myelination" as fundamentally a metabolic (molecular, biochemical) process that is developmentally regulated; hence, "dysmyelination" refers more to a biochemical aberration in myelin (as Poser viewed it) than a developmental error. Putting this aside, I would argue that while the bulk of myelination in the human cerebrum is completed by 2 years postnatally, the morphologic data derived from Weigert (myelin) stained brain sections by Flechsig and Kaes "indicate that throughout the first decade of life, myelination continues in the non-specific thalamic projections and in the association areas, and into adult life in the reticular formation and intracortical neuropil" (E. P. Richardson, Jr., 1982) and "Histologically, myelination reaches completion in early adulthood" (van der Knaap and Valk, 1995). The usual clinical onset of classical MLD, the late infantile form, is between the latter part of the first through the second year of life, precisely the developmental period when cerebral myelination is in full swing; the myelin abnormality precedes the clinical onset. Moreover, the majority of the leukodystrophies have their onsets in infancy to childhood, but most also have juvenile- and adult-onset forms (e.g., MLD, GLD, ALD). Are these later-onset forms to be considered a different class of myelin disease? Finally, myelin is not an inert substance and its biochemical components undergo a regular pattern of turnover throughout life. Is not this remodeling part of the biological process of myelination? When exactly does the "developmental" period of human myelination end? Who can say, and does it really matter? Such queries border more on the philosophical than the scientific. In ALD I believe that the myelin only becomes unstable when a sufficient amount of its abnormal fatty acid becomes incorporated into the myelin lipids and proteolipid protein. In most ALD males, this occurs at around 5 to 9 years; perhaps in the later onsets this is a slower process.

In the final analysis, I personally find the logic and classification schemes for human demyelinating and dysmyelinating diseases initiated by Adams, Kubik and Poser, while imperfect, to be prescient and far more cogent than the others. Thus, I fully endorse Poser's definition, offered in 1957, and quoted earlier: Dysmyelinating diseases are those heredofamilial disorders in which myelin is not formed properly, or in which myelin formation is delayed or arrested, or in which the maintenance of already formed myelin is disturbed. These definitional categories can be expanded or refined to include new diseases and more scientifically valid data. For example, the pathogenetic logic behind Poser's "dysmyelination" emanated from the scientific wisdom of his day: anabolic enzyme defects due to inborn errors of metabolism à la Archibald Garrod. Today, we recognize the shortcomings of his pathogenetic formulation, but this does not diminish the value of the classification.

The term leukodystrophy (leuko-white; dystroph—defective nutrition) (Bielschowsky and Henneberg, 1928), on the other hand, has traditionally been used for genetically determined, hence usually familial, and clinically progressive disorders that primarily affect CNS myelin. While all leukodystrophies are "dysmyelinating" diseases, the converse is not always true. Out of respect for historical precedent and for the sake of this present discussion leukodystrophies should have (1) a known or presumptive genetic causation, (2) a progressive clinical course, (3) a predominant and usually confluent involvement of CNS white matter, and (4) a primary lesion of myelin or myelinating cells. The latter may be manifested by either a loss or failed development of CNS white matter due to a biochemical abnormality in myelin or a molecular abnormality in myelinating cells. Those other white matter lesions that lack at least one of these diagnostic attributes can be referred to as leukoencephalopathies. This definition of a leukodystrophy may seem too restrictive to some, but it has historical precedent (briefly reviewed in van der Knaap and Valk, 1995, pp. 14–15) and the diagnosis of "leukodystrophy" has genetic and prognostic implications. Such a restricted use of "dystrophy" is not limited to diseases of CNS white matter. An analogous situation has existed in diseases of skeletal muscle with the terms "muscular dystrophy" and myopathy. In both dystrophic (i.e., myelin and muscle) situations, a primary genetic causation and somewhat predictable, often severe, clinical progression are characteristic.

The remainder of this chapter, therefore, will be confined to primary diseases of myelin and, in particular, to the major leukodystrophies (Table 28.1). It should be emphasized that Table 28.1, based on neuropathologic data, is neither all inclusive nor written in stone, but rather is an evolving process; some white matter diseases, at least presently, do not "fit" well or have debatable placements (e.g., cerebrotendinous xanthomatosis). Not all primary diseases of myelin are leukodystrophies, and some are referred to as leukoencephalopathies. For example, progressive multifocal leukoencephalopathy does not fit well into the demyelinative category and fulfills several criteria of a leukodystrophy. The JC papova virus directly infects and lyses oligodendrocytes resulting usually in a multifocal loss of CNS myelin (Fig. 28.5A) with relative sparing of axons, but usually without inflammation; it also is a progressive illness and may be confluent, such as in AIDS (Fig. 28.5B). However, it lacks the genetic element of a leukodystrophy. Some diseases also referred to as leukoencephalopathies (e.g., vacuolating megalencephalic leukoencephalopathy with subcortical cysts) have been assigned provisionally to the dysmyelinative

TABLE 28.1 Primary Diseases of Myelin

**I. DYSMYELINATING DISEASES (LEUKODYSTROPHIES)**

**Classical Dysmyelinative**

Adrenoleukodystrophy (MIM 300100)

Metachromatic leukodystrophy (MIM 250100)

Globoid cell leukodystrophy (Krabbe's disease, MIM 245200)

Sudanophilic (orthochromatic) leukodystrophies (MIM 272100)

- Simple Type
- Pigmentary Type
- With meningeal angiomatosis
- Polycystic lipomembranous osteodysplasia with sclerosing leukodystrophy (membranous lipodystrophy, Nasu-Hakola, MIM 221770)
- Neuroaxonal leukodystrophy, hereditary diffuse leukoencephalopathy with spheroids; autosomal dominant diffuse leukoencephalopathy with neuroaxonal spheroids
- Sjogren-Larsson (MIM 270200)
- Others

**Hypomyelinative**

Pelizaeus-Merzbacher disease (MIM 312080)

Alexander disease (MIM 203450)

Vanishing white matter disease/childhood ataxia with diffuse cerebral hypomyelination (MIM 603896)

Aicardi-Goutières syndrome (MIM 225750)

Cockayne syndrome (MIM 216400)

**Spongiform**

Spongy degeneration of central nervous system (Canavan or VanBogaert-Bertrand disease, MIM 271900)

Adult-onset spongiform leukodystrophy (MIM 169500)

Vacuolating megalencephalic leukoencephalopathy with subcortical cysts (Infantile-onset spongiform leukoencephalopathy, MIM 604004)

**II. MYELINOLYTIC DISEASES (SPONGY MYELINOPATHIES)**

Central pontine myelinolysis

Aminoacidurias, Organic acidurias

Mitochondrial disorders: Kearns-Sayre syndrome (MIM 530000)

Vitamin $B_{12}$ (folate) deficiency and HIV vacuolar myelopathy

Exogenous toxins: Heroin vapor, hexachlorophene and triethyl tin

**III. DEMYELINATING DISEASES (CNS)**

Multiple (disseminated) sclerosis (MIM 126200)

1. Chronic
   - a. Classical (Charcot)
   - b. Diffuse cerebral variant (Schilder)
2. Acute variants
   - a. Disseminated (Marburg)
   - b. Concentric sclerosis (Balo)
   - b. Neuromyelitis optica (Devic)

Acute disseminated encephalomyelitis

1. Classical
   - a. Postinfectious encephalomyelitis
   - b. Postvaccinal encephalomyelitis
2. Hyperacute
   - a. Acute hemorrhagic leukoencephalitis (Hurst).

Focal inflammatory demyelinating lesions with mass effect (Pseudotumor)

Infectious

1. Progressive multifocal leukoencephalopathy
2. Subacute sclerosing panencephalitis

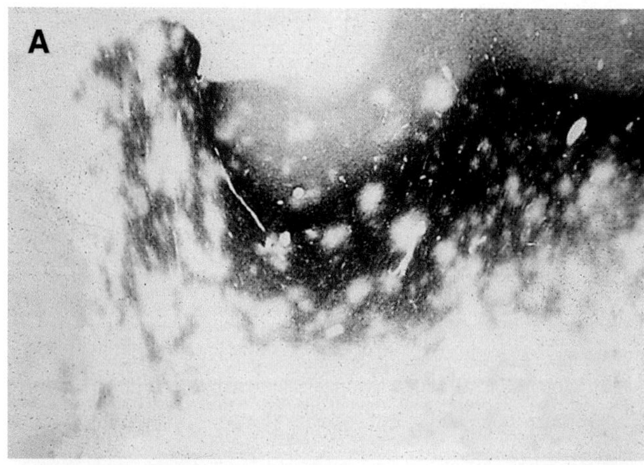


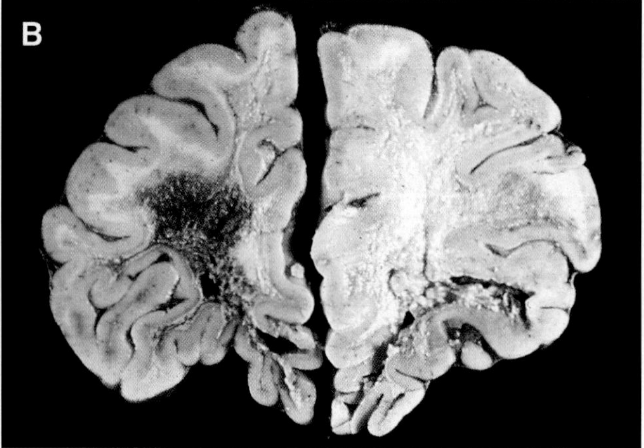


FIGURE 28.5
(A) Multifocal loss of myelin in PML. Heidenhain myelin. (B) Confluent to cavitary loss of frontal white matter in PML of AIDS patient.

disease (leukodystrophy) category, because they have shown an apparent primary lesion of myelin (van der Knaap *et al.*, 1996), in addition to the other criteria mentioned earlier. Several other familial and progressive white matter disorders have been placed provisionally in the hypomyelinative group in spite of their controversial or unknown pathogeneses: vanishing white matter disease (VWM) (van der Knaap, *et al.* 1998), Aicardi-Goutières syndrome (Razavi *et al.*, 1988), and Cockayne syndrome (reviewed in Nance and Berry, 1992), because of their similarity to Alexander disease and to the prototypic hypomyelinative leukodystrophy, Pelizaeus-Merzbacher disease (PMD), respectively. The latter calcifying disorders mimic the hypomyelinative lesions of PMD, while the cavitating quality of VWM approximates Alexander disease. Reviewing the morphology of myelin degradation and comparing and contrasting the neuropathologic features of its major types to those of other primary diseases of myelin and to each other can provide us with a neuropathologic overview of the leukodystrophies.

## MYELIN DEGRADATION

Myelin breakdown is a dynamic morphologic process in which specific cells participate in characteristic patterns for a particular disease, and the biochemical degradation of myelin can be appreciated with traditional carbohydrate and lipid stains (Adams, 1965). The galactolipids, cerebroside and sulfatide, and cholesterol are major lipid components of myelin sheaths that are liberated during myelin breakdown. Cerebroside and sulfatide contain 1, 2-glycol groups and hence are periodic acid-Schiff (PAS) positive. Sulfatide (cerebroside sulfate) has the additional property of metachromasia due to its anionic sulfate groups. A substance is metachromatic when it can produce a spectral shift, usually toward longer wavelengths such as blue to red, when stained with some basic dye (e.g., toluidine blue or cresyl violet). When an individual has normal lysosomal galactocerebrosidase and arylsulfatase A activities, the respective degradative enzymes for these substrates, the catabolic reactions are rapid and their morphologic correlates are of short duration. However, when either of these degradative enzymes is deficient, such as in globoid cell leukodystrophy (Krabbe disease; GLD) or metachromatic leukodystrophy (MLD), the PAS positivity of the nondegraded galactocerebroside or sulfatide and the metachromasia of sulfatide persist. Cholesterol is esterified primarily by macrophages that become vacuolated and have been referred to historically as gitter cells, compound granular corpuscles, or lipid-laden macrophages (lipophages). Normally the intracellular esterified cholesterol persists much longer than the galactolipids or their degradation products. Therefore, the major degradative end point of myelin in an individual with biochemically normal myelin and normal lysosomal enzymes is cholesterol ester, the neurochemist's "floating fraction" (Norton *et al.*, 1966). It is important to note that the histochemical or biochemical detection of these degradative products and particularly cholesterol esters in white matter is not restricted to primary diseases of myelin and may be seen in a variety of lesions, such as an infarct. Cholesterol esters also are detectable when myelin is being laid down by oligodendrocytes (Ramsay and Davison, 1974). Cholesterol esters within macrophages can be demonstrated with "Sudan" and other neutral lipid dyes, such as Oil Red O, in frozen sections. Hence, the end point of normal myelin degradation is referred to as sudanophilic; it is also said to be orthochromatic, because cholesterol ester does not possess metachromatic properties. Sudanophilia is typical of the major human demyelinative disease, multiple sclerosis. However, sudanophilic myelin debris also occurs in adrenoleukodystrophy (ALD), where biochemical abnormalities in both myelin lipids and proteolipid protein (PLP) have been clearly demonstrated. Comparable, but currently unrecognized, biochemical abnormalities in myelin probably underlie at least some of the "sudanophilic" (orthochromatic) leukodystrophies (SLD), the category in which ALD had been placed until the identification of its biochemical abnormality. While these histochemical reactions (Wolman, 1970) are unfolding in the classical dysmyelinative (leukodystrophies) and demyelinative diseases, myelin sheaths are generally undergoing some loss of stainability, vacuolation, and fragmentation prior to and in concert with a variable macrophage infiltration and astrocytic hypertrophy/hyperplasia eventuating in severe myelin loss, relative axonal sparing, decreased numbers of oligodendrocytes, few remaining lipophages, and chronic fibrillary astrogliosis.

## PRIMARY DISEASES OF MYELIN

As discussed earlier, primary diseases of central myelin have been divided into two major types: myelinoclastic (demyelinating/demyelinative) and dysmyelinating/dysmyelinative (Poser, 1962, 1968), and they are both characterized by a primary loss of myelin with a relative sparing of axons. Neuropathologically, this is confirmed by staining two serial sections of a white matter lesion for myelin or axons and demonstrating a loss of myelin in one and a sparing of axons in the corresponding area of the other (Fig. 28.6). A third category was added by the author, in part because those diseases shared a common light microscopic feature of spongy to vacuolated myelin (Fig. 28.7); we designated them as myelinolytic diseases or spongy myelinopathies (Powers and Horoupian, 1995) in keeping with earlier reports. The vacuoles are due to the accumulation of fluid within myelin sheaths and astrocytes; in the former they usually originate at the intraperiod line that is continuous potentially with the extracellular space (Jellinger and Seitelberger, 1970). It is difficult to determine the exact site of splits in myelin sheaths in human biopsy or autopsy specimens due to poor tissue preservation. Intramyelinic edema is considered a subtype of

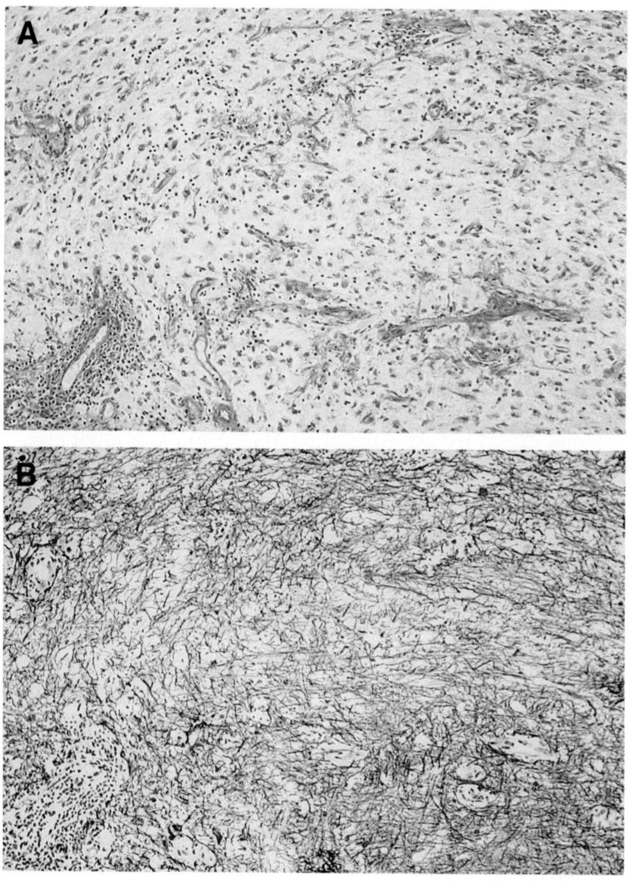

FIGURE 28.6
(A) Primary demyelination. Complete loss of myelin, reactive astrocytosis, and perivascular inflammation. Luxol fast blue—PAS myelin. (B) Slight to moderate loss of axons in the identical field of a serial section. Bodian axon.

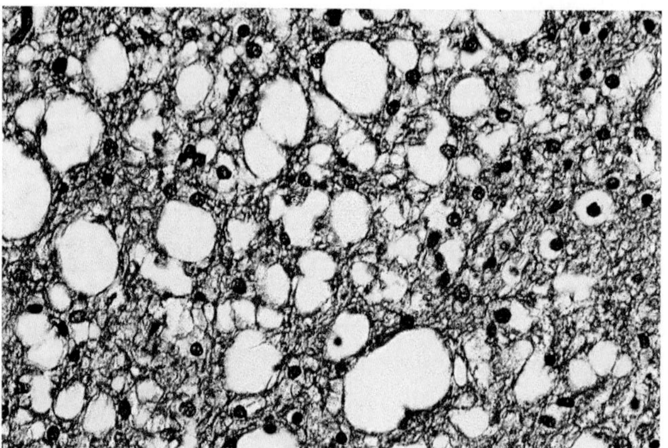

FIGURE 28.7
Spongy myelinopathy of cerebral white matter with good preservation of oligodendrocytes in Kearns-Sayre syndrome. Hematoxylin-eosin.

cytotoxic (intracellular) edema (Klatzo, 1967). Myelinolytic diseases may be either genetically transmitted or acquired; they are etiologically diverse but most often toxic or metabolic (e.g., vitamin $B_{12}$ deficiency). In many myelinolytic lesions, axonal and oligodendroglial sparing is characteristic, at least of the early stages, and inflammatory cells including macrophages do not participate to any appreciable degree; myelin debris is also sparse but is sudanophilic. Astrocytosis varies, but usually occurs. As a result and most important, the spongy myelinopathies differ from other primary diseases of myelin, particularly leukodystrophies, in that some are reversible, such as central pontine myelinolysis (Wakui *et al.*, 1991) and hexachlorophene toxicity (Kimbrough and Gaines, 1971). In some myelinolytic disorders, soluble toxins may be acting directly on myelin sheaths; in others, osmotic factors may be responsible (osmotic myelinolysis); yet in others, spongy myelin may reflect a potentially correctable metabolic dysfunction of the supporting oligodendrocytes/astrocytes. The myelin appears to be biochemically normal on the basis of its sudanophilia and biochemical analyses (Cammer *et al.*, 1975). PNS lesions are usually absent in myelinolytic diseases. One could include Canavan disease in this category because of its vacuolated myelin, a meager myelin debris-macrophage response, and the preferential involvement of subcortical arcuate fibers (Adachi *et al.*, 1973); however, its genetic defect, infantile onset, progressive clinical course, and confluent white matter lesions align it more closely to the leukodystrophies. Some aminoacidurias, organic acidurias, heritable mitochondrial disorders, and other inherited vacuolar leukoencephalopathies could fulfill the diagnostic criteria of leukodystrophies but have not yet been accorded this position.

In demyelinative diseases, such as multiple sclerosis, inflammatory cells are prominent (Fig. 28.8) and destroy biochemically normal myelin or myelinating cells (oligodendrocytes/Schwann cells). Demyelinative diseases are typically acquired, even though genetic factors also may play a role in some; their clinical progression tends to be more variable than that of the leukodystrophies. Considerable axonal sparing in the early phase of the chronic types has traditionally distinguished demyelinative diseases from the leukodystrophies (Figures 28.9A, B), but the recent demonstration of early and progressive loss of axons in the demyelinative plaques of multiple sclerosis vitiates this distinction (Trapp *et al.*, 1998). Myelin breakdown products are sudanophilic and orthochromatic. Demyelinative lesions usually do not respect the subcortical arcuate or "U" fibers, have sharp edges (Fig. 28.9A) and are usually asymmetric when bilateral. Fibrillary astrogliosis with markedly diminished myelin and oligodendrocytes (Fig. 28.9C) is the ultimate outcome of the demyelinative plaque. The prominent participation of inflammatory cells (T and B lymphocytes, macrophages, and plasma cells) and their products (cytokines and chemokines) provide convincing evidence of an immune destruction of myelin that appears to be directed against antigenic myelin proteins. Some of these proteins reside in either the CNS or PNS (e.g., the CNS PLP), and therefore the involvement of either central or peripheral myelin is typical of most demyelinative diseases.

As mentioned previously, leukodystrophies are genetically transmitted and progressive diseases in which either biochemically abnormal myelin or some molecular abnormality in

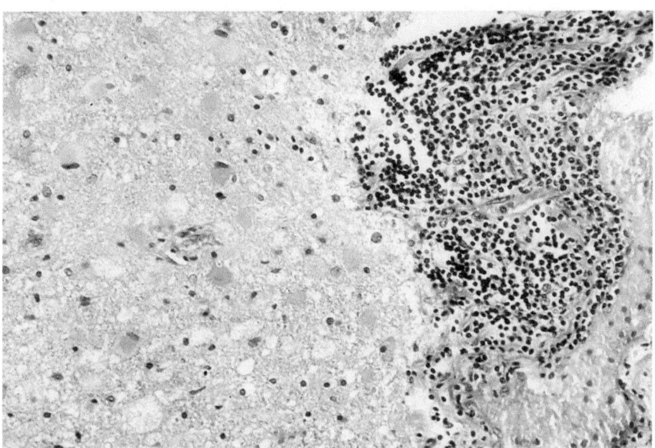

FIGURE 28.8
Prominent lymphocytic perivascular cuff in demyelinated white matter exhibiting a loss of oligodendrocytes and reactive astrocytosis in multiple sclerosis. Hematoxylin-eosin.

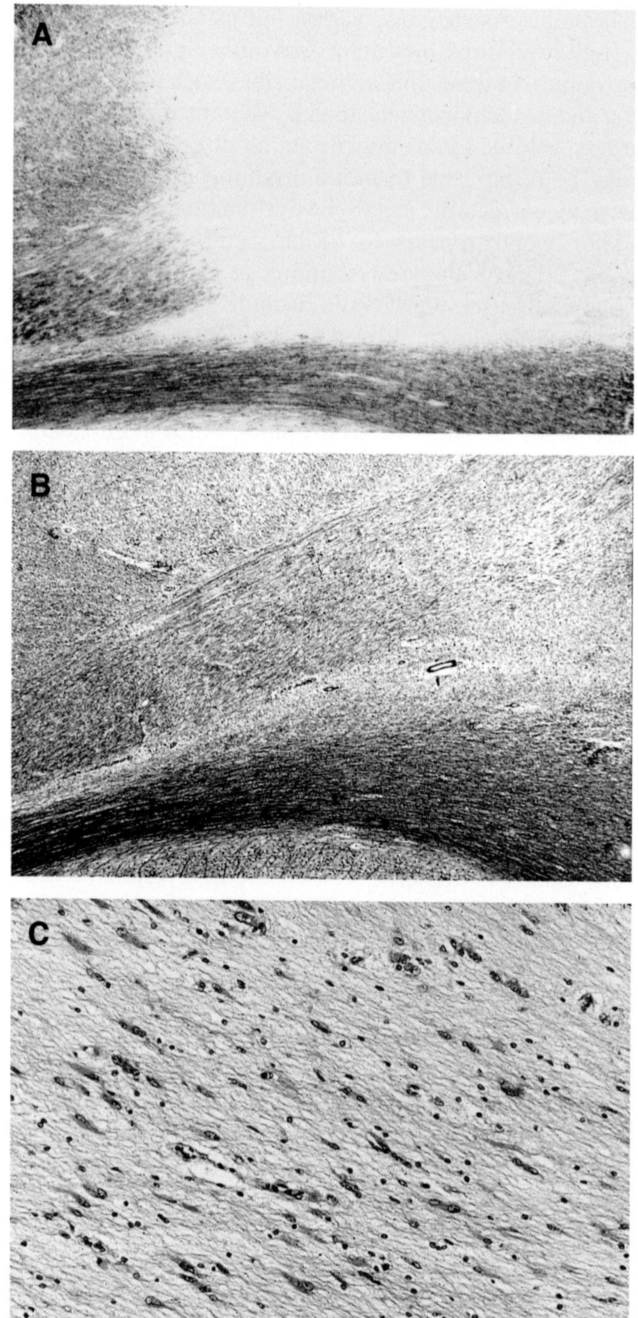


FIGURE 28.9
(A) Demyelinative plaque with sharp border in multiple sclerosis. Heidenhain myelin. (B) Axonal sparing in demyelinative plaque. Serial section of same lesion as in Figure 28.9a. Bodian axon. (C) Isomorphic fibrillary astrogliosis of chronic demyelinative plaque in multiple sclerosis. Hematoxylin-eosin.

myelinating cells has been identified. They have been classified as dysmyelinative to set them apart from demyelinative diseases. Such classical leukodystrophies include ALD, MLD, GLD, and SLD. Their biochemical/molecular defects involve myelin lipids, which are qualitatively similar in CNS and PNS; hence, the involvement of both central and peripheral myelin is typical of most classical leukodystrophies. ALD, in spite of its profound lymphocytic element that is typical of demyelinative diseases, has a firm nosological position within the dysmyelinative diseases due to the incorporation of abnormal very long chain saturated fatty acids (VLCFA) into several myelin components (reviewed in Moser, 1997). The second subgroup of dysmyelinative diseases, hypomyelinative, differs from the classical leukodystrophies in that their primary defect appears to relate more to inadequate myelinogenesis rather than myelin breakdown. At present classical/connatal X-linked PMD is the most legitimate member of this divergent group, and GLD also could call this its home. In PMD and its allelic cousin, spastic paraplegia type 2 (SP2), the molecular defect involves the PLP gene and the variable absence of myelin PLP; hence, the lesions are restricted to the CNS for all practical purposes, as is true for the others. The third subgroup, spongiform, displays the same spongy to vacuolated change in myelin that epitomizes the myelinolytic diseases (Fig. 28.7), but they are genetically determined and their primary locus is cerebral white matter that displays confluent abnormalities. PNS lesions also are not typical of spongiform leukodystrophies. One disease that doesn't fit well into this classification scheme is VWM, because it exhibits a mixed picture of hypomyelination, classical dysmyelination with some myelin breakdown and marked axonal loss, as well as spongiform changes.

## LEUKODYSTROPHIES: CLINICAL SIMILARITIES AND DISSIMILARITIES

Most leukodystrophies have similar clinical findings that reflect damage to central white matter: abnormal motor function, vision, hearing, and cognition. The specific manifestations of these system abnormalities can vary somewhat, depending on the age of the patient at the time of onset. Nevertheless, developmental delay or regression, spasticity and hypertonia or hypotonia, quadriparesis to quadriplegia, decerebrate posturing, visual and auditory agnosia, decreased visual or auditory acuity to blindness and deafness, ataxia, nystagmus, other abnormal movements, and mental retardation to dementia can be detected in patients with a leukodystrophy. Genetic transmission patterns can be autosomal recessive (e.g., MLD, 22q; GLD, 14q; Canavan disease, 17p; VWM, 3q), autosomal dominant (adult spongiform leukodystrophy, 5q) and X-linked (ALD, PMD); some are more typically sporadic (Alexander disease, SLD). The typical age of onset is also variable: infancy (GLD, Canavan disease, Alexander disease), late infancy (MLD, PMD), childhood (ALD, VWM), and adult (AMN, SLD, SP2).

## LEUKODYSTROPHIES: NEUROPATHOLOGIC SIMILARITIES AND DISSIMILARITIES

Leukodystrophies generally exhibit similar gross neuropathologic features: reduced brain size, except for the megalencephaly of Canavan and Alexander diseases, optic atrophy, ventriculomegaly, atrophy of the corpus callosum, and bilaterally symmetrical, diffuse to confluent, loss or lack of cerebral and cerebellar white matter with their replacement by firm gray to beige fibrillary astrogliosis (sclerosis) (Fig. 28.10). A patchy or tigroid myelinopathy, due to the perivascular presence of myelin, typifies PMD (Fig. 28.11) (Seitelberger, 1995); but also Cockayne syndrome (Leech *et al.*, 1985) and adult-onset spongiform leukodystrophy (Fig. 28.12) (Eldridge *et al.*, 1984). Brainstem lesions in Alexander disease often simulate the demyelinative plaques of multiple sclerosis. Preservation of subcortical "U" fibers is characteristic, except in Canavan disease (Fig. 28.13) and PMD, but severe or protracted courses can lead to their loss in the others (Fig. 28.14). Asymmetry is seen in the advancing edges of ALD, usually frontal (Schaumburg *et al.*, 1975). Cavitation of white matter due to massive axonal loss and an inadequate astrocytic reparative response rarely occurs in the classical leukodystrophies, but is characteristic of Alexander disease (Borrett and Becker, 1985) and VWM (van der Knaap *et al.*, 1997) (Fig. 28.15). The parieto-occipital lobes in ALD and late-onset GLD, the frontal lobes in Alexander disease and several late-onset leukodystrophies such as MLD, and the arcuate fibers in Canavan disease are favored early sites. Gray matter is usually not involved, except when there has been superimposed hypoxic-ischemic events

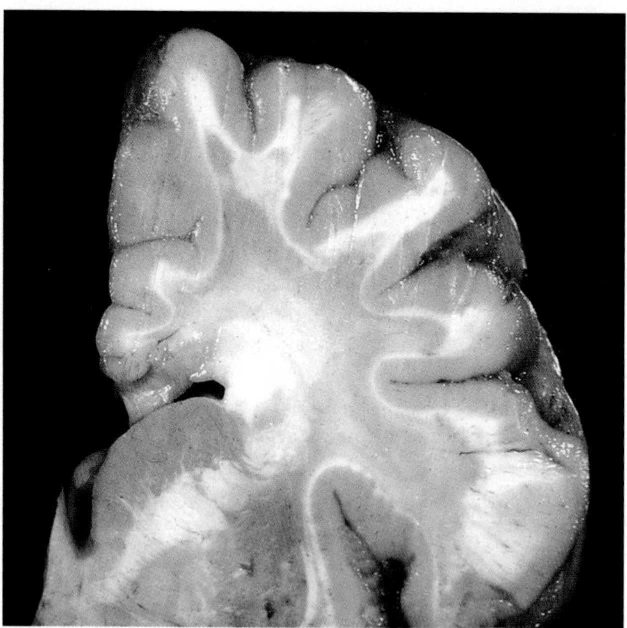

FIGURE 28.10
Confluent loss of myelin with sparing of arcuate fibers and replacement by gray-tan astrocytic tissue in frontal white matter of ALD.

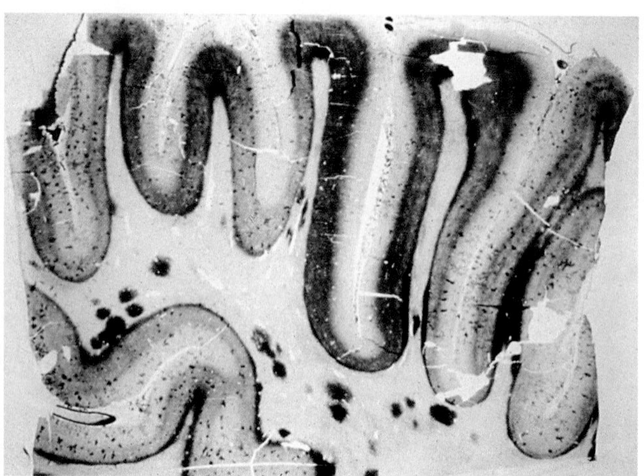

FIGURE 28.11
Absence of myelin staining, including arcuate fibers, except for small circular foci around blood vessels in PMD. Weil myelin.

or when cavitation of white matter leads to direct or transynaptic atrophy of its associated gray matter.

These same patterns of gross neuropathologic lesions now can be appreciated in living patients with modern imaging techniques, such as magnetic resonance imaging (MRI) (van der Knaap and Valk, 1995). T2-weighted images are particularly effective in demonstrating myelin abnormalities (Fig. 28.16). An MRI-pattern recognition approach has been developed and applied to unclassified white matter diseases in children with great success (van der Knaap *et al.*, 1999). MR spectroscopy (MRS), in which specific biochemical moieties within white matter lesions can be measured, also can contribute to a clinical diagnosis. Perhaps more important, MRS along with the recent modifications of magnetization transfer and diffusion anisotropy, especially when utilized in longitudinal studies of living patients and correlated with postmortem imaging and neuropathologic analysis,

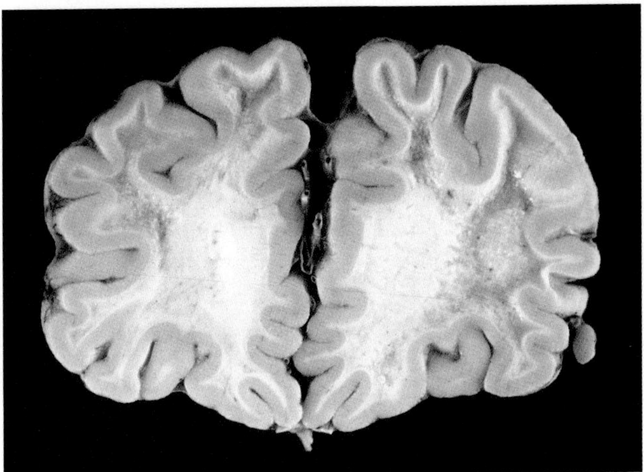

FIGURE 28.12
Confluent, but patchy, loss of myelin in frontal white matter of adult-onset spongiform leukodystrophy.

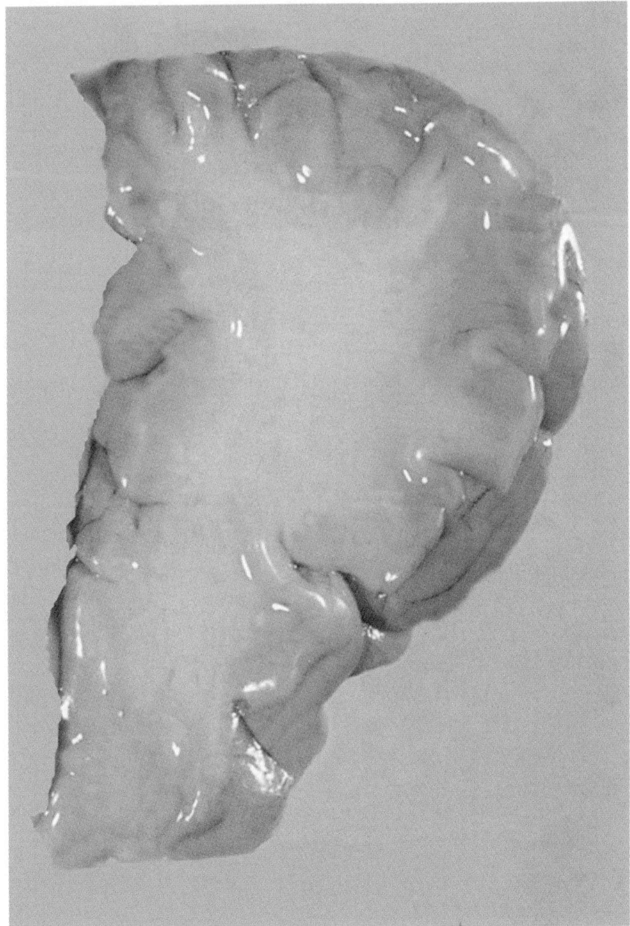

FIGURE 28.13
Mucoid appearance of arcuate fibers in swollen frontal white matter of Canavan disease.

should provide powerful pathogenetic insights (e.g., in "hypomyelination"). (The reader is referred to van der Knaap, 2001, and van der Knaap and Valk, 1995, for more specific details.)

Likewise, with the light microscope most leukodystrophies display common features: reduced myelin staining, loss of oligodendrocytes, considerable axonal loss but still a

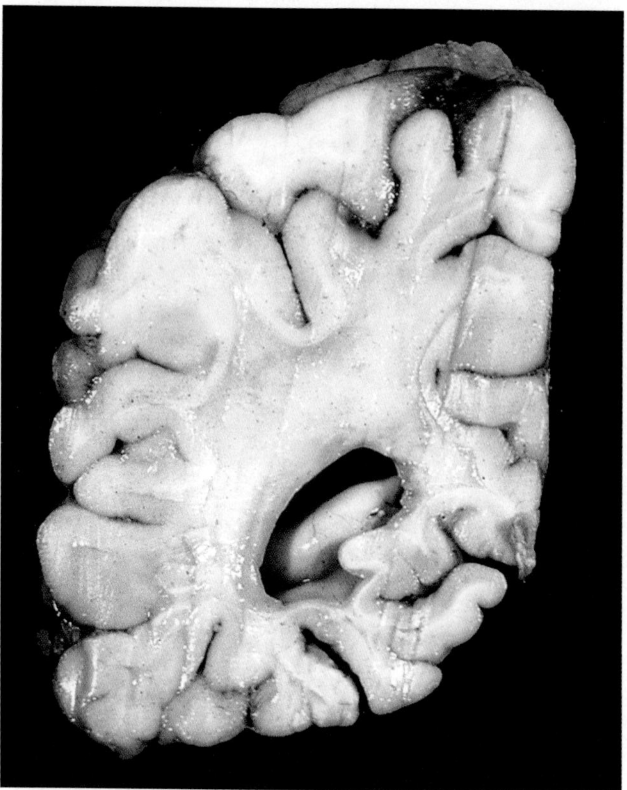

FIGURE 28.14
Confluent loss of myelin, including arcuate fibers, in occipital white matter of same ALD patient depicted in Figure 28.10.

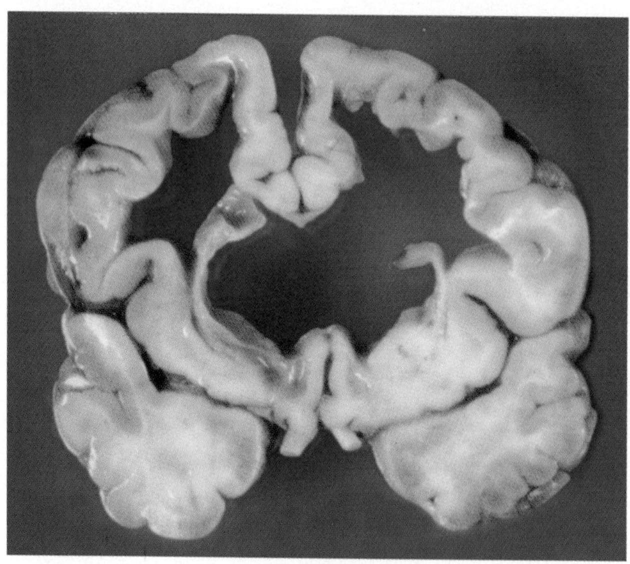

FIGURE 28.15
Cavitation of frontal white matter in Alexander disease.

relative sparing of axons and reactive astrocytosis in the early stages (Fig. 28.17A) to fibrillary astrogliosis that may be either isomorphic or anisomorphic in later stages (Fig. 28.17B). Macrophages with myelin debris are typical of the classical types but tend to be sparse in the hypomyelinative and spongiform subgroups, such as PMD and Canavan disease. Axonal loss is greater in the leukodystrophies than in the demyelinative diseases

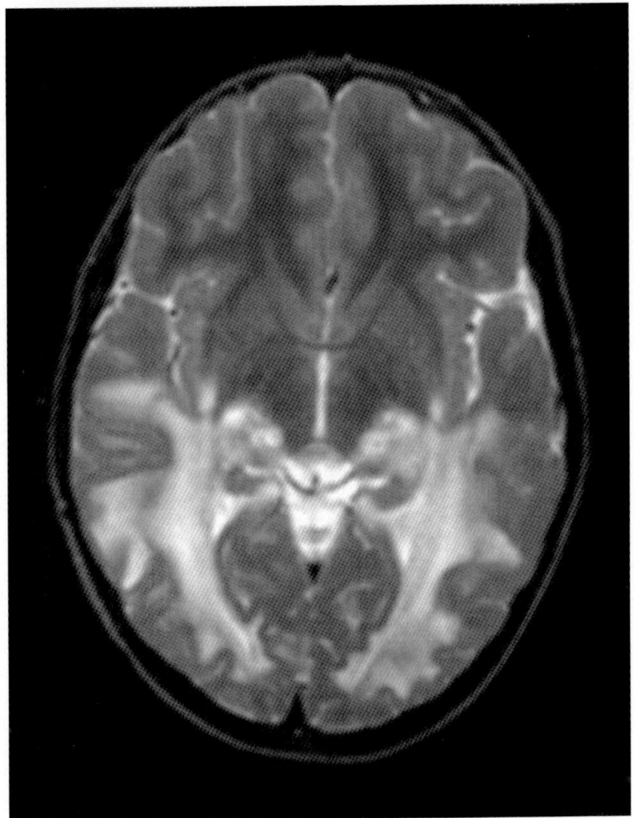

FIGURE 28.16
Confluent, bilaterally symmetrical high signal abnormalities of parieto-occipital white matter in ALD. T2-MRI.

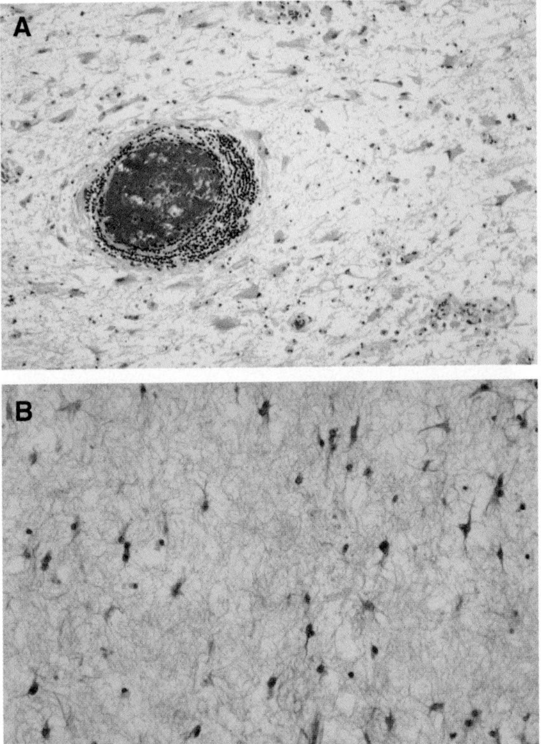


FIGURE 28.17
(A) Marked loss of myelin, axons and oligodendrocytes with reactive astrocytosis, typical of most classical leukodystrophies. Such perivascular lymphocytes are essentially restricted to ALD. Hematoxylin-eosin. (B) Fibrillary astrogliosis of demyelinated cerebral white matter in ALD. Hematoxylin-eosin.

and is particularly prominent in the cavitating lesions of VWM and Alexander disease, as well as the posterior limb of the internal capsule in ALD and GLD, characteristically leading to secondary or Wallerian-like corticospinal tract degeneration (Fig. 28.18). Other than macrophages, traditional inflammatory cells (e.g., lymphocytes) are usually inconspicuous, except in ALD (Fig. 28.19), to a mild degree in GLD, and in some early lesions of Alexander disease.

In spite of the similarities, significant differences between the leukodystrophies can be seen with both the light and electron microscopes. For example, even with a routine hematoxylin-eosin (H-E) stain, the macrophages are often distinctive because the nature and amount of myelin breakdown products are characteristic of each leukodystrophy. In the classical leukodystrophies, myelin debris is substantial during the active phase. Lipophages tend to be vacuolated in SLD, except in the pigmentary form of SLD where they are yellow-brown and granular, vacuolated and striated in ALD, coarsely granular in MLD, and epithelioid to multinucleated (globoid) in GLD (Fig. 28.20). The myelin debris is predominantly sudanophilic and orthochromatic in ALD and SLD, acid fast/PAS+, autofluorescent and variably iron positive in pigmentary SLD, metachromatic and PAS+ in MLD or PAS+, and orthochromatic in GLD (Fig. 28.21). Macrophages are diastase resistant, PAS+; so the macrophages in ALD and SLD also can be PAS+ (Fig. 28.22), but the more striated the cytoplasm in ALD the less sudanophilic. The myelin debris also displays a highly characteristic and often diagnostic ultrastructural appearance:

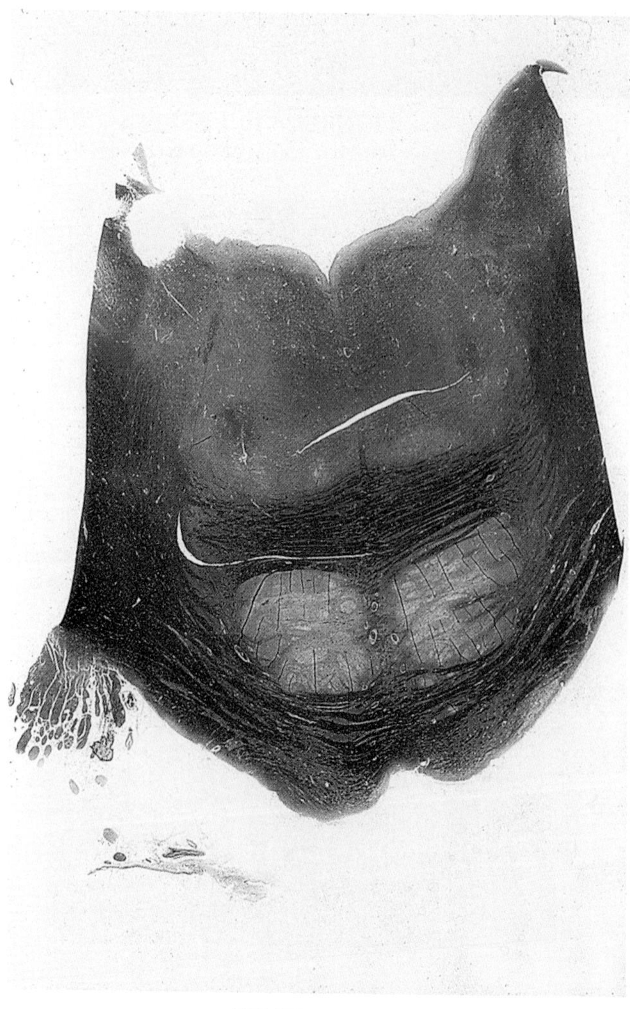

**FIGURE 28.18.**
Bilateral, secondary corticospinal tract degeneration in basis pontis of ALD. Luxol fast blue—eosin.

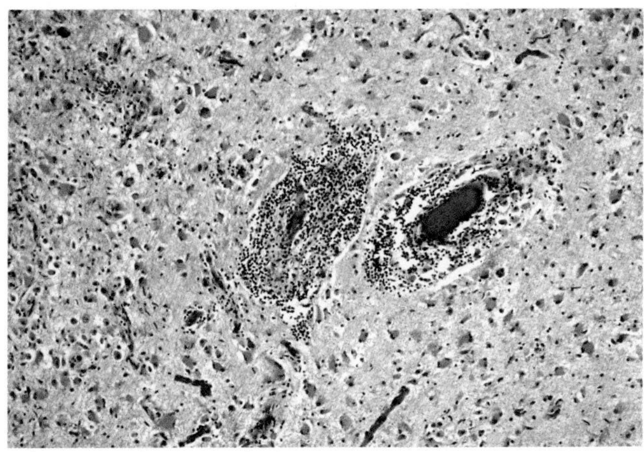

FIGURE 28.19
Prominent lymphocytic infiltrates characteristic of ALD and comparable to those of MS. Hematoxylin-eosin.

multangular crystalloids in GLD, prismatic and tuffstone bodies in MLD and lamellae and lamellar-lipid profiles in ALD. Abnormal mitochondria in Alzheimer type II astrocytes are seen in Canavan disease (Fig. 28.23), and proteinaceous Rosenthal fibers with their granular precursors in astrocytes are the hallmark of Alexander disease (Fig. 28.24). An apparent increase in the number of oligodendrocytes in the early lesions and "foamy" oligodendrocytes in later stages have been reported in VWM. Small foci of mineralization of the abnormal white matter have been noted in several leukodystrophies (Fig. 28.25) but are prominent and more widespread in Cockayne and Aicardi-Goutierès syndromes.

While the involvement of CNS white matter is constant, the association of other pathologic lesions is characteristic of specific leukodystrophies. The PNS is commonly involved in infantile GLD, late infantile MLD, and the adult ALD variant, adrenomyeloneuropathy-AMN. Concomitant neuronal storage (neurolipidosis) in subcortical sites is seen only in MLD and its variant, multiple sulfatase deficiency (mucosulfatidosis) (Fig. 28.26). Neuronal loss of the dentate nuclei, brainstem, and thalamus seems characteristic of GLD, while neuronal loss in cerebellar cortex may be conspicuous in MLD. The mineralizations mentioned earlier in Cockayne and Aicardi-Goutierès syndromes also involve gray matter, particularly the deep gray matter. Extraneural lesions are typical of ALD (adrenocortical and Leydig cells) (Fig. 28.27) and MLD (renal tubules and other epithelial cells) (Fig. 28.28). (See Harding and Surtees, 2002, Powers and DeVivo, 2002, and Suzuki and Suzuki, 2002, for further details.)

It is noteworthy that adult variants of some leukodystrophies are characterized by bilaterally symmetrical tract degenerations, such as of the optic radiations, implying a primary axonal problem rather than the dysmyelination of the pediatric patients. This is well documented in AMN where several supraspinal tracts (e.g., optic radiations and medial lemnisci) have been shown to have equivalent losses of axons and myelin, while a dominant dying-back axonopathy of the gracile, corticospinal, and spinocerebellar tracts (Fig. 28.29) is associated with atrophic dorsal root ganglion neurons containing lipidic mitochondrial inclusions (Powers *et al.*, 2000; Powers *et al.*, 2001; Schaumburg *et al.*, 1977). Similar tract lesions can be seen in juvenile-adult Alexander disease (Fig. 28.30) (personal observation), adult-onset GLD (Choi *et al.*, 1991), and perhaps SP2.

## LEUKODYSTROPHIES: PATHOGENETIC SIMILARITIES AND DISSIMILARITIES

In contrast to the common elements of their gross and microscopic neuropathologic lesions, but comparable to their distinctive morphologic features, each leukodystrophy is unique in

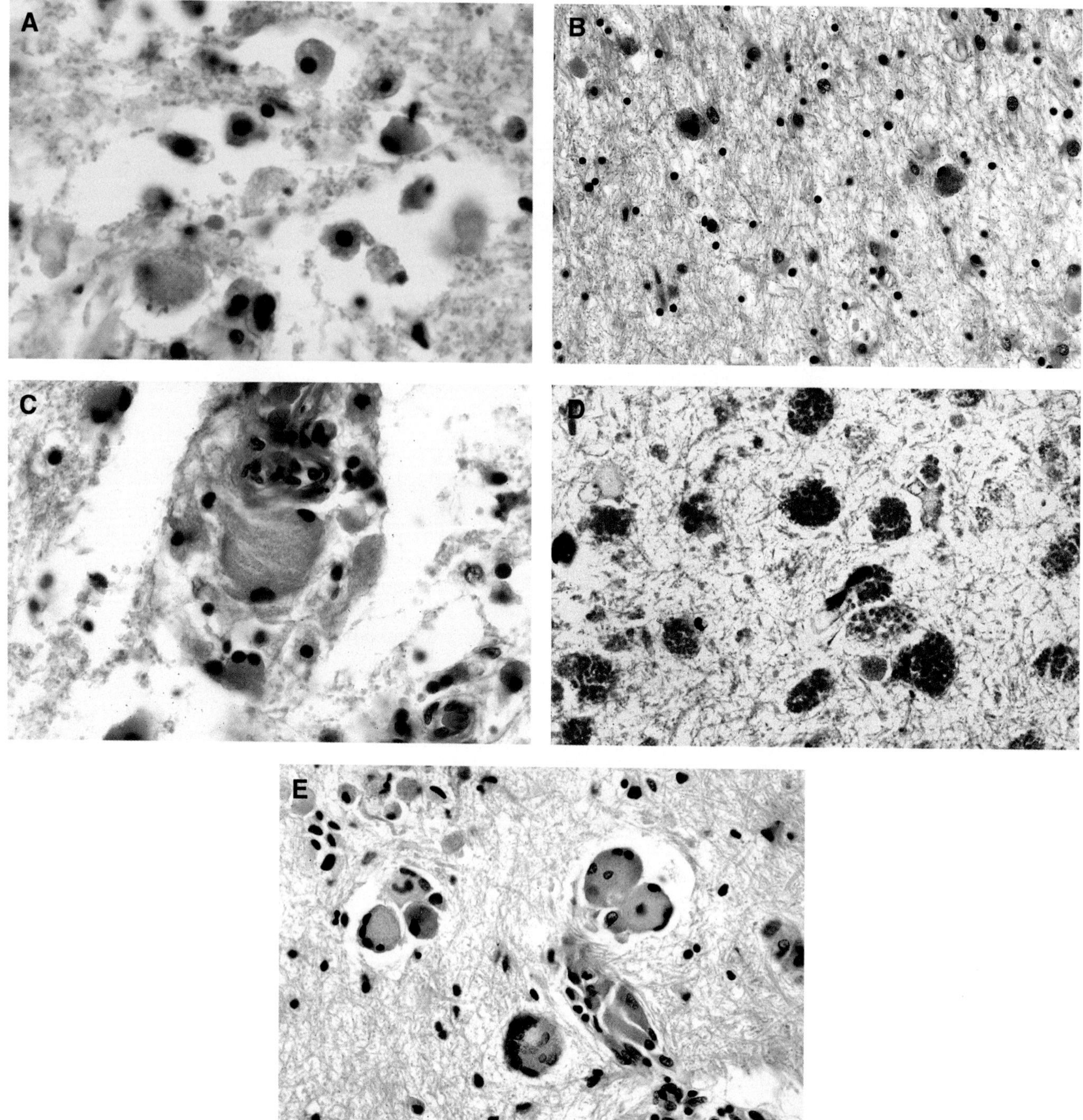


FIGURE 28.20
Macrophages. (A) Smooth to vacuolated macrophages in ALD; (B) brown macrophages in pigmentary form of SLD; (C) large striated macrophage adjacent to blood vessel in ALD; (D) coarsely granular macrophages in MLD; (E) clusters of globoid cells with single and multiple nuclei, often around blood vessels, in GLD. Hematoxylin-eosin.

its biochemical/molecular defect and, presumably, pathogenesis. In most leukodystrophies, only glimpses of their pathogenetic mechanisms exist. Genotype-phenotype correlations among the leukodystrophies are highly variable: from excellent in PMD (Hudson, 2001), to good in MLD and GLD with certain common homozygous mutations (D. Wenger, personal communication), to poor in ALD/AMN (Smith *et al.*, 1999). In spite of this season of "Light," more needs to be learned about most leukodystrophies than is known. For example, some consider the primary pathogenetic problem in VWM as glial, while others

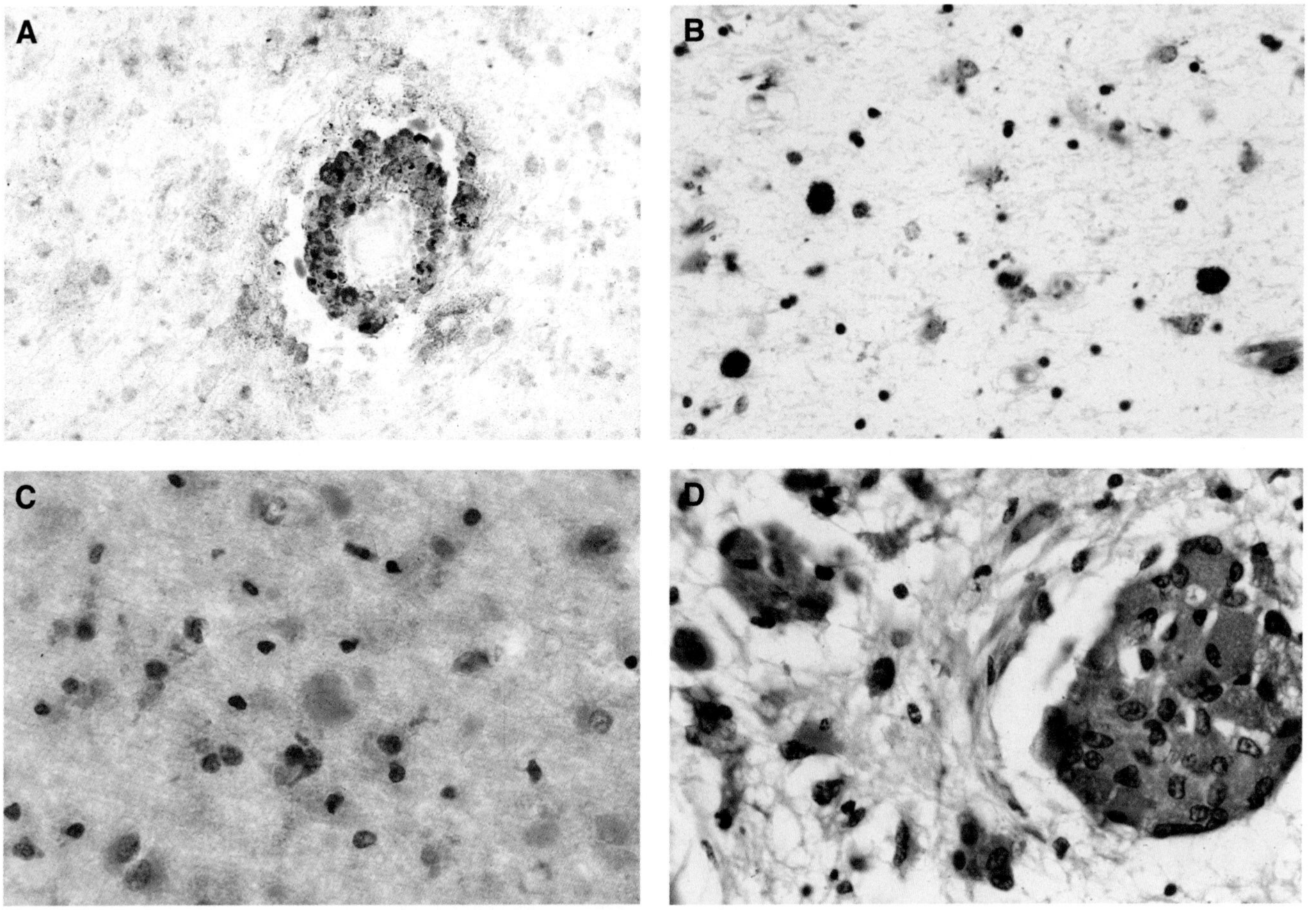

FIGURE 28.21
Myelin debris. (A) Red (sudanophilic) macrophages in ALD. frozen section, oil red 0; (B) deep red-violet macrophages in pigmentary SLD, acid fast; (C) brown-yellow metachromasia of sulfatide within macrophages of MLD, frozen section, acid-cresyl violet; (D) magenta globoid cells of GLD, PAS.

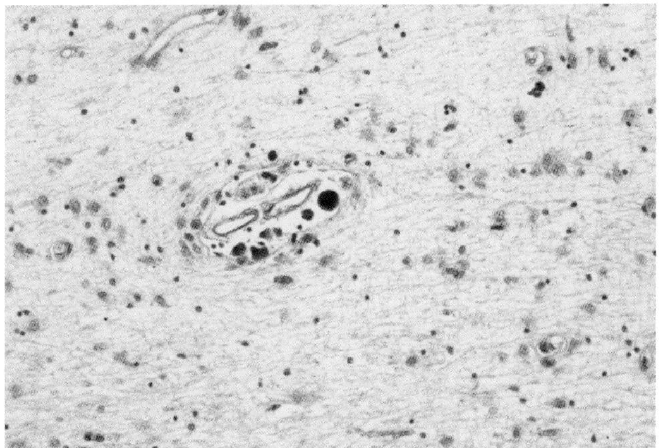

FIGURE 28.22
PAS positive macrophages around blood vessel in ALD. LFB-PAS.

see it as axonal (van der Knaap *et al.*, 1998). How the novel and revolutionary discovery of a defective translation initiation factor gene relates to this exclusively CNS white matter disorder also is a mystery at present (Leegwater *et al.*, 2001). Speaking for myself, I have been trying to understand the pathogenesis of ALD and AMN for over three decades and am still in the dark, even after the identification of the genetic defect on the X chromosome.

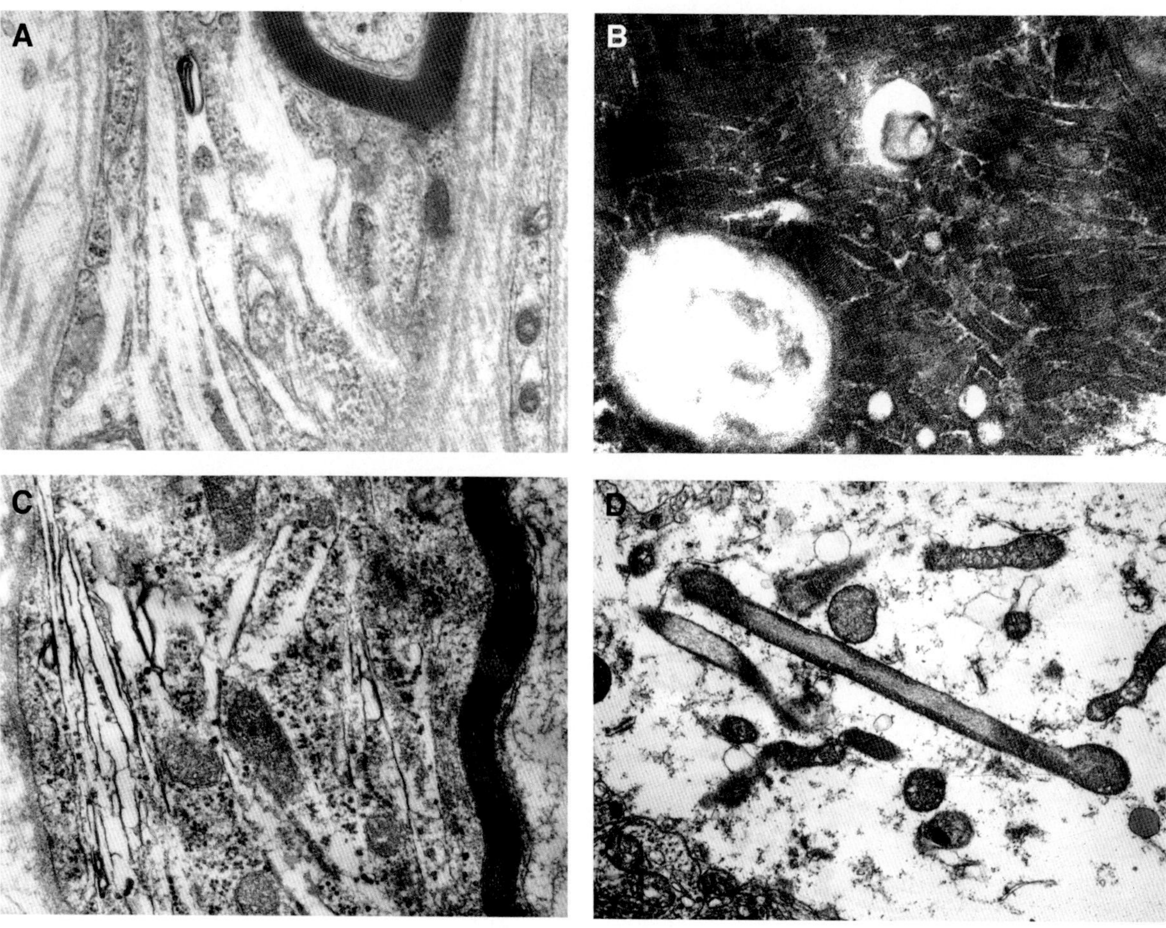

FIGURE 28.23
Ultrastructure of myelin debris. (A) Crystalloids of GLD; (B) prismatic structures of MLD; (C) lamellae and lamellar-lipid profiles of ALD; (D) abnormal mitochondria of Canavan disease.

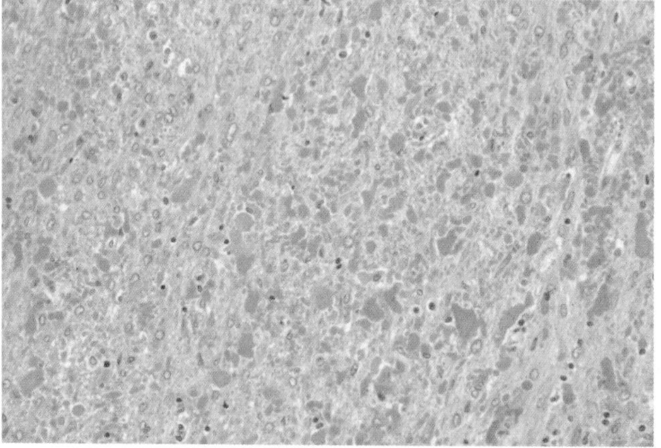

FIGURE 28.24
Countless eosinophilic Rosenthal fibers in white matter of infantile Alexander disease. Hematoxylin-eosin.

Usually the primary molecular abnormality in a leukodystrophy has been demonstrated, or assumed to be, in the oligodendrocyte, except in Alexander disease with its mutations of the astrocytic glial fibrillary acidic protein gene (Brenner *et al.*, 2001). An astrocytic and perhaps mitochondrial participation, secondary at least, may also occur in the pathogenesis of Canavan disease (Jellinger and Seitelberger, 1970) that is caused by aspartoacylase deficiency (Matalon *et al.*, 1988). Both in MLD and GLD, the enzymatic

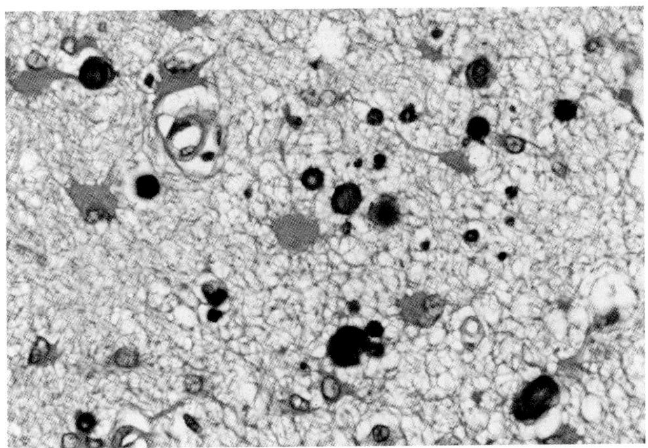

FIGURE 28.25
Round to elliptical blue mineralizations in gliotic white matter devoid of myelin and oligodendrocytes in ALD. Hematoxylin-eosin.

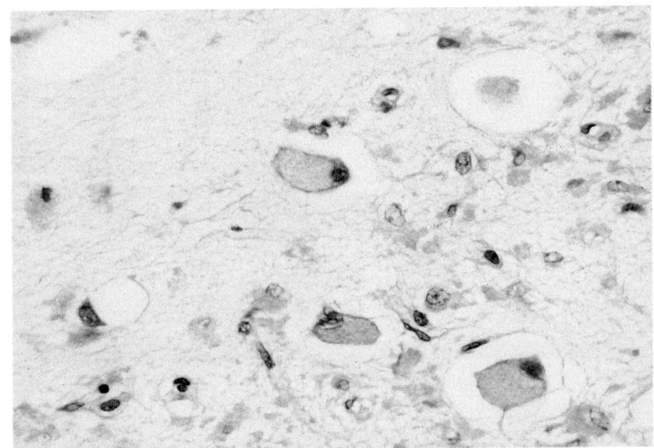

FIGURE 28.26
Neuronal storage in dentate nucleus devoid of myelin in MLD. Hematoxylin-eosin.

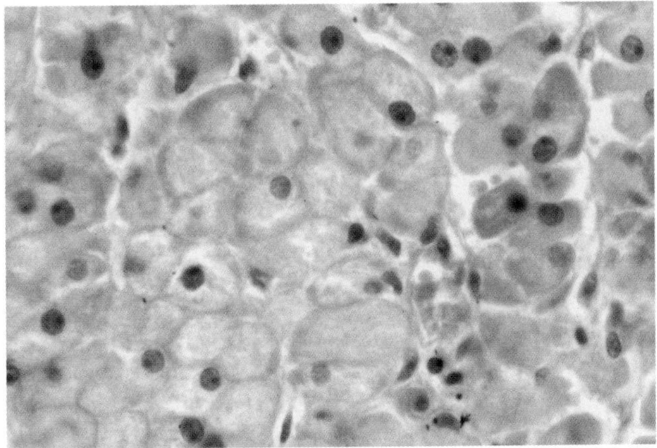

FIGURE 28.27
Pale striated and ballooned adrenocortical cells (left side of field) adjacent to normal eosinophilic counterparts in ALD.

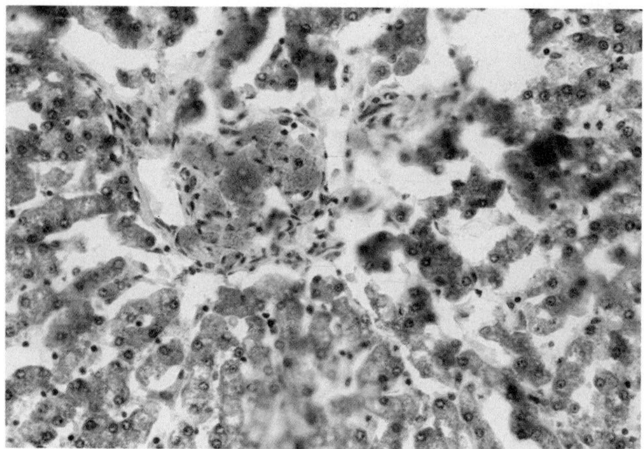

FIGURE 28.28
Brown sulfatide in biliary epithelium of MLD. Frozen section, Acid-cresyl violet.

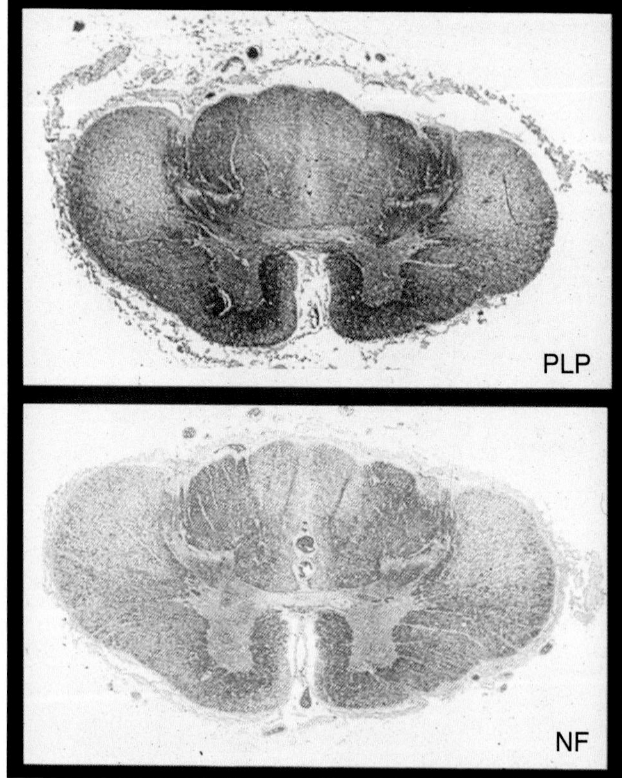


FIGURE 28.29
Comparable loss of axons (NF) and myelin (PLP) in gracile and corticospinal tracts of cervical spinal cord in AMN. Immunostains to neurofilament (NF) and proteolipid (PLP) proteins.

defect resides in the lysosome, arylsulfatase A in MLD and galactosylceramidase (galactocerebrosidase) in GLD. There is evidence that the excessive sulfatide in myelin destabilizes the sheath and leads to its breakdown in MLD (Ginsberg and Gershfeld, 1991), but a toxic effect on oligodendrocytes by lysosulfatide also has been proposed. A comparable toxic pathogenetic mechanism has considerable support in GLD, where galactosylsphingosine (psychosine) has been implicated in the death of oligodendrocytes and abortive myelination (Miyatake and Suzuki, 1972). The myelin instability model also has been suggested in the later onset and milder cases of PMD and its allelic SP2, whereas a toxic effect of mutant PLP or its alternatively spliced isoform DM20 trapped in dilated cisterns

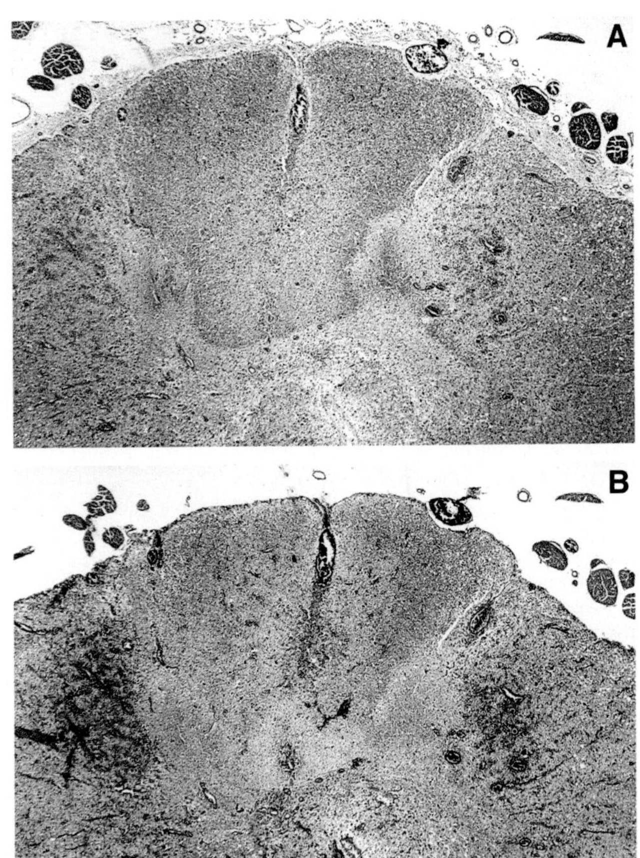


FIGURE 28.30
Similar degeneration of medial gracile and corticospinal tracts in late-onset Alexander disease evident with both (A) myelin and (B) axon stains. (A) Luxol fast blue—PAS myelin, (B) Bodian axon.

of rough endoplasmic reticulum has been proposed to cause the apoptotic death of oligodendrocytes with resultant hypomyelination in connatal and classical PMD (reviewed in Hudson, 2001). The pathogeneses of SLDs remain unknown, but the abundance of ceroid-lipofuscin and the presence of iron in the glia of its pigmentary form (Gray *et al.*, 1987) may indicate an oxidative insult. The peroxisomal (and perhaps mitochondrial) disease ALD/AMN, on the other hand, has been considered to have a more complicated two-stage pathogenetic mechanism: dysmyelination followed by inflammatory demyelination. The dysmyelinative process was originally considered to result from a toxic effect of VLCFA on oligodendrocytes, but currently a myelin instability caused by the incorporation of VLCFA into myelin lipids, particularly phosphatidylcholine and gangliosides, and into the major myelin protein PLP is favored (Ho *et al.*, 1995; Powers *et al.*, 1992; Powers *et al.*, 2000). Subsequently, a profound and rapid demyelinative (immune) destruction of myelin supervenes, in which T cells (particularly CD8 cytotoxic T cells), reactive astrocytes, macrophages, nitric oxide, TNF-$\alpha$, and CD1-mediated lipid antigen presentation participate (Ito *et al.*, 2001; Powers *et al.*, 1992). (See specific chapters in this volume and the relevant chapters in Scriver *et al.*, 2001, for further details.)

## Acknowledgments

The author thanks Tina Blazey for her usual outstanding secretarial assistance, both Jenny Smith and Nancy Dimmick for their artistic and photographic expertise, and Professor Marjo van der Knaap for Figure 28.16.

## References

Adachi, M., Schneck, L., Cara, J., and Volk, B. W. (1973). Spongy degeneration of the central nervous system (Van Bogaert and Bertrand type: Canavan disease). A review. *Hum. Pathol.* **4,** 331–347.

Adams, C. W. M. (1965). "Neurohistochemistry." pp. 437–517, Elsevier, Amsterdam.

Adams, R. D., and Kubik, C. S. (1952). The morbid anatomy of the demyelinative diseases. *Am. J. Medicine* **12,** 510–546.

Babikian, V., and Ropper, A. H. (1987). Binswanger's disease. A review. *Stroke* **18,** 2–12.

Baudrimont, M., Dubas, F., Joutel, A., Tournier-Lasserve, E., and Bousser, M. G. (1993). Autosomal dominant leukoencephalopathy and subcortical ischemic stroke. *Stroke* **24,** 122–125.

Bielschowsky, M., and Henneberg, R. (1928). Über familiare diffuse Sklerose (Leukodystrophia cerebri progressiva hereditaria). *J. Psychol. Neurol. (Lpz.)* **36,** 131–181.

Borrett, D., and Becker, L. E. (1985). Alexander's disease: A disease of astrocytes. *Brain* **108,** 367–385.

Brenner, M., Johnson, A. B., Boespflug-Tanguy, O., Rodriguez, D., Goldman, J. E., and Messing, A. (2001). Mutations in GFAP, encoding glial fibrillary acidic protein, are associated with Alexander disease. *Nature Genet.* **27,** 117–120.

Cammer, W., Rose, A. L., and Norton, W. T. (1975). Biochemical and pathological studies of myelin in hexachlorophene intoxication. *Brain Res.* **98,** 547–559.

Choi, K. G., Sung, J. H., Clark, H. B., and Krivit, W. (1991). Pathology of adult-onset globoid cell leukodystrophy (GLD) (Abstract). *J. Neuropathol. Exp. Neurol.* **50,** 336.

De Reuck, J., Crevits, L., De Coster, W., Sieben, G., and vander Eecken, H. (1980). Pathogenesis of Binswanger chronic progressive subcortical encephalopathy. *Neurology* **30,** 920–928.

Dickens, C. (1894). "A Tale of Two Cities."

Eldridge, R., Anayiotos, C. P., Schlesinger, S., Cowen, D., Bever, C., Patronas, N., and McFarland, N. (1984). Hereditary adult-onset leukodystrophy simulating chronic progressive multiple sclerosis. *N. Engl. J. Med.* **311,** 948–953.

Ginsberg, L., and Gershfeld, N. L. (1991). Membrane bilayer instability and the pathogenesis of disorders of myelin. *Neurosci. Lett.* **130,** 133–136.

Gray, F., Destee, A., Bourre, J.-M., Gherardi, R., Krivosic, I., Warot, P., and Poirier, J. (1987). Pigmentary type of orthochromatic leukodystrophy (OLD): A new case with ultrastructural and biochemical study. *J. Neuropathol. Exp. Neurol.* **46,** 585–596.

Gray, F., Dubas, F., Roullet, E., and Escourolle, R. (1985). Leukoencephalopathy in diffuse hemorrhagic cerebral amyloid angiopathy. *Ann. Neurol.* **18,** 54–59.

Harding, B. H., and Surtees, R. (2002). Metabolic and neurodegenerative diseases of childhood. *In* "Greenfield's Neuropathology" (D. I. Graham and P. L. Lantos, Eds.), 7th ed., Vol. 1, pp. 485–517. Arnold, London.

Ho, J. K., Moser, H., Kishimoto, Y., and Hamilton, J. A. (1995). Interactions of a very long chain fatty acid with model membranes and serum albumin. Implications for the pathogenesis of adrenoleukodystrophy. *J. Clin. Invest.* **96,** 1455–1463.

Hudson, L. D. (2001). Pelizaeus-Merzbacher disease and the allelic disorder X-linked spastic paraplegia type 2. *In* "The Metabolic & Molecular Bases of Inherited Disease" (C. R. Scriver, A. L. Beaudet, W. S. Sly, and D. Valle, Eds.), 8th ed., Vol. IV, pp. 5789–5805. McGraw-Hill, New York.

Ito, M., Blumberg, B. M., Mock, D. J., Goodman, A. D., Moser, A. B., Moser, H. W., Smith, K. D., and Powers, J. M. (2001). Potential environmental and host participants in the early white matter lesion of adreno-leukodystrophy: Morphologic evidence of CD8 cytotoxic T cells, cytolysis of oligodendrocytes, and CD1-mediated lipid antigen presentation. *J. Neuropathol. Exp. Neurol.* **60,** 1004–1019.

Jellinger, K., and Seitelberger, F. (1970). Spongy degeneration of the central nervous system in infancy. *Curr. Topics Pathol.* **53,** 90–159.

Joutel, A., Corpechot, C., Ducros, A., Vahedi, K., Chabriat, H., Mouton, P., Alamowitch, S., Domenga, V., Cecillion, M., Marechal, E., Maciazek, J., Vayssiere, C., Cruaud, C., Cabanis, E. A., Ruchoux, M. W., Weissenbach, J., Bach, J. F., Bousser, M. G., and Tournier-Lasserve, E. (1996). Notch3 mutations in CADASIL, a hereditary late-onset condition causing stroke and dementia. *Nature* **383,** 707–710.

Kimbrough, R. D., and Gaines, T. B. (1971). Hexachlorophene effects on the rat brain: Study of high doses by light and electron microscopy. *Arch. Environm. Hlth.* **23,** 114–118.

Klatzo, I. (1967). Neuropathological aspects of brain edema. *J. Neuropathol. Exp. Neurol.* **26,** 1–14.

Kornfeld, M., Moser, A., Moser, H., Kleinschmidt-DeMasters, B., Nolte, K., and Phelps, A. (1994). Solvent vapor abuse leukoencephalopathy. Comparison to adrenoleukodystrophy. *J. Neuropathol. Exp. Neurol.* **43,** 389–398.

Leech, R. W., Brumback, R. A., Miller, R. H., Otsuka, F., Tarone, R. E., and Robbins, J. H. (1985). Cockayne syndrome: Clinicopathologic and tissue culture studies of affected siblings. *J. Neuropathol. Exp. Neurol.* **44,** 507–519.

Leegwater, P. A., Vermeulen, G., Konst, A. A., Naidu, S., Mulders, J., Visser, A., Kersbergen, P., Mobach, D., Fonds, D., van Berkel, C. G., Lemmers, R. J., Frants, R. R., Oudejans, C. B., Schutgens, R. B., Pronk, J. C., and van der Knaap, M. S. (2001). Subunits of the translation initiation factor eIF2B are mutant in leukoencephalopathy with vanishing white matter. *Nat. Genet.* **29,** 383–388.

Ludwin, S. K. (1997). The pathobiology of the oligodendrocyte. *J. Neuropathol. Exp. Neurol.* **56,** 111–124.

Matalon, R., Michals, K., Sebesta, D., Deanching, M., Gashkoff, P., and Casanova, J. (1988). Aspartoacylase deficiency and N-acetylaspartic aciduria in patients with Canavan disease. *Am. J. Med. Genet.* **25,** 463–471.

Miyatake, T., and Suzuki, K. (1972). Globoid cell leukodystrophy. Additional deficiency of psychosine galactosidase. *Biochem. Biophys. Res. Commun.* **48,** 538–543.

Moser, H. W. (1997). Adrenoleukodystrophy: phenotype, genetics, pathogenesis, and therapy. *Brain* **120,** 1485–1508.

Nance, M. A., and Berry, S. A. (1992). Cockayne syndrome: review of 140 cases. *Am. J. Med. Genet.* **42,** 68–84.

Norton, W. T., Poduslo, S. E., and Suzuki, K. (1966). Subacute sclerosing leukoencephalitis. II. Chemical studies including abnormal myelin and an abnormal ganglioside pattern. *J. Neuropathol. Exp. Neurol.* **25,** 582–597.

Plum, F., Posner, J. B., and Hain, R. F. (1962). Delayed neurological deterioration after anoxia. *Arch. Intern. Med.* **110,** 56–63.

Poser, C. M. (1962). Concepts of dysmyelination. *In* "Cerebral Sphingolipidoses" (S. M. Aronson and B. W. Volk, eds.), pp. 141–164. Academic Press, New York.

Poser, C. M. (1968). Diseases of the myelin sheath. *In* "Pathology of the Nervous System" (J. Minckler, ed.), Vol. I, pp. 767–820. McGraw-Hill, New York.

Powers, J. M. (1996). A neuropathologic overview of the neurodystrophies and neurolipidoses. *Handbook of Clin. Neurol.* **66** *(revised series 22)*, 1–32.

Powers, J. M., DeCiero, D. P., Cox, C., Richfield, E. K., Ito, M., Moser, A. B., and Moser, H. B. (2001). The dorsal root ganglia in adrenomyeloneuropathy: Neuronal atrophy and abnormal mitochondria. *J. Neuropathol. Exp. Neurol.* **60,** 493–501.

Powers, J. M., DeCiero, D. P., Ito, M., Moser, A. B., and Moser, H. W. (2000). Adrenomyeloneuropathy: A neuropathologic review featuring its noninflammatory myelopathy. *J. Neuropathol. Exp. Neurol.* **59,** 89–102.

Powers, J. M., and De Vivo, D. C. (2002). Peroxisomal and mitochondrial disorders. *In* "Greenfield's Neuropathology" (D. I. Graham and P. L. Lantos, eds.), 7th ed., Vol. 1, pp. 737–797. Arnold, London.

Powers, J. M., and Horoupian, D. S. (1995). Central nervous system. *In* "Anderson's Pathology" (I. Damjanov and J. Linder, eds.), 10th ed., pp. 2777–2782. Mosby, Philadelphia.

Powers, J. W., Liu, Y., Moser, A. B., and Moser, H. W. (1992). The inflammatory myelinopathy of adrenoleukodystrophy. *J. Neuropathol. Exp. Neurol.* **51,** 630–643.

Prineas, J. W., McDonald, I., and Franklin, R. J. M. (2002). Demyelinating diseases. *In* "Greenfield's Neuropathology" (D. I. Graham and P. L. Lantos, eds.), 7th ed., Vol. 1, pp. 471–550. Arnold, London.

Raine, C. S. (1997). Demyelinating diseases. *In* "Textbook of Neuropathology" (R. L. Davis, D. M. Robertson, eds.), 3rd ed., pp. 627–714. Williams & Wilkins, Baltimore.

Ramsey, R. B., and Davison, A. N. (1974). Steryl esters and their relationship to normal and diseased human central nervous system. *J. Lipid Res.* **15,** 249–255.

Razavi, E. F., Larroche, J. C., and Gaillard, D. (1988). Infantile familial encephalopathy with cerebral calcifications and leukodystrophy. *Neuropediatrics* **19,** 72–79.

Richardson, E. P., Jr., (1982). Myelination in the human central nervous system. *In* "Histology and Histopathology of the Nervous System" (W. Haymaker, R. D. Adams, eds.), pp. 146–173. Charles C. Thomas, Springfield, IL.

Schaumburg, H. H., Powers, J. M., Raine, C. S., Spencer, P. S., Griffin, J. W., Prineas, J. W., and Boehme, D. M. (1977). Adrenomyeloneuropathy: A probable variant of adrenoleukodystrophy. II. General pathologic, neuropathologic, and biochemical aspects. *Neurology* **27,** 1114–1119.

Schaumburg, H. H., Powers, J. M., Raine, C. S., Suzuki, K., and Richardson, Jr., E. P. (1975). Adrenoleukodystrophy. A clinical and pathological study of 17 cases. *Arch. Neurol.* **33,** 577–591.

Scriver, C. R., Beaudet, A. L., Sly, W. S., and Valle, D. (2001). "The Metabolic & Molecular Bases of Inherited Disease," 8th ed. McGraw-Hill, New York.

Seitelberger, F. (1995). Neuropathology and genetics of Pelizaeus-Merzbacher disease. *Brain Pathol.* **5,** 267–274.

Smith, K. D., Kemp, S., Braiterman, L. T., Lu, J-F, Wei, H-M, Geraghty, M., Stetten, G., Bergin, J. S., Peysner, J., and Watkins, P. A. (1999). X-linked adrenoleukodystrophy: Genes, mutations, and phenotypes. *Neurochem. Res.* **24,** 521–535.

Suzuki, K., and Suzuki, K. (2002). Lysosomal diseases. *In* "Greenfield's Neuropathology" (D. I. Graham and P. L. Lantos, eds.), 7th ed., Vol. 1, pp. 653–735. Arnold, London.

Tournier-Lasserve, E., Joutel, A., Meilki, J., Weissenbach, J., Lathrop, G. M., Chabriat, H., Mas, J. L., Cabanis, E. A., Baudrimont, M., and Maciazek, J. (1993). Cerebral autosomal dominant arteriopathy with subcortical infarcts and leukoencephalopathy maps to chromosome 19q12. *Nat. Genet.* **3,** 256–259.

Trapp, B. D., Peterson, J., Ransohoff, R. M., Rudick, R., Mork, S., and Bo, L. (1998). Axonal transection in the lesions of multiple sclerosis. *N. Engl. J. Med.* **338,** 278–285.

van der Knaap, M. S. (2001). Magnetic resonance in childhood white-matter disorders. *Dev. Med. Child Neurol.* **43,** 705–712.

van der Knaap, M. S., Barth, P. G., Gabreels, F. J., Franzoni, E., Begeer, J. H., Stroink, H., Rotteveel, J. J., and Valk, J. (1997). A new leukoencephalopathy with vanishing white matter. *Neurology* **48,** 845–855.

van der Knaap, M. S., Barth, P. G., Vrensen, G. F. J. M., and Valk, J. (1996). Histopathology of an infantile-onset spongiform leukoencephalopathy with a discrepantly mild clinical course. *Acta Neuropathol.* **92,** 206–212.

van der Knaap, M. S., Breiter, S. N., Naidu, S., Hart, A. A. M., and Valk, J. (1999). Defining and categorizing leukoencephalopathies of unknown origin: MR imaging approach. *Radiology* **213,** 121–133.

van der Knaap, M. S., Kamphorst, W., Barth, P. G., Kraaijeveld, C. L., Gut, E., and Valk, J. (1998). Phenotypic variation in leukoencephalopathy with vanishing white matter. *Neurology* **51,** 540–547.

van der Knaap, M. S., and Valk, J. (1995). "Magnetic resonance of myelin, myelination, and myelin disorders," 2nd ed. Springer, Berlin.

Wakui, H., Nishimura, S., Watahiki, Y., Endo, Y., Nakamoto, Y, and Miura, A. B. (1991). Dramatic recovery from neurological deficits in a patient with central pontine myelinolysis following severe hyponatremia. *Jpn. J. Med.* **30,** 281–284.

Wolman, M. (1970). Histochemistry of myelination and demyelination. *In* "Handbook of Clinical Neurology" (P. J. Vinken and W. G. Bruyn, eds.), Vol. 9, pp. 24–44. North-Holland Publishing, Amsterdam.

CHAPTER

# 29

# Multiple Sclerosis Classification and Overview

*Fred D. Lublin*

## INTRODUCTION

Multiple sclerosis (MS) has been a recognized clinical entity since the latter part of the 19th century, following the clinical description by Charcot. Several pathologic descriptions preceded this one, but Charcot is credited with providing the synthesis of the clinical and pathologic pictures. Anecdotes that describe rather typical cases can be found as far back as the Middle Ages.

MS is the commonest of the demyelinating diseases and the commonest cause of neurologic disability in young adults. The prevalence of MS in North America is about 100 per 100,000 and incidence of about 6 per 100,000, increasing with latitude. Approximately 350,000 persons in the United States have MS, and this number may be an underestimate. The average age at onset is 32, and patients tend to live in excess of 35 years from time of diagnosis. Therefore, although the actual number of individuals is not large compared to some other diseases, the longevity and the potential for serious disability produce considerable economic consequences. The cost of MS in the United States is $9.6 billion per year (in 1994 dollars), around $34,000 per year for each patient, exclusive of the costs of disease-modifying agents.

The signs and symptoms of MS are the consequence of the underlying neuropathologic changes that occur in patients. The primary mechanism of injury is by inflammatory demyelination and, to a variable degree, axonal damage. Either mechanism may produce clinical features. The role of axonal damage is clear cut, disrupting conduction completely. Demyelination may result in either slowing of conduction or complete failure of transmission. The former will produce symptoms when the slowing becomes critical. As the pathologic damage may involve any area of the central nervous system (CNS), the location of the lesion(s) also plays a role in symptom production.

MS can produce any symptom or sign that might occur with damage to the CNS, especially white matter tracks. The most common findings include optic neuritis, weakness, sensory loss, ataxia, nystagmus, bladder dysfunction, and cognitive impairment, but the full list is quite long.

The progressive impairment or disability that occurs over time with MS results from one of two mechanisms. There is either stepwise worsening due to accumulated deficits from residua of exacerbations or gradual, inexorable progressive disease, independent of the exacerbations (see the fuller definition of an exacerbation presented later in the chapter). The relative role of exacerbations and progressive disease in the accumulation of deficits has been debated, but the data are clear that both impact the long-term course of the illness. Recent data from a meta-analysis of several clinical trials in MS demonstrate that residual deficit from exacerbations occurs after at least 50% of attacks. Later in the course of MS, progressive disease seems to contribute more strongly to the disability (Confavreux *et al.*, 2000).

## DIAGNOSING MS

The diagnosis of MS is based on finding clinical evidence of lesions of the CNS, disseminated in time and space. For this reason, some have referred to the illness as disseminated sclerosis. Dissemination in time implies that there is more than one episode of CNS dysfunction. Dissemination in space implies involvement of more than one area of the CNS. This is accomplished through a careful medical history and a detailed neurologic examination. Although all MS begins with a first attack, the essence of the clinical disease is the multiplicity of attacks. Several diagnostic criteria have been proposed over the past several decades, all affirming the need for dissemination, primarily white matter involvement, young age at onset (20 to 50), and an important caveat: that there be no better diagnosis.

Twenty years ago, a committee organized by the National Multiple Sclerosis Society (NMSS), developed the penultimate MS diagnostic criteria, incorporating the clinical aspects of MS, paraclinical evidence (MRI, urodynamics, evoked potentials) and cerebrospinal fluid (CSF) immunoglobulin abnormalities (Poser *et al.*, 1983). This diagnostic schema segregated patients into definite, probable, or possible MS categories and was designed primarily for clinical research protocols. The role of MRI, which was in its infancy as a diagnostic tool, was not defined. In 2000, another committee of the NMSS convened to update and revise the MS diagnostic criteria for MS, with the intention of increasing the role of MRI in the diagnostic schema. Over the past 20 years, there has been considerable knowledge of the importance of MRI in providing an *in vivo* view of the neuropathology of MS. Other objectives for this revision of the diagnostic criteria were to simplify the categories and produce guidelines that would be useful to practicing clinicians. Outside experts then reviewed the deliberations of that group. The resultant manuscript was submitted for peer review and published in the Annals of Neurology in July 2001 (McDonald *et al.*, 2001). The need for this most current revision is underscored by the development of MS disease-modifying agents (DMAs) over the past decade. Since the advent of DMAs, the need for early, accurate therapy has become extremely important as the accumulated data suggest that the earlier treatment is started, the less there is risk of accumulating impairment/disability.

The general conclusions from the new criteria are that the diagnosis of MS requires objective evidence of lesions disseminated in time and space; MRI findings may contribute to determination of dissemination in time or space; other supportive investigations include CSF and visual evoked potential (VEP); and the diagnostic categories are possible MS, MS, or not MS (the category of "probable MS," used in Poser, had little practical value for clinicians, other than suggesting more certainty than "possible," and was of no value in clinical trials). The new guidelines reaffirmed the classical approach to diagnosing MS by clinical means only: the finding of evidence of lesions of the CNS, disseminated in time and space, based on a detailed history and a complete neurological examination. This schema allows for diagnosing MS in regions of the world where there is limited access to newer technologies.

Most MS starts with an attack/relapse/exacerbation—that is, an acute episode of CNS dysfunction lasting at least 24 hours, occurring in the absence of fever or metabolic derangement. All events occurring within 30 days of such an event are considered, by convention, to be part of a single event, even though multiple areas of the CNS may be involved. The commonest clinical course of MS follows a relapsing-remitting course of multiple attacks, as will be described.

The role of MRI in the diagnosis of MS has been expanded considerably in this latest MS diagnostic guideline. After careful consideration of the various MRI studies of patients with MS, the committee determined that the criteria of Barkhof (Barkhof *et al.*, 1997), as amended by Tintore (Tintore *et al.*, 2000), provided the best combination of specificity and sensitivity, with emphasis on accuracy, as appropriate for a diagnostic guideline. For dissemination in space (Tab. 29.1), these criteria require three of the following four elements: (1) at least one gadolinium enhancing lesion or nine T2 hyperintense lesions, (2) at least one infratentorial lesion, (3) at least one juxtacortical lesion, and (4) at least three periventricular lesions. A spinal cord lesion can substitute for any of these brain lesions. If there are immunoglobulin abnormalities in the CSF, then the MRI criteria are relaxed to only two T2 lesions typical of MS.

The MRI also can be used to confirm dissemination in time (Tab. 29.2). If an MRI scan of the brain performed at 3 or more months after an initial clinical event demonstrates a new gadolinium-enhancing lesion, this would indicate a new CNS inflammatory event, as the duration of gadolinium enhancement in MS is usually less than 6 weeks. If there are no gadolinium-enhancing lesions but a new T2 lesion (presuming an MRI at the time of the initial event), then a repeat MRI scan after another 3 months is needed with demonstration of a new T2 lesion or gadolinium-enhancing lesion. The reason for the second scan to establish that a new T2 lesion has occurred relates to the inclusion of all events within 30 days of an exacerbation as part of the initial exacerbation. A new T2 lesion developing within the 30 days following an exacerbation would not count as a new event, although it would show up as new on the first 3-month scan, thus necessitating a new T2 lesion on the second 3-month scan. The 3-month interval was a consensus decision and is offered as a guideline.

Spinal fluid analysis is also useful for diagnosing MS, but not diagnostic by itself (as other conditions can produce similar abnormalities). The presence of immunoglobulin abnormalities in the CSF indicates the production of immunoglobulin within the CNS. This is best determined by the finding of oligoclonal bands of IgG present in the CSF, but not in serum. This is best determined by using the isoelectric focusing technique. The finding of an elevated IgG index (a ratio of the IgG to protein in the serum and CSF) is equally helpful. The total protein in the CSF is almost always less than 100 in MS and the finding of more than 50 WBCs in the CSF is quite uncommon.

Evoked responses can also be used to provide evidence for dissemination in space. The most valuable is the visual evoked potential (VEP). The finding of a prolonged VEP in an individual without clinical evidence of an optic nerve lesion indicates subclinical involvement of the optic nerve. The other evoked responses were not found to be discriminative or sensitive enough to provide useful diagnostic information (Gronseth and Ashman, 2000).

Putting these diagnostic guidelines into practice is rather straightforward. If the patient has had two or more attacks with objective evidence of involvement of two or more areas of the CNS, and there is no better diagnosis, then the patient has met the criteria for dissemination in time and space. In this circumstance, additional studies are not necessary, an important issue in regions where access to MRI might be limited or nonexistent. If

**TABLE 29.1** New Diagnostic Criteria for MRI Determination of Dissemination in Space (after Barkhof *et al.* and Tintore *et al.* (Tintore *et al.*, 2000))

Three out of four of the following:

- One Gd+ lesion or 9 T2 hyperintense lesions
- One infratentorial lesion
- One juxtacortical lesion
- Three periventricular lesions (One spinal cord lesion = one brain lesion)

**TABLE 29.2** New Diagnostic Criteria for MRI Determination of Dissemination in Time

- Gadolinium-enhancing lesion demonstrated in a scan done at least 3 months following onset of a clinical attack at a site different from attack/
- In the absence of gadolinium-enhancing lesions at the 3 month scan, follow-up scan after an additional 3 months showing a gadolinium-enhancing lesion or new T2 lesion.

additional studies are undertaken, such as MRI or CSF analysis, they should yield consistent results or the diagnosis should be questioned.

If there has been one attack and evidence of two lesions in the CNS, then one needs to obtain evidence for dissemination in time. This can be accomplished by either a second attack or by evidence of dissemination in time on MRI scanning (see Tab. 29.2)

If there are two or more attacks but evidence on exam of involvement of only one area of the CNS, then one needs to confirm dissemination in space. A second attack, involving a new area of the CNS or changes on subsequent MRI scan (see Tab. 29.1), will fulfill this criterion.

If there has been one attack and evidence of only one area of CNS involvement (the clinically isolated syndrome), then one need confirm dissemination in both time and space. This can be accomplished clinically or by fulfilling the MRI criteria for dissemination for each (Tabs. 29.1 and 29.2).

In the case of insidious onset and progression of neurologic dysfunction suggestive of MS (usually primary progressive MS), one needs to find positive CSF and evidence of dissemination in time by MRI or continued progression for at least 1 year and dissemination in space by MRI (see Tab. 29.1) or two or more spinal MRI abnormalities or four to eight cerebral MRI lesions and one spinal cord lesion or an abnormal VEP and four to eight cerebral lesions on MRI or an abnormal VEP and less than four cerebral lesions plus one spinal cord lesion. These criteria were adapted from those previously published by Thompson *et al.* (Thompson *et al.*, 2000). As opposed to the other guidelines, it was felt that CSF was necessary to diagnose primary progressive MS, in that the risk of alternative diagnoses was greater than for other forms of MS. There is not an abundance of demographic data on pure primary progressive MS, as currently defined. In the past, the practice of including patients with relapses, often remote, has confounded this category. Analysis of recent clinical trials of primary progressive MS should provide important additional data that can be used to support or modify the diagnostic guidelines.

These new diagnostic criteria are relatively easy to employ in clinical practice and in clinical trials. Figures 29.1 and 29.2 outline the major features of the new criteria and are available on a laminated card from the National Multiple Sclerosis Society (USA). Initial studies show that the new criteria are highly sensitive and specific, leading to earlier diagnosis. One study shows more than twice the rate of conversion from a clinically isolated syndrome to MS using the new criteria as compared to the older Poser *et al.* criteria (Dalton *et al.*, 2002). Similar results are seen in therapeutic trials of clinically isolated syndromes and early MS.

## CLINICAL SUBTYPES OF MS

The clinical course of MS, although quite variable in temporal sequence, tends to follow one of several specific courses characterized by either a relapsing pattern or a progressive course. In relapsing forms of MS, there occur multiple acute exacerbations of neurologic dysfunction lasting days to months, with a variable degree of recovery and then stability until the next exacerbation, which can occur weeks to decades later. There are at present no reliable biologic makers (either MRI or clinical laboratory) that distinguish the disease course patterns, so they were decided by consensus, based on a survey of the international MS clinical research community published in 1996 (Lublin and Reingold, 1996). The clinical course patterns can be divided into four subtypes: relapsing-remitting, primary progressive, secondary progressive, and progressive-relapsing, as outlined next.

*Relapsing-remitting.* Relapsing-remitting (RR) MS (Figs. 29.3A and B) is the commonest form at presentation and is characterized by clearly defined disease relapses with full recovery or with sequelae and residual deficit upon recovery. Periods between disease relapses are characterized by a lack of disease progression (Figs. 29.5A and B). The defining elements of RR MS are episodes of acute worsening of neurologic function followed by a variable degree of recovery, with a stable course between attacks. Approximately 85 to 90% of patients with MS start with an RR course.

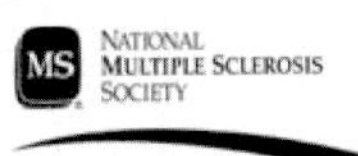


**New Multiple Sclerosis Diagnostic Criteria**

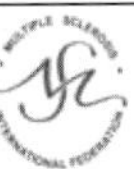

| CLINICAL (ATTACKS) | OBJECTIVE LESIONS | ADDITIONAL REQUIREMENTSTOMAKEDIAGNOSIS |
|---|---|---|
| 2 or more | 2 or more | • None;clinical evidence willsuffice (additional evidencedesirable but mustbe consistentwith MS) |
| 2 or more | 1 | • Dissemination in space by MRI ***or*** positive CSF and 2 or more MRI lesions consistentwith MS ***or*** further clinicalattack involving different site |
| 1 | 2 or more | • Dissemination in time by MRI ***or*** second clinicalattack |
| 1 mono-symptomatic | 1 | • Dissemination in space by MRI ***or*** positive CSF and 2 or more MRI lesions consistentwith MS **AND** • Dissemination in time by MRI ***or*** second clinicalattack |
| 0 (progression from onset) | 1 | • Positive CSF **AND** • Dissemination in space by MRI evidence of 9 or more T2 brain lesions ***or*** 2 ormore cord lesions ***or*** 4-8 brain and 1 cord lesion ***or*** positive VEP with 4-8 MRIlesions ***or*** positive VEP withless than4 brainlesions plus1 cordlesion **AND** • Dissemination in time by MRI ***or*** continued progressionfor 1 year |

FIGURE 29.1

**ParaclinicalEvidence in MS Diagnosis**

What is a Positive MRI?
3 out of 4of the following:
✓1 Gd-enhancing lesion ***or*** 9 T2 hyperintense lesions if no Gd-enhancing lesion
✓1 or more infratentorial lesions
✓1 or more juxtacortical lesions
✓3 or more periventricular lesions
Note: 1 cord lesion can substitute for 1 brain lesion

WhatProvides MRI Evidence of Dissemination in Time?
A Gd-enhancinglesion demonstrated in a scan done at least 3 months following onset of clinicalattack at a site different from attack, ***or***
In absence of Gd-enhancing lesions at 3 monthscan, follow-up scan after an additional 3 months showing Gd-lesion ornew T2lesion.

What is Positive CSF?
Oligoclonal IgG bandsin CSF (and not serum) ***or*** elevated IgG index

What is Positive VEP?
Delayed but well-preserved wave form



FIGURE 29.2

*Primary progressive.* Primary progressive (PP) MS (Figs. 29.4A and B) is characterized by disease progression from onset with occasional plateaus and temporary minor improvements allowed. Approximately 10% of patients have this form of MS. The essential element

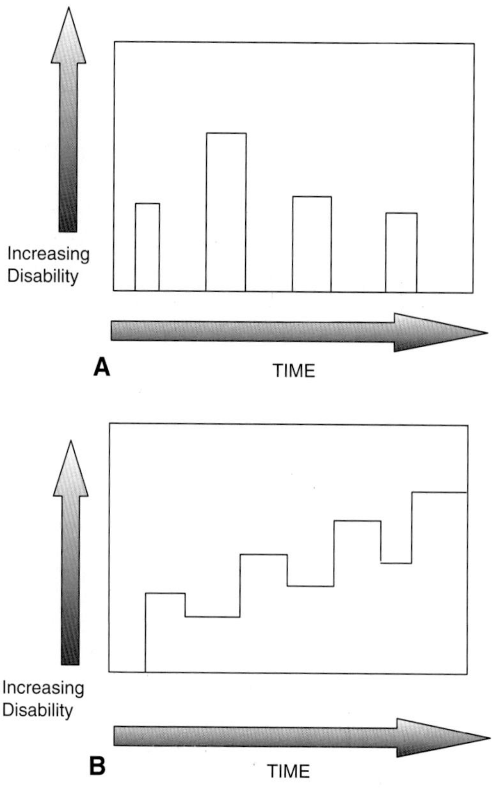


FIGURE 29.3
Relapsing-remitting (RR) MS is characterized by clearly defined acute attacks with full recovery (A) or with sequelae and residual deficit upon recover (B). Periods between disease relapses are characterized by lack of disease progression.

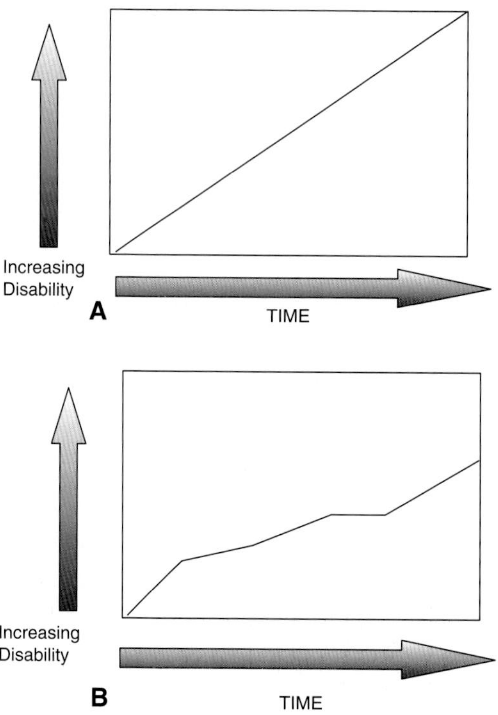


FIGURE 29.4
Primary-progressive (PP) MS is characterized by disease showing progression of disability from onset, without plateaus or remissions (A) or with occasional plateaus and temporary minor improvements (B).

in PP MS is a gradual, nearly continuously worsening baseline with minor fluctuations, but no distinct relapses. While near continuous progression is required in this definition, it was recognized that progression at a constant rate throughout disease (Fig. 29.4A) was unlikely and that accommodation must be made for variations in the rate of progression over time (Fig. 29.4B). PP MS is quite distinct from RR MS (especially the absence of any exacerbations), causing some to suggest that it may represent a different disease. However, current evidence suggests that PP is a subtype of typical MS.

*Secondary progressive.* Secondary progressive (SP) MS (Figs. 29.5A and B) is characterized by an initial relapsing-remitting disease course followed by progression with or without occasional relapses, minor remissions, and plateaus. SP MS may be seen as a long-term outcome of RR MS, in that almost all SP patients initially begin with RR disease as defined here. However, once the baseline between relapses begins to progressively worsen, the patient has switched from RR MS to SP MS. This transition from RR to SP occurs in up to 50% of RR MS patients, although it can take many years and is unpredictable.

*Progressive-relapsing.* In the progressive-relapsing (PR) form of MS (Figs. 29.6A and B), there is progressive disease from onset, with clear acute relapses, with or without recovery, with periods between relapses characterized by continuing progression. Approximately 5 to 6% of patients have this form of MS, but there are data now accruing that PP MS patients may convert to PR at a rate of almost 1% per year. This will be better understood once a large clinical trial in PP MS has completed.

The term "chronic progressive MS," used frequently in the past has been discarded in favor of one of the more descriptive progressive forms just described.

MS can also be categorized by outcome. At the extremes, MS can be designated as either benign or malignant.

Benign MS has been defined as disease that allows patients to remain fully functional in all neurologic systems 15 years after disease onset. Although this form may comprise 10 to 15% of patients, diagnosis, and thus prognosis, is difficult and by definition requires 15 years. Even then, relapses or progression can occur, sometimes as late as 25 years later.

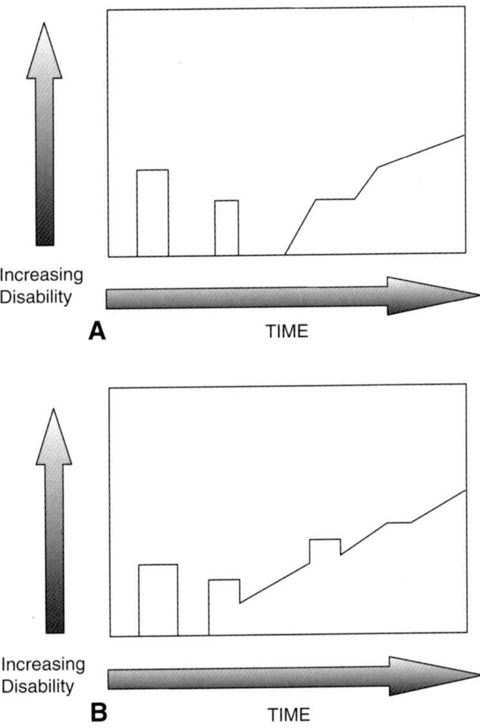


FIGURE 29.5
Secondary progressive (SP) MS begins with an initial RR course, followed by progression of variable rate (A) or may also include occasional and minor remissions (B).

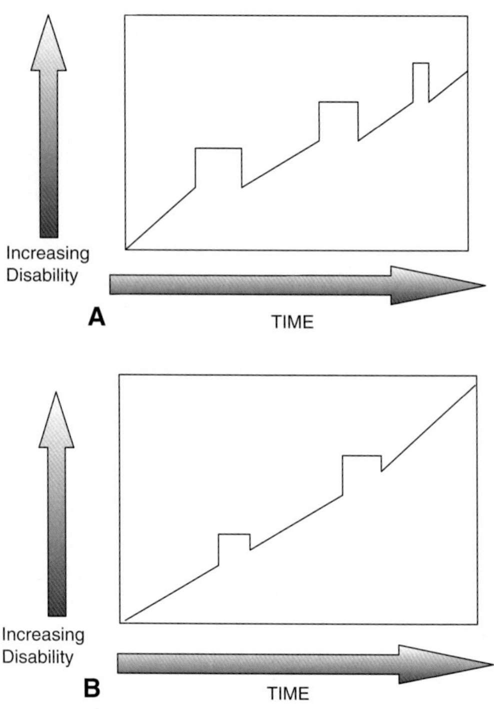


FIGURE 29.6
Progressive-relapsing (PR) MS shows progression from onset, but with clear acute relapses with (A) or without (B) full recovery.

Malignant MS is defined as disease with a rapid, progressive course, leading to significant disability in multiple neurologic systems or death in a relatively short time after disease onset. This is, fortunately, quite rare.

It is hoped that in the near future, we will have biologically based characterizations of the different MS disease courses, likely using advanced MRI metrics and possibly immunologic markers. These could improve our prognostic abilities and allow for more rational use of the various therapies available for treating MS, and perhaps provide increased insight into the complex underlying pathophysiologic aberration that is MS.

## References

Barkhof, F., Filippi, M., Miller, D. H., Scheltens, P., Campi, A., Polman, C. H., Comi, G., Ader, H. J , Losseff, N., and Valk, J. (1997). Comparison of MRI criteria at first presentation to predict conversion to clinically definite multiple sclerosis. Review. *Brain* **120,** 2059–2069.

Confavreux, C., Vukusic, S., Moreau, T., and Adeleine, P. (2000). Relapses and progression of disability in multiple sclerosis. *N. Engl. J. Med.* **343,** 1430–1438.

Dalton, C. M., Brex, P. A., Miszkiel, K. A., Hickman, S. J., MacManus, D. G., Plant, G. T., Thompson, A. J., and Miller, D. H. (2002). Application of the new McDonald criteria to patients with clinically isolated syndromes suggestive of multiple sclerosis. *Ann. Neurol.* **52,** 47–53.

Gronseth, G. S., and Ashman E. J. (2000). Practice parameter: The usefulness of evoked potentials in identifying clinically silent lesions in patients with suspected multiple sclerosis (an evidence-based review): Report of the Quality Standards Subcommittee of the American Academy of Neurology. *Neurology* **54,** 1720–1725.

Lublin, F. D., and Reingold S. C. (1996). Defining the clinical course of multiple sclerosis: Results of an international survey. National Multiple Sclerosis Society (USA) Advisory Committee on Clinical Trials of New Agents in Multiple Sclerosis. *Neurology* **46,** 907–911

McDonald, W. I., Compston, A., Edan, G., Goodkin, D., Hartung, H. P., Lublin, F. D., McFarland, H. F., Paty, D. W., Polman, C. H., Reingold, S. C., Sandberg-Wollheim, M., Sibley, W., Thompson, A., van Den, N. S., Weinshenker, B. Y., and Wolinsky, J. S. (2001). Recommended diagnostic criteria for multiple sclerosis: Guidelines from the International Panel on the diagnosis of multiple sclerosis. *Ann. Neurol.* **50,** 121–127.

Poser C. M, Paty, D. W., Scheinberg, L., McDonald W. I., Davis, F. A., Ebers, G. C., Johnson, K. P., Sibley, W. A., Silberberg, D. H., and Tourtellotte, W. W. (1983). New diagnostic criteria for multiple sclerosis: Guidelines for research protocols. *Ann. Neurol.* **13,** 227–231.

Thompson, A. J., Montalban, X., Barkhof, F., Brochet, B., Filippi, M., Miller, D. H., Polman, C.H., Stevenson, V. L., and McDonald, W. I. (2000), Diagnostic criteria for primary progressive multiple sclerosis: A position paper. *Ann. Neurol.* **47,** 831–835.

Tintore, M., Rovira, A., Martinez, M. J., Rio, J., Diaz-Villoslada, P., Brieva, L., Borras, C., Grive, E., Capellades, J., and Montalban, X .(2000). Isolated demyelinating syndromes: Comparison of different MR imaging criteria to predict conversion to clinically definite multiple sclerosis. *AJNR Am. J. Neuroradiol.* **21,** 702–706.

CHAPTER

# 30

# Genetic Susceptibility and Epidemiology

*Alastair Compston*

## THE METHODOLOGY OF EPIDEMIOLOGICAL STUDIES IN MULTIPLE SCLEROSIS

Epidemiology remains one of the most active areas of multiple sclerosis research. The emerging statistics serve several purposes: generating etiological hypotheses, establishing health care needs in the community, defining the natural history of multiple sclerosis as the basis for understanding the evolving clinical expression of tissue injury, and providing a yardstick against which the results of therapies can be compared. Because the many studies have been performed over the past 100 years in different places and at different times, comparisons—which aim to see the big epidemiological picture—are notoriously difficult. It follows that attempts to formulate reliable hypotheses using the epidemiological evidence are potentially vulnerable. Most sensitive to artifact have been the temporal and geographical trends emerging from comparisons of prevalence between regions and the serial study of individual locations.

An everyday word such as *frequency* is useful in conveying a general impression of statistics for multiple sclerosis but it lacks precision. *Cumulative frequency* or *lifetime risk* is the maximum chance that the disease will occur during the lifetime of an at-risk individual; it is around 1:400 for northern European Caucasians. Risk factors alter this rate. Their contribution to the underlying pathogenesis can be expressed as the *relative risk* (the product of the proportions of cases and controls with and without the risk factor) or the *odds ratio* (the ratio of incidence rates for individuals who have and have not been exposed to the risk factor). Relative risk is a collective descriptor and the contribution made by any one factor is the *attributable risk*. *Incidence* describes new events (the numerator) in a defined group (the denominator) over a given period. Each is liable to ascertainment error, but the impact on statistics is greater when mistakes occur in estimating the numerator. *Prevalence* describes the number of affected individuals in a population at risk on a given occasion. Ascertainment will vary inversely with size and accessibility of the at-risk population, and security of the diagnosis, and it tends to increase with repeated survey as awareness and vigilance improve among participants. The at-risk population should be demographically based. *Mortality* describes the number of individuals dying with or as a result of multiple sclerosis among the at-risk population over a given period. With the decline in autopsy rates and the trend for death certification to reflect administrative needs rather than pathological verification, mortality is a poor statistic for evaluating the epidemiology of multiple sclerosis.

Incidence, prevalence, and mortality have a close relationship. In a population not experiencing recent demographic change and where mortality returns are accurate and complete, incidence will equal mortality, and prevalence will be the product of either statistic and disease duration. In practice, changes in frequency usually arise from predictable cycles in these statistics *(regression to the mean)* and structure of the population being surveyed, rather than alteration in etiological and biological factors causing the disease. In a recent population-based study, survival was >50% at 40 years from onset with an excess of deaths from suicide and neoplasia; complications of multiple sclerosis accounted for 70% of deaths (Sumelahti *et al.*, 2002).

The difficulty of describing statistics that incorporate lifetime risk in children and young adults is addressed by quoting *age*- and *sex-specific* rates for morbidity; these relate numerators to a denominator confined to that proportion of the at-risk population, which has the same age and gender structure. One further refinement is to relate statistics to a single representative or virtual population and derive a *standardized prevalence ratio.* The 95% confidence limits (upper and lower with attention to whether or not these straddle unity) provide a statement on the likely reproducibility of a given epidemiological finding.

The easy route to answering an epidemiological problem in multiple sclerosis is to retrieve cases from an existing register, usually hospital or clinic based, of validated cases. The inclusion or exclusion of marginal cases will vary with the purpose of the survey. In seeking to identify biological features, the error should be toward inclusion of individuals who probably have the disease process even if this is not yet clinically definite. In other contexts, it is advisable to restrict the register to those who meet strict criteria (McDonald *et al.*, 2001). Most investigators segregate cases of different racial origin since sociohistoric factors may create variations in risk status across even quite small regions. However, some epidemiological questions can only be answered by comparing specifically different groups or locations. Choosing a population with a low prevalence of multiple sclerosis for the study of a rare event, such as twinning, guarantees frustration and a less than definitive result since the numerator will be low. An important genetic or biological feature may not differ significantly between groups in places where multiple sclerosis is frequent and risk factors are over-represented in the at-risk population. Paradoxically, the chance of identifying factors that are common in the at-risk population and make a major contribution to the pathogenesis is improved by surveying regions of low prevalence. Conversely, those risk factors for multiple sclerosis that are not over-represented in the normal population will be identified more easily in high prevalence regions.

## THE DISTRIBUTION OF MULTIPLE SCLEROSIS

By the beginning of the 20th century, multiple sclerosis—a disease that merited individual case reports 25 years previously—had become one of the most common reasons for admission to a neurological ward. The period 1900–1950 saw a gradual maturation of methods for accurate definition of population-based statistics. Thereafter, surveys from many parts of the world established the geography of multiple sclerosis and allowed speculation on the reasons for this pattern. Kurtzke (1975) first systematically collated published surveys of prevalence and suggested that the distribution fell into zones of low, medium, and high prevalence. The high risk band (>$30/10^5$) extended throughout northern Europe, the northern United States, Canada, southern Australia, and New Zealand. Areas of medium risk ($5\text{-}25/10^5$) were southern Europe, the southern United States, and northern Australia. Low risk (<$5/10^5$) extended to Asia and South America and was assumed in many uncharted regions. Improved methodology, alterations in classification, and enhanced investigator vigilance have all impacted on serial updating of these figures showing a rise in the absolute number of cases in almost all parts of the globe (Bauer, 1987; Lauer and Firnhaber, 1994; Kurtzke, 1993). Many of the claims for latitudinal gradients now seem less secure but multiple sclerosis does seem to show genuine variation in its distribution over quite small distances. The explanation for these patterns has been much debated in the reasonable belief that they provide important clues to the cause of the disease.

The raw statistics for prevalence are shown in Figure 30.1; these are rates per $10^5$ of the population, often rounded up or down to provide a best guess for regions subjected to

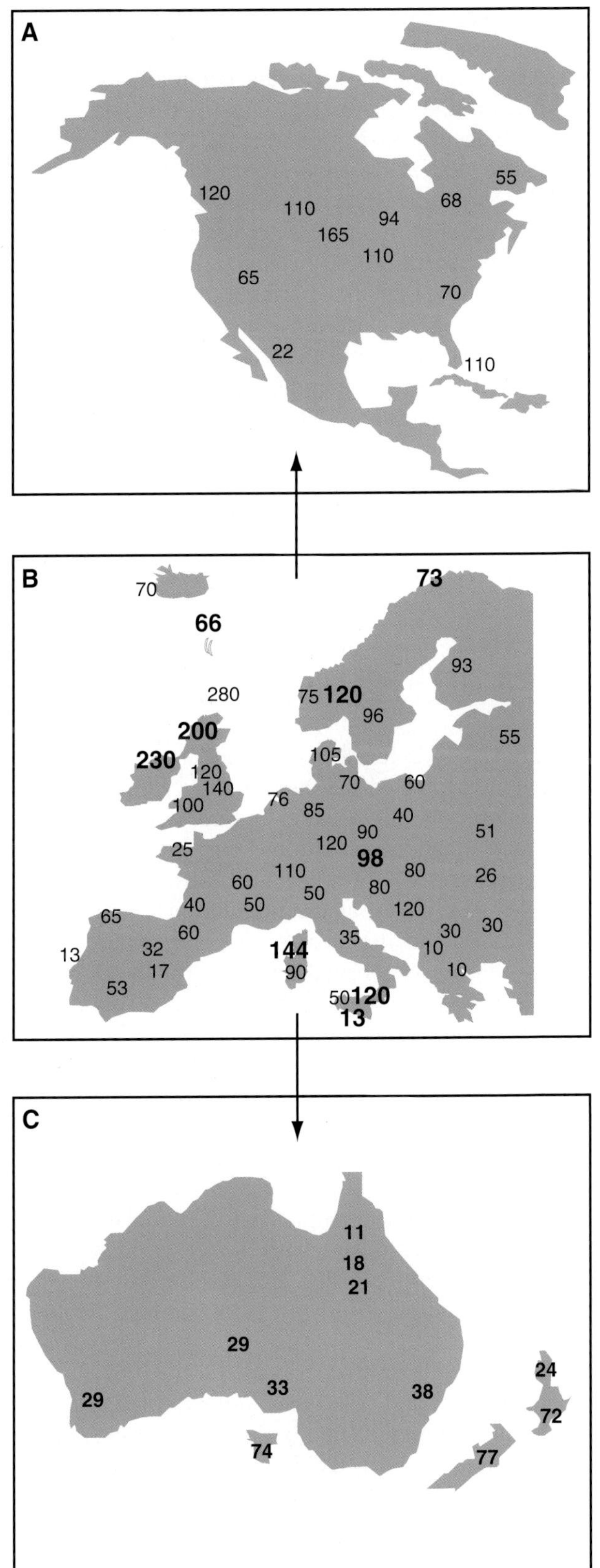


FIGURE 30.1
Prevalence rates for multiple sclerosis (per $10^5$) in Europe (B), the United States and Canada (A), and Australia & New Zealand (C). Numbers are approximations based on best available morbidity statistics. Estimates published since 1998 are shown in large font.

serial or multiple simultaneous survey; confidence intervals have not been calculated or shown for those studies in which these statistics were originally included. To summarize the situation, multiple sclerosis remains a relatively common disorder of young adults in northern Europe, continental North America, and Australasia. The indigenous peoples of the Orient, Arabian peninsula, Africa, continental South America, and India are less susceptible, although recent studies are starting to erode these differentials. Cases are now identified among small population isolates, previously considered to be absolutely protected; these include examples of multiple sclerosis in Saami, Hutterites, and African blacks, among others. In northern Europe, incidence and prevalence are higher in southern Scandinavia, northern Germany, the United Kingdom, and parts of Italy than in northern Scandinavia, France, Spain, and the eastern Mediterranean countries. Multiple sclerosis is more prevalent in northeast Scotland and the Orkney and Shetland islands than in other parts of the United Kingdom (Robertson and Compston, 1995). Differences in prevalence exist between Mediterranean regions and islands that are geographically close but differ in their genetic and cultural histories (Dean *et al.*, 2002; Rosati 1994). A diagonal gradient in frequency is seen in North America with highest rates in the Midwest and lowest in the Mississippi delta (Bulman and Ebers, 1992). A latitudinal gradient is apparent for the white Australian population with higher rates in the south than north based on definitive survey of four regions using comparable methods and working to a common prevalence date (Hammond *et al.*, 1988).

## MULTIPLE SCLEROSIS IN MIGRANTS

Populations are not stable, geographically or socially, and migrations involving relatively large numbers of people have affected the distribution of multiple sclerosis. The message from these studies of migration has been to regard multiple sclerosis as an acquired disorder triggered by environmental conditions. The contrary view, derived more from the study of stable indigenous populations, is that the distribution depends on endogenous (i.e., genetic) susceptibility easily seen at the population level and increasingly apparent from the study of individuals. But the race *versus* place, nature *versus* nurture debate is increasingly sterile given the concession that however low the threshold for susceptibility, disease processes must still be triggered; for most, there is room both for genes and the environment in considering the etiology and pathogenesis of all complex traits, including multiple sclerosis.

Comparisons of morbidity statistics for multiple sclerosis between racial groups in a single geographical setting first achieved prominence with the studies of Geoffrey Dean in South Africa from the 1950s. Dean made two influential observations. First, higher age-corrected incidence and prevalence rates were seen in immigrants from Europe compared to South African English, Afrikaners, and Cape Coloreds (with mixed African and European ancestry)—in that order—and with no cases identified in African blacks. Second, within the English-speaking white population, those moving from northern Europe to southern Africa as adults took with them the high frequency of their country of origin, whereas those migrating below the age of 15 years showed the lower rates characteristic of native-born white South Africans (Dean, 1967).

Subsequently, Geoffrey Dean and colleagues looked at the corollary to his pioneering studies from South Africa. A survey of immigrants showed prevalence rates for multiple sclerosis in the United Kingdom–born children of West Indians, Africans, and Asians approximating to those in equivalent Caucasian age groups (Elian and Dean, 1987; Elian *et al.*, 1990). Various methodological problems arise in studying ethnic minorities within a large metropolis. It is easy to miss rare events and so underestimate the numerator whereas reliable census data are available on which to base the denominator; conversely, members of ethnic minorities affected by an illness such as multiple sclerosis might tend to cluster in areas of maximum population density so as to benefit from family and other community support, thereby inflating the apparent concentration of cases. But the trawl of immigrant cases has been widespread and it is more likely that the number of patients with multiple sclerosis, born in the United Kingdom of parents who were migrants from the West Indies, Africa, or Asia, has actually been underascertained. That said, it is wise not to rush to judgment by extrapolating from studies involving a small numerator living in an unusual environment. For example, three cases were identified among a cohort of around 3400 persons born of Vietnamese mothers who came to France under the age of 20 years providing, by 1975, an age-specific prevalence of $169/10^5$ (95% CI 94-135) for the third decade (Kurtzke and Bui, 1980). Superficially, this suggests a change from the inherent low risk of multiple sclerosis in Vietnamese, but the study is confounded by the fact that having a French-born father was a requirement for immigration; genetic admixture therefore introduced a major potential bias into the study.

Another illustrative series of epidemiological studies compared the frequency of multiple sclerosis among Japanese living in Japan, Hawaii, and the West Coast of the United States. The prevalence among Japanese ($7/10^5$) in Hawaii was only one-quarter that seen in Caucasian immigrants (Alter *et al.*, 1971; Detels *et al.*, 1972; Lauer, 1994) and virtually identical to Japanese (and Caucasians) living in California (Detels *et al.*, 1977). At that time, rates quoted for native Japanese were around $2/10^5$ (Kuroiwa *et al.*, 1983), and the evidence favored a strong protective effect for Japanese irrespective of environment. But as in so many other parts of the world, subsequent surveys suggest that the baseline rates were underestimates and recent prevalence rates in Japan are higher both in the northern and in southern parts of the country. However, before reaching a final position on the frequency of multiple sclerosis in Japanese, it is important to recall that definitions have changed. The classic view was that multiple sclerosis in Japan is characterized by an opticospinal phenotype with very few cases conforming to the pattern seen in Caucasians; now, the opticospinal pattern is seen less frequently, whereas the so-called Western features are on the increase (Fukazawa *et al.*, 2000). Thus, alterations in definition and recognition may have contributed to the changing clinical and epidemiological pattern of multiple sclerosis in Japanese.

A third location where migration shows age-related differences in prevalence of multiple sclerosis is Israel. Starting from the higher prevalence in migrants from northern Europe (Ashkenazis) than Asia and Africa (Sephardis), an age-at-migration effect was apparent in Ashkenazi Jews with those arriving in Israel before adolescence underrepresented, compared to Sephardis (Alter, *et al.*, 1962; Alter, *et al.*, 1978). Age-adjusted prevalence in the Israeli-born children both of Ashkenazi and Sephardic Jews was the same as seen in the United States. Updated figures confirm these observations—although, as expected, the numbers have changed (Kahana *et al.*, 1994): after adjusting to the 1960 Israeli population and classifying on place of paternal birth, prevalences (per $10^5$) were 32 (fathers born in Israel), 38 (fathers born in Europe or North America), and 29 (fathers born in Africa or Asia) compared with 14 in immigrants. The possibility of sampling error is raised by the evidence for regional variation in these differences—with higher rates overall and less differential in Jerusalem (where ascertainment was optimized) compared to more rural areas.

Taken together, the evidence from the study of migrants supports the macroview that racially determined differences in risk for multiple sclerosis are modified by environment. Geographically more restricted movements support this hypothesis. Mortality with multiple sclerosis is higher for southern born United States citizens dying in the north ($0.68/10^5$/year) compared with those remaining in the south ($0.46/10^5$/year). For United States army veterans born in northern states but entering service from the middle and southern parts of North America, mortality ratios fall from 1.48 to 1.27 and 0.74, respectively. Taking those born in the middle states, mortality ratio decreases with entry into military service in the south and increases in the north (1.4 and 0.73, compared to baseline, respectively: Kurtzke *et al.*, 1971).

Attention needs to be directed at the Australian epidemiological studies, since these describe a large geographical area with a relatively homogenous population mix. The distribution of migrants from the United Kingdom and Ireland shows the same latitudinal gradient as for the entire population but with a bias introduced by the high prevalence for multiple sclerosis in the cohort from Hobart (Tasmania); that location apart, the rates are lower than for contemporary studies from the United Kingdom but with no differences dependent on age at migration taking 15 years as the point of stratification (Hammond *et al.*, 2000).

These studies are the epidemiological platform for suggesting a contribution from environmental factors in the etiology of multiple sclerosis, but they do not establish at what age these influences occur. The studies from South Africa and the United States argue for a critical period in childhood although it is difficult to be more precise and the Australian survey somewhat undermines this tight window of microbial opportunity.

## EPIDEMICS OF MULTIPLE SCLEROSIS

John Kurtzke has been the main protagonist for the occurrence of point source epidemics of multiple sclerosis (Kurtzke, 1993). Skeptics prefer the position that these merely follow cycles of increased ascertainment due to local enthusiasm rather than genuine changes in incidence arising from the introduction of transmissible etiological factors into virgin populations. The fact that all the better-documented examples have occurred in small island communities in the north Atlantic can be seen to support either view.

In the first survey of Iceland, 168 cases of multiple sclerosis were identified with onset between 1900 and 1975 (Kurtzke *et al.*, 1982). Incidence seemed retrospectively to have risen from about 1922, then stabilized until again increasing for around 10 years from 1945 and declining thereafter. Local observers point out the correlation between incidence and changes in health care provision with the arrival of specialists in neurology and serial reexamination of the morbidity statistics. According to this analysis, among 252 of 323 patients with onset of symptoms attributed to multiple sclerosis after January 1, 1900, who remained alive in December 1989, incidence rates were $<1/10^5$/year until the 1930s and $2.5/10^5$/year thereafter, coinciding with the arrival of two neurologists; with waning enthusiasm, there then followed a lull until 1945–1954 when incidence increased to $3.3/10^5$/year following the first systematic survey of the disease; with nine neurologists in practice from 1975, there was a further increase to a peak incidence of $4.1/10^5$/year, which has been maintained. Just as John Kurtzke takes support for a post–World War II epidemic from the lower age-at-onset between 1945 and 1954, John Benedicz holds up the long interval between onset and diagnosis, the disproportionate lack of benign cases (more easy to overlook) and overrepresentation of patients with severe multiple sclerosis before 1950 alongside the reduction in interval between onset and diagnosis after 1940 as evidence for the impact of neurological expertise on early diagnosis and improved case ascertainment making the Icelandic saga a virtual rather than a real multiple sclerosis epidemic (Benedikz *et al.*, 1994).

The epidemiology of multiple sclerosis in the Faroe Islands has assumed special significance in considering the etiology of multiple sclerosis. The story begins with the identification of fewer cases than expected from comparisons with neighboring Orkney and Shetland. Subsequently, despite diligent searches, Kurtzke was unable to identify any patient with an estimated date of onset earlier than July 1943. Among 83 individuals with multiple sclerosis resident in the Faroes during the 20th century, 55 had spent their entire life in the Faroes, or only short periods overseas, whereas 28 were either foreign born or had lived elsewhere for prolonged periods. Based on year of onset, these cases are considered to cluster into four epidemics involving 21, 10, 10, and 13 cases, and resulting from exposure between 1941–1944, 1945–1957, 1958–1970, and 1971–1983, respectively. Kurtzke has proposed that the factor determining multiple sclerosis in the Faroes was introduced by British troops between 1940 and1943, and the temporal and spatial distribution of the disease mapped nicely onto the pattern of villages where troops were billeted. The story is summarized by Kurtzke and Heltberg (2001). The Faroes hypothesis has not escaped criticism and counter-criticism with exchange of salvoes relating to validity of the diagnoses, exclusions, case ascertainment, the definition of epidemics, and the role of British occupation in triggering the putative epidemic.

Morbidity statistics for multiple sclerosis have never been higher than the rates for incidence and prevalence seen in the Orkney and Shetland Islands. Estimates of prevalence (per $10^5$) carried out on four occasions between 1954 and 1974, showed an increase from 111 to 309 in Orkney and 134 to 184 in Shetland (Cook *et al.*, 1985; Robertson and Compston, 1995). Although the overall frequency of the disease is without precedent, the evidence suggests that the incremental change in incidence and mortality are attributable to alterations in classification and ascertainment: during these decades, systematic depopulation in Orkney and Shetland left an aging population no longer at risk of multiple sclerosis; the rise in prevalence relates to increased survival (by approximately one decade) and better case recognition. Perhaps, the more recent updating of morbidity statistics does suggest significantly less multiple sclerosis in Shetland, but not Orkney, since 1965. Outside the north Atlantic, an epidemic has been claimed for Key West (south west Florida) where 37 patients with peak onset in and around 1977–1979 were identified in 1984 (prevalence 140/100,00), suggesting an exceptional frequency compared to neighboring parts of the United States not attributable to increased clinical vigilance or differential migration of symptomatic individuals to a more favorable climate (Sheremata *et al.*, 1985).

## EXOGENOUS FACTORS PREDICTING THE CLINICAL COURSE

Multiple sclerosis is almost always found to be more common in females than males in population based surveys, with a ratio of at least 2F:M in all ethnic groups. This distortion is even more marked in children with multiple sclerosis (Duquette *et al.*, 1987) but reversed in the context of late onset disease which is more common in males who show over-representation of the primary progressive phenotype. Their prognosis is less favorable that younger age-at-onset cases, females with multiple sclerosis, and cases with a phenotype characterized by infrequent sensory episodes that recover fully. There have been many attempts to categorize the course and prognosis of multiple sclerosis; this reductionist approach is tricky in the context of a disease that is notoriously fickle in its behavior, but the pattern of primary progressive multiple sclerosis in 20%, relapses with full remission in the remaining 80% of cases at onset, with conversion over time to persistent deficits and then secondary progression in 60% of this group, is a reasonable caricature. Against this background of the natural history, with all its uncertainties, various extrinsic factors have been considered that might alter the natural history either by exposing latent disease, precipitating disease activity in those with established multiple sclerosis or changing the later course of the illness.

There is no epidemiological evidence to suggest that multiple sclerosis is contagious. After correction for age and disease duration, and anticipation of the diagnosis in the second affected through enhanced awareness, Robertson *et al.* (1997) showed no clustering for year at onset in conjugal pairs, suggesting that multiple sclerosis had not been passed from one spouse to the other. A recent study purporting to provide evidence that the disease is sexually transmitted and attributable to abuse when onset is in childhood (Hawkes, 2002) is speculative, lacks scientific rigor, and is deeply offensive to many affected individuals, especially those forming part of multiplex families and their relatives.

But what is the environmental trigger? It is a rare moment in the history of research in multiple sclerosis for there not to be a current hot microbial favorite for the cause of multiple sclerosis based either on population serology, identification of particles in one tissue or another, or recovery of defined organisms from body fluids. Few have stood the test of time and most have disappeared from interest often due to the subsequent recognition of technical artifacts and as each is displaced by new and more compelling candidates. Although individual reports continue to describe an excess of antibodies to *chlamydia pneumonia* in the cerebrospinal fluid of patients with multiple sclerosis, perhaps the most telling study is a comparison between three laboratories of polymerase chain reaction detection rates for *chlamydia pneumonia* in the same samples; one (the laboratory reporting the original findings: Sriram *et al.*, 1999) found the organism in the majority of patients but few controls; the other two were unable to detect *chlamydia* in any samples (Kaufman *et al.*, 2002). HHV-6 remains a candidate (Ablashi *et al.*, 1998). Friedman *et al.* (1999) reported an excess of HHV-6 structural protein and antibody to HHV-6 in serum and brain tissue in multiple sclerosis compared to controls; Soldan *et al.* (2000) have shown increased peripheral blood lymphocyte reactivity of the neurotrophic HHV-6A variant.

The issue of vaccination has recently been resolved: three studies have shown no increase in demyelinating disorders or activity of preexisting disease in individuals undergoing hepatitis B vaccination (Ascherio *et al.*, 2001; Confavreux *et al.*, 2001; Zipp *et al.*, 1999). The United States study showed a relative risk for the onset of multiple sclerosis of 0.7 (95% CI 0.3-1.8) in the 2 years after hepatitids B vaccination (Ascherio *et al.*, 2001); the French study (Confavreux *et al.*, 2001) showed a relative risk of 0.71 (95% CI 0.40-1.26) for relapse in the 1-, 2-, or 3-month period following vaccination (mainly for hepatitis B but also tetanus and influenza).

Trauma as a trigger of disease activity in multiple sclerosis has been much considered and still features in the courts where plaintiffs may claim that an accident has provoked the first appearance of multiple sclerosis or altered the course of preexisting manifestations. Sibley *et al.* (1991) prospectively studied disease activity by questionnaire and physical examination for 8 years: taking either the 3- or 6-month period following each event as *at-risk*, only electrical trauma showed an association with new episodes; in fact, all other forms of trauma were negatively correlated both with clinical exacerbations and disease progression. Siva *et al.* (1993), using the Mayo Clinic cohort, also concluded that disease exacerbations are no more frequent in the 6 months after limb fracture than at other times.

The situation with respect to the risk from anesthesia is unresolved in that no epidemiologically based studies have been performed and the evidence is entirely anecdotal; some neurologists advise patients to avoid elective interventions while remaining sensible about treatments or procedures that justify the small risk of increasing disease activity—if it actually exists (Baskett and Armstrong, 1970; Siemkowicz, 1976).

Several authors have demonstrated prospectively that new episodes of demyelination increase after (presumed) viral exposure, but no single agent has been implicated (Anderson *et al.*, 1991; Sibley *et al.*, 1985): 9% of presumed infections are followed by relapse, and 27% of new episodes are related to infection; the relative risk for relapse in the 4-week period after upper respiratory (especially adenovirus) or gastrointestinal infections is 1.3. Most recently, Buljevac *et al.* (2002) prospectively studied 73 patients with relapsing multiple sclerosis experiencing 167 infections during 6466 patient-weeks (1.7 years) and observed a twofold increased relapse rate, and greater risk of lasting clinical deficits, during the at-risk period (−2 to +5 weeks), associated with markers of immune activation but no change in permeability of the blood brain barrier. Rather softer, but nevertheless consistent, is the evidence that new episodes of demyelination—especially optic neuritis—cluster in the spring, at least in northern Europe (Jin *et al.*, 2000).

Another attempt to link the epidemiological patterns to specific infections has recently been revisited—and with broadly similar conclusions. Compston *et al.* (1986) retrospectively compared historical and laboratory evidence for previous virus exposure in patients with multiple sclerosis and optic neuritis with HLA-DR-matched controls. Patients with demyelinating disease had a later age at infection by measles, mumps, and rubella. Martyn *et al.* (1993) later reanalyzed this series to show an even more marked effect of EBV infection; those who reported having infectious mononucleosis before the age of 18 years had a relative risk for multiple sclerosis of 7.9 (95% CI 1.7-37.9). Meanwhile, Lindberg *et al.* (1991), looking at registries for infectious mononucleosis and multiple sclerosis in Sweden, found a slight excess of demyelinating disease following EBV infection compared with controls. Haahr *et al.* (1995) used records from the Danish State Serum Institute register of EBV infections and the Danish Multiple Sclerosis Registry to identify 16 individuals who developed multiple sclerosis among 6853 experiencing EBV infection in the decade 1968–1978 (relative risk, 2.8); the median age at infection was 17 years, which did not differ from the age at infection in heterophile antibody-positive individuals who did not develop multiple sclerosis. Vaughan *et al.* (1996) used more discriminating laboratory markers and also showed an enhanced immune response to EBV, involving epitopes also expressed by other pathogens one of which appeared to cross-react with (murine) glia cells, in patients with multiple sclerosis, especially during relapse. Now, Hernan *et al.* (2001) have again shown an increased of multiple sclerosis following infectious mononucleosis (odds ratio 2.1: 95% CI 1.5-2.9) and older age-at infection by mumps and measles.

Anecdotal evidence on whether pregnancy affects the immediate or long-term course of multiple sclerosis has been supplemented by prospective surveys. A major confounder in the detailed interpretation of these studies is the decision by women with severe disability not to embark on pregnancy and the corresponding preparedness of those with mild disease to start or extend their families. Onset of multiple sclerosis does not cluster around pregnancy, and having children does not alter the long-term course of the disease, but there is an increase in relapse rate during the puerperium. The studies indicate approximately a threefold higher risk in the 3 to 6 months after term than during pregnancy and suggest that the attacks may be more severe; but since there is evidence for reduction in relapse rate during the pregnancy itself, the high puerperial rate makes for no overall increase in disease activity over the entire pregnancy year. Runmarker and Andersen (1995) studied an inception cohort in Goteborg, Sweden, and disposed of the hypothesis that the onset of multiple sclerosis is influenced by pregnancy; in fact, there was a conspicuous absence of onset bouts during pregnancy compared with nonpregnant epochs including the puerperal 8 months. Fecundity was reduced in women with multiple sclerosis, presumably by choice especially in the context of significant disability and this is the probable explanation for the conclusion that pregnancy after onset is associated with a lower risk of progression. A prospective survey (PRIMS: *PR*egnancy *I*n *M*ultiple *S*clerosis: Confavreux *et al.*, 1998) recently surveyed 222 completed European pregnancies; annualized relapse rates in the four quarters before pregnancy were 0.63, 0.74, 0.70, and 0.81, respectively, falling to 0.47, 0.58, and 0.22 during the three trimesters of pregnancy, and rising to 1.23 and 0.88 in the first 6 months of the puerperium. Confavreux *et al.* (1998) suggested that the perturbation in disease activity around the time of parturition relates to T-helper (Th)-2-like cytokine performance of the placenta.

## ANALYZING THE EPIDEMIOLOGICAL PATTERN IN MULTIPLE SCLEROSIS

The interplay of nature and nurture is reflected in the distribution of many diseases but factors determining the geography of complex traits remain to be defined. As the global pattern of multiple sclerosis has emerged, ideas have also evolved on the interplay of factors that shape the influence of race and place. At first, the accumulated evidence from serial surveys of large populations defined gradients in frequency within the high prevalence regions: northern Europe, North America, and Australia. These patterns suggested a dominant environmental effect on the etiology of multiple sclerosis. This interpretation was supported by the surveys of multiple sclerosis in migrants from northern Europe showing, with few exceptions, lower prevalence rates than the country of origin—and by the putative epidemics. But the search for an environmental cause of multiple sclerosis remains stubbornly unproductive. Systematic screening for candidate infectious agents using population serology and sophisticated methods for virus detection has not revealed the microbial cause for multiple sclerosis. And, as a result, increasingly complex alternative theories have been advanced involving the role of climate, diet, geomagnetism, sunlight, air pollutants, radioactive rocks, and toxins to account for the global pattern of the disease.

Failure to define the environmental cause therefore led others to interpret the distribution of multiple sclerosis as a function of genetic susceptibility. The geography of multiple sclerosis matches the distribution of northern Europeans. Racial groups thought to be at low risk of the disease begin to show increased frequencies as their peoples move and mix with northern Europeans (Chakraborty *et al.*, 1992). Coming at the issue of ancestry from various directions (physiognomy, social history, surname—among other indirect clues), commentators have argued for nearly 100 years that the distribution arises because multiple sclerosis is a Nordic-Celtic disease: credit should go to Davenport (1922) for the original observation, to Sutherland (1956) for the first systematic demonstration of differential rates depending on ancestry in the same geographical region, to Poser (1994) for tying this hypothesis into the rich history of the Viking sagas, and to Skegg *et al.* (1987) for the amusing trick of mapping multiple sclerosis to the density of surnames with the prefix "Mc.." in the telephone directories of New Zealand. Further support for a geo-genetic solution to the distribution of multiple sclerosis is provided by maps showing a reasonable correlation between global or regional prevalence and genetic clines for markers of susceptibility in at-risk populations (Cavalli-Svorza *et al.*, 1994). At a more micropopulation genetics level, isolates have arisen as a consequence of sociohistorical events and population migrations, leading to disproportionate concentration of susceptibility genes in small communities (with others excluded) thus adding relic groups to the global pattern that exists for many polymorphic genetic markers.

Based on the putative epidemic of multiple sclerosis in the Faroes, John Kurtzke (Kurtzke, 1993) concluded that multiple sclerosis originated in Scandinavia (central Norway or the south-central lake district of Sweden) in the early 18th century and diffused across the Baltic states and northern Europe including the British Isles over the next 100 years. From there, it was exported to North America and Australasia, to South Africa and Italy. It is an attractive hypothesis, but whereas for Kurtzke the factors being distributed are germs, for others they are genes.

## FAMILIAL MULTIPLE SCLEROSIS

The concept of genetic susceptibility to multiple sclerosis began with observations on differences in racial susceptibility and gained momentum with descriptions of familial clustering. Many interesting pedigrees were reported, but at first their collection did not follow sound epidemiological principles and the studies were therefore subject to ascertainment bias. From the 1980s, the frequency and pattern of familial multiple sclerosis has been documented in population-based samples. These large cohorts have been used systematically to document the frequency of familial clustering, thereby consolidating the case for genetic susceptibility in multiple sclerosis and illuminating many aspects of its complexity. Multiplex families can be used to assess the extent to which genetic factors determine clinical features of the disease making the distinction between susceptibility and influences on the course. Access to family pedigrees provides the opportunity for laboratory studies aimed at mapping, identifying, and describing the function of the several genes that are assumed to make a contribution based on the pattern of familial clustering, individually and through epistatic interactions. The applications of that knowledge are several: to provide recurrence risks for individual categories of relatives, to prevent the disease by intervention in high risk individuals, to understand the mechanisms of tissue injury, to predict the long term course of the illness, and to select individuals more or less likely to benefit from treatments. Of these, the most immediate and realistic application is improved understanding of the pathogenesis and the design of novel therapies. In using multiplex families to explore genetic aspects of multiple sclerosis, diagnostic criteria for inclusion may deliberately be adjusted, estimating recurrence risks and performing analyses under conditions of varying clinical stringency. For example, since the majority of patients with isolated optic neuritis eventually convert to multiple sclerosis, these may reasonably be assigned affected status in genetic studies whereas clinical phenotypes with a lower recurrence risk and a less clear relationship to multiple sclerosis should be treated differently.

Multiple sclerosis has a familial recurrence rate of approximately 15%. A summary of recurrence risks for various categories of family member is shown in Figure 30.2. Although it is usually assumed that familial aggregation is due to coinheritance of susceptibility factors, the case has to be argued and the alternative is that this results from common exposure to environmental factors in childhood. The initial study of recurrence (from

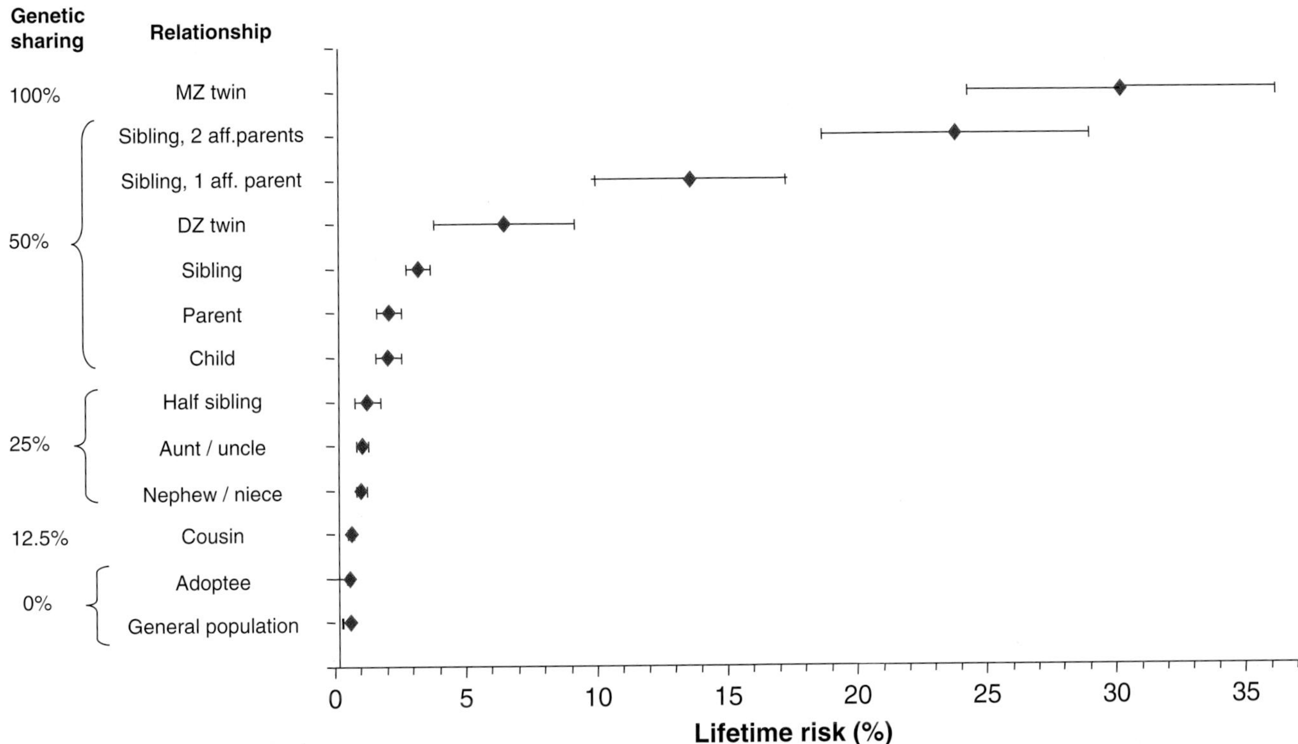


FIGURE 30.2
Age-adjusted recurrence risks for different relatives of probands with multiple sclerosis. Pooled data from population-based surveys. Estimated 95% confidence intervals are shown. Figures on left show the degree of genetic sharing between relative and proband. Kindly prepared by Dr Simon Broadley. Reproduced from Compston, D. A. S., and Coles, A. J. (2002). Multiple sclerosis: Seminar. *Lancet* **359,** 1221–1231

Canada) took as its baseline a lifetime risk of 0.2% for the entire population, and showed an increase to 3% in other first degree relatives (relative risk 20) and 1% in second degree relatives (relative risk 5.5: Sadovnick *et al.*, 1988). The United Kingdom survey confirms that the highest age-adjusted recurrence rate is for sisters (4%) and brothers (3%), compared with parents (2%) and offspring (2%). Overall, the reduction in risk changes from 3% (relative risk 9) in first-degree relatives to 1% (relative risk 3.4) and 1% (relative risk 2.9) in second- and third-degree relatives, respectively, compared with a background age-adjusted risk in this population of 0.3% (Robertson *et al.*, 1996b). In the remaining large survey from Belgium, recurrence risks were also 10-12-fold for first degree and threefold for second-degree relatives (Carton *et al.*, 1996).

With some variations in methodology, three contemporary studies have described the concordance rates for multiple sclerosis in twins identified from a population base. Surveys from Canada (Sadovnick *et al.*, 1993) and the United Kingdom (Mumford *et al.*, 1994) show a higher clinical concordance rate in monozygotic (approximately 25%) than dizygotic twin pairs (about 3%). The outlier, from France (French Research Group on Multiple Sclerosis (1992), did not identify a difference between monozygotic and dizygotic twins although this result was within the confidence limits of the two other surveys. Taken together, the relative risk for multiple sclerosis in the monozygotic twin partner of an affected proband is around 190.

Adopted individuals who subsequently develop multiple sclerosis, and probands who have themselves adopted children, provide a rare but informative resource for studying the relative contribution of genes and the environment in causing multiple sclerosis. Considering individuals with multiple sclerosis adopted in infancy, and those having adopted siblings or children, the frequency of multiple sclerosis in these social relatives matches that seen in the general at-risk population and not the recurrence rates expected for the biological first-degree relatives of index cases (Ebers *et al.*, 1995). Half-siblings share a proportion of parental genes and stratify into those reared together and apart during the period considered critical for the development of multiple sclerosis. Their age-adjusted risk of multiple sclerosis is significantly lower than for full siblings, and there is no difference in risk for half-siblings reared together and apart (Sadovnick *et al.*, 1996).

Two studies of conjugal pairs with multiple sclerosis who have children provide a special opportunity for assessing the effect of genetic loading on susceptibility. Five of 86 offspring from 45 conjugal pairs living in the United Kingdom also had multiple sclerosis, and characteristic imaging abnormalities or clinical symptoms consistent with demyelination but not meeting criteria for clinically definite disease were seen in five others (Robertson *et al.*, 1997). Ebers *et al.* (2000b) identified 23 conjugal cases among the spouses of 13,550 probands; 6 of their 49 offspring were affected providing an age-corrected recurrence risk of 30%. Although subject to ascertainment bias, the lack of an increased rate of multiple sclerosis among spouses—compared to the at-risk population—and recurrence in offspring approaching that seen in monozygotic twins emphasizes that the familial risk is genetically determined and not due to a shared environment. Although these studies favor early ascertainment, the young age at onset suggests that genetic loading does count; inheritance of factors from both parents provides evidence for epistatic effects or homogeneity in the contribution made by genetic factors.

## THE ANALYSIS OF COMPLEX TRAITS

A remarkable change in the ability to characterize the genetic basis of complex traits such as multiple sclerosis has occurred over the past two decades. In the early 1980s, activities were limited to comparing the phenotypes of those few genetic systems that were identified and known to be polymorphic—blood groups, the major histocompatibility complex, immunoglobulin isotypes, and a few others. In the mid-1980s, restriction fragment length polymorphisms opened up the opportunity to characterize genotypes at sites where genes were also known to be located. Thereafter, the cataloging and mapping of microsatellite markers widely distributed across the genome, but usually in the intervals between coding regions and made up of repeats involving two or more nucleotides increased the range and diversity of genotype definition. Widely distributed single nucleotide polymorphisms now provide a sufficient density of markers in and around genes to offer a definitive approach for indirect screens. Ultimately, coding sequence can be used to provide a direct screen for each and every gene making it no longer necessary to rely on markers, however closely placed. But the availability of reagents brings new challenges for the development of technologies needed to derive these genotypes and statistical methods for their analysis. Two methods—linkage and association—underpin the analysis of complex traits (Risch, 1990, 2000; Risch and Merikangas,1996). Their principles are illustrated in Figure 30.3. Strategies for detecting susceptibility genes have moved from case-control studies seeking associations (relatively easy to organize but vulnerable to mismatch between cases and controls) to family-based association studies comparing the distribution of alleles between affected and nonaffected first-degree relatives (usually family trios or quartets made up of cases, parents, or siblings; harder to collect in sufficient numbers and of low power given the overmatching of susceptibility factors but not vulnerable to erroneous selection of controls) to family-based linkage analysis. The choice of markers has either been driven by *a priori* guesses on the possible nature of susceptibility (candidate genes), systematic screening of whole chromosomes or the entire genome, or identification of candidates known to map within regions of chromosomal interest (positional candidates). Markers may be analyzed individually (single point analysis); alternatively, the probability that a marker is linked or associated with multiple sclerosis is corrected based on information available from juxtaposed markers (multipoint analysis). Finally, the cumulative probability that a given marker or region of interest is linked or associated with multiple sclerosis in

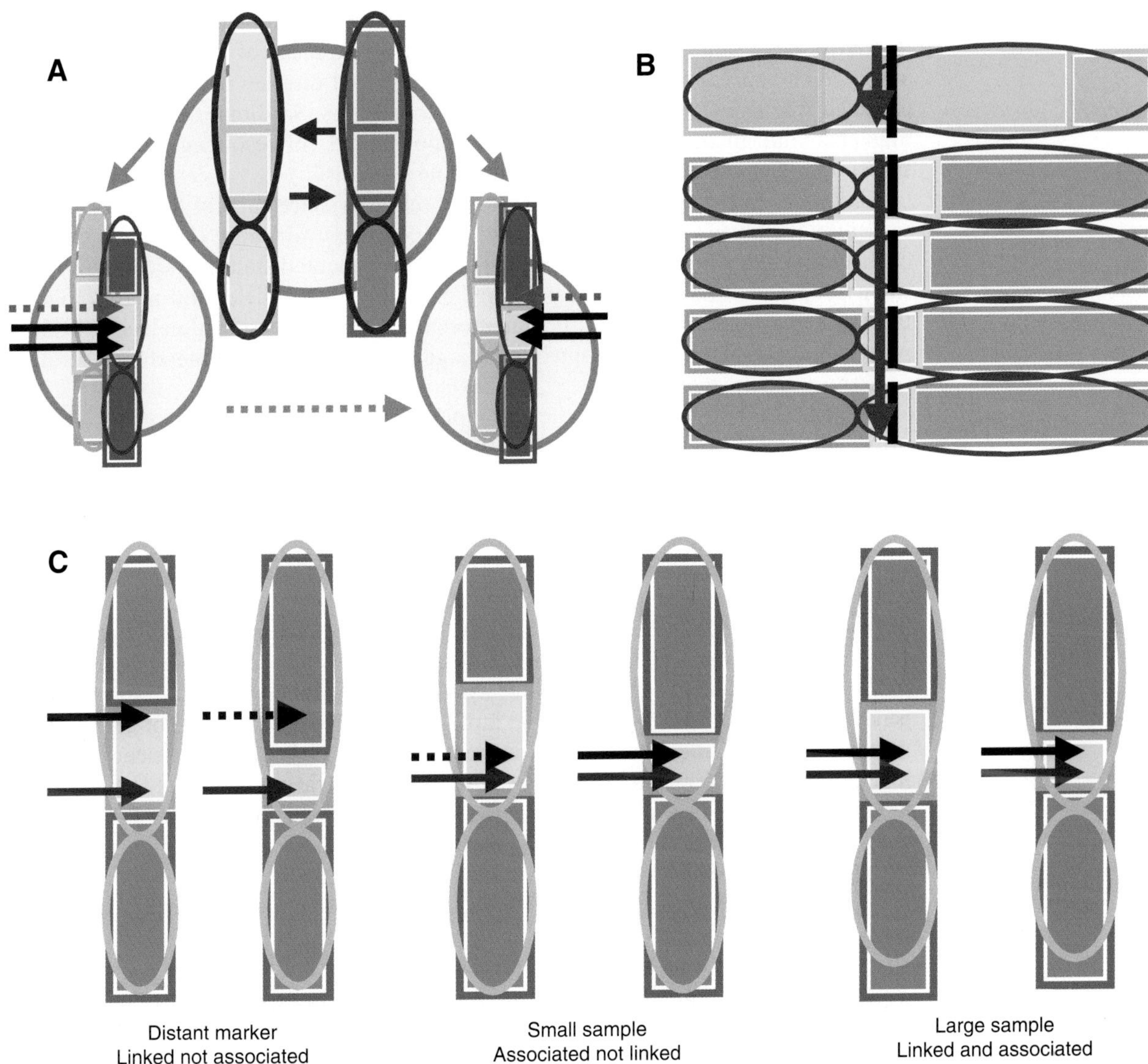


FIGURE 30.3
(A) Linkage is present when two or more affected relatives share parts of the genome encoding susceptibility genes, identified by adjacent markers, more often than expected by chance. Linkage has low statistical power but is able to track the passage of extended haplotypes. (B) Association is present when people with multiple sclerosis have a higher frequency of alleles, and markers in linkage disequilibrium, increasing susceptibility than unaffected individuals. This has higher statistical power but depends on linkage disequilibrium, which decays with genetic time (meioses) and mutation of the (microsatellite) markers. (C) Markers distant from the susceptibility gene may be linked but not associated, being outside the range of linkage disequilibrium. Markers close to the susceptibility gene may be associated but not linked if the sample size of multiplex families is small. Close markers, and disease susceptibility alleles themselves, will be linked and associated.

several studies can be formally tested by meta-analysis. Despite these advances in methodology and range of strategies, progress in identifying genes or even regions conferring susceptibility to multiple sclerosis has been slow. The lesson learned thus far is that no one gene makes a major contribution to susceptibility although collectively they determine a relative risk (for siblings) of around 20.

The classical Mendelian and biometric views of inheritance distinguish diseases attributable to the effect of single mutant alleles from those influenced by a large number of traits, each exerting only a minimal effect. Mutations are genetic variations in coding sequence occurring in <1% and polymorphisms are the alleles occurring in >1% of the population. Polymorphisms may therefore be rare or common in the population, with either category exerting trivial or substantial biological effects on disease mechanisms. It follows that disease frequency will depend on the interplay between frequency of susceptibility alleles and magnitude of their biological effects. When a small family population expands numerically in relative isolation, genetic drift can influence the frequency of mutant and polymorphic alleles. As a consequence, some genetically determined diseases may occur at higher than expected frequency. Isolated populations such as Finns, Sardinians, Icelanders, and Tasmanians could in theory provide special opportunities for resolving the issue of genetic susceptibility to complex traits such as multiple sclerosis.

Linkage is seen when two or more affected relatives share parts of the genome encoding susceptibility genes and nearby markers for a complex trait more often than expected by chance: It has low power but operates over a wide genetic distance. Association is present when people with the disorder have a higher frequency of alleles and nearby markers of factors increasing susceptibility than unaffected individuals: association has high statistical power but depends on the presence of linkage disequilibrium and therefore operates only over short genetic distances.

Linkage analysis and association mapping either select candidate genes based on a priori considerations of disease pathogenesis or perform systematic screens of the whole genome.

During meiosis, juxtaposed segments of paired chromosomes recombine such that the gametal chromosome is a mixture of the two parental copies. Linkage exploits the fact that susceptibility genes and juxtaposed markers will be carried in one or more of these recombined segments or hapotypes. The breakpoints vary with each meiosis and the size of blocks carrying the susceptibility genes will also therefore vary. Markers placed close to each susceptibility gene remain within the blocks inherited by each affected individual and so they are linked. Linkage deteriorates with distance of the marker from the susceptibility gene until it is no longer present in that family. But because the passage of genes and linked markers is being studied across very few meioses, the topographical efficiency of linkage is high and relatively few markers (i.e., relatively wide separation between those selected for a linkage screen) are needed to stand a good chance of detecting linkage. Even though the marker allele present in each family may differ, the locus remains linked to the gene influencing susceptibility in these families. However, it turns out that linkage performs poorly for genes of small biological effect and the number of families needed to show that a particular marker (allele or locus) is being inherited in multiplex families more often than expected by chance is often prohibitively large. The main failure of linkage analysis, despite economy of genotyping in the laboratory, is therefore small sample size. Where extensive genome screens fail to provide evidence for linkage, rare genes with large effects probably do not exist for that disease. The power of a linkage genome screen is critically dependent on the frequency of susceptibility alleles in the population studied and is thus expected to vary between studies. Negative studies are not necessarily definitive and linkage analysis may still be worth pursuing in locations or populations where the frequency of susceptibility alleles is more favorable for historical reasons.

Any allele actually encoding a product that causes a disease process (as in mutations of genes for Mendelian disorders) must be linked and associated with that disorder or component of the disease mechanism. But the usefulness of association lies in the fact that, for reasons of population history, susceptibility genes making even a small contribution to the disease process can also be identified by screening nearby anonymous markers making it no longer necessary to hit the disease locus itself. Association depends on the phenomenon of linkage disequilibrium. Because association and linkage refer to different aspects of genetic analysis—each providing entirely separate but complementary categories of information—it is unfortunate that the *linkage* word has crept into both definitions; this causes much confusion. When polymorphisms that increase susceptibility to disease arise in a founder group, these will necessarily be located within a large group of linked genes. This block is subject to recombination during subsequent meioses and is gradually whittled down. Markers close to the susceptibility gene are the last to become separated. It follows that the progeny of this founder continue to share segments of DNA identically by descent for many generations. Their genes are said to be in linkage disequilibrium. In time, the extent of linkage disequilibrium degrades until it is nonexistent and it is then no longer possible to detect susceptibility genes by association mapping because the population is now in linkage equilibrium.

This is the rule for older populations such the "out of Africa" races. But for younger populations that went through and survived population bottlenecks, the residual degree of linkage disequilibrium may be considerable and sufficient to use markers remote from the disease promoting polymorphism to track the genetic basis for susceptibility. However, mutation of the marker for a disease associated susceptibility allele also decays linkage disequilibrium and so reduces the ability to detect associations between that marker and the disease. Microsatellites mutate once every 1000 generations; those that mutate soon after appearance of the disease susceptibility allele will significantly reduce the number of chromosomes carrying both the marker and the susceptibility gene in the expanded present-day population, whereas more recent mutations will be much less disruptive.

Estimates for the extent of linkage disequilibrium are a moving target, but crucial in assessing the density of markers needed to explore a given region for association. At first, crude theoretical modeling of human population history suggested that variants which are common in the population as a whole will generally be very old and therefore accompanied by rather little linkage disequilibrium (Krugylak, 1999). However, empirical evidence in Europeans started to show that linkage disequilibrium is in fact much more extensive than these predictions. Initial average distances for the extent of linkage disequilibrium ranged from 60 kb to 385 kb (Collins *et al.*, 2001; Reich *et al.*, 2001) for SNPs and 0.5 Mb to 1 Mb for microsatellites (Eaves *et al.*, 2000; Kendler *et al.*, 1999). But it soon became clear that even though many parts of the genome remain to be explored, linkage disequilibrium is highly variable and therefore not uniformly accessible to association screening (Dunning *et al.*, 2000; Martin *et al.*, 2000; Taillon-Miller *et al.*, 2000). Subsequently, a different extent and structure of linkage disequilibrium in Europeans has been shown from that predicted. Recombination is not uniformly distributed, as assumed, but rather is concentrated in hot spots separating regions of marked linkage disequilibrium (Daly *et al.*, 2001; Jeffreys *et al.*, 2001). These blocks of extensive linkage disequilibrium with sharp boundaries vary in size but average around 20 kb (Daly *et al.*, 2001). It follows that the limited haplotype diversity within blocks favors testing these regions (but not the adjacent boundaries) for association with appropriately informative markers (Johnson *et al.*, 2001). A first-generation linkage disequilibrium map of human chromosome 22 in Centre d'Etude du Polymorphisme Humain (CEPH) families shows extremely variable linkage disequilibrium with blocks up 804 kb interspersed with regions of little or no detectable linkage disequilibrium. In these long blocks, 76% of human diversity could be defined using just three tagging SNPs to define the five common haplotypes; elsewhere, much more extensive typing would be needed to screen short haplotypes (Dawson *et al.*, 2002).

Association has much greater power to detect genes of small biological effect than linkage, and it is logistically easier to collect cases and controls than multiplex families. The downside of association screening is that the range of linkage disequilibrium is much narrower than for linkage; it degrades faster and the density of markers needed to cover a region of interest is necessarily much greater. For high-density screening, genotyping effort can be reduced using equal amounts of DNA from a large number of cases, controls, or parents pooled into a single sample and screened against a panel of markers (Barcellos *et al.*, 1997). Pooling introduces several additional potential sources of error in the analysis of complex traits (miscalling of alleles due to the presence of stutter bands; and the artifact of length-dependent amplification, whereby short alleles are preferentially amplified in the polymerase chain reaction skewing the apparent distribution of alleles seen with individual typing and either favoring or inhibiting the demonstration of associations resulting from short and long alleles, respectively); but allowing for these technical limitations, pooling can detect allelic frequency differences of around 5%. So association is easy on the fieldworkers but tougher on the laboratory staff. Linkage strains clinical resources for collection but is lighter on laboratory effort; off-the-shelf statistical programs are now developed for analyzing either, but their further refinements require continued biostatistical wizardry.

Associations can be demonstrated using population or family-based studies. Ethnic mismatching has proved a major limiting factor for population studies especially in large outbred populations. Family-based methods aim to show that a marker allele is transmitted to affected individuals more often than expected by chance. Transmission disequilibrium testing (TDT) uses trios consisting of single affecteds and both parents, who are usually (but need not be) unaffected. Each parental allele has a 1:2 chance of being transmitted. The test provides evidence for allelic association by demonstrating excess transmission and identifies that allele which is responsible for disequilibrium in the sample. Although not every family will be informative for this marker, those in linkage disequilibrium with susceptibility genes for multiple sclerosis will be adequately represented. One further factor limiting the extent to which a sample of family trios may not prove fully informative for a particular polymorphic locus is parental homozygosity since the transmitted allele cannot then be identified. Segregation distortion arises when a particular allele confers a survival advantage and therefore appears to be disproportionately transmitted; in fact, the allele is preferentially transmitted to all surviving offspring whether or not they have the disease in question. This issue can be resolved by studying affected and unaffected children. But a new problem then arises, which does not confuse the affected family member approach, and that is difficulty in assigning unaffected status to a young adult in a disease that may not manifest clinically until late in life, if at all, given the prevalence of pathologically verified but clinically silent disease in autopsy series.

Selecting probands from among families in which there are multiple cases increases the power and reduces the scale of the study especially in the context of rare alleles. Associations may be with a defined allele or locus. Those that are reproducible between populations carry conviction with respect to their causal relevance, but population specificity does not exclude causality. Where there is reasonable but variable linkage disequilibrium and several markers are found to be associated in separate populations, cross-cultural studies (exploiting different degrees of linkage disequilibrium) may narrow the region of interest and select the closest marker; for example, Caucasians show an association between narcolepsy and both DR and DQ alleles, but only the DQ association is found in Africans (Rogers *et al.*, 1997).

Linkage and association provide different categories of information. Assuming a reasonable sample size, any marker placed well distant from a susceptibility gene may be linked but not associated since it will lie outside the region of linkage disequilibrium. A marker that is close to a susceptibility gene may not be linked if the sample is underpowered but it may nevertheless be associated. Only the combination of a close marker tested in an adequate sample will show both linkage and association. If these conditions are met in independent tests, the candidature of a given chromosomal region is much enhanced. Many genes are mapped but have no assigned function. This is the obvious next step once a susceptibility locus has been identified (Eisenberg *et al.*, 2000). The function of genes can be assessed by computational methods using similarities and dissimilarities between the phylogenetic expression of two proteins in different organisms with fully sequenced genomes. The knowledge that two gene products are fused proteins in another species implies a generic sharing of function. Genes that are linked on the same chromosome in more than one species tend to have related functions. Those showing the same pattern of increased and decreased expression in differential displays are likely to share function providing guilt by association.

The increasing availability of reagents for distinguishing short sections of DNA, accurate mapping of these microsatellites and single nucleotide polymorphisms (SNPs) across the genome, access to extended pedigrees in which affected status can reliably be determined, the collection of large cohorts of cases and controls, and the deployment of appropriate statistical methods for assessing statistical significance across large data sets collectively have made it possible to tackle the genetics of complex traits. Meta-analysis of linkage and association screens has been explored in the expectation that this will reduce the evidence for false positive results and strengthen the candidature of those that are genuine in order to select regions for more detailed studies of positional candidates. Combining data sets from ethnically diverse groups necessarily selects for genes conferring susceptibility between populations and obscures the identification of others restricted to particular populations. For a disease that is notoriously variable in its clinical phenotype and in which a case can be made for heterogeneity in the pathogenesis, lumping all cases under the rubric of "multiple sclerosis" reduces the power to identify any one susceptibility factor and restricts the analysis to susceptibility genes ignoring those that may focus the pathological process on defined pathways, shape the clinical course, and (perhaps) determine the response to treatment. Since these distinguishing features do not segregate within families, linkage is essentially restricted to the study of susceptibility genes. Association mapping can in theory be used to reveal either susceptibility genes or those influencing the clinical course if appropriate stratifications are employed in designing the study.

## CANDIDATE GENES IN MULTIPLE SCLEROSIS

Much effort has gone into the assessment of candidate susceptibility genes chosen on the basis of prevailing ideas concerning the pathogenesis of multiple sclerosis and therefore providing a logical basis for their role in shaping the pathogenesis. It is hard to argue that progress in advancing knowledge has not been painfully slow since the burst of activity in the early 1970s, which established the range of associations with alleles of the major histocompatability complex—remarkable for its extensive linkage disequilibrium. As expected, it proved much more difficult formally to demonstrate that the region is also linked to multiple sclerosis in family studies, as of course it must be if the association is genuine. To summarize the present situation, population studies comparing unrelated cases and controls show an association between the class II major histocompatibility complex alleles DR15 and DQ6 and their underlying genotypes (DRB1*1501, DRB5*0101 and DQA1*0102, DQB2*0602) (Olerup and Hillert, 1991). This is seen in almost all populations (Caucasian, Oriental, Arab, Hispanic, Finnish, Russian, and Jewish), although the strengths of the association differ. Even those ethnic groups in which the frequency of multiple sclerosis is low, or the phenotype distinct from that usually observed in northern Europe, are now acknowledged to be DR15 associated with one regional exception. In Sardinians, there is a specifically different association with DR4 (DRB1*0405-DQA1*0301-DQB1*0302: Marrosu *et al.*, 1992). In the Canaries, the primary association is with DR15 and DQ6, but a secondary association also exists with DR4 (Coraddu *et al.*, 1998). In Turkey, there is an allelic association with both DR2 (DBR1*1501, DQA1*0102, DQB1*0602) and DR4 (DRB1*04, DQA1*03, DQB1*0302: Saruhan-Direskeneli *et al.*, 1997). Thus, there is a DR4 flavor to the association in some southern Mediterranean populations. But since this Mediterranean DR4 haplotype is not identical, opportunities exist to narrow the region. That said, most investigators assume that—based on the genetics and obvious candidature through its role in restricting the immune response—DR (or DQ) is itself the susceptibility gene encoded at 6p21. Outside the major histocompatibility complex, the list of immunologically related intelligent or positional candidates now screened includes >50 adhesion molecules, immune receptors, accessory molecules, cytokines, and chemokines and their receptors or antagonists (selected references include He *et al.*, 1998; Jacobsen et al., 2000; Kuhlman *et al.*, 2002; McDonnell *et al.*, 2000; Modin *et al.*, 2001; and Reboul *et al.*, 2000).

In the isolated population of Finns, association and linkage of susceptibility to multiple sclerosis exist for the myelin basic protein gene encoded on chromosome 18 (Tienari *et al.*, 1992). Even in this cohort from Vaasa, the effect can be traced to a subset of families with common ancestry and does not hold up in the larger cohort (Pihlaja *et al.*, 2003). But opportunities now exist for tracing the genealogy of this isolate, linking it to other regions through population history and so seeing more clearly the genetic path explaining one particular route to increased disease susceptibility. Studies of structural genes of myelin have otherwise been uninformative (Seboun *et al.*, 1999), as have efforts directed at implicating growth factors determining oligodendrocyte development and their receptors in susceptibility (Mertens *et al.*, 1998). More than 35 growth factors or genes encoding structural components of the nervous system have been assessed as candidates.

The current list of candidates is shown in Figure 30.4; those for which results are entirely negative, and therefore excluded within the limits of sample size, are distinguished from the smaller number of candidates for which a role in susceptibility or influences on the course

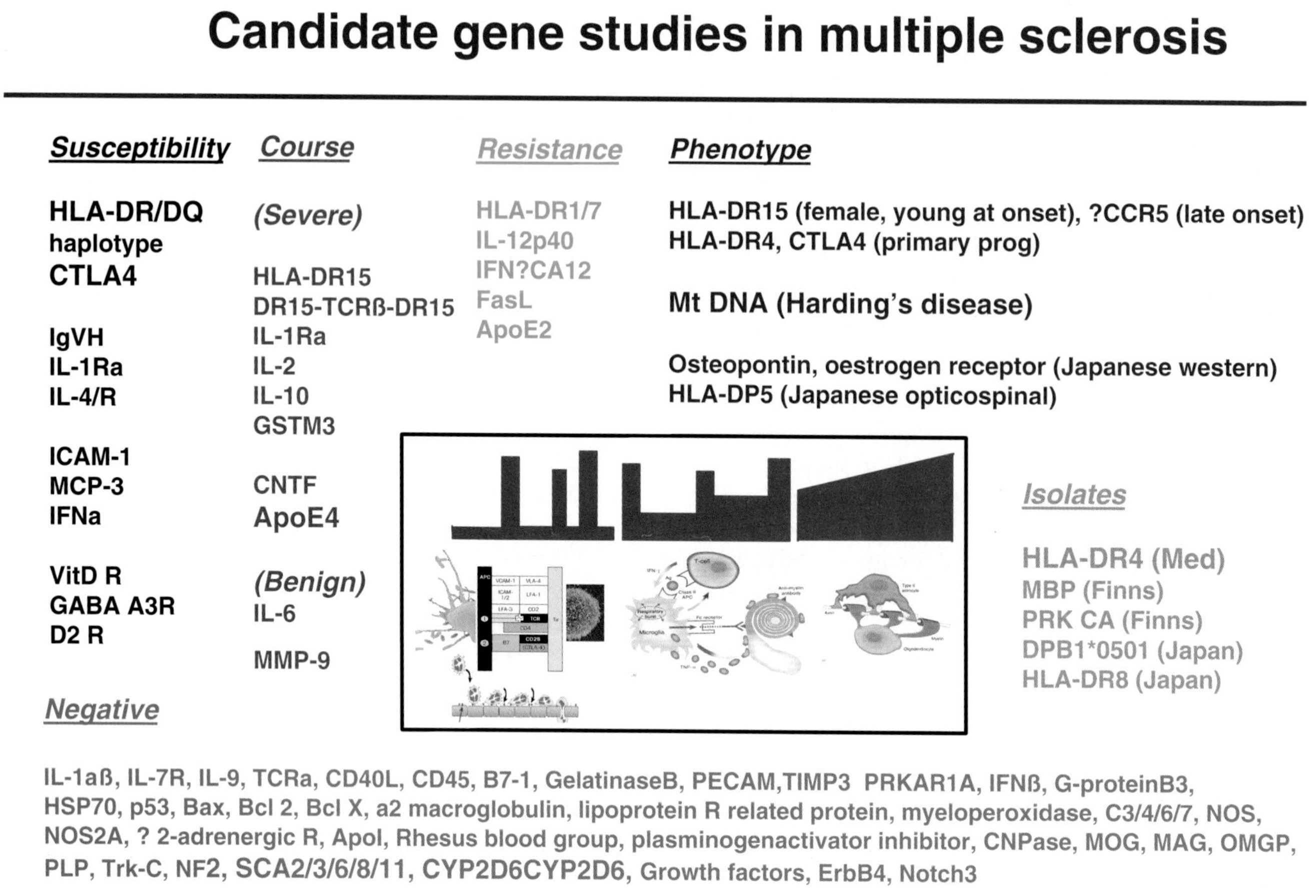

**Candidate gene studies in multiple sclerosis**

**Susceptibility**
HLA-DR/DQ haplotype
CTLA4
IgVH
IL-1Ra
IL-4/R
ICAM-1
MCP-3
IFNa
VitD R
GABA A3R
D2 R

**Course**
(Severe)
HLA-DR15
DR15-TCRß-DR15
IL-1Ra
IL-2
IL-10
GSTM3
CNTF
ApoE4
(Benign)
IL-6
MMP-9

**Resistance**
HLA-DR1/7
IL-12p40
IFN?CA12
FasL
ApoE2

**Phenotype**
HLA-DR15 (female, young at onset), ?CCR5 (late onset)
HLA-DR4, CTLA4 (primary prog)
Mt DNA (Harding's disease)
Osteopontin, oestrogen receptor (Japanese western)
HLA-DP5 (Japanese opticospinal)

**Isolates**
HLA-DR4 (Med)
MBP (Finns)
PRK CA (Finns)
DPB1*0501 (Japan)
HLA-DR8 (Japan)

**Negative**
IL-1aß, IL-7R, IL-9, TCRa, CD40L, CD45, B7-1, GelatinaseB, PECAM,TIMP3 PRKAR1A, IFNß, G-proteinB3, HSP70, p53, Bax, Bcl 2, Bcl X, a2 macroglobulin, lipoprotein R related protein, myeloperoxidase, C3/4/6/7, NOS, NOS2A, ? 2-adrenergic R, Apol, Rhesus blood group, plasminogenactivator inhibitor, CNPase, MOG, MAG, OMGP, PLP, Trk-C, NF2, SCA2/3/6/8/11, CYP2D6CYP2D6, Growth factors, ErbB4, Notch3

FIGURE 30.4
A list of candidate genes studied in multiple sclerosis. Most are neither linked nor associated (light blue), but provisional evidence is available for an effect on susceptibility (black), resistance (green), or disease progression or severity (red), population isolates (orange), and clinical phenotype (dark blue). The central panel correlates the clinical course—relapses with recovery; relapses with persistent disability and secondary progression—with the immunological interactions that disrupt normal axon-glial interactions subserving salutatory conduction and indicates potential targets for the effect of these gene products. Reproduced from Compston, D. A. S., and Coles, A. J. (2002). Multiple sclerosis: Seminar. *Lancet* **359,** 1221–1231.

of multiple sclerosis remain a possibility. The number increases weekly but with rather a poor dividend for increased knowledge. Many of the associations are negative, yet the size of the studies often leaves open the issue of whether these are type 2 errors. Others claim an association with susceptibility but the findings have proved hard to reproduce.

## LINKAGE GENOME SCREENS

If the dividend from attempting to fast-track the solution to susceptibility in multiple sclerosis has been small, the problem is also not solved by the nine whole genome linkage analyses using variable numbers of families from the United States (Haines *et al.*, 1996), Canada (Ebers *et al.*, 1996), the United Kingdom (Chataway *et al.*, 1998; Sawcer *et al.*, 1996), Finland (Kuokkanen *et al.*, 1997), Sardinia (Coraddu *et al.*, 2001), Italy (Broadley *et al.*, 2001), Turkey (Eraksoy *et al.*, 2003), Scandinavia (Akesson *et al.*, 2002), and Australia (Ban *et al.*, 2002). In the three original large and ethnically diverse populations (United States, Canada, United Kingdom), genotyping was completed on cohorts of between 21 and 225 families, together involving in excess of 1000 individuals, for each of 257 to 443 microsatellite markers. These were chosen to have an average spacing of around 10 centiMorgans giving enough power to identify regions encoding a major susceptibility gene; and the markers were sufficiently polymorphic to make a high proportion of the available families fully informative. Although several new genomic regions of interest were revealed, many are likely to be false positives. Failure to identify a major susceptibility factor may indicate that no such gene exists, that it was missed by each group, or that genetic heterogeneity obscured the picture. Other than the major histocompatability complex, several of the other new putative susceptibility loci were clearly unique to each screen. The regions of interest emerging from the United Kingdom genome screen were 1cen, 5 cen, 6p, 7p, 14q, 17q, 19q, Xp (Chataway *et al.*, 1998; Sawcer *et al.*, 1996). They were 2p, 3p, 5p, 11q, and Xp in the Canadian series (Ebers *et al.*, 1996). The United States/French consortium identified 6p, 7q, 11p, 12q, and 19q (Haines *et al.*, 1996). There were no statistically significant regions of interest in the Finnish screen, although positive lod scores were obtained for 6p21 (MHC), 5p14-p12 and 17q22-q24 (Kuokkanen *et al.*, 1997). These studies were followed by smaller screens in families from Italy (Broadley *et al.*, 2001), Sardinia (Coraddu *et al.*, 2001), and Turkey (Eraksoy *et al.*, 2003), and by surveys of comparable size from Scandinavia (Akesson *et al.*, 2002) and Australia (Ban *et al.*, 2002). Although the Italian, Sardinian, Scandinavian, and Australian linkage screens failed to provide statistically unequivocal linkages, more regions of potential interest were identified than expected on the basis of chance alone. The main positive result from the Scandinavian, Italian, and Sardinian studies, backed by an updated screen of United Kingdom families, is provisional linkage to chromosome 10p (Akesson *et al.*, 2003). Others have looked at these whole genome screens and explored regions of interest in more detail hoping to consolidate their status based on mapping but without picking out positional candidates. As a result, the linkage peak on chromosome 17q, originally identified in the United Kingdom screen, is now supported by additional positional screens from Denmark (Larsen *et al.*, 2000), Canada (Dyment *et al.*, 2001), and Finland (Saarela *et al.*, 2002). Support is also provided for chromsome 5p, 7p, and 12q based on direct evidence and synteny with genes determining susceptibility to experimental forms of demyelination (Oturai *et al.*, 1999; Xu *et al.*, 1999; 2001). Given the lack of overlap between screens and the provisional implication of different regions of interest, meta-analysis has been deployed in the expectation that this will reduce the evidence for false positive peaks and strengthen the candidature of those that are genuine, providing the best guide to shared regions of interest as the map is serially updated. By-eye analysis (Becker *et al.*, 1998) provided a start, but making the separate screens compatible has proved no trivial task. Two meta-analyses are currently available: the original United States, Canadian, and United Kingdom screen (The Transatlantic Multiple Sclerosis Genetics Cooperative, 2001), and all the published families (GAMES and The Transatlantic Multiple Sclerosis Genetics Cooperative, 2003). Superficially, these show the same peaks and troughs, but the comparison is confounded by the fact that many of the same families feature in each and the total number is dominated by the same large contributors (Fig. 30.5).

The failure of linkage genome screens reliably to identify regions of interest conferring disease susceptibility both in mixed and isolated European populations, each having a high prevalence of multiple sclerosis, has obvious implications for future genetic analyses of complex traits. Linkage data from new populations are being systematically added with the aim of confirming and excluding regions of interest; studies in progress include new cohorts from the United States and Canada. Meanwhile, continued scrutiny of the human genome map for positional candidates may shorten the search for genes that determine susceptibility and influence the course of multiple sclerosis. However, power calculations indicate that tests based on association will generally be more powerful in multiple sclerosis than those dependant on linkage, and this has led to a further switch in strategy (Risch, 1996).

## WHOLE GENOME ASSOCIATION SCREENING

Until recently, whole genome linkage disequilibrium mapping was considered impractical and dependent on chance colocalization of susceptibility genes and markers applied

**Linkage and association in multiple sclerosis: the present position:**

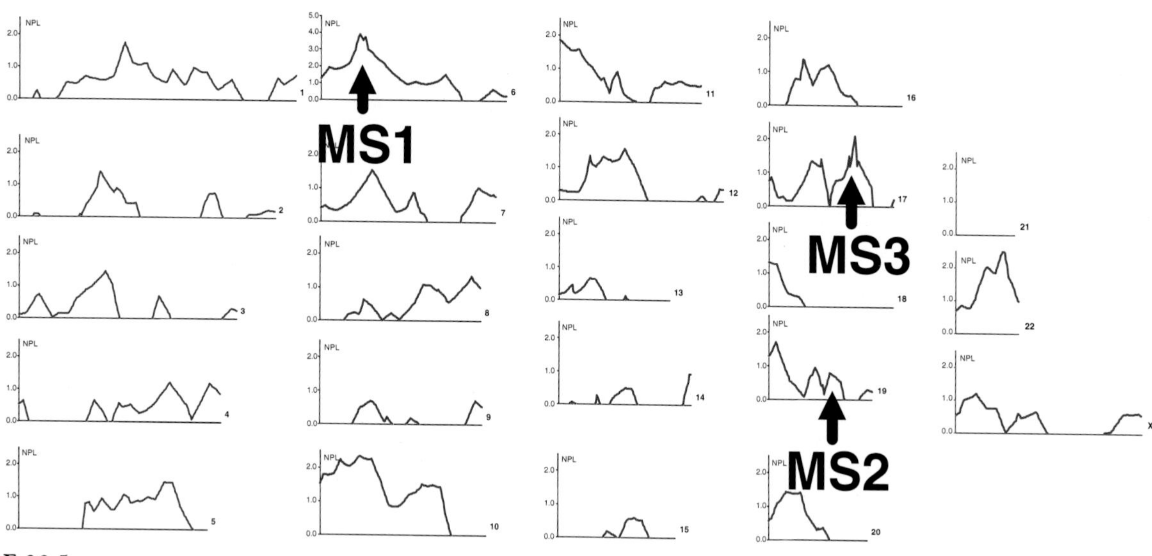


FIGURE 30.5
Whole genome linkage screening based on c600 European families is shown for each chromosome. The vertical axis shows the nonparametric likelihood (NPL) score indicating the statistical probability that a gene conferring susceptibility to multiple sclerosis is encoded at that site. Based on these results and whole genome linkage screening, a provisional list of multiple sclerosis susceptibility genes is *MS1* (6p), *2* (19q), and *3* (17q).

randomly and distributed at low density. This situation changed with the increased availability of widely distributed microsatellite markers and is set further to increase with the identification and mapping of single nucleotide polymorphisms. Both have required high throughput methods for genotyping helped by economies arising, for example, from the use of pooled DNA (Barcellos *et al.*, 1997). A first pass at screening the genome for association in multiple sclerosis has now been completed based on a 0.5 cM map of microsatellite markers and using DNA pools derived from cases with multiple sclerosis, unrelated controls and trio families (affected individuals and their parents). The initial sample came from the United Kingdom (Sawcer *et al.*, 2002), but this was the first of 19 carried out more or less simultaneously and together representing the Genetic Analysis of Multiple sclerosis in EuropeanS (GAMES). The study was designed to extend the number of families studied by linkage analysis and to place on this provisional map—assumed to show true and false positives—the location of associated markers, seeking the double hit of linkage (albeit provisional) and association. The use of pooled DNA from cases of multiple sclerosis not subject to stratification on the basis of disease course or phenotype (apart from the exclusion of primary progressive cases) restricted GAMES to the identification of susceptibility genes. The 19 populations were expected to show individual associations not necessarily replicated across the different screens. Although these domestic associations were likely to be of both local and general interest, special significance was attached to those that did survive testing in multiple populations. A highly conservative approach was adopted in defining associations emerging from testing pools for these 6000 markers. Those showing greatest deviation from the expected distribution of results were ranked. The 19 separate studies were then considered together, searching for the best ranked markers and recognizing that local associations, even if genuine, might be lost by meta-analysis. A defining and validating subset of populations was used based on typing in each of the two host laboratories. Markers showing the same allelic association in this meta-analysis and those where different alleles of the same polymorphic marker were each listed.

Finally, as a first trawl, individual typing was performed on selected markers. These offered the most likely prospect of identifying associations even though others lower down the ranking might, in time, also be shown to mark for susceptibility genes. The aim was to find regions outside the major histocompatability complex showing both linkage and association so as both to confirm the status and narrow the region of interest restricting the identification of candidate genes encoded within that region of linkage disequilibrium.

The 10 markers showing the best evidence for association with multiple sclerosis to emerge from analysis of the United Kingdom screen included three from the HLA region on chromosome 6p (D6S1615, D6S2444 and TNFa), providing a positive control for the method, four from regions previously identified by linkage analysis in United Kingdom multiplex families (two mapping to chromosome 17q: GCT6E11 and D17S1535; one to chromosome 1p: GGAA30B06; and one to 19q: D19S585), and three from novel sites with respect to linkage analysis (D1S1590 at 1q; D2S2739 at 2p; and D4S416 at 4q). These results provisionally strengthened the candidature of 6p, 17q, 19q, and 1p as regions most likely to encode susceptibility genes for multiple sclerosis. As the remaining 18 components of GAMES were completed and analyzed, many new markers were shown provisionally to be associated. All of these now need to be confirmed using individual typing in data set replications. Figure 30.4 shows the present position with respect to linked and associated markers and provides a best current estimate for the location of multiple sclerosis susceptibility genes. The number of microsatellite markers used necessarily makes GAMES a low-density screen and in many chromosomal regions quite possibly insufficient for the stochastic nature of linkage disequilibrium present in European populations. Even though it may only have covered 10% of the genome in detail and another 20% in part leaving much yet to be explored, the aim was to find some new regions outside the major histocompatibility complex showing linkage and association with multiple sclerosis not each and every such locus—and to exclude those parts of the genome not meriting further search.

Once regions of interest are mapped, the next aim is to move from whole genome screening to the identification of functional polymorphisms, which condition one component or another of the disease process and determine variations in the clinical course and features. How to reach that position is less clear and several parallel strategies have been suggested. One is to add incrementally to the number of multiplex families available for linkage until thresholds are reached for the identification of secure loci using statistical criteria for genome wide significance. An alternative is to accept that the combination of linkage and association now available is sufficient to concentrate the search for positional candidates within regions of interest. Each provisional site already offers several interesting possibilities although the number of genes encoding components of the nervous, immune and signaling systems is such as to make practically any region suggestive with respect to sensible candidates. Finally, there is the option of narrowing the region of interest—still large even if the spacing of GAMES markers has reliably identified one of the larger blocks of linkage disequilibrium—by identifying the haplotypes associated with multiple sclerosis. Sequencing one or a few genomes is a remarkable feat, but it tells us little about the rest of humankind. In time, it is expected that the whole genome will be characterized for the size, distribution, and diversity of blocks containing a restricted number of haplotypes. If the preliminary evidence holds up, it will be possible to tag the common variants within each block in populations (such as Europeans) retaining significant linkage disequilibrium and screen individuals for the susceptibility haplotype with relative economy. To date, the *hap-map* is incomplete but a start is being made on applying such topographical information as does exist to the problem of complex traits in general and multiple sclerosis in particular. Its future use is depicted in Figure 30.6.

## GENETIC INFLUENCES ON THE CLINICAL COURSE

Clinical analysis of the course and concordance for other features of the disease within pedigrees can be used to gauge the influence of genetic factors in determining the clinical

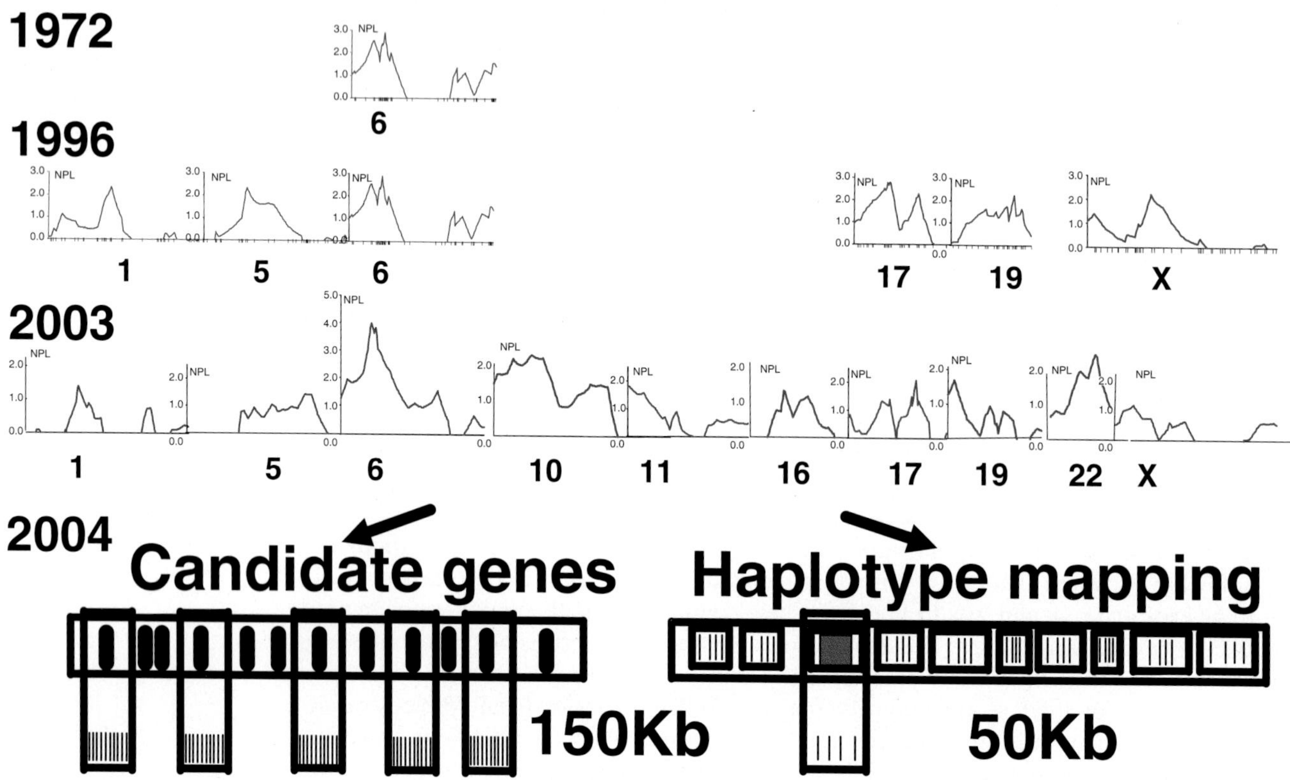


FIGURE 30.6
Association (but not linkage) between multiple sclerosis and alleles of the major histocompatibility complex was shown in 1972 and subsequently confirmed on many occasions and in many populations. Provisional linkage to novel chromosomal regions of interest was provided in 1996 by whole genome screens. Some of these regions are confirmed and others newly identified by whole genome (low-density) association mapping and updated linkage analysis. Future strategies either involve testing positional candidates suggested by reference to the human genome map or narrowing the region of interest by identifying the associated haplotype using tagged single nucleotide (SNP) markers.

phenotype of multiple sclerosis in the individual. In a large population-based sample, Ebers *et al.* (2000a) showed no differences in time to reach the later stages of disability among 206 familial cases, irrespective of relatedness to the proband, compared to sporadic multiple sclerosis although onset was earlier and the usual female predominance no longer seen in the families with most cases—providing no evidence for genetic effects on the clinical features or course. In the United Kingdom survey of conjugal pairs, there was no evidence for clinical concordance, clustering at year of onset or distortion of the expected pattern of age at onset in the second affected spouse from 33 pairs in whom these comparisons could be made (Robertson *et al.*, 1997). Statistical analysis of sibling pairs is prone to sampling bias; concordance for year at onset is much influenced by the tendency for earlier recognition of symptoms in the second individual affected in a pair through heightened awareness of the possibility of multiple sclerosis. After appropriate correction, Robertson *et al.* (1996a) found no correlation with age or year at onset, or with mode of presentation and disability, although there was a correlation with disease course, and affected siblings tended to be same-sex. The most recent assessment of concordance in coaffected siblings and parent-child pairs supports a role for genetic factors in determining eventual disability and handicap in multiple sclerosis but not the initial presentation (Chataway *et al.*, 2001). Concordant parent-child pairs show no distortion in the random distribution of male-female pairings, and neither sex nor line of inheritance influence disability, age at onset or course; however, disability is highest in the male offspring of affected fathers who more commonly follow a primary progressive course (Hupperts *et al.*, 2001). It could be argued that comparing year on age at onset and clinical features described over many years is too imprecise a method for assessing the relative contribution of genes and environmental factors in determining the development and course of multiple sclerosis in individuals; but with large numbers of siblings, artefactual correlations are reduced and useful statistical trends emerge.

Turning to specific associations, the majority of surveys investigating HLA class 2 alleles and disease course fail to confirm specifically different associations with any one of these phenotypes; the presence of DR15 is associated with younger age at diagnosis and female gender but does not distinguish features relating to disease course, outcome, specific clinical features, or paraclinical investigations (Celius *et al.*, 2000; Hensiek *et al.*, 2002 Masterman *et al.*, 2000). This suggests that DR15 exerts an effect on susceptibility rather than modifying the course of sporadic multiple sclerosis. Most recently, these observations have been extended to familial multiple sclerosis, with additional confirmation of heterogeneity since DR linkage (and concordance for early onset) are seen only in families where DR2(15) is present (The Multiple Sclerosis Genetics Group, 2002).

Some genetic studies have been confined to effects on the clinical course or prognostic factors using stratified populations (for example, Evangelou *et al.*, 1999; Giess *et al.*, 2002; Hogh *et al.*, 2000; for review, see Kantarci *et al.*, 2002); yet the stratifications are necessarily arbitrary and of doubtful provenance. Appropriately, the majority of these studies are confined to discrete populations and positive findings cannot necessarily be generalized to other groups. The example of CTLA4 serves well to illustrate the difficulty of achieving a secure position: Ligers *et al.* (1999) reported population- and family-based associations with homozygosity of the G49 allele of the CTLA4 gene in relapsing-remitting multiple sclerosis; this was confirmed by Harbo *et al.* (2000); homozygosity of the AA allele of exon 1 was then primarily associated with increased severity in Japanese patients with relapsing-remitting or secondary progressive multiple sclerosis (Fukazawa *et al.*, 1999); but Dyment *et al.* (2002) were unable to demonstrate linkage or association to susceptibility or the clinical course with a microsatellite marking exon 1 of the CTLA-4 gene in Canadian patients; Maurer *et al.* (2002) and Masterman *et al.* (2002), working from the groups that originally claimed an association to susceptibility in relapsing-remitting multiple sclerosis, then claimed a relationship with primary progressive disease; Alizadeh *et al.* (2003) identified a single nucleotide polymorphism strongly associated with susceptibility to relapsing-remitting multiple sclerosis in French and Iberian patients; finally, Roxburgh *et al.* (2003) failed to show any association in family-based studies with susceptibility or disease course.

The risk of autoimmunity is increased in the relatives of probands with multiple sclerosis. Heinzlef *et al.* (1999) studied 1971 relatives of 357 probands and identified recurrence of multiple sclerosis in 15% with another autoimmune disease in a further 8% and several disorders (Graves's disease, rheumatoid arthritis, and diabetes) occurring in 5% of pedigrees. Broadley *et al* (2000) assessed the frequency of multiple sclerosis, five definite and three putative autoimmuine disorders, and control conditions in the 1315 first degree relatives of 571 probands, compared with 375 control families. Whereas patients themselves did not have an excess of autoimmune diseases, these were over-represented in family members of individuals with multiple sclerosis. The main effect was attributed to an excess of autoimmune thyroid disease. Recurrence risk was especially high in multiplex families. Henderson *et al.* (2000) identified an odds ratio of 2.2 for recurrence of autoimmune disease in 722 first degree relatives of 117 Australian patients with multiple sclerosis. Several other disorders have been considered more frequent than expected in patients with multiple sclerosis. None of these is entirely secure, but there may be comorbidity between neurofibromatosis 1 and primary progressive multiple sclerosis; if so, this is not explained by mutation of the oligodendrocyte myelin glycoprotein gene, which maps to the same locus (Johnson *et al.*, 2000).

## HETEROGENEITY IN MULTIPLE SCLEROSIS

The existing genetic analyses are predicated on the assumption that multiple sclerosis is one disease. A major part of future genetic studies will be to resolve the question of disease heterogeneity. Even now, it is possible to dissect the disease phenotype and suggest features that may have arisen through a distinct etiology and mechanism. Furthermore, preliminary dissections of the provisional genetic descriptions suggest discrete clusters of regions forming epistatic groups.

A minority of patients who meet the clinical criteria for definite multiple sclerosis and in whom there are associated magnetic resonance imaging abnormalities and cerebrospinal fluid oligoclonal bands have an illness in which there is disproportionate involvement of the anterior visual pathway. These are commonly women with male relatives already known to be affected by Leber's hereditary optic neuropathy and they have pathological mutations of mitochondrial (mt) DNA (Harding *et al.*, 1992; Kellar Wood *et al.*, 1994). Visual involvement in multiple sclerosis may generally be associated with the haplotype J of mtDNA (Reynier *et al.*, 1999); but severe optic neuropathy occurring in the context of the Devic phenotype is not associated with mutations of mtDNA (Kalman and Mandler, 2002). Harding's disease therefore represents true heterogeneity in that a specific genotype determines a characteristic phenotype. What remains unresolved is whether the mutation of mtDNA directs the process of brain inflammation onto a particular site—constituting selective tissue vulnerability—or merely represents the chance occurrence of relatively mild multiple sclerosis and Leber's hereditary optic neuropathy. The latter seems unlikely given the number of cases of Harding's disease and the rarity of isolated Leber's hereditary optic neuropathy in women.

The distinct clinical features of demyelinating disease seen in Orientals and Africans provide another probable example of heterogeneity. The suggestion is that, in Japan, multiple sclerosis shows either a Western phenotype in which a number of sites are involved, or an opticospinal pattern in which the clinical picture is dominated by involvement of visual and spinal cord pathways having more neurodegenerative and less inflammatory activity and with a specifically different genetic background (HLA-DP*1501 rather than DRB1*1501 seen with the Western phenotype: Yamasaki *et al.*, 1999). In its extreme form, this mimics Devic's disease—a disorder that also occurs in Europeans, albeit rarely. However, as with many aspects of multiple sclerosis, the early descriptions have not always proved stable, and recent reports of multiple sclerosis in Japanese highlight the previously underreported extent of the so-called Western phenotype. Confining their analysis to patients with this Western phenotype, Kikuchi *et al.* (2003) segregated cases into two clinically indistinguishable groups defined by DR15, oligoclonal bands, and high magnetic resonance lesion load compared with patients positive for DR4 but without oligoclonal bands and having fewer magnetic resonance lesions. Demyelinating disease is considered to be extremely rare in Africans, but a number of cases are described and the phenotype is typically a severe illness dominated by one or more episodes usually affecting the anterior visual pathway and spinal cord—again combining the anatomical features of Devic's disease with the clinical course of moderately severe relapsing remitting multiple sclerosis (Dean *et al.*, 1994). Unlike Harding's disease, the evidence that this represents disease heterogeneity arising from specific genetic or environmental modification of a core pathological process remains circumstantial.

The concept of heterogeneity is further developed in the recent pathological studies using biopsy and autopsy material in which four distinct types of disease process are proposed (Luchinetti *et al.*, 2000). Allelic heterogeneity provides evidence for the functional relevance of a given locus since the probability of several different associated polymorphisms occurring at the same site in unrelated individuals would be low if this locus was altogether irrelevant. Allelic heterogeneity is suggested by detailed analysis of the most secure finding in multiple sclerosis—association with alleles of the major histocompatibility complex. In addition to the increase in DR15/DQ6 phenotype in Northern Europeans, the subsidiary association with DR3 (DR17)-DQ2 (and its associated DRB1*0301-DRB5*0101-DQA1*0501-DQB1*0201 genotype) and specifically different associations in Mediterranean populations cannot be explained by site specific similarities in sequence of the crucial peptide binding elements. The implication must be that either these alleles are in linkage disequilibrium with another (shared) susceptibility gene encoded within the major histocompatibility complex (which may or may not have a primary immunological function), or that the environmental trigger which initiates the disease process in multiple sclerosis varies and so selects specifically different at-risk populations. The evidence for genetic heterogeneity is also addressed by the analysis of primary progressive multiple sclerosis. The claim has been made that DR4 confers susceptibility and DQ7 resistance to the primary progressive form of multiple sclerosis in Scandinavian patients (Hillert *et al.*, 1992). Although there is support from a more recent study of primary progressive multiple sclerosis in Spain (de la Concha *et al.*, 1997), consensus has not been reached (McDonnell *et al.*, 1999; Weinshenker *et al.*, 1998) and definitive studies are needed. Furthermore, the opticospinal but not the Western type of multiple sclerosis is associated with DPB1$^*$0501 in northern and southern Japan, whereas the western type is DRB1$^*$1501 associated (Ma *et al.*, 1998; Yamasaki *et al.*, 1999).

Conditioning the United Kingdom genome screen for DR15 (or an extended DR15 linked haplotype also encoding alleles of TNF and the DQ locus) showed that the regions of interest on 1p, 17p, 17q, and X clustered in families that are identical by state for DR15, whereas the nonsharing group was associated with 1cen, 3p, 5cen, 7p, 14q, and 22q; in addition new regions of interest were found at 5q and 13p (DR15 sharing) and 16p and 20p (DR15 nonsharing: Chataway *et al.*, 1998; Coraddu *et al.*, 1999). As knowledge accumulates, conditioned analyses may routinely be needed in order to suggest or exclude new regions of interest or positional candidate susceptibility genes.

The presence of phenocopies is a major concern in the analysis of complex traits where diagnosis depends on pattern recognition of symptoms, signs, and laboratory investigations occurring in the absence of a test for the disease. Reassuringly, the cohort of cases included in the United Kingdom linkage genome screen was not contaminated by cases of CADASIL, spinocerebellar degenerations, or adrenoleukodystrophy in male-male pairs (Chataway *et al.*, 1998; Sawcer *et al.*, 1996). However, this search did identify a potentially important aspect of genetic heterogeneity that may have implications for selective tissue vulnerability. Although there were no individuals having an excess of triplet repeats for SCA2, the 22kb allele occurred at a higher frequency in cases than controls reported in the literature. This result prompted an assessment of transmission disequilibrium in family trios, which supported an association between multiple sclerosis and the 22kb allele (Chataway *et al.*, 1999). If confirmed, one interpretation of this finding would be that, in individuals who have a tendency for autoimmunity as a result of the interplay between genetic susceptibility and environmental factors, the inflammatory process may be targeted onto a particular system or pathway within the brain and spinal cord in those who have genetic polymorphisms exposing that pathway to tissue injury. In the case of SCA2, individuals with the 22kb allele polymorphism may have disproportionate inflammatory demyelination of the spinocerebellar pathways—similar by analogy to involvement of the anterior visual pathway in Harding's disease.

## CONCLUSIONS

To risk a summary of data that are distinctly ambiguous, genes showing some reproducibility for an effect on susceptibility are HLA DR/DQ, TNF-A, IL-1Ra, IL-4, and CTLA 4. Those apparently associated with disease protection are FAS-670 and IL-12p40. Genes that may influence the course or phenotype of multiple sclerosis include IL-10, CNTF, and ApoE4. Mutations of mitochondrial DNA may determine the phenotype. Eventually, six main categories of susceptibility gene can be predicted: genes that determine susceptibility to the process of inflammation across a range of disorders—the *autoimmune* genes; those that determine the specificity of that process for the development of multiple sclerosis—the *ubiquitous* genes; those that are relevant for the pathogenesis in isolated populations—the *domestic* genes; those that determine particular phenotypes—the *pleotropic* genes; those that determine variations in the clinical course—the *modifying* genes; and those that cluster to provide specifically different (heterogenous) contributions to the pathogenesis—the *epistatic* genes. Although perhaps overly speculative, some examples can be offered. Taken with the increased recurrence risk of autoimmunity in relatives of probands with multiple sclerosis (Broadley *et al.*, 2000; Heinzlef *et al.*, 1999, Henderson *et al.*, 2000), 10p (diabetes and multiple sclerosis: Broadley *et al.*, 2001; Coraddu *et al.*, 2001; Dyment *et al.*, 2001; Reed *et al.*, 1997),18q (diabetes, rheumatoid arthritis and multiple sclerosis: Merriman *et al.*, 2001), and 6p21 (major histocompatibility locus) may each encode genes that affect the general process of autoimmunity—*autoimmune* genes. 19q and 17q are provisionally linked and associated in several populations (Dyment *et al.*, 2001; Ebers *et al.*, 1996; Kuokkenen *et al.*, 1996; Larsen *et al.*, 2000; Saarla *et al.*, 2002; Sawcer *et al.*, 1996; Sawcer *et al.*, 2002)—*ubiquitous* multiple sclerosis genes. Myelin basic protein is linked and associated in Finns and Turks (who share their population history) with multiple sclerosis (Eraksoy *et al.*, 2003; Tiennari *et al.*, 1992)—a *domestic* gene. Mutations of mitochondrial DNA are associated with a defined phenotype, Harding's disease, in multiple sclerosis and the SCA2 association may implicate spinocerebellar pathways (Chataway *et al.*, 1999; Harding *et al.*, 1992; Kellar Wood *et al.*, 1994)—*pleotropic* genes. DR15 may be associated with earlier onset and female gender but not more severe clinical course in multiple sclerosis (Celius *et al.*, 2000; Hensiek *et al.*, 2002; Masterman *et al.*, 2000)—a *modifying* gene. Further, some regions of interest cluster within families stratified for the presence or not of DR15—*epistatic* groups. Clearly, much work lies ahead to consolidate these provisional classifications of gene effects in multiple sclerosis.

A major part of future studies will be to resolve the question of disease heterogeneity in multiple sclerosis. When eventually in place, the potential of this genetic knowledge for improved understanding of the pathogenesis of multiple sclerosis and designing novel treatments is considerable. Resolving the issues of complexity and heterogeneity in multiple sclerosis, and other complex traits, has practical dividends. Without knowledge linking etiology to pathogenesis and phenotype, putative new treatments—selected on the basis of an imperfect understanding of the pathogenesis—will continue to be screened in cohorts who may or may not have an appropriate pathological substrate for that particular intervention.

## References


Ablashi, D. V., Lapps, W., Kaplan, M., *et al.* (1998). Human herpesvirus-6 (HHV-6) infection in multiple sclerosis: A preliminary report. *Multiple Sclerosis* **4,** 490–496.

Åkesson, E., Coraddu. F., Marrosu, M., *et al.* (2003). Fine mapping of a candidate region on chromosome 10 in 449 sib-pairs with multiple sclerosis. *J. Neuroimmunology* (in press).

Åkesson, E., Oturai, A., Berg, J., *et al.* (2002). A genome-wide screen for linkage in Nordic sib-pairs with multiple sclerosis. *Genes and Immunity* **3,** 279–285,

Andersen, O., Lygner, P.-E., Berstrom, T., Andersson, M., and Vahlne, A. (1991). Viral infections trigger multiple sclerosis relapses: A prospective seroepidemiological study. *J. Neurology* **240,** 417–422.

Alizadeh M., Babron M. C., Birebent, B., *et al.* (2003). Involvement of CTLA-4 gene promoter SNP in MS genetics: A European collaborative family study *Ann. Neurol.* (in press).

Alter, M., Halpern, L., Kurland, L. T., Bornstein, V., Tikva, P., Leibowitz, U., and Silberstein, J. (1962). Multiple sclerosis in Israel: Prevalence among immigrants and native inhabitants. *Arch. Neurology* **7,** 253–263.

Alter, M., Kahana, E., and Loewenson, R. (1978). Migration and risk of multiple sclerosis. *Neurology* **28,** 1089–1093.

Alter M., Okihiro, M., Rowley, W., and Morris, T. (1971). Multiple sclerosis among Orientals and Caucasians in Hawaii. *Neurology* **2,** 122–130.

Ascherio, A., Zhang, S. M., Hernan, M. A., *et al.* (2001). Hepatitis B vaccination and the risk of multiple sclerosis. *New England J. Medicine*, **344,** 327–332.

Ban, M., Stewart, G., Bennetts, B., Heard, R., *et al.* (2002) A genome screen for linkage in Australian sibling-pairs with multiple sclerosis. *Genes and Immunity* **3**, 464–469.

Barcellos, L. F., Klitz ,W., Field, L. L., *et al.* (1997). Association mapping of disease loci using a pooled DNA genomic screen. *Am. J. Human Genetics* **61,** 734–747.

Baskett, P. J. F., and Armstrong, R. (1970). Anaesthetic problems in multiple sclerosis. *Anaesthesia* **25,** 397–401.

Bauer, H. J. (1987). Multiple sclerosis in Europe. Symposium Report. *J. Neurology* **234,** 195–206.

Becker, K. G., Simon R. M., and Bailey-Wilson, J. E. (1998). Clustering of non-major histocompatibility complex susceptibility candidate loci in human autoimmune disease. *Proceedings of the National Academy of Sciences of the USA* **95,** 9979–9984.

Benedikz, J. G., Magnusson, H., and Gudmundsson, G. (1994). Multiple sclerosis in Iceland, with observations on the alleged epidemic in the Faroe Islands. *Ann. Neurology 36 (suppl 2)*, S175–S179.

Broadley, S., Deans, J., Sawcer, S. J., *et al.* (2000). Autoimmune disease in first degree relatives of patients with multiple sclerosis in the United Kingdom. *Brain* **123,** 1102–1111.

Broadley, S., Sawcer, S., D'Alfonso, S., *et al.* (2001). A genome screen for multiple sclerosis in Italian families. *Genes and Immunity* **2,** 205–210.

Bulman, D., and Ebers, G. C. (1992). The geography of multiple sclerosis reflects genetic susceptibility. *J. Tropical and Geographical Neurology* **2,** 66–72.

Buljevac, D., Flach, H. Z., Hop, W. C. J., *et al.* (2002). Prospective study on the relationship between infections and multiple sclerosis exacerbations. *Brain* **125,** 952–960.

Carton, H., Vlietinck, R., Debruyne, J., *et al.* (1996). Recurrence risks of multiple sclerosis in relatives of patients in Flanders, Belgium. *J. Neurology Neurosurgery and Psychiatry* **62,** 329–333.

Cavalli-Sforza, L. L., Menozzi, P., and Piazza, A. (1994). "The History and Geography of Human Genes." Princeton University Press, Princeton, NJ.

Celius, E. G., Harbo, H. F., Egeland, T. *et al.* (2000). Sex and age at diagnosis are correlated with the HLA-DR2, DQ6 haplotype in multiple sclerosis. *J. Neurological Sciences* **178,** 132–135.

Chakraborty, R., Kamboh, M. I., Nwankwo, M., and Ferrell, R. E. (1992). Caucasian genes in American Blacks: New data. *Am. J. Human Genetics* **50,** 145–155.

Chataway, J., Feakes, R., Coraddu, F. *et al.* (1998). The genetics of multiple sclerosis: Principles, background and updated results of the United Kingdom systematic genome screen. *Brain* **121,** 1869–1887.

Chataway, J., Sawcer, S., Coraddu, F. *et al.* (1999). Allelic variants of the spinocerebellar ataxia genes contribute to multiple sclerosis susceptibility. *Neurogenetics* **2,** 91–96.

Chataway, S. J. S., Mander, A., Robertson, N., *et al.* (2001). Multiple sclerosis in sibling pairs: An analysis of 250 families. *J. Neurology Neurosurgery and Psychiatry* **71,** 757–761.

Collins, A., Ennis, S., Taillon-Miller, P. *et al.* (2001). Allelic association with SNPs: Metrics, populations, and the linkage disequilibrium map. *Human Mutation* **17,** 255–262.

Compston, D. A. S., Vakarelis, B.N., P. E., McDonald, W. I., Batchelor, J. R., and Mims, C. A. (1986). Viral infection in patients with multiple sclerosis and HLA-DR matched controls. *Brain* **109,** 325–344.

Confavreux, C., Hutchinson, M., Hours, M., *et al.* (1998). Rate of pregnancy-related relapse in multiple sclerosis. *The New England J. Medicine* **339,** 285–291.

Confavreux, C., Suissa, S., Saddier, P., *et al.* (2001). Vaccinations and the risk of relapse in multiple sclerosis. *The New England J. Medicine* **344,** 319–326.

Cook, S. D., Cromarty, M. B., Tapp, W., Poskanzer, D., Walker, J. D., and Dowling, P. C. (1985). Declining incidence of multiple sclerosis in the Orkney Islands. *Neurology* **35,** 545–551.

Coraddu, F., Reyes-Yanez, M. P., Aladro, Y., *et al.* (1998). HLA associations with multiple sclerosis in the Canary Islands. *J. Neuroimmunology* **87,** 130–135.

Coraddu, F., Sawcer, S., D'Alfonso, S., *et al.* (2001). A genome screen for multiple sclerosis in Sardinian multiplex families. *European J. Human Genetics* **9,** 621–626.

Coraddu, F., Sawcer, S., Feakes, R., *et al.* (1999). HLA typing in the United Kingdom multiple sclerosis genome screen. *Neurogenetics* **2,** 24–33.

Daly, M. J., Rioux, J. D., Schaffner, S. F., *et al.* (2001). High-resolution haplotype structure in the human genome. *Nature Genetics* **29,** 229–332.

Davenport, C.B. (1922). Multiple sclerosis from the standpoint of geographic distribution and race. *Arch. Neurology* **8,** 51–58.

Dawson, E., Abecasis, G. R., Bumpstead, S. *et al.* (2002) A first-generation linkage disequilibrium map of human chromosome 22. *Nature* 418, 544–548.

de la Concha, E. G., Arroyo, R., Crusius, J. B., *et al.* (1997). Combined effect of HLA-DRB1*1501 and interleukin-1 receptor antagonist gene allele 2 in susceptibility to relapsing/remitting multiple sclerosis. *J. Neuroimmunology* **80,** 172–8.

Dean, G. (1967). Annual incidence, prevalence and mortality of MS in white South African-born and in white immigrants to South Africa. *British Med. J.1* **2,** 724–730.

Dean, G., Bhighee, A. I. G., Bill, P. L. A., *et al.* (1994). Multiple sclerosis is black South Africans and Zimbabweans. *J. Neurology Neurosurgery and Psychiatry* **57,** 1064–1069.

Dean, G., Elian, M., de Bono, A. G., *et al.* (2002). Multiple sclerosis in Malta in 1998: An update. *J. Neurology Neurosurgery and Psychiatry* **73,** 256–260.

Detels, R., Brody, J. F., Edgar, A. H. (1972). Multiple sclerosis among American, Japanese and Chinese migrants to California and Washington. *J. Chronic Diseases* **25,** 3–10.

Detels, R., Visscher, B., Malmgrem, R. M., Coulson, A. H., Lucia, M. V., and Dudley, J. P. (1977). Evidence for lower susceptibility to multiple sclerosis in Japanese-Americans. *Am. J. Epidemiology* **105,** 303–310.

Duquette, P., Murray T. J., Pleines, J., Ebers, G. C., Sadovnick, D., Weldon, P., Warren, S., Paty, D. W., Upton, A., Hader, W., Nelson, R., Auty, A., Neufeld, B., and Meltzer, C. (1987). Multiple sclerosis in childhood: Clinical profile in 125 patients. *J. Pediatrics* **3,** 359–363.

Dunning, A. M., Durocher, F., Healey, C. S., *et al.* (2000). The extent of linkage disequilibrium in four populations with distinct demographic histories. *Am. J. Human Genetics* **67,** 1544–1554.

Dyment, D. A., Steckley, J. L., Willer, C. J., *et al.* (2002). No evidence to support CTLA-4 as a susceptibility gene in MS families: The Canadian Collaborative Study. *J. Neuroimmunology* **123,** 193–198.

Dyment, D. A., Willer, C. J., Scott, B., *et al.* (2001). Genetic susceptibility to MS: A second stage analysis in Canadian MS families. *Neurogenetics* **3,** 145–51.

Eaves, I. A., Merriman T. R., Barber, R. A., *et al.* (2000). The genetically isolated populations of Finland and Sardinia may not be a panacea for linkage disequilibrium mapping of common disease genes. *Nature Genetics* **25,** 320–323.

Ebers, G. C., Koopman, W. J., Hader, W., *et al.* (2000a). The natural history of multiple sclerosis: A geographically based study. *Brain* **123,** 641–649.

Ebers, G.C., Kukay, K., Bulma,n D.,*et al.* (1996). A full genome search in multiple sclerosis. *Nature Genetics* **13,** 472–476.

Ebers, G. C., Sadovnick, A. D., and Risch NJ. (1995). A genetic basis for familial aggregation in multiple sclerosis. *Nature* **377,** 150–151.

Ebers, G. C., Yee, I. M., Sadovnick, A. D., and Duquette, P. (2000b). Conjugal multiple sclerosis: Population-based prevalence and recurrence risks in offspring. Canadian Collaborative Study Group. *Ann. Neurology* **48,** 927–931.

Eisenberg, D., Marcotte, E. M., Xenaris, I., and Yeats, T. O. (2000). Protein function in the post-genome era. *Nature* **405,** 823–826.

Elian, M., and Dean, G. (1987). Multiple sclerosis among United Kingdom born children of immigrants from the West Indies. *J. Neurology, Neurosurgery and Psychiatry* **50,** 327–332.

Elian, M., Nightingale, S., and Dean, G. (1990). Multiple sclerosis among United Kingdom-born children of immigrants from the Indian subcontinent, Africa and the West Indies. *J. Neurology Neurosurgery and Psychiatry* **53,** 906–911.

Eraksoy, M., Hensiek, A., Kürtüncü, M., *et al.* (2003). A genome screen for linkage disequilibrium in Turkish multiple sclerosis. *J. Neuroimmunology* (in press).

Evangelou,, N., Jackson, M., Beeson, D., and Palace, J. (1999). Association of the APOE e4 allele with diseas activity in multiple sclerosis. *J. Neurology, Neurosurgery and Psychiatry* **67,** 203–205.

Friedman, J. E., Lyons, M. J., Cu, G., *et al.* (1999). The association of the human herpesvirus-6 and MS. *Multiple Sclerosis* **5,** 355–362.

French Research Group on Multiple Sclerosis. (1992). Multiple Sclerosis in 54 twinships: Concordance rate is independent of zygosity. *Ann. Neurology* **32,** 724–727.

Fukazawa, T., Kikuchi, S., Sasaki, H., *et al.* (2000) Genomic HLA profiles of MS in Hokkaido, Japan: Important role of DPB1*0501 allele. *J. Neurology* **247,** 175–178.

Fukazawa, T., Yanagawa, T., Kikuchi, S., *et al.* (1999). CTLA-4 gene polymorphism may modulate disease in Japanese multiple sclerosis patients. *J. Neurological Sciences* **171,** 49–55.

GAMES and The Transatlantic Multiple Sclerosis Genetics Cooperative. (2001). A meta-analysis of genome screens in multiple sclerosis. *J. Multiple Sclerosis* **7,** 3–11.

Giess, R., Maurer, M., and Pohl, D. (2002). A null mutation in the CNTF gene is associated with early onset of multiple sclerosis. *Archives of Neurology*, **59** 407–409.

Haahr, S., Koch-Henriksen, N., Moller-Larsen, A., *et al.* (1995). Increased risk of multiple sclerosis after late Epstein-Barr virus infection: A historical prospective study. *Multiple Sclerosis* **1,** 73–77.

Haines, J. L., Ter-Minassian, M., Bazyk, A., *et al.* (1996). A complete genomic screen for multiple sclerosis underscores a role for the major histocompatibility complex. *Nature Genetics* **13,** 469–471.

Hammond, S. R., English, D. R, and McLeod, J. G. (2000). The age-range of risk of developing multiple sclerosis. Evidence from a migrant population in Australia. *Brain* **123,** 968–974.

Hammond, S. R., McLeod, J. G., Millingen, K. S., Stewart-Wynne, E. G., English, D., Holland, J. T., and McCall, M. G. (1988). The epidemiology of multiple sclerosis in 3 Australian cities: Perth, Newcastle and Hobart. *Brain* **111,** 1–25.

Harbo, H. F., Celius, E. G., Vardtal, F., and Spurkland, A. (2000). CTLA4 promoter and exon 1 dimorphisms in multiple sclerosis. *Tissue Antigens* **53,** 106–110.

Harding, A. E., Sweeney, M. G., Brockington, M., *et al.* (1992). Occurrence of a multiple sclerosis-like illness in women who have a Leber's hereditary optic neuropathy mitochondrial DNA mutation. *Brain* **115,** 989–989.

Hawkes, C. H. (2002). Is multiple sclerosis a sexually transmitted infection? *J. Neurology Neurosurgery and Psychiatry* **73,** 439–443.

He, B., Xu, C., Yang, B., *et al.* (1998). Linkage and association analysis of genes encoding cytokines and myelin proteins in multiple sclerosis. *J. Neuroimmunology* **86,** 13–19.

Heinzlef, O., Alamowitch, S., Sazdovitch, V., *et al.* (1999). Autoimmune disease in families of French patients with multiple sclerosis. *Acta Neurologica Scandinavica* **100,** 1–5.

Henderson, R. D., Bain, C. J., and Pender, M. P. (2000). The occurrence of autoimmune diseases in patients with multiple sclerosis and their families. *J. Clinical Neuroscience* **7**(5), 434–437.

Hensiek, A. E., Sawcer, S. J., Feakes, R., *et al.* (2002) HLA-DR 15 is associated with female gender and younger age at diagnosis in multiple sclerosis. *J. Neurology Neurosurgery and Psychiatry* **72,** 184–187.

Hernan, M. A., Zhang, S. M., Lipworth, L., *et al.* (2001). Multiple sclerosis and age at infection with common viruses. *Epidemiology* **12,** 301–06.

Hillert, J., Gronning, M., Hyland, H., Link, H., and Olerup, O. (1992). Immunogenetic heterogeneity in multiple sclerosis. *J. Neurology Neurosurgery and Psychiatry* **55,** 887–890.

Hogh, P., Oturai, A., Schreiber, K., *et al.* (2000). Apoliprotein E and multiple sclerosis: Impact of the epsilon-4 allele on susceptibility, clinical type and progression rate. *Mutiple Sclerosis* **6,** 226–230.

Hupperts, R., Broadley, S., Mander, A., *et al.* (2001). Patterns of disease in concordant parent-child pairs with multiple sclerosis. *Neurology* **57,** 290–295.

Jacobsen, M., Schweer, D., Ziegler, A., *et al.* (2000). A point mutation in PTPRC is associated with the development of multiple sclerosis. *Nature Genetics* **26,** 495–499.

Jeffreys, A. J,. Kauppi, L., Neumann, R. (2001). Intensely punctate meiotic recombination in the class II region of the major histocompatibility complex. *Nature Genetics* **29,** 217–222.

Jin, Y.-P., de Pedro-Cuesta, J., Soderstrom, M., *et al.* (2000). Seasonal patterns in optic neuritis and multiple sclerosis: A meta-analysis. *J. Neurol. Sci.* **181**, 56–64.

Johnson, G. C., Esposito, L., Barratt B. J., *et al.* (2001). Haplotype tagging for the identification of common disease genes. *Nature Genetics* **29,** 233–237.

Johnson, M. R., Ferner, R. E., Bobrow, M., *et al.* (2000). Detailed analysis of the oligodendrocyte myelin glycoprotein gene in four patients with neurofibromatosis 1 and primary progressive multiple sclerosis. *J. Neurology, Neurosurgery and Psychiatry 68(5)*, 643–6.

Kahana, E., Zilber, N., Abramson, J. H., Biton, Y., Leibowitz, Y., and Abramsky, O. (1994). Multiple sclerosis: Genetic versus environmental aetioogy: Epidemiology in Israel updated. *J. Neurology* **241,** 341–346.

Kalman, B., and Mandler, R. N. (2002). Studies of mitochondrial DNA in Devic's disease revealed no pathogenic mutations, but polymorphisms also found in association with multiple sclerosis. *Ann. Neurology 51* **5,** 661.

Kantarci, O. H., de Andrade, M., Weinshenker, B. G. (2002) Identifying disease modifying genes in multiple sclerosis. *J. Neuroimmunology* 123, 144–159.

Kaufman, M., Gaydos, C. A., Sriram, S., *et al.* (2002). Is Chlamydia pneumoniae found in spinal fluid samples from multiple sclerosis patients? Conflicting results. *Multiple Sclerosis* **8,** 289–294.

Kellar Wood, H., Robertson, N., Govan, G. G., *et al.* (1994). Leber's hereditary optic neuropathy mitochondrial DNA mutations in multiple sclerosis. *Ann. Neurology* **36,** 109–112.

Kendler, K. S., MacLean, C. J,. Ma, Y., *et al.* (1999). Marker-to-marker linkage disequilibrium on chromosomes 5q, 6p and 8p in Irish high-density achizophreniua pedigrees. *Am. J. Human Genetics* **88,** 29–33.

Kikuchi, S., Fukazawa, T., Niino, M., *et al.* (2003). HLA-related subpopulations of MS in Japanese with and without oligoclonal bands. *Neurology* (in press).

Kruglyak, L. (1999). Prospects for whole-genome linkage disequilibrium mapping of common disease genes. *Nature Genetics* **22,** 139–144.

Kuhlmann, T., Glas, M., zum Bruch, C., *et al.* (2002). Investigation of bax, bcl-2, bcl-x and p53 gene polymorphisms in multiple sclerosis. *J. Neuroimmunology* **129,** 154–160.

Kuokkanen, S, Gschwend, M., Rioux, J. D., *et al.* (1997). Genomewide scan of multiple sclerosis in Finnish multiplex families. *Am. J. Human Genetics* **61,** 1379–1387.

Kuroiwa, Y., Shibasaki, H,. and Ikeda, M. (1983). Prevalence of multiple sclerosis and its north-south gradient in Japan. *Neuroepidemiology* **2,** 62–69.

Kurtzke, J. F. (1975). A reassessment of the distribution of multiple sclerosis. *Acta Neurologica Scandinavica* **51,** 110–136; 137–157.

Kurtzke, J. F. (1993). Epidemiologic evidence for multiple sclerosis as an infection. *Clinical Microbiology Reviews* **6,** 382–427.

Kurtzke, J. F., and Bui, Q. H. (1980). Multiple sclerosis in a migrant population to half Orientals immigrating in childhood. *Ann. Neurology* **8,** 256–260.

Kurtzke, J. F., Gudmundsson, K. R., and Bergmann, S. (1982). Multiple sclerosis in Iceland. 1. Evidence of a post-war epidemic. *Neurology* **32,** 143–150.

Kurtzke, J. F., and Heltberg, A. (2001). Multiple sclerosis in the Faroe Islands: An epitome. *J. Clinical Epidemiology* **54,** 1–22.

Kurtzke, J. F., Kurland, L. T., and Goldberg, I. D. (1971). Mortality and migration in multiple sclerosis. *Neurology* **21,** 1186–1197.

Larsen, F., Oturai, A., Ryder, L. P., *et al.* (2000). A. linkage analysis of a candidate region in Scandinavian sib pairs with multiple sclerosis reveals linkage to chromosome 17q. *Genes and Immunity* **1,** 456–459.

Lauer, K. (1994). The risk of multiple sclerosis in the USA in relation to sociogeographic features: a factor-analytic study. *J. Clinical Epidemiology* **47,** 43–48.

Lauer, K., and Firnhaber, W. (1994). Multiple sclerosis in Europe: An epidemiological update. Leuchturm-Verlag/LTV Press, Darmstadt.

Ligers, A., Xu, C., Saarinen, S., *et al.* (1999). The CTLA-4 gene is associated with multiple sclerosis. *J. Neuroimmunology* **97,** 182–190.

Lindberg, C., Andersen, O., Vahlne, A., *et al.* (1991). Epidemiological investigation of the association between infectious mononucleosis and multiple sclerosis. *Neuroepidemiology* **10,** 62–65.

Lucchinetti, C., Bruck, W., Parisi, J., *et al.* (2000). Heterogeneity for multiple sclerosis lesions: Implications for the pathogenesis of demyelination. *Annals of Neurology* **47,** 707–717.

Ma, J. J., Nishimura, M., Mine, H., *et al.* (1998). HLA-DRB1 and tumor necrosis factor gene polymorphisms in Japanese patients with multiple sclerosis. *J. Neuroimmunology* **92,** 109–112.

Masterman, T., Ligers, A., Olsson, T., *et al.* (2000). HLA-DR15 is associated with lower age at onset in multiple sclerosis. *Ann. Neurology* **48,** 211–219.

Masterman, T., Ligers, A., Zhang, Z., *et al.* (2002). *CTLA*4 polymorphisms influence disease course in multiple sclerosis. *J. Neuroimmunal.* **131**, 208–212.

Maurer, M., Ponath, A., Kruse, N., *et al.* (2002) CTLA-4 wxon 1 dimorphism is associated with primary progressive multiple sclerosis *J. Neuroimmunal.* **131**, 213–215.

McDonald, W. I., Compston, D. A. S., Edan. G., *et al.* (2001). International panel on the diagnosis of multiple sclerosis: New diagnostic criteria for multiple sclerosis. *Ann. Neurology* **50,** 121–127.

McDonnell, G. V., Kirk, C. W., Hawkins, S. A., and Graham, C. A. (2000). An evaluation of interleukin genes as susceptibility loci for multiple sclerosis. *J. the Neurological Sciences*, **176,** 4–12.

McDonnell, G. V., Mawhinney, H., Graham, C. A., *et al.* (1999). A study of the HLA-DR region in clinical subgroups of multiple sclerosis and its influence on prognosis. *J. Neurological Science* **165**(1), 77–83.

Marrosu, M. G., Muntoni, F., Murru, M. R., *et al.* (1992). HLA-DQB1 genotype in Sardinian multiple sclerosis: Evidence for a key role of DQB1. 0201 and DQB1.0302 alleles. *Neurology* **42,** 883–886.

Martin, E. R., Lai, E. H., Gilbert, J. R., *et al.* (2000). SNPing away at complex diseases: Analysis of single-nucleotide polymorphisms around APOE in Alzheimer disease. *Am. J. Human Genetics* **67,** 383–394.

Martyn, C. N., Cruddas, M., and Compston, D. A. S. (1993). Symptomatic Epstein-Barr virus infection and multiple sclerosis. *J. Neurology Neurosurgery and Psychiatry* **56,** 167–168.

Merriman, A., Cordell, H. J., Eaves, I. A., *et al.* (2001). Suggestive evidence for association of human chromosome 18q12-q21 and its orthologue on rat and mouse chromosome 18 with several autoimmune diseases. *Diabetes* **50,** 184–194.

Mertens, C., Brassat, D., Reboul, J., *et al.* (1998). A systematic study of oligodendrocyte growth factors as candidates for genetic susceptibility to multiple sclerosis. *Neurology* **51,** 748–753.

Modin, H., Dai, Y., Masterman T., *et al.* (2001). No linkage or association of the nitric oxide synthase genes to multiple sclerosis. *J. Neuroimmunology* **119,** 95–100.

The Multiple Sclerosis Genetics Group, Barcellos, L. F., Oksenberg, J. R., *et al.* (2002). Genetic basis for clinical expression in multiple sclerosis.. *Brain* **125,** 150–158.

Mumford, C. J., Wood, N. W., Kellar-Wood, H. F., *et al.* (1994). The British Isles survey of multiple sclerosis in twins. *Neurology* **44,** 11–15.

Olerup, O., and Hillert, J. (1991). HLA class II-associated genetic susceptibility in multiple sclerosis: A critical evaluation. *Tissue Antigens* **38,** 1–15.

Oturai, A., Larsen, F., Ryder, L. P., *et al.* (1999). Linkage and association analysis of susceptibility regions on chromosomes 5 and 6 in 106 Scandinavian sibling pair families with multiple sclerosis. *Annals of Neurology* **46,** 612–616.

Pihlaja, H., Rentamaki, T., Wikstrom, J., *et al.* (2003). Linkage disequilibrium between the MBP tetranucleotide repeat and multiple sclerosis is restricted to a geographically defined subpopulation in Finland. *Genes and Immunity* **4,** 138–146.

Poser, C. M. (1994). The dissemination of multiple sclerosis: A Viking saga? A historical essay. *Ann.Neurology 36 (suppl 2)*, S231–S243.

Reboul, J., Mertens, C., Levillayer, F., *et al.* (2000). Cytokines in genetic susceptibility to multiple sclerosis: A candidate gene approach. *J. Neuroimmunology* **102,** 107–12.

Reed, P., Cucca, F., Jenkins, S., *et al.* (1997). Evidence for a type 1 diabetes susceptibility locus (IDDM10) on human chromosome 10p11-q11. *Human Molecular Genetics* **6,** 1011–6.

Reich, D. E., Cargill, M., Bolk, S., *et al.* (2001). Linkage disequilibrium in the human genome. *Nature* **411,** 199–204.

Reynier, P., Pennisson-Besnier, I., Moreau, C., *et al.* (1999). MtDNA haplopgroup J: A contributing factor of optic neuritis. *European J. Human Genetics Apr.* 7(3), 404–6.

Risch, N. (1990). Linkage strategies for genetically complex traits. *Am. J. Human Genetics* **46,** 222–253.

Risch, N., and Merikangas, K. (1996). The future of genetic studies of complex human diseases. *Science* **23,** 1516–1517.

Risch, N. J. (2000). Searching for genetic determinants in the new millennium. *Nature* **405,** 847–856.

Robertson, N. P., Compston, D. A. S. (1995). Surveying multiple sclerosis in the United Kingdom. *J. Neurology Neurosurgery and Psychiatry* **58,** 2–6.

Robertson, N. P., Clayton, D., Fraser, M. B., *et al.* (1996a). Clinical concordance in sibling pairs with multiple sclerosis. *Neurology* **47,** 347–352.

Robertson, N. P., Fraser, M., Deans, J., *et al.* (1996b). Age adjusted recurrence risks for relatives of patients with multiple sclerosis. *Brain* **119,** 449–455.

Robertson, N. P., O'Riordan, J. I., Chataway, J., *et al.* (1997). Clinical characteristics and offspring recurrence rates of conjugal multiple sclerosis. *Lancet* **349,** 1587–1590.

Rogers, A. E., Meehan, J., Guilleminault, C., *et al.* (1997). HLA DR15 (DR2) and DQB1*0602 typing studies in 188 narcoleptic patients with cataplexy. *Neurology* **48,** 1550–1556.

Rosati, G. (1994). Descriptive epidemiology of multiple sclerosis in Europe in the 1980s: A critical overview. *Annals of Neurology* **36** (suppl 2), S164–S174.

Roxburgh, R., Sawcer, S., Deans, J., *et al.* (2003). Familial recurrence and genetic risk factors for autoimmune thyroid disease in patients with multiple sclerosis (submitted)

Runmarker, B., and Andersen, O. (1995). Pregnancy is associated with a lower risk of onset and a better prognosis in multiple sclerosis. *Brain* **118,** 253–261.

Saarela, J., Schoenberg Fejzo, M., Chen, D., *et al.* (2002). Fine mapping of a multiple sclerosis locus to 2.5 Mb on chromosome 17q22-q24. *Human Molecular Genetics* **11,** 2257–2267.

Sadovnick, A. D., Armstrong, H., Rice, G. P. A., *et al.* (1993). A population-based study of multiple sclerosis in twins: Update. *Annals of Neurology* **33,** 281–285.

Sadovnick, A. D., Baird, P. A., Ward, R. H. (1988). Multiple sclerosis: Updated risks for relatives. *Am. J. Medical Genetics* **29,** 533–541.

Sadovnick, A. D., Ebers, G. C., Dyment, D. A., *et al.* (1996). Evidence for genetic basis of multiple sclerosis. Lancet **347,** 1728–1730.

Saruhan-Direskeneli, G., Esin, S., Baykan-Kurt, B., *et al.* (1997). HLA-DR and -DQ associations with multiple sclerosis in Turkey. *Human Immunology* **55,** 59–65.

Sawcer, S., Jones, H. B., Feakes R., *et al.* (1996). A genome screen in multiple sclerosis reveals susceptibility loci on chromosome 6p21 and 17q22. *Nature Genetics* **13,** 464–468.

Sawcer, S., Meranian, M., Setakis, E., *et al.* (2002). A whole genome screen for linkage disequilibrium in multiple sclerosis confirms disease associations with regions previously linked to susceptibility. *Brain,* **125,** 1337–1347.

Seboun, E., Oksenberg, J. R., Rombos, A., *et al.* (1999). Linkage analysis of candidate myelin genes in familial multiple sclerosis. *Neurogenetics Sep;* **2**(3), 155–62.

Sheremata, W. A., Poskanzer, D. C., Withum, D. G., MacLeod, C. L., and Whiteside, M. E. (1985). Unusual occurrence on a tropical island of multiple sclerosis. *Lancet (letter)* **2,** 618.

Skegg, D. C. G., Corwin, P. A., Craven, R. S., Malloch, J. A., and Pollock, M. (1987). Occurrence of multiple sclerosis at the north and south of New Zealand. *J. Neurology Neurosurgery and Psychiatry* **50,** 134–139.

Sibley, W. A., Bamford, C. R., and Clark, K. (1985). Clinical viral infections and multiple sclerosis. *Lancet* **i,** 1313–1315.

Sibley, W. A., Bamford, C. R., Clark, K., Smith, M. S., and Laguna, J. F. (1991). A prospective study of physical trauma and multiple sclerosis. *J. Neurology Neurosurgery and Psychiatry* **54,** 584–589.

Siemkowicz, E. (1976). Multiple sclerosis and surgery. *Anaesthesia* **31,** 1211–1216.

Siva, A., Radhakrishnan, K., Kurland, L. T., O'Brien, P. C., Swanson, J. W., and Rodriguez, M. (1993). Trauma and multiple sclerosis: A population based cohort study from Olmsted County, Minnesota. *Neurology* **43,** 1878–1882.

Soldan, S. S., Leist, T. P., Juhng, K. N., *et al.* (2000). Increased lymphoproliferative response to human herpesvirus type 6A variant in multiple sclerosis patients. *Annals of Neurology* **47,** 306–313.

Sriram, S., Stratton, C. W., Yao, S., *et al.* (1999). Chlamydia pneumoniae infection of the central nervous system in multiple sclerosis. *Annals of Neurology* **46,** 6–14.

Sumelahti, M.-L., Tienari, P. J., Wikstrom, J., *et al.* (2002). Survival of multiple sclerosis in Finland between 1964–1993. *Multiple Sclerosis* **8,** 350–355.

Sutherland, J. M. (1956). Observations on the prevalence of multiple sclerosis in Northern Scotland. *Brain* **79,** 635–654.

Taillon-Miller, P., Bauer-Sardina, I., Saccone, N. L., *et al.* (2000). Juxtaposed regions of extensive and minimal linkage disequilibrium in human Xq25 and Xq28. *Nature Genetics* **25,** 324–328.

Tienari, P., Wikstrom, J., Sajantila, A., Palo, J., and Peltonen L. (1992). Genetic susceptibility to multiple sclerosis linked to myelin basic protein gene. *Lancet* **340,** 987–991.

The Transatlantic Multiple Sclerosis Genetics Cooperative. (2003). A meta-analysis of genome screens in multiple sclerosis. *J. Neuroimmunology* (in press).

Vaughan, J. H., Riise, T., Rhodes, G. H., *et al.* (1996). An Epstein Barr virus-related cross reactive autoimmune response in multiple sclerosis in Norway. *J. Neuroimmunology* **69,** 95–102.

Weinshenker, B. G., Santrach, P., Bissonet, A. S., *et al.* (1998). Major histocompatibility complex class II alleles and the course and outcome of MS: A population-based study. *Neurology* **51,** 742–7.

Xu, C., Dai, Y., Fredrickson, S., *et al.* (1999). Association and linkage analysis of candidate chromosomal regions in multiple sclerosis: Indication of disease genes in 12q23 and 7ptr-15. *European J. Human Genetics* **7,** 110–116.

Xu, C., Dai, Y., and Lorentzen, J. C., (2001). Linkage analysis in multiple sclerosis of chromosomal regions syntenic to experimental autoimmune disease loci. *European J. Human Genetics* **9,** 458–463.

Yamasaki, K., Horiuchi, I., Minohara, M., *et al.* (1999). HLA-DPB1*0501-associated opticospinal multiple sclerosis: Clinical, neuroimaging and immunogenetic studies. *Brain* **122,** 1689–1696.

Zipp, F., Weil, J. G., and Einhaupl, K. M. (1999). No increase in demyelinating diseases after hepatitis B vaccination. *Nature Medicine* **5,** 964–965.

CHAPTER

# 31

# Cellular Damage and Repair in Multiple Sclerosis

*Hans Lassmann*

The basic features of the pathology of multiple sclerosis (MS) were defined at the end of the 19th century (Charcot, 1868; Marburg, 1906). It is a chronic inflammatory demyelinating disease. This means that an inflammatory process of the central nervous system is associated with the formation of large lesions of primary demyelination with partial axonal preservation and reactive glial scar formation. The lesions are basically formed around small veins and venules, which show focal perivascular inflammation (Dawson, 1916; Rindfleisch, 1963). Perivenous lesions, when they enlarge, can fuse with other adjacent demyelinating areas and form large demyelinating plaques, which may reach a diameter of several centimeters. In addition, lesions can grow by radial expansion. In this case, active demyelination occurs at the periphery of the lesion, resulting in a gradual expansion of the plaque into the surrounding normal white matter.

Thus, the pathology of multiple sclerosis is defined by the presence of demyelinated plaques (Carswell, 1838; Cruveilhier, 1841, Figure 31.1). Such demyelinating lesions may occur both in the white as well as the gray matter of the central nervous system, in the latter they are, however, difficult to identify due to the low density of myelin (Brownell and Hughes, 1962; Lumsden, 1970). Although any brain or spinal cord region can be affected by the disease process, certain predilection sites are affected more frequently than others. These are the periventricular white matter, in particular the lateral angles of the lateral ventricles, the subcortical white matter, the optic nerves and chiasm, the cerebellar peduncles with the adjacent cerebellar white matter, and the spinal cord (Fog, 1950; Lumsden, 1970; Steiner, 1931). This uneven distribution of lesions in the central nervous system is due in part to their formation around small to medium-sized veins and venules. This implies that in areas with high density of drainage veins and venules, the probability for initiating an MS lesion is higher than in areas with low venous density (Lassmann, 1983).

Multiple sclerosis plaques can be easily identified by the unaided eye in the freshly dissected brain (Lumsden, 1970). They appear as sharply demarcated areas of gray discoloration within the white matter. By touching the surface of the cut brain tissue, they reveal a much higher consistency compared to the adjacent tissue. Thus, they represent multiple islets of hard "sclerotic" scar tissue within the brain and this feature is reflected by the name of the disease "multiple sclerosis." These gray, hard, and sharply demarcated lesions are old chronic plaques. Fresh lesions, which are still in the process of myelin destruction, are in contrast yellow to brown and of soft consistency. In addition, in cases with very severe disease more extensive tissue destruction may lead to cystic loss of tissue, in particular in the center of the lesions. Finally, in some multiple sclerosis patients with an acute, rapidly progressive disease course, very large lesions may appear in the hemispheric

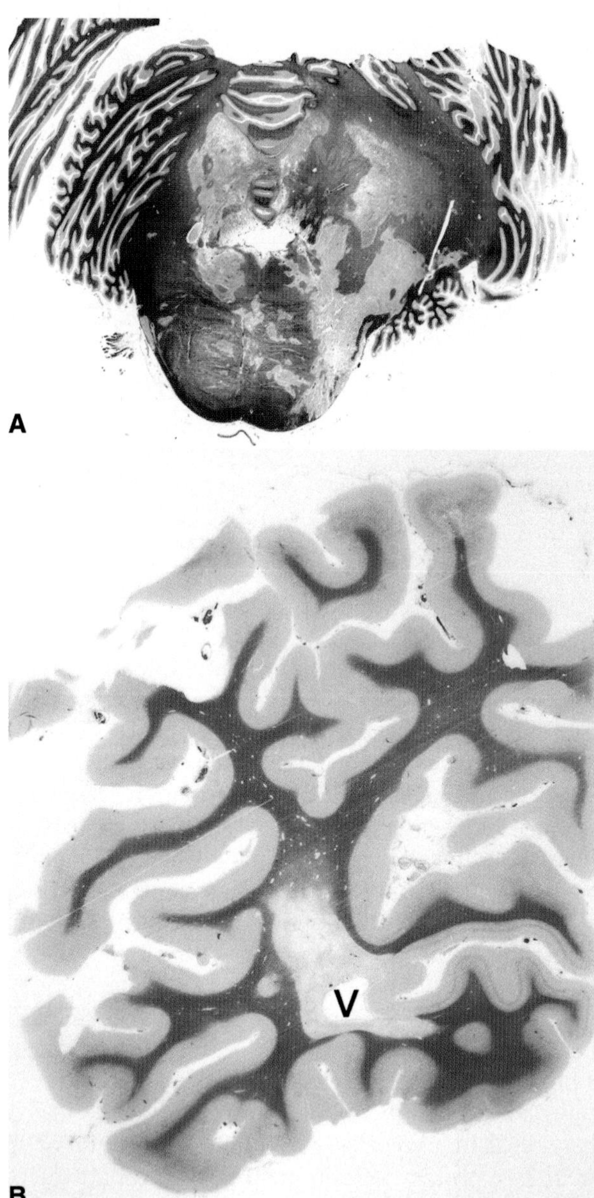


FIGURE 31.1
Demyelinated plaques in the central nervous system of MS patients. (A) acute MS (Marburg's type) with massive brain stem involvement. Demyelinated plaques are seen in the pons, the cerebellar peduncles and the cerebellar hemisphere. Two types of lesions can be differentiated: large confluent demyelinated plaques as well as small perivascular lesions, which may form finger-like extensions of the large plaques. Weigert myelin stain; × 1. (B) chronic MS with large periventricular plaque surrounding the occipital horn of the lateral ventricle (V) as well as some smaller perivenous lesions in the depth of the white matter. Weigert myelin stain, × 0.5.

white matter, which show a concentric layering of myelinated and demyelinated tissue. This variant of multiple sclerosis is called Balo's concentric sclerosis (Balo, 1928).

The hallmark of multiple sclerosis is the plaque with primary demyelination and reactive glial scar formation. Primary demyelination means that myelin sheaths are completely destroyed, while axons remain relatively well preserved in relation to the complete myelin loss. However, as stressed already in the earliest descriptions of multiple sclerosis pathology (for review, see Kornek and Lassmann, 1999), emphasis has to be laid on the term "relative." Every MS plaque has some degree of axonal injury and loss; its extent varies from plaque to plaque in a given patient but even more between plaques of different patients. The reduction of axonal density in different plaques may range from as few as

10% to as much as 90%. As noted already, in the early years of the twentieth century, the presence of lesions with a high extent of axonal loss was generally associated with poor recovery from clinical deficit in remission periods (Kornek and Lassmann, 1999).

Besides these classical plaques, the multiple sclerosis brain frequently shows areas of decreased myelin density. Such areas of partial myelin loss may be due to different underlying pathologies. They may either represent the so-called shadow plaques (Markschattenherde, Schlesinger, 1909). These shadow plaques are very similar to classical MS plaques, being sharply demarcated discolored areas in the white matter with hard sclerotic consistency and located in MS-typical distribution in the central nervous system (CNS). The major difference to classical MS plaques is that myelin is not completely lost, but present in reduced density throughout the whole lesion area. In addition, individual myelin sheaths appear unusually thin and the internode length is shortened (Prineas, 1985). As will be discussed in detail, it is now clear that such shadow plaques are areas of remyelination.

Besides the classical shadow plaques, other areas of reduced myelin density can be found, which are not sharply demarcated. They are mainly present in patients with multiple lesions at the late stage of the disease. In the brain hemispheres their location shape and distribution is irregular, but in areas of defined tract systems, such as for instance the spinal cord or the corpus callosum, these lesions follow the anatomical course of preexisting tracts. In histology, such lesions show a profound reduction in the density of myelinated axons, but the thickness of myelin in the preserved fibers is normal. These lesions represent Wallerian tract degeneration, due to axonal destruction in adjacent demyelinated plaques (Jellinger, 1969; Lumsden, 1970).

Finally, in patients with long-standing severe disease diffuse cerebral and spinal cord, atrophy is common. In this situation, the white matter volume is extensively reduced and the ventricles are enlarged. This may also be associated with atrophy of the gray matter, reflected by a narrow cortical ribbon and increased subarachnoide space (Jellinger, 1969).

All these tissue alterations occur on the background of a chronic inflammatory process (Charcot, 1868; Marburg, 1906), and it is most likely, but not definitely proven, that this inflammatory process is the primary cause of all further destructive events in the central nervous system. For this reason, anti-inflammatory, immunosuppressive, or immunomodulatory treatments are currently in the center of interest in multiple sclerosis therapy.

## THE NATURE OF THE INFLAMMATORY REACTION IN MULTIPLE SCLEROSIS

Despite the focal nature of the demyelination in multiple sclerosis, inflammation is a diffuse process, which affects the brain and spinal cord of multiple sclerosis patients as whole. The difference in inflammation between plaques and the so-called normal white matter in multiple sclerosis is quantitative, but not qualitative (Allen and McKeown, 1979; Lassmann, 1998). Thus, actively demyelinating lesions in general show more profound inflammation than inactive plaques or the "unaffected" white matter. This is not only the case for inflammatory leucocytic infiltrates in the tissue, but also for the expression of immune associated molecules, such major histocompatibility antigens, adhesions molecules or cytokines (Bo *et al.*, 1994; Cannella and Raine, 1995; Woodroofe and Cuzner, 1993). Thus, there is a diffuse process of inflammation throughout the whole CNS tissue, which is, however, accentuated within the focal lesions.

The inflammatory response consists of perivascular inflammatory infiltrates and a diffuse infiltration of the CNS tissue by leukocytes (Prineas and Wright, 1978). The inflammatory infiltrates are essentially composed of mononuclear leukocytes (Fraenkel and Jakob, 1913), which mainly include lymphocytes and macrophages (Traugott *et al.*, 1983; Figure 31.2). In addition, this inflammatory process is associated with a general activation of the local microglia cell population, which may even precede the bulk infiltration

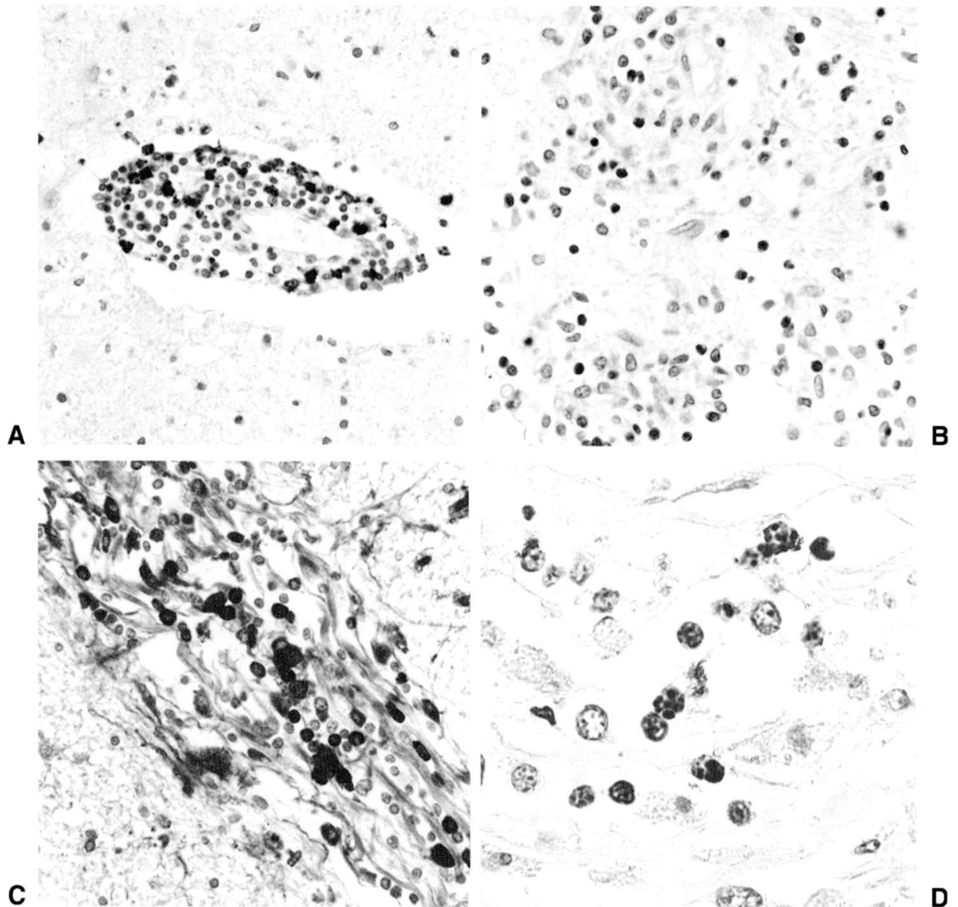


FIGURE 31.2
Inflammation in multiple sclerosis lesions. (A) Perivascular infiltrate with mononuclear cells, which mainly consist of T-cells (brown) and macrophages. Immunocytochemistry for CD3; × 400. (B) Diffuse infiltrate of T-cells (brown) in the CNS parenchyma within an actively demyelinating lesion. Immunocytochemistry for CD8; × 400. (C) Perivascular infiltrate with numerous plasma cells (brown). Immunocytochemistry for IgG; × 400. (D) Diffuse infiltrate in an actively demyelinating lesion with T-cells, expressing granzyme B (brown) in their cytotoxic granules. Immunocytochemistry for granzyme B; × 400.

of the tissue by hematogenous cells (Gay *et al.*, 1997; Trebst *et al.*, 2001). Activated macrophages and microglia cells are associated with active myelin destruction (Babinski, 1885), and their activation state, as well as their phagocytosis of myelin fragments can be used for exact staging of demyelinating activity of the lesions (Brück *et al.*, 1995). Within the lymphocyte population, T-cells outnumber B-cells (Esiri, 1980, Esiri *et al.*, 1989). In acute MS and early stages of chronic MS, T-cells are much more abundant than B-cells, generally outnumbering them by 50 to 100 times. This is different in at least a subpopulation of cases with chronic MS, in which the number of B-cells and antibody producing plasma cells may become much more prominent (Ozawa *et al.*, 1994). However, even in these cases T-cells still remain to represent the majority of the lymphocyte population.

## T-Lymphocytes

It was controversial for many years: What T-cell subpopulation dominates within MS lesions. Some authors claimed that, similar as in autoimmune encephalomyelitis, Class II MHC restricted $CD4^+$ T-lymphocytes prevailed, in particular during the stage of active demyelination (Traugott *et al.*, 1983). This was contradicted by others, who described a profound dominance of $CD8^+$ Class I MHC restricted T-cells in all lesions, irrespective their type or stage of development (Booss *et al.*, 1983). Such a discrepancy is surprising, but may be explained by several technical problems. When these studies were performed, all these markers had to be used on native frozen tissue. Such studies are inevitably restricted to small tissue samples of few patients. In addition, quantitative evaluation of $CD4^+$ T-cells is complicated by the expression of this antigen in activated microglia. Finally, some of these studies were heavily influenced by the immunological concept, that MS is, like EAE, an autoimmune disease mediated by Class II restricted T-cells.

More detailed recent studies show, that $CD8^+$ T-cells represent 60 to 80% of the total T-cell population within MS plaques (Babbe *et al.*, 2000; Gay *et al.*, 1997). This is the case in active as well as inactive lesions of acute as well as chronic MS. Furthermore, $CD8^+$ T-cells are particularly prominent in the diffuse infiltrates within the CNS tissue, while their relative number is less in the meninges and the perivascular space. It thus appears that Class I MHC restricted T-cells are concentrated within the areas where tissue damage occurs.

The mere presence of a given cell population in a lesion alone does not allow conclusions about its pathogenic role or importance in the disease process. Indirect evidence for a possible pathogenic involvement of T-cells can be obtained by determination of clonal expansion of T-cell populations. When T-cells are activated by their specific antigenic peptide together with MHC on the surface of an antigen presenting cell, they start to proliferate. If this occurs within a site of inflammation, certain T-cell clones will develop within the tissue. Thus, the degree of clonality of a T-cell population may provide an indirect evidence that they have seen a specific antigen and were stimulated to proliferate. By immunological methods, clonal expansion of T-cells within MS lesions has been shown for T-cells with $\alpha/\beta$ (Oksenberg *et al.*, 1993) and $\gamma/\delta$ T-cell receptors (Wucherpfennig *et al.*, 1992b), although this has not been reproduced for $\alpha/\beta$ T-cells in other studies (Birnbaum and Van Ness, 1992; Wucherpfennig *et al.*, 1992a). Since these studies performed T-cell receptor analysis in whole tissue extracts, the clonal expansion of individual cell populations could not be determined. This was overcome recently by applying the method of single cell PCR to analyze T-cell clonality in individual T-cells picked from defined areas of MS lesions (Babbe *et al.*, 2000). This study clearly showed that it is mainly the $CD8^+$ cell population that is present within the active and inactive lesions, which show clonal expansion, while $CD4^+$ T-cells and T-cells, which are present in the perivascular connective tissue, reveal only a low incidence of clonality. These studies suggest that Class I restricted T-cells not only numerically dominate the inflammatory infiltrate, but possibly recognize their specific antigen at the sites of CNS damage in MS.

Class I MHC restricted T-cells can either be cytotoxic T-cells, which may directly destroy antigen-containing targets, or they may be regulatory ("suppressor") cells. The question thus arises as to whether these $CD8^+$ cells are cytotoxic and involved in the pathogenic process of tissue destruction or whether they down-regulate the inflammatory response. *In vitro* studies show that these cells can directly recognize their antigen on the surface of different cells of the CNS, such as astrocytes, oligodendrocytes and neurons (Neumann *et al.*, 2002). In addition, they may induce specific cytotxicity, mediated either through the content of their cytotoxic granules or through activation of death receptors. They thus have the full potential to destroy target cells, such as oligodendrocytes, neurons, or axons, within multiple sclerosis lesions. In multiple sclerosis lesions, up-regulation of death-associated molecules, involved in T-cell cytotoxicity, such as Fas, Fas-ligand (D'Souza *et al.*, 1996; Dowling *et al.*, 1996), TNF-$\alpha$, lymphotoxin (Selmaj *et al.*, 1991), and the respective TNF receptors (Bonetti and Raine, 1997), have been described. We have recently analyzed the interaction of cytotoxic, Class I MHC restricted T-cells with local tissue elements in multiple sclerosis. We found, in particular in the lesions of acute MS, a massive expression of granzyme B in the cytotoxic granules of infiltrating T-cells and direct attachment of these granzyme B positive T-cells to oligodendrocytes and axons in actively demyelinating plaques. These data strongly suggest that $CD8^+$ T-cells play an important role in the pathogenesis of the lesions, they do, however, not rule out an additional important pro-inflammatory role of Class II MHC restricted CD4 positive T-cells in the process of inflammation in multiple sclerosis.

### B-lymphocytes and Plasma Cells

As mentioned earlier, B-lymphocytes and plasma cells are present within MS lesions, although they are much less abundant than T-cells (Esiri, 1977; Prineas and Wright, 1978). They are mainly located in perivascular and meningeal infiltrates, while T-cells are much more dispersed within the CNS tissue in the lesions. Plasma cells in multiple sclerosis brains mainly produce immunoglobulin G; the number of IgA and IgM positive B-cells and plasma cells is substantially lower in comparison to the IgG containing cells (Mussini *et al.*, 1977). Such B-cells and plasma cells are diagnostically important, since they are responsible for the intrathecal production of immunoglobulin, which is a characteristic, but nonspecific paraclinical marker used in multiple sclerosis diagnosis.

The function of B-cells and plasma cells within MS lesions is so far not clear (Archelos and Hartung, 2000). They may be functionally irrelevant cells, which are secondarily recruited into the lesions in the course of the inflammatory process. This view is supported by the fact that most of the immunoglobulins, which are intrathecally produced in MS patients, are low affinity antibodies against many different epitopes of viruses and bacteria. B-cells may, however, play a role as antigen presenting cells for T-lymphocytes, which is independent from the specificity of the antibodies they produce. Finally, some of the intrathecal B-cells and plasma cells may produce auto-antibodies, directed against myelin proteins, such as myelin basic protein (Gerritse *et al.*, 1994) and demyelinating antibodies may be involved in the pathogenesis of demyelination, at least in a subset of MS patients (Genain *et al.*, 1999; Lucchinetti *et al.*, 2000).

### Macrophages and Microglia

The vast majority of cells within actively demyelinating lesions in multiple sclerosis are macrophages (Adams and Poston, 1990; Esiri and Reading, 1987). They in general outnumber lymphocytes by at least 10 to 20 times. The show a phenotype of phagocytic macrophages and contain within their cytoplasm the remnants of myelin, which have been released in the demyelinating process (Babinski, 1885, Figure 31.3).

These myelin degradation products within macrophages are a useful tool to classify the age of a given demyelinating lesions (Brück *et al.*, 1995). When macrophages take up myelin fragments in the process of demyelination, these degradation products still contain all myelin proteins. With a few days, however, the minor myelin proteins, such as myelin oligodendrocyte glycoprotein or myelin associated glycoprotein, are degraded, while major myelin proteins like proteolipid protein are still preserved. These major myelin proteins are digested within the macrophages within one to two weeks. Thus, the presence of different myelin proteins within the digestion chambers of macrophages in MS lesions allows a fairly accurate determination of demyelinating activity and lesion age.

Macrophages are apparently instrumental in the process of myelin and tissue destruction in multiple sclerosis lesions. During active demyelination, they are closely attached to degenerating myelin sheaths and take up fragments of the dissolved myelin (Babinski, 1885). As discussed in detail in the chapter on EAE, they produce a variety of toxic products, which can destroy myelin *in vitro* and the can interact with antibodies and complement components, bound to myelin sheaths, by their Fc- and complement receptors (Ulvestad *et al.*, 1994).

Macrophages may either be derived from circulating monocytes or from the pool of resident microglia. The extent of macrophage recruitment versus microglia activation contributing to the lesion macrophages in MS is so far not determined, since no reliable markers are available, which allows the distinction of the monocyte or microglia origin of a macrophage. A detailed analysis of the dynamics of plaque formation (Woodroofe *et al.*, 1986; Gay *et al.*, 1997) and of the expression patterns of chemokine receptors within the lesions at different stages of their development (Trebst *et al.*, 2001) suggest that the majority of macrophages are derived from microglia. Although this seems to be the case in the majority of cases, there are some cases of acute MS, where hematogenous monocytes apparently play a much more important role. There, in general, granulocytes are found in addition to

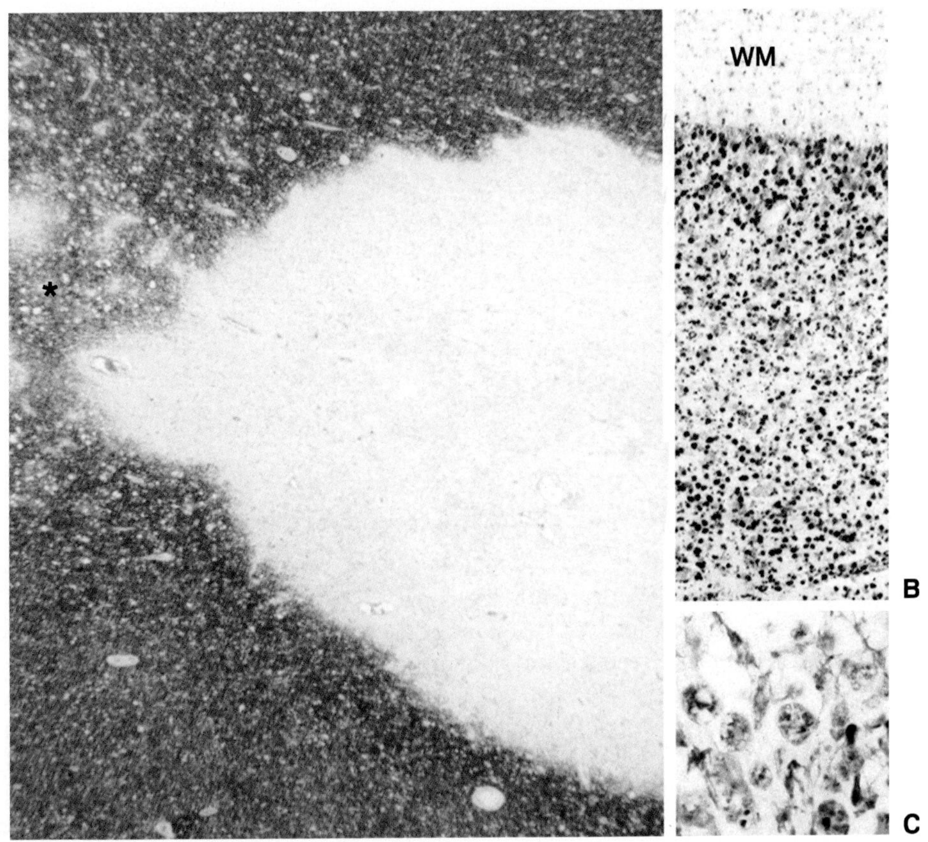


FIGURE 31.3
Active demyelination in MS. (A) Active MS plaque with complete loss of myelin and sharp demarcation from the surrounding periplaque white matter. At the left side of the plaque are perivenous areas of demyelination, which in part are in continuity with the plaque. Immunocytochemistry for MOG; × 20. (B) Edge of the plaque, stained for macrophages; numerous macrophages are present within the demyelinated lesions and there is a sharp border towards the normal periplaque white matter (WM); immunocytochemistry for CD 68; × 80. (C) Plaque edge, stained with Luxol fast blue for myelin. Only few myelin sheaths are preserved and show irregular contours (stage of myelin dissolution). In between there are macrophages, which contain small cytoplasmic granules with the same staining properties as myelin sheaths (early myelin degradation products); Luxol fast blue myelin stain, × 600.

macrophages and a large population of cells is present, which expresses an antigen that is predominately present in circulating leukocytes (MRP 14; Brück et al., 1995).

## Expression of Histocompatibility Antigens

T-lymphocytes do not recognize their specific antigenic peptide in a soluble form. For T-cell activation, antigen recognition has to occur together with MHC-molecules on the surface of antigen presenting cells. Thus, the local expression of MHC molecules is an absolute requirement for antigen recognition by T-cells. The normal CNS tissue differs from other organs by the low to absent expression of MHC antigens, which is part of the immunoprivilege of the CNS (Hayes *et al.*, 1987). Cells that contain Class I or Class II MHC antigens in the normal brain and spinal cord are perivascular and meningeal macrophages. In addition, cerebral endothelial cells express Class I MHC antigen under normal conditions. Both. Class I and Class II MHC antigens can be induced in cells after stimulation with proinflammatory cytokines, such as gamma-interferon or tumor necrosis factor alpha. Class I antigens can be present widely in all different cells of the CNS, while the expression of Class II MHC antigen is more restricted. The latter is found in the inflamed CNS tissue mainly on microglia and sometimes on astrocytes and ependymal cells.

In MS lesions the expression of MHC antigens is highly regulated by the activity of the inflammatory process. They were mainly described on microglia cells, invading leucocytes and in rare instances on astrocytes. In addition, endothelial cells consitutively express MHC Class I molecules and have also been reported in some studies to be Class II positive (Hayashi *et al.*, 1988; Ransohoff and Estes, 1991; Traugott, 1987). In principle, however, also neurons, axons, and oligodendrocytes can express Class I MHC antigens (Neumann, 2002), and such an expression has been found in other inflammatory brain diseases (Bien *et al.*, 2002). To what extent this is also the case in multiple sclerosis has to be determined.

MHC Class I and Class II antigens are responsible for the presentation of peptide antigens. The presentation of glycolipid and carbohydrate antigens, however, occurs through CD1 molecules. These molecules are similar to MHC molecules, practically absent in the normal CNS tissue. In MS lesions, however, a massive up-regulation of CD1 is found, mainly on astrocytes but sometimes also on macrophages or microglia cells (Battistini *et al.*, 1996).

### Adhesion Molecules, Chemokines and Chemokine Receptors

Migration of leukocytes from the circulation into the tissue is the prerequisite for an inflammatory response. This process is regulated by two sets of molecules, the adhesion molecules and the chemokines. Adhesion molecules are cell surface proteins, which mediate binding of cells to other cells or components of the extracellular matrix and can also be involved in intercellular signaling. In inflammatory conditions, adhesion molecules are expressed on the endothelial surface of vessels and interact with their specific binding partners on leukocytes. This interaction leads to the attachment of circulating inflammatory cells on the endothelial surface and initiates transmigration of leukocytes through the vessels wall (Springer, 1994). Different molecular classes of adhesion molecules exist, including selectins, integrins, and adhesion molecules of the immunoglobulin gene superfamily. They differ in their binding properties as well as in their ability to mediate, in addition to adhesion, intracellular signaling upon their ligation and activation.

In addition to adhesion molecules, chemokines, interacting with their specific receptors, are instrumental in leukocyte migration from the circulation to the tissue (Luster, 1998). Chemokines may act simply as chemoattractants, inducing migration of cells along their concentration gradient. In addition, they may, through intracellular signaling, enhance the binding properties of adhesions molecules and may through this mechanisms facilitate the transmigration of leukocytes through the vessel wall. There are many different chemokines, which act through a substantial number of different chemokine receptors. Importantly, different leukocyte subsets express different chemokine receptor profiles. Thus, it is the chemokines that by and large determine what types of inflammatory cells are recruited into a lesion (Luster, 1998). Both adhesion molecules and chemokines are very attractive targets for anti-inflammatory treatment, since their blockade essentially prevents the entrance of leukocytes into an inflammatory locus.

Cerebral endothelial cells in the normal brain express only very few adhesion molecules, in particular intercellular adhesion molecule 2 (ICAM-2). In contrast, in multiple sclerosis lesions, many different adhesion molecules (including selectins, integrins, and immunoglobulin family members) appear on the luminal surface of cerebral endothelial cells and their expression is related to the inflammatory activity in the lesion (Cannella and Raine, 1995; Dore Duffy *et al.*, 1993; Sobel *et al.*, 1990; Washington *et al.*, 1994). This expression is, however, not specific for MS, since very similar expression patterns are found in other inflammatory diseases of the central nervous system, being particularly similar in diseases such as virus encephalitis, which too show a T-cell and macrophage dominated inflammatory response.

A quite similar situation is found with chemokines. These molecules too, with a few exceptions, are practically absent within the normal mature CNS tissue, but they are heavily up-regulated within the inflammatory foci of multiple sclerosis. Certain members of the chemokine family, in particular those involved in the recruitment of T-cells and macrophages, are prominently expressed in the lesions, both by invading inflammatory cells as well as by astrocytes (McManus *et al.*, 1998; Simpson *et al.*, 1998; Simpson, 2000a, b; Sorensen *et al.*, 1999, 2002). In parallel with these chemokines, the respective receptors are present in MS lesions on invading lymphocytes and monocytes as well as on local microglia (Balashov *et al.*, 1999; Sorensen *et al.*, 1999, 2002; Trebst *et al.*, 2001). The expression of both, the chemokines and their receptors, is tightly associated with the activity of the lesions (both the inflammatory and the demyelinating activity), being most prominently expressed in fresh lesions.

### Cytokines

The regulation of an inflammatory process within the tissue is accomplished by cytokines, produced either by the inflammatory cells themselves or by local cells within the target tissue. Due to the similarities of the inflammatory response between multiple sclerosis and experimental autoimmune encephalomyelitis and the treatment effects of certain immunomodulatory compounds, multiple sclerosis is generally believed to be a disease, driven by cytokines of the Th-1 type. This would imply that in initial stages, when new lesions are formed, Th-1-related cytokines such as interferon-gamma, interleukin 12, interleukin 2, and tumor necrosis factor alpha dominate, while during remission Th-2-related or purely immunoregulatory cytokines such as interleukin 10 or transforming growth factor beta prevail. Studies on cytokine expression in MS lesions by immunocytochemistry or *in situ* hybridization, so far, however, were rather inconclusive. They showed, not unexpectedly, a general up-regulation of cytokine expression in MS lesions (Cannella and Raine, 1995; Merrill, 1992; Woodroofe and Cuzner, 1993). However, both pro-as well as anti-inflammatory cytokines were expressed in parallel and there was no clear-cut patterning of cytokine expression in relation to lesional activity. The source of the cytokines within the lesions are invading leukocytes (Woodroofe and Cuzner, 1993), but also local microglia (Aloisi 2001) and astrocytes (Dong and Benveniste 2001).

### Other Markers for Immune Activation

In addition, some other immune-associated molecules are expressed in MS lesions, which may play an important role in the initiation or propagation of the lesions. Antigen-specific stimulation of T-lymphocytes can be enhanced or modulated by the simultaneous signaling through co-stimulatory molecules. This may also occur directly in the lesions, since such co-stimulatory molecules, such as CD-40 and its ligand or the molecules of the B-7 family, are expressed on macrophages and lymphocytes, respectively (Gerritse *et al.*, 1996; Windhagen *et al.*, 1995). Interaction of CD40 with its ligand is a crucial step in the activation and Th1 polarization of T-cells and, thus, blockade of this pathway may be an interesting approach in anti-inflammatory therapy. The activation of CTLA-4 through B-7 molecules may be involved in down-regulation of the T-cell response. Interestingly, a genetic polymorphism in the CTLA-4 gene has been reported to be associated with multiple sclerosis susceptibility (Ligers *et al.*, 1999).

### Neurotrophins

Inflammation has for long been regarded as being deleterious for the nervous system. Recently, however, experimental studies have shown that traumatic or ischemic injury of the central nervous system can be counteracted by the presence of a moderate inflammatory response, induced by autoimmune T-cells (Moalem *et al.*, 1999). The reason for this paradox observation seems to be that inflammatory cells can be a potent source of neurotrophic factors (Moalem *et al.*, 2000). In fact, human leukocytes produce considerable amounts of bioactive BDNF when stimulated *in vitro* (Kerschensteiner *et al.*, 1999). BDNF is synthesized by many different inflammatory cells, such as T- and B-lymphocytes, macrophages, and granulocytes. Within inflammatory brain lesions of multiple sclerosis patients, massive local expression of BDNF was found in leukocytes by immunocytochemistry, the intensity of the reaction being much more prominent than in neurons

(Kerschensteiner *et al.*, 1999). In addition, the trk-B neurotrophin-(BDNF-) receptor was present on astrocytes as well as on neurons and axons (Stadelmann *et al.*, 2002). These data suggest that brain inflammation in multiple sclerosis is not always bad, but that it may also have a neuroprotective function or may play a role in the induction or glial scar formation, remyelination, and possibly also axonal sprouting.

## THE REACTION OF CEREBRAL VESSELS TO INFLAMMATION IN MULTIPLE SCLEROSIS

The normal brain is protected from the entrance of circulating toxic molecules by the blood brain barrier. A chronic inflammatory process in the central nervous system, like that in multiple sclerosis, has several major consequences on blood brain barrier integrity. During the phase of acute inflammation, when leukocytes migrate through the vessel wall, endothelial cells are partly damaged (Minagar *et al.*, 2001). This is associated with a massive disruption of blood brain barrier integrity, mediated either through a disruption of inter-endothelial junctions (Plumb *et al.*, 2002) or an increased vesicular trans-endothelial transport (Hawkins *et al.*, 1990). Endothelial damage in active MS lesions is suggested by early tracer studies, which show leakage of the blood brain barrier even in post mortem tissue (Broman, 1964). Such a leakage cannot be due to an increased active and energy dependent trans-endothelial transport, but has to reflect opening of the inter-endothelial junctions or endothelial damage. In pathology, this stage is associated with massive penetration of serum proteins into the tissue (Tavolato, 1975), associated with profound extracellular accumulation of fluid (extracellular edema). When the acute inflammatory stage passes by, the blood brain barrier function becomes partially repaired. However, it has to be emphasized that in old inactive MS plaques there is never a complete restoration of the blood brain barrier (Kwon and Prineas, 1994), but that there is in every old lesion some degree of serum protein leakage. In these vessels endothelial junctions seem to be unaffected, but the endothelial cells show increased numbers of vesicles, indicating enhanced active trans-endothelial transport (Brown, 1978). Structurally, the vessels in old inactive MS plaques are affected by profound vascular fibrosis. This means that the vessel wall is detached from the astroglial limiting membrane (Rafalowska *et al.*, 1992) and separated from it by several layers of connective tissue cells and fibers. This is sometimes associated with the formation of small perivascular channels, which by ultrastructural analysis resemble lymphatic vessels (Prineas, 1979), although they do not express markers for lymphatic endothelial cells. Whether they function as lymphatic vessels has still to be determined.

In addition to these changes in structure and function, cerebral vessels in MS plaques also increase in density. This is not only a relative increase, due to loss of tissue elements, such as myelin and axons, but a significant increase in the total number of vessels within the tissue. This is also reflected in fresh lesions by morphological signs of angiogenesis and the expression of markers for angiogenesis, such as VEGF-receptors (Ludwin *et al.*, 2001). This angiogenesis may either be stimulated by cytokines in the inflammatory environment or by hypoxia.

## SYNOPSIS OF BRAIN INFLAMMATION IN MULTIPLE SCLEROSIS

All the data, discussed so far in relation to inflammation in multiple sclerosis, are consistent with the concept that the disease is driven by a T-lymphocyte mediated inflammatory process. All molecules that are known to be important for recruitment and local activation of T-cells and macrophages are expressed in multiple sclerosis lesions and their degree and type of expression correlates well with the activity of the inflammatory process. Thus, it seems likely that in the initial stage T-cells, which are activated in the peripheral immune system, enter the CNS, where they find their specific (possibly cross reacting) antigen. This leads to reactivation of the T-cells and the production of pro-inflammatory cytokines, such as $\gamma$-IFN or TNF-$\alpha$. This in turn stimulates the production of adhesion molecules and chemokines at the site of initial inflammation, thus recruiting other T-cells as well as monocytes and activating the local microglia population. As will be discussed in the following sections in detail, tissue damage may then occur through direct T-cell cytotoxicity, through toxic products of activated macrophages and microglia cells or through additional antibodies, recognizing proteins or glycolipids on the surface of CNS cells. T-cells are locally destroyed by apoptosis, and remission of disease episodes as well as clearance of inflammation from the CNS occurs, when the rate of T-cell apoptosis in the nervous tissue exceeds the generation of new disease propagating T-cells in the peripheral lymphatic tissue and their migration into the lesions.

Although these basic principles of inflammation in multiple sclerosis are well established, there are still many open questions. The type of inflammation in multiple sclerosis is very similar to that found in other inflammatory diseases of the central nervous system, such as in particular in different forms of virus encephalomyelitis (Bauer *et al.*, 2001). In fact, so far no feature of inflammation has been reported, which is specific for MS and not found in these other diseases. Yet, in MS this inflammatory process is associated with widespread demyelination, which is largely absent in other diseases of virus-induced encephalomyelitis. Thus, there must be some pathogenetic mechanisms, which in multiple sclerosis drive the inflammatory process specifically against the myelin/oligodendroglia complex.

Another aspect, which needs further attention is the fact that nearly any immune associated molecule that has been looked for so far has been identified within MS plaques. This could mean that the immune response in a chronic inflammatory lesion is so redundant and overlapping that a therapy which targets specific immunological mechanisms is unlikely to succeed. Alternatively, there may be quantitative differences in the involvement of different immunological effector pathways, some being more and others less important in the formation of the lesions. Such possible quantitative differences have, however, so far not been identified and their possible existence has so far even not been addressed in proper studies.

Finally, it has to be considered that inflammation in multiple sclerosis is a two-edged sword. On the one hand, it induces and propagates disease and tissue damage, but on the other hand, it also may play an important role in limiting tissue destruction and in stimulating remyelination and repair. This leads to an obvious dilemma with regard to anti-inflammatory therapy.

## DEMYELINATION AND OLIGODENDROCYTE INJURY

As mentioned earlier, primary demyelination is the hallmark of multiple sclerosis pathology (Fig. 31.1). This means that myelin sheaths are completely lost, while axons are still present in high numbers within the lesions and are embedded in a dense astroglial scar tissue. This dissociation between complete myelin loss and partial or even complete preservation of axons is unique for demyelinating diseases and is the most important criterion to distinguish MS lesions from those arising in the course of other diseases. Demyelination in multiple sclerosis is a segmental process (Babinski, 1885). Thus, at the edge of established multiple sclerosis plaques, the myelin sheaths terminate with a node of Ranvier, from where the denuded axons can be traced into astrocytic scar tissue.

Active demyelination is associated with inflammation and myelin destruction occurs in close contact between degenerating myelin sheaths with activated macrophages or microglia cells (Babinski, 1885). The myelin sheaths may either be stripped from the axons by processes of phagocytic cells, which penetrate the space between myelin lamellae or the periaxonal space (Lassmann, 1983). Small fragments of myelin may also be removed from the myelinated fibers by macrophages, forming coated pits and vesicles (Prineas *et al.*, 1984). This type of myelin phagocytosis is reminiscent of a receptor mediated process, possibly involving specific anti-myelin antibodies and Fc-receptors or complement receptors on phagocytic cells. In cases with severe and rapid myelin destruction the whole myelin sheaths may be transformed into small vesicles, a process called "vesicular disruption of myelin" (Guo and Gao, 1983; Kirk, 1979). Again in other cases initial demyelination is accompanied by degenerative changes in the most distal cell processes, which is also reflected by a primary loss of those myelin proteins, which are predominantly located in these areas, such as myelin associated glycoprotein and cyclic nucleotide phosphodiesterase (CNPase). Such a pattern of demyelination is suggestive for a "distal" or "dying back" oligodendrogliopathy (Itoyama *et al.*, 1980, Rodriguez *et al.*, 1993). These data suggest, that the mechanisms of demyelination are different in plaques of different multiple sclerosis patients.

Myelin sheaths are formed by oligodendrocytes and it can therefore be expected that in a disease, where myelin is destroyed these cells are affected too. Indeed, when old chronic completely demyelinated MS plaques are analyzed, there are only very few oligodendrocytes left within the tissue (Lumsden, 1970, Prineas, 1985). As will be discussed below, there are, however, many lesions, which show partial or even complete remyelination, which implies that either oligodendrocytes have survived or that new oligodendrocytes have been recruited from progenitor cells.

The fate of oligodendrocytes in acutely demyelinating lesions has been controversial for many years. In some studies very few oligodendrocytes were found in active plaques, suggesting that these cells were lost in parallel or even prior to the myelin sheaths (Lumsden, 1970). However, many other studies showed that in freshly demyelinated plaques, the density of oligodendrocytes may be very high, sometimes even exceeding that in the periplaque white matter (Brück *et al.*, 1994; Prineas *et al.*, 1984; Raine *et al.*, 1981). This controversy has recently been resolved in a systematic study on a very large sample of cases and lesions. This study showed a profound intra-individual heterogeneity with respect to oligodendrocyte destruction and loss in multiple sclerosis plaques (Lucchinetti *et al.*, 1999). In some patients there was a massive loss of oligodendrocytes already at the earliest stages of demyelination, and there was also no hint for a recruitment of new oligodendrocytes from the pool of progenitor cells. Such patients only had completely demyelinated lesions without remyelination. In most of the patients, however, there was, as described before by Prineas (1985), an initial loss of oligodendrocytes of variable extent in acute lesions, while new oligodendrocytes, apparently derived from progenitor cells, appeared in more advanced plaques. In other patients and lesions, only a minor loss of oligodendrocytes was found in the initial stages of demyelination, which was followed by a progressive loss of these cells at later stages of lesion development (Fig. 31.4).

The mode of cell death of oligodendrocytes within actively demyelinating lesions has been described to resemble either necrosis or apoptosis. Again, when a large sample of lesions from different MS patients was analyzed, it became clear that there are major inter-individual differences in the patterns of oligodendrocyte destruction (Lucchinetti *et al.*, 1999).

Within the demyelinated plaque, two essentially different populations of oligodendrocytes can be found (Wolswijk, 2000). One, which is present at the time when myelin falls apart and then gradually disappears, is a small round cell with little or no cell processes, which expresses myelin oligodendrocyte glycoprotein on its surface. It is negative for most other myelin and oligodendrocyte antigens and does not or only in a limited degree contain mRNA for major myelin proteins. It is suggested that these cells represent mature oligodendrocytes, which have survived the demyelinating attack. These cells disappear at later stages of plaque formation, but it is not clear, whether they are removed by programmed cell death or whether they may dedifferentiate and reenter the pool of remyelinating cells. The other cell type is a large and activated cell with elaborate cell processes, which contains abundant mRNA for myelin proteins. It expresses different myelin proteins, including MBP, CNPase, and MAG in its cytoplasm, but shows a low and variable expression of myelin oligodendrocyte glycoprotein on its surface. These cells apparently are immature myelinating cells. It is likely, but so far not definitely proven, that these cells are derived from progenitor cells and are the prime candidates, mediating remyelination in the lesions.

Summarizing the patterns of myelin and oligodendrocyte damage in multiple sclerosis, it becomes clear that there is a major heterogeneity in the patterns of demyelination between different MS lesions, in particular, when lesions of different patients are analyzed (Lucchinetti *et al.*, 1996). This strongly argues in favor for an inter-individual variability in

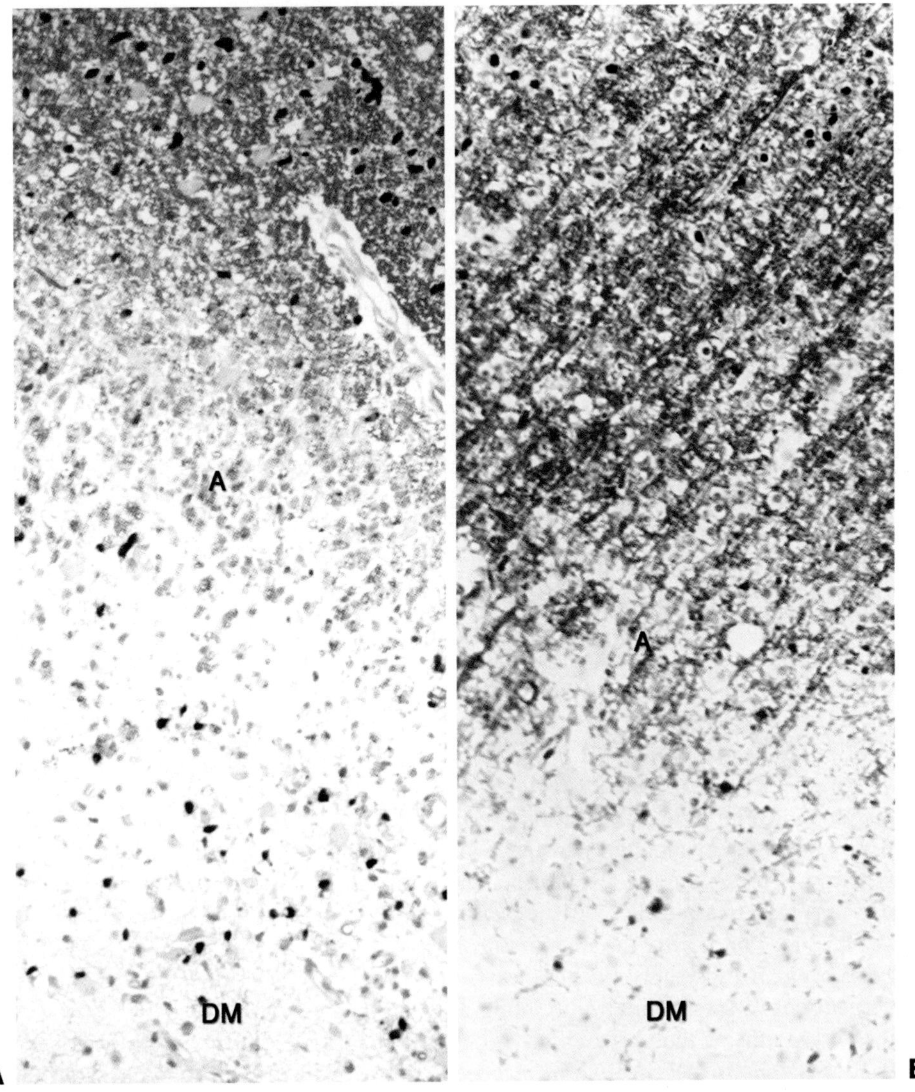


FIGURE 31.4
Oligodendrocytes in active multiple sclerosis lesions. (A) Actively demyelinating lesion in chronic MS with oligodendrocytes (black cells) in the periplaque white matter. These cells are absent in the zone of active demyelination (A), but reappear within the demyelinated areas (DM) of the plaque. (B) Actively demyelinating chronic MS lesion with extensive loss of oligodendrocytes (black cells). These cells can be seen in the periplaque white matter, but are nearly completely lost at the actively demyelinating plaque edge (A) and within the demyelinated center of the plaque (DM). *In situ* hybridization for PLP mRNA (black cells) and immunocytochemistry for PLP protein (red); × 200.

the mechanisms of demyelination and tissue destruction in this disease. The data further show that at least in the early stages of disease and lesion formation, there are high numbers of oligodendrocytes within the tissue, and this is associated with extensive remyelination. However, with increasing chronicity of lesions and disease, this remyelinating potential is gradually lost.

## OLIGODENDROCYTE PROGENITORS AND REMYELINATION IN MULTIPLE SCLEROSIS LESIONS

In chronic multiple sclerosis in patients with long-standing disease the typical lesion in the central nervous system is the completely demyelinated sclerotic plaque. There remyelination is sparse and restricted to a very small rim at the border to the adjacent periplaque white matter. It has therefore been believed for long time that remyelination and reparation of tissue damage does not occur in multiple sclerosis. The situation, however, is different when cases of acute or rapidly progressive MS are analyzed. Paradoxically, in this most severe clinical subtype of multiple sclerosis, remyelination is extensive and may lead to complete repair of myelin in plaques of several centimeters in diameter (Lassmann, 1983). Such lesions are called "Markschattenherde" or shadow plaques (Fig. 31.5). They were first described by Schlesinger (1912) as sharply demarcated areas of reduced myelin density and reactive gliosis. Schlesinger interpreted these lesions as areas or incomplete demyelination, although possible remyelination was already suggested earlier by Marburg (1906). With the use of ultrastructural techniques and by the analysis of myelin protein and mRNA synthesis, such lesions now can clearly be classified as remyelinated plaques. Remyelination is, however, not restricted to patients with acute MS, but also occurs in patients with classical chronic disease (Prineas *et al.*, 1993a, 1993b). Such lesions contain nerve fibers with unusually thin myelin sheaths and shortened myelin internodes (Prineas, 1985). In addition, the oligodendrocytes within these plaques are increased in size, show signs of metabolic activation, and contain high amounts of mRNAs for diverse myelin proteins (Ozawa *et al.*, 1994). At the peak of remyelination even the myelin proteins, such as myelin basic protein or myelin associated glycoprotein, are present within the perinuclear cytoplasm of these cells (Prineas *et al.*, 1984, 1989). Remyelination may be quite extensive in actively demyelinating, but not in inactive plaques even in patients with long-standing chronic disease. As with demyelination and oligodendrocyte damage, however, the presence and extent of remyelination is highly variable in lesions of different MS patients (Lucchinetti *et al.*, 1999; Ozawa *et al.*, 1994).

Not unexpectedly, oligodendrocyte progenitor cells have been identified in large numbers in remyelinating MS lesions (Wolswijk, 2000). However, such cells, are even present in chronic demyelinated plaques, which do not show any signs of ongoing myelin repair. They are present in highest numbers in lesions, which still contain macrophages and decrease in number in parallel with the extent of macrophage infiltration of the plaques (Wolswijk, 2002) and with the age of the lesion (Chang *et al.*, 2002; Wolswijk, 2002). However, even in most chronic plaques, some progenitor cells are present, in spite of complete absence of remyelination (Chang *et al.*, 2002).

Thus, in summary there is a high potential for remyelination in multiple sclerosis lesions, but it fails to be effective in a large proportion of lesions and patients. Overall remyelination is much more effective in early stages of the disease and in actively demyelinating lesions than at later stages or in inactive plaques, although there are additional major differences in the remyelinating capacity between different MS patients (Lucchinetti *et al.*, 1999).

There are several different explanations for this complex situation. First, the extent of remyelination may depend on the mechanism of demyelination, which vary between different patients (Lucchinetti *et al.*, 2000). Apparently in many patients the destructive process involves mature myelin and oligodendrocytes, leaving progenitor cells unaffected. In such a situation, new remyelinating oligodendrocytes can be recruited and remyelination can be accomplished (Prineas, 1993b). In some patients, however, progenitor cells seem to be affected together with mature oligodendrocytes and myelin. Certain macrophage toxins—such as, for instance, excitotoxins—affect progenitor cells more effectively than mature oligodendrocytes (Fern and Moller, 2000). Thus, when demyelination is mediated through such toxins, both the mature and immature oligodendrocytes will be lost. In addition, some patients develop antibodies, which are directed against the AN-2/NG-2 epitope (Niehaus *et al.*, 2000). Such antibodies may selectively destroy progenitor cells within an inflammatory demyelinating lesion and thus reduce the number of cells capable for remyelination of the lesions.

Another mechanism may involve demyelinating antibodies. When they are present in high titers, they may directly inhibit remyelination (Seil *et al.*, 1975) or destroy remyelinating oligodendrocytes at the moment when they express their respective target antigen, such as, for instance, myelin oligodendrocyte glycoprotein. In such lesions the remyelination

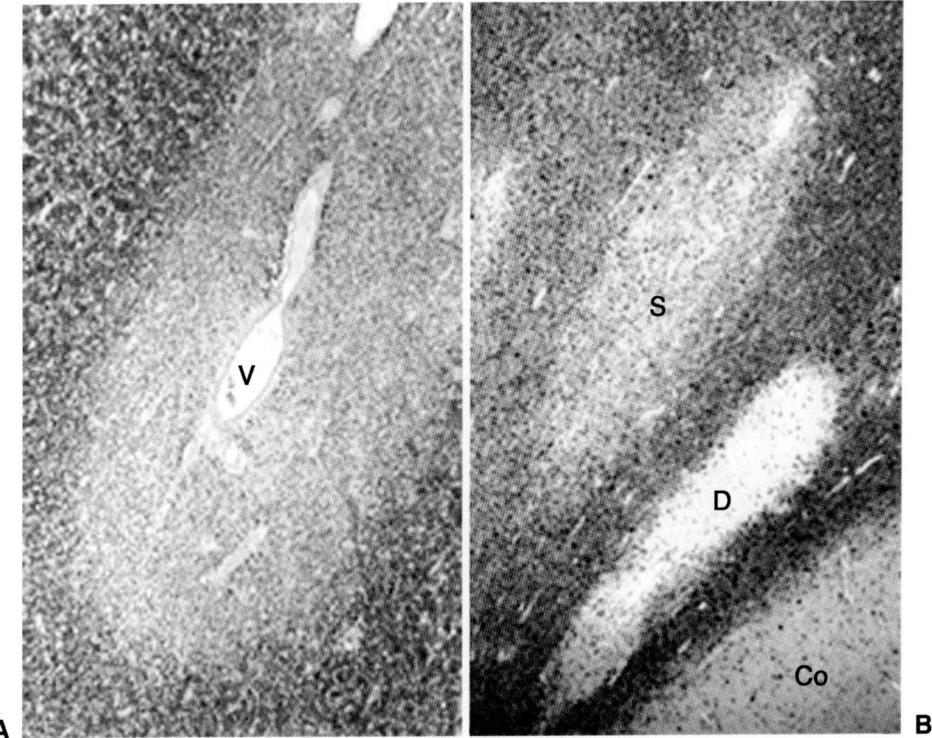


FIGURE 31.5
Remyelinated, shadow plaques in multiple sclerosis. (A) Sharply demarcated plaque with reduced myelin staining intensity, oriented around a central vein (V). Luxol fast blue myelin stain; × 20. (B) Sharply demarcated remyelinated shadow plaque (S) and a demyelinated plaque (D) without remyelination located side by side. Within the remyelinated area and the periplaque white matter there are numerous oligodendrocytes. In the demyelinated plaque these cells are only present at the plaque margin; Co: Cortex; *in situ* hybridization for PLP mRNA (black) and PLP protein (red); × 10.

program is started, but new myelin and oligodendrocytes are quickly removed during maturation (Storch *et al.*, unpublished).

Remyelination may also be impaired due to multiple demyelinating episodes, occurring in the same brain area. Remyelinated MS plaques may frequently become the target of new demyelinating attacks (Prineas *et al.*, 1993b; Figure 31.6), possibly due to the disturbed integrity of the blood brain barrier within these areas. In experimental models, it has been shown that repeated demyelinating episodes in the same area may decrease the capacity for remyelination (Linington *et al.*, 1992; Ludwin, 1980). It is thus feasible that in MS demyelination occurs in a given area, which is followed by remyelination. During one of the next bouts of the disease, the same area becomes affected with a new demyelinating episode, which again is followed by remyelination (Prineas *et al.*, 1993b). When this happens several times, the pool of progenitor cells may be depleted and remyelination may be severely compromised.

Finally, it has to be taken into account that in some chronic, persistently demyelinated lesions oligodendrocyte progenitor cells are present, which, however, fail to start the remyelinating process. It has been suggested that in such lesions, axons may be defect in a way that they are unable to initiate the remyelinating program (Chang *et al.*, 2002). Alternatively, progenitor cells may require stimulation by trophic factors, which are produced by the inflammatory cells and in particular by macrophages. Indeed, depletion of macrophages impairs remyelination in experimental models (Kotter *et al.*, 2001). In both, acute as well as chronic MS lesions remyelination is most prominent during and immediately following the stage of acute demyelination and the extent of remyelination correlates with the degree of macrophage infiltration in the lesions. Thus, lack of remyelination in chronic inactive MS plaques may in part be due to the lack of "beneficial" inflammation.

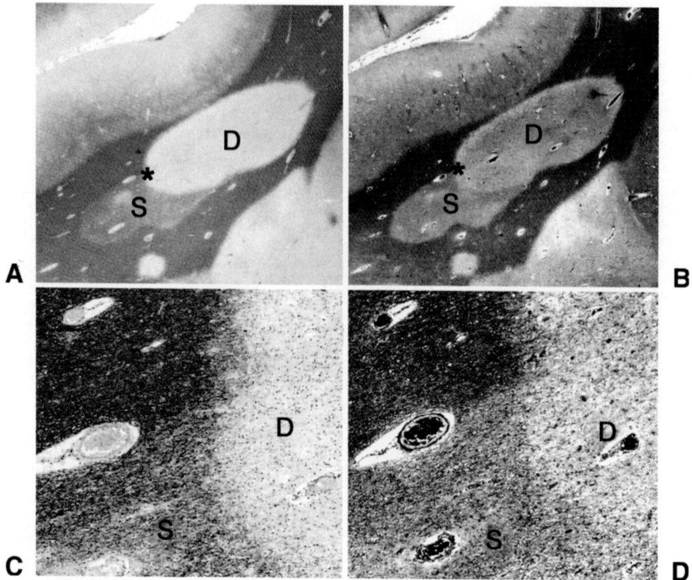


FIGURE 31.6
Repeated demyelination in the same area of the CNS. One demyelinated plaque without remyelination (D) overlaps with a remyelinated shadow plaque (S). This suggests that an old remyelinated plaque partially became demyelinated again during the formation of the new demyelinated plaque. Axonal staining in Figures B and D shows reduction of axonal density in both plaques, being more pronounced in the area of overlap. (A, C) Immunocytochemistry for MOG. (B, D) Bielschowsky silver impregnation; C and D are higher magnification images of the areas labeled by * in Figures A and B; A and B: × 20; Cc and D: × 180.

## THE NEURODEGENERATIVE COMPONENT IN MULTIPLE SCLEROSIS: NEURONAL AND AXONAL INJURY IN INFLAMMATORY DEMYELINATING LESIONS

Primary demyelination is the key feature of multiple slcerosis pathology. This means that in comparison to the complete destruction and loss of myelin sheaths axons are relatively spared within the plaques (Charcot, 1868, for review see Kornek and Lassmann, 1999). The term "relative," however, implies that axons are not completely unaffected and that in every MS lesion there is some degree of axonal injury and loss (Marburg, 1906). Its extent is variable between different plaques in the same MS patient and even more variable between plaques of different patients (Fig. 31.7). In addition, MS lesions are not restricted to the white matter but may also affect gray matter areas, such as for instance the cortex. Gray matter lesions too are defined by demyelination, but neuronal and axonal injury is profound (Peterson *et al.*, 2001). Axonal injury in plaques is associated with secondary Wallerian degeneration, affecting tracts that pass through the demyelinated areas (Evangeou *et al.*, 2000a). Furthermore, it may result in anterograde or retrograde neuronal degeneration, which may further contribute to neuronal and axonal loss (Evangelou *et al.*, 2001). As a result of all these neurodegenerative events, multiple sclerosis in patients with long-standing and severe disease is generally associated with brain atrophy, affecting both the gray and white matter (Lumsden, 1970).

All these neurodegenerative features have been noticed and carefully described in the earliest reports of multiple sclerosis pathology (Kornek and Lassmann, 1999), but have not been appreciated very much during past decades. Only recently magnetic resonance imaging studies brought these feature back into the center of interest, since these studies suggest that it is this neurodegenerative component, which plays an important role in the establishment of permanent functional deficit and irreversible clinical disease (see the chapter on MRI).

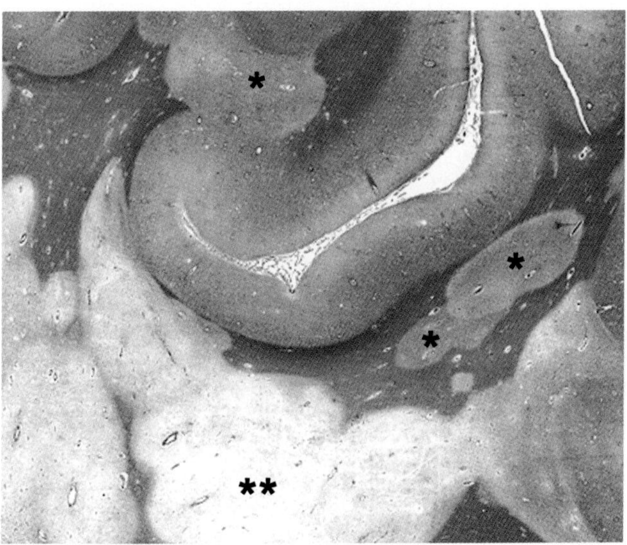

FIGURE 31.7
Axonal loss in multiple sclerosis lesions. Chronic active multiple sclerosis with multiple plaques in the subcortical white matter. Axonal staining shows profound differences in axonal density within different lesions. In some lesions, reduction of staining intensity is moderate (*), while in others there is nearly complete loss of tissue integrity (**). Bielschowsky silver impregnation; × 10.

## Axonal Injury in Demyelinated Plaques

In comparison to the adjacent normal periplaque, white matter the density of axons is always reduced in demyelinated plaques of MS patients (Lassmann, 1998). This reduction of axonal density is highly variable, ranging from less than 10% to up to 90%. A decreased axonal density not necessarily has to reflect true axonal loss, since it may also occur when axons are separated from each other by pronounced tissue edema and the infiltrating leukocytes. Thus, in acute plaques it is in general more pronounced in very early stages of demyelination than in later ones, where inflammation and edema have partially been cleared.

Quantitative assessment of true axonal loss is difficult to perform in the human central nervous system and is therefore restricted so far to defined tract areas, such as for instance the spinal cord, where total numbers of axons of a given tract can be counted (Bjatmar *et al.*, 2000). This study showed an average of true axonal loss between 60 and 70%, which is quite comparable to the data obtained by evaluating relative axonal density in brain lesions (Mews *et al.*, 1998). In addition, clinico-pathological correlation suggests that overt clinical deficit requires a profound loss of axons in a given tract system, which is in the range of 40 to 50%. This means that there is a very high reserve capacity in the human brain and spinal cord, which allows functional compensation of a loss of nearly half of the axons in a functionally important system such as the pyramidal tract.

Axonal loss in the spinal cord is not restricted to the demyelinated plaques, but occurs in quite similar extent also in white matter areas, devoid of demyelinated plaques (Bjartmar *et al.*, 2001; Ganter *et al.*, 1999; Lovas *et al.*, 2000). Since demyelinated plaques in MS patients may affect all levels of the cord, the most reasonable explanation for this observation is that axonal loss in myelinated areas of the spinal cord reflects tract degeneration due to demyelinating lesions in upper or lower spinal cord segments. Such a mechanism may also explain the rather diffuse atrophy of the cord, seen in MRI images of MS patients, which is apparently not related to the location of individual demyelinated lesions. Such tract degeneration has also convincingly been shown to occur in the corpus callosum in relation to deep white matter lesions (Evangelou *et al.*, 2000b).

Acute axonal injury results in a disturbance of axonal transport, which is reflected by focal axonal swelling and the accumulation of amyloid precursor protein (Fig. 31.8). Both features can be used to identify acutely injured axons in multiple sclerosis lesions (Ferguson *et al.*, 1997; Trapp *et al.*, 1998). Acute axonal injury is most pronounced in

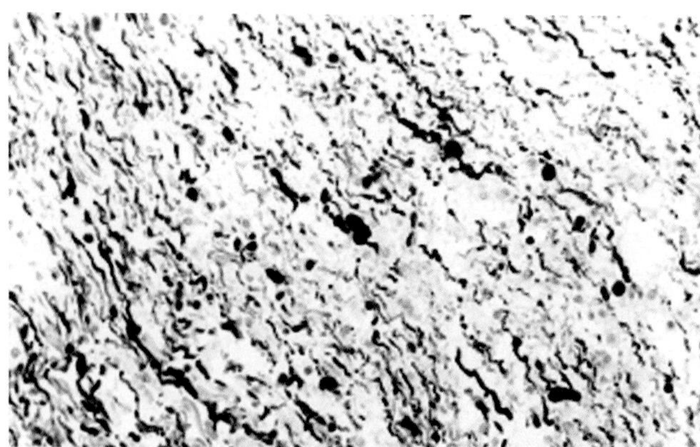

FIGURE 31.8
Axonal pathology in actively demyelinating plaque in multiple sclerosis. Reduced axonal density and multiple axons with focal enlargements of their diameter (axonal spheroids), suggesting acute disturbance of axonal transport. Immuncytochemistry for phosphorylated neurofilament; × 300.

actively demyelinating MS lesions (Ferguson *et al.*, 1997; Kornek *et al.*, 2000; Trapp *et al.*, 1998). In addition, however, there is a low density of acutely injured axons also in chronic established demyelinated plaques, which do not show any signs of ongoing destruction of myelin (Kornek *et al.*, 2000). This slow burning axonal degeneration in old lesions is not seen in remyelinated shadow plaques. Thus, in MS axonal destruction seems to occur in two different steps. Many axons are injured during a limited period of time, spanning the phase of active demyelination. In addition, there seems to be a slow process of axonal injury, which occurs in inactive plaques and may progress for months or years.

Little is known so far about the mechanisms of axonal damage in multiple sclerosis. Within the lesions as well as in the "normal" white matter, small fibers are more severely affected than thick axons (Evangelou *et al.*, 2000a, 2001). The extent of acute axonal injury correlates with the number of activated macrophages (Ferguson *et al.*, 1997) and—much less significantly—with the density of cytotoxic T-cells in the lesions (Bitsch *et al.*, 2000). This is not only the case in acute lesions, but also in inactive demyelinated "silent" plaques (Kornek *et al.*, 2000). It is thus likely that toxic mediators, produced by activated macrophages and microglia cells, play a key role in the induction of axonal death. Macrophage produced proteases (Anthony *et al.*, 1998) and nitric oxide radicals (Smith and Lassmann, 2001) are first line candidates for such an effect. Further axonal disintegration may be due to calcium influx into the axolemma and subsequent activation of calcium dependent proteases (Kornek *et al.*, 2001).

## Gray Matter Lesions/Cortical Plaques

Multiple sclerosis is generally regarded as a disease affecting the white matter. This is due to the fact that white matter lesions in this disease can easily be seen by pathologists and are distinctly visible in magnetic resonance images. However, gray matter areas are frequently affected in this disease, as for instance in cases with brain stem and spinal cord involvement. In addition, cortical plaques are abundant in patients with chronic multiple sclerosis. In some patients up to 60% of all hemispheric lesions involve the cortex (Brownell and Hughes, 1962; Lumsden, 1970).

As in white matter lesions, those in the gray matter and in particular cortical plaques are defined by the demyelinating process (Lumsden, 1970). Thus, myelin sheaths are completely lost, while other structures of the cortex are relatively well preserved. According to their shape and distribution, several types of cortical lesions can be distinguished (Kidd *et al.*, 1999; Peterson *et al.*, 2001). One type is defined as a subcortical white matter plaque, which extends into the cortex. Other lesions are sharply demarcated perivascular intracortical lesions, which, however, do not reach the subcortical white matter. The third type is oriented toward the outer surface of the cortex. It is generally large, affecting one or more gyri as a whole and extending from the outer surface into the three to four outer layers of the cortex. Thus, in such lesions there is demyelination from the molecular to the inner granular layer of the cortex, while myelin in the deeper cortical layers remains intact (Peterson *et al.*, 2001). Since the density of myelin sheaths in the normal cortex is low, such cortical plaques are difficult to identify and generally require for their detection very sensitive myelin stains.

Gray mater lesions and in particular cortical plaques differ in several aspects from those arising in the white matter (Peterson *et al.*, 2001). Although also in cortical lesions inflammation by lymphocytes and macrophages as well as microglia activation are present, the density of macrophages and microglia cells even in actively demyelinating lesions is about 10 times lower than in white matter plaques. In addition, large foamy macrophages with myelin degradation products, the hallmark of active white matter lesions are hardly detectable in active cortical plaques, remnants of myelin sheaths can mainly be found in small ramified activated microglia cells. Similar as in white matter plaques there is profound axonal injury in cortical lesions but in addition, neuronal damage can also be seen. Some neurons within the lesions show DNA fragmentation and sometimes the neuronal expression of activated caspase 3 as a marker for apoptotic cells death can be seen. Oligodendrocyte injury in cortical plaques is reflected by accumulation of the complement component C4d in their cytoplasm (Schwab and McGeer, 2002).

Thus, cortical lesion can be abundant in MS patients and may in such patients contribute to a major extent to the clinical disease burden. These lesions are mainly found in patients with progressive MS at late disease stages, but are rare in the early stages of the disease and nearly absent in patients with Marburg's type of acute MS (Lassmann, unpublished). In comparison to white matter plaques, the extent of the inflammatory response is less, but in addition to demyelination, neurodegeneration is prominent.

All these neurodegenerative changes within the central nervous system of MS patients finally lead to extensive brain changes and atrophy, denominated "MS-encephalopathy" (Jellinger, 1969). Brain atrophy affects both, the white and the gray matter, although in general the white matter is more severely damaged (Prineas and McDonald, 1997). White matter atrophy is diffuse and affects all portions of the hemispheres, some areas, such as the corpus callosum, however, are more severely affected than others. It is characteristically associated with dilatation of the cerebral ventricles. Gray matter, and in particular the cortex too can show some degree of atrophy, reflected by a widening of cerebral sulci and a thinning of the cortical ribbon. It is, however, much less extensive than that in the white matter and is found, when at all, mainly in patients with very severe chronic disease of long duration. Atrophy cannot only be seen in pathology, but is quantifiable in magnetic resonance images and thus became a useful quantitative indicator for progression of brain damage in multiple sclerosis patients (Fisher *et al.*, 2000).

## MECHANISMS OF DEMYELINATION AND TISSUE DAMAGE IN MULTIPLE SCLEROSIS LESIONS

There is little doubt that multiple sclerosis lesions develop on the background of a T-lymphocyte driven inflammatory response in the central nervous system (Noseworthy *et al.*, 2000). Some data suggest that the inflammatory response is due to an autoimmune reaction against central nervous system antigens (Martino and Hartung, 1999). Arguments in favor of the autoimmune concept are that all attempts to transmit the disease to animals so far failed, that immune suppression has a beneficial effect on disease development, and that autoimmune reactions, both on the level of T-cells as well as of antibodies, have been found in multiple sclerosis patients. Proof for a pathogenic autoimmunity in MS patients is indirect; current evidence does not rule out the involvement of an infectious agent at some time points in disease development (Noseworthy *et al.*, 2000). Indeed, epidemiological data argue in favor of an exogenous agents being involved in the induction of the disease.

The induction and development of disease in MS is, however, to a large extent determined by the host's genes. Although the genetic contribution to disease development is high, there is not a single gene responsible for this effect. In fact, multiple genes are involved in the control of this disease and the genetic risk factors appear to differ between patient subgroups. MS is thus a chronic disease with complex pathogenetic background, determined by multiple genes as well as by environmental factors (Kalman and Lublin, 1999; Noseworthy *et al.*, 2000).

The pathology of multiple sclerosis apparently reflects a common basic mechanism of inflammatory tissue damage, which is principally mediated by T-lymphocytes and activated macrophages or microglia cells. This basic pathology can then in different patients be modified by additional immune reactions, which may amplify disease and tissue damage. In addition, the genetic susceptibility of the target tissue may to a major extent influence the extent and type of tissue damage within the lesions (Lassmann *et al.*, 2001). Based on this concept of pathogenesis, different patterns of active demyelination, occurring in different subgroups of MS patients, have recently been defined (Lucchinetti *et al.*, 2000).

## The Basic Pattern of T-cell Mediated Inflammatory Tissue Damage

The basic inflammatory reaction within the CNS is similar in all MS patients, irrespective of the severity or the clinical course of the disease. It consists of an infiltration, dominated by cytotoxic Class I MHC restricted T-lymphocytes, which is associated with recruitment of hematogenous macrophages and a massive activation of local microglia (Babbe *et al.*, 2000; Gay *et al.*, 1997). Demyelination and tissue destruction in such lesions apparently is mediated by the cytotoxic T-cells themselves, as well as by activated macrophages. Several different effector pathways may be involved. For cytotoxic T-cells, it may be either the direct action of cytotoxic granules, destroying the target tissue through perforin and granzymes, or the activation of so-called death receptors, such as the Fas- or the TNF receptors (Neumann *et al.*, 2002). In addition to T-cells, however, activated macrophages and microglia cells seem to play a major role. These cells can destroy local target cells through various toxins (see the chapter on experimental autoimmune encephalomyelitis).

Many cytotoxic molecules have been identified in multiple sclerosis lesions, mainly produced by activated macrophages and microglia cells or some of them also by astrocytes, and their possible function in MS lesions has been extensively reviewed.

### *Proteolytic Enzymes*

Proteases, and in particular matrix metallproeinases and their inhibitors are highly expressed in actively demyelinating multiple sclerosis lesions (Cuzner *et al.*, 1996; Maeda and Sobel, 1996), but are absent in normal human brain. They are mainly present in activated macrophages and in part in lymphocytes. They may play a major role in the inflammatory cascade by promoting leukocyte migration into the lesions (Cuzner and Opdenakker, 1999). When released in the lesions in high concentration, they may also induce myelin and axonal damage, although, due to the poor selectivity of tissue damage induced by proteases, they are unlikely to be responsible for the large areas of primary demyelination in MS (Anthony *et al.*, 1998)

### *Tumor Necrosis Factor*

Members of the TNF family are present predominantly in active MS lesions, but to a lower extent they are also present in inactive plaques. Lymphotoxin-alpha is mainly found in lymphocytes and microglia, while TNF-$\alpha$ dominates in macrophages, microglia and some astrocytes. (Hofman *et al.*, 1989; Selmaj *et al.*, 1991). Oligodendrocytes and microglia cells express the respective TNF-receptors (TNF-R1 and TNF-R2; Bonetti and Raine, 1997). TNF, is a pro-inflammatory cytokine, which appears to be involved in the recruitment of leukocytes into the lesions. In addition, oligodendrocytes are particularly vulnerable for the induction of TNF-mediated cell death *in vitro* and *in vivo* (Probert *et al.*, 2000).

### *Reactive Oxygen and Nitrogen Specie (ROS and RNI)*

Direct visualization of ROS and RNI within tissue sections is so far not possible. However, the enzymes involved in their synthesis as well as downstream footprints of oxidative and nitrative damage have been identified in actively demyelinating multiple sclerosis lesions. The cellular source within the lesions are macrophages, microglia cells, and possibly astrocytes (Smith *et al.*, 1999; Smith and Lassmann 2002). Tissue damage induced by ROS and RNIs is mostly accomplished in cooperation—for instance, by the formation of peroxynitrite. They may play different roles in the pathogenesis of multiple sclerosis lesions. They may increase blood brain barrier permeability and are cytotoxic for oligodendrocytes and neurons. In addition, they can block axonal function and induce axonal degeneration (for details see Smith and Lassmann, 2002).

### *Excitotoxins*

Macrophages are a potent source of excitotoxins (Lipton, 1998). Since oligodendrocytes as well as neurons and axons are highly susceptible to excitotoxic injury, such a mechanism may in part be responsible for tissue damage in an inflammatory demyelinating disease (Pitt *et al.*, 2000; Smith *et al.*, 2000). An imbalanced glutamate homeostasis has recently been suggested to occur in multiple sclerosis lesions, reflected by increased glutaminase expression in macrophages or microglia and reduced expression of glutamate dehydrogenase in oligodendrocytes (Werner *et al.*, 2001).

### *Complement Components*

Activated complement, in particular activation of the terminal lytic complement complex, is present in a subset of MS cases, located on myelin at sites of active demyelination (Compston *et al.*; 1989; Prineas *et al.*; 2001; Storch *et al.*, 1998). Its activation on myelin may either occur nonspecifically or through specific antibodies, bound to the myelin surface. Myelin and oligodendrocytes are particularly vulnerable to the toxic effects of complement activation (Benn *et al.*, 2001).

### *General Significance of Macrophage Mediated Tissue Injury in MS Lesions*

The previously discussed data provide compelling evidence that macrophage toxins may play a crucial role in demyelination and tissue damage in multiple sclerosis. However, macrophages and microglia cells are nonspecific cells of the defense system and do not recognize specific antigenic targets. It is thus surprising that an inflammatory reaction, which induces tissue damage through activated macrophages, is able to mediate selective primary demyelination. The reason for this appears to reside in a differential vulnerability of different target cells and structures for macrophage mediated damage. Overall, *in vitro* studies show that there is a differential vulnerability of different brain cells to most macrophage toxins, oligodendrocytes and myelin being the most susceptible, followed by neurons and axons, astrocytes, and, as the least susceptible cell, the microglia or macrophage itself (Benn *et al.*, 2001). Thus, direct application of macrophage toxins on CNS tissue *in vitro* or *in vivo* leads at low concentration to selective primary demyelination, while higher concentration increasingly also destroy other cell types. However, there are many virus-induced diseases of the nervous system that show similar inflammation and macrophage activation in the lesions, but lack primary demyelination. Thus, there has to be some specific mechanism that drives the process in MS so selectively against myelin sheaths and oligodendrocytes. Whether this is accomplished by specific cytotoxic T-cells or autoantibodies has to be determined.

A question of major importance for the design of new therapeutic strategies is, what macrophage or microglia toxin is the most relevant in the pathogenesis of multiple sclerosis lesions? Studies in the model of EAE show that in principle all different molecules are involved in the destructive process, their relative importance varies between different models (see the chapter on experimental autoimmune encephalomyelitis). In MS lesions, all these molecules are expressed and detailed quantitative studies on their level of expression in different MS patients are not available. Thus, in a situation like this, a prediction regarding the best therapeutic target is difficult. Two key players as cytotoxic effector molecules in inflammatory tissue damage are either tumor necrosis factor alpha or nitrogen and oxygen radicals. Both of them seem to be involved at several steps of the injury cascade in inflammatory demyelinating lesions. Yet experimental studies aimed to therapeutically block these molecules in EAE revealed controversial results. Indeed, in many studies disease was not ameliorated but rather augmented. The reason for this dilemma is that such macrophage toxins are not only involved in inflammatory tissue damage, but are also essential for the elimination of pathogenic T-lymphocytes and thus for the termination of the inflammatory response (Probert *et al.*, 2000; Smith and Lassmann, 2002; Willenborg *et al.*, 1999).

## Modulation of T-Cell Mediated Inflammation by Antibodies

In a subgroup of MS patients, specific antibodies seem to be involved in demyelination and tissue injury (Lucchinetti *et al.*, 2000). Active lesions in such cases show profound deposition of immunoglogulin and activated complement on the surface of myelin sheaths and oligodendrocytes at the sites where myelin is falling apart (Prineas and Graham, 1981; Storch *et al.*, 1998; Figure 31.9). This may be associated with the interaction of macrophages with myelin fragments through coated pits and vesicles, suggestive of a receptor mediated phagocytosis (Prineas *et al.*, 1984). Whether the antibodies that are bound to degenerating myelin are really directed against myelin oligodendrocyte glycoprotein, as suggested in one study (Genain *et al.*, 1999), has to await confirmation. Possible other targets for demyelinating antibodies are, in particular, glycolipids, such as galactocerebroside (Dubois-Dalq *et al.*, 1970). Besides demyelination, specific antibodies could also play other roles in the pathogenesis of MS lesions. In a subgroup of MS patients, circulating antibodies against oligodendrocyte progenitor cells have been detected, which could, when they reach the lesion, destroy these cells and impair remyelination (Niehaus *et al.*, 2000). In other patients, massive immunoglobulin and complement deposition is found in vessel walls, which may indicate additional antibody mediated vasculitis as a potentiation factor of inflammation (Lucchinetti *et al.*, 2002).

Within the spectrum of multiple sclerosis patients, the most intense antibody involvement can be found in cases with Devic's type of neuromyelitis optica (Luchinetti *et al.*, 2002). In these patients, the massive complement activation is also associated with an inflammatory infiltrate, which contains significant numbers of granulocytes, including eosinophilic granulocytes. This granulocyte component, which is also observed in the cerebrospinal fluid of the respective patients, can be diagnostically useful. It may further help in the therapeutic decision to concentrate on immunosuppressive strategies, which in particular ameliorate B-lymphocyte and antibody responses.

## Modification of MS Lesions by Hypoxia-Like Tissue Damage

In some MS patients, active myelin destruction follows a structural pattern, which is closely reflected in acute lesions of white matter stroke (Lassmann *et al.*, 2001). This type of demyelination is in its initial phases characterized by a loss of myelin associated glycoprotein and cyclic nucleotide phosphodiesterase, while other myelin proteins, such as myelin basic protein, proteolipid protein, or myelin oligodendrocytes glycoprotein, initially remain preserved (Itoyama *et al.*, 1980). This process is associated with nuclear condensation and fragmentation of oligodendrocytes, structurally resembling apoptotic cell death (Lucchinetti *et al.*, 2000). When the oligodendrocytes are subsequently destroyed, myelin sheaths completely fall apart and are taken up by macrophages or microglia cells. Active lesions, which are demyelinated by this type of injury, differ in several aspects from the previously described MS plaques. They are ill demarcated from the surrounding periplaque white matter, and in some instances they may show a concentric, rim-like pattern of demyelination. In addition, inflamed vessels in the center of the lesions are frequently surrounded by a rim of preserved myelin (Fig. 31.10).

These changes of myelin are closely similar to those occurring in initial stages of ischemic myelin damage in white matter stroke lesions. In addition, this pattern of

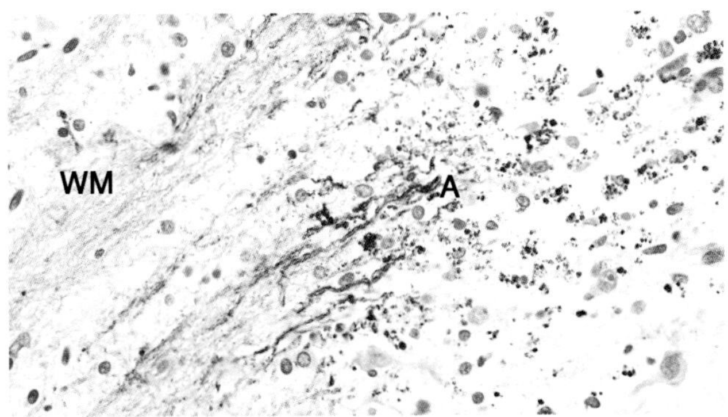


FIGURE 31.9
Active demyelination in a multiple sclerosis patient with antibody mediated demyelination. Massive deposition of activated complement (C9neo-antigen) on damaged myelin sheaths and in myelin degradation products within macrophages in the areas of demyelinating activity (A); very little deposition of activated complement in the surrounding normal white matter (WM). Immunocytochemistry for C9neo-antigen; × 900.

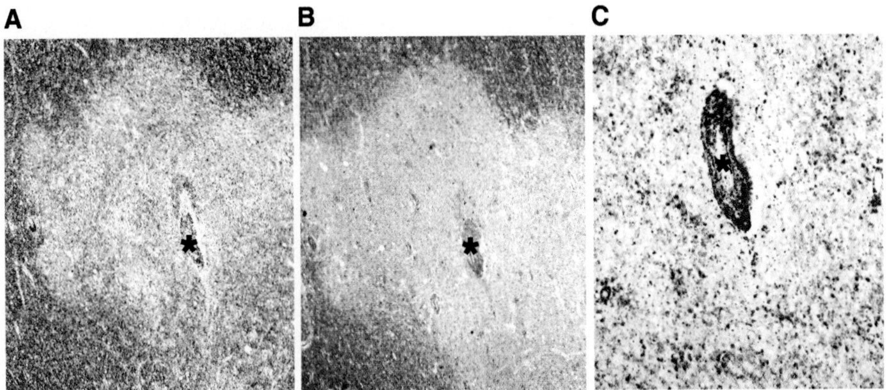


FIGURE 31.10
Actively demyelinating lesion in a patient with acute multiple sclerosis and a pattern of demyelination, resembling hypoxia/ischemia. In contrast to other MS lesions, these plaques are not sharply demarcated; MOG (Fig. A) is partially preserved, while other myelin components are lost (Fig. B, stained with Luxol fast blue); the central vessel in the plaque (*) shows a perivascular cuff of inflammatory cells, but is surrounded by a rim of preserved myelin. Within the lesion there is massive perivascular inflammation (Fig. C), but the diffuse tissue infiltration with macrophages or activated microglia cells is less profound compared to MS lesions, following other types of demyelination (see Figure 31.3). (A) Immunocytochemistry for MOG; × 50. (B) Luxol fast blue myelin stain; × 50. (C) Immunocytochemistry for CD68; × 100.

demyelination, being present in ischemia or in multiple sclerosis lesions, is always associated with increased expression and nuclear translocation of hypoxia inducible factor 1 alpha, which is a sensitive and specific sensor for decreased oxygen tension in the tissue (Lassmann, unpublished).

Hypoxia-like tissue damage can be induced in inflammatory brain lesions by a variety of different mechanisms. It may just occur as a consequence of edema in tissues, which are constrained in swelling by connective tissue or bone barriers, as they exist in the spinal cord or the optic nerve (Prineas and McDonald, 1997). Such an edema-induced increase in tissue pressure may result in disturbance of microcirculation with subsequent ischemia. Hypoxia and ischemia could also be induced through vasculitic reactions, which may lead to thrombotic occlusion of cerebral vessels in MS plaques (Wakefield *et al.*, 1994). Vasculitis in brain inflammation can either be mediated by cytotoxic T-cells or by specific antibodies, both recognizing their specific antigens within the vessel wall. Finally, hypoxia-like tissue injury can also be induced by toxic inflammatory mediators. Toxicity of nitric oxide radicals is at least in part mediated by a blockade of mitochondrial function within the respective target cells (Bolanos *et al.*, 1997). Mitochondrial failure will lead to a hypoxia-like metabolic tissue injury even under normoxic conditions.

Hypoxia-like tissue injury is frequently observed in patients with Marburg's type of acute multiple sclerosis, but is rare in the lesions of patients with classical chronic MS. Interestingly, all MS lesions with concentric demyelinating lesions of Balo's disease type follow in their acute stage the pattern of hypoxia-like demyelination.

### Differential Susceptibility of the Target Tissue for Inflammatory Demyelination in Multiple Sclerosis Patients

In addition to the quality and quantity of the immune response, the genetic susceptibility of the target tissue may influence the outcome of inflammatory demyelinating lesions. This has been shown in the model of autoimmune encephalomyelitis, in which, for instance, a deficiency of ciliary neurotrophic factor in the CNS may augment demyelination and oligodendrocyte destruction (Linker *et al.*, 2002).

In multiple sclerosis too, the genetic properties of the target tissue may modify the pathology of the lesions. In some patients, demyelination and oligodendrocyte destruction is significantly more severe compared to other patients with identical quality and quantity of the inflammatory response (Lucchinetti *et al.*, 2000). Similarly, the extent of axonal destruction and neurodegeneration is highly variable between patients, in spite of very similar patterns of inflammation (Lassmann, 1998).

Genetic studies in large cohorts of multiple sclerosis patients revealed various different candidate genes, which may modify the course of multiple sclerosis. They have no major influence on the global disease incidence, but they are associated with more severe disease or with specific atypical features of the disease. As examples, deficiency of CNTF has been described to be associated with earlier onset and more severe disease (Giess *et al.*, 2002). Other gene defects or polymorphisms that are associated with certain atypical features of the disease are related to genes for apolipoprotein E (Fazekas *et al.*, 2000) or mitochondrial DNA (Mojon *et al.*, 1999). The specific pathological substrate of this modification of multiple sclerosis is so far not known, but it is expected that it may be related to the degree of demyelination, oligodendrocyte destruction, and axonal injury, but may also affect the topography of the lesions.

## CONCLUSIONS

Numerous very elaborate studies of the central nervous system in multiple sclerosis patients have defined an inflammatory demyelinating disease process as the basic pathological process. Inflammation is apparently driven by a T-lymphocyte mediated immune response, which may be directed against one or more autoantigens of the nervous system, although the additional contribution of unknown infectious agents cannot be excluded. Demyelination is associated with a variable extent of axonal and neuronal injury, which may lead to secondary degeneration of respective tracts or projection areas. The mechanisms of demyelination and tissue destruction is complex and heterogeneous between patients. This heterogeneity is most likely controlled by genes of the patients, influencing qualitatively and quantitatively the type of the immune response that is responsible for tissue injury. In addition, genetic factors appear to control the susceptibility of the target tissue for immune-mediated injury and to determine the capacity of the tissue for remyelination and repair. MS is thus not unlike other chronic immunological diseases, in which an exogenous trigger initiates a cascade of events, which in their quantity and quality are determined by the genetic background of the patient. The complexity of such a disease, however, explains, why curative therapies are so difficult to establish. Since the immune system is armed with many different effector mechanisms, which in many situations of immune defense or autoimmunity work in parallel, treatments focusing on a single mechanism are unlikely to succeed. In addition, the heterogeneity in the mechanisms of demyelination between different MS patients implies that different patient subgroups will require different therapeutic strategies.

Apart from these complications, there are other implications for therapy from the data reviewed here. Obviously in an inflammatory demyelinating disease, inflammation is one of the prime targets for intervention. In this case, however, it has to be considered that inflammation in the CNS is not only bad, but can also through the production of neurotrophins limit damage and stimulate remyelination or tissue repair. Thus, a modulatory therapy, changing the quality of the inflammatory reaction, may be the better choice than global immune suppression. In addition, other therapies should be developed, aimed to stimulate remyelination and to prevent axonal and neuronal degeneration. Remyelination in MS plaques seems to be instrumental to prevent further axonal degeneration in established lesions. Finally, axonal protection appears to be crucial. Functional deficit, induced by inflammation and demyelination, is potentially reversible, while that due to axonal loss is irreversible. Since the final pathway of axonal injury and destruction seems to be similar in inflammatory conditions like MS and other pathologies such as stroke or trauma, it can be expected that neuroprotective therapies developed in the latter conditions will also be beneficial in multiple sclerosis patients.

## References


Adams, C. W., and Poston, R. N. (1990). Macrophage histology in paraffin-embedded multiple sclerosis plaques is demonstrated by the monoclonal pan-macrophage marker HAM-56: Correlation with chronicity of the lesion. *Acta. Neuropathol. (Berl)* 80, 208–211.

Allen, I. V., and McKeown, S. R. (1979). A histological, histochemical and biochemical study of the macroscopically normal white matter in multiple sclerosis. *J. Neurol. Sci.* **41,** 81–91.

Aloisi, F. (2001). Immune function of microglia. *Glia* **36,** 165–179.

Anthony, D. C., Miller, K. M., Fearn, S., Townsend, M. J., Opdenakker, G., Wells, G. M., Clements, J. M., Chandler, S., Gearing, A. J., and Perry, V. H. (1998). Matrix metalloproteinase expression in an experimentally-induced DTH model of multiple sclerosis in the rat CNS. *J. Neuroimmunol.* **87,** 62–72.

Archelos, J. J., and Hartung, H. P. (2000). Pathogenetic role of autoantibodies in neurological disease. *Trends Neurosci.* **23,** 317–327.

Babbe, H., Roers, A., Waisman, A., Lassmann, H., Goebels, N., Hohlfeld, R., Friese, M., Schröder, R., Deckert, M., Schmidt, S., Ravid, R., and Rajewsky, K. (2000). Clonal expansion of CD8+ T cells dominate the T cell infiltrate in active multiple sclerosis lesions as shown by micromanipulation and single cell polymerase chain reaction. *J. Exp. Med.* **192,** 393–404.

Babinski, J. (1885). Recherches sur l'anatomie pathologique de la sclerose en plaque et etude comparative des diverses varietes de la scleroses de la moelle. *Arch. Physiol.* (Paris) **5–6,** 186–207.

Balashov, K. E., Rottman, J. B., Weiner, H. L., and Hancock, W. W. (1999). CCR5(+) and CXCR3(+) T cells are increased in multiple sclerosis and their ligands MIP-1alpha and IP-10 are expressed in demyelinating brain lesions. *Proc. Natl. Acad. Sci. U.S.A.* **96,** 6873–6878.

Balo, J. (1928). Encephalitis periaxialis concentrica. *Arch. Neurol.* **19,** 242–264.

Battistini, L., Fischer, F. R., Raine, C. S., and Brosnan, C. F. (1996). CD1b is expressed in multiple sclerosis lesions. *J. Neuroimmunol.* **67,** 145–151.

Bauer, J., Rauschka, H., and Lassmann, H. (2001). Inflammation in the nervous system: The human perspective. *Glia* **36,** 235–243.

Benn, T., Halfpenny, C., and Scolding, N. (2001). Glial cells as targets for cytotoxic immune mediators. *Glia* **36,** 200–211.

Bien, C. G., Bauer, J., Deckwerth, T. L., Wiendl, H., Deckert, M., Wiestler, O. D., Schramm, J., Elger, C. E., and Lassmann, H. (2002). Destruction of neurons by cytotoxic T cells: A new pathogenic mechanism in Rasmussen's encephalitis. *Ann. Neurol.* **51,** 311–318.

Birnbaum, G., and van Ness, B. (1992) Quantitation of T-cell receptor V beta chain expression on lymphocytes from blood, brain, and spinal fluid in patients with multiple sclerosis and other neurological diseases. *Ann. Neurol.* **32,** 24–30.

Bitsch, A., Schuchardt, J., Bunkowski, S., Kuhlmann, T., and Bruck, W. (2000). Acute axonal injury in multiple sclerosis. Correlation with demyelination and inflammation. *Brain 2000* **123,** 1174–83.

Bjartmar, C., Kidd, G., Mork, S., Rudick, R., and Trapp, B. D. (2000). Neurological disability correlates with spinal cord axonal loss and reduced N-acetyl aspartate in chronic multiple sclerosis patients. *Ann. Neurol.* **48,** 893–901.

Bjartmar, C., Kinkel, R. P., Kidd, G., Rudick, R. A., and Trapp, B. D. (2001). Axonal loss in normal-appearing white matter in a patient with acute MS. *Neurology* **57,** 1248–52.

Bo, L., Mork, S., Nyland, H., Pardo, C. A., and Trapp, B. D. (1994). Detection of MHC class II antigens on macrophages and microglia, but not on astrocytes and endothelia in active multiple sclerosis lesions. *J. Neuroimmunol.* **51,** 135–146.

Bolanos, J. P., Almeida, A., Stewart, V., Peuchen, S., Land, J. M., Clark, J. B., and Heales, S. J. (1997). Nitric oxide-mediated mitochondrial damage in the brain: Mechanisms and implications for neurodegenerative diseases. *J. Neurochem.* **68,** 2227–40.

Bonetti, B., and Raine, C. S. (1997). Multiple sclerosis: Oligodendrocytes display cell death-related molecules in situ but do not undergo apoptosis. *Ann. Neurol.* **42,** 74–84.

Booss, J., Esiri, M. M., Tourtellotte, W. W., and Mason, D. Y. (1983). Immunohistological analysis of T lymphocyte subsets in the central nervous system in chronic progressive multiple sclerosis. *J. Neurol. Sci.* **62,** 219–232.

Broman, T. (1964). Blood brain barrier damage in multiple sclerosis. Supra-vital test observations. *Acta. Neurol. Scand.* **10,** 21–24.

Brown, W. J. (1978). The capillaries in acute and subacute multiple sclerosis plaques: A morphometric analysis. *Neurology* **28,** 84–92.

Brownell, B., and Hughes, J. T. (1962). The distribution of plaques in the cerebrum in multiple scleosis. *J. Neurol. Neurosurg. Psychiat.* **25,** 315–320.

Brück, W., Porada, P., Poser, S., Riechmann, P., Hanefeld, F., Kretschmar, H-A., and Lassmann, H. (1995). Monocyte/macrophage differentiation in early multiple sclerosis lesions. *Ann. Neurol.* **38,** 788–796.

Brück, W., Schmied, M., Suchanek, G., Brück, Y., Breitschopf, H., Poser, S., Piddlesden, S., and Lassmann, H. (1994). Oligodendrocytes in the early course of multiple sclerosis. *Ann. Neurol.* **35,** 65–73.

Cannella, B., and Raine, C. S. (1995). The adhesion molecule and cytokine profile of multiple sclerosis lesions. **Ann. Neurol. 37,** 424–435.

Carswell, R. (1838). "Pathological Anatomy: Illustrations on Elementary Forms of Disease." Longman, London.

Chang, A., Tourtellotte, W. W., Rudick, R., and Trapp, B. D. (2002). Premyelinating oligodendrocytes in chronic lesions of multiple sclerosis. *New Engl. J. Med.* **346,** 165–173.

Charcot, J. M. (1868). Histologie de la sclerose en plaque. *Gaz Hopital* (Paris) **41,** 554–566.

Compston, D. A., Morgan, B. P., Campbell, A. K., Wilkins, P., Cole, G., Thomas, N. D., and Jasani, B. (1989). Immunocytochemical localization of the terminal complement complex in multiple sclerosis. *Neuropathol. Appl. Neurobiol.* **15,** 307–16.

Cruveilhier, J. (1829–1842). "Anatomie pathologique du corps humain." JB Bailliere, Paris.

Cuzner, M. L., Gveric, D., Strand, C., Loughlin, A. J., Paemen, L., Opdenakker, G., and Newcombe, J. (1996). The expression of tissue-type plasminogen-activator, matrix metalloproteinases and endogenous inhibitors in the central nervous system in multiple sclerosis: Comparison of stages of lesion evolution. *J. Neuropathol. Exp. Neurol.* **55,** 1194–1204.

Cuzner, M. L., and Opdenakker, G. (1999). Plasminogen activators and matrix metalloproteinases, mediators of extracellular proteolysis in inflammatory demyelination of the central nervous system. *J. Neuroimmunol.* **94,** 1–14

D'Souza, S. D., Bonetti, B., Balasingam, V., Cashman. N. R., Barker, B. A., Troutt, A. B., Raine, C. S., and Antel, J. P. (1996). Multiple sclerosis: Fas signaling in oligodendrocyte death. *J. Experimental Medicine* **184,** 2361–2370.

Dawson, J. W. (1916). The histology of disseminated sclerosis. *Trans. R. Soc.* **50,** 517–540.

Dong, Y., and Benveniste, E. N. (2001). Immune function of astrocytes. Glia **36,** 180–190.

Dore-Duffy, P., Washington, R., and Dragovic, L. (1993). Expression of endothelial cell activation antigens in microvessels from patients with multiple sclerosis. *Adv. Exp. Med. Biol.* **331,** 243–248.

Dowling, P., Shang, G., Raval, S., Menona, J., Cook, S., and Husar, W. (1996). Involvement of the CD95 (APO1/Fas) receptor/ligand system in multiple sclerosis brain. *J. Exp. Med.* **184,** 1513–1518.

Dubois-Dalcq, M., Niedieck, B., and Buyse, M. (1970). Action of anti-cerebroside sera on myelinated nervous tissue cultures. *Pathologica Europea* **5,** 331–347.

Esiri, M. M. (1977). Immunoglobulin-containing cells in multiple sclerosis plaques. *Lancet* **2,** 478–480.

Esiri, M. M., and Reading, M. C. (1987). Macrophage populations associated with multiple sclerosis plaques. *Neuropathol. Appl. Neurobiol.* **13,** 451–465.

Esiri, M. M., Reading, M. C., Squier, M. V., and Hughes, J. T. (1989). Immunocytochemical characterization of the macrophage and lymphocyte infiltrate in the brain in six cases of human encephalitis. *Neuropathol. Appl. Neurobiol.* **15,** 289–305.

Esiri, M. M. (1980). Multiple sclerosis: A quantitative and qualitative study of immunoglobulin-containing cells in the central nervous system. *Neuropathol. Appl. Neurobiol.* **6,** 9–21.

Evangelou, N., Esiri, M. M., Smith, S., Palace, J., and Matthews, P. M. (2000a). Quantitative pathological evidence for axonal loss in normal appearing white matter in multiple sclerosis. *Ann. Neurol.* **47,** 391–5.

Evangelou, N., Konz, D., Esiri, M. M., Smith, S., Palace, J., and Matthews, P. M. (2000b). Regional axonal loss in the corpus callosum correlates with cerebral white matter lesion volume and distribution in multiple sclerosis. *Brain* **123,** 1845–9.

Evangelou, N., Konz, D., Esiri, M. M., Smith, S., Palace, J., and Matthews, P. M. (2001). Size-selective neuronal changes in the anterior optic pathways suggest a differential susceptibility to injury in multiple sclerosis. *Brain* **124,** 1813–20.

Fazekas, F., Strasser Fuchs, S., Schmidt, H., Enzinger, C., Ropele, S., Lechner, A., Flooh, E., Schmidt, R., and Hartung, H. P. (2000). Apolipoprotein E genotype related differences in brain lesions of multiple sclerosis. *J. Neurol. Neurosurg. Psychiat.* **69,** 25–28.

Ferguson, B., Matyszak, M. K., Esiri, M. M., and Perry, V. H. (1997). Axonal damage in acute multiple sclerosis lesions. *Brain* **120,** 393–9.

Fern, R., and Moller, T. (2000). Rapid ischemic cell death in immature oligodendrocytes: A fatal glutamate release feedback loop. *J. Neurosci.* **20,** 34–42.

Fisher, E., Rudick, R. A., Cutter, G., Baier, M., Miller, D., Weinstock-Guttman, B., Mass, M. K., Dougherty, D. S., and Simonian, N. A. (2000). Relationship between brain atrophy and disability: An 8-year follow-up study of multiple sclerosis patients. *Mult. Scler.* **6,** 373–7.

Fog, T. (1950). Topographic distribution of plagues in the spinal cord in multiple sclerosis. *A.M.A. Arch Neurol Psychiat* **63,** 382–414.

Fraenkel, M., and Jakob, A. (1913). Zur Pathologie der multiplen Sklerose mit besonderer Berücksichtigung der akuten Formen. *Z. Neurol.* **14,** 565–603.

Ganter, P., Prince, C., and Esiri, M. M. (1999). Spinal cord axonal loss in multiple sclerosis: A post-mortem study. *Neuropathol. Appl. Neurobiol.* **25,** 459–67.

Gay, F. W., Drye, G. W., Dick, G. W. A., and Esiri, M. M. (1997). The application of multifactorial cluster analysis in the staging of plaques in early multiple sclerosis: Identification and characterization of the primary demyelinating lesion. *Brain* **120,** 1461–1483.

Genain, C. P., Cannella, B., Hauser, S. L., and Raine, C. S. (1999). Autoantibodies to MOG mediate myelin damage in MS. *Nat. Med.* **5,** 170–175.

Gerritse, K., Deen, C., Fasbender, M., Ravid, R., Boersma, W., and Claassen, E. (1994). The involvement of specific anti myelin basic protein antibody-forming cells in multiple sclerosis immunopathology. *J. Neuroimmunol* **49,** 153–159.

Gerritse, K., Laman, J. D., Noelle, R. J., Aruffo, A., Ledbetter, J. A., Boersma, W. J., and Claassen,-E. (1996). CD40-CD40 ligand interactions in experimental allergic encephalomyelitis and multiple sclerosis. *Proc. Natl. Acad. Sci. U.S.A.* **93,** 2499–504.

Giess, R., Maurer, M., Linker, R., Gold, R., Warmuth-Metz, M., Toyka, K. V., Sendtner, M., and Rieckmann, P. (2002). Association of a null mutation in the CNTF gene with early onset of multiple sclerosis. *Arch. Neurol.* **59,** 407–9.

Guo, Y. P., and Gao, S. F. (1983). Concentric sclerosis. *In* "Clinical and Experimental Neurology. Proc Australian Association of Neurologists," (J. H. Tyrer and M. J. Eadie, eds.), 19; pp. 67–76. Adis Health Science Press Sydney.

Hawkins, C. P., Munro, P. M., MacKenzie, F., Kesselring, J., Tofts, P. S., du-Boulay, E. P., Landon, D. N., and McDonald, W. I. (1990). Duration and selectivity of blood-brain barrier breakdown in chronic relapsing experimental allergic encephalomyelitis studied by gadolinium-DTPA and protein markers. *Brain* **113,** 365–78.

Hayashi, T., Morimoto, C., Burks, J. S., Kerr, C., and Hauser, S. L. (1988). Dual-label immunocytochemistry of the active multiple sclerosis lesion: Major histocompatibility complex and activation antigens. *Ann. Neurol.* **24,** 523–31.

Hayes, G. M., Woodroofe, M. N., and Cuzner, M. L. (1987). Microglia are the major cell type expressing MHC class II in human white matter. *J. Neurol. Sci.* **80,** 25–37.

Hofman, F. M., Hinton, D. R., Johnson, K., and Merrill, J. E. (1989). Tumor necrosis factor identified in multiple sclerosis brain. *J. Exp. Med.* **170,** 607–612.

Itoyama, Y., Sternberger, N. H., Webster, H. deF., Quarles, R. H., Cohen, S. R., and Richardson, E. P., Jr. (1980). Immunocytochemical observation on the distribution of myelin-associated glycoprotein and myelin basic protein in multiple sclerosis lesions. *Ann. Neurol.* **7,** 167–177.

Jellinger, K. (1969). Einige morphologische Aspekte der Multiplen Sklerose. *Wien Z Nervenheilk* (Suppl) **II,**12–37.

Kalman, B., and Lublin, F. D. (1999). The genetics of multiple sclerosis. A review. *Biomed. Pharmacother.* **53,** 358–70.

Kerschensteiner, M., Gallmeier, E., Behrens, L., Leal, V. V., Misgeld, T., Klinkert, W. E., Kolbeck, R., Hoppe, E., Oropeza-Wekerle, R. L., Bartke, I., Stadelmann, C., Lassmann, H., Wekerle, H., and Hohlfeld, R. (1999). Activated human T cells, B cells, and monocytes produce brain-derived neurotrophic factor in vitro and in inflammatory brain lesions: A neuroprotective role of inflammation? *J. Exp. Med.* **189,** 865–70.,

Kidd, T., Barkhof, F., McConnell, R., Algra, P. R., Allen, I. V., and Revesz, T. (1999). Cortical lesions in multiple sclerosis. *Brain* **122,** 17–26.

Kirk, J. (1979). The fine structure of the CNS in multiple sclerosis. Vesicular demyelination in an acute case. *Neuropathol. Appl. Neurobiol.* **5,** 289–294.

Kornek, B., and Lassmann, H. (1999). Axonal pathology in multiple sclerosis: A historical note. *Brain Pathol.* **9,** 651.656.

Kornek, B., Storch, M. K., Bauer, J., Djamshidian, A., Weissert, R., Wallstrom, E., Stefferl, A., Zimprich F., Olsson, T., Linington, C., Schmidbauer, M., and Lassmann, H. (2001). Distribution of calcium channel subunit in dystrophic axons in multiple sclerosis and experiemntal autoimmune encephalomyelitis. *Brain* **124,** 1114–1124.

Kornek, B., Storch, M., Weissert, R., Wallstroem, E., Stefferl, A., Olsson, T., Linington C., Schmidbauer, M., and Lassmann, H. (2000). Multiple sclerosis and chronic autoimmune encephalomyelitis: A comparative quantitative study of axonal injury in active, inactive and remyelinated lesions. *Amer. J. Pathol.* **157,** 267–276.

Kotter, M. R., Setzu, A., Sim, F. J., Van-Rooijen, N., and Franklin, R. J. (2001). Macrophage depletion impairs oligodendrocyte remyelination following lysolecithin-induced demyelination. *Glia.* **35,** 204–12.

Kwon, E. E., and Prineas, J. W. (1994). Blood brain barrier abnormalities in longstanding multiple sclerosis lesions. An immunohistochemical study. *J. Neuropath. Exp. Neurol.* **53,** 625–636.

Lassmann, H. (1983). Comparative neuropathology of chronic experimental allergic encephalomyelitis and multiple sclerosis. *Springer Schriftenr. Neurol.* **25:**1–135.

Lassmann, H. (1998). Pathology of multiple sclerosis. *In* "McAlpine's Multiple Sclerosis" (A. Compston, ed.), pp323–358. Churchill Liningstone, London.

Lassmann, H., Brück, W., and Lucchinetti, C. (2001). Heterogeneity of multiple sclerosis pathogenesis: Implications for diagnosis and therapy. *Trends Mol. Med.* **7,** 115–121.

Ligers, A., Xu, C., Saarinen, S., Hillert, J., and Olerup, O. (1999). The CTLA-4 gene is associated with multiple sclerosis. *J. Neuroimmunol.* **97,** 182–190.

Linington, C., Engelhardt, B., Kapocs, G., and Lassmann, H. (1992). Induction of persistently demyelinated lesions in the rat following the repeated adoptive transfer of encephalitogenic T cells and demyelinating antibody. *J. Neuroimmunol.* **40,** 219–24.

Linker, R. A., Maurer, M., Gaupp, S., Martini, R., Holtmann, B., Giess, R., Rieckmann, P., Lassmann, H., Toyka, K. V., Sendtner, M., and Gold, R. (2002). CNTF is a major protective factor in demyelinating CNS disease: A neurotrophic cytokine as modulator in neuroinflammation. *Nat. Med.* **8,** 620–4.

Lipton, S. A. (1998). Neuronal injury associated with HIV-1: Approaches and treatment. *Annu. Rev. Pharmacol. Toxicol.* **38,** 159–177.

Lovas, G., Szilagyi, N., Majtenyi, K., Palkovits, M., and Komoly, S. (2000). Axonal changes in chronic demyelinated cervical spinal cord plaques. *Brain* **123,** 308–17.

Lucchinetti, C., Brück, W., Parisi, J., Scheithauer, B., Rodriguez, M., and Lassmann, H. (2000). Heterogeneity of multiple sclerosis lesions: Implications for the pathogenesis of demyelination. *Ann. Neurol.* **47,** 707–717.

Lucchinetti, C., Brück, W., Parisi, J., Scheithauer, B., Rodriguez, M., and Lassmann, H. (1999). A quantitative analysis of oligodendrocytes in multiple sclerosis lesions. A study of 117 cases. *Brain* **122,** 2279–2295.

Lucchinetti, C. F., Brück, W., Rodriguez, M., and Lassmann, H. (1996). Distinct patterns of multiple sclerosis pathology indicates heterogeneity in pathogenesis. *Brain Pathol.* **6,** 259–274.

Lucchinetti, C. F., Mandler, R., McGavern, D., Brück, W., Gleich, G., Ransohoff, R. M., Trebst, C., Weinshenker, B., Wingerchuck, D., Parisi, J., and Lassmann, H. (2002). A role for humoral mechanisms in he pathogenesis of Devic's neuromyelitis optica. *Brain* (in press).

Ludwin, S. K. (1980). Chronic demyelination inhibits remyelination in the central nervous system. An analysis of contributing factors. *Lab. Invest.* **43,** 382–387.

Ludwin, S. K., Henry, J. M., McFarland, H. (2001). Vascular proliferation and angiogenesis in multiple sclerosis: Clinical and pathogenetic implications. *J. Neuropathol. Exp. Neurol.* **60,** 505.

Lumsden, C. E. (1970) The neuropathology of multiple sclerosis. In "Handbook of clinical Neurology" (Vinken, P. I., Bruyn, and G. W., eds.), Vol. 9, pp. 217–309. Elsevier, New York.

Luster, A. D. (1998). Chemokines — chemotactic cytokines that mediate inflammation. *N. Engl. J. Med.* **338,** 436–445.

Maeda, A., and Sobel, R. A. (1996). Matrix metalloproteinases in the normal human central nervous system, microglia nodules and multiple sclerosis lesions. *J. Neuropathol. Exp. Neurol.* **55,** 300–309.

Marburg, O. (1906). Die sogenannte "akute Multiple Sklerose" Jahrb *Psychiatrie* **27,** 211–312.

Martino, G., and Hartung, H. P. (1999). Immunopathogenesis of multiple sclerosis: The role of T cells. *Curr. Opin. Neurol.* **12,** 309–321.

McManus, C., Berman, J. W., Brett, F. M., Staunton, H., Farrell, M., and Brosnan, C. F. (1998). MCP-1, MCP-2 and MCP-3 expression in multiple sclerosis lesions: An immunohistochemical and in situ hybridization study. *J. Neuroimmunol.* **86,** 20–9.

Merrill, J. E. (1992). Proinflammatory and antiinflammatory cytokines in multiple sclerosis and central nervous system acquired immunodeficiency syndrome. *J Immunother.* **12,** 167–170.

Mews, I., Bergmann, M., Bunkowski, S., Gullotta, F., and Brück, W. (1998). Oligodendrocyte and axon pathology in clinically silent multiple sclerosis lesions. *Multiple Sclerosis* **4,** 55–62.

Minagar, A., Jy, W., Jimenez, J. J., Sheremata, W. A., Mauro, L. M., Mao, W. W., Horstman, L L., and Ahn, Y. S. (2001). Elevated plasma endothelial microparticles in multiple sclerosis. *Neurology.* **56,** 1319–24.

Moalem, G., Gdalyahu, A., Shani, Y., Otten, U., Lazarovici, P., Cohen, I. R., and Schwartz, M. (2000). Production of neurotrophins by activated T cells: Implications for neuroprotective autoimmunity. *J. Autoimmun.* **15,** 331–45.

Moalem, G., Leibowitz-Amit, R., Yoles, E., Mor, F., Cohen, I. R., and Schwartz, M. (1999). Autoimmune T cells protect neurons from secondary degeneration after central nervous system axotomy. *Nat. Med.* **5,** 49–55.

Mojon, D., Fujihara, K., Hirano, M., Miller, C., Lincoff, N., Jacobs, D., and Greenberg, S. (1999). Leber's hereditary optic neuropathy mitochondrial DNA mutations in familial multiple sclerosis. *Graefes Arch. Clin. Exp. Ophtalmol.* **237,** 348–350.

Mussini, J. M., Hauw, J. J., and Escourolle, R. (1977). Immunofluorescence studies of intra cytoplasmatic immunoglobulin binding lymphoid cells in the central nervous system. Report of 32 cases including, 19 multiple sclerosis. *Acta. Neuropathol. (Berl.)* **40,** 227–232.

Neumann, H., Medana, I., Bauer, J., and Lassmann, H. (2002). Cytotoxic T lymphocytes in autoimmune and degenerative CNS diseases. *Trend Neurosci.* **25,** 313–319.

Niehaus, A., Shi, J., Grzenkowski, M., Diers-Fenger, M., Hartung, H. P,. Toyka, K., Bruck, W., and Trotter, J. (2000). Patients with active relapsing-remitting multiple sclerosis synthesize antibodies recognizing oligodendrocyte progenitor cell surface protein: Implications for remyelination. *Ann. Neurol.* **48,** 362–71.

Noseworthy, J. H., Lucchinetti, C., Rodriguez, M., and Weinshenker, B. G. (2000). Multiple sclerosis. *New Engl. J. Med.* **343,** 938–952.

Oksenberg, J. R., Panzara, M. A., Begovich, A. B., Mitchell, D., Ehrlich, H. A., Murray, R. S., Shimonkevitz, R., Sherritt, M., Rothbard, J., and Bernard, C. C. (1993). Selection for T-cell receptor V beta-D beta-J beta gene rearrangements with specificity for a myelin basic protein peptide in brain lesions of multiple sclerosis. *Nature* **362,** 68–70.

Ozawa, K., Suchanek, G., Breitschopf, H., Brück, W., Budka, H., Jellinger, K., and Lassmann, H. (1994). Patterns of oligodendroglia pathology in multiple sclerosis. *Brain* **117,** 1311–1322.

Peterson, J. W., Bo, L., Mork, S., Chang, A., and Trapp, B. D. (2001). Transected neurites, apoptotic neurons and reduced inflammation in cortical multiple sclerosis lesions. *Ann. Neurol.* **50,** 389–400.

Pitt, D., Werner, P., Raine, C. S. (2000). Glutamate excitotoxicity in a model of multiple sclerosis. *Nature Med.* **6,** 67–70.

Plumb, J., McQuaid, S., Mirakhur, M., and Kirk, J. (2002). Abnormal endothelial tight junctions in active lesions and normal appearing white matter in multiple sclerosis. *Brain Pathol.* **12,**, 199–211.

Prineas, J. W. (1979). Multiple sclerosis: Presence of lymphatic capillaries and lymphoid tissue in the brain and spinal cord. *Science* **203,** 1123–1125.

Prineas, J. W. (1985). The neuropathology of multiple sclerosis. In "Handbook of Clinical Neurology" (J. C. Koetsier, ed.), Vol. 47, pp. 337–395. Elsevier, New York.

Prineas, J. W., Barnard, R. O., Kwon, E. E, Sharer, L. R., and Cho, E. S. (1993a). Multiple sclerosis: Remyelination of nascent lesions. *Ann. Neurol.* **33,** 137–151.

Prineas, J. W., Barnard, R. O., Revesz, T., Kwon, E. E., Sharer, L., and Cho, E. S. (1993b). Multiple sclerosis: Pathology of recurrent lesions. *Brain* **116,** 681–693.

Prineas, J. W., and Graham, J. S. (1981). Multiple sclerosis: Capping of surface immunoglobulin G on macrophages engaged in myelin breakdown. *Ann. Neurol.* **10,** 149–158.

Prineas, J. W., Kwon, E. E., Cho, E. S., and Sharer, L. R. (1984). Continual breakdown and regeneration of myelin in progressive multiple sclerosis plaques. *Ann. NY Acad. Sci.* **436,** 11–32.

Prineas, J. W., Kwon, E. E., Cho, E. S., Sharer, L. R., Barnett, M. H., Oleszak, E. L., Hoffman, B., and Morgan, B. P. (2001). Immunopathology of secondary-progressive multiple sclerosis. *Ann. Neurol.* **50,** 646–657.

Prineas, J. W., Kwon, E. E., Goldenberg, P. Z., Ilyas, A. A., Quarles, R. H., Benjamins, J. A., and Sprinkle, T. J. (1989). Multiple sclerosis: Oligodendrocyte proliferation and differentiation in fresh lesions. *Lab. Invest.* **61,** 489–503.

Prineas, J. W., and McDonald, I. W. (1997). Demyelinating diseases. In "Greenfield's Neuropathology" (D. I. Graham and P. L. Lantos, eds.), 6th ed., pp. 813–896. Arnold, London, Sidney, Auckland.

Prineas, J. W., and Wright, R. G. (1978). Macrophages, lymphocytes, and plasma cells in the perivascular compartment in chronic multiple sclerosis. *Lab. Invest.* **38,** 409–421.

Probert, L., Eugster, H. P., Akassoglou, K., Bauer, J., Frei, K., Lassmann, H., and Fontana, A. (2000). TNFR1 signalling is critical for the development of demyelination and the limitation of T-cell responses during immune-mediated CNS disease. *Brain* **123,** 2005–19.

Rafalowska, J., Krajewski, S., Dolinska, E., and Dziewulska, D. (1992). Does damage to perivascular astrocytes in multiple sclerosis participate in blood brain barrier permeability. *Neuropathol. Pol.* **30,** 73–80.

Raine, C. S., Scheinberg, L., and Waltz, J. M. (1981). Multiple sclerosis: Oligodendrocyte survival and proliferation in an active established lesion. *Lab. Invest.* **45,** 534–546.

Ransohoff, R. M., and Estes, M. L. (1991). Astrocyte expression of major histocompatibility complex gene products in multiple sclerosis brain tissue obtained by stereotactic biopsy. *Arch. Neurol.* **48,** 1244–6

Rindfleisch, E. (1863). Histologisches Detail zur grauen Degeneration von Gehirn und Rückenmark. *Arch. Pathol. Anat. Physiol. Klin. Med. (Virchow)* **26,** 474–483.

Rodriguez, M., Scheithauer, B. W., Forbes, G., and Kelly, P. J. (1993) Oligodendrocyte injury is an early event in lesions of multiple sclerosis. *Mayo Clin. Proc.* **68,** 627–636.

Schlesinger, H. (1909). Zur Frage der akuten multiplen Sklerose und der encephalomyelitis disseminata im Kindesalter. *Arb. Neurol. Inst. (Wien)* **17,** 410–432.

Schwab, C., and McGeer, P. L. (2002). Complement activated C4d immunoreactive oligodendrocytes delineate small cortical plaques in multiple sclerosis. *Exp. Neurol.* **174,** 81–88.

Seil, F. J., Smith, M. E., Leiman, A. L., and Kelly, J. M. (1975). Myelination inhibiting neuroelectric blocking factors in experimental allergic encephalomyelitis. *Science* **187,** 951–953.

Selmaj, K., Raine, C. S., Cannella, B., and Brosnan, C. F. (1991). Identification of lymphotoxin and tumor necrosis factor in multiple sclerosis lesions. *J. Clin. Invest.* **87,** 949–954.

Simpson, J., Rezaie, P., Newcombe, J., Cuzner, M. L., Male, D., and Woodroofe, M. N. (2000b). Expression of the beta-chemokine receptors CCR2, CCR3 and CCR5 in multiple sclerosis central nervous system tissue. *J. Neuroimmunol.* **108,** 192–200.

Simpson, J. E., Newcombe, J., Cuzner, M. L., and Woodroofe, M. N. (1998). Expression of monocyte chemoattractant protein-1 and other beta-chemokines by resident glia and inflammatory cells in multiple sclerosis lesions. *J. Neuroimmunol.* **84,** 238–49.

Simpson, J. E., Newcombe, J., Cuzner, M. L., and Woodroofe, M. N. (2000a). Expression of the interferon-gamma-inducible chemokines IP-10 and Mig and their receptor, CXCR3, in multiple sclerosis lesions. *Neuropathol. Appl. Neurobiol.* **26,** 133–42.

Smith, K. J., and Lassmann, H. (2002). The role of nitric oxide in multiple sclerosis. *Lancet Neurology* **1,** 232–241.

Smith, K. J., Kapoor, R., and Felts, P. A. (1999). Demyelination: The role of reactive oxygen and nitrogen species. *Brain Pathol.* **9,** 69–92.

Smith, T., Groom, A., Zhu, B., and Turski, L. (2000). Autoimmune encephalomyelitis ameliorated by AMPA antagonists. *Nature Med.* **6,** 62–66.

Sobel, R. A., Mitchell, M. E., and Fondren, G. (1990). Intercellular adhesion molecule-1 (ICAM-1) in cellular immune reactions in the human central nervous system. *Am. J. Pathol.* **136,** 1309–1316.

Sorensen,T. L., Tani, M., Jensen, J., Pierce, V., Lucchinetti, C., Folcik, V. A., Qin, S., Rottman, J., Sellebjerg, F., Strieter, R. M., Frederiksen, J. L., and Ransohoff, R. M. (1999). Expression of specific chemokines and chemokine receptors in the central nervous system of multiple sclerosis patients. *J. Clin. Invest.* **103,** 807–15.

Sorensen, T. L., Trebst, C., Kivisakk, P., Klaege, K. L., Majmudar, A., Ravid, R, Lassmann, H., Olsen, D. B., Strieter, R. M., Ransohoff, R. M., and Sellebjerg, F. (2002). Multiple sclerosis: A study of CXCL10 and CXCR3 co-localization in the inflamed central nervous system. *J. Neuroimmunol.* **127,** 59–68

Springer, T. A. (1994). Traffic signals for lymphocyte recirculation and leucocyte emigration: The multistep paradigm. *Cell* **76,** 301–314.

Stadelmann, C., Kerschensteiner, M., Misgeld, T, Brück, W., Hohlfeld, R., and Lassmann, H. (2002). BDNF and gp145trkB in multiple sclerosis brain lesions: Neuroprotective interactions between immune cells and neuronal cells? *Brain* **125,** 75–85.

Steiner, G. (1931). Regionale Verteilung der Entmarkungsherde in ihrer Bedeutung für die Pathogenese der multiplen Sklerose. In "Krankheitserreger und Gewebsbefund bei multipler Sklerose," pp. 108–120. Springer, Berlin.

Storch, M. K., Piddlesden, S., Haltia, M., Iivanainen, M., Morgan, P., and Lassmann, H. (1998). Multiple sclerosis: In situ evidence for antibody and complement mediated demyelination. *Ann. Neurol.* **43,** 465–471.

Tavolato, B. (1975). Immunoglobulin G distribution in multiple sclerosis brain. An immunofluorescence study. *J. Neurol. Sci.* **24,** 1–11.

Trapp, B. D., Peterson, J., Ransohoff, R. M., Rudick, R., Mork, S., and Bo, L. (1998). Axonal transection in the lesions of multiple sclerosis. *N. Engl. J. Med.* **338,** 278–85.

Traugott, U. (1987). Multiple sclerosis: Relevance of class I and class II MHC-expressing cells to lesion development. *J. Neuroimmunol.* **16,** 283–302.

Traugott, U., Reinherz, E. L., and Raine, C. S. (1983). Multiple sclerosis: Distribution of T cells, T cell subsets and Ia-positive macrophages in lesions of different ages. *J. Neuroimmunol.* **4,** 201–221.

Trebst, C., Sorensen, T. L., Kivisakk, P., Cathcart, M. K., Hesselgesser, J., Horuk, R., Sellebjerg, F., Lassmann, H., and Ransohoff, R. M. (2001). CCR1+/CCR5+ mononuclear phagocytes accumulate in the central nervous system of patients with multiple sclerosis. *Am. J. Pathol.* **159,** 1701–10.

Ulvestad, E., Williams, K., Vedeler, C., Antel, J., Nyland, H., Mork, S., and Matre, R. (1994). Reactive microglia in multiple sclerosis lesions have an increased expression of receptors for the Fc part of IgG. *J. Neurol. Sci.* **121,** 125–131.

Wakefield, A. J., More, L. J., Difford, J., and McLaughlin, J. E. (1994). Immunohistochemical study of vascular injury in acute multiple sclerosis. *J. Clin. Pathol.* **47,** 129–133.

Washington, R., Burton, J., Todd, R. F., 3rd, Newman, W., Dragovic, L., and Dore-Duffy, P. (1994). Expression of immunologically relevant endothelial cell activation antigens on isolated central nervous system microvessels from patients with multiple sclerosis. *Ann. Neurol.* **35,** 89–97.

Werner, P., Pitt, P., and Raine, C. S. (2001). Multiple sclerosis: Altered glutamate homeostasis in lesions correlates with oligodendrocyte and axonal damage. *Ann. Neurol.* **50,** 169–180.

Willenborg, D. O., Staykova, M. A., and Cowden, W. B. (1999). Our shifting understanding of the role of nitric oxide in autoimmune encephalomyelitis: A review. *J. Neuroimmunol.* **100,** 21–35.

Windhagen, A., Newcombe, J., Dangond, F., Strand, C., Woodroofe, M. N., Cuzner, M. L., and Hafler, D. A. (1995). Expression of costimulatory molecules B7–1 (CD80), B7–2 (CD86), and interleukin 12 cytokine in multiple sclerosis lesions. *J. Exp. Med.* **182,** 1985–96.

Wolswijk, G. (2000) Oligodendrocyte survival, loss and birth in lesions of chronic-stage multiple sclerosis. *Brain* **123,** 105–115.

Wolswijk, G. (2002). Oligodendrocyte precursor cells in the demyelinated multiple sclerosis spinal cord. *Brain* **125,** 338–349.

Woodroofe, M. N., Bellamy, A. S., Feldmann, M., Davison, A. N., and Cuzner, M. L. (1986). Immunocytochemical characterisation of the immune reaction in the central nervous system in multiple sclerosis. Possible role for microglia in lesion growth. *J. Neurol. Sci.* **74,** 135–52.

Woodroofe, M. N., and Cuzner, M. L. (1993). Cytokine mRNA expression in inflammatory multiple sclerosis lesions: Detection by nonradioactive in situ hybridization. *Cytokine* **5,** 583–588.

Wucherpfennig, K. W., Newcombe, J., Li, H., Keddy, C., Cuzner, M. L., and Hafler, D. A. (1992a). Gamma delta T-cell receptor repertoire in acute multiple sclerosis lesions. *Proc. Natl. Acad. Sci.* (USA) **89,** 4588–4592.

Wucherpfennig, K. W., Newcombe, J., Li, H., Keddy, C., Cuzner, M. L., and Hafler, D. A. (1992b). T-cell receptor V alpha-V beta repertoire and cytokine gene expression in active multiple sclerosis lesions. *J. Exp. Med.* **175,** 993–1002.

CHAPTER

# 32

# MRI Visualization of Multiple Sclerosis

*Alberto Cifelli, D. L. Arnold, and P. M. Matthews*

## INTRODUCTION

Magnetic resonance imaging (MRI) and related techniques make possible the noninvasive visualization of structural, biochemical, and functional changes in the brain (Gadian, 1995; Hashemi and Bradley, 1997; Jezzard *et al.*, 2001). This visualization of pathological changes *in vivo* has had a profound impact on the clinical management of patients with multiple sclerosis (MS) and on the understanding of the disease and its treatment (Miller *et al.*, 1997). MRI has substantially changed the way the *diagnosis* of MS is made (Arnold and Matthews, 2002). Diagnosis with high confidence now is possible very early in the course of disease (McDonald *et al.*, 2001). More accurate information regarding *prognosis* is available, e.g., for patients presenting with clinically isolated syndromes, MRI data help to estimate the risk of progression to MS and for patients early in the course of MS it provides information relevant to predicting disease severity (Brex *et al.*, 2002). MRI and related techniques also have been able to shed considerable light on the natural history of the pathology of MS (Miller *et al.*, 1998) and its responses to treatments (Arnold and Matthews, 2002; Rovaris and Filippi, 1999). This has improved the efficiency of trial designs, particularly for the earlier stages of evaluation of new drugs.

MRI provides a range of techniques for visualizing the central nervous system (CNS) in patients with MS, each of which is sensitive to different aspects of pathological change (Arnold and Matthews, 2002). The application of these MRI techniques to MS thus can be viewed in a similar way to the application of different staining techniques to post-mortem material by the pathologist. Each MR-based technique allows visualization of particular characteristics of the pathology (Barkhof and van Walderveen, 1999). By integration of data from multiple MR techniques, a usefully comprehensive view of the disease emerges (Rovaris and Filippi, 2000b). With greater understanding of the genesis of the pathological changes, neurobiologically driven hypotheses regarding disease evolution or the effects of interventions now can be tested by observations during life. The relationship between changes in MS and in animal models of CNS inflammatory disease also can be evaluated directly, enhancing the information available from the models (Hawkins *et al.*, 1990).

This chapter outlines the basic principles of MRI and related techniques. MRI techniques define pathology on the basis of changes in biophysical parameters of tissue. With an understanding of these biophysical parameters, it can be appreciated that they have variably specific relations with pathological features as defined using traditional methods.

The chapter then reviews several contributions of MRI and related techniques to the understanding of MS and to pathology. MR and related techniques have been important particularly in emphasizing that much pathological change is subclinical, the diffuse nature of pathology, the prominence of gray matter involvement, and the role of neurodegeneration, even in the early stages of disease evolution. Together these observations provide a remarkably comprehensive view of key features essential for understanding the way MS progresses.

## BASIC PRINCIPLES OF MRI

### Conventional Magnetic Resonance Imaging Techniques

MRI and related techniques are based on the weak interaction between the proton nuclear magnetic dipole and a strong, homogeneous applied magnetic field. The conventional MRI techniques used to study MS patients produce images that reflect primarily the physicochemical state of protons in brain water. Contrast in such images is derived from tissue-specific differences in (1) water content, (2) spin-spin relaxation time (*i.e.*, the time constant for the decay of magnetization in the plane perpendicular to the magnetic field, referred to as $T_2$), and (3) spin-lattice relaxation time (*i.e.*, the time constant for the recovery of magnetization along the axis of the magnetic field, referred to as $T_1$) (for reviews of MRI theory and applications see, for example, Gadian, 1995; Hashemi and Bradley, 1997; Jezzard *et al.*, 2001). Conventional MRI techniques include (1) $T_2$-weighted imaging, (2) proton-density-weighted imaging, (3) fluid-attenuated inversion-recovery (FLAIR) imaging, (4) standard $T_1$-weighted imaging, and (5) gadolinium-enhanced $T_1$-weighted imaging (Fig. 32.1).

#### $T_2$-Weighted Imaging

MR images are $T_2$-weighted by allowing more time for $T_2$ relaxation to occur during a relatively-long echo time (*i.e.*, the time between radio-frequency excitation and subsequent acquisition of the signal from a "spin-echo", referred to as TE). Signals from water protons located in tissues associated with longer $T_2$ values decay less during a long TE; because of this, such tissues appear hyperintense on $T_2$-weighted images relative to tissues that have shorter $T_2$ relaxation times.

The T2 relaxation *rate* (the reciprocal of the relaxation *time*) is determined both by local static magnetic interactions and by interactions that fluctuate at the resonance (Larmor) frequency. The resonance frequency is determined by an unchanging physical property of the nuclear magnetic moment of the proton (the gyromagnetic ratio) and the strength of

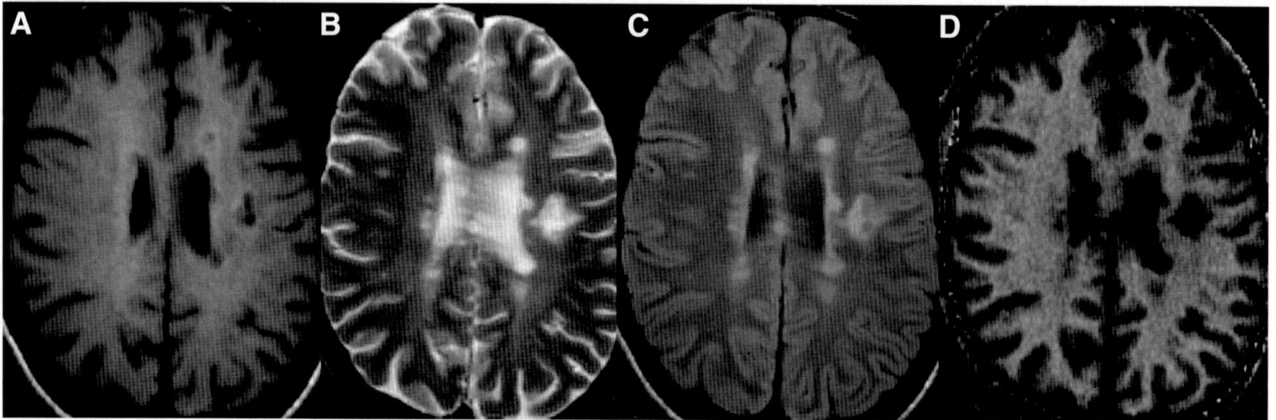


FIGURE 32.1
Use of different MRI pulse sequences allows contrast to be generated on the basis of different biophysical parameters. These have different sensitivities to histopathological change. (A) A T1-weighted image defines areas of substantial demyelination, axonal loss, and matrix destruction as hypointense volumes. (B) A T2-weighted image more sensitively identifies pathology associated with multiple sclerosis, but shows T2-hyperintense signal change nonspecifically for edema, demyelination, and gliosis. (C) A proton density-weighted image has a similar relative lack of pathological specificity, but can be useful particularly for identifying the extent of lesions in the periventricular regions because CSF is hypointense, in contrast to the hyperintensity of MS lesions. (D) A magnetization transfer ratio (MTR) image shows decreased intensity in areas of demyelination and axonal loss. This technique thus defines lesion distribution similarly to T2-weighted imaging, although the latter is more sensitive to edema.

the applied magnetic field. At 1.5T, this is in the radiofrequency range at 62 MHz. Because the T2 relaxation rate depends on both static and Larmor frequency interactions, it is very sensitive to even small changes in the nature and extent of the association between water and local macromolecules in tissue. T2 therefore is highly sensitive to changes in tissue water content and to the nature and concentration of tissue macromolecules.

A practical problem with T2-weighted brain images for the quantitative characterization of MS pathology is that both CSF and focal lesions are hyperintense, so the precise extent of periventricular lesions often cannot be defined clearly. The FLAIR sequence is a T2-weighted imaging sequence modified to "null" signal from the CSF compartment: it is often used with (or in preference to) a simple T2-weighting.

### $T_1$-Weighted Imaging

$T_1$-weighted images are produced by shortening the time between repetitions of a pulse sequence (TR), allowing less time for water to regain its equilibrium magnetization. Water protons in tissues with a relatively short $T_1$ relaxation time recover more quickly and generate more signal with a shorter TR than do those in tissues with a longer $T_1$. Protons in bulk water (*e.g.*, in CSF or in tissue that is associated with edema or a loss of structural integrity) have a long $T_1$ and appear hypointense on $T_1$-weighted sequences. The T1 relaxation rate is determined by interactions only at the resonance frequency, giving T1-weighted imaging changes less sensitivity but greater specificity to pathological phenomena. $T_1$-weighted images are less sensitive to variations in either the matrix water- or myelin content than are $T_2$-weighted images, for example.

### Proton Density-Weighted Imaging

Contrast in conventional MRI arises from differences in water content, as well as intrinsic relaxation characteristics between different tissues or between normal and pathological tissue. Signal intensity in images acquired with a very long inter-pulse interval (TR) and a very short delay before data acquisition (TE) is related directly to the concentration of tissue water protons. This type of image would be a true proton density (PD) image. In practice, so-called PD-weighted images are obtained with relatively long TR and relatively short TE, such that CSF is hypointense and lesions are hyperintense.

Both PD- and T2-weighted MRI provide qualitatively similar pathological information in MS. In practice, PD-weighted images (and FLAIR images) are more useful for identification of lesions adjacent to the ventricles, because the CSF in their proximity is hypointense (i.e., darker than lesions) (Fig. 32.1).

### Gadolinium-Enhanced $T_1$-Weighted Imaging

As reviewed by Rovaris and Filippi (Rovaris and Filippi, 2000a), the sensitivity of lesion detection in $T_1$-weighted imaging can be increased selectively with the injection of gadolinium-diethylenetriaminepentacetate (Gd-DTPA), a chelated form of gadolinium (Gd) (Fig. 32.2). Gd is one of the lanthanide elements and has strong paramagnetic properties, so that in its nontoxic chelate with DTPA it changes the local rate of water MR relaxation. Gd-DTPA facilitates both longitudinal (T1) and transverse (T2) water proton relaxation in proportion to its concentration in local tissue water (Tofts and Kermode, 1991). As water proton T1 is 5-10 times longer than T2 in most tissues, the relaxation time shortening effects of Gd-DTPA are more pronounced on T1 than on T2. Normally, Gd-DTPA in serum does not cross the blood-brain barrier (BBB) and would enhance only signal in blood vessels. However, when BBB integrity is compromised, Gd-DTPA can enter the CNS and, with shortening of T1, increases signal intensity on T1-weighted images selectively at the sites of BBB breakdown.

## "Nonconventional" MR Imaging Techniques

Several "nonconventional" MR imaging measures can be defined arbitrarily on the basis of their lack of integration into routine clinical practice at present. Each generates image contrast based on different biophysical parameters. In combination with conventional

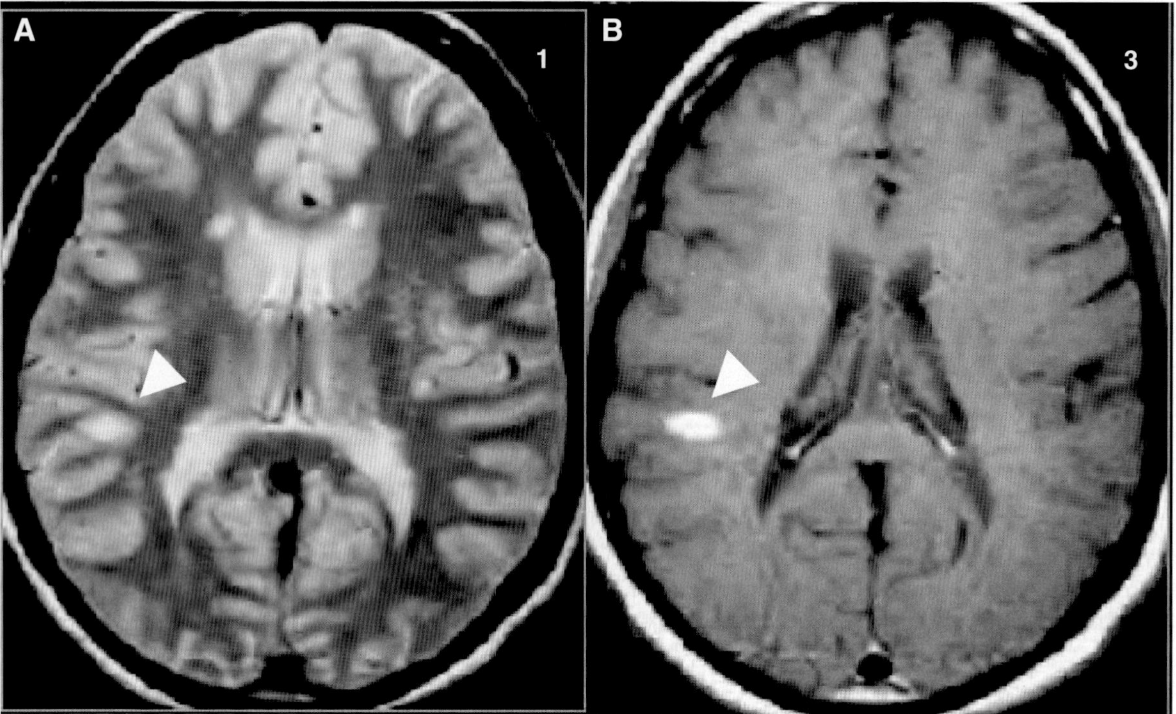


FIGURE 32.2
Gd-enhancement can identify focal breakdown of the blood brain barrier (BBB). (A) This T2-weighted MRI scan from a patient with multiple sclerosis demonstrates multiple T2-hyperintense lesions. Acute and chronic lesions cannot be distinguished on the basis of the T2-weighted MRI signal alone. (B) This gadolinium-enhanced T1-weighted image shows focal hyperintense signal (arrowhead) in one of the lesions identified as T2-hyperintense in (A). This lesion is an acute or subacute lesion, distinguishing it from the other T2-hyperintense lesions as shown in (A). Together, images in (A) and (B) provide evidence for dissemination of lesions in both space and time.

measures, they can enhance the specificity and allow more precise quantification of pathological changes.

*Magnetization Transfer Imaging*

Magnetization transfer (MT) images are created by applying a selective radiofrequency irradiation that saturates the signal from protons in macromolecules not normally visualized by conventional MRI (Grossman, 1999; McGowan, 1999) (Fig. 32.3). When this saturation is subsequently transferred to the bulk water pool that is normally visualized by MRI, the bulk water MR signal decreases by an amount that depends on (1) the density of the macromolecules at a given location and (2) the nature of their interactions with bulk water. The extent of the effect can be quantified conveniently as the magnetization transfer ratio (MTR), which is defined as the percent decrease in signal between the image with the saturating irradiation of macromolecule protons and that without their saturation. A greater magnetization transfer between macromolecules and associated water (giving a higher MTR) implies a greater or stronger interaction between water and macromolecular protons. Loss of macromolecular density or structure (as occurs with demyelination) will reduce the MTR.

As conventionally applied, the MTR does not specifically probe any particular class of macromolecules. However, because the relative abundance of myelin proteins in the brain is so high, changes in myelin content dominate MTR changes in MS. Even aside from technical factors related to variations in the efficiency of macromolecule saturation, MTR is not completely specific for changes in magnetization transfer, as it is also influenced by T1 changes associated with severe edema. This limitation may be circumvented by quantifying magnetization transfer, rather than relying simply on the ratio. Such quantification is nontrivial, but is being pursued in a number of laboratories since it may improve the pathological specificity of the technique (Brass *et al.*, 2002a, 200b; Dalton *et al.*, 2002; Levesque *et al.*, 2002; Ramani *et al.*, 2001; Ropele *et al.*, 2002; Santos *et al.*, 2002).

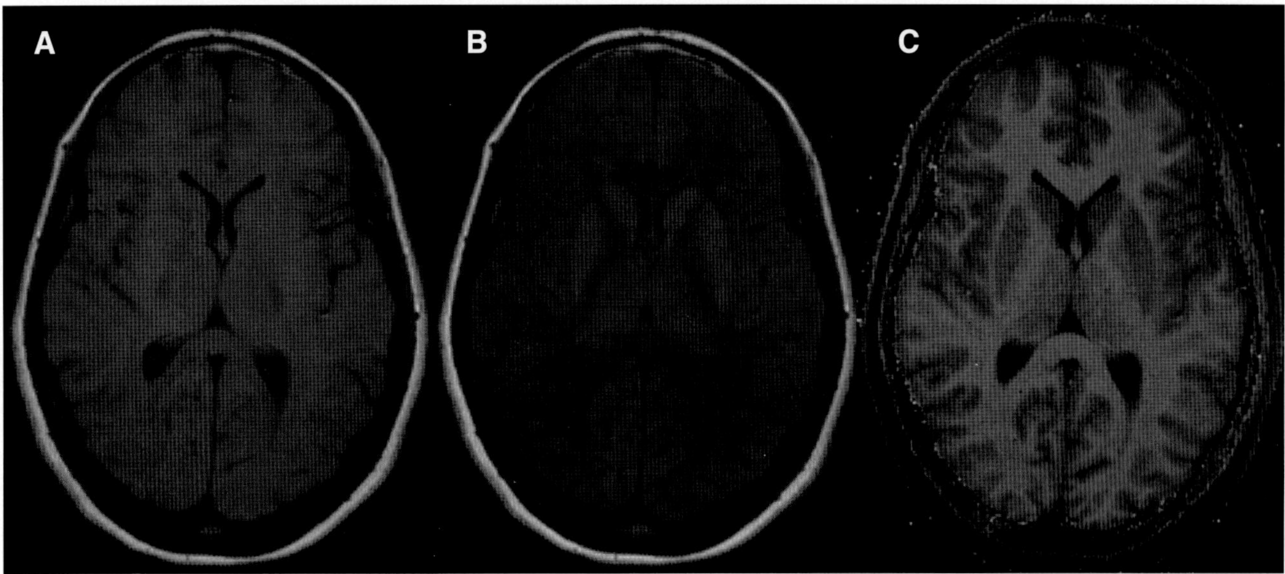


FIGURE 32.3
Magnetization transfer imaging generates contrast on the basis of relaxation interactions between tissue water and macromolecules. (A) Image acquired without off-resonance irradiation to saturate macromolecular protons. (B) An image from the same level with off-resonance irradiation to fully saturate the macromolecule protons. The intensity is diminished in (B) relative to (A) because of transfer of saturation from macromolecule protons to tissue water. (C) A magnetization transfer ratio (MTR) image in which the contrast expresses the signal in (B) relative to (A). The white matter is bright because of the strong cross-relaxation effects of myelin proteins on tissue water.

### *Diffusion-Weighted Imaging*

Application of high magnetic field gradients during the imaging sequence can make it sensitive to the diffusion of water (Cercignani and Horsfield, 2001; Cercignani *et al.*, 1999). Diffusion properties of water in tissue can be expressed without regard to direction, as an apparent diffusion coefficient (ADC), or with respect to the relative anisotropy, either as a simple measure, such as the fractional anisotropy (FA), or as a full diffusion tensor, defining the direction of anisotropy explicitly in three-dimensional space. Water diffusion in healthy white matter is highly anisotropic because of the oriented axons and myelin, along the axes of which water diffusion distances are greatest. Although the relative contributions of water in myelin and axons to diffusion anisotropy measurements are not well defined, it is clear that factors associated with demyelination and an increase in the extracellular space markedly decrease diffusion anisotropy.

### *Magnetic Resonance Spectroscopy and Spectroscopic Imaging*

Proton magnetic resonance spectroscopy (MRS) is fundamentally different from the water-proton-based MRI techniques described earlier in that it records signals that arise from protons in CNS metabolites (Rudkin and Arnold, 1999). Because the concentration of such tissue metabolites is approximately one-thousandth that of tissue water, the signal-to-noise ratio and image resolution of these metabolite-based images is much lower than in water-based images. Nevertheless, the resulting metabolite images can provide chemico-pathological specificity that is not possible with conventional water-based images.

As shown in Figure 32.4, the water-suppressed, localized proton MRS spectrum of the normal human brain that is recorded at relatively long echo times (i.e., TE of 136 or 272 ms) reveals three major resonance peaks [the locations of which are expressed as the difference in parts per million (ppm) between the resonance frequency of the compound of interest and that of a standard compound (i.e., tetramethylsilane)]. The three major peaks are ascribed to choline (Cho), creatine (Cr), and N-acetylaspartate (NAA). The Cho peak at 3.2 ppm arises from tetramethyl amines, which are mainly found in choline-containing phospholipids participating in membrane synthesis and degradation. The Cr peak, which resonates at 3.0 ppm, arises from both creatine and phosphocreatine (Cr). The

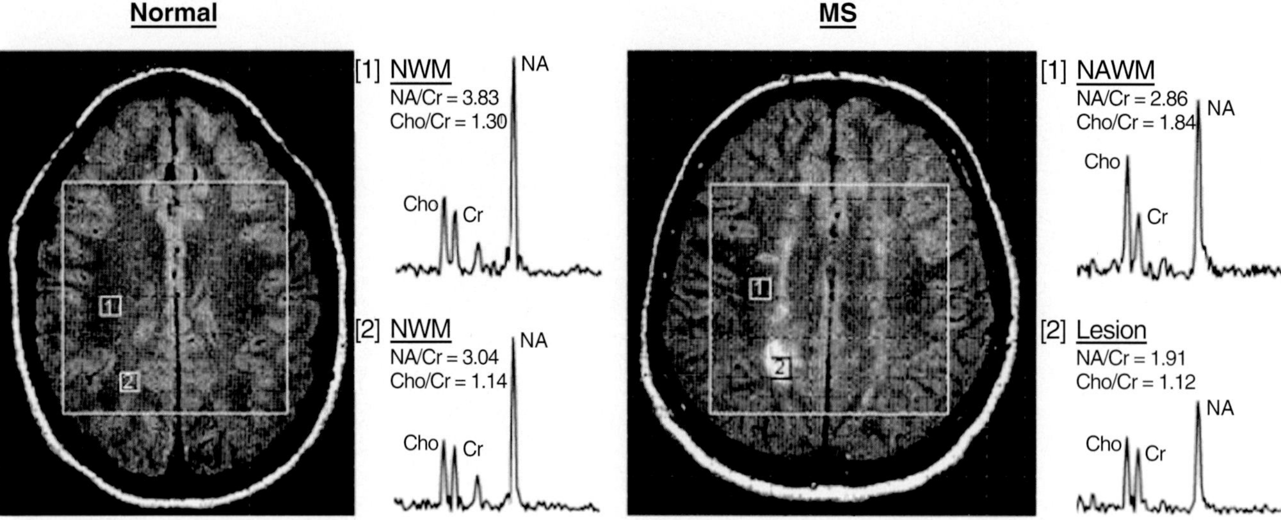


FIGURE 32.4
Proton-density-weighted magnetic resonance images through the centrum semiovale and the results of proton MRSI in a patient with multiple sclerosis and in a normal control subject. The superimposed grid in each image represents individual $^{1}$H-MRSI voxels, and the large white box represents the entire proton MRSI volume of interest for that individual. The smaller, numbered boxes represent voxels of normal-appearing white matter (NAWM) and lesional brain tissue in the patient and normal white matter (NWM) in the normal control subject. The $^{1}$H-MRSI spectra from within each of these voxels are shown to the right of each image. The areas under the NA and Cho peaks (normalized to Cr) are shown above each spectrum. The spectra have been scaled so that the Cr peak in each of them has the same height.

N-acetylaspartate resonance at 2.0 ppm originates from N-acetyl groups (NA), which, in the brain, are found primarily in the neuronally localized compound N-acetylaspartate (NAA). A fourth peak, which is attributed to the methyl resonance of lactate (LA) and resonates at 1.3 ppm, is normally only barely visible above the baseline noise; in certain pathological conditions, it may increase many-fold and a methyl resonance from lipids may also be detected in the same region of the spectrum.

The resonance intensity that is ascribed to NAA is, arguably, the most important proton MRS signal in the characterization of MS pathology, because NAA is localized within neurons and neuronal processes such as axons and dendrites (Bitsch *et al.*, 1999; Bjartmar *et al.*, 2000; Moffett *et al.*, 1991; Simmons *et al.*, 1991; Wujek *et al.*, 2002).

MRS can acquire biochemical data from a single volume of tissue (single-voxel spectroscopy) or from multiple voxels simultaneously, thereby generating an image based on the distribution of a selected proton resonance (magnetic resonance spectroscopic imaging or MRSI) (Salibi and Brown, 1998).

### *Functional Magnetic Resonance Imaging*

FMRI is a magnetic resonance technique based on monitoring blood oxygen level dependent (BOLD) contrast (Jezzard *et al.*, 2001). Neuronal activity is associated with an increased local synaptic activity. The increased metabolism is associated with an increase of blood flow and oxygen consumption. The relative increment in blood flow is greater than the increase in oxygen consumption. This leads to a boost of the oxyhaemoglobin/deoxyhaemoglobin ratio. Contrast changes arise because the effects of (diamagnetic) oxyhaemoglobin and (paramagnetic) deoxyhaemoglobin on local water relaxation times are different. Increased oxyhaemoglobin levels lead to a relatively longer T2 relaxation time for water in and around blood vessels, resulting in an enhancement of the MR signal (0.5–1.5% at 1.5 T). This signal change can be visualized by subtracting images acquired during a period of greater neural activation (e.g., during a movement) from images acquired during a relative resting state (Fig. 32.5). FMRI measures neural activation only *indirectly* by sampling the relative changes in microvascular (mainly venular) blood oxygenation. Albeit a young technique (Ogawa *et al.*, 1993), fMRI already has been found application in a vast array of research and clinical settings.

## MRI VISUALIZATION OF MULTIFOCAL LESIONS FOR EARLY DIAGNOSIS OF MS

MRI has substantially increased the sensitivity for detection of pathological changes associated with MS and allows the diagnosis of MS to be made much earlier than in the past, when it was based to a greater extent on clinical manifestations of the disease (McDonald *et al.*, 2001). Although CT changes can be seen with MS (Hershey *et al.*, 1979), most lesions are not highlighted by contrast and abnormalities on unenhanced scans are typically apparent only with very large acute lesions or in the later stages of the disease. Even then, CT abnormalities have limited specificity. In contrast, characteristic patterns of lesions are found on MRI in approximately 95% of MS patients (Paty *et al.*, 1988) and in the vast majority of patients with clinically isolated syndromes (initial attacks) suggestive of MS, who will go on to develop additional episodes or MRI lesions that would be sufficient to make a diagnosis (Brex *et al.*, 2002).

A number of studies have defined criteria with different sensitivity and specificity for interpretation of MRI in the context of suspected MS (Barkhof *et al.*, 1997; Fazekas *et al.*, 1988; Gean-Marton *et al.*, 1991; Horowitz *et al.*, 1989; Paty *et al.*, 1988; Tas *et al.*, 1995; Tintore *et al.*, 2000) (Tab. 32.1). Further specificity arises from gadolinium enhancement of lesions defining acute to subacute blood brain barrier (BBB) breakdown due to inflammation. The currently recommended criteria for use of MRI in the diagnosis of MS (McDonald *et al.*, 2001) are shown in Table 32.2. They are relatively stringent in order to increase the specificity of the MRI findings (Barkhof *et al.*, 1997; Tintore *et al.*, 2000). Although other pathologies also can give rise to multiple T2 hyperintense lesions, these have rather different characteristics, often allowing them to be discriminated on the basis of imaging alone (Arnold and Matthews, 2002; Barkhof and Scheltens, 2002).

Additional information can come from spinal cord imaging (Simon, 2000). However, spinal cord MRI is much less sensitive to the pathological changes of MS than is brain (Bergers *et al.*, 2002).

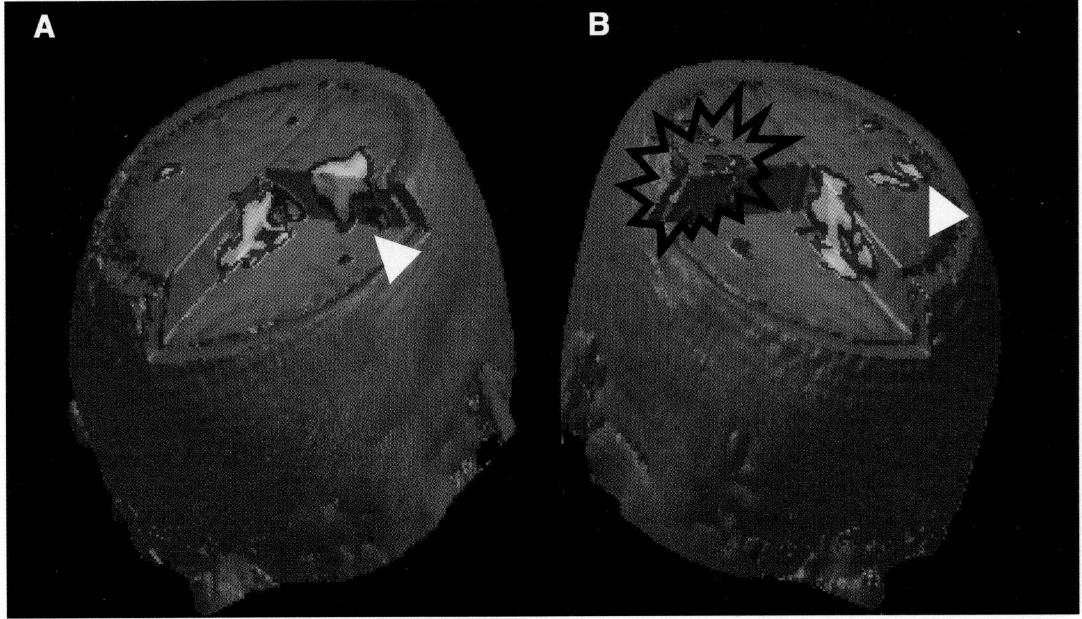


FIGURE 32.5
Functional magnetic resonance imaging (fMRI) can define altered patterns of brain activation associated with sensory, motor, or cognitive tasks in patients with multiple sclerosis. (A) The pattern of activation in the superior aspect of the brain from a healthy control during simple hand flexion-extension movements is shown. The contralateral primary sensorimotor area (large arrow), the midline supplementary motor area and a small region in the ipsilateral premotor cortex show activation. (B) In a patient with multiple sclerosis, activation in the contralateral primary sensorimotor area may be diminished with significantly increased activation in the ipsilateral motor cortex (black borders). This relative recruitment of ipsilateral motor cortex for a simple action is potentially adaptive, limiting disability in the patients.

TABLE 32.1 Interpretation of MRI in the Diagnosis of Multiple Sclerosis

| Reference | Definition | Study design | Sensitivity (%) | Specificity (%) |
|---|---|---|---|---|
| Fazekas *et al.*, 1988 | ≥3 lesions with two of<br>1. An infratentorial lesion<br>2. A periventricular lesion<br>3. A lesion >6 mm | Retrospective | 88 | 100 |
| Paty *et al.*, 1988 | ≥ four lesions, or three lesions of which one is periventricular | Prospective (following from first presentation) | 94 | 57 |
| Tas *et al.*, 1995 | ≥1 Gd[a]-enhancing lesion and ≥ one nonenhancing lesion | Prospective | 59 | 80 |
| Barkhof *et al.*, 1997[b,c] | At least 1 Gd-enhancing lesion or 9 T2-hyperintense lesions including<br>1. At least one juxtacortical lesion<br>2. At least three periventricular lesions<br>3. At least one infratentorial lesion | Prospective | 82 | 78 |

[a]Gd = gadolinium-DTPA.
[b]According to Tintore' *et al* (2000), if three out of four criteria are fulfilled, the highest accuracy and best compromise between sensitivity and specificity are achieved.
[c]McDonald *et al.* (2001) allow the substitution of one spinal cord lesion for one brain lesion.
Adapted from Barkhof *et al.*, 1997.

TABLE 32.2 McDonald (McDonald *et al.*, 2001) Criteria for Diagnosis of Multiple Sclerosis

| Clinical (attacks) | Objective lesions | Additional requirements to make diagnosis |
|---|---|---|
| Two or more | Two or more | None: Clinical evidence will suffice (additional evidence is desirable but must be consistent with MS) |
| Two or more | One | Dissemination in *space* by MRI *or* CSF+[a] and two or more MRI lesions consistent with MS *or* further clinical attack involving different site |
| One | Two or more | Dissemination in *time* by MRI *or* second clinical attack |
| One (monosymptomatic) | One | Dissemination in *space* by MRI *or* CSF+ and two or more MRI lesions consistent with MS *And* dissemination in *time* by MRI *or* second clinical attack |
| Zero (progression from onset) | One | CSF+ *And* dissemination in space with MRI evidence of nine or more brain lesions *or* two or more cord lesions *or* four to eight brain and one cord lesion<br>*Or* positive VEP[b] with four to eight MRI lesions<br>*Or* positive VEP with less than four brain lesions plus one cord lesion<br>*And* dissemination in *time* by MRI *or* continued progression for one year |

[a]CSF+ = Presence in the cerebrospinal fluid of oligoclоclonal bands different from any such bands in serum or of a raised IgG index.
[b]VEP = Visual evoked potentials.

When patients present with their first symptoms suggestive of MS, it is important to be able to predict the risk of developing another attack (which would qualify the patient for a diagnosis of MS) and also the risk of significant future disability. MRI data cannot yet be used to predict disability reliably. However, the presence of asymptomatic lesions in the brain at the time of initial presentation is a strong predictor that the patient will eventually develop clinically definite MS (Brex *et al.*, 2002). An increased proportion of T1 hypointense changes within chronic lesions is associated with more severe disease, although specific criteria for this have not been evaluated yet (Fazekas *et al.*, 2000).

## MRI VISUALIZATION OF THE PROGRESSION OF MS LESIONS

While progression of lesions in MS has long been inferred on the basis of variations in pathology at post-mortem, longitudinal MRI studies have provided a direct view of the dynamics of evolution of individual lesions (Grossman *et al.*, 1988; Kermode *et al.*, 1990a; Thompson *et al.*, 1992). A basic model has developed in which the earlier stages of evolution are associated with blood brain barrier (BBB) breakdown, followed by later inflammatory changes leading to demyelination, axonal loss, and gliosis. With more severe

TABLE 32.3 Pathological Correlations in MS for MR-based Imaging Changes

| Technique | Findings | Pathological correlates |
|---|---|---|
| *Conventional T2-weighted imaging* | Hyperintensity | Inflammation, oedema, demyelination, gliosis, remyelination, axonal loss |
| *Conventional T1-weighted images* | Acute hypointensity | Oedema |
| | Chronic hypointensity | Demyelination, axonal loss, and matrix destruction |
| | Gd[a]-enhancement | Blood brain barrier disruption |
| | Cerebral (or spinal cord) atrophy | Demyelination, axonal loss and gliosis (relative contributions uncertain) |
| *Conventional PD*[b] -weighted images | Hyperintensity | As for T2-weighted imaging, but better contrast between lesions and CSF[c] |
| *Magnetic resonance spectroscopy (MRS) or spectoscopic imaging (MRSI)* | N-acetyl-aspartate (NAA) decrease | Atrophy, metabolic dysfunction, or loss of axons or neurons |
| | Increased macromolecule (lipid) resonances | Early myelin damage |
| | Increased choline resonances | Myelin breakdown and inflammatory cell infiltration |
| | Increased lactate resonance | Acute inflammation |
| | Decreased creatine resonances | Glial changes |
| | Increased *myo*-inositol resonance | Inflammatory or glial response |
| *Magnetisation transfer (MT) imaging* | Reduced magnetisation transfer ratio (MTR) | Demyelination and axonal loss |
| *Diffusion weighted imaging (DWI)*[d] | Increased water diffusivity and decreased diffusion anisotropy | Oedema, demyelination, and axonal loss |
| *Functional MRI* | Altered patterns of cerebral activation during sensory, motor, or cognitive tasks | Systems-level, potentially adaptive functional reorganization |

[a]Gd = Gadolinium-DTPA.
[b]PD = Proton density.
[c]CSF = Cerebrospinal fluid.
[d]No pathological evidence from human studies available.

inflammation, substantial matrix destruction and local axonal damage can occur. However, as will be discussed subsequently, important refinements to this model continue to be made.

## Visualization of Blood Brain Barrier Breakdown with Contrast-Enhanced T1-Weighted MRI

BBB disruption is an early event in the pathogenesis of an MS lesion. The BBB refers to several mechanisms that restrict free exchange of non-lipid soluble molecules between blood and the CSF space. The BBB includes both active (energy-requiring) processes (e.g., amino-acid transporters) and passive mechanisms (e.g., endothelial tight junctions) that regulate the physiological environment in the central nervous system (CNS). Anatomical barriers contributing to the BBB include the capillary endothelium, with its tight junctions, adjacent glia, and components of the extracellular matrix.

Intravenous injection of an exogenous contrast agent that is normally excluded from the CNS space, but can enter with damage to the integrity of the BBB, allows MRI to visualize breakdown of the BBB (Fig. 32.2). The contrast agent in most common use is Gd-DTPA. Local Gd-enhancement is associated with active lesions in MS (Table 32.3) Movement of Gd-DTPA across the BBB can be shown to be driven by altered endothelial pinocytotic transport in animal models, as well as possibly by loss of the integrity of tight junctions between endothelial cells, as suggested by a study of post-mortem MS brains (Plumb *et al.*, 2002). Rare observations have provided additional, direct histopathological correlations of Gd-enhancement in MS as well. These were first described in a study of a secondary progressive (SP) MS patient scanned first at 4 weeks and then at 10 days prior to death (Katz *et al.*, 1990, 1993). Enhancing lesions were extensively demyelinated and contained abundant perivascular cuffs with lymphocytes, macrophages, and plasma cells. Within areas of enhancement were multiple small areas of demyelination centered around a perivascular cuff and bordered by macrophages filled with undigested myelin debris.

Active lesions are highly likely to show Gd-enhancement. In a study based on both biopsy and autopsy material (Nesbit *et al.*, 1991), *all* of the histologically active lesions showed enhancement whereas none of the inactive lesions did. Not surprisingly, Gd-enhancement is associated with clinical relapses (Miller *et al.*, 1988). A majority of patients in relapse with focal neurological symptoms will show Gd-enhancement in lesions anatomically localized to account for new symptoms (Miller *et al.*, 1988). However, most enhancing lesions are asymptomatic. This likely reflects the variable severity of the associated conduction block or axonal injury, as well as the fact that many areas of brain do not eloquently express deficits from smaller lesions. Gd-enhancement of lesions is 5 to 10 times higher than the number of clinical exacerbations. Activity can be high even in the early RR phase of the disease (Harris *et al.*, 1991). Most lesions enhance for less than 1 month. Enhancement for greater than 6 months is rare (McFarland *et al.*, 1992). Gd-enhancement thus is a useful marker of acute to subacute inflammatory activity.

Dynamic contrast studies follow the time course of signal changes with a rapidly acquired series of images after Gd-DTPA injection. In a dynamic study of RR MS (Kermode *et al.*, 1990b), images acquired 2 to 4 minutes after injection of Gd-DTPA showed a variable extent of enhancement, which was typically smaller than the corresponding volumes on unenhanced scans and frequently had the appearance of confluent rings. This ring enhancement likely reflects acute inflammation at the border of chronic active demyelinating lesions. By 16 to 20 minutes after injection, most lesions enhanced homogeneously. Over several hours after the injection the initially hypointense center of many of the ring lesions then became brighter than the periphery. By 5 hours post-injection, the enhancing volumes enlarged to the full size of the corresponding T2 hyperintense lesions. The mean time to the peak enhancement of lesions was just under 30 minutes, but newer lesions tended to show peak enhancement earlier than older ones, suggesting that time course may provide a marker of the timing of inflammation. Dynamic contrast studies are not performed routinely, however. As a practical guide, the optimal timing to maximize the sensitivity to enhancement of active lesions after contrast injection is between 10 and 30 minutes with conventional techniques (Kermode *et al.*, 1990b; Silver *et al.*, 1997). Most clinical Gd-enhanced scans are begun 5 minutes after the injection, in the interest of time efficiency.

The extent of contrast enhancement for a specific lesion is determined by the dose of contrast agent injected, as well as the time delay after administration before imaging. Use of triple dose gadolinium can increase the frequency of detection of enhancing lesions by 66 to 75% (Filippi *et al.*, 1996b; Silver *et al.*, 1997).

The primary application of Gd-enhancement is for assessment of lesion activity. In conjunction with conventional T2-weighted or PD-weighted imaging, it can increase overall lesion detection, but the benefits are modest. The gain in sensitivity is greatest for lesions at cortical-subcortical junctions (Miller *et al.*, 1993).

Gd-enhancement is highly variable between patients. However, in a fairly large group of relapsing-remitting patients studied monthly three consecutive times 78% had evidence of BBB breakdown on at least one MRI (Stone *et al.*, 1995). There is a rather cyclical trend to the variation in frequency of Gd-enhancement in individual patients (McFarland *et al.*, 1992). Gd-enhancing lesion number or volume is predictive of relapse frequency in RR MS (Smith *et al.*, 1993). The frequency of Gd-enhancing lesions also may be predictive of subsequent development of disability (Khoury *et al.*, 1994; Koudriavtseva *et al.*, 1997; Losseff *et al.*, 1996a; Smith *et al.*, 1993).

Although there is a strong relationship between histopathologically defined active lesions and Gd-enhancement, it is not clear that all lesions visible by T2-weighted MRI necessarily evolve through an early, Gd-enhancing phase (Bruck *et al.*, 1997). There are discrepancies between patterns of Gd-enhancement and T2-hyperintense lesions, for example. The rate of Gd-enhancing lesion appearance may decrease in later stages of the disease, without an associated decrease in T2-hyperintense lesion accumulation rates (Filippi *et al.*, 1997). The rate of enhancing lesion formation in SP MS patients can be significantly lower than in RR patients, despite comparable increments in the rates of increase of the unenhanced lesion load and in disability. A possible explanation for this was provided by Lee *et al.* (1999), who demonstrated that the spatial *distributions* of T2-hyperintense and Gd-enhancing lesions were different across cerebral white matter in a population of patients with established MS. There was a much higher probability for T2-hyperintense lesions to be periventricular than for Gd-enhancing lesions, which tended to be more peripheral in the white matter. This implies that the periventricularly localized component of the T2 hyperintense lesion burden less frequently involves an early stage of BBB breakdown that could be detected using Gd-enhancement. T2-signal changes in the periventricular area may, at least in part, reflect gliosis secondary to the Wallerian degeneration of descending fibers transected in more peripheral lesions.

#### *Proton Density and T2-Weighted MRI Allows Visualization of Inflammation, Demyelination, and Gliosis*

T2- and PD-weighted images allow discrimination of MS lesions from the surrounding normal appearing white matter because of lesional changes in the water proton T2 relaxation time and content. These techniques are very sensitive to pathology; even direct inspection of unfixed brains at post-mortem examination does not reveal all the lesions seen on T2-weighted images of the same specimens (Newcombe *et al.*, 1991), for example.

The sensitivity of the proton density or T2-weighted image for MS lesions is important for diagnosis, but as a routine follow-up implement it is pathologically nonspecific. Histopathological studies of biopsy material show that areas of hyperintense signal on T2-weighted MRI define the whole spectrum of MS lesion evolution from pathologically early active, through late active to chronic inactive and including remyelinating lesions (Bruck *et al.*, 1997; van Waesberghe *et al.*, 1999).

While both acute and chronic lesions show contrast changes with PD- or T2-weighted imaging, the underlying pathological correlations may vary (Table 32.3). Consider the pathological changes potentially associated with increased signal on PD-weighted images, for example. Acute lesions show increased water content with breakdown of the BBB and associated transudation of soluble serum proteins. Chronic lesions have increased water content with reduced myelin lipids and changes in cellularity with a greater glial component. These different mechanisms and the differences in the extent of associated increases in water content lead to subtle, time-dependent changes in lesion appearance. Lesions that are less than approximately 30 days old, for example, have a pattern of central hyperintensity in the PD-weighted image. Around 2 to 3 months of age, approximately 60% of lesions acquire a ring-like appearance with a darker central core and brighter periphery. This may correspond with more extensive demyelination and other chronic changes centrally, and with active inflammation at the lesion rim (Guttmann *et al.*, 1995).

Similarly, quantitatively different changes in T2 relaxation might define differences in pathology more specifically. Early active lesions, for example, have a border of decreased intensity contrasting with a brighter center (Bruck *et al.*, 1997). More recent studies with direct measurement of T2 relaxation times eventually might allow this specificity to be applied to discrimination of different lesions types (Santos *et al.*, 2002), although at present the spatial resolution for these T2 relaxometric techniques is substantially lower than for the structural images, limiting their practical application.

Serially acquired T2-weighted images emphasize that the pathology of MS is evolving continuously (Fig. 32.6); clinical relapses identify only a minority of new lesions. In general, there may be as much as a 10-fold greater activity defined by T2-weighted MRI than from clinical course (Miller *et al.*, 1997). Asymptomatic lesions may either be in noneloquent parts of the CNS, represent less destructive pathology, or develop slowly enough that functional adaptation may occur to prevent their expression.

### T1-Weighted MRI Allows Visualization of Matrix Destruction in Lesions

As noted earlier, T2- or PD-weighted hyperintense lesions are pathologically nonspecific. An attractive approach to improving specificity is to combine definitions of pathology

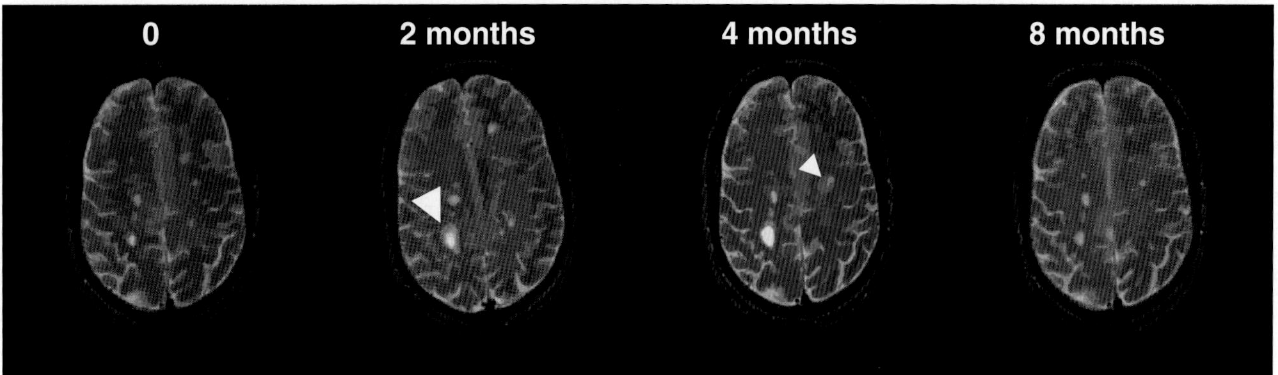


FIGURE 32.6
MRI demonstrates dynamic changes in T2 hyperintense lesion size and distribution. These serially acquired T2-weighted MRI scans from the same level of the brain of a patient with multiple sclerosis demonstrate both lesion growth (large arrow) and lesion shrinkage (small arrow) over time.

based on T2-weighted imaging with a different range of pathological sensitivity acquired using different pulse sequences. One of the most practical efforts toward this integration is the study of T1 hypointensity, arising from increases in water T1 or an increased proportion of free water in lesions. Uhlenbrock and Sehlen (1989) described focal T1-hypointensities or "black holes" in some T2-hyperintense lesions in brains of patients with MS. They postulated that they represented regions of axonal loss and gliosis (Table 32.3). This was confirmed for chronic lesions by post-mortem studies (Bruck *et al.*, 1997; van Walderveen *et al.*, 1998; van Waesberghe *et al.*, 1999). T1 hypointensity in acute lesions may be less pathologically specific as it is significantly influenced by the acute edema.

Axonal loss is the major determinant of chronic disability (Matthews *et al.*, 1998). Not surprisingly, therefore, increases in the volume of chronic T1-hypointensity are related to progression of disability. In a pioneering study (Truyen *et al.*, 1996), T1 lesion load was found to be more strongly correlated with disability than the less pathologically specific T2 hyperintense lesion load. Objective definition of focal T1 lesions using voxel-by-voxel T1-mapping has confirmed that the volume of the most abnormally prolonged T1 is correlated strongly with disability (Parry *et al.*, 2002a). These observations have led to increasingly widespread use of the chronic T1-hypointense lesion volume as a measure of the progression of pathology relevant to disability.

## Visualization of Focal Demyelination

Myelin is a primary target of tissue damage in MS. Understanding the dynamics of myelin loss and its repair by remyelination therefore is an important goal for *in vivo* pathological studies of MS. The lack of specificity of T1 and T2 relaxation time changes limits their usefulness as MR-based indices of myelin damage.

MT imaging defines changes in biophysical parameters that are altered by myelin loss more selectively than are water proton T1 or T2 (McGowan, 1999) (Table 32.3). The most direct evidence for this has come from correlative pathological and imaging studies of a primate model (Brochet and Dousset, 1999). In this EAE model, there is a close correlation between MTR changes prior to sacrifice and histopathological changes of demyelination post-mortem.

An alternative and promising newer technique for myelin visualization is selective imaging of the component of water with a very short T2 relaxation time (about 20 msec), which includes water trapped between the layers of myelin (Fig. 32.7) (Laule *et al.*, 2002; Webb *et al.*, 2002). This short T2 water may be more specific for myelin than water associated with macromolecules in general and correlates extremely well with myelin content on histological examination (Gareau *et al.*, 2000). MacKay and his coworkers (MacKay *et al.*, 1994) have spatially mapped the amount of this "myelin water" in the brains of patients with MS. Post-mortem studies confirmed an association between loss of the short T2 component and

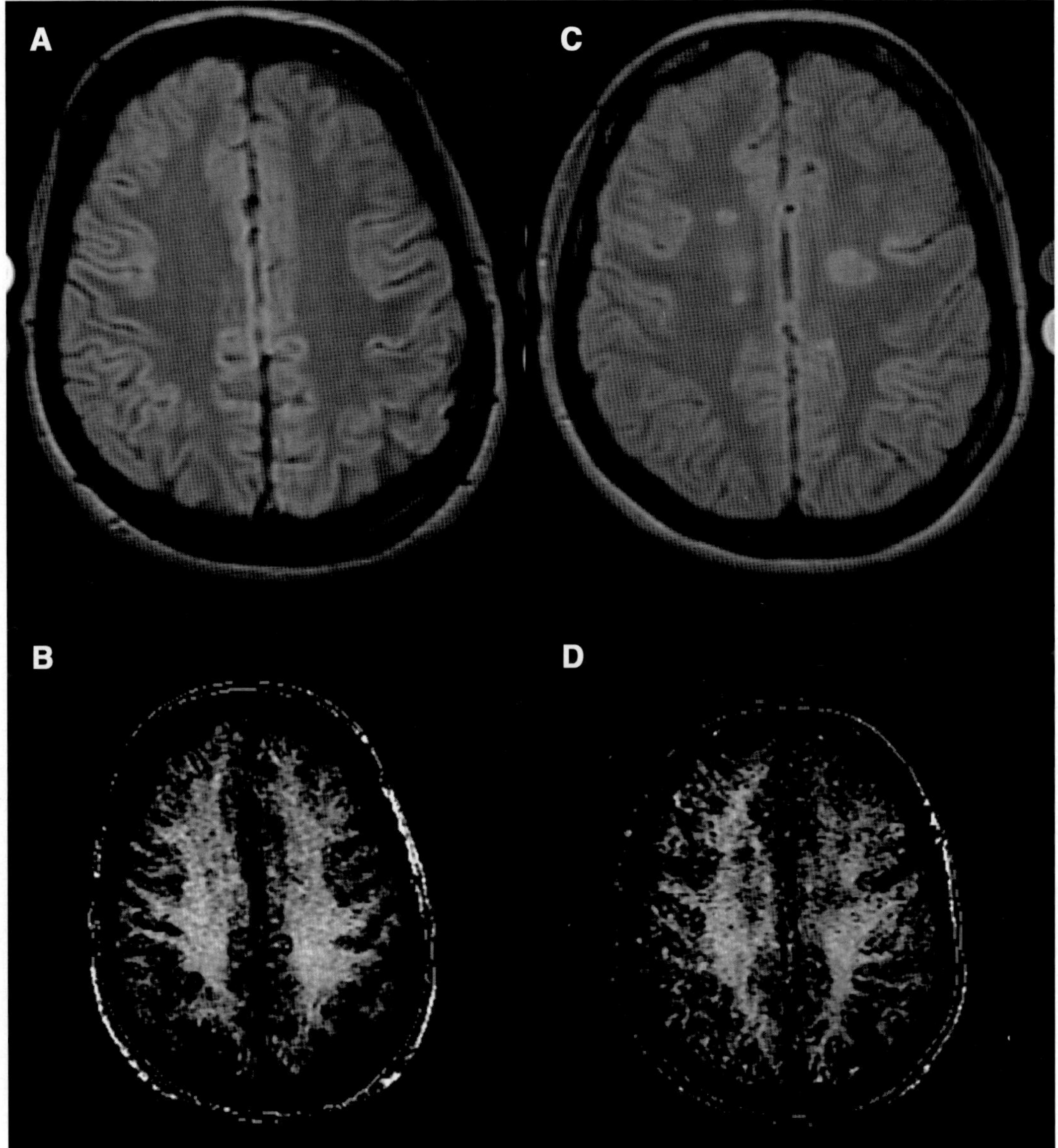


FIGURE 32.7
Mapping the distribution of the short T2-relaxation time component of the tissue water relaxation decay curve for the brain may help to identify myelin distribution. Water associated with myelin may have the shortest T2 relaxation time of any brain water compartment. In a normal brain (A) the water short T2 relaxation time component distribution is relatively evenly distributed over the central white matter (B). In contrast, in a patient with multiple sclerosis and focal white matter lesions (C), the short T2 component is reduced particularly in areas of focal lesions, suggesting demyelination. (Images courtesy of C. Laule and A. McKay, University of British Columbia).

demyelination (Moore *et al.*, 2000). The myelin-associated water content may be more than 50% lower in lesions than in the surrounding white matter (Laule *et al.*, 2002). A limitation to the technique at present is the long time necessary for acquisition of the full relaxation time dataset, as well as the hardware and analytical demands for measuring such short relaxation time components of the total water relaxation accurately.

There is a general problem with the interpretation of changes in MT or myelin-associated water exclusively in terms of demyelination, as myelin and axonal loss usually occur concomitantly (Arnold *et al.*, 1992; van Waesberghe *et al.*, 1999). Thus, while MT is sensitive to demyelination, it is difficult in practice to quantitatively assess the extent of demyelination independent of axonal loss using MT alone (Filippi, 1999).

Quantitative evaluation of myelin integrity also suggests that not all the pathology in MS is confined to focal lesions. In the extra-lesional white matter there are in fact changes relative to healthy white matter, although these are more modest than in focal lesions. T2 compartmentation studies, for example, suggest an increase in total water content of about 2% and a reduction in myelin-associated water content of approximately 15% in the so-called normal-appearing white matter (NAWM) (Laule *et al.*, 2002).

## MRI VISUALIZATION OF DIFFUSE WHITE MATTER INVOLVEMENT IN MS

Pathologists traditionally have focused attention on the plaques of MS. An important general contribution of MRI techniques has been to emphasize the importance of pathology outside of the lesions. It is becoming increasingly clear that in established MS *all* white matter shows some evidence of pathological change if techniques with appropriate sensitivity are used. A compelling reason to be interested in these diffuse changes is that the focal lesion load in a typical MS brain constitutes at most a few percent of the total white matter volume: the bulk of changes occurs diffusely.

### Magnetic Resonance Spectroscopy for Assessment of Diffuse Axonal Injury and Loss

None of the MRI techniques that measure signals from water are able to directly detect and quantify the dysfunction of neurons and their axonal processes. However, this information can be obtained from MRS or MRSI (Rudkin and Arnold, 1999).

In one of the earliest MRS reports (Arnold *et al.*, 1992), N-acetylaspartate (NAA) was shown to be decreased in MS patients when a large central brain volume of interest was used for acquisition of the proton spectrum. N-acetylaspartate is a specific marker of axonal integrity in the adult central nervous system (Clark, 1998; Matthews and Arnold, 2001; Simmons *et al.*, 1991; Trapp *et al.*, 1998; Tsai and Coyle, 1995) (Table 32.3). As the volume of lesions within the large spectroscopic volume was small, the bulk of changes must have occurred diffusely in the normal-appearing tissue, which was predominantly NAWM. A diffuse decrease of white matter NAA has been subsequently observed in many studies (Cucurella *et al.*, 2000; De Stefano *et al.*, 2001; Fu *et al.*, 1998; Husted *et al.*, 1994; Leary *et al.*, 1999; Sarchielli *et al.*, 1999; Tedeschi *et al.*, 2002). The extent of the diffuse reduction of NAA measured by MRS is at least approximately consistent with the relative loss of axons measured directly in white matter projection volumes using histopathological methods. The relative contribution of extra-lesional NAA decrease is different in patients with RR and SP disease and accounts for the axonal injury and loss that correlates best with the progression of disability (Matthews *et al.*, 1996).

Later studies directly contrasted the relative concentrations of NAA within lesions and in surrounding white matter. Decreases are most marked in lesions, but smaller reductions also occur outside of plaques. It remains unclear how much of the diffuse loss is due to secondary consequences of axonal transection in focal lesions (anterograde or retrograde degeneration), diffuse inflammation, or a more primary neurodegenerative process. The extent of this NAA reduction decreases with the distance from the core of a lesion (Arnold *et al.*, 1992), consistent with the notion that the diffuse changes are at least in part related to dying back of axons transected (Trapp *et al.*, 1998) within plaques. There is also a correlation between the extent of diffuse axon loss and local lesion load suggested both by spectroscopic imaging (Matthews *et al.*, 1996) and direct histopathological observations (Evangelou *et al.*, 2000).

Although retrograde or anterograde changes resulting from focal lesions contribute to the diffuse abnormalities, other factors may be involved. Diffusible toxins such as proteolytic enzymes, cytokines and nitric oxide, and other free radicals may damage axons and glial cells outside, and sometimes at a considerable distance from, the focal lesions. Immunoglobulins directed against both neurons and oligodendroylial cells may cause damage or dysfunction (Bauer *et al.*, 2001; Rieckmann and Smith, 2001).

## Brain and Spinal Cord Atrophy: Measures of Neuronal and Glial Changes

Diffuse damage also is demonstrated by atrophy of brain and spinal cord. Many measures of atrophy based on imaging have been proposed. Although these vary in sensitivity to change and to some extent in their regional specificity, they commonly demonstrate enhanced rates of loss of CNS parenchyma in MS. Rates of volume change are in general well correlated with the progression of disability in later stages of MS (Losseff *et al.*, 1996b).

A striking finding from recent longitudinal MRI studies has been that brain and spinal cord atrophy begins early in the disease. RR patients with mild disability may have substantially increased rates of brain substance loss, both in the white and the gray matter (Chard *et al.*, 2002). Significant cerebral atrophy reflected in lateral ventricular enlargement can occur even in the interval between the first clinical presentation and clinical diagnosis of MS (Brex *et al.*, 2000).

The specific tissue changes that contribute to the genesis of this atrophy remain uncertain (Miller *et al.*, 2002). These likely include axonal loss and demyelination in the white matter, as well as glial changes in chronic lesions. In gray matter changes in myelin content and axonal loss are also found, as well as atrophy of dendritic arborisations and loss of neurons. It is likely, but not well established, that the relative contributions of atrophy in different tissue compartments may change during the course of the disease. The primary utility of atrophy as a marker of disease progression lies in the extent to which its magnitude and rate of increase reflect irreversible nervous system injury and are correlated with disability and its worsening (Edwards *et al.*, 1999; Losseff *et al.*, 1996b; Nijeholt *et al.*, 1998). As atrophy can be measured from serially acquired T1-weighted images entirely automatically (Stevenson *et al.*, 2002), it also provides a measure that is reasonably sensitive to change and not very demanding of special hardware or analysis capabilities.

There is evidence that the rate of atrophy may be related to inflammatory activity, at least in the RR stage of MS. The number of Gd-enhancing lesions at baseline in the placebo arm of an interferon-beta trial predicted the relative extent of atrophy over the subsequent 2-year period (Simon *et al.*, 1998), a finding supported by cross-sectional (Lin and Blumhardt, 2001) and longitudinal (Leist *et al.*, 2001) studies. However, this relationship may either be variable or potentially confounded by other factors (Paolillo *et al.*, 2000; Rudick *et al.*, 1999; Saindane *et al.*, 2000). One factor likely to contribute is time after injury, perhaps because demyelinated axons are chronically deprived of the trophic support of myelin. A recent study has shown that optic nerve atrophy continues for more than two years after an episode of optic neuritis (Hickman *et al.*, 2002). However, whether some degree of ongoing, subclinical inflammatory activity might contribute to this apparent progressive axonal degeneration is at present unresolved.

## Other Quantitative Techniques That Show Diffuse White Matter Abnormalities

Other quantitative measures provide further evidence for diffuse pathology. The MTR is diffusely low in white matter of patients with MS (Catalaa *et al.*, 2000; Cercignani *et al.*, 2001; Ge *et al.*, 2002; Guo *et al.*, 2001; Siger-Zajdel and Selmaj, 2001). Water proton relaxation time measurements also show diffuse changes in the NAWM (Miller *et al.*, 1989; Ormerod *et al.*, 1986). Recent data from a novel, rapid T1 mapping technique have defined changes in the T1 relaxation time histogram for extra-lesional white matter that are strongly correlated with disability (Parry *et al.*, 2002a). T2-relaxation times may be similarly diffusely prolonged in white matter of MS patients (Barbosa *et al.*, 1994). Finally, diffusion anisotropy measurements also show significant increases in white matter that appears normal on conventional imaging (Bammer *et al.*, 2000; Cercignani *et al.*, 2000; Christiansen *et al.*, 1993; Ciccarelli *et al.*, 2001; Filippi *et al.*, 2000, 2001; Guo *et al.*, 2001; Horsfield *et al.*, 1996; Rocca *et al.*, 2000; Werring *et al.*, 1999, 2001).

Recent histopathological studies have confirmed the substantial diffuse damage in the white matter suggested by imaging studies (Allen *et al.*, 2001). Ferguson and coworkers (1997) noted that the expression of amyloid precursor protein (APP), a marker of axonal injury, was abnormally elevated around active chronic lesions. Trapp *et al.* (1998) have reported abnormal hypophosphorylated neurofilaments in axons outside of lesions. More recent work has directly measured the diffuse axonal loss and matrix changes distant from plaques. Ganter and coworkers (1999) noted that the density of axons in cervical thoracic spinal cord outside of lesions was reduced up to 42% relative to controls. Further work by Evangelou *et al.* (Evangelou *et al.*, 2000) showed that in the corpus collosum, a brain region ideal for axon quantification because of the highly oriented structure, axonal density was reduced by approximately 35% outside of lesions. An important observation in this study was that both axonal density and the cross-sectional area of the corpus collosum decrease in MS patients, suggesting that independent measures of either brain volume or axonal density changes underestimate the total injury in the diffuse white matter.

## MRI VISUALIZATION OF GRAY MATTER PATHOLOGY IN MS

Lesions have long been described in gray matter (Brownell and Hughes, 1962; Lumsden, 1970). The relative lack of previous appreciation for the importance of gray matter abnormalities arose because traditional pathological approaches (Peterson *et al.*, 2001) are relatively insensitive to cortical lesions. Conventional T2-weighted imaging also is insensitive to these gray matter changes (Kidd *et al.*, 1999; Miller *et al.*, 1998). For example, in a post-mortem imaging study of unfixed brains, out of 54 gray matter lesions identified histologically, only 2 were detected by T2-weighted MRI (Newcombe *et al.*, 1991). FLAIR imaging increases the sensitivity for cortical lesions, particularly those that are juxtacortical (Bakshi *et al.*, 2001; Boggild *et al.*, 1996; Filippi *et al.*, 1996a; Gawne-Cain *et al.*, 1997), but is still relatively insensitive to the majority of lesions, which are intracortical.

The small sizes of the discrete cortical lesions, and differences in the nature of the inflammatory changes in gray matter lesions and in the structure of gray relative to white matter, likely account for the insensitivity of conventional MRI to gray matter lesions (Peterson *et al.*, 2001). It is also possible that imaging characteristics of gray matter lesions may be fundamentally different from plaques in the white matter. Bakshi *et al.* (2002) have reported that T2-*hypo*intense lesions can be defined in most gray matter regions in patients with established MS. The hypointensity may be related to T2-shortening with deposition of paramagnetic iron in the lesions, a finding associated nonspecifically with neurodegeneration in other contexts.

As more sensitive techniques begin to be applied, it is likely that the contribution of gray matter to the total brain pathology in MS will be shown to be substantial (Chard *et al.*, 2002). Peterson *et al.* (2001) have emphasized that large, confluent volumes of hypomyelination in neocortex are common. While these have not yet been visualized using MRI, imaging suggests that gray matter atrophy may be substantial. Chard *et al.* (2002) demonstrated that as much as 50% of total brain atrophy could be ascribed to neocortical atrophy in RR MS. Because gray matter constitutes well over 50% of brain volume, gray matter atrophy contributes profoundly to total brain volume changes. However, these changes are difficult to measure, because the neocortex is so thin. Recent work by Chen *et al.* (2002) has attempted to more precisely define the loss of neocortex in different stages of multiple sclerosis. Substantial loss was shown both in early RR and later SP stages. Although the sample was limited, the data suggested that the relative contribution of the neocortical volume loss to total brain atrophy was substantially greater in RR than in the SP patients. In fact, loss of neocortex accounted for most of the total brain atrophy in patients in the earlier stages of the disease.

MRS measurements have shown significant decreases in NAA in the neocortex of MS patients, consistent with neuronal or axonal injury (Kapeller *et al.*, 2001; Presciutti *et al.*, 2000). This NAA reduction, however, could also be explained by a retraction of dendritic arborisation in the gray matter (Tseng and Hu, 1996). Interpretation of these findings is confounded by the concomitant development of atrophy and partial volume effects.

This problem was addressed by Cifelli and coworkers (2002), who studied neurodegeneration in the thalamus using either MRS or histopathological methods for similar SP MS cohorts. Because the thalamus does not include sulcal CSF spaces, its MRS investigation can be performed without the confound of partial volume effects. Using a specially tailored MRI sequence that defined the borders of the thalamus well, Cifelli *et al.* (2002) demonstrated a mean 17% loss of thalamic volume in patients with SP MS (Fig. 32.8). This was associated with a 19% decrease in the relative NAA concentration (a measure of the loss of neuronal or axonal density) to suggest a total neuronal loss of about 30%. In a parallel histopathological study with comparable post-mortem specimens, they measured a similar volume loss in the mediodorsal nucleus of the thalamus directly and showed that this was associated with a 22% loss of neuronal density, a 21% loss of volume and thus a total loss of neurons of about 35%, which is comparable to the decrease defined *in vivo*. Just as in the earlier studies of axonal loss in the corpus callosum, both neuronal density loss and tissue volume loss contributed to estimation of the total change. More recently, this work was extended to patients with RR MS, who showed similar changes, the magnitude of which was related to the duration of disease (Wylezinska *et al.*, 2003).

Together, these MRS and atrophy studies emphasize that gray matter pathology contributes a substantial proportion of the load of disease in MS. Differences in gray matter pathology could account for the apparent lack of a consistent association between measures of focal white matter disease and disability across different clinical subtypes of MS. The differences in sensitivity of MR measures to gray and white matter abnormalities emphasize the need to use multiple MR-based techniques simultaneously in order to describe the full range of pathology in this disease.

## VISUALIZATION OF "PRELESIONAL" CHANGES

Although all focal lesion changes may not be initiated by a phase of increased BBB permeability, until recently Gd-enhancement was the earliest focal change that could be

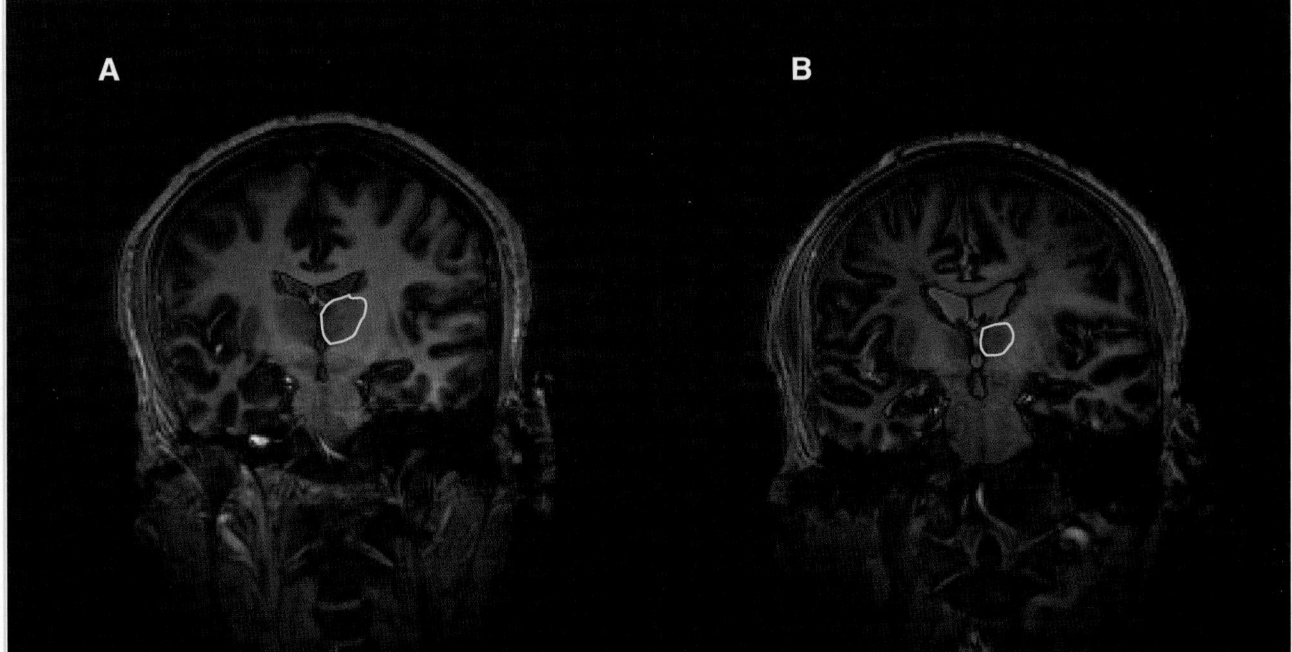


**FIGURE 32.8**
The acquisition parameters of these MRI images have been optimized by means of simulations in order to achieve high contrast between central gray matter and surrounding white matter. Moderate enlargement of both lateral and third ventricles can be noted in the MS patient (B). Volume loss of the thalamic gray matter can also be observed in the patient as compared with the normal control (A).

detected in the evolution of new lesions. However, other, quantitative MR techniques reveal focal changes in NAWM that precede Gd-enhancement and the appearance of T2-weighted hyperintensity. Spectroscopy acquisitions at short TE can reveal signals from mobile macromolecules (which arise mainly from lipids): they become MRS-visible due to increases in mobility associated with demyelination. In their longitudinal study, Narayana and his colleagues (1998) found examples of the focal appearance of lipid peaks in regions that later developed new T2-hyperintense lesions. De Stefano and colleagues (2001) found a focal increase in Cho preceding the development of new T2 lesions. This suggests that low-grade, focal myelin pathology may antedate the development of acute, severe inflammation.

Focal MTR changes also can occur prior to the appearance of T2-hyperintense lesions. Filippi's group (1998) serially studied RR patients over 3 months and outlined the contours of new enhancing lesions. These regions then were mapped onto coregistered MT images acquired at previous time points. Even before lesion development, MTR was focally reduced in these volumes. Changes were progressive and proportionally higher in the month preceding enhancement. Similar findings have been described by others (Goodkin *et al.*, 1998). A more recent study (Pike *et al.*, 2000) based on less frequent scanning over a much longer period demonstrated subtle MTR changes predating the development of T2 lesions by years. The rates of change of MTR were remarkably consistent before and after lesion appearance, suggesting that the pathology associated with MTR decline is continuous and accelerates only transiently during the acute inflammation associated with Gd-enhancement and new T2 lesion formation.

## ADAPTIVE REORGANIZATION CAN BE VISUALIZED USING FUNCTIONAL MAGNETIC RESONANCE IMAGING (FMRI)

### Forms of Adaptive Reorganization after Brain Injury in MS

Recovery from the brain injury of MS involves several mechanisms that can be visualized by MR-based techniques. Resolution of the primary inflammation and repair of myelin must have a role, which can be demonstrated as reduction of Gd-enhancement and resolution of T2-hyperintensity, respectively. Also, impairment (and partial restoration) of axonal and neuronal metabolic function takes place and can be monitored by changes in NAA. However, an increasingly strong case can be made for the importance of adaptive cerebral plasticity, which can occur at a number of levels:

1. Axonal, with expression of new sodium channels (Waxman, 2001)
2. Neuronal, with enhanced dendritic arborisation from surviving neurons (Jones and Schallert, 1992)
3. Synaptic, with changes in synapse number or distribution with respect to the soma
4. Systems organization, with altered recruitment of parallel processing pathways or other "latent connections" (Jacobs and Donoghue, 1991)

FMRI is proving useful in defining the systems-level changes directly. Animal studies have shown a direct correlation between behavior and electrophysiologically defined changes in the cortical representations for movement or sensation in primary motor cortex around focal lesions. For example, after an ischaemic lesion of the hand area in the motor cortex of an adult squirrel monkey, the hand movement representation changed over time after infarction (Nudo *et al.*, 1996). However, while with injury alone the hand representation decreased by at least 25%, if aggressive physiotherapy was used the representation could *increase* by 10%. The increased representation in some areas occurs at the expense of neighboring regions and is correlated with improved function. Cortical reorganization also can occur at a distance from a focal lesion. Dendritic remodeling is stimulated in homotopic neocortex contralateral to a focal injury. Immobilization of the paretic limb prevents the dendritic growth and impairs functional recovery (Kozlowski *et al.*, 1996).

## Functional Magnetic Resonance Imaging (FMRI): Imaging Functional Reorganization of the Human Brain after Injury from MS

FMRI allows patterns of brain activation associated with sensory, motor or cognitive tasks to be mapped with greater sensitivity than was possible before (Matthews, 2001). FMRI demonstrates a widely distributed network of regions involved in the control of even a simple hand movement, for example. Differences in the patterns of activity in such a network can be defined between patients and healthy controls (Rocca *et al.*, 2002a, 2002b). One of the most consistent findings has been relatively increased ipsilateral motor cortex activation (Lee *et al.*, 2000; Pantano *et al.*, 2002). Just as has been demonstrated with white matter ischaemic disease (Reddy *et al.*, 2002a), in MS there is a strong correlation between increasing disease burden and the extent of the functional changes (Lee *et al.*, 2000; Pantano *et al.*, 2002; Rocca *et al.*, 2002a).

The functional changes identified also appear to be dynamic, just like the pathology of MS. In a case report based on the study of a relapsing-remitting MS patient with a very large demyelinating lesion of the left hemisphere and resolving right hemiplegia, Reddy *et al.* (2000b) correlated serially acquired measures of clinical evolution, lesion size assessed from conventional MRI, biochemical pathology defined with magnetic resonance spectroscopic imaging (MRSI), and relative cortical activation during a finger-thumb opposition paradigm with fMRI over the 6 months following presentation of the lesion. The NAA concentrations in the corticospinal tract increased in parallel with recovery from functional impairment. Abnormal patterns of fMRI activation were found throughout the period of study. Although the extent of the abnormality was greatest when the lesion was largest and NAA in the corticospinal tracts was lower fMRI activation remained abnormal even after apparent clinical recovery of motor function. Together, these observations are consistent with the hypothesis that the changes are functionally adaptive, although often only incompletely so.

In some cases, cortical areas related to polymodal or higher levels of processing may become more involved with injury to primary pathways in sensory system. Werring *et al.* (2000) made the intriguing observation that patients who had suffered from optic neuritis showed reduced primary visual cortical activation with photic stimulation, but increased activation of extra-striate visual areas, including polymodal sensory areas such as the claustrum. The apparent relationship to primary tissue injury was demonstrated by a correlation between delay in the P100 visual evoked potential peak and extent of extra-striate activations.

## Adaptive Change May Limit the Clinical Expression of Deficits in MS

A common concern in the interpretation of imaging studies of brain plasticity is that the activation changes observed might not be due to adaptive phenomena, but instead could simply result from differences in performance between the patients and healthy subjects. Performance cannot be easily controlled for in studies of movement. Even if behavior is similar, the relative difficulty or "effortfulness" may not be well matched (Lee *et al.*, 2000). One partial solution to this conundrum is the study of patients without any clinical deficits for the movement under examination. Reddy and colleagues (Reddy *et al.*, 2000a), for example, studied MS patients without any clinically evident motor or sensory impairment in the upper limbs with a finger flexion-extension paradigm. Even in these patients (whose behavior was well matched with the healthy controls), there was a strong correlation between the extent of ipsilateral sensorimotor cortex activation and concentration of NAA in voxels localized to the descending corticospinal tract.

An alternative approach is to use a task that reports on elements of relevance to motor control but that is intrinsically well matched between patients and healthy controls. Because of the rich, reciprocal innervations between motor and sensory cortex, passive movement of the hand activates cortical regions that would be active with a similar, active movement (Reddy *et al.*, 2001, 2002c). Comparison of fMRI activation patterns associated with active and passive hand movements in patients and healthy controls confirmed that differences in patterns of activation related to disease burden can be found even when performance and its difficulty is matched (Reddy *et al.*, 2002b).

However, disease burden is just one factor that may contribute to determining the extent of functional reorganization with MS. A recent study attempted to test whether altered patterns of limb use have a distinct and *direct* influence on patterns of brain organization. Three groups of MS patients with different degrees of disability and white matter disease burden as assessed from brain atrophy and NAA decreases were studied (Reddy *et al.*, 2002b). One group had no evidence of either substantial injury or functional impairment, a second group had significant white matter injury but no upper limb impairment, and the final group had a similar burden of brain injury but showed substantial upper limb impairment. Contrast of patients with no hand impairment, but with reduced or normal white matter NAA, showed significant activation increases in the ipsilateral premotor cortex and the supplementary motor area bilaterally. To assess whether disability itself can alter patterns of cortical activation associated with hand weakness, a contrast was made between patients with decreased NAA and either impaired or unimpaired hand function. This contrast demonstrated greater bilateral primary and secondary somatosensory cortex activation with greater limb disability. The authors concluded that the pattern of cerebral activity with finger movements changes independently both with increasing injury and with increasing disability. It was hypothesized that the changes related to disability may be caused by altered patterns of use.

Potentially adaptive functional changes also may occur with purely cognitive processes. In a study of MS patients with mild neuropsychological deficits, Staffen *et al.* demonstrated that patients show abnormal, increased recruitment of prefrontal cortex (corresponding approximately to Brodman areas 6, 8, and 9) during a visual serial addition task. Parry *et al.* (2002b) identified abnormally increased activity in a similar region of frontopolar cortex in MS patients performing the Stroop task, a test of executive function, and demonstrated that the extent of recruitment of this region is increased with greater disease burden (Fig. 32.9).

Functional imaging has the potential to identify regions that may be critical for the genesis of symptoms difficult to localize using conventional strategies. Filippi's group (Filippi *et al.*, 2002) applied a simple hand movement paradigm to distinguish brain activity changes associated with MS-related fatigue. MS patients with fatigue showed relative increases in brain activity in several brain regions, including the thalamus, intraparietal sulcus, and rolandic operculum. The extent of the increases in these regions were correlated with fatigue scores, suggesting that activity in these areas may contribute to the genesis of symptoms.

## CONCLUSIONS

MRI and related MR-based techniques offer an increasingly comprehensive view of the pathology of MS. Because these methods are noninvasive and well tolerated, longitudinal studies have allowed the dynamics of pathological changes to be defined directly. Such studies have emphasized that clinical expression has a complex relation to the underlying dynamics of the pathological change, suggesting that maybe the latter should be targeted directly in neurobiologically driven, rational treatment strategies.

While inflammatory demyelination may be the most obvious histological feature of MS, imaging studies have led to a shift in focus toward associated pathologies. It has become clear that axonal and neuronal loss, rather than the damage to myelin, is responsible for the irreversible progression of disability. One important consequence of this concept is that it links strategies for limiting disability in MS to those for control of progression in the broad range of primary neurodegenerative diseases.

With the advent of functional imaging methods, it may be expected that better characterization of previously poorly understood symptoms such as fatigue, attentional, and memory impairments will be possible. In general, by allowing clear relationships to be

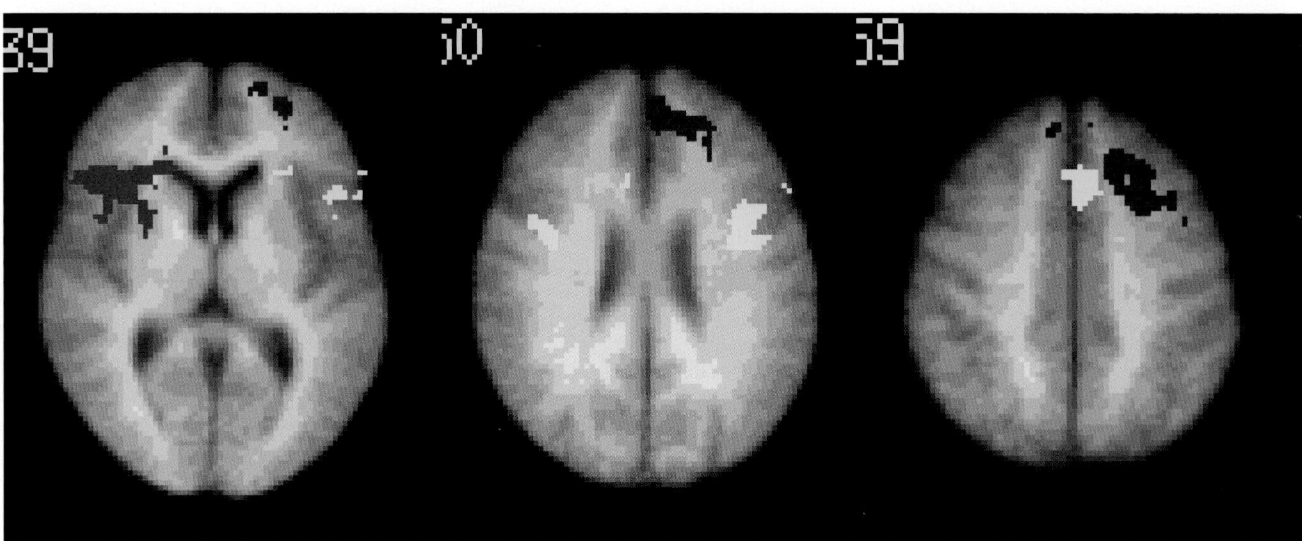


FIGURE 32.9
Functional magnetic resonance imaging can define altered patterns of brain activation with cognitive tasks in patients with multiple sclerosis. The Stroop paradigm is a test of executive function demanding inhibition of a preferred response. The counting Stroop task, for example, demands subjects to report the number of words presented on a screen. The words may be either neutral words (e.g., cat, dog) or number words (e.g., three, four). Response times for the latter are prolonged relative to the former, because of the need to suppress answers based on the words' meaning rather than their number. In healthy controls, this produces activation in multiple areas (red and yellow). Patients with multiple sclerosis activate similar areas (yellow), but fail to show significant activation in the right inferior frontal cortex (red). Unlike controls, they show significant activation in predominantly left frontopolar areas (blue). Activation in the frontopolar areas relative to the right inferior frontal area is related directly to disease burden.

established between structural, functional, and behavioral changes in *individual* patients, imaging is ushering in an exciting new era of MRI-based pathology that should play a critical role in relieving suffering from this disease.

## Acknowledgments

AC and PMM thank the MS Society of Great Britain and Northern Ireland and the Medical Research Council, and DLA thanks the MS Society of Canada and the Canadian Institutes of Health Research for support. All of us acknowledge the considerable assistance we have received over the years from our many collaborators, particularly those within the Brain Imaging Laboratory Linkage.

## References

Allen, I. V., McQuaid, S., Mirakhur, M., and Nevin, G. (2001). Pathological abnormalities in the normal-appearing white matter in multiple sclerosis. *Neurol. Sci.* **22,** 141–144.

Arnold, D. L., and Matthews, P. M. (2002). MRI in the diagnosis and management of multiple sclerosis. *Neurology* **58,** S23-S31.

Arnold, D. L., Matthews, P. M., Francis, G. S., O'Connor, J., and Antel, J. P. (1992). Proton magnetic resonance spectroscopic imaging for metabolic characterization of demyelinating plaques. *Ann. Neurol.* **31,** 235–241.

Bakshi, R., Ariyaratana, S., Benedict, R. H., and Jacobs, L. (2001). Fluid-attenuated inversion recovery magnetic resonance imaging detects cortical and juxtacortical multiple sclerosis lesions. *Arch. Neurol.* **58,** 742–748.

Bakshi, R., Benedict, R. H., Bermel, R. A., Caruthers, S. D., Puli, S. R., Tjoa, C. W., Fabiano, A. J., and Jacobs, L. (2002). T2 hypointensity in the deep gray matter of patients with multiple sclerosis: A quantitative magnetic resonance imaging study. *Arch. Neurol.* **59,** 62–68.

Bammer, R., Augustin, M., Strasser-Fuchs, S., Seifert, T., Kapeller, P., Stollberger, R., Ebner, F., Hartung, H. P., and Fazekas, F. (2000). Magnetic resonance diffusion tensor imaging for characterizing diffuse and focal white matter abnormalities in multiple sclerosis. *Magn Reson. Med.* **44,** 583–591.

Barbosa, S., Blumhardt, L. D., Roberts, N., Lock, T., and Edwards, R. H. (1994). Magnetic resonance relaxation time mapping in multiple sclerosis: normal appearing white matter and the "invisible" lesion load. *Magn. Reson. Imaging*. **12,** 33–42.

Barkhof, F., Filippi, M., Miller, D. H., Scheltens, P., Campi, A., Polman, C. H., Comi, G., Ader, H. J., Losseff, N., and Valk, J. (1997). Comparison of MRI criteria at first presentation to predict conversion to clinically definite multiple sclerosis. *Brain* **120** (Pt. 11), 2059–2069.

Barkhof, F., and van Walderveen, M. (1999). Characterization of tissue damage in multiple sclerosis by nuclear magnetic resonance. *Philos. Trans. R. Soc. Lond B Biol. Sci.* **354,** 1675–1686.

Barkhof, F., and Scheltens, P. (2002). Imaging of white matter lesions. *Cerebrovasc. Dis.* **13 Suppl 2,** 21–30.

Bauer, J., Rauschka, H., and Lassmann, H. (2001). Inflammation in the nervous system: The human perspective. *Glia* **36,** 235–243.

Bergers, E., Bot, J. C., van, d., V, Castelijns, J. A., Nijeholt, G. J., Kamphorst, W., Polman, C. H., Blezer, E. L., Nicolay, K., Ravid, R., and Barkhof, F. (2002). Diffuse signal abnormalities in the spinal cord in multiple sclerosis: direct postmortem in situ magnetic resonance imaging correlated with in vitro high-resolution magnetic resonance imaging and histopathology. *Ann. Neurol.* **51,** 652–656.

Bitsch, A., Bruhn, H., Vougioukas, V., Stringaris, A., Lassmann, H., Frahm, J., and Bruck, W. (1999). Inflammatory CNS demyelination: histopathologic correlation with in vivo quantitative proton MR spectroscopy. *AJNR Am. J. Neuroradiol.* **20,** 1619–1627.

Bjartmar, C., Kidd, G., Mork, S., Rudick, R., and Trapp, B. D. (2000). Neurological disability correlates with spinal cord axonal loss and reduced N-acetyl aspartate in chronic multiple sclerosis patients. *Ann. Neurol.* **48,** 893–901.

Boggild, M. D., Williams, R., Haq, N., and Hawkins, C. P. (1996). Cortical plaques visualised by fluid-attenuated inversion recovery imaging in relapsing multiple sclerosis. *Neuroradiology* **38 Suppl 1,** S10-S13.

Brass, S. D., Santos, A. C., Francis, S. J., Caramanos, Z., Parrilla, G., Lapierre, Y., Levesque, I., Narayanan, S., Sled, J. G., Pike, G. B., and Arnold, D. L. (2002a). Regional variations of quantitative magnetisation transfer imaging parameters in normal-appearing gray matter and normal-appearing white matter in multiple sclerosis. *Proc. Int. Soc. Magn. Reson. Med.* **10,** 1178.

Brass, S. D., Santos, A. C., Francis, Caramanos, Z., Parrilla, G., Lapierre, Y., Levesque, I., Narayanan, S., Sled, J. G., Pike, G. B., and Arnold, D. L. (2002b). Quantitative magnetization transfer imaging parameters in white matter, grey matter, and lesions in patients with multiple sclerosis compared to normal controls. *Proc. Int. Soc. Magn. Reson. Med.* **10,** 1179.

Brex, P. A., Ciccarelli, O., O'Riordan, J. I., Sailer, M., Thompson, A. J., and Miller, D. H. (2002). A longitudinal study of abnormalities on MRI and disability from multiple sclerosis. *N. Engl. J. Med.* **346,** 158–164.

Brex, P. A., Jenkins, R., Fox, N. C., Crum, W. R., O'Riordan, J. I., Plant, G. T., and Miller, D. H. (2000). Detection of ventricular enlargement in patients at the earliest clinical stage of MS. *Neurology* **54,** 1689–1691.

Brochet, B., and Dousset, V. (1999). Pathological correlates of magnetization transfer imaging abnormalities in animal models and humans with multiple sclerosis. *Neurology* **53,** S12-S17.

Brownell, B., and Hughes J. T. (1962). The distribution of plaques in the cerebrum in multiple sclerosis. *J. Neurol. Neurosurg. Psychiat.* **25,** 315–320.

Bruck, W., Bitsch, A., Kolenda, H., Bruck, Y., Stiefel, M., and Lassmann, H. (1997). Inflammatory central nervous system demyelination: correlation of magnetic resonance imaging findings with lesion pathology. *Ann. Neurol.* **42,** 783–793.

Catalaa, I., Grossman, R. I., Kolson, D. L., Udupa, J. K., Nyul, L. G., Wei, L., Zhang, X., Polansky, M., Mannon, L. J., and McGowan, J. C. (2000). Multiple sclerosis: Magnetization transfer histogram analysis of segmented normal-appearing white matter. *Radiology* **216,** 351–355.

Cercignani, M., Bozzali, M., Iannucci, G., Comi, G., and Filippi, M. (2001). Magnetisation transfer ratio and mean diffusivity of normal appearing white and grey matter from patients with multiple sclerosis. *J. Neurol. Neurosurg. Psychiatry* **70,** 311–317.

Cercignani, M., and Horsfield, M. A. (2001). The physical basis of diffusion-weighted MRI. *J. Neurol. Sci.* **186 Suppl 1,** S11-S14.

Cercignani, M., Iannucci, G., and Filippi, M. (1999). Diffusion-weighted imaging in multiple sclerosis. *Ital. J. Neurol. Sci.* **20,** S246-S249.

Cercignani, M., Iannucci, G., Rocca, M. A., Comi, G., Horsfield, M. A., and Filippi, M. (2000). Pathologic damage in MS assessed by diffusion-weighted and magnetization transfer MRI. *Neurology* **54,** 1139–1144.

Chard, D. T., Griffin, C. M., Parker, G. J., Kapoor, R., Thompson, A. J., and Miller, D. H. (2002). Brain atrophy in clinically early relapsing-remitting multiple sclerosis. *Brain* **125,** 327–337.

Chen, J. T., Smith, S. M., Arnold, D. L., and Matthews, P. M. (2002). Quantification of change in cortical grey matter thickness in multiple sclerosis. *Proc. Int. Soc. Magn. Reson. Med.* **10,** 351.

Christiansen, P., Gideon, P., Thomsen, C., Stubgaard, M., Henriksen, O., and Larsson, H. B. (1993). Increased water self-diffusion in chronic plaques and in apparently normal white matter in patients with multiple sclerosis. *Acta Neurol. Scand.* **87,** 195–199.

Ciccarelli, O., Werring, D. J., Wheeler-Kingshott, C. A., Barker, G. J., Parker, G. J., Thompson, A. J., and Miller, D. H. (2001). Investigation of MS normal-appearing brain using diffusion tensor MRI with clinical correlations. *Neurology* **56,** 926–933.

Cifelli, A., Arridge, M., Jezzard, P., Esiri, M. M., Palace, J., and Matthews, P. M. (2002). Thalamic neurodegeneration in multiple sclerosis. *Ann. Neurol. (in press).*

Clark, J. B. (1998). N-acetyl aspartate: a marker for neuronal loss or mitochondrial dysfunction. *Dev. Neurosci.* **20,** 271–276.

Cucurella, M. G., Rovira, A., Rio, J., Pedraza, S., Tintore, M. M., Montalban, X., and Alonso, J. (2000). Proton magnetic resonance spectroscopy in primary and secondary progressive multiple sclerosis. *NMR Biomed.* **13,** 57–63.

Dalton, C. M., Ramani, A., Wheeler-Kingshott, C., Barker, G. J., Miller, D. H., and Tofts, P. S. (2002). Bound water magnetization transfer measurements in patients with multiple sclerosis: a pilot study. *Proc. Int. Soc. Magn. Reson. Med.* **10,** 1180.

De Stefano, N., Narayanan, S., Francis, G. S., Arnaoutelis, R., Tartaglia, M. C., Antel, J. P., Matthews, P. M., and Arnold, D. L. (2001). Evidence of axonal damage in the early stages of multiple sclerosis and its relevance to disability. *Arch. Neurol.* **58,** 65–70.

Edwards, S. G., Gong, Q. Y., Liu, C., Zvartau, M. E., Jaspan, T., Roberts, N., and Blumhardt, L. D. (1999). Infratentorial atrophy on magnetic resonance imaging and disability in multiple sclerosis. *Brain* **122** (Pt. 2), 291–301.

Evangelou, N., Konz, D., Esiri, M. M., Smith, S., Palace, J., and Matthews, P. M. (2000). Regional axonal loss in the corpus callosum correlates with cerebral white matter lesion volume and distribution in multiple sclerosis. *Brain* **123** (Pt. 9), 1845–1849.

Fazekas, F., Offenbacher, H., Fuchs, S., Schmidt, R., Niederkorn, K., Horner, S., and Lechner, H. (1988). Criteria for an increased specificity of MRI interpretation in elderly subjects with suspected multiple sclerosis. *Neurology* **38,** 1822–1825.

Fazekas, F., Strasser-Fuchs, S., Schmidt, H., Enzinger, C., Ropele, S., Lechner, A., Flooh, E., Schmidt, R., and Hartung, H. P. (2000). Apolipoprotein E genotype related differences in brain lesions of multiple sclerosis. *J. Neurol. Neurosurg. Psychiatry* **69,** 25–28.

Ferguson, B., Matyszak, M. K., Esiri, M. M., and Perry, V. H. (1997). Axonal damage in acute multiple sclerosis lesions. *Brain* **120 (Pt 3),** 393–399.

Filippi, M. (1999). Magnetization transfer imaging to monitor the evolution of individual multiple sclerosis lesions. *Neurology* **53,** S18–S22.

Filippi, M., Cercignani, M., Inglese, M., Horsfield, M. A., and Comi, G. (2001). Diffusion tensor magnetic resonance imaging in multiple sclerosis. *Neurology* **56,** 304–311.

Filippi, M., Iannucci, G., Cercignani, M., Assunta, R. M., Pratesi, A., and Comi, G. (2000) A quantitative study of water diffusion in multiple sclerosis lesions and normal-appearing white matter using echo-planar imaging. *Arch. Neurol.* **57,** 1017–1021.

Filippi, M., Rocca, M. A., Martino, G., Horsfield, M. A., and Comi, G. (1998). Magnetization transfer changes in the normal appearing white matter precede the appearance of enhancing lesions in patients with multiple sclerosis. *Ann. Neurol.* **43,** 809–814.

Filippi, M., Rocca, M. A., Martino, G., Horsfield, M. A., and Comi, G. (1998). Magnetization transfer changes in the normal appearing white matter precede the appearance of enhancing lesions in patients with multiple sclerosis. *Ann. Neurol.* **43,** 809–814.

Filippi, M., Rossi, P., Campi, A., Colombo, B., Pereira, C., and Comi, G. (1997). Serial contrast-enhanced MR in patients with multiple sclerosis and varying levels of disability. *AJNR Am. J. Neuroradiol.* **18,** 1549–1556.

Filippi, M., Yousry, T., Baratti, C., Horsfield, M. A., Mammi, S., Becker, C., Voltz, R., Spuler, S., Campi, A., Reiser, M. F., and Comi, G. (1996a). Quantitative assessment of MRI lesion load in multiple sclerosis. A comparison of conventional spin-echo with fast fluid-attenuated inversion recovery. *Brain* **119** (Pt. 4), 1349–1355.

Filippi, M., Yousry, T., Campi, A., Kandziora, C., Colombo, B., Voltz, R., Martinelli, V., Spuler, S., Bressi, S., Scotti, G., and Comi, G. (1996b). Comparison of triple dose versus standard dose gadolinium-DTPA for detection of MRI enhancing lesions in patients with MS. *Neurology* **46,** 379–384.

Filippi, M., Rocca, M. A., Colombo, B., Falini, A., Codella, M., Scotti, G., and Comi, G. (2002). Functional magnetic resonance imaging correlates of fatigue in multiple sclerosis. *Neuroimage.* **15,** 559–567.

Fu, L., Matthews, P. M., De Stefano, N., Worsley, K. J., Narayanan, S., Francis, G. S., Antel, J. P., Wolfson, C., and Arnold, D. L. (1998). Imaging axonal damage of normal-appearing white matter in multiple sclerosis. *Brain* **121** (Pt. 1), 103–113.

Gadian, D. G. (1995). "NMR and Its Applications to Living Systems." Oxford University Press, Oxford, UK.

Ganter, P., Prince, C., and Esiri, M. M. (1999). Spinal cord axonal loss in multiple sclerosis: a post-mortem study. *Neuropathol. Appl. Neurobiol.* **25,** 459–467.

Gareau, P. J., Rutt, B. K., Karlik, S. J., and Mitchell, J. R. (2000). Magnetization transfer and multicomponent T2 relaxation measurements with histopathologic correlation in an experimental model of MS. *J. Magn Reson. Imaging* **11,** 586–595.

Gawne-Cain, M. L., O'Riordan, J. I., Thompson, A. J., Moseley, I. F., and Miller, D. H. (1997). Multiple sclerosis lesion detection in the brain: a comparison of fast fluid-attenuated inversion recovery and conventional T2-weighted dual spin echo. *Neurology* **49,** 364–370.

Ge, Y., Grossman, R. I., Udupa, J. K., Babb, J. S., Mannon, L. J., and McGowan, J. C. (2002). Magnetization transfer ratio histogram analysis of normal-appearing gray matter and normal-appearing white matter in multiple sclerosis. *J. Comput. Assist. Tomogr.* **26,** 62–68.

Gean-Marton, A. D., Vezina, L. G., Marton, K. I., Stimac, G. K., Peyster, R. G., Taveras, J. M., and Davis, K. R. (1991). Abnormal corpus callosum: a sensitive and specific indicator of multiple sclerosis. *Radiology* **180,** 215–221.

Goodkin, D. E., Rooney, W. D., Sloan, R., Bacchetti, P., Gee, L., Vermathen, M., Waubant, E., Abundo, M., Majumdar, S., Nelson, S., and Weiner, M. W. (1998). A serial study of new MS lesions and the white matter from which they arise. *Neurology* **51,** 1689–1697.

Grossman, R. I. (1999). Application of magnetization transfer imaging to multiple sclerosis. *Neurology* **53,** S8–11.

Grossman, R. I., Braffman, B. H., Brorson, J. R., Goldberg, H. I., Silberberg, D. H., and Gonzalez-Scarano, F. (1988). Multiple sclerosis: serial study of gadolinium-enhanced MR imaging. *Radiology* **169,** 117–122.

Guo, A. C., Jewells, V. L., and Provenzale, J. M. (2001). Analysis of normal-appearing white matter in multiple sclerosis: comparison of diffusion tensor MR imaging and magnetization transfer imaging. *AJNR Am. J. Neuroradiol.* **22,** 1893–1900.

Guttmann, C. R., Ahn, S. S., Hsu, L., Kikinis, R., and Jolesz, F. A. (1995). The evolution of multiple sclerosis lesions on serial MR. *AJNR Am. J. Neuroradiol.* **16,** 1481–1491.

Harris, J. O., Frank, J. A., Patronas, N., McFarlin, D. E., and McFarland, H. F. (1991). Serial gadolinium-enhanced magnetic resonance imaging scans in patients with early, relapsing-remitting multiple sclerosis: implications for clinical trials and natural history. *Ann. Neurol.* **29,** 548–555.

Hashemi, R. H., and Bradley, W. G. (1997). "MRI: The Basics." Lippincott, Williams & Wilkins, Baltimore.

Hawkins, C. P., Munro, P. M., Mackenzie, F., Kesselring, J., Tofts, P. S., Du Boulay, E. P., Landon, D. N., and McDonald, W. I. (1990). Duration and selectivity of blood-brain barrier breakdown in chronic relapsing experimental allergic encephalomyelitis studied by gadolinium-DTPA and protein markers. *Brain* **113** (Pt .2), 365–378.

Hershey, L. A., Gado, M. H., and Trotter, J. L. (1979). Computerized tomography in the diagnostic evaluation of multiple sclerosis. *Ann. Neurol.* **5,** 32–39.

Hickman, S. J., Brierley, C. M., Brex, P. A., MacManus, D. G., Scolding, N. J., Compston, D. A., and Miller, D. H. (2002). Continuing optic nerve atrophy following optic neuritis: a serial MRI study. *Mult. Scler.* **8,** 339–342.

Horowitz, A. L., Kaplan, R. D., Grewe, G., White, R. T., and Salberg, L. M. (1989). The ovoid lesion: A new MR observation in patients with multiple sclerosis. *AJNR Am. J. Neuroradiol.* **10,** 303–305.

Horsfield, M. A., Lai, M., Webb, S. L., Barker, G. J., Tofts, P. S., Turner, R., Rudge, P., and Miller, D. H. (1996). Apparent diffusion coefficients in benign and secondary progressive multiple sclerosis by nuclear magnetic resonance. *Magn Reson. Med.* **36,** 393–400.

Husted, C. A., Goodin, D. S., Hugg, J. W., Maudsley, A. A., Tsuruda, J. S., de Bie, S. H., Fein, G., Matson, G. B., and Weiner, M. W. (1994). Biochemical alterations in multiple sclerosis lesions and normal-appearing white matter detected by in vivo 31P and 1H spectroscopic imaging. *Ann. Neurol.* **36,** 157–165.

Jacobs, K. M., and Donoghue, J. P. (1991). Reshaping the cortical motor map by unmasking latent intracortical connections. *Science* **251,** 944–947.

Jezzard, P., Matthews, P. M., and Smith, S. (Eds.). (2001). "Functional Magnetic Resonance Imaging: An Introduction to Methods." Oxford: Oxford University Press.

Jones, T. A., and Schallert, T. (1992). Overgrowth and pruning of dendrites in adult rats recovering from neocortical damage. *Brain Res.* **581,** 156–160.

Kapeller, P., McLean, M. A., Griffin, C. M., Chard, D., Parker, G. J., Barker, G. J., Thompson, A. J., and Miller, D. H. (2001). Preliminary evidence for neuronal damage in cortical grey matter and normal appearing white matter in short duration relapsing-remitting multiple sclerosis: A quantitative MR spectroscopic imaging study. *J. Neurol.* **248,** 131–138.

Katz, D., Taubenberger, J., Raine, C., McFarlin, D., and McFarland, H. (1990). Gadolinium-enhancing lesions on magnetic resonance imaging: Neuropathological findings. *Ann. Neurol.* **28,** 243.

Katz, D., Taubenberger, J. K., Cannella, B., McFarlin, D. E., Raine, C. S., and McFarland, H. F. (1993). Correlation between magnetic resonance imaging findings and lesion development in chronic, active multiple sclerosis. *Ann. Neurol.* **34,** 661–669.

Kermode, A. G., Thompson, A. J., Tofts, P., MacManus, D. G., Kendall, B. E., Kingsley, D. P., Moseley, I. F., Rudge, P., and McDonald, W. I. (1990a). Breakdown of the blood-brain barrier precedes symptoms and other MRI signs of new lesions in multiple sclerosis. Pathogenetic and clinical implications. *Brain* **113** (Pt. 5), 1477–1489.

Kermode, A. G., Tofts, P. S., Thompson, A. J., MacManus, D. G., Rudge, P., Kendall, B. E., Kingsley, D. P., Moseley, I. F., Du Boulay, E. P., and McDonald, W. I. (1990b). Heterogeneity of blood-brain barrier changes in multiple sclerosis: An MRI study with gadolinium-DTPA enhancement. *Neurology* **40,** 229–235.

Khoury, S. J., Guttmann, C. R., Orav, E. J., Hohol, M. J., Ahn, S. S., Hsu, L., Kikinis, R., Mackin, G. A., Jolesz, F. A., and Weiner, H. L. (1994). Longitudinal MRI in multiple sclerosis: Correlation between disability and lesion burden. *Neurology* **44,** 2120–2124.

Kidd, D., Barkhof, F., McConnell, R., Algra, P. R., Allen, I. V., and Revesz, T. (1999). Cortical lesions in multiple sclerosis. *Brain* **122** (Pt. 1), 17–26.

Koudriavtseva, T., Thompson, A. J., Fiorelli, M., Gasperini, C., Bastianello, S., Bozzao, A., Paolillo, A., Pisani, A., Galgani, S., and Pozzilli, C. (1997). Gadolinium enhanced MRI predicts clinical and MRI disease activity in relapsing-remitting multiple sclerosis. *J. Neurol. Neurosurg. Psychiatry* **62,** 285–287.

Kozlowski, D. A., James, D. C., and Schallert, T. (1996) Use-dependent exaggeration of neuronal injury after unilateral sensorimotor cortex lesions. *J. Neurosci.* **16,** 4776–4786.

Laule, C., Vavasour, I. M., Oger, J., Paty, D. W., Li, D. K. B., and MacKay, A. L. (2002). T2 relaxation measurements of in-vivo water content and myelin water content in normal appearing white matter and lesions in multiple sclerosis. *Proc. Intl. Soc. Mag. Reson. Med.* **10,** 185.

Leary, S. M., Davie, C. A., Parker, G. J., Stevenson, V. L., Wang, L., Barker, G. J., Miller, D. H., and Thompson, A. J. (1999). 1H magnetic resonance spectroscopy of normal appearing white matter in primary progressive multiple sclerosis. *J. Neurol.* **246,** 1023–1026.

Lee, M., Reddy, H., Johansen-Berg, H., Pendlebury, S., Jenkinson, M., Smith, S., Palace, J., and Matthews, P. M. (2000). The motor cortex shows adaptive functional changes to brain injury from multiple sclerosis. *Ann. Neurol.* **47,** 606–613.

Lee, M. A., Smith, S., Palace, J., Narayanan, S., Silver, N., Minicucci, L., Filippi, M., Miller, D. H., Arnold, D. L., and Matthews, P. M. (1999). Spatial mapping of T2 and gadolinium-enhancing T1 lesion volumes in multiple sclerosis: evidence for distinct mechanisms of lesion genesis? *Brain* **122** (Pt. 7), 1261–1270.

Leist, T. P., Gobbini, M. I., Frank, J. A., and McFarland, H. F. (2001). Enhancing magnetic resonance imaging lesions and cerebral atrophy in patients with relapsing multiple sclerosis. *Arch. Neurol.* **58,** 57–60.

Levesque, I., Sled J. G., Brass S. D., Santos, A. C., Narayanan, S., Francis, S. J., Arnold, D. L., and Pike, G. B. (2002). Comparison of MTR and qMT imaging of multiple sclerosis lesions. *Proc. Int. Soc. Magn. Reson. Med.* **10,** 1183

Lin, X., and Blumhardt, L. D. (2001). Inflammation and atrophy in multiple sclerosis: MRI associations with disease course. *J. Neurol. Sci.* **189,** 99–104.

Losseff, N. A., Kingsley, D. P., McDonald, W. I., Miller, D. H., and Thompson, A. J. (1996a). Clinical and magnetic resonance imaging predictors of disability in primary and secondary progressive multiple sclerosis. *Mult. Scler.* **1,** 218–222.

Losseff, N. A., Wang, L., Lai, H. M., Yoo, D. S., Gawne-Cain, M. L., McDonald, W. I., Miller, D. H., and Thompson, A. J. (1996b). Progressive cerebral atrophy in multiple sclerosis. A serial MRI study. *Brain* **119** (Pt. 6), 2009–2019.

Lumsden, C. E. (1970). The neuropathology of multiple sclerosis. *In* "Multiple Sclerosis and Other Demyelinating Diseases. Handbook of Clinical Neurology" (P. J. Vinken and G. W. Bruyn, eds.), Vol. 9, pp. 217–309. North-Holland, Amsterdam.

MacKay, A., Whittall, K., Adler, J., Li, D., Paty, D., and Graeb, D. (1994). In vivo visualization of myelin water in brain by magnetic resonance. *Magn Reson. Med.* **31,** 673–677.

Matthews, P. M. (2001). An introduction to functional magnetic resonance imaging. *In* "Functional Magnetic Resonance Imaging: An Introduction to Methods" (P., Jezzard, P. M. Matthews, and S. Smith, Eds.). Oxford: Oxford University Press.

Matthews, P. M., and Arnold, D. L. (2001). Magnetic resonance imaging of multiple sclerosis: new insights linking pathology to clinical evolution. *Curr. Opin. Neurol.* **14,** 279–287.

Matthews, P. M., Pioro, E., Narayanan, S., De Stefano, N., Fu, L., Francis, G., Antel, J., Wolfson, C., and Arnold, D. L. (1996). Assessment of lesion pathology in multiple sclerosis using quantitative MRI morphometry and magnetic resonance spectroscopy. *Brain* **119** (Pt. 3), 715–722.

Matthews, P. M., De Stefano, N., Narayanan, S., Francis, G. S., Wolinsky, J. S., Antel, J. P., and Arnold, D. L. (1998). Putting magnetic resonance spectroscopy studies in context: Axonal damage and disability in multiple sclerosis. *Semin. Neurol.* **18,** 327–336.

McDonald, W. I., Compston, A., Edan, G., Goodkin, D., Hartung, H. P., Lublin, F. D., McFarland, H. F., Paty, D. W., Polman, C. H., Reingold, S. C., Sandberg-Wollheim, M., Sibley, W., Thompson, A., van den, N. S., Weinshenker, B. Y., and Wolinsky, J. S. (2001). Recommended diagnostic criteria for multiple sclerosis: Guidelines from the International Panel on the diagnosis of multiple sclerosis. *Ann. Neurol.* **50,** 121–127.

McFarland, H. F., Frank, J. A., Albert, P. S., Smith, M. E., Martin, R., Harris, J. O., Patronas, N., Maloni, H., and McFarlin, D. E. (1992). Using gadolinium-enhanced magnetic resonance imaging lesions to monitor disease activity in multiple sclerosis. *Ann. Neurol.* **32,** 758–766.

McGowan, J. C. (1999). The physical basis of magnetization transfer imaging. *Neurology* **53,** S3-S7.

Miller, D. H., Barkhof, F., Frank, J. A., Parker, G. J., and Thompson, A. J. (2002). Measurement of atrophy in multiple sclerosis: Pathological basis, methodological aspects and clinical relevance. *Brain* **125,** 1676–1695.

Miller, D. H., Barkhof, F., and Nauta, J. J. (1993). Gadolinium enhancement increases the sensitivity of MRI in detecting disease activity in multiple sclerosis. *Brain* **116** (Pt. 5), 1077–1094.

Miller, D. H., Grossman, R. I., Reingold, S. C., and McFarland, H. F. (1998). The role of magnetic resonance techniques in understanding and managing multiple sclerosis. *Brain* **121** (Pt. 1), 3–24.

Miller, D. H., Johnson, G., Tofts, P. S., MacManus, D., and McDonald, W. I. (1989). Precise relaxation time measurements of normal-appearing white matter in inflammatory central nervous system disease. *Magn Reson. Med.* **11,** 331–336.

Miller, D. H., Kesselring, J., McDonald, W. I., Paty, D. W., and Thompson, A. J. (1997). "Magnetic Resonance in Multiple Sclerosis." Cambridge University Press, Cambridge, United Kingdom.

Miller, D. H., Rudge, P., Johnson, G., Kendall, B. E., MacManus, D. G., Moseley, I. F., Barnes, D., and McDonald, W. I. (1988) Serial gadolinium enhanced magnetic resonance imaging in multiple sclerosis. *Brain* **111** (Pt. 4), 927–939.

Moffett, J. R., Namboodiri, M. A., Cangro, C. B., and Neale, J. H. (1991). Immunohistochemical localization of N-acetylaspartate in rat brain. *Neuroreport* **2,** 131–134.

Moore, G. R., Leung, E., MacKay, A. L., Vavasour, I. M., Whittall, K. P., Cover, K. S., Li, D. K., Hashimoto, S. A., Oger, J., Sprinkle, T. J., and Paty, D. W. (2000). A pathology-MRI study of the short-T2 component in formalin-fixed multiple sclerosis brain. *Neurology* **55,** 1506–1510.

Narayana, P. A., Doyle, T. J., Lai, D., and Wolinsky, J. S. (1998). Serial proton magnetic resonance spectroscopic imaging, contrast-enhanced magnetic resonance imaging, and quantitative lesion volumetry in multiple sclerosis. *Ann. Neurol.* **43,** 56–71.

Nesbit, G. M., Forbes, G. S., Scheithauer, B. W., Okazaki, H., and Rodriguez, M. (1991). Multiple sclerosis: Histopathologic and MR and/or CT correlation in 37 cases at biopsy and three cases at autopsy. *Radiology* **180,** 467–474.

Newcombe, J., Hawkins, C. P., Henderson, C. L., Patel, H. A., Woodroofe, M. N., Hayes, G. M., Cuzner, M. L., MacManus, D., Du Boulay, E. P., and McDonald, W. I. (1991). Histopathology of multiple sclerosis lesions detected by magnetic resonance imaging in unfixed postmortem central nervous system tissue. *Brain* **114** (Pt. 2), 1013–1023.

Nijeholt, G. J., van Walderveen, M. A., Castelijns, J. A., van Waesberghe, J. H., Polman, C., Scheltens, P., Rosier, P. F., Jongen, P. J., and Barkhof, F. (1998). Brain and spinal cord abnormalities in multiple sclerosis. Correlation between MRI parameters, clinical subtypes and symptoms. *Brain* **121** (Pt. 4), 687–697.

Nudo, R. J., Wise, B. M., SiFuentes, F., and Milliken, G. W. (1996). Neural substrates for the effects of rehabilitative training on motor recovery after ischemic infarct. *Science* **272,** 1791–1794.

Ogawa, S., Menon, R. S., Tank, D. W., Kim, S. G., Merkle, H., Ellermann, J. M., and Ugurbil, K. (1993). Functional brain mapping by blood oxygenation level-dependent contrast magnetic resonance imaging. A comparison of signal characteristics with a biophysical model. *Biophys. J.* **64,** 803–812.

Ormerod, I. E., Johnson, G., MacManus, D., Du Boulay, E. P., and McDonald, W. I. (1986). Relaxation times of apparently normal cerebral white matter in multiple sclerosis. *Acta Radiol. Suppl* **369,** 382–384.

Pantano, P., Iannetti, G. D., Caramia, F., Mainero, C., Di Legge, S., Bozzao, L., Pozzilli, C., and Lenzi, G. L. (2002). Cortical motor reorganization after a single clinical attack of multiple sclerosis. *Brain* **125,** 1607–1615.

Paolillo, A., Pozzilli, C., Gasperini, C., Giugni, E., Mainero, C., Giuliani, S., Tomassini, V., Millefiorini, E., and Bastianello, S. (2000). Brain atrophy in relapsing-remitting multiple sclerosis: relationship with 'black holes', disease duration and clinical disability. *J. Neurol. Sci.* **174,** 85–91.

Parry, A., Clare, S., Jenkinson, M., Smith, S., Palace, J., and Matthews, P. M. (2002a). White matter and lesion T1 relaxation times increase in parallel and correlate with disability in multiple sclerosis. *J. Neurol. (in press).*

Parry, A. M. M., Scott, R. B., Palace, J., Smith, S. M., and Matthews, P. M. (2002b). Potentially adaptive functional changes for cognitive processing in multiple sclerosis. *Submitted for publication.*

Paty, D. W., Oger, J. J., Kastrukoff, L. F., Hashimoto, S. A., Hooge, J. P., Eisen, A. A., Eisen, K. A., Purves, S. J., Low, M. D., Brandejs, V., Robertson, W. D. and Li, D. K. B. (1988). MRI in the diagnosis of MS: A prospective study with comparison of clinical evaluation, evoked potentials, oligoclonal banding, and CT. *Neurology* **38,** 180–185.

Peterson, J. W., Bo, L., Mork, S., Chang, A., and Trapp, B. D. (2001). Transected neurites, apoptotic neurons, and reduced inflammation in cortical multiple sclerosis lesions. *Ann. Neurol.* **50,** 389–400.

Pike, G. B., De Stefano, N., Narayanan, S., Worsley, K. J., Pelletier, D., Francis, G. S., Antel, J. P., and Arnold, D. L. (2000). Multiple sclerosis: Magnetization transfer MR imaging of white matter before lesion appearance on T2-weighted images. *Radiology* **215,** 824–830.

Plumb, J., McQuaid, S., Mirakhur, M., and Kirk, J. (2002). Abnormal endothelial tight junctions in active lesions and normal-appearing white matter in multiple sclerosis. *Brain Pathol.* **12,** 154–169.

Presciutti, O., Sarchielli, P., Gobbi, G., Tarducci, R., Pelliccioli, G. P., Chiarini, P., Gentile, E., and Gallai, V. (2000). $^1$H MRS study in occipital gray matter of multiple sclerosis patients. *Proc. Int. Soc. Magn. Reson. Med.* **8,** 627.

Ramani, A., Barker, G. J., and Tofts, P. S. (2001). Fast measurement of quantitative MT parameters in fixed multiple sclerosis brain. *Proc. Int. Soc. Magn. Reson. Med.* **9,** 259.

Reddy, H., Bendahan, D., Lee, M. A., Johansen-Berg, H., Donaghy, M., Hilton-Jones, D., and Matthews, P. M. (2002c). An expanded cortical representation for hand movement after peripheral motor denervation. *J. Neurol. Neurosurg. Psychiatry.* **72,** 203–210.

Reddy, H., De Stefano, N., Mortilla, M., Federico, A., and Matthews, P. M. (2002a). Functional reorganization of motor cortex increases with greater axonal injury from CADASIL. *Stroke* **33,** 502–508.

Reddy, H., Floyer, A., Donaghy, M., and Matthews, P. M. (2001). Altered cortical activation with finger movement after peripheral denervation: comparison of active and passive tasks. *Exp. Brain Res.* **138,** 484–491.

Reddy, H., Narayanan, S., Arnoutelis, R., Jenkinson, M., Antel, J., Matthews, P. M., and Arnold, D. L. (2000a). Evidence for adaptive functional changes in the cerebral cortex with axonal injury from multiple sclerosis. *Brain* **123** (Pt. 11), 2314–2320.

Reddy, H., Narayanan, S., Matthews, P. M., Hoge, R. D., Pike, G. B., Duquette, P., Antel, J., and Arnold, D. L. (2000b). Relating axonal injury to functional recovery in MS. *Neurology* **54,** 236–239.

Reddy, H., Narayanan, S., Woolrich, M., Mitsumori, T., Lapierre, Y., Arnold, D. L., and Matthews, P. M. (2002b). Functional brain reorganisation for hand movements in patients with multiple sclerosis: defining distinct effects of injury and disability. *Brain (in press).*

Rieckmann, P., and Smith, K. J. (2001). Multiple sclerosis: More than inflammation and demyelination. *Trends Neurosci.* **24,** 435–437.

Rocca, M. A., Cercignani, M., Iannucci, G., Comi, G., and Filippi, M. (2000). Weekly diffusion-weighted imaging of normal-appearing white matter in MS. *Neurology* **55,** 882–884.

Rocca, M. A., Falini, A., Colombo, B., Scotti, G., Comi, G., and Filippi, M. (2002a) Adaptive functional changes in the cerebral cortex of patients with nondisabling multiple sclerosis correlate with the extent of brain structural damage. *Ann. Neurol.* **51,** 330–339.

Rocca, M. A., Matthews, P. M., Caputo, D., Ghezzi, A., Falini, A., Scotti, G., Comi, G., and Filippi, M. (2002b). Evidence for widespread movement-associated functional MRI changes in patients with PPMS. *Neurology* **58,** 866–872.

Ropele, S., Strasser-Fuchs, S., Seifert, T., Enzinger, C., and Fazekas, F. (2002). Development of active multiple sclerosis lesions: A quantitative MT study. *Proc. Int. Soc. Magn. Reson. Med.* **10,** 180.

Rovaris, M., and Filippi, M. (1999). Magnetic resonance techniques to monitor disease evolution and treatment trial outcomes in multiple sclerosis. *Curr. Opin. Neurol.* **12,** 337–344.

Rovaris, M., and Filippi, M. (2000a). Contrast enhancement and the acute lesion in multiple sclerosis. *Neuroimaging Clin. N. Am.* **10,** 705–716.

Rovaris, M., and Filippi, M. (2000b). The value of new magnetic resonance techniques in multiple sclerosis. *Curr. Opin. Neurol.* **13,** 249–254.

Rudick, R. A., Fisher, E., Lee, J. C., Simon, J., and Jacobs, L. (1999) Use of the brain parenchymal fraction to measure whole brain atrophy in relapsing-remitting MS. Multiple Sclerosis Collaborative Research Group. *Neurology* **53,** 1698–1704.

Rudkin, T. M., and Arnold, D. L. (1999). Proton magnetic resonance spectroscopy for the diagnosis and management of cerebral disorders. *Arch. Neurol.* **56,** 919–926.

Saindane, A. M., Ge, Y., Udupa, J. K., Babb, J. S., Mannon, L. J., and Grossman, R. I. (2000). The effect of gadolinium-enhancing lesions on whole brain atrophy in relapsing-remitting MS. *Neurology* **55,** 61–65.

Salibi, N., and Brown, M. A. (1998). "Clinical MR Spectroscopy. First Principles." Wiley-Liss: New York.

Santos, A. C., Sled, J. G., Narayanan, S., Francis, S. J., Brass, S. D., Levesque, I., Caramanos, Z., Pike, G. B., and Arnold, D. L. (2002). Quantitative magnetisation transfer for assessment of tissue damage in individual multiple sclerosis lesions. *Proc. Int. Soc. Magn. Reson. Med.* **10,** 1177.

Sarchielli, P., Presciutti, O., Pelliccioli, G. P., Tarducci, R., Gobbi, G., Chiarini, P., Alberti, A., Vicinanza, F., and Gallai, V. (1999). Absolute quantification of brain metabolites by proton magnetic resonance spectroscopy in normal-appearing white matter of multiple sclerosis patients. *Brain* **122** (Pt. 3), 513–521.

Siger-Zajdel, M., and Selmaj, K. (2001). Magnetisation transfer ratio analysis of normal appearing white matter in patients with familial and sporadic multiple sclerosis. *J. Neurol. Neurosurg. Psychiatry* **71,** 752–756.

Silver, N. C., Good, C. D., Barker, G. J., MacManus, D. G., Thompson, A. J., Moseley, I. F., McDonald, W. I., and Miller, D. H. (1997). Sensitivity of contrast enhanced MRI in multiple sclerosis. Effects of gadolinium dose, magnetization transfer contrast and delayed imaging. *Brain* **120** (Pt. 7), 1149–1161.

Simmons, M. L., Frondoza, C. G., and Coyle, J. T. (1991). Immunocytochemical localization of N-acetyl-aspartate with monoclonal antibodies. *Neuroscience* **45,** 37–45.

Simon, J. H. (2000). The contribution of spinal cord MRI to the diagnosis and differential diagnosis of multiple sclerosis. *J. Neurol. Sci.* **172,** Suppl 1, S32–S35.

Simon, J. H., Jacobs, L. D., Campion, M., Wende, K., Simonian, N., Cookfair, D. L., Rudick, R. A., Herndon, R. M., Richert, J. R., Salazar, A. M., Alam, J. J., Fischer, J. S., Goodkin, D. E., Granger, C. V., Lajaunie, M., Martens-Davidson, A. L., Meyer, M., Sheeder, J., Choi, K., Scherzinger, A. L., Bartoszak, D. M., Bourdette, D. N., Braiman, J., Brownscheidle, C. M., and Whitham, R. H. (1998). Magnetic resonance studies of intramuscular interferon beta-1a for relapsing multiple sclerosis. The Multiple Sclerosis Collaborative Research Group. *Ann. Neurol.* **43,** 79–87.

Smith, M. E., Stone, L. A., Albert, P. S., Frank, J. A., Martin, R., Armstrong, M., Maloni, H., McFarlin, D. E., and McFarland, H. F. (1993). Clinical worsening in multiple sclerosis is associated with increased frequency and area of gadopentetate dimeglumine-enhancing magnetic resonance imaging lesions. *Ann. Neurol.* **33,** 480–489.

Stanisz, G. J., and Webb, S. (2002). Understanding the MT, T1 and T2 changes during demyelination and inflammation. *Proc. Int. Soc. Magn. Reson. Med.* **10,** 183.

Stevenson, V. L., Smith, S. M., Matthews, P. M., Miller, D. H., and Thompson, A. J. (2002). Monitoring disease activity and progression in primary progressive multiple sclerosis using MRI: sub-voxel registration to identify lesion changes and to detect cerebral atrophy. *J. Neurol.* **249,** 171–177.

Stone, L. A., Smith, M. E., Albert, P. S., Bash, C. N., Maloni, H., Frank, J. A., and McFarland, H. F. (1995). Blood-brain barrier disruption on contrast-enhanced MRI in patients with mild relapsing-remitting multiple sclerosis: Relationship to course, gender, and age. *Neurology* **45,** 1122–1126.

Tas, M. W., Barkhol, F., van Walderveen, M. A., Polman, C. H., Hommes, O. R., and Valk, J. (1995). The effect of gadolinium on the sensitivity and specificity of MR in the initial diagnosis of multiple sclerosis. *AJNR Am. J. Neuroradiol.* **16,** 259–264.

Tedeschi, G., Bonavita, S., McFarland, H. F., Richert, N., Duyn, J. H., and Frank, J. A. (2002). Proton MR spectroscopic imaging in multiple sclerosis. *Neuroradiology* **44,** 37–42.

Thompson, A. J., Miller, D., Youl, B., MacManus, D., Moore, S., Kingsley, D., Kendall, B., Feinstein, A., and McDonald, W. I. (1992). Serial gadolinium-enhanced MRI in relapsing/remitting multiple sclerosis of varying disease duration. *Neurology* **42,** 60–63.

Tintore, M., Rovira, A., Martinez, M. J., Rio, J., Diaz-Villoslada, P., Brieva, L., Borras, C., Grive, E., Capellades, J., and Montalban, X. (2000). Isolated demyelinating syndromes: Comparison of different MR imaging criteria to predict conversion to clinically definite multiple sclerosis. *AJNR Am. J. Neuroradiol.* **21,** 702–706.

Tofts, P. S., and Kermode, A. G. (1991). Measurement of the blood-brain barrier permeability and leakage space using dynamic MR imaging. 1. Fundamental concepts. *Magn Reson. Med.* **17,** 357–367.

Trapp, B. D., Peterson, J., Ransohoff, R. M., Rudick, R., Mork, S., and Bo, L. (1998). Axonal transection in the lesions of multiple sclerosis. *N. Engl. J. Med.* **338,** 278–285.

Truyen, L., van Waesberghe, J. H., van Walderveen, M. A., van Oosten, B. W., Polman, C. H., Hommes, O. R., Ader, H. J., and Barkhof, F. (1996). Accumulation of hypointense lesions ("black holes") on T1 spin-echo MRI correlates with disease progression in multiple sclerosis. *Neurology* **47,** 1469–1476.

Tsai, G., and Coyle, J. T. (1995). N-acetylaspartate in neuropsychiatric disorders. *Prog. Neurobiol.* **46,** 531–540.

Tseng, G. F., and Hu, M. E. (1996). Axotomy induces retraction of the dendritic arbor of adult rat rubrospinal neurons. *Acta Anat.(Basel)* **155,** 184–193.

Uhlenbrock, D., and Sehlen, S. (1989). The value of T1-weighted images in the differentiation between MS, white matter lesions, and subcortical arteriosclerotic encephalopathy (SAE). *Neuroradiology* **31,** 203–212.

van Waesberghe, J. H., Kamphorst, W., De Groot, C. J., van Walderveen, M. A., Castelijns, J. A., Ravid, R., Nijeholt, G. J., van, d., V, Polman, C. H., Thompson, A. J., and Barkhof, F. (1999). Axonal loss in multiple sclerosis lesions: Magnetic resonance imaging insights into substrates of disability. *Ann. Neurol.* **46,** 747–754.

van Walderveen, M. A., Kamphorst, W., Scheltens, P., van Waesberghe, J. H., Ravid, R., Valk, J., Polman, C. H., and Barkhof, F. (1998). Histopathologic correlate of hypointense lesions on T1-weighted spin-echo MRI in multiple sclerosis. *Neurology* **50,** 1282–1288.

Waxman, S. G. (2001). Acquired channelopathies in nerve injury and MS. *Neurology* **56,** 1621–1627.

Webb, S., Munro, C. A., Midha, R., and Stanisz, G. J. (2002). Is quantitative T2 a good measure of myelin content in white matter pathologies? *Proc. Int. Soc. Magn. Reson. Med.* **10,** 184.

Werring, D. J., Bullmore, E. T., Toosy, A. T., Miller, D. H., Barker, G. J., MacManus, D. G., Brammer, M. J., Giampietro, V. P., Brusa, A., Brex, P. A., Moseley, I. F., Plant, G. T., McDonald, W. I., and Thompson, A. J. (2000). Recovery from optic neuritis is associated with a change in the distribution of cerebral response to visual stimulation: a functional magnetic resonance imaging study. *J. Neurol. Neurosurg. Psychiatry* **68,** 441–449.

Werring, D. J., Clark, C. A., Barker, G. J., Thompson, A. J., and Miller, D. H. (1999). Diffusion tensor imaging of lesions and normal-appearing white matter in multiple sclerosis. *Neurology* **52,** 1626–1632.

Werring, D. J., Clark, C. A., Droogan, A. G., Barker, G. J., Miller, D. H., and Thompson, A. J. (2001). Water diffusion is elevated in widespread regions of normal-appearing white matter in multiple sclerosis and correlates with diffusion in focal lesions. *Mult. Scler.* **7,** 83–89.

Wujek, J. R., Bjartmar, C., Richer, E., Ransohoff, R. M., Yu, M., Tuohy, V. K., and Trapp, B. D. (2002). Axon loss in the spinal cord determines permanent neurological disability in an animal model of multiple sclerosis. *J. Neuropathol. Exp. Neurol.* **61,** 23–32.

Wylezinska, M., Cifelli, A., Jezzard, P., Palace, J., Alecci, M., and Matthews, P. M. (2002a). Thalamic neurodegeneration in relapsing-remitting multiple sclerosis *Neurology* **60,** 1949–1959.

Wylezinska, M., Cifelli, A., Matthews, P., Palace, J., and Jezzard, P. (2002b). Neuronal damage in thalamic grey matter in relapsing-remitting multiple sclerosis. *Proc. Int. Soc. Magn. Reson. Med.* **10,** 592.

Zorzon, M., De Masi, R., Nasuelli, D., Ukmar, M., Mucelli, R. P., Cazzato, G., Bratina, A., and Zivadinov, R. (2001). Depression and anxiety in multiple sclerosis. A clinical and MRI study in 95 subjects. *J. Neurol.* **248,** 416–421.

CHAPTER

# 33

# Multiple Sclerosis: Therapy

*Jack Antel and Amit Bar-Or*

## INTRODUCTION

The clinical and pathologic features of multiple sclerosis (MS) began to be described in the mid-1800s and by the 1870s had been synthesized into a recognizable entity by Charcot and colleagues. Charcot emphasized the loss of the myelin sheath with relative, but not absolute, preservation of axons. He referred to the observation by Reinfleisch in 1863 of inflammation around a vessel in the center of MS plaques; this can be viewed as the beginning of the continuing debate of the relative contributions of immune mediated versus "neurodegenerative" processes as a basis for the disease pathology (Hoeber, 1922; Murray, 2000). As reviewed in other chapters, since that time there have been major advances in our understanding of the clinical, pathologic and imaging aspects of the disease.

Charcot had stated in his lectures that the time had not yet come to consider therapy for the disorder (Charcot, 1877). Over the ensuing years, multiple therapeutic interventions were attempted, often based on the ideas of the time regarding disease pathogenesis or on availability of therapies for other diseases. The National Multiple Sclerosis Society, through the various editions of its publication *Therapeutic Claims in Multiple Sclerosis*, has compiled a comprehensive list of such therapies (National Multiple Sclerosis Society, 1982; *Therapeutic Claims in Multiple Sclerosis*, 1992). Expert committees were used to evaluate therapeutic claims in the era that preceded the controlled clinical trial supported by magnetic resonance (MR) based imaging. Examples of therapies listed as in use prior to 1935 include arsenic, belladonna, fever therapy, and hypnotism; between 1935 and 1950, dicoumaral, histamine, and vitamins B12, D, E, and K were among those mentioned. Theories of disease pathogenesis that generated associated therapies between 1950 and 1965 included those directed at nutritional status (including vitamin supplementation), metabolic status (with carbohydrate and fat supplements), vascular abnormalities (using either anticoagulants or vasodilators), and infectious etiologies (including antispirochete therapies). None of these interventions were judged to have demonstrated efficacy. Candidate infectious agents such as chlamydia, Epstein-Barr virus, and human herpes virus type 6 continue to be evaluated (Kaufman *et al.*, 2002; Moore *et al.*, 2002; Talbot *et al.*, 2001).

The postulate that immune-mediated mechanisms underlie the pathogenesis of MS has been raised since the initial descriptions of MS and has dominated thinking in the past several decades, as discussed in other chapters. As they became available, an array of anti-inflammatory (e.g., corticosteroids) and immune-suppressive agents (e.g., cyclophosphamide) were tested on patients with MS (reviewed in Antel *et al.*, 2003, and Smith *et al.*, 1998). The results of modern clinical/MRI trials indicate the limitations of the study designs used in these early studies—for example, length of study, number of patients, phase of disease, placebo control, primary end point. A number of the immune modulators for which there were uncertain conclusions in the 1982 edition of *MS Therapeutic Claims*, such as azathioprine and cyclophosphamide, have been and are being reexamined in light of results with current therapies and insights regarding the immunobiology of MS. Some therapies have been abandoned for toxicity reasons (lymphoid irradiation), although greater risks may now be acceptable in specific patient groups (e.g., those who fail currently approved therapies.)

The major themes considered in this chapter relate to defining the relationship between the clinical phenotypes of MS and their underlying immunobiologic and neurobiologic substrates and explaining results of or predicting outcomes of past, current, and future clinical trials in the context of the underlying disease process. Although many of the clinical features of MS were described in the early writings, recent natural history and large-scale epidemiologic studies have provided a more solid source of information, as reviewed in separate chapters in this book. The insights into immunobiology have been derived from pathologic analyses of MS tissues, *in vivo* imaging, largely using MR techniques, and animal models. All of these are also reviewed in separate chapters. The results of clinical trials conducted on well-defined subtypes of MS provide further insights and identify new challenges regarding the biologic substrates that underlie the various phases of the MS disease process.

## IMMUNOBIOLOGY OF THE CLINICAL FEATURES OF MS

As described in chapter 29, the clinical phenotypes can be summarized into four major categories although overlaps exist. These include relapsing-remitting (RR), secondary progressive (SP), primary progressive (PP), and progressive-relapsing.(PR). Natural history studies indicate that more than 50% of RR cases will evolve into the SP phenotype over about 15 years with such evolution being almost inevitable once fixed motor deficits become evident (reviewed in (Paty and Ebers, 1997)). A meaningful number, albeit a minority of MS patients do, however, follow a relatively benign course, with autopsy-defined cases being reported in which no clinical manifestations were ever evident ((McAlpine, 1961; Paty and Ebers, 1997)).

### Clinically Isolated Syndrome (CIS)

Most cases of MS begin with a discrete neurologic event consistent with demyelination within the CNS. Common examples would include optic neuritis, brain stem dysfunction, or transverse myelitis. If the individual is seen at this time, the condition is referred to as a clinically isolated syndrome (CIS). CIS may occur with or with or without multifocal lesions on MRI. The MRI findings are now shown to be very significant predictors of future disease course. The risk of recurrent disease in cases of CIS with multifocal MRI abnormalities approaches 80% over the subsequent 10 years but is only 5 to 10% in cases with normal MRIs (Brex *et al.*, 2002). New definitions of MS attempt to incorporate recurrent MR-defined lesions as being sufficient to accept the diagnosis of the disease (McDonald *et al.*, 2001). An unresolved question is whether CIS with and without multifocal lesions have a common underlying pathogenesis.

The clinical disorder acute disseminated encephalomyelitis (ADEM) provides a prototype of an immune mediated demyelinating disorder that affects the CNS. The disorder is characterized by a uniphasic course followed by a variable degree of recovery. MRI data confirm the multifocal involvement of the CNS. Pathologic analysis shows multiple perivascular demyelinating lesions, associated with inflammation. All are of the same age. This disorder was first described after Pasteur introduced a neural tissue containing vaccine as a therapy for rabies. It should be noted that, unlike MS, peripheral nervous system involvement is described in >50% of cases (Swamy *et al.*, 1984). The frequency of post-rabies vaccine–associated ADEM has declined with introduction of vaccines prepared in the absence of neural tissues. ADEM is also recognized to occur after exposure to an array of viral infections. Viral infection is also an established risk factor for disease exacerbation in relapsing MS. Recurrent forms of ADEM have been described in children (an age in which typical MS is unusual); the relationship of this disorder to MS remains to be established (Gusev *et al.*, 2002; Murthy *et al.*, 2002; Tourbah *et al.*, 1999). The Pasteur vaccine complication was initially reproduced in animals by immunization with neural tissue, resulting in an inflammatory demyelinating disorder termed experimental autoimmune encephalomyelitis (EAE). The disorder can now also be induced by means of adoptive transfer of myelin-reactive pro-inflammatory $CD4^+$ T cells into the systemic circulation. Of note, direct injection of such autoreactive T cells into the CNS does not produce EAE. Distinct phenotypes of EAE can be induced that have characteristic regional involvement such as spinal cord or optic nerve. Relapsing and chronic disease forms of EAE can be obtained by means of selection of precise myelin antigen, strain of inbred animal, and immunization regimen. The overlap of acute and chronic/relapsing syndromes in the EAE model raise the issue of overlapping pathogenic mechanisms of uniphasic, recurrent, and chronic phenotypes in the human.

Initiation of the MS disease process, by analogy with EAE, has been attributed to CNS-directed autoreactive T cells. Such autoreactive T cells can, however, be derived from the circulation of normal individuals, as well as MS patients. There is an apparent increase in the frequency in the latter, particularly if one considers only cells that show evidence of previous activation by antigen (Bieganowska *et al.*, 1997). Whether this increased frequency in MS reflects a unique exposure to a specific antigen or a defect in immune regulation remains speculative. One possible explanation for antigen exposure in MS patients invokes the concept of molecular mimicry. This refers to shared antigenicity between autoantigens (such as myelin constituents) and exogenous antigens (infectious agents) (Wucherpfennig, 2002). The recognition that cross reactivity among peptide antigens is determined by the very limited number of amino acids that make the crucial contact with the receptor on specific T cells predicts that the possibilities for cross reactivity are extremely high (Lang *et al.*, 2002). Results of studies in which myelin reactive T cell clones have been exposed to combinatorial libraries of peptides demonstrate that optimal reactivity of such clones is more likely to be induced by a nonmyelin peptide (Sung *et al.*, 2002). In the EAE model, almost always performed in inbred animal strains, the actual autoantigen and the actual encephalitogenic peptide portion thereof varies from strain to strain.

Additional models of immune mediated CNS demyelination involve those in which a persistent viral infection in the CNS results in generation of autoreactive T cells. Generation of such cells presumably develops in response to myelin antigens released as a consequence of viral induced neural cell injury (Miller *et al.*, 2001). T cell sensitization could occur either within the CNS or in regional draining lymph nodes. Support for the former is derived from observations that lymphocyte trafficking is ongoing in the CNS even under physiologic conditions and that perivascular and parenchymal microglia have the capacity to serve as competent antigen presenting cells (reviewed in Becher *et al.*, 2000). The documentation that CNS-released antigens are transported back to regional lymph nodes also implicates this site for generation of the putative disease relevant immune response.

Entry of autoreactive T cells into the CNS requires a number of molecular events to occur at the level of the blood brain barrier (BBB) and within the CNS parenchyma (Prat *et al.*, 2001). These include the processes of immune cell—endothelial cell adhesion, chemoattraction, and proteolytic digestion of the basement membrane that comprises the BBB and of the extracellular matrix (see other chapters for detailed discussion). Using a Boyden chamber model in which the dual compartments are divided by a porous fibronectin-coated membrane on which are grown human brain endothelial cells (HBECs), we have found that lymphocyte migration rates are increased in patients during times of relapses compared to times of clinically stable disease (Prat *et al.*, 2002).

Once antigen reactive T cells enter a tissue, their persistence is dependent on being presented with antigen by competent antigen presenting cells. Animal model studies show that T cells reactive with either neural (MBP reactive) or non-neural (ovalbumin) antigens can transmigrate into the CNS but that only the former will persist (Owens *et al.*, 1998). As mentioned, perivascular and parenchymal microglia are competent APCs. An issue to consider both in the experimental model and in MS is what is the source of antigen that is being presented to the T cells in the CNS of a previously healthy individual. Only now are the techniques becoming available to determine what, if any, peptides are sitting within the MHC class II groove of microglia under "physiologic conditions" (Santambrogio *et al.*, 2001). One speculates whether there is sufficient turnover of myelin under even normal conditions so that its processed peptides are expressed in APCs in the CNS. If tissue injury has occurred, greater amounts of peptide would be expected to be available. Perhaps the initial wave of activated cells that enters the CNS induces sufficient injury via release of pro-inflammatory molecules to result in antigen release. The initial autoreactive T cells interacting with the resident neural cells could initiate a cascade of events that would lead to the tissue injury characteristic of MS (see other chapters).

### Remission: Basis for Recovery

The basis of clinical recovery following immune mediated tissue injury with resultant neurologic dysfunction appears to involve cessation of the injury process and functional recovery by the injured tissue. The former could result from a relatively passive process in which the infiltrating disease relevant immune cells can no longer sustain their activation state. The process may also be impacted by active immune regulatory mechanisms that can involve functionally distinct cell subsets acting via cell-cell contact or release of soluble anti-inflammatory mediators (Anderton *et al.*, 1999; Kohm *et al.*, 2002). Recovery of function of injured tissue could reflect restoration of impaired axonal function or by remyelination. Restoration of axonal function may occur as a result of redistribution of sodium channels on demyelinated nerve segments (Waxman, 2001). Remyelination could arise from previously myelinating mature oligodendrocytes or, as suggested by most experimental studies, from progenitor cells that have differentiated into oligodendrocytes, as discussed later (Chari *et al.*, 2002). Functional recovery, as most clearly shown by functional MRI activation studies, can also reflect the recruitment of additional brain regions to mediate the functions previously associated with the actual sites of injury (Reddy *et al.*, 2000).

### Recurrence of Neurologic Episodes

Relapses in MS have been empirically defined as the appearance or reappearance of one or more neurologic abnormalities persisting for at least 24 to 48 hours and occurring 30 days or more after any previous relapse. The requirement that the symptoms or signs persist for at least 1 to 2 days is used to distinguish new pathologic events from transient physiological dysfunction that often occurs in previously damaged tissue. The interval of a month is an arbitrary attempt to define whether repeated events belong to one ongoing relapse or to different relapses. As discussed in detail in chapter 32, the MRI correlate of the relapse is a new T2 defined lesion generally associated with gadolinium enhancement on T1, indicating a local breakdown of the blood brain barrier. The rate of new MRI lesion formation is approximately tenfold greater than the clinical relapse rate. New MRI lesion formation without clinical features is common and as mentioned has been incorporated into the McDonald diagnostic criteria. The best pathologic correlate of the acute relapse and new MRI lesion is perivascular inflammation with extension into the parenchyma.

Analysis of cells recovered from the CNS of animals with recurrent forms of EAE suggests that such recurrences can reflect expansion of the immune response over time with development of T cell populations that are reactive with CNS antigens other than those used to initially induce the disease (Tuohy *et al.*, 2000). This is referred to as epitope spreading. Although this phenomenon has been demonstrated to occur in MS patients using functional *in vitro* measures of frequency of circulating myelin reactive T cells (limiting dilution, ELISPOT) (Pelfrey *et al.*, 2000), stronger confirmation is to be expected with advances in methodology (e.g., MHC class II tetramers). Such methodology should also help address the heterogeneity of autoantigens involved initially in any individual cases. Reactivation or expansion of a disease relevant immune response could occur either in the systemic compartment or within the CNS.

### Secondary Progression

As stated, approximately 50 to 60% of RR patients will evolve into a secondary progressive (SP) phase of disease after 10 to 15 years. Features of the SP phase of the disease include dysfunction at all levels of the neuraxis including cognitive impairment. Significant difficulty walking (EDSS >4) correlates most closely with spinal cord involvement. In approximately 10 to 15% of cases the disease is progressive from onset with or without intermixed relapses—primary progressive (PP) and progressive relapsing (PR). Whether the basis for progression in these clinical phenotypes is identical to that which accounts for the more common SP form of disease remains speculative. As will be noted, there is an apparent significant lack of efficacy of systemic immunomodulatory and immunosuppressive therapies in the progressive forms or phases of MS compared to the relapsing forms. Progressive forms of disease can also be induced in the EAE model dependent on animal strain and immunization regimen. In both the progressive MS case and the animal model, the pathology is characterized by extensive tissue destruction within the lesion with loss of oligodendrocytes and axons. At the lesion edge there is accumulation of activated microglia/macrophage with evidence of continued myelin breakdown. Lymphocyte accumulation is less evident. There is little ongoing remyelination. These features are consistent with MRI findings of expanded total lesion burden with reduction in the number of gadolinium enhancing lesions.

The basis for the evolution of the lesion in MS over time remains to be defined. The activated microglia/macrophages are sources of potential effector molecules that could induce tissue injury. Furthermore, uptake of tissue debris serves as means of activation of these cells. Removal of CNS tissue debris by invading macrophages may be necessary for optimal tissue repair. We have proposed that the end-stage loss of oligodendrocytes in the later phases of MS could reflect the increased vulnerability of initial sublethally injured oligodendrocytes to effector molecules derived from inflammatory cells present in the chronic inflammatory lesion (Wosik *et al.*, 2001). We showed that human oligodendrocytes experimentally injured by transfection with sublethal levels of p53 up-regulated expression of death receptors on the cells making them vulnerable to programmed cell death mediated by death receptor ligands including Fas-ligand and TRAIL. One further speculates whether the lack of remyelination reflects failure of progenitor cells due to such cells themselves being targets of immune mediated injury (Niehaus *et al.*, 2000) or that these cells or that these cells exhaust their capacity to replace destroyed oligodendrocytes/myelin. As regards axonal/nerve cell injury, initial transection of axons would result in extensive Wallerian degeneration of distal segments and loss of cell bodies if the initial injury were close to the cell body. In parallel with observations made at the neuromuscular junction in cases of post-polio syndrome, failure of compensatory synapses over time may also be expected (Cashman *et al.*, 1995).

## THERAPY AND MS

One might consider this issue in terms of those therapies directed at the immune system and those that are directed at the nervous system. The former therapies are aimed at halting disease development or progression; therapies targeting the nervous system are aimed at protecting tissue from injury, promoting recovery, or enhancing function.

A consideration of therapeutic claims in MS needs to take into account the actual design of the clinical studies from which relevant data were generated and how widely the results can be extrapolated across the different clinical phenotypes and phases of the disease. Trials in which stringent clinical trial methodology has been applied are the easiest to evaluate. A major dilemma is how to relate results of short-term studies to the long-term natural history of MS. The pivotal phase 3 studies leading to drug approval have been powered to assess effects on relapse rate and short-term progression. Most current and proposed immune-directed phase 2 studies are powered to generate MRI rather than clinical evidence of potential treatment efficacy.

## IMMUNOMODULATORY AND IMMUNE SUPPRESSIVE TREATMENT

Trials with these agents are based on the immune mediated hypothesis of MS pathogenesis; conversely, results of these trials provide support for the hypothesis. These therapies can be divided into those aimed at limiting the severity of relapses and those that prevent them.

## TREATMENT OF RELAPSES

Glucocorticoid therapy has become an accepted means to reduce the severity and shorten the duration of clinical attacks of MS, although the lack large-scale clinical trials makes it difficult to quantitate the magnitude of the effect (reviewed in Goodin *et al.*, 2002). Existing data do suggest the superiority of a short course of high dose intravenous therapy compared to relatively low and more protracted doses of oral therapy. A single study implicating a deleterious short-term effect of low dose therapy has not yet been confirmed (Beck *et al.*, 1993). Definitive data on high dose oral therapy are awaited. There seems to be little long-term beneficial impact on the course of the illness. The apparent limited magnitude of benefit of IV Ig and plasma exchange therapy for relapses of MS, coupled with the complexity or expense of administering these therapies, limit their use for the usual clinical situation. An open label study suggested that patients who have a very severe attack of fulminant demyelinating disease (not only MS) and who are unresponsive to high-dose glucocorticoids may benefit from a course of plasma exchange (Weinshenker *et al.*, 1999). Phase 2 clinical trials using an anti-VLA-4 adhesion molecule antibody (Natalizumab, Antegren) indicated that this therapy produced significant results with regard to reducing new MRI lesion frequency and clinical relapse rate (Miller *et al.*, 2003). A phase 3 clinical trial with this agent is currently in progress.

## TREATMENTS DIRECTED AT MODIFYING THE COURSE OF MS—RRMS

### *Immunomodulatory Treatment of RRMS*

Two families of molecules, interferon β (IFNβ) and glatiramer acetate (GA), have undergone large-scale clinical trials in patients with established RRMS. These trials have used both clinical and MR-based measures to demonstrate that the therapies reduced disease activity or development of further neurologic disability. Although the trials share many principles of design, it remains hazardous to do comparative analyses in the absence of head-to-head trials.

**Interferon β** —***Interferon beta-1β*** (IFN***β***-1***b***, ***Betaseron, Betaferon)*** The results of a large, multicenter, placebo-controlled trial using IFNβ-1b were reported in 1993 (The IFNB Multiple Sclerosis Study Group, 1993) and demonstrated that compared to treatment with placebo, treatment with 8 million international units (MIU) of IFNβ-1b injected subcutaneously (sc) every other day (qod) reduced the annual clinical attack rate (- 34%; $p = 0.0001$), rapidly reduced MRI activity as assessed by the number of newly forming gadolinium enhancing lesions (- 59%; $p = 0.0089$), and decreased the volume of developing white matter disease seen on MRI (- 20%; $p = 0.001$). This trial also showed a trend toward reduction in confirmed 1-point EDSS progression rate (- 29%; $p = 0.16$). Treatment with 1.6 mIU sc qod of IFNβ-1b (Betaseron) was also better than placebo on several outcome measures but was, in general, not as beneficial as the higher dose. The approved dose of Betaseron is 8 MIU, sc, qod.

***IFNβ-1a (Avonex)*** The placebo-controlled clinical trial, published in 1996 (Jacobs *et al.*, 1996), involved administration of 30 μg (6 mIU) of IFNβ-1a intramuscularly weekly for up to 2 years to relatively mildly affected patients (EDSS 1 – 3.5). The treatment produced a reduction in the clinical attack rate (- 18%; $p = 0.04$), MRI gadolinium activity (- 52%; $p = 0.05$) and confirmed 1-point EDSS progression rate (- 37%; $p = 0.02$). The total volume of white matter disease seen on MRI may also have been reduced in the treated group (- 6.7%; $p = 0.36$). A subsequent clinical trial comparing 30 and 60 μg concluded there was no significant dose related effect (Clanet *et al.*, 2001). 30 μg remains the recommended dose; this would be considered as the lowest dose of currently used IFNβs.

***IFNβ-1a (Rebif)*** The PRISMS trial, published in 1998 (PRISMS Study Group, 1998), demonstrated that compared with placebo, sc injection of 44 μg (12 mIU) of IFNβ-1a (Rebif) three times a week was associated with a reduction in clinical attack rate (- 33%; $p < 0.005$), the confirmed 1-point EDSS progression rate (- 30%; $p = 0.01$), the number of newly forming gadolinium enhancing lesions on MRI (- 78%; $p < 0.0001$), and the volume of white matter disease seen on MRI (-14.7%; $p < 0.0001$). Treatment with 22 μg sc three times a week was also effective on each of these outcome measures. The high-dose IFNβ-1a (Rebif) appeared to do better than the lower dose on each of the four main outcome measures, though these differences were not statistically significant; 44 μg sc, three times a week is the only approved dose in Europe.

The neuroimaging and pathological studies that underscore that damage occurs early in the CNS of patients have sparked an interest in the potential of immunomodulators to change the disease course more effectively if administered at the time of the initial clinical event. The CHAMPS study (Jacobs *et al.*, 2000) reported that IFNβ-1a (Avonex), used in patients with clinically isolated syndromes (CIS) and multifocal MRI abnormalities significantly delayed the progression to clinically definite MS compared with placebo. The ETOMS study (Comi *et al.*, 2000) reported similar findings when IFNβ-1a (Rebif) was used to treat selected patients with CIS. These observations further support the use of IFNβ therapies early in the course of disease. The bulk of evidence suggests that there is a dose response effect of IFNβ on the rate of new lesion formation in the MS disease process, as measured by short-term studies of relapse rate (EVIIDENCE) (Panitch H *et al.*, 2002). However, even at the highest IFNβ doses used currently, the therapeutic benefits seem to approach a plateau. As a result, it seems unlikely that clinical relapse rate will ever be reduced by more than 30 to 40% using IFNβ alone.

IFNβ therapies are thought to reduce new lesion formation by acting at several levels of the putative immune cascade that underlies development of such lesions (see Fig. 33.1). These include suppressing T cell activation, inhibiting pro-inflammatory cytokine production, inducing IL-l0 production, and inhibiting the expression of adhesion molecules (Fig. 33.1, step 2) and tissue breaking enzymes (Fig. 33.1, step 4). Because of the latter, interferons would be expected to have an important impact at the level of the blood brain barrier, which is indeed reflected by the consistent demonstration of significant and early suppression of gadolinium enhancement across all IFNβ trials.

How significant an impact the initial reduction on lesion formation has on subsequent development of long-term neurologic disability remains to be established. A complicating factor regarding long-term efficacy of IFNβ therapy relates to generation of anti-IFNβ antibodies during the course of treatment (Bertolotto *et al.*, 2002; Coles, 2002; Pozzilli *et al.*, 2002). Such antibodies may interfere with the beneficial action of the medication in some patients. Generation of antibodies may reflect the relative dose or preparation (and hence the immunogenicity) of the IFNβ used.

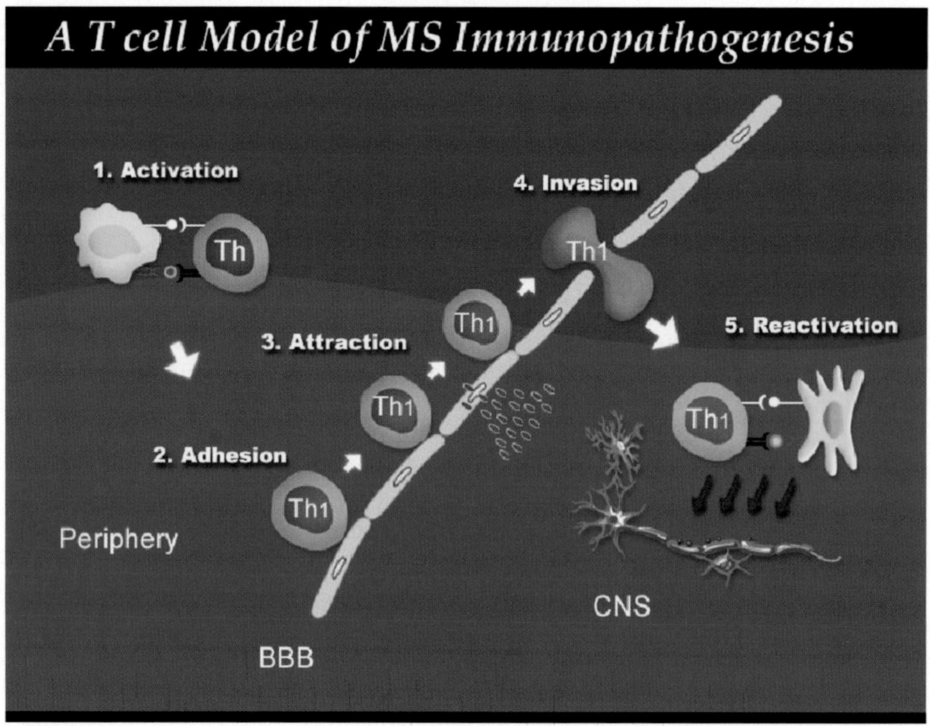


FIGURE 33.1
Potential sites of action of immunomodulatory therapies in MS. In MS, immune cells activated in the periphery (step 1) are thought to migrate across the blood brain barrier (BBB) through a series of molecular interactions involving adhesion (step 2), chemoattraction, (step 3) and transendothelial invasion (step 4). Once in the central nervous system (CNS), tissue directed immune cells may become reactivated (step 5) and participate in the local disease process. Available, and experimental, therapies for MS are likely to mediate their effects, in part, by acting on these potential targets.

Little data exist to date comparing the impact of current IFNβ therapies on quality-of-life measures. Although in all of the preceding trials, a high proportion of patients were able to meet the study end point, the array of side effects associated with IFNβ therapy, particularly the systemic "flu-like symptoms" and injection site reactions, do impact on patient decisions to accept or continue with therapy in the clinical situation. The rate of discontinuation of IFNβ therapy in clinical practice approaches 35 to 40% over 1 to 2 years).

*Glatiramer Acetate* (Copaxone, GA) is a copolymer comprised of four randomly assembled amino acids. In a multicenter, placebo-controlled trial published in 1995 (54), daily 20 mg sc injections of GA were associated with a reduction in the clinical attack rate over a 2-year period (- 29%; $p = 0.007$). The confirmed 1-point EDSS progression rate also appeared to be slightly reduced (- 13%; ns). In a subsequent short-duration trial, specifically directed toward MRI outcome measures, both the number of newly forming gadolinium enhancing lesions and the volume of white matter disease accumulation seen on MRI, were reduced in the group receiving GA, compared to placebo (Comi *et al.*, 2001). The effects on MRI reached statistical significance between 6 to 7 months after initiation of therapy. These MRI results contrast with the rapid suppression of new gadolinium enhancing lesions seen with IFNβ therapies. These results would be consistent with current data indicating that GA acts via inducing a deviation of the immune response in a Th2 direction, rather than by blocking lymphocyte trafficking across the blood brain barrier (Neuhaus *et al.*, 2001). Thus, the presence or absence of gadolinium enhancement per se does not directly inform us about the pathologic state of the CNS tissue within that lesion. GA therapy can be associated with localized skin reactions, hives, and occasional episodes of immediate post-injection reactions. Flu-like symptoms and fatigue are not an expected side effect. The conclusion from a recent clinical trial with an oral form of Copaxone was that no efficacy was apparent at the dose being studied.

*Glucocorticoids* Chronic oral steroid therapy has been abandoned as a treatment strategy. A recent trial of regular 3 monthly pulses of high dose I-V corticosteroids concluded that such therapy reduced the development of long-term disability and inhibited development of brain atrophy (Zivadinov *et al.*, 2001). These data raise the issue of the corticosteroids acting via a neuroprotective mechanism.

*IVIg* Several studies have reported that IVIg therapy reduces the frequency of clinical relapses (summarized in 39). To date, however, the effects of IVIg on disability or on the accumulation of MRI lesion burden have not been firmly established.

*Campath-1* This lympholytic anti-T cell antibody has been shown to virtually eliminate relapse rate and MRI new lesion formation but without an apparent effect on disease progression (Paolillo *et al.*, 1999). These data again raise the issue as to whether some of the progressive component of MS reflects pathophysiologic mechanisms that are distinct from those underlying the relapsing-remitting elements of the disease. Also of concern is identifying when the progressive process begins. When Campath was initially used, transient worsening of patients was observed that could be prevented by corticosteroid therapy. This effect was shown to be due to release of cytokines and nitric oxide (NO) and was reproduced *in vitro* by showing conduction block with NO.

**_Treatments That Aggravate Disease Activity_ (reviewed in Owens et al., 2001, and Wiendl et al., 2002)**

Systemic IFN $\gamma$ therapy was reported to increase symptoms in MS patients with RR disease. This study was conducted in the pre-MRI era leaving open the question whether the exacerbation of neurologic deficits reflected actual new inflammatory lesion formation or physiologic dysfunction of previously demyelinated axons, in parallel with results seen with initial use of Campath-1. Systemic therapies aimed at reducing TNF levels, namely anti-TNF antibody and soluble TNF receptor increased MRI and clinically defined disease activity. The mechanisms accounting for these results remains to be explained. The deleterious effects of systemic IFN$\gamma$ and anti-TNF directed therapies in MS were not predicted by results obtained in the EAE model.

**_Future Directions_ (see Fig. 33.1)**

Based on growing insights into the immune pathophysiology of MS and the presumed mechanisms of action of the currently approved therapies, a variety of new immunomodulators are being introduced into early phase clinical trials. The process of T cell stimulation (Fig. 33.1, step 1) is being targeted with the development of molecules such as CTLA4-Ig and anti-CD40 antibody that block costimulatory signals required for T cell activation (Laman *et al.*, 1998; Racke *et al.*, 2000). Other molecules including an altered peptide ligand (APL) of myelin basic protein (MBP) have been designed to shift responses of activated T cells from pro-inflammatory to anti-inflammatory response profiles (Bielekova *et al.*, 2000; Kappos *et al.*, 2000). Administration of mixtures of myelin antigens or myelin encoding DNA vaccines are being tested as means to eliminate autoreactive T cells recognizing these antigens via high dose tolerance (Robinson *et al.*, 2002). Studies continue with T cell vaccines using whole T cells, autoreactive T cells, or peptides encoded by T cell receptor V-beta genes whose products are implicated as recognizing disease relevant autoantigens (Vandenbark *et al.*, 1996; Zhang *et al.*, 2002). The anti-VLA-4 antibody (Antegren) noted earlier targets immune cell adhesion to endothelial cells (Fig. 33.1, step 2) and thus prevents entry of inflammatory cells into the CNS. Additional molecules are being designed to limit immune cell infiltration by targeting chemokine-chemokine receptor interactions (Fig. 33.1, step 3) and by suppressing the ability of immune cells to release tissue-breaking enzymes (Fig. 33.1, step 4).

### Immunomodulatory Treatment of SPMS

The European trial with IFNβ-1b (Betaferon) for SPMS reported benefit of treatment over placebo in significantly delaying time to sustained progression of disability, with additional benefits on relapse rate and MRI variables (European Study Group on interferon beta-1b in secondary progressive MS, 1998). The North American study of IFNβ-1b (Betaseron) in SPMS and the recently completed trial of IFNβ-1a (Rebif) in SPMS both failed to demonstrate a significant reduction in the confirmed 1-point EDSS progression (the predefined primary endpoint of both trials) (randomized controlled trial of interferon-beta-1a in secondary progressive MS: Clinical results, 2001; Goodkin *et al.*, 2000). Both reported significant reductions in clinical attack rate, MRI gadolinium activity, and MRI accumulation of white matter disease. The apparent discrepancy between these two trials and the earlier IFNβ-1b (Betaferon) trial would appear to relate to the variable inclusion in these trials of progressive patients with concomitant relapses. The use of a 1-point EDSS change to define disease progression, and differences in the entry EDSS between trial populations, may have also contributed to the disparate results. A trial with Avonex reported a beneficial effect on the newly developed MSFC scale but not on the EDSS (Li *et al.*, 2001). While IFNβ therapies may therefore have a role in the treatment of patients with progressive MS who also have relapses, there is currently no firm evidence to support the use of this family of immunomodulators in patients with SPMS without relapses. IVIg also has no proven efficacy in the progressive forms of MS.

### Immunosuppressive Treatments

In the past several decades, there has been considerable interest in the potential use of immunosuppressive agents for patients with MS, particularly those who fail the currently approved therapies described earlier. With the exception of mitoxantrone (recently approved in Europe and by the FDA for use in selected patients with MS), these therapies remain either "off label" in MS (to be considered only in select circumstances with careful review of toxicity profiles) or strictly experimental. Multiple agents have been tested including methotrexate, cyclosporine A, and cladribine (Goodkin *et al.*, 1995; Rice *et al.*, 2000; Zhao *et al.*, 1997). Described next are those agents that remain in active clinical use or that provide particular insights into the basis of disease development.

#### *Azathioprine*

Meta-analysis of published trials (mainly SPMS) suggests that this agent is marginally effective (Fernandez *et al.*, 2002; Palace *et al.*, 1997). It is generally administered at a total daily dose of 2 to 3 mg per kg with the goal of lowering the white blood cell count to between 3500 and 4000 cells/μL.

#### *Cyclophosphamide*

This alkylating agent has potent cytotoxic and immunosuppressive effects. Short-term side effects include alopecia and hemorrhagic cystitis, and longer-term toxicities include infertility and a potential increase in the risk of bladder cancer. The Northeast Cooperative Treatment Group reported a benefit of "pulse" therapy on clinical disease stabilization at 24 months though this effect was no longer seen at 36 months (Hauser *et al.*, 1983; Smith *et al.*, 1998). The Canadian Cooperative MS Study did not show a benefit of cyclophosphamide therapy on disease progression in an older cohort with more advanced disease (Noseworthy *et al.*, 1991). These apparently contrasting results can be viewed as supporting the concept that early lesion formation in MS reflects an immune-mediated process that is responsive to systemic immune directed therapies, whereas the later progressive phase is more dependent on neurobiologic variables that are resistant to systemic immune therapies.

A current focuses of immunosuppressive therapy in MS is on patients with frequent relapses or those who are transitioning into a progressive course despite the use of approved immunomodulating therapies. Treatment protocols involving immunosuppressive induction regimes at disease outset are also being investigated.

#### *Mitoxantrone* (Novantrone)

This anti-neoplastic agent intercalates with DNA and potently suppresses cellular and humoral immune responses. An initial clinical trial involved intravenous (IV) infusion of doses of 12 mg per $m^2$ or 5 mg per $m^2$ every 3 months for 2 years to both RRMS and SPMS patients (Edan *et al.*, 1997; van de Wyngaert *et al.*, 2001). The high-dose mitoxantrone resulted in significant reductions in the clinical attack rate ($P = 0.0002$), the MRI development of new gadolinium enhanced lesions ($P < 0.05$), and the total MRI lesion accumulation ($P < 0.05$), as well as a benefit in time to reach a 1-point EDSS change ($P = 0.04$). It has been approved by the FDA for the treatment of SPMS patients and may also be considered in severe, refractory relapses. Because of concerns regarding cardiac toxicity, the recommended total lifetime dose of mitoxantrone is limited, and the proposed regimen is generally offered for only 2 years. Such a limitation will be problematic for patients expected to require treatment over many years

*Chronic corticosteroid* use, including repeated pulse therapy, in SPMS has been evaluated in several studies that, for the most part, have not demonstrated sustained benefits. *Total lymphoid irradiation* is considered too risky for the marginal benefit it may provide. *Plasmapheresis* in SPMS has not been shown to be effective.

#### *Intense Immunoablation Followed by Autologous Stem Cell Rescue*

Early unblinded studies in advanced patients have had mixed results, with "'remissions" reported in some but not all patients and a small but real risk of mortality. A Canadian trial is under way in relatively early aggressive patients who are refractory to conventional therapies. The rational is that such patients may have more to gain and be at lower risk of serious complications.

Overall, immunomodulatory and immunosuppressive therapies appear to provide their greatest benefit early in the disease, during a period in which inflammatory responses are major contributors to tissue injury. As progressive disease sets in and irreversible axonal injury becomes the major process underlying clinical deterioration, the relative contribution of inflammation to ongoing injury may diminish and with it the role of anti-inflammatory therapies. This underscores the importance of initiating therapy early in the disease.

## NEURAL DIRECTED THERAPY

These can be considered in terms of therapies that mediate neuroportection or repair and those that improve function of the damaged nervous system (i.e., symptomatic therapy).

#### *Neurprotection/Regeneration*

To date there are no significant definitive trials or approved therapies related to this category. IFNβ itself is shown to increase NAA (a magnetic resonance spectroscopy marker of axonal integrity) after a 6-month delay (Narayanan *et al.*, 2001). Short-term systemic GA therapy is reported to accelerate recovery from experimental acute CNS traumatic lesions, an effect attributed to pro-inflammatory GA reactive cells that access the injury site. Neuroprotective therapies such as those used in ALS eg the gltutamate inhibitor Riluzole are being explored (Miller *et al.*, 2002). IV Ig therapy failed to promote functional recovery in MS patients (Noseworthy *et al.*, 2001). Initial clinical proof-of-principal trials using myelin forming cell transplants and gene transfer of neurotrophic agents are under way.

## SYMPTOMATIC TREATMENT IN MS

MS produces an array of symptoms that, if effectively treated, would have major impact on the affected individual's quality of life. The symptoms considered next represent those that presumably arise directly consequent to CNS demyelination and axonal injury.

### *Focal Weakness*

fMRI studies confirm the positive effects on neural plasticity and functional reorganization achieved by rehabilitation programs.

### *Fatigue*

Fatigue remains a very common and often very debilitating symptom for patients with MS. Potential biologic correlates of this symptom include critical lesion sites such as brain stem, release of cytokines, and ineffective neural transmission consequent to demyelination. Pharmacologic strategies to combat the fatigue of MS include pemoline, amantadine, and modafinil. All have demonstrated significant albeit small benefits in clinical trials.

The potassium channel blockers (e.g., 4-aminopyridine, 10 to 40 mg per day; and 3,4-diaminopyridine, 40 to 80 mg per day) may help some MS symptoms (especially heat-sensitive symptoms). These drugs presumably work by prolonging the duration of the nerve action potential. This would facilitate conduction through demyelinated fibers. At high doses, they may also cause seizures for similar reasons.

### *Spasticity*

This symptom reflects interruption of transmission along corticospinal tracts. Forty percent of patients rate their spasticity as moderate to severe. Nonpharmacologic approaches to the management of spasticity include physical therapy and exercise. Pharmacologic agents for reducing both spasticity and relalted spasms include baclofen (Lioresal), 20 to 120 mg per day; diazepam (Valium), 2 to 40 mg per day; and tizanidine (Zanaflex), 8 to 32 mg per day. Clonazepam (Klonopin, Rivotril) can be useful, particularly at bedtime, to decrease spasticity and improve sleep quality in some patients. Other medications less well established to provide benefit for patients with spasticity include carbamazepine, phenytoin, gabapentin, tetrahydrocannabinol, barbiturates, and alcohol. When the spasticity is particularly severe and the patient already has limited use of the lower extremities, a surgically implanted baclofen pump can often provide substantial relief. Destructive procedures such as selective rhyzotomy, tenotomy, myotomy, and phenol injections are reserved for only the most extreme situations.

### *Paroxysmal Symptoms*

Several different paroxysmal syndromes occur in MS. These syndromes are distinguished by brief duration (30 seconds to 2 minutes); high frequency of occurrence (5 to 40 paroxysms per day; lack of any alteration of consciousness or change in background electroencephalogram during the events); and a self-limited nature (generally lasting only months and then subsiding). They may be precipitated by hyperventilation or movement. These syndromes include the familiar Lhermitte's sign (electric shock-like sensations induced by neck flexion), tonic seizures, paroxysmal dysarthria/ataxia, paroxysmal sensory disturbances, and several other less well characterized syndromes. These syndromes are also distinguished by their marked responsiveness to very low dosages of anticonvulsant medications such as carbamazepine (Tegretol), 50 to 400 mg per day; phenytoin (Dilantin), 50 to 300 mg per day; or acetazolamide (Diamox), 200 to 600 mg per day.

### *Pain*

Pain is an under-appreciated symptom in MS. More than half of patients with MS complain of pain and, in a substantial fraction, the pain is described as severe, at least at times. An improved understanding of the mechanisms that produce pain of central origin has produced several successful approaches to its management, including the anticonvulsant drugs such as carbamazepine, 100 to 1000 mg per day, phenytoin, 300 to 600 mg per day, or gabapentin (Neurontin), 300 to 4800 mg per day; the antidepressant drugs such as amitriptyline, 25 to 150 mg per day, nortriptyline, 25 to 150 mg per day, desipramine, 100 to 300 mg per day, or venlafaxine, 75 to 225 mg per day; or the antiarrhythmic drugs such as mexiletine (Mexitil), 300 to 900 mg per day.

### *Ataxia or Tremor*

Ataxia or tremor is a relatively common and often intractable symptom in MS that is difficult to treat effectively. Some medications are occasionally helpful including clonazepam (Klonopin, Rivotril), 1.5 to 20 mg per day; primidone (Mysoline), 50 to 250 mg per day; propranolol (Inderal), 40 to 200 mg per day; and on dansetron (Zofran), 8 to 16 mg per day. For the most part, however, the success of such therapy is limited. Recently, there has been interest in the use thalamotomy or the placement of deep brain stimulators to control tremor. However, the response to this intervention, even when performed by a highly qualified surgeon, is often partial, the response rates are limited (< 50%), and the duration of any therapeutic benefit is unknown. Moreover, the surgical procedure itself carries risk.

## References


Anderton, S., Burkhart, C., Metzler, B., and Wraith, D. Mechanisms of central and peripheral T-cell tolerance: lessons from experimental models of multiple sclerosis. *Immunol. Rev.* **169,** 123–137. 1999.

Antel, J. P. and Bar-Or, A. Multiple sclerosis. (R. E. Rakel and E. T. Bope, eds.). "Conn's Current Therapy." 55th. 1-1-2003. W. B. Saunders Company.

Becher, B., Prat, A., and Antel, J. P. Brain-immune connection: Immuno-regulatory properties of CNS-resident cells. *Glia* **29**(4), 293–304. 2-15-2000.

Beck, R. W., Cleary, P. A., Trobe, J. D., Kaufman, D. I., Kupersmith, M. J., Paty, D. W., and Brown, C. H. The effect of corticosteroids for acute optic neuritis on the subsequent development of multiple sclerosis. The Optic Neuritis Study Group. *N. Engl. J. Med.* **329**(24), 1764–1769. 12-9-1993.

Bertolotto, A., Malucchi, S., Sala, A., Orefice, G., Carrieri, P. B., Capobianco, M., Milano, E., Melis, F., and Giordana, M. T. Differential effects of three interferon betas on neutralising antibodies in patients with multiple sclerosis: a follow up study in an independent laboratory. *J. Neurol. Neurosurg. Psychiatry* **73**(2), 148–153. 2002.

Bieganowska, K. D., Ausubel, L. J., Modabber, Y., Slovik, E., Messersmith, W., and Hafler, D. A. Direct ex vivo analysis of activated, Fas-sensitive autoreactive T cells in human autoimmune disease. *J. Exp. Med.* **185**(9), 1585–1594. 5-5-1997.

Bielekova, B., Goodwin, B., Richert, N., Cortese, I., Kondo, T., Afshar, G., Gran, B., Eaton, J., Antel, J., Frank, J. A., McFarland, H. F., and Martin, R. Encephalitogenic potential of the myelin basic protein peptide (amino acids 83–99) in multiple sclerosis: Results of a phase II clinical trial with an altered peptide ligand. *Nat. Med.* **6**(10), 1167–1175. 2000.

Brex, P. A., Ciccarelli, O., O'Riordan, J. I., Sailer, M., Thompson, A. J., and Miller, D. H. A longitudinal study of abnormalities on MRI and disability from multiple sclerosis. *N. Engl. J. Med.* **346**(3), 158–164. 1-17-2002.

Cashman, N. R. and Trojan, D. A. Correlation of electrophysiology with pathology, pathogenesis, and anticholinesterase therapy in post-polio syndrome. *Ann. N. Y. Acad. Sci.* **753,** 138–150. 5-25-1995.

Charcot J. M. Lectures on diseases of the nervous system. translated by G. Sigerson. 158–222. 1877. The New Sydenham Society, London.

Chari, D. M., and Blakemore, W. F. New insights into remyelination failure in multiple sclerosis: Implications for glial cell transplantation. *Mult. Scler.* **8**(4), 271–277. 2002.

Clanet, M., Raduc, E. W., Kappos, L., Hartung, H. P., Hohlfeld, R., Sandberg-Wollheim, M., Kooijmans-Coutinho, M. F., Tsao, E. C., Sandrock, A. W. (2002). A randomized, double blind, dose-comparison study of weekly interferon beta-1a in relapsing MS. *J. Neurol.* **59** (10), 1507–1517.

Coles, A. J. Neutralising antibodies to the beta interferons. *J. Neurol. Neurosurg. Psychiatry* **73**(2), 110–111. 2002.

Comi, G., Filippi, M., Barkhof, F., Durelli, L., Edan, G., Fernandez, O., Hartung, H., Seeldrayers, P., Sorensen, P. S., Rovaris, M., Martinelli, V., Hommes, O. R. (2001). Effect of early interferon treatment on conversion to definite multiple sclerosis: a randomised study. *Lancet* **357** 1576–1582.

Comi, G., Filippi, M., and Wolinsky, J. S. European/Canadian multicenter, double-blind, randomized, placebo-controlled study of the effects of glatiramer acetate on magnetic resonance imaging—measured disease activity and burden in patients with relapsing multiple sclerosis. European/Canadian Glatiramer Acetate Study Group. *Ann. Neurol.* **49**(3), 290–297. 2001.

Edan, G., Miller, D., Clanet, M., Confavreux, C., Lyon-Caen, O., Lubetzki, C., Brochet, B., Berry, I., Rolland, Y., Froment, J. C., Cabanis, E., Iba-Zizen, M. T., Gandon, J. M., Lai, H. M., Moseley, I., and Sabouraud, O. Therapeutic effect of mitoxantrone combined with methylprednisolone in multiple sclerosis: A randomised multicentre study of active disease using MRI and clinical criteria. *J. Neurol. Neurosurg. Psychiatry* **62**(2), 112–118. 1997.

European Study Group on Interferon Beta-1b in Secondary Progressive MS. Placebo-controlled multicentre randomised trial of interferon beta-1b in treatment of secondary progressive multiple sclerosis. *Lancet* **352**(9139), 1491–1497. 11-7-1998.

Fernandez, O., Guerrero, M., Mayorga, C., Munoz, L., Lean, A., Luque, G., Hervas, M., Fernandez, V., Capdevila, A., and De Ramon, E. Combination therapy with interferon Beta-1b and azathioprine in secondary progressive multiple sclerosis: A two-year pilot study. *J. Neurol.* **249**(8), 1058–1062. 2002.

Goodin, D. S., Frohman, E. M., Garmany, G. P., Jr., Halper, J., Likosky, W. H., Lublin, F. D., Silberberg, D. H., Stuart, W. H., and van den, Noort S. Disease modifying therapies in multiple sclerosis: Report of the Therapeutics and Technology Assessment Subcommittee of the American Academy of Neurology and the MS Council for Clinical Practice Guidelines. *Neurology* **58**(2), 169–178. 1-22-2002.

Goodkin, D., and the North American Study Group on Interferon beta-1b in Secondary Progressive MS. Interferon beta-1b in secondary progressive MS: clinical and MRI results of a 3-year randomized controlled trial. *Neurology* 54, 2352. 2000.

Goodkin, D. E., Rudick, R. A., VanderBrug, Medendorp S., Daughtry, M. M., Schwetz, K. M., Fischer, J., and Van Dyke, C. Low-dose (7.5 mg) oral methotrexate reduces the rate of progression in chronic progressive multiple sclerosis. *Ann. Neurol.* **37**(1), 30–40. 1995.

Gusev, E., Boiko, A., Bikova, O., Maslova, O., Guseva, M., Boiko, S., Vorobeichik, G., and Paty, D. The natural history of early onset multiple sclerosis: comparison of data from Moscow and Vancouver. *Clin. Neurol. Neurosurg.* **104**(3), 203–207. 2002.

Hauser, S. L., Dawson, D. M., Lehrich, J. R., Beal, M. F., Kevy, S. V., Propper, R. D., Mills, J. A., and Weiner, H. L. Intensive immunosuppression in progressive multiple sclerosis. A randomized, three-arm study of high-dose intravenous cyclophosphamide, plasma exchange, and ACTH. *N. Engl. J. Med.* **308**(4), 173–180. 1-27-1983.

Hoeber, Paul B. Association for Research in Nervous and Mental Disease: Multiple Sclerosis (disseminated sclerosis). [1). 1922. New York.

Interferon Beta-1b Is Effective in Relapsing-Remitting Multiple Sclerosis. I. Clinical results of a multicenter, randomized, double-blind, placebo-controlled trial. The IFNB Multiple Sclerosis Study Group. *Neurology* **43**(4), 655–661. 1993.

Jacobs, L. D., Beck, R. W., Simon, J. H., Kinkel, R. P., Brownscheidle, C. M., Murray, T. J., Simonian, N. A., Slasor, P. J., and Sandrock, A. W. Intramuscular interferon beta-1a therapy initiated during a first demyelinating event in multiple sclerosis. CHAMPS Study Group. *N. Engl. J. Med.* **343**(13), 898–904. 9-28-2000.

Jacobs, L. D., Cookfair, D. L., Rudick, R. A., Herndon, R. M., Richert, J. R., Salazar, A. M., Fischer, J. S., Goodkin, D. E., Granger, C. V., Simon, J. H., Alam, J. J., Bartoszak, D. M., Bourdette, D. N., Braiman, J., Brownscheidle, C. M., Coats, M. E., Cohan, S. L., Dougherty, D. S., Kinkel, R. P., Mass, M. K., Munschauer, F. E., III, Priore, R. L., Pullicino, P. M., Scherokman, B. J., Whitham, R. H., and Intramuscular interferon beta-1a for disease progression in relapsing multiple sclerosis. The Multiple Sclerosis Collaborative Research Group (MSCRG). *Ann. Neurol.* **39**(3), 285–294. 1996.

Kappos, L., Comi, G., Panitch, H., Oger, J., Antel, J., Conlon, P., and Steinman, L. Induction of a non-encephalitogenic type 2 T helper-cell autoimmune response in multiple sclerosis after administration of an altered peptide ligand in a placebo-controlled, randomized phase II trial. The Altered Peptide Ligand in Relapsing MS Study Group. *Nat. Med.* **6**(10), 1176–1182. 2000.

Kaufman, M., Gaydos, C. A., Sriram, S., Boman, J., Tondella, M. L., and Norton, H. J. Is Chiamydia pneumoniae found in spinal fluid samples from multiple sclerosis patients? Conflicting results. *Mult. Scler.* **8**(4), 289–294. 2002.

Kohm, A. P., Carpentier, P. A., Anger, H. A., and Miller, S. D. Cutting Edge: CD4(+)CD25(+) Regulatory T Cells Suppress Antigen-Specific Autoreactive Immune Responses and Central Nervous System Inflammation During Active Experimental Autoimmune Encephalomyelitis. *J. Immunol.* **169**(9), 4712–4716. 11-1-2002.

Laman, J. D., Maassen, C. B., Schellekens, M. M., Visser, L., Kap, M., de Jong, E., van Puijenbroek, M., van Stipdonk, M. J., van Meurs, M., Schwarzler, C., and Gunthert, U. Therapy with antibodies against CD40L (CD154) and CD44-variant isoforms reduces experimental autoimmune encephalomyelitis induced by a proteolipid protein peptide. *Mult. Scler.* **4**(3), 147–153. 1998.

Lang, H. L., Jacobsen, H., Ikemizu, S., Andersson, C., Harlos, K., Madsen, L., Hjorth, P., Sondergaard, L., Svejgaard, A., Wucherpfennig, K., Stuart, D. I., Bell, J. I., Jones, E. Y., and Fugger, L. A functional and structural basis for TCR cross-reactivity in multiple sclerosis. *Nat. Immunol.* **3**(10), 940–943. 2002.

Li, D. K., Zhao, G. J., and Paty, D. W. Randomized controlled trial of interferon-beta-1a in secondary progressive MS: MRI results. *Neurology* **56**(11), 1505–1513. 6-12-2001.

McAlpine D. The benign form of multiple sclerosis. a study based on 241 cases seen within 3 years of onset and followed up until the 10th year or more of the disease. *Brain* 84, 186–203. 1961.

McDonald, W. I., Compston, A., Edan, G., Goodkin, D., Hartung, H. P., Lublin, F. D., McFarland, H. F., Paty, D. W., Polman, C. H., Reingold, S. C., Sandberg-Wollheim, M., Sibley, W., Thompson, A., van den Noort S., Weinshenker, B. Y., and Wolinsky, J. S. Recommended diagnostic criteria for multiple sclerosis: Guidelines from the International Panel on the diagnosis of multiple sclerosis. *Ann. Neurol.* **50**(1), 121–127. 2001.

Miller, D. H., Khan, O. A., Sheremata, W. A., Blumbardt, L. D., Rice, G. P., Libonati, M. A., Willmer-Hulme, A. J. Dalton, C. M., Miszkiel, K. A., O'Connor, P. W. (2003). A controlled trial of natalizumab for relapsing multiple sclerosis. *N. Engl. J. Med.* **348**, 15–23.

Miller, R. G., Mitchell, J. D., Lyon, M., and Moore, D. H. Riluzole for amyotrophic lateral sclerosis (ALS)/motor neuron disease (MND). *Cochrane. Database. Syst. Rev.* (2), CD001447. 2002.

Miller, S. D., Katz-Levy, Y., Neville, K. L., and Vanderlugt, C. L. Virus-induced autoimmunity: Epitope spreading to myelin autoepitopes in Theiler's virus infection of the central nervous system. *Adv. Virus Res.* 56, 199–217. 2001.

Moore, F. G., and Wolfson, C. Human herpes virus 6 and multiple sclerosis. *Acta Neurol. Scand.* **106**(2), 63–83. 2002.

Murray T. J., Burks, J. S., and Johnson, K. P. "Multiple Sclerosis: Diagnosis, Medical Management, and Rehabilitation," (1), 1–34. 2000. Demos Medical Publishing, New York.

Murthy, S. N., Faden, H. S., Cohen, M. E., and Bakshi, R. Acute disseminated encephalomyelitis in children. *Pediatrics* **110** (2 Pt 1), e21. 2002.

Narayanan, S., De Stefano, N., Francis, G. S., Arnaoutelis, R., Caramanos, Z., Collins, D. L., Pelletier, D., Arnason, B. G. W., Antel, J. P., and Arnold, D. L. Axonal metabolic recovery in multiple sclerosis patients treated with interferon beta-1b. *J. Neurol.* **248**(11), 979–986. 2001.

National Multiple Sclerosis Society. "Therapeutic Claims in Multiple Sclerosis," 1st. ed. 1982. New York.

Neuhaus, O., Farina, C., Wekerle, H., and Hohlfeld, R. Mechanisms of action of glatiramer acetate in multiple sclerosis. *Neurology* **56**(6), 702–708. 3-27-2001.

Niehaus, A., Shi, J., Grzenkowski, M., Diers-Fenger, M., Archelos, J., Hartung, H. P., Toyka, K., Bruck, W., and Trotter, J. Patients with active relapsing-remitting multiple sclerosis synthesize antibodies recognizing oligodendrocyte progenitor cell surface protein: implications for remyelination. *Ann. Neurol.* **48**(3), 362–371. 2000.

Noseworthy, J. H., O'Brien, P. C., Petterson, T. M., Weis, J., Stevens, L., Peterson, W. K., Sneve, D., Cross, S. A., Leavitt, J. A., Auger, R. G., Weinshenker, B. G., Dodick, D. W., Wingerchuk, D. M., and Rodriguez, M. A randomized trial of intravenous immunoglobulin in inflammatory demyelinating optic neuritis. *Neurology* **56**(11), 1514–1522. 6-12-2001.

Noseworthy, J. H., Vandervoort, M. K., Penman, M., Ebers, G., Shumak, K., Seland, T. P., Roberts, R., Yetisir, E., Gent, M., and Taylor, D. W. Cyclophosphamide and plasma exchange in multiple sclerosis. *Lancet* **337**(8756), 1540–1541. 6-22-1991.

Owens, T., Tran, E., Hassan-Zahraee, M., and Krakowski, M. Immune cell entry to the CNS–a focus for immunoregulation of EAE. *Res. Immunol.* **149**(9), 781–789. 1998.

Owens, T., Wekerle, H., and Antel, J. Genetic models for CNS inflammation. *Nat. Med.* **7**(2), 161–166. 2001.

Palace, J., and Rothwell, P. New treatments and azathioprine in multiple sclerosis. *Lancet* **350**(9073), 261. 7-26-1997.

Panitch, H., Goodin, D. S., Francis, G., Chang, P., Coyle, P. K., O'Connor, P., Monaghan, E., Li, D., Weinsberkar, B. (2002). Randomized, comparative study of interferon beta-1a treatment regimens in MS: the evidence trail. *Neurology* **59**(10), 1496–1506.

Paolillo, A., Coles, A. J., Molyneux, P. D., Gawne-Cain, M., MacManus, D., Barker, G. J., Compston, D. A., and Miller, D. H. Quantitative MRI in patients with secondary progressive MS treated with monoclonal antibody Campath 1H. *Neurology* **53**(4), 751–757. 9-11-1999.

Paty, D., and Ebers, G. C. "Multiple Sclerosis." 1997.F. A. Davis Company, Philadelphia.

Pelfrey, C. M., Rudick, R. A., Cotleur, A. C., Lee, J. C., Tary-Lehmann, M., and Lehmann, P. V. Quantification of self-recognition in multiple sclerosis by single-cell analysis of cytokine production. *J. Immunol.* **165**(3), 1641–1651. 8-1-2000.

Pozzilli, C., Antonini, G., Bagnato, F., Mainero, C., Tomassini, V., Onesti, E., Fantozzi, R., Galgani, S., Pasqualetti, P., Millefiorini, E., Spadaro, M., Dahlke, F., and Gasperini, C. Monthly corticosteroids decrease neutralizing antibodies to IFNbeta1 b: A randomized trial in multiple sclerosis. *J. Neurol.* **249**(1), 50–56. 2002.

Prat, A., Biernacki, K., Lavoie, J. F., Poirier, J., Duquette, P., and Antel, J. P. Migration of multiple sclerosis lymphocytes through brain endothelium. *Arch. Neurol.* **59**(3), 391–397. 2002.

Prat, A., Biernacki, K., Wosik, K., and Antel, J. P. Glial cell influence on the human blood-brain barrier. *Glia* **36**(2), 145–155. 2001.

PRISMS (Prevention of Relapses and Disability by Interferon beta-1a Subcutaneously in Multiple Sclerosis) Study Group. Randomised double-blind placebo-controlled study of interferon beta-1a in relapsing/remitting multiple sclerosis. *Lancet* **352**(9139), 1498–1504. 11-7-1998.

Racke, M. K., Ratts, R. B., Arredondo, L., Perrin, P. J., and Lovett-Racke, A. The role of costimulation in autoimmune demyelination. *J. Neuroimmunol.* **107**(2), 205–215. 7-24-2000.

Randomized controlled trial of interferon-beta-1a in secondary progressive MS: Clinical results. *Neurology* **56**(11), 1496–1504. 6-12-2001.

Reddy, H., Narayanan, S., Arnoutelis, R., Jenkinson, M., Antel, J., Matthews, P. M., and Arnold, D. L. Evidence for adaptive functional changes in the cerebral cortex with axonal injury from multiple sclerosis. *Brain* **123** (Pt. 11), 2314–2320. 2000.

Rice, G. P., Filippi, M., and Comi, G. Cladribine and progressive MS: Clinical and MRI outcomes of a multi-center controlled trial. Cladribine MRI Study Group. *Neurology* **54**(5), 1145–1155. 3-14-2000.

Robinson, W. H., Garren, H., Utz, P. J., and Steinman, L. Millennium Award. Proteomics for the development of DNA tolerizing vaccines to treat autoimmune disease. *Clin. Immunol.* **103**(1), 7–12. 2002.

Santambrogio, L., Belyanskaya, S. L., Fischer, F. R., Cipriani, B., Brosnan, C. F., Ricciardi-Castagnoli, P., Stern, L. J., Strominger, J. L., and Riese, R. Developmental plasticity of CNS microglia. *Proc. Natl. Acad. Sci. USA* **98**(11), 6295–6300. 5-22-2001.

Smith, D. R., Olek, M. J., Balashov, K. E., Khoury, S. J., Hafler, D. A., and Weiner, H. L. Principles of immunotherapy. "Clinical Neuroimmunology" (J. P. Antel, G. Birnbaum, and H-P Hartung), (7), 92–104. 1998. Blackwell Science, Oxford.

Sung, M. H., Zhao, Y., Martin, R., and Simon, R. T-cell epitope prediction with combinatorial peptide libraries. *J. Comput. Biol.* **9**(3), 527–539. 2002.

Swamy, H. S., Shankar, S. K., Chandra, P. S., Aroor, S. R., Krishna, A. S., and Perumal, V. G. Neurological complications due to beta-propiolactone (BPL)-inactivated antirabies vaccination. Clinical, electrophysiological and therapeutic aspects. *J. Neurol. Sci.* **63**(1), 111–128. 1984.

Talbot, P. J., Arnold, D., and Antel, J. P. Virus-induced autoimmune reactions in the CNS. *Curr. Top. Microbiol. Immunol.* **253,** 247–271. 2001.

"Therapeutic Claims in Multiple Sclerosis." 3rd. ed. Sibley, W. 1992. Demo Publications, New York.

Tourbah, A., Gout, O., Liblau, R., Lyon-Caen, O., Bougniot, C., Iba-Zizen, M. T., and Cabanis, E. A. Encephalitis after hepatitis B vaccination: recurrent disseminated encephalitis or MS? *Neurology* **53**(2), 396–401. 7-22-1999.

Tubridy, N., Behan, P. O., Capildeo, R., Chaudhuri, A., Forbes, R., Hawkins, C. P., Hughes, R. A., Palace, J., Sharrack, B., Swingler, R., Young, C., Moseley, I. F., MacManus, D. G., Donoghue, S., and Miller, D. H. The effect of anti-alpha4 integrin antibody on brain lesion activity in MS. The UK Antegren Study Group. *Neurology* **53**(3), 466–472. 8-11-1999.

Tuohy, V. K., and Kinkel, R. P. Epitope spreading: a mechanism for progression of autoimmune disease. *Arch. Immunol. Ther. Exp. (Warsz).* **48**(5), 347–351. 2000.

van de Wyngaert, F. A., Beguin, C., D'Hooghe, M. B., Dooms, G., Lissoir, F., Carton, H., and Sindic, C. J. A double-blind clinical trial of mitoxantrone versus methylprednisolone in relapsing, secondary progressive multiple sclerosis. *Acta Neurol. Belg.* **101**(4), 210–216. 2001.

Vandenbark, A. A., Chou, Y. K., Whitham, R., Mass, M., Buenafe, A., Liefeld, D., Kavanagh, D., Cooper, S., Hashim, G. A., and Offner, H. Treatment of multiple sclerosis with T-cell receptor peptides: Results of a double-blind pilot trial. *Nat. Med.* **2**(10), 1109–1115. 1996.

Waxman, S. G. Acquired channelopathies in nerve injury and MS. *Neurology* **56**(12), 1621–1627. 6-26-2001.

Weinshenker, B. G., O'Brien, P. C., Petterson, T. M., Noseworthy, J. H., Lucchinetti, C. F., Dodick, D. W., Pineda, A. A., Stevens, L. N., and Rodriguez, M. A randomized trial of plasma exchange in acute central nervous system inflammatory demyelinating disease. *Ann. Neurol.* **46**(6), 878–886. 1999.

Wiendl, H., and Hohlfeld, R. Therapeutic approaches in multiple sclerosis: Lessons from failed and interrupted treatment trials. *BioDrugs.* **16**(3), 183–200. 2002.

Wosik, K., Antel, J., Kuhlmann, T., Bruck, W., Massie, B., and Nalbantoglu, J. (2003). Oligodendrocyte injury in multiple sclerosis: a role for p53. *J. Neurochem.* **85**(3), 635–644.

Wucherpfennig, K. W. Infectious triggers for inflammatory neurological diseases. *Nat. Med.* **8**(5), 455–457. 2002.

Zhang, J. Z., Rivera, V. M., Tejada-Simon, M. V., Yang, D., Hong, J., Li, S., Haykal, H., Killian, J., and Zang, Y. C. T cell vaccination in multiple sclerosis: Results of a preliminary study. *J. Neurol.* **249**(2), 212–218. 2002.

Zhao, G. J., Li, D. K., Wolinsky, J. S., Koopmans, R. A., Mietlowski, W., Redekop, W. K., Riddehough, A., Cover, K., and Paty, D. W. Clinical and magnetic resonance imaging changes correlate in a clinical trial monitoring cyclosporine therapy for multiple sclerosis. The MS Study Group. *J. Neuroimaging* **7**(1), 1–7. 1997.

Zivadinov, R., Rudick, R. A., De Masi, R., Nasuelli, D., Ukmar, M., Pozzi-Mucelli, R. S., Grop, A., Cazzato, G., and Zorzon, M. Effects of IV methylprednisolone on brain atrophy in relapsing-remitting MS. *Neurology* **57**(7), 1239–1247. 10-9-2001.

CHAPTER

34

# Adrenoleukodystrophies

*Hugo W. Moser*

## HISTORY

The disorder now referred to as X-linked adrenoleukodystrophy (X-ALD) was first described by Siemerling and Creutzfeldt in 1923 (Siemerling and Creutzfeldt, 1923). They reported a 7-year-old boy who had been well until age 3 or 4, when he was first noted to be hyperpigmented. At 61/2 years he became disturbed, and his speech and gait deteriorated. He became spastic, unable to walk or swallow, and died at 7 years. Postmortem examination showed adrenal atrophy and extensive demyelination combined with perivascular accumulation of lymphocytes and plasma cells in the central nervous system. They referred to this condition as Bronzekrankheit und Skelosierendc Encephalomyelitis, and noted the resemblance of the neuropathological features to the encephalitis periaxialis diffusa described by Paul Schilder in 1912 and in 1913. In retrospect it is now clear that the case reported by Haberfeld and Spieler in 1910, and studied neuropathologically by Schilder (Schilder, 1924), had the same condition, in view of the fact that the clinical history and neuropathological findings were similar and the note in the case history that the patient had become hyperpigmented, even though adrenal pathology was not commented on. Additional cases were reported by Pfister (1936), Hampel (1937), Adams and Kubic (Adams and Kubic, 1952), Gagnon (1959), Lichenstein and Rosenbluth (1959), Brun and Voigt (1960), Hoefnagel and Van Den Noort (1962), Fanconi *et al.* (1963), and Blaw *et al.* (1964). The cases were referred to variously as "Diffuse Hirnsklerose" (Pfister, 1936), "Morbus Addisonii und Skleroriesiende Erkrankung" (Hampel, 1937), "Sclerose Cerebrale diffuse avec Melanoderme et atrophie surrenale" (Gagnon, 1959), "Entzundlische cerebrale Sklerose mit Nebenniereninsuffizienz" (Brun and Voigt, 1960), and "Addison's disease and diffuse sclerosi" (Hoefnagel and Van Den Noort, 1962). It has also been referred to as Addison-Schilder disease, and less specifically as Schilder's disease. The designation adrenoleukodystrophy was introduced by Blaw in 1970 (Blaw, 1970) and is now used worldwide. On the basis of pedigree analysis Fanconi *et al.* proposed in 1963 (Fanconi *et al.*, 1963) that the disorder had an X-linked recessive mode of inheritance, and this has been confirmed. In 1976 and in 1977, Budka *et al.* and Griffin *et al.* independently described X-ALD adult patients with progressive paraparesis and primary adrenal insufficiency (Budka *et al.*, 1976; Griffin *et al.*, 1977). This entity is now referred to as adrenomyeloneuropathy (AMN). AMN has now been shown to have the same biochemical and genetic basis as the childhood forms of X-ALD and they often co-occur in the same family. We recommend that the designation X-linked adrenoleukodystrophy (X-ALD) be applied to encompass all of the phenotypic variants listed in Table 34.1. X-ALD must be distinguished sharply from the entity referred to as connatal adrenoleukodystrophy (Ulrich *et al.*, 1978) or neonatal adrenoleukodystrophy (NALD) (Kelley *et al.*, 1986). Although NALD shares certain biochemical and pathological features

TABLE 34.1 Phenotypes in Males and Females

**Phenotypes in Males**

| Phenotype | Description | Estimated relative frequency |
|---|---|---|
| Childhood cerebral (CCER) | Onset at 3–10 years of age. Progressive behavioral, cognitive and neurologic deficit, often leading to total disability within 3 years. Inflammatory brain demyelination | 31–35% |
| Adolescent | Like childhood cerebral. Onset age 11–21 years. Somewhat slower progression. | 4–7% |
| Adrenomyeloneuropathy (AMN) | Onset 28 ± 9 years, progressive over decades. Involves spinal cord mainly, distal axonopathy inflammatory response mild or absent. Approximately 40% have or develop cerebral involvement with varying degrees of inflammatory response and more rapid progression. | 40–46% |
| Adult cerebral | Dementia, behavioral disturbances. Sometimes focal deficits, without preceding AMN. White matter inflammatory response present. Progression parallels that of childhood cerebral form. | 2–5% |
| Olivo-ponto-cerebellar | Mainly cerebellar and brainstem involvement in adolescence or adulthood. | 1–2% |
| Aaddison-only@ | Primary adrenal insufficiency without apparent neurologic involvement. Onset common before 7.5 years. Most eventually develop AMN. | Varies with age. Up to 50% in childhood. |
| Asymptomatic | Biochemical and gene abnormality without demonstrable adrenal or neurologic deficit. Detailed studies often show adrenal hypofunction or subtle signs of AMN. | Diminishes with age. Common < 4 years. Very rare > 40 years |

**Phenotypes in Female X-ALD Carriers**

| Phenotype | Description | Estimated relative frequency |
|---|---|---|
| Asymptomatic | No evidence of adrenal or neurologic involvement | Diminishes with age. Most women < 30 years neurologically uninvolved. |
| Mild myelopathy | Increased deep tendon reflexes and distal sensory changes in lower extremities with absent or mild disability. | Increases with age. Approximately 50% > 40 years. |
| Moderate to severe myeloneuropathy | Symptoms and pathology resemble AMN, but milder and later onset. | Increases with age. Approximately 15% > 40 years. |
| Cerebral involvement | Rarely seen in childhood and slightly more common in middle age and later. | Approximately 2%. |
| Clinically evident adrenal insufficiency | Rare at any age. | Approximately 1%. |

with X-ALD, it is fundamentally distinct. It is a disorder of peroxisome biogenesis with an autosomal recessive mode of inheritance (Gould *et al.*, 2001). The discussion in this chapter will be confined to X-ALD.

A key advance about the understanding of X-ALD was achieved at the Albert Einstein College of Medicine in New York between 1973 and 1976 when Powers and Schaumburg (1973) demonstrated characteristic inclusions in the adrenal cortical cells and brain macrophages and Igarashi *et al.* (1976b) showed that these inclusions contained large amounts of cholesterol esterified with saturated unbranched very long chain fatty acids (VLCFA). These VLCFA consisted mainly of tetracosanoic (C24:0) and hexacosanoic (C26:0) acids. This led to the recognition that X-ALD is a lipid storage disease. In 1980 and 1981, Moser *et al.* showed that VLCFA levels were also increased in cultured skin fibroblasts and plasma. The plasma VLCFA assay is the most widely used diagnostic assay and has led to the identification of thousands of patients (Moser *et al.*, 1999). In 1984 Singh *et al.* (1984b) showed that white blood cells and cultured skin fibroblasts had an impaired capacity to degrade VLCFA. This led to the conclusion that the basic biochemical defect in X-ALD is the impaired capacity to degrade VLCFA. Two laboratories (Lazo *et al.*, 1988; Wanders *et al.*, 1988) reported that the biochemical defect involved the impaired capacity to form the coenzyme derivative of VLCFA, a reaction catalyzed by the peroxisomal enzyme VLCFA synthetase (VLCS). This conclusion had been generally accepted, but has been thrown into question recently by the studies of McGuinness (McGuinness *et al.*, 2003), which indicate that the earlier report of Tsuji *et al.* (1981a) that VLCFA synthesis is increased in patients with X-ALD must also be considered as a factor in the pathogenesis of the VLCFA accumulation.

The gene that is defective in X-ALD was mapped to Xq28 in 1981 (Migeon *et al.*, 1981). Mosser *et al.* identified the defective gene by positional cloning (Mosser *et al.*, 1993). It is now referred to as ABCD1. The gene product has no homology to VLCS, but codes for a peroxisomal membrane protein (ALDP) that is a member of the ATP binding cassette (ABC) transporter protein family (Higgins, 1992). The mechanism through which the ALDP deficiency leads to the accumulation of VLCFA or to the adrenal and brain pathology is not yet understood. Mouse models of X-ALD by targeted inactivation of ABCD1 were developed in 1997 (Forss-Petter *et al.*, 1997; Kobayashi *et al.*, 1997; Lu *et al.*, 1997).

## CLINICAL FEATURES

X-ALD has been observed in all ethnic groups and affects approximately 1:20,000 males (Bezman *et al.*, 2001). The pattern of inheritance is X-linked recessive. The clinical manifestations of X-ALD vary widely and for reasons that are still unknown the various phenotypes often co-occur within the same family. Table 34.1 shows the subgroupings that have been established and their relative frequency. Figure 34.1 shows a survival analysis for the cerebral phenotypes.

### Childhood Cerebral X-ALD

The designation of childhood cerebral X-ALD (CCER) is applied to boys who develop evidence of neurologic involvement before 10 years of age. Prenatal, perinatal, and early postnatal development are entirely normal. In a 1987 survey (Moser *et al.*, 1987), we found the mean age of onset of neurologic symptoms to be 7.2 $\pm$ 1.0 years with a range of 2.75 to 10 years, but recently we became aware of a patient who became symptomatic at 21 months of age. Table 34.2 lists the initial symptoms in a series of 180 patients. Most commonly, the first neurologic symptoms are in the behavioral sphere and are often mistaken for hyperactivity attention deficit disorder. The child may also exhibit emotional lability, withdrawn behavior, or school failure or combination of the three. The behavioral disturbances vary with the location of the demyelinating lesions on MRI. In approximately 80%, the initial lesions involve the parieto-occipital white matter (Kumar *et al.*, 1987) and manifest as disturbances of visuospatial or auditory perception and spatial orientation. Difficulty in understanding speech in a noisy room or over the telephone are common early symptoms and reflect impaired auditory discrimination, often with retention in normal pure tone perception. Visual impairment is an early symptom in approximately one-third of the patients and often is due to a combination of optic nerve, optic tract, and occipital lobe involvement. Visual field cuts and impaired visual acuity are common. In approximately 15% of patients, the initial lesion involves the frontal lobes. These patients often present with disinhibited behavior and other behavioral disturbances without the focal neuropsychological deficits that occur in patients with the parieto-occipital lesions. Shapiro and collaborators have described a series of neuropsychologic tests that are particularly relevant to the evaluation of children with leukodystrophies (Shapiro *et al.*, 1995, 2000; Shapiro and Klein, 1994). These tests assess the five major domains of language, visual perception, visual/constructional function, memory, and executive function. They are of value in assessing disease progression and prognosis and for the selection of patients who are candidates for bone marrow transplantation (Shapiro *et al.*, 2000).

Apart from the neuropsychological, auditory and visual disturbances, early neurologic symptoms may include impaired sport performance, unsteady gait, poor handwriting,

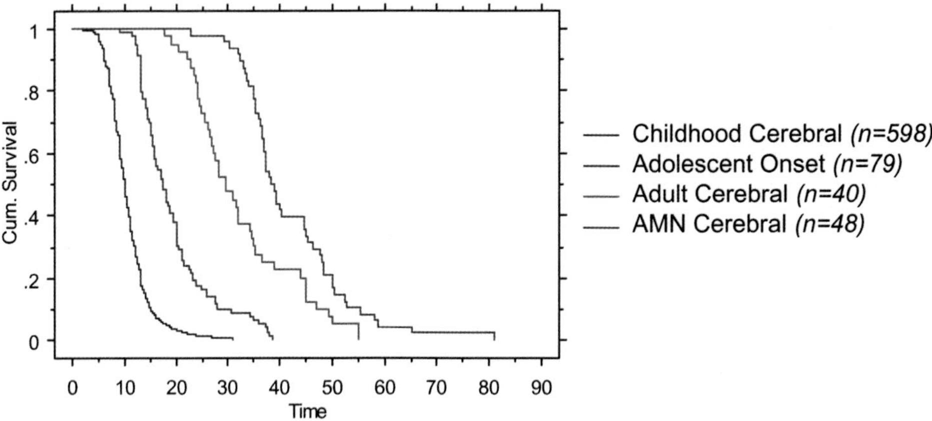


FIGURE 34.1
Time is age in years. See Table 34.1 for definition of phenotypes. Note that the rapid downward slopes for each of the cerebral phenotypes are approximately equal. As noted in the sections on pathology and pathogenesis, the rapid progression of X-ALD is due the inflammatory cerebral demyelination. Most commonly, this response manifests in childhood. Less commonly, it manifests in adolescence or adulthood, but once it commences the rate of progression is approximately the same, irrespective of age. The approximately equal downward slope of the survival curves of each of the cerebral phenotypes demonstrates this.

TABLE 34.2 Initial Symptoms in 160 Patients with the Childhood Cerebral Form of Adrenoleukodystrophy

| Symptom | Percentage |
|---|---|
| School difficulty | 16 |
| Behavioral disturbances | 13 |
| Impaired vision | 11 |
| Impaired hearing | 8 |
| Poor coordination | 8 |
| Dementia | 7 |
| Seizure | 7 |
| Hyperactivity | 6 |
| Squint, double vision | 5 |
| Difficulty walking | 4 |
| Speech difficulty | 4 |
| Limb weakness | 3 |
| Poor handwriting | 2 |
| Headaches | 2 |
| Loss of athletic ability | 1 |
| Urinary incontinence | 1 |
| Tics | 1 |
| Fecal incontinence | 0.3 |
| Increased intracranial pressure | 0.3 |
| Difficulty swallowing | 0.3 |
| Coma | 0.3 |

strabismus, and seizures. A seizure was the first neurologic manifestation in 7% of the patients (Table 34.2). Once the neurologic symptoms become manifest, progression often is rapid. In the 1987 Kennedy Krieger Institute series (Moser *et al.*, 1987) that involved 167 patients with CCER, the mean interval between first neurologic symptoms and an apparently vegetative state was 1.9 $\pm$ 2 years (range 0.5 to 10.5 years). In this state, the child is bedridden, is unable to speak or see, and is fed via nasogastric tube or gastrostomy. Ability to interact may be retained to a variable extent that may be difficult to assess. The child or adolescent may remain in this apparently vegetative state for several years, in some instances more than 5 years. The mean age at death in the childhood form was 9.4 $\pm$ 2 years.

Recent follow-up studies at the Kennedy Krieger Institute have shown that information of prognostic significance can be obtained by subdividing the patients in accordance with age and degree of MRI abnormality (Moser *et al.*, 2000). Eighteen subgroups were established. The purpose of the study was to determine whether the presence or absence of brain MRI abnormality at a given age correlates with outcome. The MRI involvement was assessed with the 34-point scale developed specifically for X-ALD by Loes *et al.* (1994). As demonstrated in Figures 34.2A and 34.2B, the correlation in some of the age groups was striking. In the 7-to-10-year age group, all of the 22 patients with normal MRI (Loes score $< 1$) survived and remained neurologically intact, whereas half of the patients with MRI score $> 3$ died during the follow-up period. Table 34.3 summarizes the results.

### Adolescent Cerebral ALD

In one series (Moser *et al.*, 1987) of 837 patients, there were 42 patients in whom first symptoms occurred between age 11 and 21. Symptoms resemble those in CCER.

### Adrenomyeloneuropathy

Adrenomyeloneuropathy (AMN) is a disorder that involves the spinal cord mainly. It is now subdivided into "pure AMN," where neuropathological changes are confined to the spinal cord and peripheral nerves (Powers *et al.*, 2000), and "AMN-cerebral," in which there is also diffuse involvement of cerebral white matter (Schaumburg *et al.*, 1975). As discussed in the section on pathogenesis, the distinction between AMN and the cerebral forms of the disease is fundamental. Kumar *et al.* (1995) found that the brain MRI is normal in 54% of AMN patients. Some degree of cerebral involvement coexists in 46%. In a 10-year follow-up study, van Geel *et al.* found that, 19% of pure AMN patients developed cerebral involvement during that period (van Geel *et al.*, 2001).

Typically, a man with pure AMN had been neurologically normal, often with good athletic skills, until his twenties when he noted stiffness or clumsiness in his legs. Adrenocortical insufficiency is demonstrable in at least 50% of AMN patients (Brennemann *et al.*, 1996). The neurologic disability is slowly progressive, so that within the next to 15 years, the gait disturbance becomes severe and requires the use of a cane or a wheelchair. Urinary disturbances and sexual dysfunction are noted in the twenties or thirties. The somatosensory and brainstem auditory evoked responses are nearly always abnormal. Visual evoked and peripheral nerve abnormalities occur less frequently. Neuropsychologic function in patients with pure AMN is normal or only minimally impaired (Edwin *et al.*, 1996).

### AMN-Cerebral Phenotype

Griffin *et al.* noted already in 1977 (Griffin *et al.*, 1977) that some pure AMN patients develop diffuse cerebral involvement. In a cross sectional study, Kumar *et al.* (1995) found that 46% of AMN patients had some degree of cerebral involvement. The cerebral involvement may already be present when AMN is first diagnosed, or it may develop later in patients with pure AMN. The inflammatory cerebral pathology may not begin until the fifth decade (van Geel *et al.*, 2001), but once it manifests it may progress as rapidly as in patients with CCER.

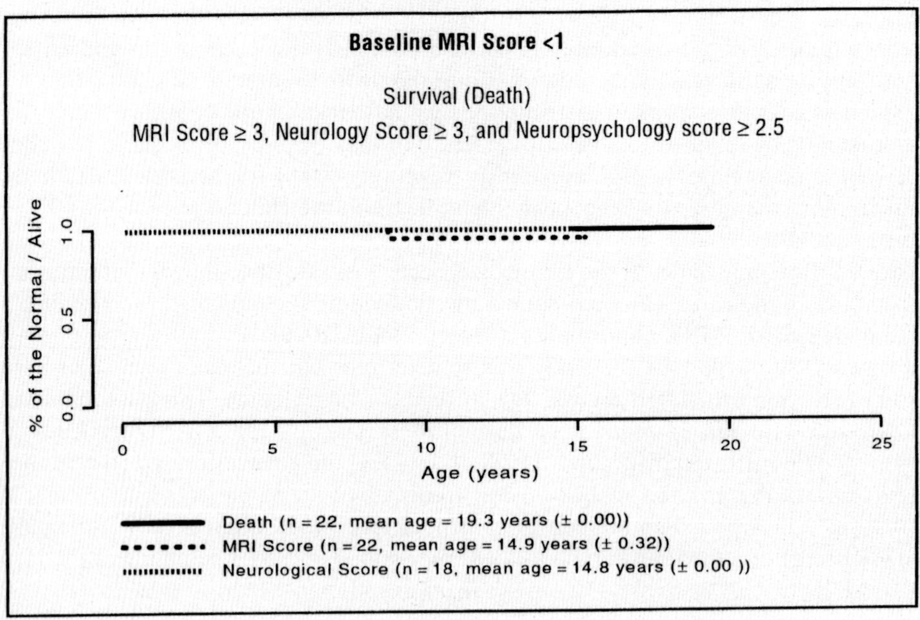


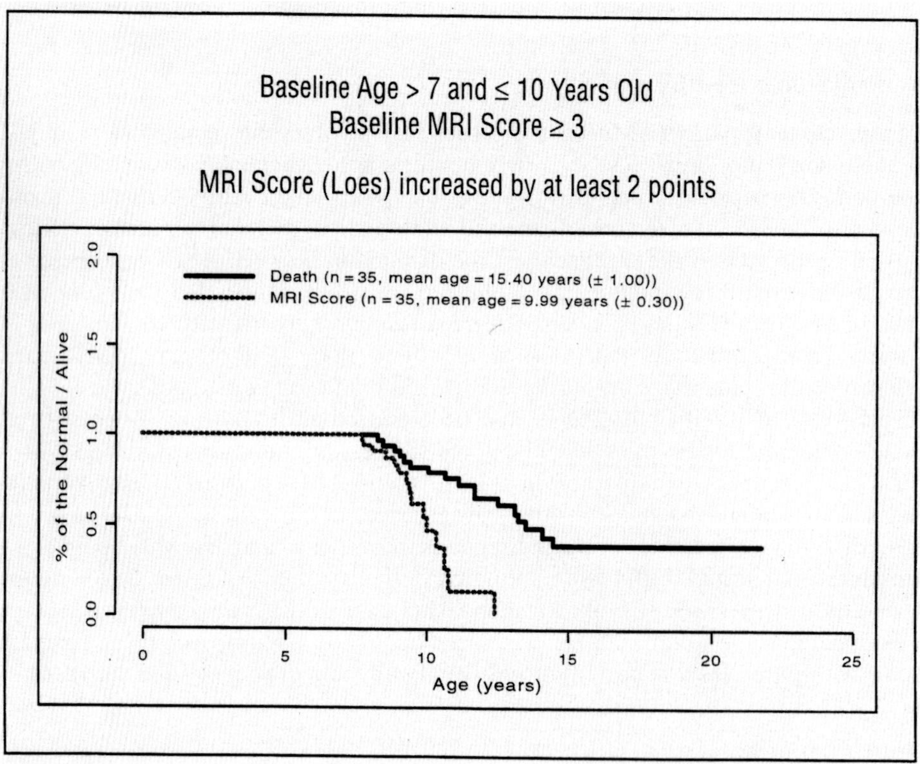


FIGURES 34.2A AND 34.2B

MRI score is based on the 34-point scale developed by Loes *et al.* (1994) specifically for X-ALD. A score of < 1 is classified as within normal limits. The figures show that for the 7 to 10 years age group, the MRI score is highly predictive. If a 7- to 10-year-old boy has an MRI score that is greater than three, he has a 50% chance of dying in the next 5 years. None of the boys in this age group who had a normal MRI died during that period. However, they will most likely develop the milder AMN in adulthood.

TABLE 34.3 X-ALD Prognosis as a Function of Age and MRI Score at First Encounter

| |
|---|
| MRI score > 3: 70–80% worsen irrespective of age; |
| 8/80 remain neurological stable |
| MRI score 1–3: 60% worsen irrespective of age; |
| Longer survival |
| MRI score < 1: Age 3–7: 30% develop cerebral involvement; |
| Ages 7–10: 10% develop cerebral involvement |
| Age > 10: Cerebral involvement rare |

## Adult Cerebral X-ALD

The term "adult cerebral X-ALD" is applied to patients with the biochemical defect of X-ALD who develop cerebral symptoms after 21 years of age, but who do not have signs of spinal cord involvement; that is, they do not have evidence of AMN. This form is relatively rare. Twenty-three cases have been reported (Moser *et al.*, 2000). Age of onset ranged from the early twenties to the fifties. Symptoms resembled schizophrenia with dementia or there may be a focal neurological deficit that led to suspicion of a brain tumor (Bresnan and Richardson, 1979). The most common initial psychiatric manifestations are signs of hypomania including disinhibition, impulsivity, increased spending, hypersexuality, loudness, and perserveration (Garside *et al.*, 1999). Adult cerebral X-ALD has a serious prognosis. The mean interval between first neurologic symptom and an apparently vegetative state or death was 3 to 4 years.

## Presentation AS Olivocerebellar Atrophy

There are eight reports of patients who presented with clinical manifestations of olivopontocerebellar atrophy (Kurihara *et al.*, 1993). Age at presentation ranged from 5 years to adulthood. Cerebellar and pontine atrophy was present in all patients in whom imaging studies were performed and may be the only demonstrable abnormality initially. The illness was progressive and cerebral white matter abnormalities became evident later in all instances.

## Addison Disease Only

X-ALD patients are assigned to the "Addison only" phenotype category if they have adrenal insufficiency without demonstrable evidence of nervous system involvement. X-ALD is one of the causes of Addison disease. Lauretti *et al.* (1996) reported it as the cause of adrenal insufficiency in 35% of male patients who had previously been diagnosed as having primary idiopathic adrenocortical insufficiency. They noted that none of the X-ALD patients had adrenocortical antibodies. Analogous results were obtained by Jorge *et al.* (1994), who demonstrated X-ALD as the cause of Addison disease in 5 of 24 patients. Statistical analysis indicated that the likelihood of X-ALD as the cause is age dependent. It is most likely when Addison manifests before the age of 7.5 years. Most patients with the Addison-only phenotype later develop neurologic involvement. Van Geel *et al.* (2001) found that during a 10-year follow-up period this occurred in 50%.

## Asymptomatic Male X-ALD Patients

While many young X-ALD patients are asymptomatic, most develop either neurologic or adrenal involvement or both at some time and we are not aware of any male patients who remained asymptomatic after age 60.

### Manifesting Heterozygotes

Some degree of neurologic involvement occurs frequently in women who are heterozygous for X-ALD. In a series of 104 women who attended the annual meeting of the United Leukodystrophy Foundation, 61% had some neurologic abnormalities that resembled pure AMN (Moser *et al.*, 1991). It is likely that this group was reasonably representative of the overall X-ALD heterozygote population because most of the women attended the conference because of concern about their sons rather than their own health. Their mean age was 32 years. Disability was severe in 14%. Twenty percent had slight to moderate symptoms, while another 22% had not complained of symptoms but were found to have hyperreflexia and impaired vibration sense in the lower extremities. The mean age of onset of neurologic symptoms was 37.8 $\pm$ 14.8 years. Restuccia *et al.* (1999) demonstrated abnormalities of motor and sensory evoked responses in 12 of, 191 heterozygotes. The pure AMN-like neurologic symptoms are progressive and are present in more than 50% heterozygous women in late middle age or later. Less than 1% of heterozygous women develop Addison disease or cerebral involvement. Naidu *et al.* (1997) have proposed that these rare occurrences are associated with skewed X-inactivation patterns in which the normal allele is not expressed. Maier *et al.* (2002) reported recently that neurologically symptomatic women are more likely to have skewed X-inactivation patterns. Hershkovitz (Hershkovitz *et al.*, 2002) have reported a 9-year-old girl with cerebral involvement as severe as in boys with CCER. She had a pathogenic X-ALD mutation on the maternally derived X-chromosome combined with a de-novo deletion of Xq28 on the paternally derived X, and thus was totally deficient in the X-ALD gene.

## PATHOLOGY

It is of key importance to note that the pathology of the cerebral forms of X-ALD differs fundamentally from that of pure AMN. The cerebral forms are associated with an inflammatory response in the cerebral white matter. Pure AMN is mainly a distal axonopathy (Powers *et al.*, 2000), and the inflammatory response is absent or mild.

### *Pathology of the Cerebral Forms*

The gray matter is usually intact, but the centrum semiovale is consistently firm (sclerotic) and replaced by large areas of brown to gray translucent tissue. The loss of myelin is confluent, usually asymmetric, and most prominent in the parieto-occipital regions with caudorostral progression. Several less common patterns has been reported, including the forms in which the demyelinative process starts in the frontal region or in the cerebellum and pons (Kurihara *et al.*, 1993). Cavitation and calcification of white mater may be seen in severe cases. Arcuate fibers are relatively spared. In the most common form with posterior presentation, the posterior cingulum, corpus callosum, fornix, hippocampas commissure, posterior limb of the internal capsule, and optic systems are typically involved. The cerebellar white matter usually exhibits a similar but milder, confluent loss of myelin and sclerosis. Secondary corticospinal tract degeneration extending down through the peduncles, basis pontis, medullary pyramids, and spinal cord is characteristic. The spinal cord is spared in the CCER phenotype except for the descending tract degeneration. Histopathologically there is a marked loss of myelinated axons (Myelin > axons) and oligodendrocytes in association with hypertrophic reactive astrocytosis. The advancing active edges of myelin loss are sites of intense perivascular inflammation and lipid-laden macrophages. Diffuse infiltration of macrophages and large perivascular collections of mononuclear cells, particularly lymphocytes, are highly characteristic of areas of early myelin breakdown. Recent studies have revealed that most of the lymphocytes are CD8 cytotoxic cells (Ito *et al.*, 2001).

### *Pathology of Pure AMN*

The spinal cord bears the brunt of the disease process in men with pure AMN and also in neurologically symptomatic heterozygous women. Loss of myelinated axons and a milder loss of oligodendrocytes is observed in the long ascending and descending tracts of the spinal cord, especially the fasciculus gracilis and the lateral corticospinal tracts. The pattern of fiber loss is consistent with a distal axonopathy in that the greatest losses are observed in the distal segments—that is, in the cervical region for the ascending fasciculus gracilis and the descending corticospinal tract. Recent pathological studies of the dorsal root ganglia in AMN patients (Powers *et al.*, 2001) provide further support for this formulation. Powers *et al.* point out that a dying-back pattern of axonal degeneration such as seen in Friedreich's ataxia, and AMN could be due either to neuronal death or to axonal damage. The former is the case in Friedreich's ataxia, where there is neuronal loss and nodules of Nageoti are prominent (Hughes *et al.*, 1968). In contrast, in the AMN patients the number of dorsal root ganglion cells was not reduced, there was no evidence of necrosis or apoptosis, and nodules of Nageoti were not observed. This points toward axonal pathology as the primary event. Two other findings were of interest: even though the total number of neurons was not reduced, there was a reduction of the number of large neurons and ultrastructural studies of the neurons revealed electron-dense lipidic inclusions. The implications of these findings will be discussed in the section on pathogenesis.

#### *Peripheral Nerves*

Peripheral nerve lesions in AMN are variable and mild compared to the myelopathy. Sural and peroneal nerves have displayed loss of large and small diameter myelinated fibers, endoneurial fibrosis, and thin myelin sheaths (Julien *et al.*, 1981; Martin *et al.*, 1980). Chaudhry *et al.* (1996) studied 13 variables of peripheral nerve function in 99 men with AMN and 37 heterozygous women. At least one variable was abnormal in 87% of the men and 67% of the women. Abnormalities were more common in the men than the women. They concluded that the abnormalities represented a mixture of axonal loss and multifocal demyelination. Van Geel *et al.* (1996) studied 18 men with AMN and five neurologically symptomatic heterozygotes. Sixty-five percent of the patients had a polyneuropathy with predominantly axonal sensorimotor features, and they concluded that primary axonal degeneration is the principal abnormality. Only two (9%) of the patients fulfilled the electrodiagnostic criteria for primary demyelination.

#### *Adrenal Cortex and Testis*

Adrenocortical cells, particularly those of the inner fasciculata-reticularis, become ballooned and striated due to accumulations of lamellae, lamellar lipid-laden profiles, and fine lipid clefts (Fig. 34.3). The striated material, which contains cholesterol esters esterified with VLCFA, appears to lead to cell dysfunction, atrophy, and death (Powers and Schaumburg, 1974). Inflammatory cells are only rarely observed. Ultimately primary atrophy of the adrenal cortex ensues. In fetuses affected by X-ALD, the fetal adrenal zone is already severely involved (Powers *et al.*, 1982). In the testes, lamellae and lamellar-lipid profiles are present in the interstitial cells of Leydig and their precursors. Degenerative changes in the seminiferous tubules and Sertoli cells are observed in AMN (Powers and Schaumburg, 1981), and may eventually lead to azoospermia (Aversa *et al.*, 1998). It should be noted, however, that many X-ALD patients have fathered children. The Kennedy Krieger Institute records include 964 children fathered by 336 X-ALD patients.

## BIOCHEMICAL ABNORMALITIES

### Accumulation of Very Long Chain Fatty Acids

Very long chain fatty acids (VLCFA) are defined as saturated and unsaturated fatty acids with carbon chain lengths longer than 22 atoms. Rezanka (1989) reviewed the literature about VLCFA up to 1989 and points out that they are almost omnipresent in the animal and plant kingdoms, varying from 0343.1% to 10% of total fatty acids. Normally saturated VLCFA occur in highest concentration in myelin lipids and red blood cell sphingomyelin. They occur in much lower concentration in other tissues. The accumulation of very long

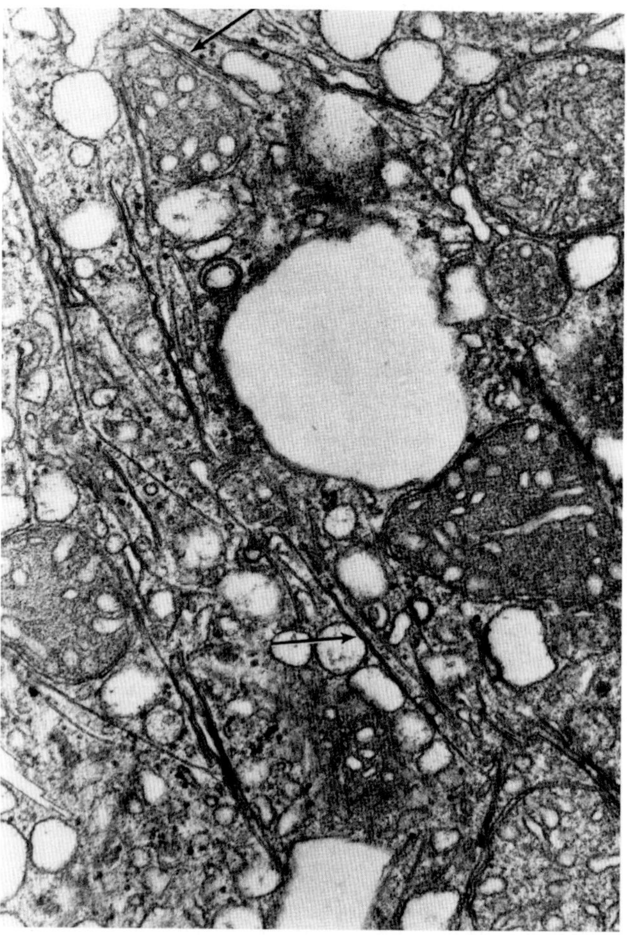

FIGURE 34.3
This adrenocortical cell contains both unilamellate and multilammete inclusions, which are both free in the cytoplasm and are attached to various organelles (arrows). (Magnification X 23,625.) Electron micrograph was taken from uranyl acetate-lead citrate-stained thin sections. From CRC critical reviews of *Neurobiology* **3**, 29–88 1987, with permission

chain fatty acids is the principal biochemical abnormality in X-ALD. This was demonstrated first in post-mortem brain tissue and adrenal gland by Igarashi *et al.* (1976b), where these fatty acids accounted for 11 to 40% of fatty acids in the cholesterol ester fraction, whereas they were virtually absent from similar fractions in control tissues. The excess of VLCFA in postmortem brain tissue has been confirmed in numerous subsequent studies (Brown *et al.*, 1983; Menkes and Corbo, 1977; Molzer *et al.*, 1981; Ramsey *et al.*, 1979; Reinecke *et al.*, 1985; Taketomi *et al.*, 1987; Theda *et al.*, 1992; Wilson and Sargent, 1993). The VLCFA that accumulate in X-ALD are saturated and unbranched, and involve mainly those with a carbon chain length of 26 (hexacosanoic acid, C26:0) or 24 (tetracosanoic acid, C24:0).

The accumulation of VLCFA in X-ALD brain has a specific pattern. While some degree of excess is present in most tissues, the most striking increases are found in the cholesterol ester fractions of the brain and the adrenal glands. The VLCFA excess in the brain cholesterol ester fraction correlates with histopathology. The greatest enrichment (approximately 40%) is found in actively demyelinating areas, whereas it was similar to control (6%) in the cholesterol ester fraction of histologically normal brain regions, and two and a half times normal (15%) in a gliotic region (Theda *et al.*, 1992). VLCFA levels are also increased in the proteolipid fraction (Bizzozero *et al.*, 1991) and in gangliosides. VLCFA of brain gangliosides in X-ALD patients account for 25 to 40% of their total fatty acids, compared to less than 1% in controls. Brown *et al.* (1983) examined the lipid composition of purified myelin from three X-ALD patients. Unlike the controls, the lipids of this preparation included 8.9% cholesterol ester. This may have been due to contamination with a low-density fraction from regions where myelin had been destroyed. While this cholesterol ester fraction contained tenfold C26:0 increase, the C26:0 increase in the cerebroside, sulfatide, and sphingomyelin fractions was less than twofold. VLCFA levels are increased also in the total lipid fractions of plasma (Moser *et al.*, 1981, 1999) and in the erythrocyte membrane sphingomyelin fraction (Antoku *et al.*, 1987; Tsuji *et al.*, 1981c). Measurement of VLCFA levels in plasma (Moser *et al.*, 1981, 1999) or red blood cells (Antoku *et al.*, 1987; Tsuji *et al.*, 1981c) are the most commonly used diagnostic assays.

The mechanisms responsible for the VLCFA accumulation will be discussed in the section on pathogenesis.

## GENE DEFECT

ABCD1, the gene that is defective in X-ALD, was mapped to Xq28 in 1981 (Migeon *et al.*, 1981) and isolated and cloned by positional cloning in 1993 (Mosser *et al.*, 1993). It occupies approximately 26 kb of genomic DNA. It is composed of 10 exons and encodes an mRNA of 4.3 kb and a predicted protein (ALDP) of 745 amino acids (Sarde *et al.*, 1994). ALDP, contrary to earlier expectations (see section on pathogenesis), has no sequence homology to any of the VLCS, but instead was found to be a member of the ATP binding cassette (ABC) transmembrane transporter superfamily that transport a wide variety of substrates, including ions, sugars, amino acids, proteins, and lipids (Higgins, 1992). Forty-eight mammalian ABC transporters are estimated to exist (Dean *et al.*, 2001). Mammalian ABC transporter proteins typically consist of two hydrophobic transmembrane domains and two hydrophobic nucleotide-binding folds encoded by a single gene. Peroxisomal ABC transporters have been designated as subgroup (D), which at this time includes four members that are listed in Table 34.4. ABCD1 is the gene that is defective in X-ALD. ABCD2 codes for ALDR (adrenoleukodystrophy related protein). ALDR maps to 12q11 has 66 homology to ALDP (Lombard-Platet *et al.*, 1996) and its exon structure is similar to that of ALDP (Broccardo *et al.*, 1998). The ABCD2 expression patterns differs from that of ABCD1. ABCD1 is expressed strongly in glia and the adrenal cortex, and ABCD2 in neurons and the adrenal medulla (Dubois-Dalq *et al.*, 1999). ABCD3 codes for PMP70 (Kamijo *et al.*, 1990) and ABCD4 for PMP70/69R (Holzinger *et al.*, 1997; Shani *et al.*, 1997). They are all encoded as half-transporters with a single transporter domain and a single binding fold (Dean *et al.*, 2001). They function as dimers, either as homodimers or as heterodimers with other members of the ABCD group (Liu *et al.*, 1999; Smith *et al.*, 1999).

### Mutation Analyses

Figure 34.4 shows a topographic model of ALDP. The Kennedy Krieger Institute and the Laboratory for Genetic Metabolic Disease at the Academic Medical Center in Amsterdam have established a website (www.x-ald.nl), which lists and updates the mutations that have been identified worldwide. Four-hundred-six mutations had been defined by 2001 (Kemp *et al.*, 2001). Their nature and location in respect to exons and domains is shown in Figure 34.5. Two-hundred-thirty-four (57.6%) of the mutations are nonrecurrent and unique to a kindred. Of all the mutations, 227 (55.9%) are missense, 110 (27.1%) are nonsense, 16 (3.9%) are small in-frame amino acid insertions or deletions, and 16 (3.9%) are large deletions of one or more exons. Figure 34.4 shows that disease-causing mutations are distributed throughout the gene, but the distribution is not even. There is clustering of mutations in the transmembrane domain (40%), in the ATP binding domain (30%) and in exon 5 (14%). A hotspot has been identified on exon 5 (Kemp *et al.*, 1994; Kok *et al.*, 1995). This mutation involves the deletion of two nucleotides (AG) at cDNA position 1415–1416. This results in a frame shift at amino acid residue Glu 471 (fs E471) and a premature stop codon at position 554. The predicted ALDP lacks the ALDP-binding

TABLE 34.4 Peroxisomal ABC Half-Transporters

| Protein | Percentage identity to ALDP | Chromosomal location |
|---|---|---|
| ALD | 100 | Xq28 |
| ALDR | 66 | 12q11 |
| PMP70 | 38 | 1p21 |
| P70R (PMP69) | 27 | 14q24 |

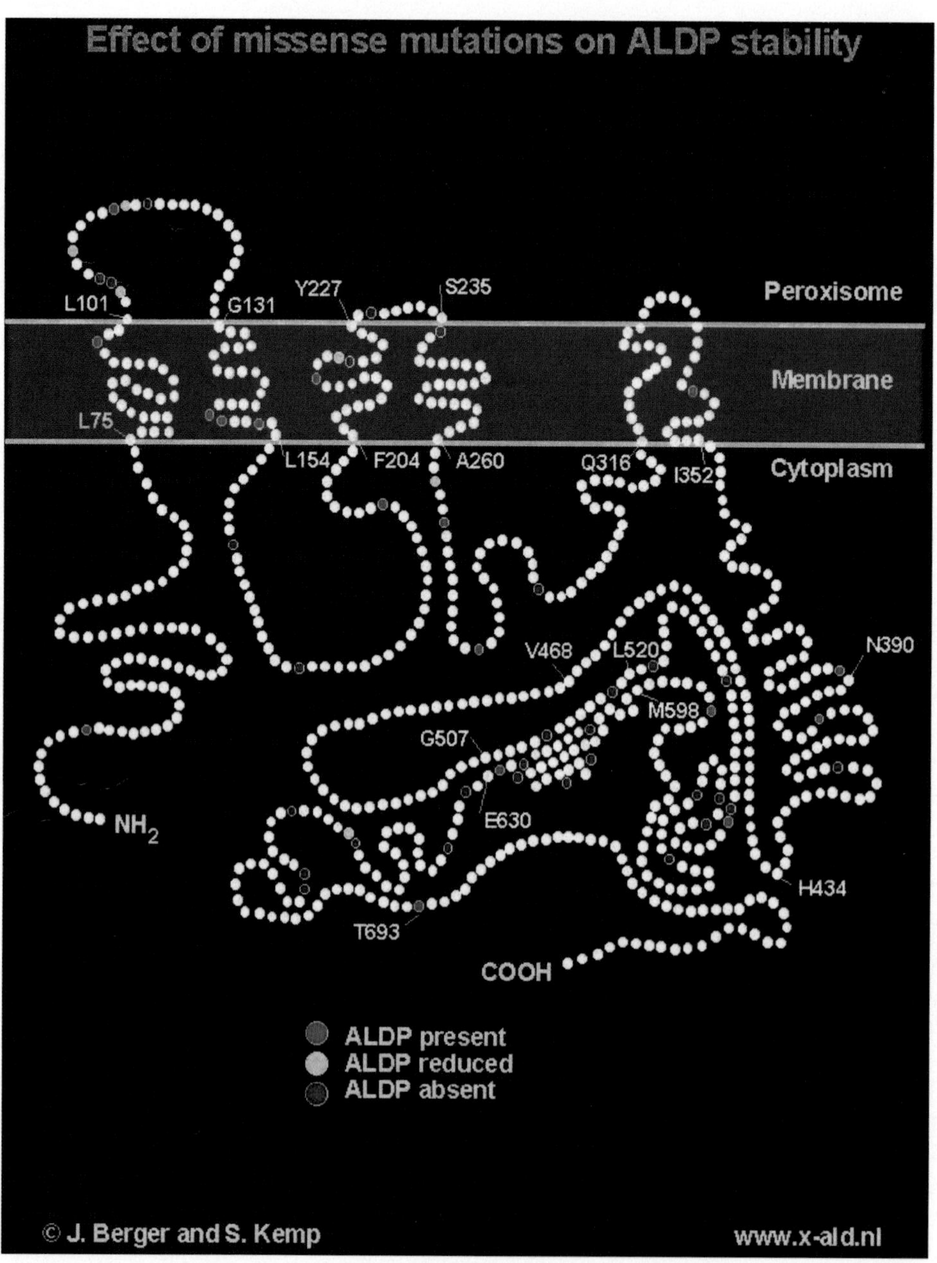


FIGURE 34.4

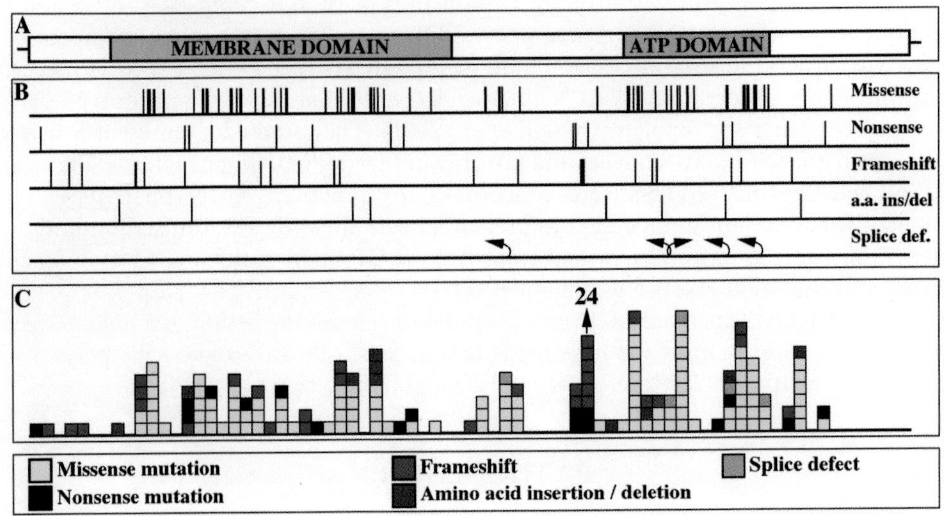


FIGURE 34.5
Graphic presentations of mutations in the X-ALD gene identified worldwide up to 1998. Schematic presentation of the open reading frame. The putative transmembrane and ATP-binding domain are shown in A. B. Distribution of nonrecurrent mutations in the X-ALD gene. Each vertical bar represents the location of a "private" mutation. Mutations are grouped by type. The density of missense mutations is greatest in the transmembrane and ATP-binding domains. The arrows in the splice defect columns indicate whether the defect affects the splice donor or spice acceptor site. C. Presentation of all mutations identified in the ALD gene other than the 15 large chromosomal deletions that had been identified by 1998. The common dinucleotide deletion (415delAG) that was observed in 24 families is not to scale. From Archives of *Neurology* **56,** 273–275 1999, with permission.

domain and is both unstable and inactive. This deletion has been found in 10.3% (42/406) of X-ALD kindreds. Haplotype analysis has excluded a founder effect (Kemp *et al.*, 1994).

Combined mutation and ALDP expression data (Feigenbaum *et al.*, 1996; Watkins *et al.*, 1995) were available in 216 X-ALD cell lines as of June 2001 (Kemp *et al.*, 2001). ALDP was not immunologically detectable in 178 (82.4%). The 216 informative cell lines included 78 non-recurrent mutations. Sixty of these (79.5%) result in the absence of detectable protein levels. Normal levels of ALDP expression were found in 38 (17.6%). In these 38 cell lines, 16 different missense mutations were identified. All ABCD1 mutations other than missense mutations resulted in unstable and therefore non-detectable levels of protein. Expression data was available on 137 missense mutations, which included 52 that were unique. Only 31% of the nonrecurrent mutations failed to affect expression of ALDP. Of these, 11% resulted in strongly reduced expression, and 58% in unstable or absent levels. Missense mutations located around the ATP-binding cassette are more likely to affect protein stability. Liu *et al.* (1999) demonstrated that amino acids near the carboxyl site, which includes this region, are important for the dimerization of ALDP with itself, with ALDRP, or with PMP70. The disease-causing effect of some these missense mutations thus may be due to the inhibition of dimer formation.

## Genotype-Phenotype Correlations

It has not been possible to establish genotype-phenotype correlations so far. Mild phenotypes have been observed in patients with large deletions (Mosser *et al.*, 1993) and in a large number of mutations that result in absence of protein, and conversely severe phenotypes have been associated with missense mutations in which ALDP is expressed. The mutation 1415 del AG has been identified in patients with all possible X-ALD phenotypes

(Kemp *et al.*, 1994). Another striking demonstration of the complexity of genotype-phenotype correlation is the presence of five different phenotypes in six members of a family with a destabilizing missense mutation P 484R (Berger *et al.*, 1994). However, a recent intriguing observation by O'Neill *et al.* suggests that genotype-phenotype correlation may exist in some families (O'Neill *et al.*, 2001). They studied a family in which the phenotype pattern is highly unusual and possibly unique in that all nine affected males and affected heterozygous women were concordant for the pure AMN phenotype. They demonstrated a so far unique mutation that affects an ABCD1 translation-initiation codon, which results in an N-terminal truncated ALDP missing the first 65 amino acids. Possibly this mutation exerts a dominant effect.

The frequent co-occurrence of diverse phenotypes suggest the action of a modifier gene. Genetic segregation support the hypothesis that at least one autosomal gene plays a role (Maestri and Beaty, 1992; Moser *et al.*, 1992; Smith *et al.*, 1991).

## PATHOGENESIS

### Pathogenesis of VLCFA Accumulation

#### *Impaired Peroxisomal Beta Oxidation in X-ALD Fibroblasts, White Blood Cells, and Amniocytes: Recent Controversy*

In 1984, Singh *et al.* (1984b) demonstrated that the capacity to oxidize C24:0 was reduced to 20 to 30% of control in cultured skin fibroblasts and in white blood cells of patients with X-ALD. This finding has been confirmed in three other laboratories (Kemp *et al.*, 1998; Poulos *et al.*, 1986; Rizzo *et al.*, 1984; Wanders *et al.*, 1987). The defect has also been demonstrated in cultured skin fibroblasts of the X-ALD mouse model (Kemp *et al.*, 1998; Lu *et al.*, 1997) and in cultured human X-ALD amniocytes and in one instance in an adrenal biopsy sample from an X-ALD patient (Singh *et al.*, 1981). The oxidation of VLCFA takes place in the peroxisome (Singh *et al.*, 1984a) by a series of biochemical reactions that differ from those used for fatty acid oxidation in the mitochondrion (Hashimoto, 1996). These results had led to the generally accepted conclusion that the accumulation of VLCFA is due to defective VLFA oxidation in the peroxisome.

However, this conclusion was recently challenged by McGuinness *et al.* (2003). While their studies in the X-ALD mouse model confirmed that VLCFA oxidation in fibroblasts was impaired, they reported the surprising finding that VLCFA oxidation the brain, adrenal, heart, liver, and kidney did not differ from control even though VLCFA levels were increased in all of these tissues. There is no explanation at this time for the difference in VLCFA oxidation in fibroblasts in mice and humans and in human white blood cells and amniocytes versus those in X-ALD mouse tissues. Comparable studies in human X-ALD tissues are not available, except for the earlier study of Singh *et al.* of the adrenal biopsy sample of one X-ALD patient (Singh *et al.*, 1981), in which VLCFA beta-oxidation was reduced. McGuinness *et al.* carried out an extensive investigation of the mechanism of VLCFA accumulation, which also included studies of the effects of pharmacological agents such as 4-phenylbutyrate and studies of VLCFA oxidation in cell lines of patients with various mitochondrial disorders. They present evidence that the gene defect in X-ALD affects the interaction between peroxisomes and mitochondria, with the primary defect involving the oxidation of long chain fatty acids in mitochondria. They found that increased levels of saturated long chain fatty acids (C16:0) impair peroxisomal VLCFA oxidation in both normal and in X-ALD fibroblasts. They propose that an increase in long chain fatty acid levels is a primary event and that increased VLCFA levels are secondary. They postulate that in X-ALD mouse tissues there is an imbalance between the rate of incorporation VLCFA into complex lipids and the rate of complex lipid degradation, with a shift toward synthesis in X-ALD. Consistent with this finding are the earlier reports of Tsuji *et al.* (1981a) that the rate of C26:0 synthesis is increased in X-ALD fibroblasts.

The discrepancy between these recent findings of McGuinness *et al.* in X-ALD mouse tissues and the previously generally accepted conclusion that the VLCFA accumulation in fibroblasts and white blood cells is due to impaired peroxisomal VLCFA oxidation is unresolved at this time. Intuitively it seems unlikely that different mechanisms would be the cause of VLCFA in fibroblasts and the tissues. However, as noted in the next section, the VLCFA CoA synthetases, enzymes involved in peroxisomal beta oxidation, have tissue specificity, and this could contribute to differences in the mechanism of VLCFA accumulation in various tissues. In any case, the recent data of McGuinness *et al.* indicate that the previous conclusion that the VLCFA excess is fully accounted for by a defect in VLCFA oxidation must be reexamined.

### *VLCFA CoA Synthetases Involved in Peroxisomal Beta Oxidation*

In 1984, Singh *et al.* (1984a) demonstrated that C24:0 is oxidized mainly in the peroxisome. Peroxisomal beta oxidation shortens VLCFA by a series of cycles each of which shortens the fatty acid by two carbons. Each cycle involves four enzymatic reactions (Hashimoto, 1996). The first of these involves the formation of the thioester with Coenzyme A. Three groups have reported that this reaction is deficient in X-ALD (Hashmi *et al.*, 1986; Lazo *et al.*, 1988; Wanders *et al.*, 1988). The reaction is catalyzed by VLCFA CoA synthetase (VLCS). The family of proteins that have VLCS activity includes six members (Watkins *et al.*, 1999) that differ in regard to substrate specificity, species and tissue distribution. One is involved mainly in bile acid metabolism (Mihalik *et al.*, 2002; Steinberg *et al.*, 2000a). Most are localized to the peroxisomes and microsomes. The VLCS (VLCS 1) that has been studied in greatest detail in respect to ALD was the first to be purified (Heinzer *et al.*, 2002) and cloned (Uchiyama *et al.*, 1996). The human and murine enzymes have 83% identity contain 620 amino acids and contain both peroxisomal and microsomal targeting sequences with most activity found in the peroxisome. All of the VLCS activate also long chain fatty acids such as C16:0 in addition to VLCFA, with the activation of long chain fatty acids being greater than that of VLCFA. They have two highly conserved motifs. Motif 1 is an AMP-binding domain that is also present in other acyl-CoA synthetases, suggesting that the reaction involves the hydrolysis of ATP to AMP and pyrophosphate. The second motif, the function of which is still unknown, was unique to the VLCS that had been identified by, 1997 (Black *et al.*, 1997). VLCS1 is expressed in human and mouse fibroblasts. In the mouse VLCS1 RNA is most abundant in the liver and kidney. It is also present in the brain and the adrenal, but only at approximately one fifth the level of that in the liver (Heinzer *et al.*, 2002).

Recently, a newly identified VLCS has attracted interest in regard to X-ALD. This enzyme was first identified in a Drosophila Melanogaster neurodegenerative mutant that accumulates neuronal lipids that under the microscope look like bubblegum. Brain VLCFA levels were increased (Min and Benzer, 1999). The enzyme that is deficient in this mutant was found to have VLCS activity and is referred to as bubblegum. Human bubblegum has been cloned (Steinberg *et al.*, 2000b). While it has VLCS activity, it does not contain the Motifs associated with all of the other mammalian VLCS that has been identified up to 1999 (Watkins *et al.*, 1999). It also differs from the other VLCS in that it is localized to the cytosol and plasma membrane rather than the peroxisome. However, it is of interest in relation to X-ALD because, unlike the other VLCS, it is expressed primarily in the brain (Steinberg *et al.*, 2000b) and also in the adrenal gland and testis (Watkins, P., personal communication), the tissues that are involved in X-ALD.

### *VLCS Has No Direct Role in X-ALD*

When deficient VLCS activity was demonstrated in X-ALD fibroblasts in 1984, it was considered likely that the gene defect in X-ALD would be found to involve this enzyme. However, when the defective gene was cloned in 1993, it was found to code for a peroxisomal membrane protein (ALDP) that is a member of the ATP binding cassette (ABC) transporter superfamily (Higgins, 1992) and the gene product has no homology to VLCS. VLCS activity and localization in the mouse model of X-ALD is normal (Heinzer *et al.*, 2002) and a VLCS1 mouse knockout model does not show accumulation of VLCFA or any other features of X-ALD (Heinzer, A., unpublished observation).

It is thus clear that VLCS deficiency is not the primary biochemical defect in X-ALD. Nevertheless, some interactions between ALDP, the gene product that is deficient in X-ALD, and VLCS have been described and will be discussed in the section on the physiological role of ALDP.einze

### *VLCFA Synthesis and Its Relation to X-ALD*

Synthesis of fatty acids with chain length greater than 16 carbons is carried out by the fatty acid elongating system. The system occurs in both mitochondria and microsomes. The microsomal system appears to be more active and to have greater physiological significance (Murad and Kishimoto, 1978).

The stoichiometry of the reaction is as follows:

$$\text{Palmitoyl CoA} + \text{Malonyl CoA} + \text{NADPH} + \text{H}|\text{stearoyl CoA} + \text{CO2} + \text{NADP+} \\ \text{CoA} + \text{H2O}$$

With this reaction, a C16:0 fatty acid (palmitic) is elongated to C18:0 (stearic acid). VLCFA synthesis is achieved by repeated additions of malonyl CoA, so that two carbon units are added until the desired chain length is achieved. Fatty acid synthesis and elongation are complex and highly regulated processes involving multiple enzymes and acyl carrier proteins (Volpe and Vagelos, 1976). The maturational changes in activity of the brain microsomal fatty acid elongating system correlate with the deposition of myelin (Murad and Kishimoto, 1978). Formation of saturated VLCFA was first demonstrated in rat sciatic nerve (Cassagne *et al.*, 1978). The factors that control the rate of elongation are still poorly understood. The chain length of the substrate is an important factor. In a study utilizing swine cerebral microsomes, it was found that elongation of C20:0 CoA yielded C22:0 and 24:0 concomitantly, whereas elongation of C22:0 CoA yielded only negligible amounts of C24:0. Kinetic studies in this system suggested that elongation of C20:0 CoA and of C22:0 CoA are carried out through two separate pathways with that for the C20:0 substrate more active (Yoshida and Takeshita, 1987). Bourre *et al.* concluded that a single enzyme is responsible for the elongation of behenic acid (2w23:0) and its monounsaturated counterpart erucic acid (22:1) (Bourre *et al.*, 1976). This presumably is the basis for the striking lowering of the levels of saturated VLCFA when patients with X-ALD are treated with a 4.1 mixture of glyceryl trioleate and trierucate (Lorenzo's Oil), the active component of which is erucic acid (Rizzo *et al.*, 1989) (see section on therapy).

Further study of the elongating system in X-ALD is indicated for three reasons:

(1) studies in which deuterated water was administered orally to a patient with X-ALD demonstrated substantial incorporation of deuterium into VLCFS, indicating that there was substantial endogenous synthesis (Moser *et al.*, 1983); (2) administration of a 4:1 glyceryl trioleate and glyceryl trieuricate mixture, which is thought to act by inhibiting VLCFA synthesis, leads to a striking reduction in plasma VLCFA levels (Rizzo *et al.*, 1989); )and 3) kinetic studies in cultured skin fibroblasts of X-ALD patients conducted by Tsuji and associates indicate that the activity of the fatty acid elongating system that forms C26:0 is increased (Koike *et al.*, 1991; Tanaka, 1988; Tsuji *et al.*, 1981b). Further discussion of this topic is presented in the next section.

### *Physiological Role of ALDP*

The physiological role of ALDP is not yet understood. ALDP has been localized to the peroxisomal membrane in human fibroblasts (Mosser *et al.*, 1994) with the hydrophylic carboxyl-terminal domain oriented toward the cytoplasm (Watkins *et al.*, 1995). That ALDP does have a role in VLCFA metabolism is indicated by the demonstration in several laboratories that overexpression of ALDP increases VLCFA oxidation in cultured fibroblasts of X-ALD patients (Braiterman *et al.*, 1998; Flavigny *et al.*, 1999; Kemp *et al.*, 1998; Netik *et al.*, 1999). See Figure 34.7. Note that addition of the other peroxisomal ABC transporter proteins (ALDRP and PMP 70) also had this stimulatory effect. The mechanism of this effect is not known. ALDP does not have VLCS activity (Steinberg, S. J., and Watkins, P. A., unpublished data, 1998). In view of the transport function of the ABC proteins, it has been postulated that ALDP is involved in the anchoring or transport of VLCS into the peroxisomal membrane (Contreras *et al.*, 1994; Mosser *et al.*, 1993). The subsequent studies of Steinberg *et al.* (1999) make this unlikely. They cloned VLCS and showed by immunocytochemical studies that VLCS in X-ALD fibroblasts is localized in the peroxisome in an amount indistinguishable from that in controls. They also conducted topographical studies, which showed that VLCS in both X-ALD and control cells faces the peroxisomal surface of the membrane. If ALDP is required for VLCS translocation into the peroxisome, then VLCS would have been expected to be found on the exterior of the organelle in the X-ALD cells. They also studied the effect of overexpression of either ALDP or VLCS in SV 40 transformed human X-ALD fibroblasts. As noted previously, ALDP overexpression improved VLCFA oxidation, but it did not increase VLCS activity. VLCS overexpression did not alter VLCFA oxidation. However, combined overexpression of ALDP and VLCS showed a synergistic effect that was statistically significant. The mechanism of this effect is not known. Braiterman *et al.* (1999) proposed that ALDP plays a role in the trafficking of VLCFA between microsomes and peroxisomes. This aspect has not been examined experimentally, but deserves study in view of the earlier reports by Tsuji *et al.* (Tsuji *et al.*, 1981a) that VLCFA synthesis is increased in fibroblasts of X-ALD patients (Koike *et al.*, 1991). The possibility exists that in the absence of ALDP, VLCFA do not enter the peroxisome at the normal rate and that the microsomal elongation pathway is favored. McGuinness *et al.* have proposed recently that the primary effect of ALDP is on mitochondrial metabolism (McGuinness *et al.*, 2003). They propose that ALDP facilitates the interaction between peroxisomes and mitochondria, resulting in increased VLCFA levels when ALDP is deficient.

## Pathogenesis of the Nervous System Lesions

In this section we consider separately the pathogenesis of the noninflammatory myelopathy of adrenomyeloneuropathy (AMN) and the inflammatory white matter response in the cerebral forms of the disease (CCER, adolescent and adult cerebral ALD, and AMN-cerebral). The severe inflammatory white matter demyelinative sets X-ALD apart from the other leukodystrophies. It is the cause of rapid progression and rapidly fatal outcome. It is most common in childhood. However, approximately 40% of male patients and 99% of heterozygous women escape the inflammatory form of the disease. We hypothesize that all affected males and 50% of heterozygous women would develop the noninflammatory AMN syndrome in adulthood, but that approximately 40% of males die in childhood or adolescence due to the inflammatory brain disease before AMN manifests. It should be noted, however, that while the clinical and pathological differences between childhood cerebral X-ALD and pure AMN are striking, the difference is not absolute. Detailed neuropathological studies may show mild inflammatory response in some pure AMN patients.

### *Pathogenesis of Pure Adrenomyeloneuropathy*

The previously cited studies of Powers *et al.* (2000 and 2001) provide strong evidence that the primary disease process in AMN is a distal axonopathy. It is hypothesized that this is caused by impaired membrane stability and function secondary to the accumulation of VLCFA based upon the following observations:

1. VLCFA accumulation is the principal biochemical abnormality in X-ALD (Bizzozero *et al.*, 1991; Brown *et al.*, 1983; Igarashi *et al.*, 1976b; Menkes and Corbo, 1977; Molzer *et al.*, 1981; Ramsey *et al.*, 1979; Reinecke *et al.*, 1985; Taketomi *et al.*, 1987; Theda *et al.*, 1992; Wilson and Sargent, 1993).
2. VLCFA accumulation alters the biophysical properties and function of cell membranes.
   a. The desorption rate constant of saturated fatty acids from phospholipid membranes of VLCFA is much lower than that of shorter length fatty acids. The constant for C26:0 is 10,000 times lower than that for C16:0.
   b. While albumin has six or more high or low affinity binding sites for fatty acids with 12 to 18 carbon chain length (Hamilton *et al.*, 1991), it has only a single low affinity

binding site for C26:0 (Ho *et al.*, 1995). Recent structural studies have shown that C26:0 cannot be accommodated in the binding groove of the high affinity binding sites (Ho *et al.*, 2002).

c. The viscosity of red cell membranes in X-ALD and AMN patients is increased (Knazek *et al.*, 1983). Normalization of VLCFA levels with "Lorenzo's oil" (see section on therapy) also normalizes red blood cell membrane viscosity (HW Moser, unpublished observation).
d. Microcalometric studies have shown that the inclusion of C26:0 in a model membrane disrupts membrane structure (Ho *et al.*, 1995).
e. VLCFA excess impairs function in cultured human adrenal cells. Whitcomb *et al.* (1988) assessed ACTH-stimulated cortisol release in cultured human adrenocortical cells. The addition of C26:0 or C24:0 to the culture medium in concentrations equivalent to those in X-ALD plasma increased microviscosity of adrenocortical cell membranes and decreased ACTH-stimulated cortisol secretion.

It has also been hypothesized that gangliosides that contain excess VLCFA play a role in the axonal dysfunction in AMN (Powers *et al.*, 2000). In gangliosides isolated from X-ALD brain fatty acids with chain lengths greater than C22:0 account for 28 to 50% of total fatty acids compared to 2.5% in controls (Igarashi *et al.*, 1976a). Gangliosides are present in high concentration in plasma membranes and play a role in cell function (Zeller and Marchase, 1992). It is of interest that gangliosides containing ganglioside $GT1_b$ appear to be restricted to the axolemma (Sheikh *et al.*, 1999). Excess VLCFA content may alter ganglioside function. For instance, gangliosides that contain VLCFA have less immunosuppressive activity than those with fatty acids. It is this ganglioside fraction that has the highest proportion of VLCFA (Igarashi *et al.*, 1976a).

At this time the evidence that the axonopathy in AMN is a consequence of VLCFA in excess is still indirect and conjectural and other pathogenetic mechanisms must be considered. As noted, McGuinness *et al.* (2003) and Ito *et al.* (2001) have demonstrated the existence of mitochondrial abnormalities in X-ALD and energy deficiencies or accumulation of oxygen radicals could contribute to axon dysfunction. Furthermore, since the function of ALDP is not yet understood, there may be disease mechanisms that have not yet been considered.

#### *Pathogenesis of the Inflammatory Response*

The most generally accepted concept for the pathogenesis of the inflammatory responses is that the accumulation of VLCFA has an adverse impact on myelin, and oligodendrocyte stability and function, which renders them vulnerable to various other adverse events (a "second hit"), which then initiate a destruction cascade that results in the death of oligodendrocytes and rapid breakdown of myelin (Dubois-Dalcq *et al.*, 1999; Feigenbaum *et al.*, 2000; Ito *et al.*, 2001; Powers *et al.*, 1992). In the absence of a "second hit," the nervous system pathology is mainly the distal axonopathy of AMN. Cytokines and immune mechanisms have been postulated to play a role in the initiation of the destructive cascade. Definitive conclusions are hampered by the lack of an animal model of the X-ALD inflammatory demyelination.

Several investigators have implicated the role of cytokines in the inflammatory cascade associated with the cerebral forms of X-ALD. Powers *et al.* (1992) emphasized the presence of tumor necrosis factor alpha (TNF) in the astrocytes at the active edge of the lesion. TNF produced by stimulated astrocytes has been shown to be toxic to oligodendrocytes (Robbins *et al.*, 1987). Immunocytochemical studies demonstrated increased interleukin-1 and ICAM-1 expression in astrocytes and microvessels at the edge and within the lesion. However, a study in which cytokine gene expression patterns in X-ALD were considered by reverse transcriptase polymerase chain reaction showed only small increases and less than those in multiple sclerosis (McGuinness *et al.*, 1997).

Feigenbaum *et al.* (2000) reported apoptosis in the oligodendrocytes of actively demyelinating lesions of X-ALD patients and postulated that this was triggered or enhanced by inflammatory cells.

Ito *et al.* (2001) reexamined the pathogenesis of the inflammatory with the aid of recently developed antibodies. They demonstrated that most of the perivascular lymphocytes in the acute demyelinating lesions were CD8 cytotoxic T-cells, many of which showed strong immunoreactivity for granzyme B and CD44 and often showed intimate topographical association with oligodendrocytes. There was severe loss of oligodendrocytes. However, contrary to the previously cited findings of Feigenbaum *et al.* (2000), these authors concluded that in most instances the mechanisms of oligodendrocyte death was lytic/cytolytic rather than apoptotic. An intriguing new finding is that there was strong CD1 immunoreactivity (particularly CD1b and CD1c) in astrocytes and microglia. CD1 molecules are antigen presenting surface glycoproteins that are encoded on chromosome 1, and unlike the MHC complex proteins can present self-lipid antigens to T-cells (Moody *et al.*, 1999). This finding is of particular interest in respect to X-ALD, since these lipid antigens may contain VLCFA such as those associated with the mycobacterium tuberculosis. CD1d has a molecular conformation in which there is a hydrophobic groove that optimally accommodates lipid of approximately 32 carbon chain length. The authors postulate that CD1-lipid presentation may play a key role in the destructive cascade in cerebral X-ALD. As before, they consider that the primary event is biochemical membrane instability due to the VLCFA excess associated with the gene defect, and that this results in predisposition to some degree of spontaneous breakdown. They state that "prior to the second stage of fulminant inflammatory demyelination at least 3 additional events occur: the cytolytic killing of oligodendrocytes by CD8 cytotoxic T-cells, the MCH class 11-restricted presentation of peptide antigens by microglia, and the CD1-restricted presentation of lipid antigens" (Ito *et al.*, 2001). These additional events then lead to the rapidly progressive demyelinative cascade. The CD1-lipid presentation may play a key role in this process. The presence of CD1b, c, and d in X-ALD suggests that several VLCFA-containing lipid classes are being presented. It is also of interest that gangliosides that contain VLCFA fatty acids bind eight times more avidly to anti-gangliosidase antibodies than those that contain 18 to 20 chain length fatty acids (Tagawa *et al.*, 2002).

## ANIMAL MODELS OF X-ALD

Mice with targeted inactivation of the X-ALD gene have been produced independently in three laboratories (Forss-Petter *et al.*, 1997; Kobayashi *et al.*, 1997; Lu *et al.*, 1997). All showed the same features. VLCFA levels were increased in the same tissue distribution, but somewhat less markedly than in the human disease. Excess was greatest in the brain and adrenal, with smaller increases in other tissues. Unlike the human disease, plasma VLCFA levels are normal in the X-ALD mouse (A. Moser, unpublished observation). Beta oxidation of VLCFA is decreased to the same extent as in the human disease, and the animal shows the characteristic needle-like inclusions in the adrenal cortex, testis and ovaries. During the first year the growth, motor function, behavior and brain structure of the mouse model is entirely normal. However, at 15 months and later, the animals show impaired rotarod performance, moderately impaired nerve conduction velocity, and histological abnormalities of myelin and axons in the spinal cord and sciatic nerve, but not the brain (Pujol *et al.*, 2002). It is concluded that the mouse presents a relatively mild model of "pure adrenomyeloneuropathy." There has been no clinical evidence of adrenal insufficiency. The severe inflammatory brain disease has never been observed in the mouse model in spite of repeated attempts to induce it. This limits the value of the X-ALD mouse to serve as a model to test the effectiveness of therapeutic interventions.

## DIAGNOSIS OF X-ALD

The diagnosis of X-ALD will be discussed in four different settings: (1) symptomatic patients, (2) screening of at-risk family members, (3) prenatal diagnosis, and (4) mass neonatal screening. Measurements of VLCFA is a key diagnostic technique in all four settings. Mutation analysis, when available, is of great value in settings 1 to 3, and of key importance for the identification of heterozygotes. Neuroimaging studies are important in the first setting. The plasma assay of VLCFA is the most commonly used diagnostic technique (Moser *et al.*, 1999). It is reliable for the identification of affected males, irrespective of age, but false negative or borderline results are obtained in approximately 20% of heterozygotes. Mutation analysis is the most accurate method for the identification of heterozygotes (Boehm *et al.*, 1999). As noted previously, more than 400 different mutations have been identified and often are unique to one kindred. Mutation analysis is now available on a service basis. The initial characterization of the mutation in a kindred requires approximately 4 to 6 weeks and is relatively expensive. It can be performed on blood samples of affected males or obligate heterozygotes. Once the family mutation has been identified, at-risk family members can be screened for the presence of this mutation with a shorter turn around time and at lesser cost. Prenatal identification of affected male fetuses can be accomplished by measuring VLCFA levels in cultured amniocytes or chorion villus cells. A series of 255 studies performed at the Kennedy Krieger Institute up to 1998 identified 63 affected male fetuses without known false negatives, subject to the caution that long-term follow-up was not available for some of the samples with normal results (Moser and Moser, 1999). However, the literature includes two reports of false negative results in male fetuses later found to have been affected (Carey *et al.*, 1994; Gray *et al.*, 1995). When the family mutation has been defined, the risk of false negatives can be minimized by performing mutation analysis in the fetal cells, and this procedure is recommended.

### Diagnosis of Symptomatic Patients

The diagnosis of X-ALD must be considered in boys with various neurological syndromes that manifest after 3 years of age. These include acquired attention deficit disorders, or hyperactivity, progressive behavioral deficits and progressive school failure, seizure disorders, disorders of vision or hearing, and progressive incoordination. An abnormal brain MRI study is often the initial reason for suspecting the diagnosis, with the MRI not infrequently having been performed for another reason, such as ruling out brain damage following an injury. The MRI abnormality precedes clinical manifestations, and abnormalities can be extensive even when clinical manifestations are mild. Approximately 80% of patients with the childhood cerebral form of X-ALD have the classical posterior patterns (Fig. 34.6) with symmetrical involvement of the parieto-occipital lobes and the splenium of the corpus callosum and contrast enhancement at the margins of the lesion (Kumar *et al.* 1987; Loes *et al.* in press). In 15% of the patients, the initial involvement is in the frontal lobes. Less common patterns are those with initial cerebellopontione involvement. Cerebral lesions may be unilateral and when this occurs have been mistaken for brain tumor. Even when the radiological pattern is classical, it is not specific for X-ALD and the diagnosis must be confirmed by biochemical assay. A more complete discussion of the differential diagnosis is provided in a recent review article (Moser *et al.*, 2000).

A progressive myelopathy with paraparesis and sphincter disturbances in adults is the other common clinical presentation of X-ALD. When this presentation is combined with adrenal insufficiency, adrenomyeloneuropathy (AMN) is by far the most common cause and readily confirmed by biochemical assay. However, in approximately 30% of patients with AMN, adrenal function is not demonstrably abnormal or is only mild. Under these circumstances, the diagnosis is often not made and patients may be misdiagnosed as having progressive multiple sclerosis. We recommend that plasma levels of VLCFA be measured in all patients with progressive myelopathy. The diagnosis of the AMN-like syndrome in women heterozygous for X-ALD is a challenge. Less than 1% have adrenal insufficiency, it presents most commonly in middle age or later, and it must be distinguished from many other causes of myelopathy. Furthermore, the biochemical abnormality in plasma is not as marked as in affected males. False negative tests occur in approximately 20% of heterozygotes. Most of the women with this syndrome have been identified because they were

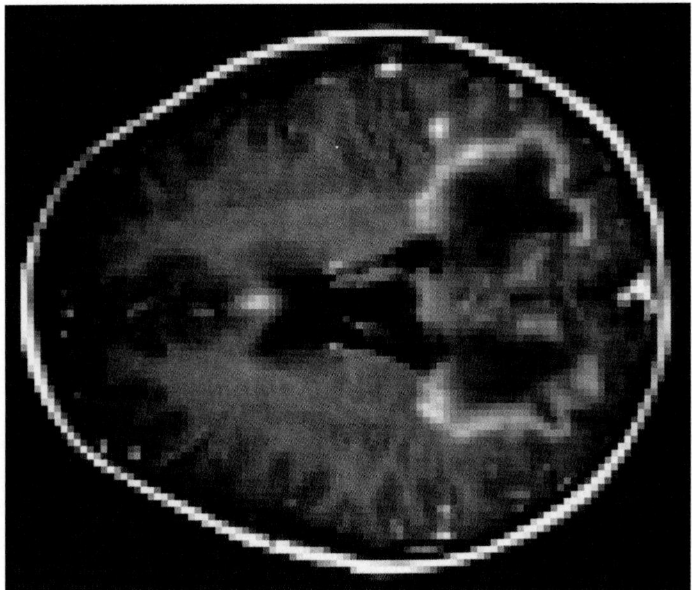

FIGURE 34.6
"Classical" MRI pattern in a patient with the childhood cerebral form of X-ALD. T-1 weighted image obtained following intravenous injection of pentaacetic acid. The symmetric regions of decreased signal intensity in the parieto-occipital regions are indicative of loss of myelin and gliosis. The garland of increased signal density that surrounds these regions is the zone in which the gadolinium contrast material has accumulated due to the breakdown of the blood-brain barrier associated with the inflammatory response. From *Radiology* **165**, 496, 1987, with permission

relatives of affected male patients. However, as awareness about this syndrome has increased, more women without known affected relatives are being diagnosed. This is important because it increases the opportunity for genetic counseling.

Primary adrenal insufficiency without neurological involvement, the "Addison-only" phenotype is the third mode of clinical presentation of X-ALD. It cannot be distinguished clinically from other forms of primary adrenocortical insufficiency. It has been estimated that X-ALD is the cause of adrenal insufficiency in 35% patients with idiopathic Addison disease that manifested before 7.5 years of age) (Jorge *et al.*, 1993; Laureti *et al.*, 1996). It is recommended that plasma VLCFA levels be measured in all males with adrenal insufficiency of unknown cause.

### Extended Family Screening

Extended family screening programs have identified many asymptomatic males with X-ALD and many heterozygous women. This is clinically important, since many of the asymptomatic males have unrecognized adrenal insufficiency and can be started on appropriate hormone replacement therapy before they develop clinical symptoms. Furthermore, as discussed in the next section, current therapy for the neurological manifestations (bone marrow transplantation) is most effective when it is initiated when involvement is still mild, and dietary therapy in young asymptomatic patients appears to reduce the risk of developing the childhood cerebral disease. Identification of heterozygotes is of key importance for genetic counseling. Bezman *et al.* (2001) used the plasma VLCFA assay to screen 4169 at-risk members of the extended families of known X-ALD patients and identified 594 affected males, 250 of whom were asymptomatic, and 1270 heterozygous women.

### Prenatal Diagnosis

Prenatal identification can be achieved by VLCFA analysis in cultured amniocytes or chorion villus cells (Moser and Moser, 1999). The risk of false negatives can be reduced by immunofluorescence assay (Ruiz *et al.*, 1997). Mutation analysis is the preferred procedure when the mutation in an affected member of the family has been defined.

### Mass Neonatal Screening

Plasma VLCFA levels in affected males are increased already on the day of birth (Moser *et al.*). Studied to determine the feasibility of screening all newborn males with tandem mass spectrometry techniques are now in progress.

## TREATMENT

The design of therapy of the neurological manifestation X-ALD is hampered by the incomplete understanding of its pathogenesis: The function of the defective gene product, ALDP, is still not understood, nor is the pathogenesis of the inflammatory demyelination that causes the rapid disease progression. The development of an animal model that displays the inflammatory demyelination would enhance greatly the capacity to design and evaluate therapeutic intervention. This section will begin with an appraisal of the therapies that are in current use and cite briefly to therapies that have been proposed for the future. It should be noted that the development of mass neonatal screening, which may become available during the next 5 years, would have a profound effect on therapeutic strategies: nervous system function in X-ALD patients does not become abnormal until 2 to 3 years of age, and often considerably later. Neonatal screening thus has the potential of detecting all affected males years before they develop nervous system dysfunction and therapeutic approaches could then focus on the prevention of nervous system damage.

### Adrenal Steroid Replacement Therapy

Adrenal steroid replacement therapy is mandatory and life saving. Even though relatively simple, this form of therapy is often not properly implemented, and preventable deaths due to adrenal crisis continues to occur. Glucocorticoid dose requirements are generally those used for other forms of adrenal insufficiency. Most patients do not require mineralocorticoid replacement. While the adrenal steroid replacement therapy can improve strength and well being, it generally does not appear to alter progression of neurological disability. However, neurologic improvement coincident with glucocorticoid replacement has been reported in some cases (Peckham *et al.*, 1982; Zhang and Moser, 2003).

### Bone Marrow Transplantation-Benefit in Patients with Early Cerebral Involvement

It has been shown that allogeneic bone marrow transplantation (BMT) can prevent further progression and occasionally reverse deficits in children and adolescents with cerebral X-ALD who received the transplant when brain involvement was still relatively mild (Aubourg *et al.*, 1990; Malm *et al.*, 1997; Shapiro *et al.*, 2000). Some of the patients have now been followed for 10 years and have normal cognitive function and the brain MRI abnormality has remained stable, and in one patient it disappeared (Aubourg *et al.*, 1990; Shapiro *et al.*, 2000). However, when the cerebral involvement is already advanced, the effect of BMT is not favorable. The deficit may increase during the days and weeks following the transplant, and this may lead to fatal outcome. When long-term stabilization occurs in patients with advanced disability, the quality of life often is impaired to such an extent that the ethical justification for the procedure is questionable. It is not known whether BMT has a favorable effect in adult patients with AMN, the noninflammatory form of X-ALD. It has not been performed in pure AMN patients because the risk of graft versus host disease (GVH) is higher than in children and adolescents, and in view of the slow progression of AMN, the risk/benefit ratio is not favorable. A point of key interest will be whether the children who had been transplanted successfully for cerebral ALD will develop AMN in adulthood. While there is no doubt that BMT is the most effective therapy currently available for children and adolescents, and possibly young adults with cerebral X-ALD, patients must be selected with great care so that advantage is taken of the relatively small "window of opportunity." This window can be identified by serial MRI and neuropsychological studies. The most favorable patients are those who show evidence of relatively mild but progressive MRI abnormalities and still have a performance intelligence quotient (PIQ) of 80 or above (Shapiro *et al.*, 2000). These conditions are encountered most often in the follow-up of asymptomatic patients identified by family screening. Unfortunately, many children and adolescents who are identified because of clinically identified abnormalities already have such advanced disabilities that they are no longer considered to be candidates for BMT.

The mechanism of the favorable effect of BMT is not yet clear. The BMT-derived cells have the capacity to metabolize VLCFA (Moser *et al.*, 1984), and the plasma VLCFA levels are reduced, although not normalized (Shapiro *et al.*, 2000). Unlike the lysosomal disorders, where the normal gene product is excreted by donor cells and can be taken up by host cells, this is not applicable to X-ALD because the transfer of a peroxisomal membrane protein from donor to host cells is not possible. The favorable effect in X-ALD brain may result from the donor-derived microglia. Microglia are bone marrow derived at least in part (Hickey and Kimura, 1988), and BMT-derived cells do enter the nervous system (Unger *et al.*, 1993). The donor-derived microglia may have a favorable effect on local brain metabolism. Microglia have a slow turnover rate (Hickey *et al.*, 1992). This could account for the findings that BMT beneficial effects are not observed until 6 to 12 months after BMT and may continue to increase thereafter (Aubourg *et al.*, 1990).

An alternative or additive mechanism for the favorable effect of BMT may be due to the immunosuppression that forms part of the preparative regimen. So far, the beneficial effects of BMT have been documented only in patients with inflammatory demyelination. BMT has been shown to abolish the accumulation of contrast material in MRI studies, which is an index of the inflammatory response (Charnas, L., unpublished observation). Were this to be the case, then an immunosuppressive regimen alone could be beneficial. Against this hypothesis is that immunosuppressive regimens tested so far have not been beneficial (discussed later), and that no improvement was observed in a patient who received a BMT who had been immunosuppressed but failed to engraft (Nowaczyk *et al.*, 1997).

### Reduction of VLCFA Levels by Dietary Therapy

Oral administration of a 4:1 mixture of glyceryl-trioleate, and glyceryl-trierucate, also referred to as "Lorenzo's oil," when combined with reduction of fat intake, normalizes plasma VLCFA levels in X-ALD patients within 4 weeks (Odone and Odone, 1989; Rizzo *et al.*, 1989), probably by competitive inhibition with the microsomal elongating system for saturated long chain fatty acids (Bourre *et al.*, 1976). In spite of this striking biochemical effect, it does not appear to alter disease progression in patients who already are neurologically symptomatic (Aubourg *et al.*, 1993; Kaplan *et al.*, 1993; Uziel *et al.*, 1991; van Geel *et al.*, 1999). The lack of clinical benefit has been attributed to the apparently low rate of entry of erucic acid, the active component of Lorenzo's oil" into the brain (Poulos *et al.*, 1994; Rasmussen *et al.*, 1994). This clinical experience in several clinical centers combined with the observation that about 30% of treated patients developed moderate thrombocytopenia (Zinkham *et al.*, 1993) and a lesser incidence of other side effects (van Geel *et al.*, 1999) led to the consensus that this therapy is not indicated in patients who are already symptomatic.

An international multicenter study to evaluate the preventive effect of Lorenzo's oil has been conducted. Enacted since 1989, the study involves five centers in the United States and two in Europe and included a total of 104 boys who all had proven X-ALD, were less than 6 years old, and had normal neurological examination and MRI. They received Lorenzo's oil in accordance with a previously described protocol. Lorenzo's oil therapy combined with reduced fat intake from other sources, was initiated between 1 and 6 years of age using a regimen that has been described previously (Moser and Borel, 1995). Outcome measurements were the time of development of neurologic and MRI abnormalities, which were evaluated separately independently by standardized criteria. An open study rather than a randomized placebo-controlled study design was selected after ethical advice because of the devastating nature of childhood cerebral X-ALD combined with the possibility that clinical benefit might result from reduction of plasma VLCFA levels. Two criteria were used to evaluate preventive effect: (1) comparison of age of onset of neurologic symptoms in the treated group (1989–1999) with that in historical controls; and (2) correlation between neurologic outcome and MRI progression and the degree of reduction of plasma VLCFA levels, a measure of compliance. Analysis of these data is complex because of the nonrandomized study design and incomplete information about historical controls. Preliminary appraisal of the data by Hugo Moser and Ann Moser presented at a meeting on peroxisomal diseases in 2002 (Moser and Moser, 2003) indicated that the oil diminished the subsequent risk of neurological involvement. However, additional analysis of the data is required for definitive conclusion.

It was recommended that this therapy be offered to boys in this category, subject to the caution that the benefit may represent a delay in disease onset rather than prevention and that some patients did develop neurological involvement in spite of good control of plasma levels. It was emphasized that the therapy be supervised by a multidisciplinary team to help assure normal growth and development and prevent complications such as reduction of platelet count. Adrenal function must be monitored and deficiency treated by adrenal steroid therapy. Levels of essential and polyunsaturated fatty acids, including docosahexaenoic acid, must be monitored and appropriate supplementation provided. Finally, it is of crucial importance that brain MRI be monitored so that those patients who can benefit from bone marrow transplant be identified in a timely manner.

### Phenylbutyrate—Favorable Biochemical Effect in X-ALD Mouse Model

Kemp *et al.* (1998) reported that 4-phenylbutyrate (4PB) normalizes VLCFA levels and restores VLCFA oxidation in cultured skin fibroblasts of patients with X-ALD and of X-ALD mice. They also made the important observation that oral administration to X-ALD mice reduced substantially levels of VLCFA in the brain and adrenal glands of these animals. The mechanism of this effect is not yet fully understood. The authors made the intriguing observation that 4PB increased the expression of ALDR (ABCD2), a homologue of ABCD1 (the gene that is defective in X-ALD). ALDR can substitute at least in part for the effects of ALDP on VLCFA metabolism in X-ALD cells (Fig. 34.7) (Kemp *et al.*, 1998; Netik *et al.*, 1999). In their initial publication, these authors suggested that 4PB therapy here could be an example of pharmacological gene therapy made possible by the existence of gene redundancy. However, later studies by the same group led them to conclude that this is not the mechanism (McGuinness *et al.*, 2001), based on their observation that the effect on VLCFA levels preceded the increased expression of ALDR. The authors found that 4PB has a rapid but as yet not fully understood effects on both peroxisomal and mitochondrial fatty acid oxidation and that the reduction of VLCFA levels in X-ALD cells appears to be a consequence of this effect.

4PB therapy has not been evaluated systematically in X-ALD patients. Moser *et al.* (unpublished observation) conducted a phase I study in six men with AMN who received oral 4PB at a dose of 20 grams per day for two 6-week periods. While platelet VLCFA levels were reduced by approximately 50%, levels of VLCFA in plasma and red cells were unchanged. VLCFA oxidation in white blood cells and the expression of ALDR were not increased in white blood cells. There were no adverse effects. Clinical findings were not changed, but this was not expected over such a short time in patients with the slowly progressive pure AMN. Systematic long-term clinical trials of 4PB therapy in X-ALD have not been conducted.

### Immunosuppression

The aim of immunosuppression therapy is to abolish the inflammatory response in cerebral X-ALD and thus convert this rapidly progressive form into the milder pure AMN pheno-

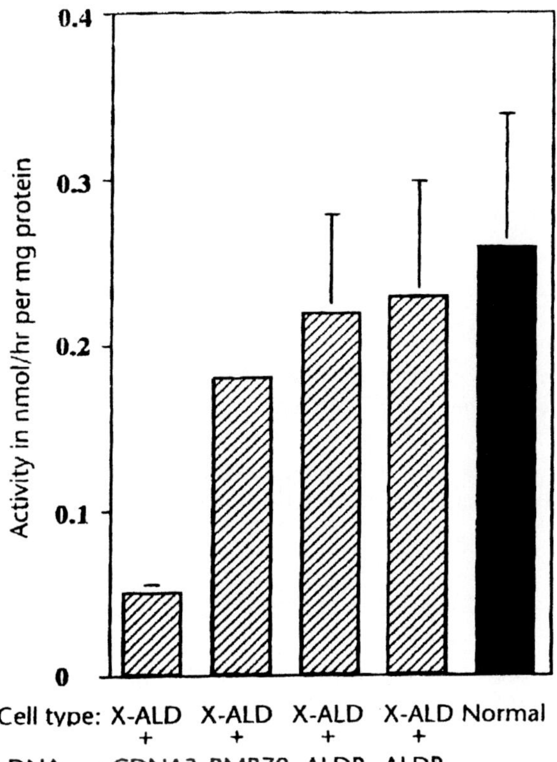


FIGURE 34.7
Peroxisomal ABC half-transporter complementation of C24:0 ß-oxidation. Human X-ALD fibroblasts transformed with SV40T antigen were transfected with recombinant expression vector (pCDNA3) alone or with vector-containing cDNA for PMP70, ALDP, or ALDRP (hatched bars). The rates of C24:0 ß-oxidation in the transfected cells were corrected for the fraction of cells expressing the transgene, as determined by immunofluorescence staining of the transgene. The adjusted rates were compared with the rates of C24:0 ß-oxidation determined in transformed fibroblasts from normal individuals (filled bar). The indicated values are the mean and standard deviation for pCDNA3 (n = 6); ALDP (n = 5); ALDRP (n = 4); and normal m (n = 5). PMP70, n = 1. From *Nature Medicine* **4,** 1261, 1998.

type. Agents tested so far are cyclophophamide (Naidu *et al.*, 1988; Stumpf *et al.*, 1981), beta interferon (Korenke *et al.*, 1997), and Rolipram (Netik *et al.*, 1999). They have not been successful. Other recently developed approaches that have shown promise in the treatment of multiple sclerosis, such as the alpha 4 integrin antagonist Natalizumab (Miller *et al.*, 2003), have not been tested. Better understanding of the pathogenesis of the inflammatory response in X-ALD may lead to more effective immunosuppressive therapies, and in view of the devastating effect of the inflammatory response, this represents a high priority.

## Lovastatin

Singh and associates have proposed lovastatin as a possible therapeutic agent. They have shown that lovastatin increases the capacity of cultured X-ALD cells to metabolize tetracosanoic acid (C24:0) and that it normalized the levels of VLCFA in these cells (Singh *et al.*, 1998). Oral administration of lovastatin in a dosage of 40 mg per day lowered the levels of VLCFA in the plasma of X-ALD patients (Pai *et al.*, 2000; Singh *et al.*, 1998), but the lowering is not as consistent as that achieved with Lorenzo's oil (Moser, A. B., unpublished observation). Lovastatin administration in X-ALD mice did not reduce VLCFA levels in their brain (Cartier *et al.*, 2000; Yamada *et al.*, 2000). Weinhofer *et al.* have shown that lowering cholesterol leads to activation of sterol regulatory element binding protein and increased expression of the ABCD2 gene and reduced VLCFA accumulation in cultured

ABCD1 cells. This may account for the VLCFA lowering action of lovastatin (Weinhofer *et al.*, 2002). Lovastatin has another action, which may be relevant to X-ALD. It has been shown to reduce the inflammatory demyelination in experimental allergic encephalitis in Lewis rats (Stanislaus *et al.*, 1999), at least in part due to its induction of nitric oxide synthase (Pahan *et al.*, 1997). Nitric oxide synthase induction appears to play a role in the pathogenesis of the inflammatory response in X-ALD (Gilg *et al.*, 2000). Lovastatin did not appear to alter neurologic progression in brief noncontrolled clinical trials (Pai, *et al.*, 2000), but longer-term controlled trials have not been conducted.

### Gene Replacement Therapy

Retroviral transfer of the X-ALD gene into C34+ cells of X-ALD patients has been achieved (Doerflinger *et al.*, 1998). A higher and more persistent transduction has been achieved with lenti-virus (Aubourg, P., personal communication) and warrants consideration of *ex vivo* therapy with bone marrow derived cells. However, such trials must be deferred until the safety of this vector has been examined in greater detail.

## PREVENTION OF X-ALD

In spite of emerging therapies, X-ALD is a devastating experience to the patients and families. The importance of disease prevention through genetic counseling cannot be overemphasized.

## References

Adams R. D., and Kubik C. S. (1952). The morbid anatomy of the demyelinative diseases. *Am J Med* **12,** 510–546.

Antoku Y., Sakai T., Tsukamoto K., Imanishi K., Ohtsuka Y., Iwashita H., and Goto I. (1987). A simple diagnostic method of adrenoleukodystrophy: Total fatty acid analysis of erythrocyte membranes. *Clin Chim Acta* **169,** 121–125.

Aubourg P., Adamsbaum C., Lavallard-Rousseau M. C., Rocchiccioli F., Cartier N., Jambaque I., Jakobezak C., Lemaitre A., Boureau F., Wolf C., and Bougneres, P. F. (1993). A two-year trial of oleic and erucic acids ("Lorenzo's oil") as treatment for adrenomyeloneuropathy. *N Engl J Med* **329,** 745–752.

Aubourg P., Blanche S., Jambaque I., Rocchiccioli F., Kalifa G., Naud-Saudreau C., Rolland M. O., Debre M., Chaussain J. L., Griscelli C., Fischer, A., and Bougneres, P. F. (1990). Reversal of early neurologic and neuroradiologic manifestations of X-linked adrenoleukodystrophy by bone marrow transplantation. *N Engl J Med* **322,** 1860–1866.

Aversa A., Palleschi S., Cruccu G., Silvestroni L., Isidori A., and Fabbri A. (1998). Rapid decline of fertility in a case of adrenoleukodystrophy. *Hum Reprod* **13,** 2474–2479.

Berger J., Molzer B., Fae I., and Bernheimer H. (1994). X-linked adrenoleukodystrophy (ALD).: A novel mutation of the ALD gene in 6 members of a family presenting with 5 different phenotypes. *Biochem Biophys Res Commun* **205,** 1638–1643.

Bezman L., Moser A. B., Raymond G. V., Rinaldo P., Watkins P. A., Smith K. D., Kass N. E., and Moser H. W. (2001). Adrenoleukodystrophy: Incidence, new mutation rate, and results of extended family screening. *Ann Neurol* **49,** 512–517.

Bizzozero O. A., Zuniga G., and Lees M. B. (1991). Fatty acid composition of human myelin proteolipid protein in peroxisomal disorders. *J Neurochem* **56,** 872–878.

Black P. N., Zhang Q., Weimar J. D., and DiRusso C. C. (1997). Mutational analysis of a fatty acyl-coenzyme A synthetase signature motif identifies seven amino acid residues that modulate fatty acid substrate specificity. *J Biol Chem* **272,** 4896–4903.

Blaw M. E. (1970). Melanodermic type leucodystrophy (adrenoleukodystrophy). *In* "Leucodystrophies and Poliodystrophies" (Vinken P. J., and Bruyn G. W. E., eds.), pp. 128–133. North Holland Publishing Company, Amsterdam.

Blaw M. E., Osterberger K., Kozak P., and Nelson E. (1964). Sudanophilic leukodystrophy and adrenal cortical atrophy. *Arch Neurol* **11,** 626–631.

Boehm C. D., Cutting G. R., Lachtermacher M. B., Moser H. W., and Chong S. S. (1999). Accurate DNA-based diagnostic and carrier testing for X-linked adrenoleukodystrophy. *Mol Genet Metab* **66,** 128–136.

Bourre J. M., Daudu O., and Baumann N. (1976). Nervonic acid biosynthesis by erucyl-CoA elongation in normal and quaking mouse brain microsomes. Elongation of other unsaturated fatty acyl-CoAs (mono and poly-unsaturated). *Biochim Biophys Acta* **424,** 1–7.

Braiterman L. T., Watkins P. A., Moser A. B., and Smith K. D. (1999). Peroxisomal very long chain fatty acid beta-oxidation activity is determined by the level of adrenodeukodystrophy protein (ALDP). expression. *Mol Genet Metab* **66,** 91–99.

Braiterman L. T., Zheng S., Watkins P. A., Geraghty M. T., Johnson G., McGuinness M. C., Moser A. B., and Smith K. D. (1998). Suppression of peroxisomal membrane protein defects by peroxisomal ATP binding cassette (ABC). proteins. *Hum Mol Genet* **7,** 239–247.

Brennemann W., Kohler W., Zierz S., and Klingmuller D. (1996). Occurrence of adrenocortical insufficiency in adrenomyeloneuropathy. *Neurology* **47,** 605.

Bresnan M. J., and Richardson E. P. (1979). Case records of the Massachusetts General Hospital. Weekly clinicopathological exercises. Case 18–1979. *N Engl J Med* **300,** 1037–1045.

Broccardo C., Troffer-Charlier N., Savary S., Mandel J. L., and Chimini G. (1998). Exon organisation of the mouse gene encoding the Adrenoleukodystrophy related protein (ALDRP). *Eur J Hum Genet* **6,** 638–641.

Brown F. R. 3rd, Chen W. W., Kirschner D. A., Frayer K. L., Powers J. M., Moser A. B., and Moser H. W. (1983). Myelin membrane from adrenoleukodystrophy brain white matter–biochemical properties. *J Neurochem* **41,** 341–348.

Brun A., and Voigt G. E. (1960). Entzundliche cerebrale sklerose mit nebenniereninsuffizienz. *Deutsche Zellschrift F. Nervenheilkunde* **180,** 654–664.

Budka H., Sluga E., and Heiss W. D. (1976). Spastic paraplegia associated with Addison's disease: Adult variant of adreno-leukodystrophy. *J Neurol* **213,** 237–250.

Carey W. F., Poulos A., Sharp P., Nelson P. V., Robertson E. F., Hughes J. L., and Gill A. (1994). Pitfalls in the prenatal diagnosis of peroxisomal beta-oxidation defects by chorionic villus sampling. *Prenat Diagn* **14,** 813–819.

Cartier N., Guidoux S., Rocchiccioli F., and Aubourg P. (2000). Simvastatin does not normalize very long chain fatty acids in adrenoleukodystrophy mice. *FEBS Lett* **478,** 205–208.

Cassagne C., Darriet D., and Bourre J. M. (1978). Biosynthesis of very long chain fatty acids by the sciatic nerve of the rabbit. *FEBS Lett* **90,** 336–340.

Chaudhry V., Moser H. W., and Cornblath D. R. (1996). Nerve conduction studies in adrenomyeloneuropathy. *J Neurol Neurosurg Psychiatry* **61,** 181–185.

Cox R. D. (1972). Regression models and life tables. *J Royal Statistics Society* **34,** 187.

Dean M., Hamon Y., and Chimini G. (2001). The human ATP-binding cassette (ABC). transporter superfamily. *J Lipid Res* **42,** 1007–1017.

Doerflinger N., Miclea J. M., Lopez J., Chomienne C., Bougneres P., Aubourg P., and Cartier N. (1998). Retroviral transfer and long-term expression of the adrenoleukodystrophy gene in human CD34+ cells. *Hum Gene Ther* **9,** 1025–1036.

Dubois-Dalcq M., Feigenbaum V., and Aubourg P. (1999). The neurobiology of X-linked adrenoleukodystrophy, a demyelinating peroxisomal disorder. *Trends Neurosci* **22,** 4–12.

Edwin D., Speedie L. J., Kohler W., Naidu S., Kruse B., and Moser H. W. (1996). Cognitive and brain magnetic resonance imaging findings in adrenomyeloneuropathy. *Ann Neurol* **40,** 675–678.

Fanconi V. A., Prader A., Isler W., Luthy F., and Siebenmann R. (1963). Morbus Addison mit hirnsklerose im kindesalter–Ein hereditares syndrom mit X-chromosomaler vererbung? *Helv Paediatr Acta* **18,** 480–501.

Feigenbaum V., Gelot A., Casanova P., Daumas-Duport C., Aubourg P., and Dubois-Dalcq M. (2000). Apoptosis in the central nervous system of cerebral adrenoleukodystrophy patients. *Neurobiol Dis* **7,** 600–612.

Feigenbaum V., Lombard-Platet G., Guidoux S., Sarde C. O., Mandel J. L., and Aubourg P. (1996). Mutational and protein analysis of patients and heterozygous women with X-linked adrenoleukodystrophy. *Am J Hum Genet* **58,** 1135–1144.

Flavigny E., Sanhaj A., Aubourg P., and Cartier N. (1999). Retroviral-mediated adrenoleukodystrophy-related gene transfer corrects very long chain fatty acid metabolism in adrenoleukodystrophy fibroblasts: Implications for therapy. *FEBS Lett* **448,** 261–264.

Forss-Petter S., Werner H., Berger J., Lassmann H., Molzer B., Schwab M. H., Bernheimer H., Zimmermann F., and Nave K. A. (1997). Targeted inactivation of the X-linked adrenoleukodystrophy gene in mice. *J Neurosci Res* **50,** 829–843.

Gagnon J. L. R. (1959). Sclerose cerebral diffuse avec melanodermie et atrophie surrenale. *Union Med Canada* **88,** 392–418.

Garside S., Rosebush P. I., Levinson A. J., and Mazurek M. F. (1999). Late-onset adrenoleukodystrophy associated with long-standing psychiatric symptoms. *J Clin Psychiatry* **60,** 460–468.

Gilg A. G., Singh A. K., and Singh I. (2000). Inducible nitric oxide synthase in the central nervous system of patients with X-adrenoleukodystrophy. *J Neuropathol Exp Neurol* **59,** 1063–1069.

Gould S. J., Raymond G. V., and Valle D. (2001). The Peroxisome Biogenesis Disorders. *In* "The Metabolic and Molecular Bases of Inherited Diseases" (Scriver C. R., Beaudet A. L., Sly W. S., and Valle D., eds.), pp. 3181–3217. McGraw Hill, New York.

Gray R. G., Green A., Cole T., Davidson V., Giles M., Schutgens R. B., and Wanders R. J. (1995). A misdiagnosis of X-linked adrenoleukodystrophy in cultured chorionic villus cells by the measurement of very long chain fatty acids. *Prenat Diagn* **15,** 486–490.

Griffin J. W., Goren E., Schaumburg H., Engel W. K., and Loriaux L. (1977). Adrenomyeloneuropathy: A probable variant of adrenoleukodystrophy. I. Clinical and endocrinologic aspects. *Neurology* **27,** 1107–1113.

Hamilton J. A., Era S., Bhamidipati S. P., and Reed R. G. (1991). Locations of the three primary binding sites for long-chain fatty acids on bovine serum albumin. *Proc Natl Acad Sci U S A* **88,** 2051–2054.

Hampel E. (1937). Morbus Addisonii und sklerosierende erkrankung des hemispharenmarks. Beitrag zu den hirnveranderungen beim morbus Addisonii und Zum kapitel der diffusen sklerosen. *Dtsch Z Nervenheilk* **142,** 186–208.

Hashimoto T. (1996). Peroxisomal beta-oxidation: Enzymology and molecular biology. *Ann N Y Acad Sci* **804,** 86–98.

Hashmi M., Stanley W., and Singh I. (1986). Lignoceroyl-CoASH ligase: Enzyme defect in fatty acid beta-oxidation system in X-linked childhood adrenoleukodystrophy. *FEBS Lett* **196,** 247–250.

Heinzer A. K., Kemp S., Lu J. F., Watkins P. A., and Smith K. D. (2002). Mouse very long-chain acyl-CoA synthetase in X-linked adrenoleukodystrophy. *J Biol Chem* **277,** 28765–28773.

Hershkovitz E., Narkis G., Shorer Z., Moser A. B., Watkins P. A., Moser H. W., and Manor E. (2002). Cerebral X-linked adrenoleukodystrophy in a girl with Xq27-ter deletion. *Ann Neurol* **52,** 234–237.

Hickey W. F., and Kimura H. (1988). Perivascular microglial cells of the CNS are bone marrow-derived and present antigen in vivo. *Science* **239,** 290–292.

Hickey W. F., Vass K., and Lassmann H. (1992). Bone marrow-derived elements in the central nervous system: An immunohistochemical and ultrastructural survey of rat chimeras. *J Neuropathol Exp Neurol* **51,** 246–256.

Higgins C. F. (1992). ABC transporters: From microorganisms to man. *Annu Rev Cell Biol* **8,** 67–113.

Ho J. K., Duclos R. I. Jr and Hamilton J. A. (2002). Interactions of acyl carnitines with model membranes: A (13).C-NMR study. *J Lipid Res* **43,** 1429–1439.

Ho J. K., Moser H., Kishimoto Y., and Hamilton J. A. (1995). Interactions of a very long chain fatty acid with model membranes and serum albumin. Implications for the pathogenesis of adrenoleukodystrophy. *J Clin Invest* **96,** 1455–1463.

Hoefnagel D., and Van Den Noort S. (1962). Diffuse cerebral sclerosis with endocrine abnormalities in young males. *Brain* **85,** 553–568.

Holzinger A., Kammerer S., and Roscher A. A. (1997). Primary structure of human PMP69, a putative peroxisomal ABC-transporter. *Biochem Biophys Res Commun* **237,** 152–157.

Hughes J. T., Brownell B., and Hewer R. L. (1968). The peripheral sensory pathway in friedreich's ataxia. An examination by light and electron microscopy of the posterior nerve roots, posterior root ganglia, and peripheral sensory nerves in cases of friedreich's ataxia. *Brain* **91,** 803–18.

Igarashi M., Belchis D., and Suzuki K. (1976a). Brain gangliosides in adrenoleukodystrophy. *J Neurochem* **27,** 327–328.

Igarashi M., Schaumburg H. H., Powers J., Kishmoto Y., Kolodny E., and Suzuki K. (1976b). Fatty acid abnormality in adrenoleukodystrophy. *J Neurochem* **26,** 851–860.

Ito M., Blumberg B. M., Mock D. J., Goodman A. D., Moser A. B., Moser H. W., Smith K. D., and Powers J. M. (2001). Potential environmental and host participants in the early white matter lesion of adreno-leukodystrophy: Morphologic evidence for CD8 cytotoxic T cells, cytolysis of oligodendrocytes, and CD1-mediated lipid antigen presentation. *J Neuropathol Exp Neurol* **60,** 1004–1019.

Jorge P., Quelhas D., and Nogueira A. (1993). Characterization of X-linked adrenoleukodystrophy in different biological specimens from ten Portuguese families. *J Inherit Metab Dis* **16,** 55–62.

Jorge P., Quelhas D., Oliveira P., Pinto R., and Nogueira A. (1994). X-linked adrenoleukodystrophy in patients with idiopathic Addison disease. *Eur J Pediatr* **153,** 594–597.

Julien J. J., Vallat J. M., Vital C., Lagueny A., Ferrer X., and Darriet D. (1981). Adrenomyeloneuropathy: Demonstration of inclusions at the level of the peripheral nerve. *Eur Neurol* **20,** 367–373.

Kamijo K., Taketani S., Yokota S., Osumi T., and Hashimoto T. (1990). The 70-kDa peroxisomal membrane protein is a member of the Mdr (P-glycoprotein).-related ATP-binding protein superfamily. *J Biol Chem* **265,** 4534–4540.

Kaplan P. W., Tusa R. J., Shankroff J., Heller J., and Moser H. W. (1993). Visual evoked potentials in adrenoleukodystrophy: A trial with glycerol trioleate and Lorenzo oil. *Ann Neurol* **34,** 169–174.

Kelley R. I., Datta N. S., Dobyns W. B., Hajra A. K., Moser A. B., Noetzel M. J., Zackai E. H., and Moser H. W. (1986). Neonatal adrenoleukodystrophy: New cases, biochemical studies, and differentiation from Zellweger and related peroxisomal polydystrophy syndromes. *Am J Med Genet* **23,** 869–901.

Kemp S., Ligtenberg M. J., van Geel B. M., Barth P. G., Wolterman R. A., Schoute F., Sarde C. O., Mandel J. L., van Oost B. A., and Bolhuis P. A. (1994). Identification of a two base pair deletion in five unrelated families with adrenoleukodystrophy: A possible hot spot for mutations. *Biochem Biophys Res Commun* **202,** 647–653.

Kemp S., Pujol A., Waterham H. R., van Geel B. M., Boehm C. D., Raymond G. V., Cutting G. R., Wanders R. J., and Moser H. W. (2001). ABCD1 mutations and the X-linked adrenoleukodystrophy mutation database: Role in diagnosis and clinical correlations. *Hum Mutat* **18,** 499–515.

Kemp S., Wei H. M., Lu J. F., Braiterman L. T., McGuinness M. C., Moser A. B., Watkins P. A., and Smith K. D. (1998). Gene redundancy and pharmacological gene therapy: Implications for X-linked adrenoleukodystrophy. *Nat Med* **4,** 1261–1268.

Knazek R. A., Rizzo W. B., Schulman J. D., and Dave J. R. (1983). Membrane microviscosity is increased in the erythrocytes of patients with adrenoleukodystrophy and adrenomyeloneuropathy. *J Clin Invest* **72,** 245–248.

Kobayashi T., Shinnoh N., Kondo A., and Yamada T. (1997). Adrenoleukodystrophy protein-deficient mice represent abnormality of very long chain fatty acid metabolism. *Biochem Biophys Res Commun* **232,** 631–636.

Koike R., Tsuji S., Ohno T., Suzuki Y., Orii T., and Miyatake T. (1991). Physiological significance of fatty acid elongation system in adrenoleukodystrophy. *J Neurol Sci* **103,** 188–194.

Kok F., Neumann S., Sarde C. O., Zheng S., Wu K. H., Wei H. M., Bergin J., Watkins P. A., Gould S., Sack G., Moser, H., Mandel, J-L., and Smith, K. D. (1995). Mutational analysis of patients with X-linked adrenoleukodystrophy. *Hum Mutat* **6,** 104–115.

Korenke G. C., Christen H. J., Kruse B., Hunneman D. H., and Hanefeld F. (1997). Progression of X-linked adrenoleukodystrophy under interferon-beta therapy. *J Inherit Metab Dis* **20,** 59–66.

Kumar A. J., Kohler W., Kruse B., Naidu S., Bergin A., Edwin D., and Moser H. W. (1995). MR findings in adult-onset adrenoleukodystrophy. *AJNR Am J Neuroradiol* **16,** 1227–1237.

Kumar A. J., Rosenbaum A. E., Naidu S., Wener L., Citrin C. M., Lindenberg R., Kim W. S., Zinreich S. J., Molliver M. E., Mayberg H. S., and Moser, H. W. (1987). Adrenoleukodystrophy: Correlating MR imaging with CT. *Radiology* **165,** 497–504.

Kurihara M., Kumagai K., Yagishita S., Imai M., Watanabe M., Suzuki Y., and Orii T. (1993). Adrenoleukomyeloneuropathy presenting as cerebellar ataxia in a young child: A probable variant of adrenoleukodystrophy. *Brain Dev* **15,** 377–380.

Laureti S., Casucci G., Santeusanio F., Angeletti G., Aubourg P., and Brunetti P. (1996). X-linked adrenoleukodystrophy is a frequent cause of idiopathic Addison's disease in young adult male patients. *J Clin Endocrinol Metab* **81,** 470–474.

Lazo O., Contreras M., Hashmi M., Stanley W., Irazu C., and Singh I. (1988). Peroxisomal lignoceroyl-CoA ligase deficiency in childhood adrenoleukodystrophy and adrenomyeloneuropathy. *Proc Natl Acad Sci U S A* **85,** 7647–7651.

Lichtenstein B. W., and Rosenbluth P. R. (1959). Schilder's disease with melanoderma. *J Neuropathol Exp Neurol* **18,** 384–396.

Liu L. X., Janvier K., Berteaux-Lecellier V., Cartier N., Benarous R., and Aubourg P. (1999). Homo- and heterodimerization of peroxisomal ATP-binding cassette half-transporters. *J Biol Chem* **274,** 32738–32743.

Loes D. J., Fatemi A., Melhem E. R., Gupte N., Bezman L., Moser H. W., and Raymond G. V. (in press). Brain MRI patterns and their predictive role in cerebral X-linked adrenoleukodystrophy. *Neurology.*

Loes D. J., Hite S., Moser H., Stillman A. E., Shapiro E., Lockman L., Latchaw R. E., and Krivit W. (1994). Adrenoleukodystrophy: A scoring method for brain MR observations. *AJNR Am J Neuroradiol* **15,** 1761–1766.

Lombard-Platet G., Savary S., Sarde C. O., Mandel J. L., and Chimini G. (1996). A close relative of the adrenoleukodystrophy (ALD). gene codes for a peroxisomal protein with a specific expression pattern. *Proc Natl Acad Sci U S A* **93,** 1265–1269.

Lu J. F., Lawler A. M., Watkins P. A., Powers J. M., Moser A. B., Moser H. W., and Smith K. D. (1997). A mouse model for X-linked adrenoleukodystrophy. *Proc Natl Acad Sci U S A* **94,** 9366–9371.

Maestri N. E., and Beaty T. H. (1992). Predictions of a 2-locus model for disease heterogeneity: Application to adrenoleukodystrophy. *Am J Med Genet* **44,** 576–582.

Maier E. M., Kammerer S., Muntau A. C., Wichers M., Braun A., and Roscher A. A. (2002). Symptoms in carriers of adrenoleukodystrophy relate to skewed X inactivation. *Ann Neurol* **52,** 683–688.

Malm G., Ringden O., Anvret M., von Dobeln U., Hagenfeldt L., Isberg B., Knuutila S., Nennesmo I., Winiarski J., and Marcus C. (1997). Treatment of adrenoleukodystrophy with bone marrow transplantation. *Acta Paediatr* **86,** 484–492.

Martin J. J., Ceuterick C., and Libert J. (1980). Skin and conjunctival nerve biopsies in adrenoleukodystrophy and its variants. *Ann Neurol* **8,** 291–5.

McGuinness M. C., Lu J. F., Zhang H. P., Dong G. X., Heinzer A. K., Watkins P. A., Powers J., and Smith K. D. (2003). Role of ALDP (ABCD1)., and Mitochondria in X-Linked Adrenoleukodystrophy. *Mol Cell Biol* **23,** 744–753.

McGuinness M. C., Powers J. M., Bias W. B., Schmeckpeper B. J., Segal A. H., Gowda V. C., Wesselingh S. L., Berger J., Griffin D. E., and Smith K. D. (1997). Human leukocyte antigens and cytokine expression in cerebral inflammatory demyelinative lesions of X-linked adrenoleukodystrophy and multiple sclerosis. *J Neuroimmunol* **75,** 174–182.

McGuinness M. C., Zhang H. P., and Smith K. D. (2001). Evaluation of pharmacological induction of fatty acid beta-oxidation in X-linked adrenoleukodystrophy. *Mol Genet Metab* **74,** 256–263.

Menkes J. H., and Corbo L. M. (1977). Adrenoleukodystrophy. Accumulation of cholesterol esters with very long chain fatty acids. *Neurology* **27,** 928–932.

Migeon B. R., Moser H. W., Moser A. B., Axelman J., Sillence D., and Norum R. A. (1981). Adrenoleukodystrophy: Evidence for X linkage, inactivation, and selection favoring the mutant allele in heterozygous cells. *Proc Natl Acad Sci U S A* **78,** 5066–5070.

Mihalik S. J., Steinberg S. J., Pei Z., Park J., Kim do G., Heinzer A. K., Dacremont G., Wanders R. J., Cuebas D. A., Smith K. D., and Watkins P. A. (2002). Participation of two members of the very long-chain acyl-CoA synthetase family in bile acid synthesis and recycling. *J Biol Chem* **277,** 24771–24779.

Miller D. H., Khan O. A., Sheremata W. A., Blumhardt L. D., Rice G. P., Libonati M. A., Willmer-Hulme A. J., Dalton C. M., Miszkiel K. A., and O'Connor P. W. (2003). A controlled trial of natalizumab for relapsing multiple sclerosis. *N Engl J Med* **348,** 15–23.

Min K. T., and Benzer S. (1999). Preventing neurodegeneration in the Drosophila mutant bubblegum. *Science* **284,** 1985–1988.

Molzer B., Bernheimer H., Budka H., Pilz P., and Toifl K. (1981). Accumulation of very long chain fatty acids is common to 3 variants of adrenoleukodystrophy (ALD). "Classical" ALD, atypical ALD (female patient)., and adrenomyeloneuropathy. *J Neurol Sci* **51,** 301–310.

Moody D. B., Besra G. S., Wilson I. A., and Porcelli S. A. (1999). The molecular basis of CD1-mediated presentation of lipid antigens. *Immunol Rev* **172,** 285–296.

Moser A. B., Kreiter N., Bezman L., Lu S., Raymond G. V., Naidu S., and Moser H. W. (1999). Plasma very long chain fatty acids in 3,000 peroxisome disease patients and 29,000 controls. *Ann Neurol* **45,** 100–110.

Moser A. B., and Moser H. W. (1999). The prenatal diagnosis of X-linked adrenoleukodystrophy. *Prenat Diagn* **19,** 46–48.

Moser H. W., and Borel J. (1995). Dietary management of X-linked adrenoleukodystrophy. *Annu Rev Nutr* **15,** 379–397.

Moser H. W., Loes D. J., Melhem E. R., Raymond G. V., Bezman L., Cox C. S., and Lu S. E. (2000). X-Linked adrenoleukodystrophy: Overview and prognosis as a function of age and brain magnetic resonance imaging abnormality. A study involving 372 patients. *Neuropediatrics* **31,** 227–239.

Moser H. W., Moser A. B. (2003). Evaluation of the preventive effect of glyceryl trioleate-trierucate (Lorenzo's oil). therapy in asymptomatic X-linked adrenoleukodystrophy: Results of two concurrent studies. *Peroxisomal Disorders and Regulation of Genes*. Frank Roels (Ed). Kluwer Academic, Plenum Publishers, London, in press.

Moser H. W., Moser A. B., Frayer K. K., Chen W., Schulman J. D., O'Neill B. P., and Kishimoto Y. (1981). Adrenoleukodystrophy: Increased plasma content of saturated very long chain fatty acids. *Neurology* **31,** 1241–1249.

Moser H. W., Moser A. B., Naidu S., and Bergin A. (1991). Clinical aspects of adrenoleukodystrophy and adrenomyeloneuropathy. *Dev Neurosci* **13,** 254–261.

Moser H. W., Moser A. B., Smith K. D., Bergin A., Borel J., Shankroff J., Stine O. C., Merette C., Ott J., Krivit W., and Shapiro, E. (1992). Adrenoleukodystrophy: Phenotypic variability and implications for therapy. *J Inherit Metab Dis* **15,** 645–664.

Moser H. W., Naidu S., Kumar A. J., and Rosenbaum A. E. (1987). The adrenoleukodystrophies. *Crit Rev Neurobiol* **3,** 29–88.

Moser H. W., Pallante S. L., Moser A. B., Rizzo W. B., Schulman J. D., and Fenselau C. (1983). Adrenoleukodystrophy: Origin of very long chain fatty acids and therapy. *Pediatr Res* **17,** 293A.

Moser H. W., Smith K. D., Watkins P. A., Powers J., and Moser A. B. (2000). X-linked adrenoleukodystrophy. *In* "The Metabolic and Molecular Bases of Inherited Disease" (Scriver C. R., Beaudet A. L., Sly W. S., and Valle D., eds.), pp. 3257–3301. McGraw Hill, New York.

Moser H. W., Tutschka P. J.; Brown F. R. III; Moser A. B.; Yeager A. M.; Singh I.; Mark S. A.; Kumar A. A. J.; McDonnell J. M.; White C. L. III; Maumenee I. H.; Green W. R.; Powers J. M.; and Santos G. W. (1984). Bone marrow transplant in adrenoleukodystrophy. *Neurology* **34,** 1410–1417.

Mosser J., Douar A. M., Sarde C. O., Kioschis P., Feil R., Moser H., Poustka A. M., Mandel J. L., and Aubourg P. (1993). Putative X-linked adrenoleukodystrophy gene shares unexpected homology with ABC transporters. *Nature* **361,** 726–730.

Mosser J., Lutz Y., Stoeckel M. E., Sarde C. O., Kretz C., Douar A. M., Lopez J., Aubourg P., and Mandel J. L. (1994). The gene responsible for adrenoleukodystrophy encodes a peroxisomal membrane protein. *Hum Mol Genet* **3,** 265–271.

Murad S., and Kishimoto Y. (1978). Chain elongation of fatty acid in brain: A comparison of mitochondrial and microsomal enzyme activities. *Arch Biochem Biophys* **185,** 300–306.

Naidu S., Bresnan M. J., Griffin D., O'Toole S., and Moser H. W. (1988). Childhood adrenoleukodystrophy. Failure of intensive immunosuppression to arrest neurologic progression. *Arch Neurol* **45,** 846–848.

Naidu S., Washington C., Thirumalai S., Smith K. D., Moser H. W., and Watkins P. A. (1997). X-chromosome inactivation in symptomatic heterozygotes of X-linked adrenoleukodystrophy. *Ann Neurol* **42,** 498a.

Netik A., Forss-Petter S., Holzinger A., Molzer B., Unterrainer G., and Berger J. (1999). Adrenoleukodystrophy-related protein can compensate functionally for adrenoleukodystrophy protein deficiency (X-ALD): Implications for therapy. *Hum Mol Genet* **8,** 907–913.

Nowaczyk M. J., Saunders E. F., Tein I., Blaser S. I., and Clarke J. T. (1997). Immunoablation does not delay the neurologic progression of X-linked adrenoleukodystrophy. *J Pediatr* **131,** 453–455.

O'Neill G. N., Aoki M., and Brown R. H. Jr (2001). ABCD1 translation-initiator mutation demonstrates genotype-phenotype correlation for AMN. *Neurology* **57,** 1956–1962.

Odone A., and Odone M. (1989). Lorenzo's oil. *J Pediatr Neurosci* **5,** 55.

Pahan K., Sheikh F. G., Namboodiri A. M., and Singh I. (1997). Lovastatin and phenylacetate inhibit the induction of nitric oxide synthase and cytokines in rat primary astrocytes, microglia, and macrophages. *J Clin Invest* **100,** 2671–2679.

Pai G. S., Khan M., Barbosa E., Key L. L., Craver J. R., Cure J. K., Betros R., and Singh I. (2000). Lovastatin therapy for X-linked adrenoleukodystrophy: Clinical and biochemical observations on 12 patients. *Mol Genet Metab* **69,** 312–322.

Peckham R. S., Marshall M. C. Jr, Rosman P. M., Farag A., Kabadi U., and Wallace E. Z. (1982). A variant of adrenomyeloneuropathy with hypothalamic-pituitary dysfunction and neurologic remission after glucocorticoid replacement therapy. *Am J Med* **72,** 173–176.

Pfister R. (1936). Beitrag sur kenntnis der diffusen kirnsklerose. *Archiv fur Psychiatrie* **105,** 1–16.

Poulos A., Gibson R., Sharp P., Beckman K., and Grattan-Smith P. (1994). Very long chain fatty acids in X-linked adrenoleukodystrophy brain after treatment with Lorenzo's oil. *Ann Neurol* **36,** 741–746.

Poulos A., Singh H., Paton B., Sharp P., and Derwas N. (1986). Accumulation and defective beta-oxidation of very long chain fatty acids in Zellweger's syndrome, adrenoleukodystrophy and Refsum's disease variants. *Clin Genet* **29,** 397–408.

Powers J. M., DeCiero D. P., Cox C., Richfield E. K., Ito M., Moser A. B., and Moser H. W. (2001). The dorsal root ganglia in adrenomyeloneuropathy: Neuronal atrophy and abnormal mitochondria. *J Neuropathol Exp Neurol* **60,** 493–501.

Powers J. M., DeCiero D. P., Ito M., Moser A. B., and Moser H. W. (2000). Adrenomyeloneuropathy: A neuropathologic review featuring its noninflammatory myelopathy. *J Neuropathol Exp Neurol* **59,** 89–102.

Powers J. M., Liu Y., Moser A. B., and Moser H. W. (1992). The inflammatory myelinopathy of adreno-leukodystrophy: Cells, effector molecules, and pathogenetic implications. *J Neuropathol Exp Neurol* **51,** 630–643.

Powers J. M., Moser H. W., Moser A. B., and Schaumburg H. H. (1982). Fetal adrenoleukodystrophy: The significance of pathologic lesions in adrenal gland and testis. *Hum Pathol* **13,** 1013–1019.

Powers J. M., and Schaumburg H. H. (1973). The adrenal cortex in adreno-leukodystrophy. *Arch Pathol* **96,** 305–310.

Powers J. M., and Schaumburg H. H. (1974). Adreno-leukodystrophy (sex-linked Schilder's disease). A pathogenetic hypothesis based on ultrastructural lesions in adrenal cortex, peripheral nerve and testis. *Am J Pathol* **76,** 481–491.

Powers J. M., and Schaumburg H. H. (1981). The testis in adreno-leukodystrophy. *Am J Pathol* **102,** 90–98.

Pujol A., Hindelang C., Callizot N., Bartsch U., Schachner M., and Mandel J. L. (2002). Late onset neurological phenotype of the X-ALD gene inactivation in mice: A mouse model for adrenomyeloneuropathy. *Hum Mol Genet* **11,** 499–505.

Ramsey R. B., Banik N. L., and Davison A. N. (1979). Adrenoleukodystrophy brain cholesteryl esters and other neutral lipids. *J Neurol Sci* **40,** 189–196.

Rasmussen M., Moser A. B., Borel J., Khangoora S., and Moser H. W. (1994). Brain, liver, and adipose tissue erucic and very long chain fatty acid levels in adrenoleukodystrophy patients treated with glyceryl trierucate and trioleate oils (Lorenzo's oil). *Neurochem Res* **19,** 1073–1082.

Reinecke C. J., Knoll D. P., Pretorius P. J., Steyn H. S., and Simpson R. H. (1985). The correlation between biochemical and histopathological findings in adrenoleukodystrophy. *J Neurol Sci* **70,** 21–38.

Restuccia D., Di Lazzaro V., Valeriani M., Oliviero A., Le Pera D., Barba C., Cappa M., Bertini E., Di Capua M., and Tonali P. (1999). Neurophysiologic follow-up of long-term dietary treatment in adult-onset adrenoleukodystrophy. *Neurology* **52,** 810–816.

Rezanka T. (1989). Very-long-chain fatty acids from the animal and plant kingdoms. *Prog Lipid Res* **28,** 147–187.

Rizzo W. B., Avigan J., Chemke J., and Schulman J. D. (1984). Adrenoleukodystrophy: Very long-chain fatty acid metabolism in fibroblasts. *Neurology* **34,** 163–169.

Rizzo W. B., Leshner R. T., Odone A., Dammann A. L., Craft D. A., Jensen M. E., Jennings S. S., Davis S., Jaitly R., and Sgro J. A. (1989). Dietary erucic acid therapy for X-linked adrenoleukodystrophy. *Neurology* **39,** 1415–1422.

Robbins D. S., Shirazi Y., Drysdale B. E., Lieberman A., Shin H. S., and Shin M. L. (1987). Production of cytotoxic factor for oligodendrocytes by stimulated astrocytes. *J Immunol* **139,** 2593–2597.

Ruiz M., Coll M. J., Pampols T., and Giros M. (1997). ALDP expression in fetal cells and its application in prenatal diagnosis of X-linked adrenoleukodystrophy. *Prenat Diagn* **17,** 651–656.

Sarde C. O., Mosser J., Kioschis P., Kretz C., Vicaire S., Aubourg P., Poustka A., and Mandel J. L. (1994). Genomic organization of the adrenoleukodystrophy gene. *Genomics* **22,** 13–20.

Schaumburg H. H., Powers J. M., Raine C. S., Suzuki K., and Richardson E. P. Jr (1975). Adrenoleukodystrophy. A clinical and pathological study of 17 cases. *Arch Neurol* **32,** 577–591.

Schilder P. (1924). Die encephalitis periaxilis. Difusa. *Arch Psychiatr Nervenkr* **71,** 327–356.

Shani N., Jimenez-Sanchez G., Steel G., Dean M., and Valle D. (1997). Identification of a fourth half ABC transporter in the human peroxisomal membrane. *Hum Mol Genet* **6,** 1925–1931.

Shapiro E., Krivit W., Lockman L., Jambaque I., Peters C., Cowan M., Harris R., Blanche S., Bordigoni P., Loes D., Ziegler R., Crittenden M., Ris D., Berg B., Cox C., Moser H., Fischer A., and Aubourg P. (2000). Long-term effect of bone-marrow transplantation for childhood-onset cerebral X-linked adrenoleukodystrophy. *Lancet* **356,** 713–718.

Shapiro E. G., and Klein K. A. (1994). Dementiq in childhood: Issues in neuropsychological assessment with application to the natural history and treatment of degenerative storage diseases. *In* "Advances in Child Neuropsychology" (Tramontana M. G., and Hooer S. R., eds.), pp. 119–171. Springer Verlag, New York.

Shapiro E. G., Lockman L. A., Balthazor M., and Krivit W. (1995). Neuropsychological outcomes of several storage diseases with and without bone marrow transplantation. *J Inherit Metab Dis* **18,** 413–429.

Sheikh K. A., Deerinck T. J., Ellisman M. H., and Griffin J. W. (1999). The distribution of ganglioside-like moieties in peripheral nerves. *Brain* **122 (Pt 3),** 449–60.

Siemerling E., and Creutzfeldt H. G. (1923). Bronzekrankheit und Sklerosierende Encephalomyelitis. *Arch Psychiatr Nervenkr* **68,** 217–244.

Singh I., Khan M., Key L., and Pai S. (1998). Lovastatin for X-linked adrenoleukodystrophy. *N Engl J Med* **339,** 702–703.

Singh I., Moser A. E., Goldfischer S., and Moser H. W. (1984a). Lignoceric acid is oxidized in the peroxisome: Implications for the Zellweger cerebro-hepato-renal syndrome and adrenoleukodystrophy. *Proc Natl Acad Sci U S A* **81,** 4203–4207.

Singh I., Moser A. E., Moser H. W., and Kishimoto Y. (1984b). Adrenoleukodystrophy: Impaired oxidation of very long chain fatty acids in white blood cells, cultured skin fibroblasts, and amniocytes. *Pediatr Res* **18,** 286–290.

Singh I., Moser H. W., Moser A. B., and Kishimoto Y. (1981). Adrenoleukodystrophy: Impaired oxidation of long chain fatty acids in cultured skin fibroblasts an adrenal cortex. *Biochem Biophys Res Commun* **102,** 1223–1229.

Singh I., Pahan K., and Khan M. (1998). Lovastatin and sodium phenylacetate normalize the levels of very long chain fatty acids in skin fibroblasts of X-adrenoleukodystrophy. *FEBS Lett* **426,** 342–346.

Smith K. D., Kemp S., Braiterman L. T., Lu J. F., Wei H. M., Geraghty M., Stetten G., Bergin J. S., Pevsner J., and Watkins P. A. (1999). X-linked adrenoleukodystrophy: Genes, mutations, and phenotypes. *Neurochem Res* **24,** 521–535.

Smith K. D., Sack G., Beaty T., Bergin A., Naidu S., Moser A., and Moser H. (1991). A genetic basis for multiple phenotypes of X-ALD. *Am J Hum Genet* **49**(Suppl)., 865.

Stanislaus R., Pahan K., Singh A. K., and Singh I. (1999). Amelioration of experimental allergic encephalomyelitis in Lewis rats by lovastatin. *Neurosci Lett* **269,** 71–74.

Steinberg S. J., Kemp S., Braiterman L. T., and Watkins P. A. (1999). Role of very-long-chain acyl-coenzyme A synthetase in X-linked adrenoleukodystrophy. *Ann Neurol* **46,** 409–412.

Steinberg S. J., Mihalik S. J., Kim D. G., Cuebas D. A., and Watkins P. A. (2000a). The human liver-specific homolog of very long-chain acyl-CoA synthetase is cholate:CoA ligase. *J Biol Chem* **275,** 15605–15608.

Steinberg S. J., Morgenthaler J., Heinzer A. K., Smith K. D., and Watkins P. A. (2000b). Very long-chain acyl-CoA synthetases. Human "bubblegum" represents a new family of proteins capable of activating very long-chain fatty acids. *J Biol Chem* **275,** 35162–35169.

Stumpf D. A., Hayward A., Haas R., Frost M., and Schaumburg H. H. (1981). Adrenoleukodystrophy. Failure of immunosuppression to prevent neurological progression. *Arch Neurol* **38,** 48–49.

Tagawa Y., Laroy W., Nimrichter L., Fromholt S. E., Moser A. B., Moser H. W., and Schnaar R. L. (2002). Anti-ganglioside antibodies bind with enhanced affinity to gangliosides containing very long chain fatty acids. *Neurochem Res* **27,** 847–855.

Taketomi T., Hara A., Kitazawa N., Takada K., and Nakamura H. (1987). An adult case of adrenoleukodystrophy with features of olivo-ponto-cerebellar atrophy: II. Lipid biochemical studies. *Jpn J Exp Med* **57,** 59–70.

Tanaka Y. A. S. T. S. M. T. (1988). Enhanced synthesis of hexacosanoic acid in the cultured fibroblasts from patients with adrenoleukodystrophy. *Biomed Res* **9,** 451–456.

Theda C., Moser A. B., Powers J. M., and Moser H. W. (1992). Phospholipids in X-linked adrenoleukodystrophy white matter: Fatty acid abnormalities before the onset of demyelination. *J Neurol Sci* **110,** 195–204.

Tsuji S., Sano T., Ariga T., and Miyatake T. (1981a). Increased synthesis of hexacosanoic acid (C23:0). by cultured skin fibroblasts from patients with adrenoleukodystrophy (ALD)., and adrenomyeloneuropathy (AMN). *J Biochem (Tokyo)*. **90,** 1233–1236.

Tsuji S., Sano T., Ariga T., and Miyatake T. (1981b). Increased synthesis of hexacosanoic acid (C26:0). by cultured skin fibroblasts from patients with adrenoleukodystrophy (ALD)., and adrenomyeloneuropathy (AMN). *Biochem J (Tokyo)*. **90,** 1233–1236.

Tsuji S., Suzuki M., Ariga T., Sekine M., Kuriyama M., and Miyatake T. (1981c). Abnormality of long-chain fatty acids in erythrocyte membrane sphingomyelin from patients with adrenoleukodystrophy. *J Neurochem* **36,** 1046–1049.

Uchiyama A., Aoyama T., Kamijo K., Uchida Y., Kondo N., Orii T., and Hashimoto T. (1996). Molecular cloning of cDNA encoding rat very long-chain acyl-CoA synthetase. *J Biol Chem* **271,** 30360–30365.

Ulrich J., Herschkowitz N., Heitz P., Sigrist T., and Baerlocher P. (1978). Adrenoleukodystrophy. Preliminary report of a connatal case. Light- and electron microscopical, immunohistochemical and biochemical findings. *Acta Neuropathol (Berl)*. **43,** 77–83.

Unger E. R., Sung J. H., Manivel J. C., Chenggis M. L., Blazar B. R., and Krivit W. (1993). Male donor-derived cells in the brains of female sex-mismatched bone marrow transplant recipients: A Y-chromosome specific in situ hybridization study. *J Neuropathol Exp Neurol* **52,** 460–470.

Uziel G., Bertini E., Bardelli P., Rimoldi M., and Gambetti M. (1991). Experience on therapy of adrenoleukodystrophy and adrenomyeloneuropathy. *Dev Neurosci* **13,** 274–279.

van Geel B. M., Assies J., Haverkort E. B., Koelman J. H., Verbeeten B. Jr, Wanders R. J., and Barth P. G. (1999). Progression of abnormalities in adrenomyeloneuropathy and neurologically asymptomatic X-linked adrenoleukodystrophy despite treatment with "Lorenzo's oil". *J Neurol Neurosurg Psychiatry* **67,** 290–299.

van Geel B. M., Bezman L., Loes D. J., Moser H. W., and Raymond G. V. (2001). Evolution of phenotypes in adult male patients with X-linked adrenoleukodystrophy. *Ann Neurol* **49,** 186–194.

van Geel B. M., Koelman J. H., Barth P. G., and Ongerboer de Visser B. W. (1996). Peripheral nerve abnormalities in adrenomyeloneuropathy: A clinical and electrodiagnostic study. *Neurology* **46,** 112–118.

Volpe J. J., and Vagelos P. R. (1976). Mechanisms and regulation of biosynthesis of saturated fatty acids. *Physiol Rev* **56,** 339–417.

Wanders R. J., van Roermund C. W., van Wijland M. J., Heikoop J., Schutgens R. B., Schram A. W., Tager J. M., van den Bosch H., Poll-The B. T., Saudubray J. M., *et al.* (1987). Peroxisomal very long-chain fatty acid beta-oxidation in human skin fibroblasts: Activity in Zellweger syndrome and other peroxisomal disorders. *Clin Chim Acta* **166,** 255–263.

Wanders R. J., van Roermund C. W., van Wijland M. J., Schutgens R. B., van den Bosch H., Schram A. W., and Tager J. M. (1988). Direct demonstration that the deficient oxidation of very long chain fatty acids in X-linked adrenoleukodystrophy is due to an impaired ability of peroxisomes to activate very long chain fatty acids. *Biochem Biophys Res Commun* **153,** 618–624.

Watkins P. A., Gould S. J., Smith M. A., Braiterman L. T., Wei H. M., Kok F., Moser A. B., Moser H. W., and Smith K. D. (1995). Altered expression of ALDP in X-linked adrenoleukodystrophy. *Am J Hum Genet* **57,** 292–301.

Watkins P. A., Pevsner J., and Steinberg S. J. (1999). Human very long-chain acyl-CoA synthetase and two human homologs: Initial characterization and relationship to fatty acid transport protein. *Prostaglandins Leukot Essent Fatty Acids* **60,** 323–328.

Weinhofer I., Forss-Petter S., Zigman M., Berger J. (2002). Cholesterol regulates ABCD2 expression: Implications for the therapy of X-linked adrenoleukodystrophy. *Hum Mol Genet* **11,** 2701–2708.

Whitcomb R. W., Linehan W. M., and Knazek R. A. (1988). Effects of long-chain, saturated fatty acids on membrane microviscosity and adrenocorticotropin responsiveness of human adrenocortical cells in vitro. *J Clin Invest* **81,** 185–188.

Wilson R., and Sargent J. R. (1993). Lipid and fatty acid composition of brain tissue from adrenoleukodystrophy patients. *J Neurochem* **61,** 290–297.

Yamada T., Shinnoh N., Taniwaki T., Ohyagi Y., Asahara H., Horiuchi and Kira J. (2000). Lovastatin does not correct the accumulation of very long-chain fatty acids in tissues of adrenoleukodystrophy protein-deficient mice. *J Inherit Metab Dis* **23,** 607–614.

Yoshida S., and Takeshita M. (1987). Analysis of the condensation step in elongation of very-long-chain saturated and tetraenoic fatty acyl-CoAs in swine cerebral microsomes. *Arch Biochem Biophys* **254,** 170–179.

Zeller C. B., and Marchase R. B. (1992). Gangliosides as modulators of cell function. *Am J Physiol* **262,** C1341–55.

Zhang and Moser H. W. (2003). *Arch Neurol* in press.

Zinkham W. H., Kickler T., Borel J., and Moser H. W. (1993). Lorenzo's oil and thrombocytopenia in patients with adrenoleukodystrophy. *N Engl J Med* **328,** 1126.

CHAPTER

# 35

# Krabbe Disease

*Kunihiko Suzuki*

## HISTORY

In 1916, a Danish physician, Knud Krabbe, described clinical and pathological findings in five infants from two families who died of an "acute infantile familial diffuse brain sclerosis" (Krabbe, 1916). These infants developed episodes of violent crying and irritability beginning at age 4 to 6 months, followed by progressive muscular rigidity, tonic spasms evoked by such stimuli as noise, light, and touching. Death occurred between 11 months to 1.5 years. He provided a detailed description of the globoid cells, the histologic hallmark of the disease. Thus, the first description of the disease is credited to Krabbe. Retrospectively, however, similar abnormal cells in the white matter had been described in neuropathological literature. Collier and Greenfield (1924) first used the term "globoid cells" to describe the PAS-positive macrophages unique in this disease. In 1970, deficiency in the activity of a lysosomal enzyme, galactosylceramidase, was identified as the underlying genetic cause (Suzuki and Suzuki, 1970) that made noninvasive antemortem diagnosis possible (Suzuki and Suzuki, 1971). Prenatal diagnosis of an affected fetus was first accomplished in 1971 (Suzuki *et al.*, 1971). Toxic effect of a related metabolite, galactosylsphingosine (psychosine), was first proposed in 1972 as critical in the biochemical pathogenesis (Miyatake and Suzuki, 1972). The psychosine hypothesis has since been generally substantiated both in the human disease and in animal models (Suzuki, 1998). In 1990, the gene encoding galactosylceramidase was mapped to human chromosome 14 (Zlotogora *et al.*, 1990). Human galactosylceramidase cDNA was cloned in 1993–1994 (Chen *et al.*, 1993; Sakai *et al.*, 1994), and more than 60 disease causing mutations have been identified (Wenger *et al.*, 2001).

## INCIDENCE, GENETICS, AND CLINICAL FORMS

Globoid cell leukodystrophy is inherited as an autosomal recessive trait with a wide geographical distribution. Until enzymatic diagnosis became feasible, the diagnosis was made on the basis of the characteristic neuropathology. Since the gene was cloned, recently described cases have enzymatic as well as molecular diagnosis. Typical infantile patients develop first clinical signs and symptoms at 3 to 6 months after birth, but there are cases of very early or late onset with atypical clinical manifestations. The incidence of the typical infantile form is estimated as 1 in 100,000 births in the United States, 2 in 100,000 births in Sweden, and 0.5 to 1 in 100,000 births in Japan. There are pockets of populations where the incidence is unusually high; for example, the Druze community in Israel has an incidence of 6 in 1000 births. In contrast, no Jewish patients have ever been reported. Late-onset and adult forms of the disease are even rarer but are being reported in increasing frequency. Since definitions of "late-onset" and "adult" forms are not necessarily standardized, precise incidence of the later-onset forms is difficulty to assess. In contrast to the infantile form, which appears to have somewhat higher incidence in Nordic countries, patients with the late-onset form appear to be more common in Southern Europe (Barone *et al.*, 1996; Fiumara *et al.*, 1990). The frequency of late-onset cases was estimated to be approximately 10% of the nearly 350 GLD patients diagnosed by Wenger (Wenger *et al.*, 2001).

## CLINICAL MANIFESTATIONS

### Infantile GLD

Clinical phenotype of the classical infantile Krabbe disease is relatively stereotypic. Hagberg *et al.* (Hagberg *et al.*, 1963) divided the steady and rapidly progressive clinical course into three stages. The general clinical picture is that of a progressive white matter disorder. Stage I is characterized by generalized hyperirritability, hyperesthesia, episodic fever of unknown origin, and some stiffness of the limbs. The child, apparently normal for the first few months after birth, becomes hypersensitive to auditory, tactile, or visual stimuli and begins to cry frequently without apparent cause. Slight retardation or regression of psychomotor development, vomiting with feeding difficulty, and convulsive seizures may occur as initial clinical symptoms. The cerebrospinal fluid protein level is already highly increased. In stage II, rapid and severe motor and mental deterioration develops. There is marked hypertonicity, with extended and crossed legs, flexed arms, and the backward-bent head. Tendon reflexes are hyperactive. Minor tonic or clonic seizures occur. Optic atrophy and sluggish pupillary reactions to light are common. Stage III is the "burnt-out" stage, sometimes reached within a few weeks or months. The infant is decerebrate and blind and has no contact with the surroundings. Deafness may appear. Patients rarely survive for more than 2 years.

Clinical examination may not always reveal neuropathy, especially in the early stages, because symptoms and signs of central nervous system involvement are overwhelming. Krabbe (1916), however, noted in his original five patients that kneejerks could not be elicited and that stiffness passed into a flaccid state toward the end of the disease. The typical pathology is always present in the peripheral nerves, and careful clinical examination combined with appropriate electrophysiological studies should reveal presence of PNS involvement. Spinal fluid protein is invariably highly elevated in patients with infantile GLD. The symptoms and signs are, for all practical purposes, confined to the nervous system. No visceromegaly is present.

### Late-Onset GLD

Earlier, patients with late-onset globoid cell leukodystrophy were often misdiagnosed during life, and the definite diagnosis could be established only by histological examination. Since the advent of the enzymatic diagnosis, late-onset GLD has been reported in increasing frequency. Most patients develop initial clinical signs and symptoms by 10 years of age, but some may develop neurological signs after 40 years of age. Late-onset GLD is often divided into two types; late infantile (or early childhood) and juvenile (late childhood). In the late infantile group (onset 6 months to 3 years), irritability, psychomotor regression, stiffness, ataxia, and loss of vision are frequent initial symptoms. The course is progressive resulting in death approximately in 2 to 3 years after the onset. In the juvenile group (onset 3 to 8 years), patients commonly develop loss of vision, together with hemiparesis, ataxia, and psychomotor regression. Most patients with the juvenile form show rapid deterioration initially, followed by a more gradual progression possibly lasting for years. The number of reports on adult cases is also increasing steadily. Adult patients may develop slowly progressive spastic paraparesis or slow, unsteady stiff- and wide-based gait during life. Progressive and generalized neurological deterioration may not be observed until 40 years of age. Some adult patients may have a normal life span. The cerebrospinal fluid protein is normal or only mildly elevated in the juvenile or adult type patients. Peripheral nerve conduction velocity is generally reduced in late infantile patients but may be normal in juvenile patients with some exceptions.

## PATHOLOGY

Pathology is, for all practical purposes, limited to the nervous system (Suzuki and Suzuki, 2002). In the most common infantile type, the brain is atrophic with firm rubbery gliotic white matter. At the terminal stage, loss of myelin is nearly complete with possible exception of the subcortical intergyral arcuate U-fibers. Microscopically, marked paucity of myelin with some axonal degeneration is present throughout the brain. Extensive fibrillary gliosis and infiltration of numerous macrophages, often multinucleated ("globoid cells"), are the unique features. The globoid cells are abundant in the region of active demyelination and often clustered around blood vessels. Oligodendrocytes are markedly reduced. Correlative MRI and neuropathological studies showed that the areas of marked hyper-intensity on the T2-weighted MRI images corresponded to the areas of demyelination with globoid cell infiltration (Percy *et al.*, 1994). Globoid cells contain PAS-positive storage materials. On the ultrastructural level, the globoid cells contain tubular and filamentous structures with polygonal cross sections that are structurally identical with chemically pure galactosylceramide (Yunis and Lee, 1970). In long surviving cases, the white matter may be totally gliotic and devoid of macrophages. The optic nerves are usually atrophic but, in some cases, they are markedly enlarged with extensive gliosis. The peripheral nerves are often grossly enlarged and firm with marked endoneurial fibrosis, segmental demyelination, and evidence of remyelination process with onion bulb formation. Quantitative analyses demonstrated a severe loss of large myelinated fibers without loss of unmyelinated fibers. Endoneurial macrophages and also Schwann cells contain tubular inclusions similar to those in the globoid cells in the cerebral white matter. Neuropathological reports of late onset cases, however, are limited. In a meeting abstract, Choi *et al.* described the neuropathology of the adult onset GLD in 18-year-old twins. Their clinical symptoms developed 12 and 7 months prior to their death, respectively. Both died of severe graft-versus-host disease 2 months after allogeneic bone marrow transplantation. The brains showed degeneration of the optic radiation and frontoparietal white matter with corticospinal tract degeneration. Multiple necrotic foci with calcium deposits were found within the lesion. Globoid cell infiltration was present in actively degenerating white matter. In the peripheral nerves, loss of myelinated fibers, disproportionately thin myelin sheaths and inclusions in Schwann cells were described.

## ANALYTICAL BIOCHEMISTRY

The genetic cause of all so far known human patients with Krabbe disease is deficient activity of galactosylceramidase (Fig. 35.1). Galactosylceramidase is a degradative enzyme with an acid ph optimum localized in the lysosome. Thus, the disease conceptually belongs to the category of genetic disorders, the lysosomal disease as originally defined by Hers (Hers, 1966). Essentially all lysosomal diseases are "storage diseases," in which subtrates of the genetically defective enzymes accumulate to abnormally high levels. The enzyme is fairly specific for glycolipids with a terminal galactose moiety in a β anomeric configuration. Quantitatively, by far the major natural substrate is galactosylceramide, which is highly localized in the myelin sheath. Other known natural substrates are psychosine (galactosylsphingosine), monogalactosyldiglyceride, and the precursor of seminolipid (1-alkyl, 2-acyl-, 3-galactosyl glycerol). *In vivo* degradation of these substrates requires, in addition to the enzyme, galactosylceramidase, an activator protein, saposin A. In addition, the two lysosomal ß-galactosidases, galactosylceramide and GM1-ganglioside ß-galactosidase,

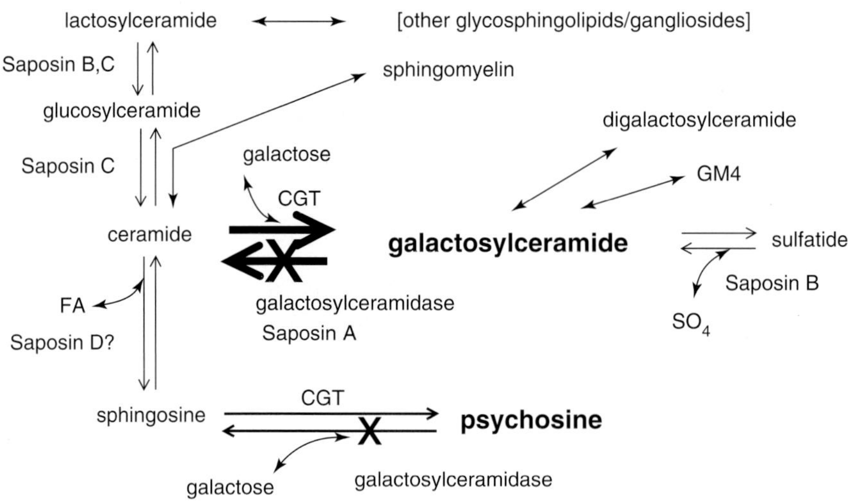


FIGURE 35.1
Metabolic pathways pertinent to galactosylceramide and related compounds. In the synthetic pathway, sphingosine is first acylated to ceramide, which in turn is galactosylated by UDP-galactose:ceramide galactosyltransferase (CGT) to form galactosylceramide. The same enzyme can galactosylate sphingosine directly to generate psychosine. Both galactosylceramide and psychosine are degraded by galactosylceramidase, which is genetically deficient in Krabbe disease. *In vivo* degradation of galactosylceramide requires, in addition to the enzyme, a sphingolipid activator protein, saposin A. Galactosylceramide is further sulfated to form sulfatide. Both galactosylceramide and sulfatide are characteristic myelin glycolipids.

share lactosylceramide as their common substrate. The unique biochemical characteristic of Krabbe disease is lack of abnormal accumulation of galactosylceramide in the brain, contrary to what is expected from the enzymatic defect (Svennerholm *et al.*, 1980; Vanier and Svennerholm, 1975). This paradoxical phenomenon results from the unique localization of galactosylceramide in the myelin sheath and very rapid and early disappearance of the myelinating cells in the process of the disease. Since the myelinating cells disappear at a very early stage of myelination and since no further synthesis of galactosylceramide occurs, it does not accumulate beyond the level attained at the early stage of myelination. Instead, however, a related toxic metabolite, psychosine (galactosylsphingosine), does accumulate abnormally and is considered the key compound in the pathogenesis of the disease (discussed later) (Miyatake and Suzuki, 1972; Vanier and Svennerholm, 1976). Although there is no abnormal accumulation of galactosylceramide in the brain tissue as a whole, there is clear evidence to indicate that localized accumulation of galactosylceramide does occur within the characteristic globoid cells. Biochemical analysis of a fraction enriched with the characteristic globoid cells contained a relatively large amounts of galactosyceramide (Austin, 1963). Galactosylceramide has unique capacity to elicit infiltration of globoid cells when it is implanted into the brain (Austin and Lehfeldt, 1965) and such experimentally induced globoid cells appear morphologically identical to those seen in patients with Krabbe disease (Andrews and Menkes, 1970; Suzuki, 1970). Biochemical abnormalities are essentially limited to the nervous system, at least in human patients (see Chapter 45, "Models of Krabbe Disease".

## PATHOPHYSIOLOGY

### Metabolism of Myelin and Its Galactolipids

Galactosylceramide has a uniquely restricted tissue distribution. It is mostly, but not exclusively, localized in the myelin sheath and thus almost exclusively synthesized within the oligodendrocytes and the Schwann cells. Its sulfate ester, sulfatide, is synthesized only by sulfation of galactosylceramide (Fig. 35.1). Thus, both galactosylceramide and sulfatide are characteristically the glycolipids of the myelin sheath and are virtually absent in the brain before myelination and are present at abnormally low concentrations in any pathologic conditions where severe loss of myelin occurs. The amount of total brain galactosylceramide correlates precisely with the amount of myelin that can be isolated from the brain, whereas amounts of other lipids do not (Norton and Poduslo, 1973). It is practically absent in systemic organs except in the kidney, which normally contains appreciable amounts of galactosylceramide, although much less than in the nervous system. Myelin of adult mammalian brain generally contains galactosylceramide at a concentration of 15 to 18% of total lipid. The sum of galactosylceramide and sulfatide makes up to 20% of the dry weight of myelin. The content of galactosylceramide in myelin from the peripheral nerve is somewhat less than that of CNS myelin. In view of the unusually high concentrations of galactosylceramide and sulfatide in the myelin sheath, metabolic diseases involving these lipids (Krabbe disease and metachromatic leukodystrophy) would be expected to manifest themselves primarily as disorders of white matter and peripheral nerves.

The most significant metabolic features of CNS myelin are its high rate of formation and turnover during a relatively short period of brain development and its slow turnover in the adult brain. The period of most active myelination in humans probably extends from the perinatal period to about age 18 months. Myelination does not stop after this period, and in the human brain, it may not be complete until age 20 years. The amount of galactosylceramide in immature brain is very low. Activity of galactosylceramide synthase, UDP-galactose:ceramide galactosyltransferase (CGT), peaks sharply at 20 to 25 days after birth in rodent brains well correlating with the most active period of myelination (Costantino-Ceccarini and Morell, 1972). The recent cloning of the rat and mouse CGT confirmed that the peak levels of the corresponding mRNA occur during the period of most active myelination and that relatively high mRNA levels are found in the brain and kidney (Stahl *et al.*, 1994). Synthesis and turnover of galactosylceramide occurs at much lower rates in the adult brain.

## Pathogenesis

Some aspects of the chemistry and metabolism of galactosylceramide should be kept in mind when the pathogenetic mechanism of GLD is considered. (1) Galactosylceramide consists of sphingosine, fatty acid, and galactose. (2) Galactosylceramide is the precursor of sulfatide. (3) Both galactosylceramide and sulfatide are highly concentrated in the myelin sheath. (4) Galactosylceramidase degrades galactosylceramide to ceramide and galactose. (5) A few related galactolipids also serve as substrates for galactosylceramidase, including psychosine, monogalactosyldiglyceride, seminolipid precursor, and lactosylceramide. (6) Biosynthesis of galactosylceramide reaches a peak, coincident with the maximum period of myelination (during the first year and a half in humans), when myelin also turns over relatively rapidly. (7) Once formed, adult myelin is relatively stable metabolically, although there is some turnover. (8) Galactosylceramide is uniquely capable of inducing infiltration of globoid cells when implanted into the brain but does not appear toxic, while another normally insignificant substrate, psychosine, is highly cytotoxic.

### *Two Separate but Related Pathogenetic Mechanisms?*

Three of the most characteristic pathological features of Krabbe disease are (1) the infiltration of macrophages that are often multinucleated and contain strongly PAS-positive materials ("globoid cells"), (2) the rapid and almost complete disappearance of the oligodendrocytes, and (3) lack of abnormal tissue accumulation of the primary substrate of the defective enzyme, galactosylceramide, contrary to what is expected in a "storage disease" due to genetic defect in degradative enzymes. These phenotypic characteristics must be explained as consequences of the underlying genetic defect. Defective degradation of two substrates, galactosylceramide and psychosine (galactosylsphingosine), appears to play critical roles in the pathogenesis. While these mechanisms are fundamentally distinct from each other, they are closely intertwined to result in the unique phenotype of the disease.

*Globoid cells* The genetic defect in degradation of galactosylceramide clearly is a major factor for the unique pathological feature of the disease, the globoid cells. It has long been known that free galactosylceramide has a specific capacity to elicit infiltration of macrophages into the brain (Austin and Lehfeldt, 1965; Suzuki *et al.*, 1976). Once in the brain, they phagocytize galactosylceramide and are transformed to multinucleated globoid cells. The characteristic inclusions in the globoid cells have morphological appearance identical to galactosylceramide itself (Yunis and Lee, 1970). No other agent is known to have a similar capacity *in vivo*. The globoid cell reaction can be reconstructed in the following way. Once the active period of myelination begins, turnover of already formed myelin also begins. In patients' brains, however, galactosylceramide cannot be degraded due to the underlying galactosylceramidase deficiency. Free galactosylceramide thus generated elicits infiltration of macrophophages, which become the characteristic PAS-positive, often multinucleated globoid cells.

*Psychosine hypothesis* On the other hand, the devastating early destruction of the myelin-forming cells is difficult to explain on the basis of undegradable galactosylceramide because galactosylceramide implanted in the brain does not exhibit any functionally detrimental capacity other than eliciting the globoid cell reaction. There is no experimental evidence that galactosylceramide is a metabolic toxin. On the other hand, a closely related metabolite, psychosine (galactosylsphingosine), is highly cytotoxic (Taketomi and Nishimura, 1964) and causes fatal hemorrhagic infarct when implanted into the brain (Miyatake and Suzuki, 1972). At least in mammalian tissues, psychosine can be generated only by galactosylation of sphingosine by galactosylceramide synthase, UDP-galactose:ceramide galactosyltransferase (CGT), but not by de-acylation of galactosylceramide. Since CGT is nearly exclusively localized in the myelin-forming cells, synthesis of psychosine should also occur only in the oligodendrocytes and Schwann cells. Psychosine is detectable in normal brain with highly sensitive analytical methods but its concentration is minuscule (less than 10 picomoles/mg protein). It appears to be a dead-end product, which is normally degraded immediately. However, psychosine is degraded also by galactosylceramidase. Therefore, patients with Krabbe disease cannot degrade psychosine. A hypothesis, known as the psychosine hypothesis, was first proposed on the basis of this enzymological consideration (Miyatake and Suzuki, 1972), and then its abnormal accumulation was analytically demonstrated in the brain of patients (Svennerholm *et al.*, 1980; Vanier and Svennerholm, 1976) and in canine and murine models (Igisu and Suzuki, 1984). The psychosine hypothesis postulates that, in globoid cell leukodystrophy, not only the primary substrate of the defective enzyme, galactosylceramide, but also the toxic metabolite, galactosylsphingosine (psychosine), cannot be degraded and the consequent abnormal accumulation of psychosine causes the uniquely rapid destruction of the myelin-forming cells. The hypothesis initially met considerable skepticism but has survived the intervening 30 years (Suzuki, 1998). In fact, the basic premise of the hypothesis has been extended to other sphingolipidoses (Hannun and Bell, 1987). For varieties of reasons, however, its plausibility for other disorders is not as firm as it is for GLD, with possible exceptions of neuronopathic form of Gaucher disease and Niemann-Pick type A disease.

*Overall pathogenesis* Close interactions of these two pathogenetic mechanisms can explain the most important aspects of the characteristic phenotype of Krabbe disease (Fig. 35.2). The fundamental cause of the disease is the genetic defect in galactosyceramidase activity. Since galactosylceramide synthesis is limited to actively myelinating cells, the disease process does not begin until the active myelination period. Once myelination begins, its metabolic turnover also starts. This generates free galactosylceramide in the brain of patients because of the inability to degrade galactosylceramide, which in turn elicits the characteristic globoid cell reaction. Galactosylceramide synthase also synthesizes psychosine within the actively myelinating cells. Normally, it is immediately degraded and never reaches beyond a barely detectable levels. In Krabbe disease, however, an abnormal accumulation of psychosine occurs to the level toxic to cellular metabolism. This causes the other characteristic feature of the disease, a rapid and almost complete disappearance of

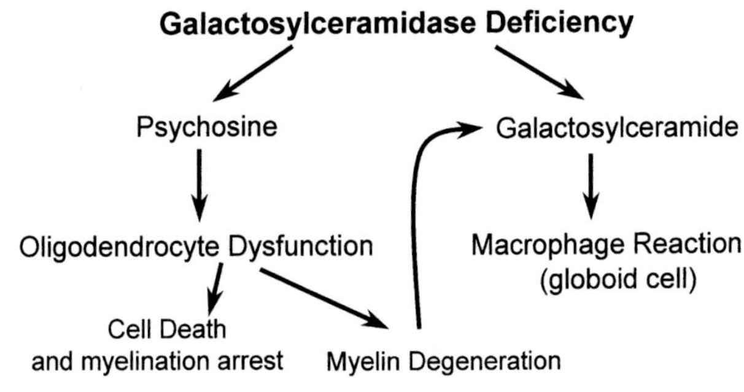


FIGURE 35.2
Pathogenetic mechanisms operating in Krabbe disease. See text for explanation.

the oligodendrocytes. Psychosine is as potent an apoptosis inducer as C6 ceramide (Tohyama *et al.*, 2001). The cellular death results in further destruction of already formed myelin, which contributes more free galactosylceramide that in turn further elicits the globoid cell infiltration. On the other hand, myelination ceases at a very early stage due to the near-complete loss of the oligodendrocytes. This explains the paradoxical characteristics of the disease that the primary substrate of the defective enzyme, galactosylceramide, does not accumulate abnormally.

## MOLECULAR GENETICS

### Gene Structure

Human galactosylceramidase gene, *galc* (GenBank database Accession No. 119970), was localized to the region of 14q24.3-q32.1 by linkage analysis (Oehlmann *et al.*, 1993) and later further narrowed to 14q31 by *in situ* hybridization (Cannizzaro *et al.*, 1994). Using N-terminal amino acid sequence information, the human cDNA was cloned in 1993–1994 (Chen *et al.*, 1993; Sakai *et al.*, 1994). The full-length cDNA consists of 3795 bp, including 2007 bp of the coding region, 47 base pairs of 5′ untranslated sequence and 1741 bp of 3′ untranslated sequence. The base and amino acid sequences have no similarities and thus no suggestion of evolutionary relationship with the other β-galactosidases or any other known genes. The encoded protein consists of 669 amino acids with six potential glycosylation sites. The first 26-amino acids have the characteristic of a leader sequence. The precursor protein is approximately 80-85 kD, which is processed to 50–52 kD and 30 kD subunits. The coding sequence for the 50–52 kD subunit is at the 5′ end and the 30 kD subunit is at the 3′ end of the coding region. The organization of the human gene was characterized in 1995 (Luzi *et al.*, 1995). It consists of 17 exons spread over about 56 kb. Other than exons 1 and 17, the other exons range in size from 39 to 181 nucleotides. The 200 nucleotides preceding the initiation codon and the 5′ end of intron 1 are GC-rich, including 13 GGC trinucleotides. The 5′ flanking region includes a YYI element and one potential SP1 binding site. No consensus TATA box or CAAT box is present among the 800 nucleotides preceding the initiation codon. A construct containing nucleotides −176 to −24 had the strongest promoter activity. However, evidence for inhibitory sequences was found just upstream of the promoter region and also at the 5′ end of intron 1. There is another potential initiation codon located 48 nucleotides upstream; however, there is no evidence that it is utilized or if it might play a role in tissue specific expression.

### Disease-Causing Mutations

More than 60 disease-causing missense, nonsense mutations, deletions, and insertions have been identified in the human galactosylceramidase gene (Wenger *et al.*, 2001). A major deletion of 30-kb from the middle of intron 10 to beyond the end of the gene that always occurs on a 502T polymorphic background (502T/del) is common among patients from Northern Europe and the United States, including those with Mexican ancestry. The 30 kb deletion eliminates all of the coding region for the 30 kD subunit and about 15% of the coding region for the 50–52 kD subunit. A survey conducted among patients within the Dutch population and from other parts of Europe confirmed that 502T/del mutation makes up about 50% of the total mutant alleles. In infantile Swedish patients, this mutation makes up 75% of the mutant alleles. This mutation probably initially occurred in Sweden and was transmitted from there throughout Europe, Near Asia, and the United States. It has not been found among Japanese patients. Two other mutations (C1538T and A1652C) make up an additional 10 to 15% of the mutant alleles in infantile patients with European ancestry. Three mutations (635del+ins, A198G, and T1853C) have been found in multiple unrelated Japanese patients. In Israel there are two populations with an extremely high carrier rate for Krabbe disease, and they have different mutations. All infantile patients in the Druze population in Northern Israel are homozygous for the T→G transversion at nucleotide 1748 (I583S), and patients from a Moslem village near Jerusalem are homozygous for the G→A transition at nucleotide 1582 (D528N).

### Polymorphisms

There is a relatively broad range of galactosylceramidase activities in the "normal" population and among the obligate heterozygotes. This makes enzyme-based carrier testing in the general population nearly impossible. Also, there are normal individuals, including obligate heterozygotes, who have galactosylceramidase activity sufficiently low for diagnosis for Krabbe disease but who are clinically normal. These phenomena can be explained at least partially by the presence of polymorphisms in the galactosylceramidase gene that result in amino acid substitutions. The C502T polymorphism is widespread but the A865G polymorphism has been reported only among Japanese. These polymorphisms generate galactosylceramidase proteins that are less active than the most common type. It has been observed by several groups that these polymorphisms occur on the same alleles as disease-causing mutations at a higher than expected frequency. Some "disease-causing" mutations may in fact be deleterious only when the polymorphism is present on the same allele. Polymorphisms may also play a role in the development of clinical disease when inherited either in multiple copies, on the same allele with another mutation, or together with a known disease-causing mutation on the other chromosome.

## TREATMENT

Only supportive care is available for patients with the classical infantile form of the disease, who are diagnosed too late for hematopoietic stem cell transplantation. For patients with either late-onset, slowly progressive disease or infantile disease prior to the onset of neurological manifestations, clinical improvements can occur by bone marrow transplantation (Krivit *et al.*, 1998).

## ANIMAL MODELS

Genetic galactosylceramidase deficiency (Krabbe disease) occurs naturally in the mouse (twitcher), sheep, dogs (West Highland white terriers and Cairn terriers; blue-tick hound and beagles), and Rhesus monkeys. Clinical and pathological features of these models are similar to those of the human disease. Galactosylceramidase cDNA was cloned and disease-causing mutations have been identified in the mouse (Sakai *et al.*, 1996), West Highland and Cairn terriers (Victoria *et al.*, 1996), and the Rhesus monkey (Luzi *et al.*, 1997). More details about animal models are found elsewhere in this volume (see Section V, "Animal Models of Human Disease").

## References


Andrews, J. M., and Menkes, J. H. (1970). Ultrastructure of experimentally produced globoid cells in the rat. *Exp. Neurol.* **29,** 483–493.

Austin J. H. (1963). Studies in globoid (Krabbe) leukodystrophy II. Controlled thin-layer chromatographic stuides of globoid body fractions in seven patients. *J. Neurochem.* **10,** 921–930.

Austin, J. H., and Lehfeldt, D. (1965). Studies in globoid (Krabbe) leukodystrophy. III. Significance of experimentally-produced globoid-like elements in rat white matter and spleen. *J. Neuropathol. Exp. Neurol.* **24,** 265–289.

Barone, R., Brühl, K., Stoeter, P., Fiumara, A., Pavone, L., and Beck, M. (1996). Clinical and neuroradiological findings in classic infantile and late-onset globoid-cell leukodystrophy (Krabbe disease). *Am. J. Med. Genet.* **63,** 209–217.

Cannizzaro, L. A., Chen, Y. Q., Rafi, M. A., and Wenger, D. A. (1994). Regional mapping of the human galactocerebrosidase gene (GALC) to 14q31 by in situ hybridization. *Cytogenet. Cell Genet.* **66,** 244–245.

Chen, Y. Q., Rafi, M. A., De Gala, G., and Wenger, D. A. (1993). Cloning and expression of cDNA encoding human galactocerebrosidase, the enzyme deficient in globoid cell leukodystrophy. *Hum. Mol. Genet.* **2,** 1841–1845.

Collier, J., and Greenfield, J. G. (1924). The encephalitis periaxialis of Schilder: A clinical and pathological study with an account of two cases, one of which as diagnosed during life. *Brain* **47,** 489–519.

Costantino-Ceccarini, E., and Morell, P. (1972). Biosynthesis of brain sphingolipids and myelin accumulation in the mouse. *Lipids* 7, 656–659.

Fiumara, A., Pavone, L., Siciliano, L., Tine, A., Parano, E., and Innico, G. (1990). Late-onset globoid cell leukodystrophy. Report on seven new patients. *Childs. Nerv. Syst.* **6,** 194–197.

Hagberg, B., Sourander, P., and Svennerholm, L. (1963). Diagnosis of Krabbe's infantile leukodystrophy. *J. Neurosurg. Psychiat.* **26,** 195–204.

Hannun, Y. A., and Bell, R. M. (1987). Lysosphingolipids inhibit protein kinase C: Implications for the sphingolipidoses. *Science* **235,** 670–674.

Hers, H. G. (1966). Inborn lysosomal disease. *Gastroenterology* **48,** 625–633.

Igisu, H., and Suzuki, K. (1984). Progressive accumulation of toxic metabolite in a genetic leukodystrophy. *Science* **224,** 753–755.

Krabbe, K. (1916). A new familial, infantile form of diffuse brain sclerosis. *Brain* **39,** 74–114.

Krivit, W., Shapiro, E. G., Peters, C., Wagner, J. E., Cornu, G., Kurtzberg, J., Wenger, D. A., Kolodny, E. H., Vanier, M. T., Loes, D. J., Dusenbery, K., and Lockman, L. A. (1998). Hematopoietic stem-cell transplantation in globoid-cell leukodystrophy. *N. Engl. J. Med.* **338,** 1119–1126.

Luzi, P., Rafi, M. A., Victoria, T., Baskin, G. B., and Wenger, D. A. (1997). Characterization of the rhesus monkey galactocerebrosidase (GALC) cDNA and gene and identification of the mutation causing globoid cell leukodystrophy (Krabbe disease) in this primate. *Genomics* **42,** 319–324.

Luzi, P., Rafi, M. A., and Wenger, D. A. (1995). Structure and organization of the human galactocerebrosidase (GALC) gene. *Genomics* **26,** 407–409.

Miyatake, T., and Suzuki, K. (1972). Globoid cell leukodystrophy: Additional deficiency of psychosine galactosidase. *Biochem. Biophys. Res. Commun.* **48,** 538–543.

Norton, W. T., and Poduslo, S. E. (1973). Myelination in rat brain: changes in myelin composition during brain maturation. *J. Neurochem.* **21,** 759–773.

Oehlmann, R., Zlotogora, J., Wenger, D. A., and Knowlton, R. G. (1993). Localization of the Krabbe disease gene (GALC) on chromosome 14 by multipoint linkage analysis. *Am. J. Hum. Genet.* **53,** 1250–1255.

Percy, A. K., Odrezin, G. T., Knowles, P. D., Rouah, E., and Armstrong, D. D. (1994). Globoid cell leukodystrophy: Comparison of neuropathology with magnetic resonance imaging. *Acta Neuropathol. (Berl)* **88,** 26–32.

Sakai, N., Inui, K., Fujii, N., Fukushima, H., Nishimoto, J., Yanagihara, I., Isegawa, Y., Iwamatsu, A., and Okada, S. (1994). Krabbe disease: Isolation and characterization of a full-length cDNA for human galactocerebrosidase. *Biochem. Biophys. Res. Commun.* **198,** 485–491.

Sakai, N., Inui, K., Tatsumi, N., Fukushima, H., Nishigaki, T., Taniike ,M., Nishimoto, J., Tsukamoto, H., Yanagihara, I., Ozone, K., and Okada, S. (1996). Molecular cloning and expression of cDNA for murine galactocerebrosidase and mutation analysis of the twitcher mouse, a model of Krabbe's disease. *J. Neurochem.* **66,** 1118–1124.

Stahl, N., Jurevics, H., Morell, P., Suzuki, K., and Popko, B. (1994). Isolation, characterization, and expression of cDNA clones that encode rat UDP-galactose:ceramide galactosyltransferase. *J. Neurosci. Res.* **38,** 234–242.

Suzuki, K. (1970). Ultrastructural study of experimental globoid cells. *Lab. Invest.* **23,** 612–619.

Suzuki, K. (1998). Twenty five years of the psychosine hypothesis: A personal perspective of its history and present status. *Neurochem. Res.* **23,** 251–259.

Suzuki, K., Schneider, E. L., and Epstein, C. J. (1971). I*n utero* diagnosis of globoid cell leukodystrophy. *Biochem. Biophys. Res. Commun.* **45,** 1363–1366.

Suzuki, K., and Suzuki, K. (2002). Lysosomal disease. *In* "Greenfield's Neuropathology" (Graham, D. I., and Lantos, P. L., eds.), pp. 653–735. Edward Arnold, London.

Suzuki, K., and Suzuki, Y. (1970). Globoid cell leucodystrophy (Krabbe's disease): Deficiency of galactocerebroside ß-galactosidase. *Proc. Natl. Acad. Sci., USA* **66,** 302–309.

Suzuki, K., Tanaka, H., and Suzuki, K. (1976). Studies on the pathogenesis of Krabbe's leukodystrophy: Cellular reaction of the brain to exogenous galactosylsphingosine, monogalactosyl diglyceride and lactosylceramide. *In* "Current Trends in Sphingolipidoses and Allied Disorders" (Volk, B. W., and Schneck, L., eds.), pp. 99–113. Plenum Press, New York.

Suzuki, Y., and Suzuki, K. (1971). Krabbe's globoid cell leukodystrophy: Deficiency of galactocerebrosidase in serum, leukocytes, and fibroblasts. *Science* **171,** 73–75.

Svennerholm, L., Vanier, M.-T., and Månsson, J.-E. (1980). Krabbe disease: A galactosylsphingosine (psychosine) lipidosis. *J. Lipid Res.* **21,** 53–64.

Taketomi, T., and Nishimura, K. (1964). Physiological activity of psychosine. *Jap. J. Exp. Med.* **34,** 255–265.

Tohyama, J., Matsuda, J., and Suzuki, K. (2001). Psychosine is as potent an inducer of cell death as C6-ceramide in cultured fibroblasts and in MOCH-1 cells. *Neurochem. Res.* **26,** 667–671.

Vanier, M.-T., and Svennerholm, L. (1975). Chemical pathology of Krabbe's disease. III. Ceramide hexosides and gangliosides of brain. *Acta Paediat. Scand.* **64,** 641–648.

Vanier, M.-T., and Svennerholm, L. (1976). Chemical pathology of Krabbe disease: The occurrence of psychosine and other neutral sphingoglycolipids. *In* "Current Trends in Sphingolipidoses and Allied Disorders" (Volk, B. W., and Schneck, L., eds.), pp. 115–126. Plenum Press, New York.

Victoria, T., Rafi, M. A., and Wenger, D. A. (1996). Cloning of the canine GALC cDNA and identification of the mutation causing globoid cell leukodystrophy in west highland white and cairn terriers. *Genomics* **33,** 457–462.

Wenger, D. A., Suzuki, K., Suzuki, Y., and Suzuki, K. (2001). Galactosylceramide lipidosis: Globoid cell leukodystrophy (Krabbe disease). *In* "The Metabolic and Molecular Basis of Inherited Disease" (Scriver, C. R., Beaudet, A. L., Sly, W. S., and Valle, D., eds.), pp. 3669–3694. McGraw-Hill, New York.

Yunis, E. J., and Lee, R. E. (1970). Tubules of globoid cell leukodystrophy: A right-handed helix. *Science* **169,** 64–66.

Zlotogora, J., Chakraborty, S., Knowlton, R. G., and Wenger, D. A. (1990). Krabbe disease locus mapped to chromosome 14 by genetic linkage. *Am. J. Hum. Genet.* **47,** 37–44.

CHAPTER

# 36

# Alexander Disease

*Albee Messing and James E. Goldman*

## EARLY HISTORY AND CLINICAL PRESENTATIONS

In 1949, W. S. Alexander described a boy who died at 16 months of age with a history of megalencephaly, hydrocephalus, and psychomotor retardation (Alexander, 1949). A striking feature of the neuropathology in this child was the accumulation of Rosenthal fibers within astrocytes, and an associated degeneration or failure of myelination. During the ensuing 15 years, several similar patients were reported and given such descriptive diagnoses as fibrinoid degeneration of astrocytes, dysmyelogenic leukodystrophy, leukodystrophy with megalobarencephaly, fibrinoid leukodystrophy, and megalencephaly with hyaline pan-neuropathy. When Friede described the sixth case in 1964, he also provided relief from the growing chaos in nomenclature by coining the eponym Alexander disease to refer to this fascinating but mysterious childhood disease (Friede, 1964).

Subsequently, other patients were described who, despite sharing the common neuropathologic feature of prominent accumulation of Rosenthal fibers, differed markedly in age of onset, clinical presentation, and distribution of lesions (Borrett and Becker, 1985; Johnson, 1996; Pridmore *et al.*, 1993; Russo *et al.*, 1976). Hence, presently three main forms of Alexander disease are recognized: infantile, juvenile, and adult (Russo *et al.*, 1976). There has been considerable debate about whether these are different manifestations of the same disease or fundamentally different disorders (Herndon, 1999), though recent genetic studies now shed light on this issue (discussed later). There is no sex predilection, and the disease occurs in diverse ethnic groups.

The infantile form, with onset between birth and about 2 years of age, is the most common (Arend *et al.*, 1991; Deprez *et al.*, 1999; Klein and Anzil, 1994; Neal *et al.*, 1992; Townsend *et al.*, 1985; Wohlwill *et al.*, 1959). It is usually accompanied by megalencephaly, but this is not invariantly present (Rodriguez *et al.*, 2001). Seizures and developmental delay or regression are commonly found. Motor function gradually deteriorates to quadriparesis and spasticity. Hydrocephalus is often present, and though found occasionally along with stenosis of the cerebral aqueduct (Ni *et al.*, 2002; Sherwin and Berthrong, 1970), there is no direct evidence that the stenosis results from Rosenthal fiber accumulation. There is often profound mental retardation, but other patients have been described with only late, minimal, or even no cognitive difficulties. Survival varies from only a few weeks to several years, with some patients surviving into their early teens. Nearly all cases are sporadic. A few putative sib ships have been described (discussed later), and two examples are known of monozygotic twins where both were affected (Brenner *et al.*, unpublished observations; Meins *et al.*, 2002). Some investigators have argued for a distinct early-onset or neonatal form that is rapidly fatal and where seizures and elevated intracranial pressure are the predominant signs without spasticity (Springer *et al.*, 2000).

The juvenile form shows a later onset and initial signs may not be seen until the mid-teens (Deprez *et al.*, 1999; Neal *et al.*, 1992). Especially prominent are bulbar signs, with difficulties in swallowing or speech and vomiting, often accompanied by lower limb spasticity and incoordination. There may be some slow loss of intellectual function. The juvenile form generally progresses more slowly than the infantile, but the brain stem involvement can be life threatening. Some patients presented with signs resembling those of brain stem tumors, with the confusion resolved only by biopsy (Duckett *et al.*, 1992).

Adult-onset Alexander disease is the most variable and the least common form (Honnorat *et al.*, 1993; Howard *et al.*, 1993; Martidis *et al.*, 1999; Okamoto *et al.*, 2002; Rizzuto *et al.*, 1980; Schwankhaus *et al.*, 1995; Seil *et al.*, 1968). Sometimes it mimics the juvenile form, but with a later onset and slower progression. Other times it may simulate multiple sclerosis. Some cases exhibit palatal myoclonus and there may be abnormal eye movements (Martidis *et al.*, 1999). Three reports exist of apparent autosomal dominant inheritance. These individuals developed symptoms late and lived well into reproductive age (Howard *et al.*, 1993; Okamoto *et al.*, 2002; Schwankhaus *et al.*, 1995). Okanoto, *et al.* (2002) describe a heterozygous *GFAP* mutation in parent and children (discussed later).

## PATHOLOGY

Alexander disease is usually grouped among the leukodystrophies because of the pronounced white matter deficiency seen in children with this disorder. Infants, who typically have rapid clinical courses, do not myelinate appropriately and manifest widespread destruction of white matter, even to the point of cavitation (Klein and Anzil, 1994; Schochet *et al.*, 1968). Young patients typically show megalencephaly. Older children, who have a longer clinical course, show less white matter degeneration, although in long-standing cases glio-vascular scars with little myelin are seen in the deep white matter. In addition, older children show prominent involvement of the brain stem. Myelination in arcuate fibers is relatively spared, as is the case in many leukodystrophies. Patients with adult forms of the disease may show only patchy zones of myelin pallor or cavitation (Honnorat *et al.*, 1993; Schwankhaus *et al.*, 1995; Spalke and Mennel, 1982) or more widespread myelin loss (Walls *et al.*, 1984). Presumably, infants with early forms of the disorder never myelinate properly to begin with, while children and adults with later onset forms may myelinate and then demyelinate focally as the disease progresses. Rare reports of defects in PNS myelin are not convincing (Terao *et al.*, 1983).

Effects on neurons have also been observed, but have not been investigated thoroughly. A loss of axons has been reported as variable, ranging from none to severely diminished, particularly in the more gliotic regions (Borrett and Becker, 1985; Schochet *et al.*, 1968). It is not clear when axonal degeneration begins during the evolution of the Alexander pathology, nor what causes axonal loss. Even when axonal degeneration is present, the myelin loss is far more severe (Walls *et al.*, 1984). Similarly, neuronal somatal pathology has occasionally been reported. For example, Russo *et al.* (1976) described neuronal loss and chromatolytic changes in the brain stem. A number of authors have noted a paucity of oligodendrocytes in affected areas, but oligodendrocyte death has not been carefully studied.

The most characteristic finding in the Alexander brain is the presence of enormous numbers of Rosenthal fibers. These astrocytic inclusions appear by routine staining as eosinophilic, refractile, often rod-shaped bodies, varying in size from less than 1 micron to dozens of microns in length (Fig. 36.1). Although Rosenthal fibers are distributed in all regions of the CNS, they are particularly concentrated in astrocytic processes in the deep white matter, at the glial limitans and periventricular zones, in spinal white matter and intracranial regions of the optic nerve, and in the brain stem, particularly at the medullary level, where they accumulate in tegmental and ventral regions. Thalamic and basal ganglionic astrocytes can also accumulate large numbers of Rosenthal fibers (Towfighi *et al.*, 1983).

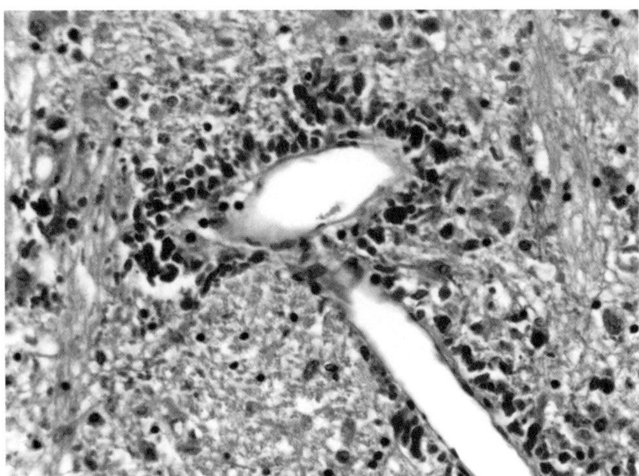

FIGURE 36.1
Rosenthal fibers concentrated in the astrocytic endfeet surrounding a blood vessel in the brain stem of a 1-year-old child with Alexander disease. Hematoxylin and eosin stain, paraffin section. Reprinted with permission from Elsevier (*Lancet Neurology*, 2003, 2, 75).

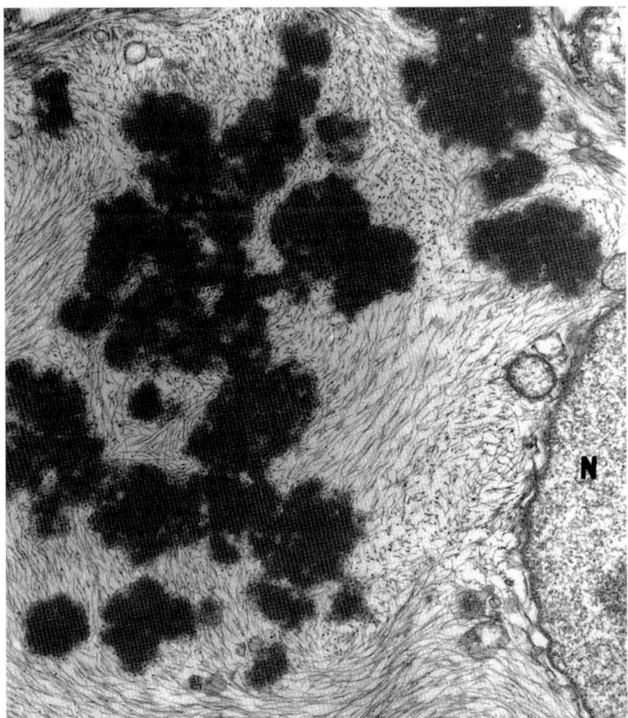


FIGURE 36.2
Rosenthal fibers in an astrocyte cell body from a 17-month-old child with Alexander disease, viewed by electron microscopy. Reprinted from Eng *et al.*, 1998, with permission of Wiley-Liss, Inc., a subsidiary of John Wiley & Sons, Inc.

Although astrocytes in cortical gray matter do not seem as prone to develop Rosenthal fibers, small inclusions are often found by careful observation. Examination of autopsies and biopsies of infants, or of children in the early stages of the disease, reveals small Rosenthal fibers in cell bodies (Borrett and Becker, 1985; Townsend *et al.*, 1985). During the course of the disease, the Rosenthal fibers enlarge and eventually come to reside in astrocyte processes and endfeet, hence the pronounced subpial and perivascular localization typically seen.

Ultrastructural examination of Rosenthal fibers reveals intracellular osmiophilic deposits in intimate contact with bundles of intermediate filaments (Fig. 36.2) (Herndon *et al.*,

1970; Seil *et al.*, 1968). Rosenthal fibers are not enclosed by membranes and show no lamellar features. The filaments contain GFAP (Johnson and Bettica, 1989) and vimentin (Tomokane *et al.*, 1991), both normally expressed by astrocytes. The osmiophilic matrix contains GFAP as well as two members of the small heat shock protein (hsp) family, αB-crystallin (Iwaki *et al.*, 1989) and hsp 27 (Iwaki *et al.*, 1993) and likely other components yet to be defined. A fraction of the αB-crystallin is ubiquitinated (Goldman and Corbin, 1991). Other post-translational modifications reportedly associated with Rosenthal fibers include lipid peroxidation adducts (Castellani *et al.*, 1998) and advanced glycation end products (Castellani *et al.*, 1997).

The amount of inflammation in the Alexander brain is variable. Some cases show appreciable lymphocytic accumulation around blood vessels, particularly in the brain stem (Russo *et al.*, 1976; Towfighi *et al.*, 1983), while others show little. It is not known what produces an inflammatory response or if this response contributes to the pathology.

Several patients who have not manifested any neurological signs or symptoms have been found at autopsy to have widespread accumulation of Rosenthal fibers in their brains (Mastri and Sung, 1973; Riggs *et al.*, 1988). This accumulation was not accompanied by demyelination, however. All of these patients suffered such systemic illnesses as lymphoma, ovarian carcinoma, cardiac and respiratory insufficiency, diabetes, and myocardial infarction. Whether these individuals should be considered to have a form of Alexander disease is dubious, and whether there is a causal relationship between their illnesses and the deposition of Rosenthal fibers, is not clear (Herndon, 1999).

Finally, we note that while most patients with Alexander disease exhibit widespread pathology in the CNS, there are individuals with focal lesions, particularly in bulbar regions (Duckett *et al.*, 1992; Goebel *et al.*, 1981; Russo *et al.*, 1976; Soffer and Horoupian, 1979). Localized brain stem pathology can be confused with pilocytic astrocytomas. Indeed, astrocytes in the Alexander brain can show a moderate degree of nuclear and cytoplasmic pleomorphism, thus compounding this rare diagnostic dilemma. Another consideration is that Rosenthal fibers are not specific to Alexander disease; for example, sporadic Rosenthal fibers can be found in the context of old glial scars, in pilocytic astrocytomas, or in the walls of syrinx cavities where they were first described (Rosenthal, 1898).

## CLINICAL DIAGNOSIS

Until recently there has been no definitive laboratory diagnostic test for Alexander disease (but see the discussion of a new genetic analysis, presented later in the chapter). It is important to rule out other more common leukodystrophies and to differentiate Alexander disease from other causes of megalencephaly (Matalon *et al.*, 1996). In particular, Canavan disease is indicated by a positive test for urinary N-acetylaspartic acid, very low activity of aspartoacylase in skin fibroblasts, or detection of known mutations in the aspartoacylase gene (Kaul *et al.*, 1993). One infantile patient presented with clinical signs and laboratory results indicative of Leigh's encephalopathy, with elevations in serum pyruvate and lactate and CSF pyruvate, but was subsequently found on autopsy to have Alexander disease (Gingold *et al.*, 1999). Brain lactate was also elevated in a patient with biopsy-proven Alexander disease as determined by MR spectroscopy (Kang *et al.*, 2001). Some have proposed evaluating CSF levels of HSP27 or αB-crystallin as indicators of Rosenthal fiber accumulation, but these findings are likely to be nonspecific (Takanashi *et al.*, 1998).

Radiology, especially MR imaging, are the current standard tools in the diagnosis of Alexander disease for both the infantile and juvenile forms (Hess *et al.*, 1990; Takanashi *et al.*, 1998; van der Knaap and Valk, 1995; van der Knaap *et al.*, 2001). Typical cases show bilateral frontal predominance of white matter changes with relative sparing of the posterior and parietal lobes (Fig. 36.3). They also show abnormalities of the basal ganglia, especially the caudate and sometimes the thalami, and a periventricular rim of abnormal signal

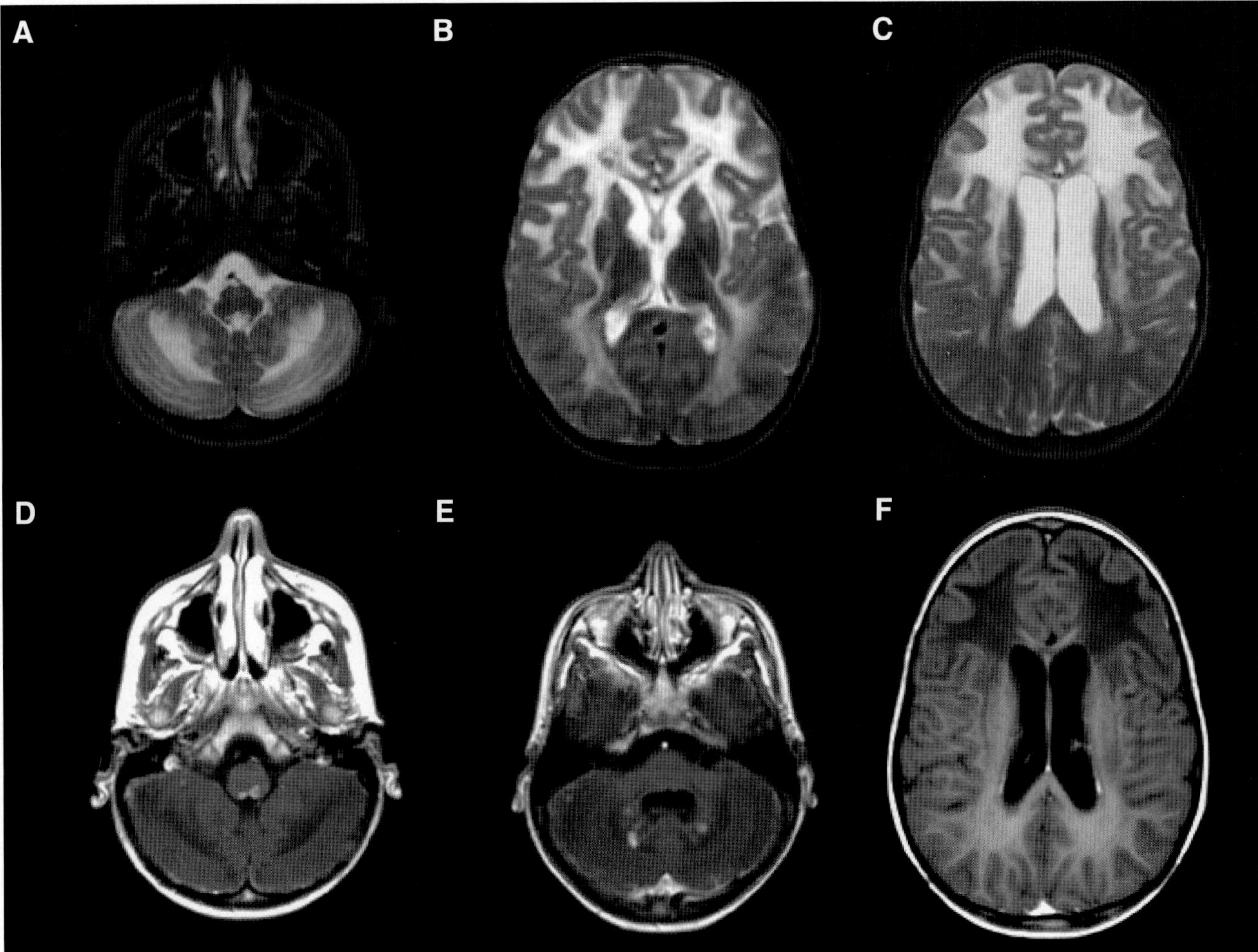


FIGURE 36.3
MR images of a 10-year-old boy with Alexander disease. The axial T2-weighted images (A–C) show extensive abnormalities of the cerebral white matter with frontal predominance. The parieto-occipital white matter is partially spared (B, C). There is a thin periventricular rim of low signal intensity (B, C). The basal ganglia and thalamus show some signal changes and are mildly atrophic (B). The cerebellar white matter is abnormal, and there is a lesion in the dorsal medulla (A). After contrast administration, enhancement is seen of the lesion in the medulla (D), the dentate nucleus (E), the cerebellar surface (D, E), and parts of the ependymal lining of the lateral ventricles (F). Generously provided by Dr. Marjo van der Knaap.

intensity, particularly around the frontal horns. Sometimes the medulla and brain stem show changes, and less commonly the cerebellum. The white matter changes show decreased signal in T1-weighted images, but increased signal on T2-weighted images. Often there is swelling of the periventricular rim, with abnormal contrast enhancement. Other advanced imaging techniques such as PET (Bobele *et al.*, 1990; Sawaishi *et al.*, 1999) and NMR spectroscopy (Kang *et al.*, 2001; Shiroma *et al.*, 2001) have been used occasionally, showing reduced metabolism in white matter and low NAA/creatinine ratios, but have not significantly aided in the diagnosis. Using the criteria of van der Knaap *et al.* (2001), diagnostic accuracy approaches 90% based on comparison with subsequent pathological analyses of the same patients. In atypical cases, however, pathological analysis of biopsy or autopsy samples is still essential for definitive diagnosis of Alexander disease.

## GFAP MUTATIONS

Although a genetic basis for Alexander disease had been speculated for some time, the rarity and sporadic nature of the disorder precluded traditional linkage analysis and few candidate genes were considered. As described earlier, the primary constituents of Rosenthal fibers include GFAP, αB-crystallin, and hsp 27. A reasonable supposition is that an abnormality in one of these components might cause Alexander disease. Indeed, αB-crystallin was sequenced to investigate this possibility for two patients, but with negative results (Iwaki *et al.*, 1992a). GFAP would be an even more attractive candidate, as it is expressed almost exclusively in astrocytes, the apparent focus for the disease. In fact, Becker and Teixiera (1988) suggested GFAP as a candidate gene more than a decade ago. However, it was the accidental discovery that transgenic mice engineered to constitutively overexpress GFAP developed a fatal encephalopathy with formation of bona fide Rosenthal fibers that gave new impetus to this idea (Messing *et al.*, 1998). This discovery provided strong evidence that a primary alteration in the expression of GFAP could lead to the hallmark feature of Alexander disease.

Prompted by these findings, Brenner *et al.* (2001) evaluated the GFAP coding region and proximal promoter in DNA from 13 patients who had died of biopsy-or autopsy-proven Alexander disease. Nonconservative, heterozygous point mutations were found in 11 of 12 infantile cases and in the single older patient examined (who had onset at 10 years with survival to 48 years). These mutations were found to alter seven different nucleotides, predicting changes in five different amino acids (all arginines). Following this initial report, a number of other studies have now confirmed and extended these findings (Aoki *et al.*, 2001; 2002; Gorospe *et al.*, 2002; Meins *et al.*, 2002; Okamoto *et al.*, Rodriguez, 2001; Sawaishi *et al.*, 2002; Shiihara *et al.*, 2002; Shiroma *et al.*, 2001). A diagram showing the location of all published mutations in relation to the protein domains of GFAP and variant of Alexander disease is shown in Fig. 36.4, and detailed discussion of these mutations and other polymorphisms in GFAP can be found in the review by Li *et al.* (2002). Websites that will continue to provide current updates on GFAP mutations can be found at the University of Wisconsin-Madison (www.waisman.wisc.edu/alexander) and the Human Intermediate Filament Mutation Database (www.interfil.org).

As of fall 2002, the GFAP gene has been evaluated in more than 60 Alexander disease patients. Mutations were present in nearly all (~95%) cases of infantile Alexander disease and in at least a certain proportion of juvenile and adult cases. Remarkably, mutations at only two amino acids, Arg79 or Arg239, account for nearly half of all cases. All of the mutations are heterozygous, presumably acting in an autosomal dominant fashion. For all of the infantile and juvenile cases where parents were available for testing, the parents were normal (i.e., did not have the mutation present in their child), confirming that the mutations occurred *de novo*. The one example of a GFAP mutation being inherited occurred in a family of adult-onset cases where a mother and two adult children were affected and carried the same mutation (Okamoto *et al.*, 2002). The penetrance also approaches 100%, the only exceptions being two children whose initial evaluation for other problems led to MRI diagnoses of leukodystrophy, with subsequent genetic analysis revealing GFAP mutations (Gorospe *et al.*, 2002), and one of these children is now showing signs.

The finding of GFAP mutations in nearly all cases of Alexander disease, and of diverse types, supports a uniform underlying mechanism for the disease. However, the same data do not provide a strong case for genotype-phenotype correlations. For instance, two children with the juvenile form (onset at 4 and 10 years of age) have the same R416W mutation previously found in two infantile patients (Brenner *et al.*, 2001; Gorospe *et al.*, 2002). Rodriquez *et al.* have argued that the R79 mutations may cause a relatively mild phenotype compared to the R239 mutations (Rodriguez *et al.*, 2001). The mutation associated with the single adult onset family, V87G (Okamoto *et al.*, 2002), has not yet been found in any other patients, but more adult-onset cases need to be tested.

Many of the GFAP mutations occur within an amino acid sequence that is highly conserved among intermediate filament proteins (Quinlan *et al.*, 1995). Mutations at the homologous sites of other intermediate filament proteins are associated with human diseases involving skin blistering, cataracts, cardiomyopathies, and muscular dystrophies (reviewed by Quinlan, 2001). However, although homologous sites are affected, most of these other mutations lead to a dominant *loss* of function, whereas the GFAP mutations appear to produce a dominant *gain* of function. For example, a loss of function is indicated

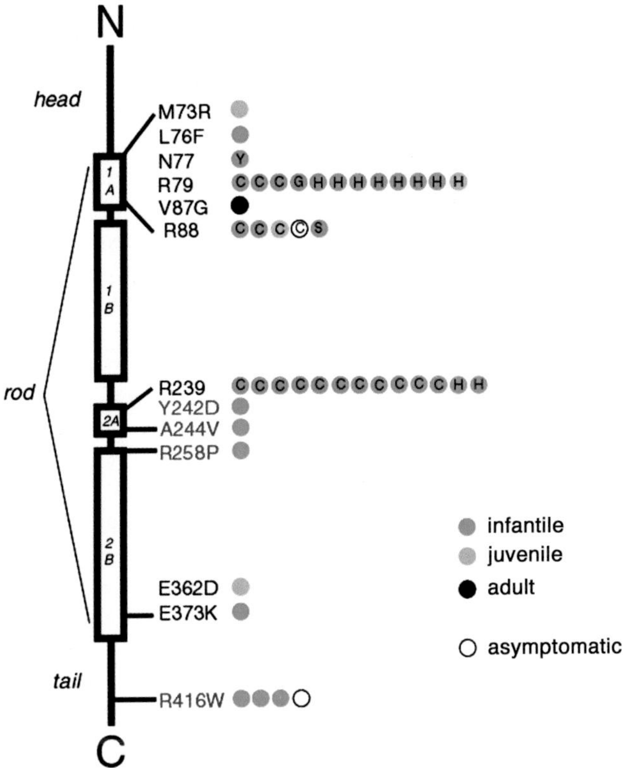


FIGURE 36.4
Location of Alexander's disease-associated mutations in *GFAP* mutations in relation to protein domain structure of intermediate filaments. Like other intermediate filaments, the structure of GFAP consists of randomly coiled N-terminal and C-terminal regions flanking four segments of an α-helical rod (shown by boxes) that are interconnected by nonhelical linkers. Mutations that are homologous to disease-causing mutations in other intermediate filaments are shown in black, whereas those that currently appear unique to GFAP are shown in red. Multiple independent cases with a given mutation are indicated by the number of symbols shown to the right (a single symbol is used for the set of cases from a single family). Classification of each case by age of onset is indicated by the color of the symbol (infantile = teal; juvenile = orange; adult = black; asymptomatic = open). N = N-terminal, C = C terminal. Adapted and updated from Figure 36.1 of Li *et al.*, 2002.

for keratin mutations because both heterozygous mutations in humans and null mutations of the homologous gene in mice disrupt the keratin filament network and produce a similar blistering disease (reviewed by Fuchs and Cleveland, 1998). In contrast, GFAP filaments are present in Alexander disease patients, and GFAP null mice are fully viable and their pathology does not resemble Alexander disease (Gomi *et al.*, 1995). Thus, the GFAP mutations do not appear to be acting by reducing or eliminating normal GFAP function, but rather by producing a new, deleterious, activity.

The GFAP mutations could arise either in the developing embryo or in the germ cells of one of the parents. If the mutation arose early in development, all astrocytes might be affected. However, if the mutation arose after the first several cellular divisions of the embryo, it is possible that not all cells or CNS areas would be involved, and that the disease could be more or less severe depending on when in development the mutation occurred. Focal lesions, such as those mimicking brain stem gliomas, might be explained by such a mechanism.

Finally, it is important to keep in mind that GFAP mutations have not been found in all cases of pathologically proven Alexander disease, suggesting that there could be other genetic or nongenetic causes for this disease. Since Rosenthal fibers appear to form in response to chronic overexpression of GFAP, another potential cause is increased synthesis due to a mutation in the transcriptional control region or to gene duplication. Gene duplication has been found to cause other human neurological disorders (Lupski *et al.*,

1991; Sistermans *et al.*, 1998). However, we have found no evidence yet for duplication of *GFAP* in any patients (Hagemann, unpublished observations). There are a number of methodological and conceptual reasons that could explain these negative findings, and for the purpose of genetic counseling one must stress that this absence of information is simply that, and is unfortunately noninformative. GFAP mutations may also eventually be found associated with disorders other than Alexander disease—at present there is no hint as to what those disorders might be.

The immediate clinical benefit derived from the close association of GFAP mutations with Alexander disease is that invasive diagnostic procedures such as brain biopsy have now been replaced by rapid and accurate DNA analysis. In addition, parents now have the option of fetal testing for subsequent pregnancies.

## FAMILIAL CASES

For many years, Alexander disease was speculated to be a genetic disorder and likely autosomal recessive given the apparent normalcy of the parents (for instance, see discussion in Pridmore *et al.*, 1993). In part, this speculation was fueled by occasional reports of families with more than one affected sibling. Given the significance attributed to these sib ships, and the understandable concern of parents regarding the risk of having other affected children and the need for guidance in genetic counseling, a careful review of these reports is warranted. The first was by Wohlwill *et al.* (1959), who described a family of nine children in which one sister and three brothers died between the ages of 3 and 6 years with macrocephaly and hydrocephalus. An autopsy of the last child revealed Alexander disease (though not so named at the time), but autopsies were not performed on any of the other children. Two subsequent reports appeared of infantile sibling pairs produced from consanguineous marriages, strongly implying a recessive genetic trait. However, all four of these patients were diagnosed as having Alexander disease based on clinical signs, progression, and radiology, without any pathological confirmation (Barbieri *et al.*, 1980; Springer *et al.*, 2000).

Three other reports exist of sibling pairs with later onset or very slow course of Alexander disease. In the first and best-documented pair, Duckett *et al.* (1992) describe a brother and sister who developed symptoms at ages 11 and 26 years, respectively. Although the initial considerations pointed toward gliomas of the posterior fossa, biopsies of the brain stem (brother) and cerebellum (sister) instead revealed Rosenthal fibers without any evidence of a tumor. A second pair, reported as a personal communication to V. McKusick (McKusick, 2001), presented at the ages of 11 and 13 years with nonprogressive macrocephaly, developmental delay, and radiological evidence of a leukodystrophy. Both of these patients are still alive in their twenties (P. Pearl, personal communication). The third pair (Klein *et al.*, 1988) is very unusual in that both siblings had early onsets (birth to 6 months) but are known to have lived into their mid-twenties, with one still alive at the age of 26. The latter two pairs lack pathological confirmation of the diagnosis.

These sibships lack absolute certainty that all are affected with Alexander disease. Nevertheless, it is worth considering how such familial cases could occur given the findings described earlier emphasizing heterozygous *de novo* mutations in *GFAP*. If the mutation arose in a parental germinal stem cell instead of in the patient, multiple gametes could carry the defect. Although highly unusual as a pattern of inheritance (Vogel and Motulsky, 1997), such gonadal mosaicism could account for the rare sibships described here. Thus, it will be of considerable interest to determine if affected sibs have GFAP mutations and, if so, if the same mutation is found in each affected family member. In addition, although all known GFAP mutations appear to act in the heterozygous state, and thus fit with mechanisms known from other intermediate filament disease, it remains possible on theoretical grounds that some GFAP mutations could act in an autosomal recessive fashion to cause Alexander disease.

Finally, three reports describe adult-onset syndromes in families in which more than one generation was affected. All noted similar clinical signs of palatal myoclonus, ataxia, and paresis or paraplegia. These are the only examples of Alexander disease in which any of the parents have been affected. In the first family, a father developed signs in his early thirties and died after a 15-year course, whereupon autopsy revealed numerous Rosenthal fibers (Seil *et al.*, 1968). Subsequently, Schwankhaus *et al.* (1995) reported that three of his five children developed similar neurological signs beginning in their twenties to forties, and one was autopsy-confirmed as Alexander disease. In a second family, Howard *et al.* (1993) reported that three of ten adult sibs developed similar syndromes in their twenties, with one having a biopsy showing Rosenthal fibers. Their mother, maternal aunt, and two of four children of the aunt were reported by family members to have had similar neurological problems. Although the authors of this report distinguished their patients from what had been described as adult Alexander disease, the striking similarities between this family and that of Schwankhaus *et al.* suggest that these two families suffered from the same disease. Most recently, Okamoto *et al.* (2002) described a family of three individuals in which a mother and one adult child developed palatal myoclonus, spastic paraparesis, and atrophy of the caudal brain stem and spinal cord in their fifties and thirties, respectively, with another adult child showing subtle neurological signs in his early thirties. Subsequent genetic analysis of this family indicated that all three shared the same mutation, thus supporting the concept that infantile, juvenile, and adult forms of adult Alexander disease can share a common etiology. The adult-onset families are consistent with the autosomal dominant pattern of inheritance predicted from the heterozygous nature of the GFAP mutations observed in Alexander disease.

## OTHER CANDIDATE GENES

As previously noted, a small subset of Alexander disease patients do not have *GFAP* mutations. Alexander disease might theoretically arise from alterations in proteins that interact with GFAP. There is precedent for the involvement of such genes in several other disorders associated with intermediate filament mutations. These include epidermolysis bullosa simplex, which can result from either mutations in keratins or the interacting plectin protein (Fuchs and Cleveland, 1998); Emery-Dreifuss muscular dystrophy, which can be produced by mutation in either nuclear lamins or the interacting emerin protein (Raffaele Di Barletta *et al.*, 2000); and desmin-related myopathy, which can be produced either by mutations in desmin (Goldfarb *et al.*, 1998) or the associated αB-crystallin (Vicart *et al.*, 1998).

αB-crystallin interacts with GFAP as well as with desmin (Nicholl and Quinlan, 1994; Wisniewski and Goldman, 1998) and thus remains a candidate gene for patients in whom a GFAP mutation is not present (the two patients whose αB-crystallin gene was sequenced were among those subsequently found to have GFAP mutations). Although none of the Alexander disease patients has been reported to have either the cataracts or myopathies observed in the one αB-crystallin mutation family documented (Vicart *et al.*, 1998), different mutations in the protein might lead to different phenotypes. In the normal mammalian brain, αB-crystallin is expressed at low levels in astrocytes and oligodendrocytes (Iwaki *et al.*, 1990), but accumulates in glia and neurons in a variety of neurological disorders (Iwaki *et al.*, 1992b). In most of these examples, Rosenthal fibers do not form, suggesting that its elevation per se does not trigger Rosenthal fiber formation. On the contrary, αB-crystallin appears to decrease filament aggregation, probably by inhibiting interactions between filaments (Koyama and Goldman, 1999; Perng *et al.*, 1999). Thus, Rosenthal fibers may form because conditions prevent αB-crystallin from organizing a normal intermediate filament network. Such conditions could include the presence of excess or mutant GFAP protein or a defect in the αB-crystallin itself.

Another candidate gene for Alexander disease is *NDUFV1*, which encodes a component of mitochondrial complex I. In 1999, Schuelke and colleagues (Schuelke *et al.*, 1999) described a young girl with mitochondrial complex I deficiency and clinical signs resembling Alexander disease. Sequencing of the *NDUFVI* open reading frame revealed homozygosity for a nonconservative mutation in the coding region. Both parents were confirmed as heterozygotes, supporting a recessive mode of transmission. In the absence of pathological confirmation, it cannot be certain that the diagnosis of Alexander disease in this child is accurate. If correct, however, this case would suggest a link to mitochondrial dysfunction as a pathway of injury in Alexander disease (Castellani *et al.*, 1998), as also suggested by the patient initially thought to have Leigh's encephalopathy mentioned earlier (Gingold *et al.*, 1999).

## POSSIBLE DISEASE MECHANISMS

GFAP missense mutations have been found in a high proportion of cases of Alexander disease. A strong argument can be made that these mutations are responsible for the disease based on their homology to known disease-causing mutations in other intermediate filament genes, and the finding that they arose de novo in all instances that parental DNAs were analyzed (the probability of this occurring at random is miniscule). Formal proof that the GFAP mutations cause Alexander disease must await demonstration that their introduction into mice reproduces the salient features of the disease, or direct demonstration of a biological effect of mutant protein. Mice are being engineered with point mutations of GFAP that correspond to the most common mutations found in Alexander disease patients, and preliminary analysis indicates that these mutations are indeed sufficient to induce formation of Rosenthal fibers in brain (Hagemann, unpublished observations).

How might GFAP mutations lead to Alexander disease? One approach to this question is to look for a common feature among instances in which Rosenthal fibers form; for example, in response to chronic gliosis, in the GFAP transgenic mice, and as a result of GFAP mutations. In the first two conditions there is a sustained elevation of GFAP. Elevated levels of GFAP may also be instrumental in Alexander disease, as Rosenthal fibers are typically found in patients at sites where GFAP is normally highly expressed, such as the glial limitans, white matter, and the subependymal zone (which might also explain why pathology is not seen in nonastrocytic cells that are known to express GFAP, albeit at much lower levels, such as nonmyelinating Schwann cells or lens epithelium). Thus, one possible mechanism by which the GFAP mutations might cause the disease is by raising levels of the protein; for example, by increasing its stability.

However, the mutations might instead cause accumulation of a particular form of GFAP that compromises astrocyte function, rather than by increasing the amount of total GFAP. For example, the mutant protein could assume a conformation, or receive a modification, that occurs less frequently for the wild type protein and that leads to an abnormal association with other cellular constituents (possibly itself). Such a scenario has been reported for α-synuclein, a protein found in the Lewy bodies of Parkinson's disease, and which is mutated in several familial cases of this disease (Dawson, 2000). Aggregation of α-synuclein is promoted either by increasing its level of expression or by the presence of the Parkinson's disease–associated mutations (Conway *et al.*, 1998; Dawson, 2000; Giasson *et al.*, 1999; Narhi *et al.*, 1999).

Another way that the mutations could lead to accumulation of a toxic form of GFAP is by interfering with its usual polymerization into filaments. It was noted earlier that homologous mutations in other intermediate filament proteins disrupt their incorporation into normal filament networks. Although typical intermediate filaments are observed in Alexander disease, it is possible that they form with reduced efficiency, resulting in the accumulation of GFAP oligomers that react to form toxic products. Such side reactions might also be promoted by GFAP accumulation resulting from overexpression.

It is unclear whether the Rosenthal fiber itself compromises astrocyte function, or whether it instead is formed as a protective mechanism to sequester aberrant GFAP-containing complexes. In addition, the distribution of Rosenthal fibers in the brain does not always coincide with the location of the most severe myelin defects (perhaps implying a pathogenic role for toxic soluble forms of GFAP, as discussed earlier). Recent evidence suggests that the protein aggregates associated with several other diseases may indeed be benign or protective, including the Lewy bodies of Parkinson's disease (Mizuno *et al.*, 1999), the inclusions found in Huntington's disease (Kim *et al.*, 1999), and the Mallory bodies present in liver cirrhosis (Zatloukal *et al.*, 2000). It should also be borne in mind that there is no evidence for destruction of astrocytes in Alexander disease; instead, a primary clinical feature is hypomyelination or demyelination. Apparently the GFAP mutations lead to aberrant interactions between astrocytes and oligodendrocytes.

However, Alexander disease astrocytes do display characteristics of physiological stress, as evidenced by the elevation of the small hsps αB-crystallin and hsp 27 (Head *et al.*, 1993). Interestingly, these same stress proteins are increased in the GFAP overexpressing mice (Messing *et al.*, 1998). Additional evidence for stress, and a suggestion that it may involve oxidative damage, is the association of lipid peroxidation products with Rosenthal fibers (Castellani *et al.*, 1998). On the other hand, the components of Rosenthal fibers are readily dissociated by SDS or urea (Goldman and Corbin, 1988), and so do not display the extensive cross-linking that is found in many other disease-associated protein aggregates and that has been attributed to oxidative damage (Giasson *et al.*, 2000). What consequences the stress response of Alexander disease astrocytes have for the functions of these cells and their interactions with other CNS cells remains to be determined.

Whatever the triggering mechanism, once the disease process begins, it would likely lead to a catastrophic positive feedback loop. Almost any insult to astrocytes prompts a reactive response, which includes a strong upregulation of GFAP synthesis. Robustly reactive astrocytes are abundant in the GFAP overexpressing mice, and if GFAP mutations provoke a similar reactive response in humans, levels of the mutant protein would be further increased, reactivity further stimulated, and so on in a noxious spiral. Another positive feedback loop might operate through effects on protein degradation. It has been recently suggested that the intermediate filament network may play a role in organizing degradative complexes that remove aberrant protein (Garcia-Mata *et al.*, 1999; Johnston *et al.*, 1998), and if this function were compromised by the mutant GFAP, another spiral of increasing levels of mutant GFAP would ensue.

Finally, although the presence of GFAP mutations in Alexander disease suggests that this is a primary disorder of astrocytes, the clinical and pathological features suggest that there must also be significant dysfunction of oligodendrocytes and perhaps neurons as well. For instance, patients with Alexander disease display either lack of proper myelin development (as in infants) or loss of myelination (as in older patients) at many levels of the CNS, including optic nerves, subcortical white matter, cerebellum, and spinal cord. We are therefore faced with a situation in which the expression of a mutated gene in one cell type (the astrocyte) has deleterious effects on the functions of another cell type (the oligodendrocytes). What mechanism might underlie these effects? One possibility is that astrocytes expressing a mutant GFAP undergo a stress response, possibly due to the accumulation of intermediate filaments, and as part of that response, secrete factors that are toxic to oligodendrocytes. These compounds could include TNF-α, a known stress protein that at least under some conditions induced oligodendrocyte cell death (Selmaj and Raine, 1988). A second possibility based on astrocyte toxicity is a secondary loss of axons, which would in turn prevent or cause loss of myelination. Axonal loss has not been demonstrated in Alexander disease, although clearly it takes place in severe cavitating lesions or in children with long-term clinical courses.

Whether the broader features of the Alexander phenotype truly reflect secondary effects of astrocyte dysfunction alone remains an open question. Clearly there is abundant evidence for how astrocytes might regulate the properties of both oligodendrocytes and neurons, but one should also consider the possibility that GFAP expression (and hence effects of mutant GFAPs) might not strictly be limited to astrocytes. Brenner (1994) reviewed the transcriptional regulation of GFAP, and there are several isoforms about which much less is known than the major GFAPα species of mRNA. A recently identified isoform, termed GFAPε, arises by alternative splicing and produces a protein that interacts with presenilin, although the precise cell in which GFAPε is expressed is not yet clear (Nielsen *et al.*, 2002). Transcriptional infidelity might also lead to markedly abnormal forms of GFAP, some of which may be expressed in neurons (Hol *et al.*, 2001; van Leeuwen *et al.*, 1998). Finally, considerable evidence now suggests that either GFAP is expressed at low levels in a multipotential stem cell (Doetsch *et al.*, 1999; Johansson *et al.*, 1999; Laywell *et al.*, 2000; Zhuo *et al.*, 2001), or that radial glia (which in primates do express GFAP) regularly give rise to neurons as a normal pathway of differentiation (Campbell and Gotz, 2002; Malatesta *et al.*, 2000; Noctor *et al.*, 2001). If mutant GFAPs were to exert their effects at the level of such stem cells, the defects could then manifest in a diverse population of cellular progeny.

## SUMMARY

Prior to finding that GFAP mutations underlie many cases of Alexander disease, it was unclear whether the disease originated in astrocytes or if the formation of Rosenthal fibers was a response to an external insult. It was also unclear whether the etiology of the disease was environmental or genetic. For many cases of Alexander disease, these questions have now been answered. An immediate clinical benefit of this discovery is the possibility of diagnosing most cases of Alexander disease through analysis of patient DNA samples, rather than resorting to brain biopsy. In addition, fetal testing is now an option for parents who have had an Alexander disease child with an identified mutation and who wish to have additional children. For the future, these mutations should provide a unique window for illuminating the mechanism of the disease, for further understanding the role of astrocytes and GFAP in myelination, and eventually for suggesting means of treatment.

### Acknowledgments

We thank our collaborators, especially Michael Brenner, all the Alexander patients, and their families who have participated in this research, and Marjo van der Knaap for contributing MRI images. This work was supported by grants from the NIH (NS-22475, NS-41803, and NS17125). This chapter is adapted and updated from a review published in the *Journal of Neuropathology & Experimental Neurology* (60:563, 2001).

### References

Alexander, W. S. (1949). Progressive fibrinoid degeneration of fibrillary astrocytes associated with mental retardation in a hydrocephalic infant. *Brain* **72,** 373–381.

Aoki, Y., Haginoya, K., Munakata, M., Yokoyama, H., Nishio, T., Togashi, N., Ito, T., Suzuki, Y., Kure, S., Iinuma, K., Brenner, M., and Matsubara, Y. (2001). A novel mutation in glial fibrillary acidic protein gene in a patient with Alexander disease. *Neurosci. Lett.* **312,** 71–74.

Arend, A. O., Leary, P. M., and Rutherfoord, G. S. (1991). Alexander's disease: A case report with brain biopsy, ultrasound, CT scan and MRI findings. *Clinical Neuropathology* **10,** 122–126.

Barbieri, F., Filla, A., De Falco, F. A., and Buscaino, G. A. (1980). Alexander's disease. A clinical study with computerized tomographic scans of the first two Italian cases. *Acta Neurologica* **2,** 1–9.

Becker, L. E., and Teixeira, F. (1988). Alexander's disease. *In* "The Biochemical Pathology of Astrocytes" (M. D. Norenberg, L. Hertz, and A. Schousboe, eds.), pp. 179–190. Alan R. Liss, New York.

Bobele, G. B., Garnica, A., Schaefer, G. B., Leonard, J. C., Wilson, D., Marks, W. A., Leech, R. W., and Brumback, R. A. (1990). Neuroimaging findings in Alexander's disease. *Journal of Child Neurology* **5,** 253–258.

Borrett, D., and Becker, L. E. (1985). Alexander's disease. A disease of astrocytes. *Brain* **108,** 367–385.

Brenner, M. (1994). Structure and transcriptional regulation of the GFAP gene. *Brain Pathol.* **4,** 245–257.

Brenner, M., Johnson, A. B., Boespflug-Tanguy, O., Rodriguez, D., Goldman, J. E., and Messing, A. (2001). Mutations in *GFAP*, encoding glial fibrillary acidic protein, are associated with Alexander disease. *Nature Genet.* **27,** 117–120.

Campbell, K., and Gotz, M. (2002). Radial glia: Multi-purpose cells for vertebrate brain development. *Trends Neurosci.* **25,** 235–238.

Castellani, R. J., Perry, G., Harris, P. L. R., Cohen, M. L., Sayre, L. M., Salomon, R. G., and Smith, M. A. (1998). Advanced lipid peroxidation end-products in Alexander's disease. *Brain Res.* **787,** 15–18.

Castellani, R. J., Perry, G., Harris, P. L. R., Monnier, V. M., Cohen, M. L., and Smith, M. A. (1997). Advanced glycation modification of Rosenthal fibers in patients with Alexander disease. *Neurosci. Lett.* **231,** 79–82.

Conway, K. A., Harper, J. D., and Lansbury, P. T. (1998). Accelerated in vitro fibril formation by a mutant alpha-synuclein linked to early-onset Parkinson disease. *Nature Med.* **4,** 1318–1320.

Dawson, T. M. (2000). New animal models for Parkinson's disease. *Cell* **101,** 115–118.

Deprez, M., D'Hooghe, M., Misson, J. P., de Leval, L., Ceuterick, C., Reznik, M., and Martin, J. J. (1999). Infantile and juvenile presentations of Alexander's disease: A report of two cases. *Acta Neurologica Scandinavica* **99,** 158–165.

Doetsch, F., Caille, I., Lim, D. A., Garcia-Verdugo, J. M., and Alvarez-Buylla, A. (1999). Subventricular zone astrocytes are neural stem cells in the adult mammalian brain. *Cell* **97,** 703–716.

Duckett, S., Schwartzman, R. J., Osterholm, J., Rorke, L. B., Friedman, D., and McLellan, T. L. (1992). Biopsy diagnosis of familial Alexander's disease. *Pediatr. Neurosurg.* **18,** 134–138.

Eng, L. F., Lee, Y. L., Kwan, H., Brenner, M., and Messing, A. (1998). Astrocytes cultured from transgenic mice carrying the added human glial fibrillary acidic protein gene contain Rosenthal fibers. *J. Neurosci. Res.* **53,** 353–360.

Friede, R. L. (1964). Alexander's disease. *Arch. Neurol.* **11,** 414–422.

Fuchs, E., and Cleveland, D. W. (1998). A structural scaffolding of intermediate filaments in health and disease. *Science* **279,** 514–519.

Garcia-Mata, R., Bebok, Z., Sorscher, E. J., and Sztul, E. S. (1999). Characterization and dynamics of aggresome formation by a cytosolic GFP-chimera. *J. Cell Biol.* **146,** 1239–1254.

Giasson, B. I., Duda, J. E., Murray, I. V. J., Chen, Q. P., Souza, J. M., Hurtig, H. I., Ischiropoulos, H., Trojanowski, J. Q., and Lee, V. M. Y. (2000). Oxidative damage linked to neurodegeneration by selective alpha-synuclein nitration in synucleinopathy lesions. *Science* **290,** 985–989.

Giasson, B. I., Uryu, K., Trojanowski, J. Q., and Lee, V. M. (1999). Mutant and wild type human alpha-synucleins assemble into elongated filaments with distinct morphologies in vitro. *J. Biol. Chem.* **274,** 7619–7622.

Gingold, M. K., Bodensteiner, J. B., Schochet, S. S., and Jaynes, M. (1999). Alexander's disease: Unique presentation. *Journal of Child Neurology* **14,** 325–329.

Goebel, H. H., Bode, G., Caesar, R., and Kohlschutter, A. (1981). Bulbar palsy with Rosenthal fiber formation in the medulla of a 15-year-old girl. Localized form of Alexander's disease? *Neuropediatrics* **12,** 382–391.

Goldfarb, L. G., Park, K. Y., Cervenakova, L., Gorokhova, S., Lee, H. S., Vasconcelos, O., Nagle, J. W., Seminomora, C., Sivakumar, K., and Dalakas, M. C. (1998). Missense mutations in desmin associated with familial cardiac and skeletal myopathy. *Nature Genet.* **19,** 402–403.

Goldman, J. E., and Corbin, E. (1988). Isolation of a major protein component of Rosenthal fibers. *Am. J. Pathol.* **130,** 569–578.

Goldman, J. E., and Corbin, E. (1991). Rosenthal fibers contain ubiquitinated alpha B-crystallin. *Am. J. Pathol.* **139,** 933–938.

Gomi, H., Yokoyama, T., Fujimoto, K., Ideka, T., Katoh, A., Itoh, T., and Itohara, S. (1995). Mice devoid of the glial fibrillary acidic protein develop normally and are susceptible to scrapie prions. *Neuron* **14,** 29–41.

Gorospe, J. R., Naidu, S., Johnson, A. B., Puri, V., Raymond, G. V., Jenkins, S. D., Pedersen, R. C., Lewis, D., Knowles, P., Fernandez, R., De Vivo, D., van der Knaap, M. S., Messing, A., Brenner, M., and Hoffman, E. P. (2002). Molecular findings in symptomatic and pre-symptomatic Alexander disease patients. *Neurology* **58,** 1494–1500.

Head, M. W., Corbin, E., and Goldman, J. E. (1993). Overexpression and abnormal modification of the stress proteins alpha B-crystallin and HSP27 in Alexander disease. *Am. J. Pathol.* **143,** 1743–1753.

Herndon, R. M. (1999). Is Alexander's disease a nosologic entity or a common pathologic pattern of diverse etiology? *Journal of Child Neurology* **14,** 275–276.

Herndon, R. M., Rubinstein, L. J., Freeman, J. M., and Mathieson, G. (1970). Light and electron microscopic observations on Rosenthal fibers in Alexander's disease and in multiple sclerosis. *J. Neuropathol. Exp. Neurol.* **29,** 524–551.

Hess, D. C., Fischer, A. Q., Yaghmai, F., Figueroa, R., and Akamatsu, Y. (1990). Comparative neuroimaging with pathologic correlates in Alexander's disease. *Journal of Child Neurology* **5,** 248–252.

Hol, E. M., Roelofs, R. F., Moraal, M., Sonnemans, M. A., Sluijs, J. A., van Tijn, P., Proper, E. A., de Graan, P. N., and van Leeuwen, F. W. (2001). Expression of novel splice variants of GFAP in human brain and neuronal accumulation of mutant GFAP protein in Alzheimer patients. Society for Neuroscience 429.10. Abstract.

Honnorat, J., Flocard, F., Ribot, C., Saint-Pierre, G., Pineau, D., Peysson, P., and Kopp, N. (1993). [Alexander's disease in adults and diffuse cerebral gliomatosis in 2 members of the same family]. [French]. *Revue Neurologique* **149,** 781–787.

Howard, R. S., Greenwood, R., Gawler, J., Scaravilli, F., Marsden, C. D., and Harding, A. E. (1993). A familial disorder associated with palatal myoclonus, other brainstem signs, tetraparesis, ataxia and Rosenthal fibre formation. *J. Neurol. Neurosurg. Psychiatry* **56,** 977–981.

Iwaki, A., Iwaki, T., Goldman, J. E., Ogomori, K., Tateishi, J., and Sakaki, Y. (1992a). Accumulation of alpha B-crystallin in brains of patients with Alexander's disease is not due to an abnormality of the 5′-flanking and coding sequence of the genomic DNA. *Neurosci. Lett.* **140,** 89–92.

Iwaki, T., Iwaki, A., Tateishi, J., Sakaki, Y., and Goldman, J. E. (1993). Alpha B-crystallin and 27-kd heat shock protein are regulated by stress conditions in the central nervous system and accumulate in Rosenthal fibers. *Am. J. Pathol.* **143,** 487–495.

Iwaki, T., Kume-Iwaki, A., and Goldman, J. E. (1990). Cellular distribution of alpha B-crystallin in non-lenticular tissues. *Journal of Histochemistry & Cytochemistry* **38,** 31–39.

Iwaki, T., Kume-Iwaki, A., Liem, R. K. H., and Goldman, J. E. (1989). αB-Crystallin is expressed in non-lenticular tissues and accumulates in Alexander's disease brain. *Cell* **57,** 71–78.

Iwaki, T., Wisniewski, T., Iwaki, A., Corbin, E., Tomokane, N., Tateishi, J., and Goldman, J. E. (1992b). Accumulation of alpha B-crystallin in central nervous system glia and neurons in pathologic conditions. *Am. J. Pathol.* **140,** 345–356.

Johansson, C. B., Momma, S., Clarke, D. L., Risling, M., Lendahl, U., and Frisén, J. (1999). Identification of a neural stem cell in the adult mammalian central nervous system. *Cell* **96,** 25–34.

Johnson, A. B. (1996). Alexander disease. *In* "Handbook of Clinical Neurology" (H. G. Moser, ed.), Vol. 22 (66): Neurodystrophies and Neurolipidoses, pp. 701–710. Elsevier, Amsterdam.

Johnson, A. B., and Bettica, A. (1989). On-grid immunogold labeling of glial intermediate filaments in epoxy-embedded tissue. *Am. J. Anat.* **185,** 335–341.

Johnston, J. A., Ward, C. L., and Kopito, R. R. (1998). Aggresomes: A cellular response to misfolded proteins. *J. Cell Biol.* **143,** 1883–1898.

Kang, P. B., Hunter, J. V., and Kaye, E. M. (2001). Lactic acid elevation in extramitochondrial childhood neurodegenerative diseases. *Journal of Child Neurology* **16,** 657–660.

Kaul, R., Ping Gao, G., Balamurugan, K., and Matalon, R. (1993). Cloning of the human aspartoacylase cDNA and a common missense mutation in Canavan disease. *Nature Genet.* **5,** 118–123.

Kim, M., Lee, H. S., LaForet, G., McIntyre, C., Martin, E. J., Chang, P., Kim, T. W., Williams, M., Reddy, P. H., Tagle, D., Boyce, F. M., Won, L., Heller, A., Aronin, N., and DiFiglia, M. (1999). Mutant huntingtin expression in clonal striatal cells: Dissociation of inclusion formation and neuronal survival by caspase inhibition. *J. Neurosci.* **19,** 964–973.

Klein, E. A., and Anzil, A. P. (1994). Prominent white matter cavitation in an infant with Alexander's disease. *Clin. Neuropathol.* **13,** 31–38.

Klein, S. K., Goulden, K. J., and Rapin, I. (1988). Evidence for autosomal recessive transmission of Alexander's disease. *Annals of Neurology* **24,** 302. Abstract.

Koyama, Y., and Goldman, J. E. (1999). Formation of GFAP cytoplasmic inclusions in astrocytes and their disaggregation by αB-crystallin. *Am. J. Pathol.* **154,** 1563–1572.

Laywell, E. D., Rakic, P., Kukekov, V. G., Holland, E. C., and Steindler, D. A. (2000). Identification of a multipotent astrocytic stem cell in the immature and adult mouse brain. *Proc. Natl. Acad. Sci. USA* **97,** 13883–13888.

Li, R., Messing, A., Goldman, J. E., and Brenner, M. (2002). GFAP mutations in Alexander disease. *Int. J. Dev. Neurosci.* **20,** 259-268.

Lupski, J. R., Montes de Oca-Luna, R., Slaugenhaupt, S., Pentao, L., Guzzetta, V., Trask, B. J., Saucedo-Cardenas, O., Barker, D. F., Killian, J. M., Garcia, C. A., Chakravarti, A., and Patel, P. I. (1991). DNA duplication associated with Charcot-Marie-Tooth disease type 1A. *Cell* **66,** 219–232.

Malatesta, P., Hartfuss, E., and Götz, M. (2000). Isolation of radial glial cells by fluorescent-activated cell sorting reveals a neuronal lineage. *Development* **127,** 5253–5263.

Martidis, A., Yee, R. D., Azzarelli, B., and Biller, J. (1999). Neuro-ophthalmic, radiographic, and pathologic manifestations of adult-onset Alexander disease. *Arch. Ophthalmol.* **117,** 265–267.

Mastri, A. R., and Sung, J. H. (1973). Diffuse Rosenthal fiber formation in the adult: A report of four cases. *J. Neuropathol. Exp. Neurol.* **32,** 424–436.

Matalon, R., Michals, K., and Kaul, R. (1996). Canavan disease. *In* "Handbook of Clinical Neurology," (H. G. Moser, ed.), Vol. 22 (66): Neurodystrophies and Neurolipidoses, pp. 661–669. Elsevier, Amsterdam.

McKusick, V. A. Alexander disease. OMIM. 2001. Electronic Citation.

Meins, M., Brockmann, K., Yadav, S., Haupt, M., Sperner, J., Stephani, U., and Hanefeld, F. (2002). Infantile Alexander disease: A *GFAP* mutation in monozygotic twins and novel mutations in two other patients. Neuropediatrics. In press.

Messing, A., Head, M. W., Galles, K., Galbreath, E. J., Goldman, J. E., and Brenner, M. (1998). Fatal encephalopathy with astrocyte inclusions in GFAP transgenic mice. *Am. J. Pathol.* **152,** 391–398.

Mizuno, Y., Hattori, N., and Mori, H. (1999). Genetics of Parkinson's disease. *Biomedicine & Pharmacotherapy* **53,** 109–116.

Narhi, L., Wood, S. J., Steavenson, S., Jiang, Y., Wu, G. M., Anafi, D., Kaufman, S. A., Martin, F., Sitney, K., Denis, P., Louis, J. C., Wypych, J., Biere, A. L., and Citron, M. (1999). Both familial Parkinson's disease mutations accelerate alpha-synuclein aggregation [published erratum appears in J Biol Chem 1999 May 7;274(19):13728]. *J. Biol. Chem.* **274,** 9843–9846.

Neal, J. W., Cave, E. M., Singhrao, S. K., Cole, G., and Wallace, S. J. (1992). Alexander's disease in infancy and childhood: A report of two cases. *Acta Neuropathol. (Berl.)* **84,** 322–327.

Ni, Q., Johns, G. S., Manepalli, A., Martin, D. S., and Geller, T. J. (2002). Infantile Alexander's disease: Serial neuroradiologic findings. *J. Child Neurol.* **17,** 463–466.

Nicholl, I. D., and Quinlan, R. A. (1994). Chaperone activity of α-crystallins modulates intermediate filament assembly. *EMBO J.* **13,** 945–953.

Nielsen, A. L., Holm, I. E., Johansen, M., Bonven, B., Jørgensen, P., and Jørgensen, A. L. (2002). A new splice variant of glial fibrillary acidic protein, GFAPε, interacts with the presenilin proteins. *J. Biol. Chem.* **277,** 29983–29991.

Noctor, S. C., Flint, A. C., Weissman, T. A., Dammerman, R. S., and Kriegstein, A. R. (2001). Neurons derived from radial glial cells establish radial units in neocortex. *Nature* **409,** 714–720.

Okamoto, Y., Mitsuyama, H., Jonosono, M., Hirata, K., Arimura, K., Osame, M., and Nakagawa, M. (2002). Autosomal dominant palatal myoclonus and spinal cord atrophy. *J. Neurol. Sci.* **195,** 71–76.

Perng, M. D., Cairns, L., van den IJssel, P., Prescott, A., Hutcheson, A. M., and Quinlan, R. A. (1999). Intermediate filament interactions can be altered by HSP27 and αB-crystallin. *J. Cell Sci.* **112,** 2099–2112.

Pridmore, C. L., Baraitser, M., Harding, B., Boyd, S. G., Kendall, B., and Brett, E. M. (1993). Alexander's disease: Clues to diagnosis. *J. Child. Neurol.* **8,** 134–144.

Quinlan, R. (2001). Cytoskeletal catastrophe causes brain degeneration. *Nature Genet.* **27,** 10–11.

Quinlan, R., Hutchison, C., and Lane, B. (1995). Intermediate filament proteins. *Protein Profile* **2,** 801–952.

Raffaele Di Barletta, M., Ricci, E., Galluzzi, G., Tonali, P., Mora, M., Morandi, L., Romorini, A., Voit, T., Orstavik, K. H., Merlini, L., Trevisan, C., Biancalana, V., Housmanowa-Petrusewicz, I., Bione, S., Ricotti, R., Schwartz, K., Bonne, G., and Toniolo, D. (2000). Different mutations in the LMNA gene cause autosomal dominant and autosomal recessive Emery-Dreifuss muscular dystrophy. *Am. J. Hum. Genet.* **66,** 1407–1412.

Riggs, J. E., Schochet, S. S. J., and Nelson, J. (1988). Asymptomatic adult Alexander disease: Entity or nosological misconception? *Neurology* **38,** 152–154.

Rizzuto, N., Ferrari, G., and Piscioli, A. (1980). Diffuse Rosenthal fiber formation in adults. A case report. *Acta Neuropathol. (Berl.)* **50,** 237–240.

Rodriguez, D. (2001). Infantile Alexander disease: Spectrum of GFAP mutations and genotype-phenotype correlation (vol 69, pg 1134, 2001). *Am. J. Hum. Genet.* **69,** 1413.

Rodriguez, D., Gauthier, F., Bertini, E., Bugiani, M., Brenner, M., N'guyen, S., Goizet, C., Gelot, A., Surtees, R., Pedespan, J.-M., Hernandorena, X., Troncoso, M., Uziel, G., Messing, A., Ponsot, P., Pham-Dinh, D., Dautigny, A., and Boespflug-Tanguy, O. (2001). Infantile Alexander disease: Spectrum of GFAP mutations and genotype-phenotype correlation. *Am. J. Hum. Genet.* **69,** 1134–1140.

Rosenthal, W. (1898). Über eine eigenthümliche, mit syringomyelie complicirte geschwulst des rückenmarks. *Bietr. Pathol. Anat.* **23,** 111–143.

Russo, L. S., Jr., Aron, A., and Anderson, P. J. (1976). Alexander's disease: A report and reappraisal. *Neurology* **26,** 607–614.

Sawaishi, Y., Hatazawa, J., Ochi, N., Hirono, H., Yano, T., Watanabe, Y., Okudera, and Takada, G. (1999). Positron emission tomography in juvenile Alexander disease. *J. Neurol. Sci.* **165,** 116–120.

Sawaishi, Y., Yano, T., Takaku, I., and Takada, G. (2002). Juvenile Alexander's disease with a novel mutation in glial fibrillary acidic protein gene. *Neurology* **58,** 1541–1543.

Schochet, S. S., Lampert, P. W., and Earle, K. M. (1968). Alexander's disease: A case report with electron microscopic observations. *Neurology* **18,** 543–549.

Schuelke, M., Smeitink, J., Mariman, E., Loeffen, J., Plecko, B., Trijbels, F., Stockler-Ipsiroglu, S., and van den Heuvel, L. (1999). Mutant NDUFV1 subunit of mitochondrial complex I causes leukodystrophy and myoclonic epilepsy. *Nature Genet.* **21,** 260–261.

Schwankhaus, J. D., Parisi, J. E., Gulledge, W. R., Chin, L., and Currier, R. D. (1995). Hereditary adult-onset Alexander's disease with palatal myoclonus, spastic paraparesis, and cerebellar ataxia. *Neurology* **45,** 2266–2271.

Seil, F. J., Schochet, S. S. J., and Earle, K. M. (1968). Alexander disease in an adult. Report of a case. *Arch. Neurol.* **19,** 494–502.

Selmaj, K. W., and Raine, C. S. (1988). Tumor necrosis factor mediates myelin and oligodendrocyte damage in vitro. *Ann. Neurol.* **23,** 339–346.

Sherwin, R. M., and Berthrong, M. (1970). Alexander disease with sudanophilic leukodystrophy. *Archives of Pathology & Laboratory Medicine* **89,** 321–328.

Shiihara, T., Kato, M., Honma, T., Ohtaki, S., Sawaishi, Y., and Hayasaka, K. (2002). Fluctuation of computed tomographic findings in white matter in Alexander's disease. *Journal of Child Neurology* **17,** 227–230.

Shiroma, N., Kanazawa, N., Izumi, M., Sugai, K., Fukumizu, M., Sasaki, M., Hanaoka, S., Kaga, M., and Tsujino, S. (2001). Diagnosis of Alexander disease in a Japanese patient by molecular genetic analysis. *Journal of Human Genetics* **46,** 579–582.

Sistermans, E. A., Decoo, R. F. M., Dewijs, I. J., and Vanoost, B. A. (1998). Duplication of the proteolipid protein gene is the major cause of Pelizaeus-Merzbacher disease. *Neurology* **50,** 1749–1754.

Soffer, D., and Horoupian, D. S. (1979). Rosenthal fibers formation in the central nervous system. Its relation to Alexander's disease. *Acta Neuropathol. (Berl.)* **47,** 81–84.

Spalke, G., and Mennel, H. D. (1982). Alexander's disease in an adult: Clinicopathologic study of a case and review of the literature. *Clinical Neuropathology* **1,** 106–112.

Springer, S., Erlewein, R., Naegele, T., Becker, I., Auer, D., Grodd, W., and Krageloh-Mann, I. (2000). Alexander disease - Classification revisited and isolation of a neonatal form. *Neuropediatrics* **31,** 86–92.

Takanashi, J., Sugita, K., Tanabe, Y., and Niimi, H. (1998). Adolescent case of Alexander disease: MR imaging and MR spectroscopy. *Pediatr. Neurol.* **18,** 67–70.

Terao, Y., Ishi, M., Hamada, T., and Murata, R. (1983). [Ultrastructural changes of skin nerve in Alexander's disease]. [Japanese]. *Nippon Hifuka Gakkai Zasshi - Japanese Journal of Dermatology* **93,** 1533–1535.

Tomokane, N., Iwaki, T., Tateishi, J., Iwaki, A., and Goldman, J. E. (1991). Rosenthal fibers share epitopes with alpha B-crystallin, glial fibrillary acidic protein, and ubiquitin, but not with vimentin. Immunoelectron microscopy with colloidal gold. *Am. J. Pathol.* **138,** 875–885.

Towfighi, J., Young, R., Sassani, J., Ramer, J., and Horoupian, D. S. (1983). Alexander's disease: Further light-, and electron-microscopic observations. *Acta Neuropathol. (Berl.)* **61,** 36–42.

Townsend, J. J., Wilson, J. F., Harris, T., Coulter, D., and Fife, R. (1985). Alexander's disease. *Acta Neuropathol. (Berl.)* **67,** 163–166.

van der Knaap, M. S., Naidu, S., Breiter, S. N., Blaser, S., Stroink, H., Springer, S., Begeer, J. C., Van Coster, R., Barth, P. G., Thomas, N. H., Valk, J., and Powers, J. M. (2001). Alexander disease: Diagnosis with MR imaging. *Am. J. Neuroradiol.* **22,** 541–552.

van der Knaap, M. S., and Valk, J. (1995). Magnetic Resonance of Myelin, Myelination, and Myelin Disorders. In Magnetic Resonance of Myelin, Myelination, and Myelin Disorders (Berlin: Springer-Verlag), pp. 259–264.

van Leeuwen, F. W., Burbach, J. P., and Hol, E. M. (1998). Mutations in RNA: A first example of molecular misreading in Alzheimer's disease. [Review] [48 refs]. *Trends Neurosci.* **21,** 331–335.

Vicart, P., Caron, A., Guicheney, P., Li, Z. L., Prevost, M. C., Faure, A., Chateau, D., Chapon, F., Tome, F., Dupret, J. M., Paulin, D., and Fardeau, M. (1998). A missense mutation in the alphaB-crystallin chaperone gene causes a desmin-related myopathy. *Nature Genet.* **20,** 92–95.

Vogel, F., and Motulsky, A. G. (1997). Human Genetics: Problems and Approaches. (Berlin: Springer), pp. pg. 409–410.

Walls, T. J., Jones, R. A., Cartlidge, N., and Saunders, M. (1984). Alexander's disease with Rosenthal fibre formation in an adult. *J. Neurol. Neurosurg. Psychiatry* **47,** 399–403.

Wisniewski, T., and Goldman, J. E. (1998). αB-crystallin is associated with intermediate filaments in astrocytoma cells. *Neurochem. Res.* **23,** 385–392.

Wohlwill, F. J., Bernstein, J., and Yakovlev, P. I. (1959). Dysmyelinogenic leukodystrophy: Report of a case of a new, presumably familial type of leukodystrophy with megalobarencephaly. *J. Neuropathol. Exp. Neurol.* **18,** 359–383.

Zatloukal, K., Stumptner, C., Lehner, M., Denk, H., Baribault, H., Eshkind, L. G., and Franke, W. W. (2000). Cytokeratin 8 protects from hepatotoxicity, and its ratio to cytokeratin 18 determines the ability of hepatocytes to form mallory bodies. *Am. J. Pathol.* **156,** 1263–1274.

Zhuo, L., Theis, M., Willecke, K., Brenner, M., and Messing, A. (2001). hGFAP-cre transgenic mice for manipulation of glial and neuronal function in vivo. *genesis* **31,** 85–94.

CHAPTER

# 37

# Pelizaeus-Merzbacher Disease

*Lynn D. Hudson, James Y. Garbern, and John A. Kamholz*

## A HISTORICAL PERSPECTIVE OF PELIZAEUS-MERZBACHER DISEASE (PMD)

In 1885, Friedrich Pelizaeus described a family with an unusual inherited disease that now bears his name. In this description he also noted "that the disease is passed on by the mother but does not hurt her" (Pelizaeus, 1885) consistent with an X-linked mode of inheritance (Boulloche and Aicardi, 1986; Seitelberger, 1970). Twenty-five years later, Ludwig Merzbacher reinvestigated 12 affected individuals from the same family and performed a detailed pathological analysis of the brain of one of its members. In this analysis he identified the widespread loss of myelin in the cortical white matter (Merzbacher, 1910). In his exhaustive clinical description, Merzbacher noted that the disease began in early neonatal life with aimless, wandering eye movements, followed by nystagmus. Infants failed to develop normal head control and displayed tremors or shaking movements of the head. The disease was slowly progressive, with additional signs including bradylalia, scanning speech, ataxia and intention tremor of the upper limbs, spastic contractions of the lower limbs, athetotic movements, and cognitive impairment (Merzbacher, 1910; Pelizaeus, 1885).

A disorder with pathology similar to that described by Merzbacher was reported by Franz Seitelberger in 1954 (Seitelberger, 1954). In this condition, however, there was nearly complete absence of myelin sheaths and a profound loss of myelin-forming oligodendrocytes. Seitelberger suggested that this disease, which he called the connatal form of PMD, was similar to that described by Pelizaeus and Merzbacher, which he designated the classical form of PMD. In addition, he noted that in both disorders the absence of myelin was the primary biochemical defect, suggesting that both were leukodystrophies. Zeman and coworkers subsequently suggested that the defect in PMD resided in the proteolipid protein (PLP; also known as lipophilin or Folch-Lees protein), the major protein component of myelin (Zeman *et al.*, 1964), a hypothesis verified by the sequencing of mutations in the *PLP* gene of several patients with the disease a quarter of a century later (Gencic *et al.*, 1989; Hudson *et al.*, 1989; Trofatter *et al.*, 1989). In the early 1990s, Boespflug-Tanguy and collaborators found genetic linkage of spastic paraparesis type 2 to the Xq22 region where PMD also mapped, suggesting that *PLP1* mutations could produce this syndrome. Then these researchers identified several patients with *PLP1* mutations who presented with spastic paraplegia without the other signs of PMD (Saugier-Veber *et al.*, 1994; reviewed in Nave and Boespflug-Tanguy, 1996). Evaluation of additional patients with X-linked spastic paraplegia and mutations in the *PLP1* gene showed that this syndrome could exist as either a "complicated" or a milder "pure" form in which the clinical phenotype is confined to lower limb spasticity. The detection of families in which PMD and SPG2 coexist emphasize the broad clinical continuum of these disorders (Tab. 37.1), all of which

TABLE 37.1 Spectrum of *PLP*-Related Disorders

| Phenotype | Age of onset | Neurologic findings | Ambulation | Speech | Lifespan |
|---|---|---|---|---|---|
| Connatal PMD | Neonatal period | *Nystagmus at birth<br>*Pharyngeal weakness<br>*Stridor<br>*Hypotonia<br>*Severe spasticity<br>* ± Seizures<br>*Cognitive impairment | Never achieved | Absent | Death in childhood to third decade |
| Classic PMD | First year | *Nystagmus in first two months<br>*Initial hypotonia<br>*Spastic quadriparesis<br>*Ataxia titubation<br>* ± Dystonia, athetosis<br>*Cognitive impairment | With assistance if achieved; lost in childhood/adolescence | Usually present | Death in 3rd to 7th decade |
| *PLP1* null syndrome | First 1–5 years | *No nystagmus<br>*Mild spastic quadriparesis<br>*Ataxia<br>*Peripheral neuropathy<br>*Mild to moderate cognitive impairment | Present | Present; usually worsens after adolescence | Death in 5th to 7th decade |
| Complicated spastic paraplegia (SPG2) | First 1–5 years | ± Nystagmus<br>*Ataxia<br>*Autonomic dysfunction (spastic urinary bladder)<br>*Spastic gait<br>*Little or no cognitive impairment | + | Present | Normal |
| Pure spastic paraplegia (SPG2) | First 1–5 years | *Autonomic dysfunction (spastic urinary bladder)<br>*Spastic gait<br>*Normal cognition | + | Present | Normal |

share a phenotype of spasticity and hypomyelination (Cambi, F *et al.*, 1996; Bond *et al.*, 1997; Kobayashi *et al.*, 1994; Osaka *et al.*, 1995).

## GENETICS OF PMD/SPG2

### The Proteolipid Protein (PLP) Gene Is Mutated in PMD and SPG2

Proteolipid protein (PLP), the predominant protein of CNS myelin (reviewed in Chapter 16) is one of nature's most hydrophobic proteins. What gives this integral membrane protein extra hydrophobic character is an unusual degree of fatty acid acylation. Six fatty acid chains are covalently linked to a PLP molecule (Weimbs and Stoffel, 1992), and those fatty acids attached to the intracellular loop of PLP have been proposed to mediate the association of PLP with the adjacent lipid leaflet in compact myelin (Sporkel *et al.*, 2002, see Fig. 3B in Chapter 16). Acylation occurs autocatalytically at a stage following translation of PLP mRNA (Bizzozero *et al.*, 1987; Ross and Braun, 1988), a temporal pattern consistent with a role for this post-translational modification in the stabilization or compaction of myelin. PLP is synthesized in the rough endoplasmic reticulum as a tetraspan intrinsic membrane protein with both termini on the cytoplasmic face (Gow *et al.*, 1997; Wahle and Stoffel, 1998) and subsequently transported through the Golgi complex, where other myelin lipid constituents such as cholesterol and galactocerebroside associate with PLP in "rafts" (Simons *et al.*, 2000). Raft formation is one of the initial stages of myelin assembly and is followed by the vesicular transport of PLP to the myelin membrane.

The exceptional nature of PLP as a protein is echoed in the gene, which is extremely well conserved. *PLP* gene structure is preserved among tetrapods and readily discernible in the primordial gene of the lipophilin family present in invertebrates (Stecca *et al.*, 2000). Mammals share a nearly identical coding capacity for *PLP* (reviewed in Chapter 16). Moreover, no amino acid polymorphisms have been detected in the thousands of coding regions sequenced in the human *PLP* gene. PLP is encoded by a single gene, composed of seven exons located on the X chromosome (Xq22.2) (Diehl *et al.*, 1986; Ikenaka *et al.*, 1988; Macklin *et al.*, 1987; Stoffel *et al.*, 1984) (see Fig. 1, Chapter 16). The first exon ends one base after the initiator methionine, which is cleaved off the nascent protein. An additional exon with the potential of encoding an alternate amino terminus was reported in mouse (Bongarzone *et al.*, 1999) but is not present in the human gene. The third exon contains an internal donor splice site, which is used to generate transcripts encoding the smaller (20 kDa) DM20 isoform. While identical to PLP in topology, DM20 is missing part of the intracellular loop that contains two acylation sites, an absence which may account for the altered conformation and physical properties observed for DM20 (Gow *et al.*, 1997; Helynck *et al.*, 1983; Skalidis *et al.*, 1986). Like PLP, DM20 is abundantly produced, estimably at 60% of the level of PLP (Schindler *et al.*, 1990), and the two proteins can form heteromers (McLaughlin *et al.*, 2002).

PLP and DM20 perform distinct roles in the maintenance of myelin structure, as DM20 cannot fully compensate for a loss of PLP in myelin (Sporkel *et al.*, 2002; Stecca *et al.*, 2000). Other functions have been proposed for PLP/DM20 based on features of these lipophilin family members resembling channel proteins, the detection of secreted fragments of PLP/DM20, and the expression in other glial cells as well as outside of the nervous system (reviewed in Chapter 16). The intriguing hypothesis that PLP acts as a sensor in transmitting information across the lipid bilayer (Gow and Lazzarini, 1996) was validated by the discovery that PLP, but not DM20, interacts with $\alpha_V$-integrin as part of a signaling complex (Gudz *et al.*, 2002). Apart from oligodendrocytes, the PLP gene is transcriptionally active in the nervous system in olfactory ensheathing cells (Dickinson *et al.*, 1997), satellite cells (Griffiths *et al.*, 1995), and Schwann cells (Garbern *et al.*, 1997; Griffiths *et al.*, 1989; Puckett *et al.*, 1987), where the predominant isoform expressed is DM20 (Pham-Dinh *et al.*, 1991). Schwann cell expression of PLP/DM20 is an order of magnitude lower than that observed in oligodendrocytes, and most of the proteins produced are not normally incorporated into the myelin sheath (Anderson *et al.*, 1997; Garbern *et al.*, 1997). A low level of PLP/DM20 expression also occurs outside of the nervous system, in the heart (Campagnoni *et al.*, 1992), fetal thymus, spleen (Pribyl *et al.*, 1996), thyroid, testes, and skin (Skoff, unpublished). In general, cells other than myelinating oligodendrocytes tend to favor the synthesis of DM20 over PLP. Even in oligodendrocytes, the DM20 expression profile is not always coincident with myelination, as immature oligodendrocytes selectively express DM20 (Ikenaka *et al.*, 1992; Schindler *et al.*, 1990; Timsit *et al.*, 1992; Timsit *et al.*, 1995; Yu *et al.*, 1994).

## Mutations Result in Overexpression, Loss-of-Function, or Gain-of-Function of PLP

In keeping with the conserved nature of the *PLP* gene, all types of mutations at the *PLP* locus have discernible effects in humans. Most frequently encountered are duplications of the *PLP* gene, which have been estimated to account for 60 to 70% of cases (Inoue *et al.*, 1996; Mimault *et al.*, 1999; Sistermans *et al.*, 1998; Wang *et al.*, 1997), as depicted in Figure 37.1. *PLP* duplications are typically tandem in nature, involving a large genomic segment that includes neighboring genes (Inoue *et al.*, 1996; Inoue *et al.*, 1999a; Woodward *et al.*, 1998). Striking variation in the position of the breakpoints occurs in different PMD families (Inoue *et al.*, 1999a; Woodward *et al.*, 1998), unlike the situation with other inherited duplications such as Charcot-Marie-Tooth disease type 1A (CMT1A) (reviewed in Inoue and Lupski, 2002). The duplicated segment can be as large as three megabases (Mb), more than 150 times the size of the *PLP* locus (Inoue *et al.*, 1999a). Therefore, not only will PLP be overexpressed in these patients, a number of other X-linked genes will be inappropriately expressed. Only a fraction of genes are sensitive to dosage effects, and in the segments of the X chromosome duplicated in the PMD patients, *PLP* is apparently the sole gene for which changes in copy number spawn phenotypic aberrations. Not that the families with duplications display a uniform phenotype (Inoue *et al.*, 1999a; Sistermans *et al.*, 1998; Woodward *et al.*, 1998), as the position of the breakpoints can disrupt other X-linked genes, which if haplo-insufficient could contribute to the overall phenotype. That *PLP* is a gene subject to dosage control is reinforced by the description of possibly three copies of the *PLP* gene in patients with a more severe form of PMD (Harding *et al.*, 1995; Woodward *et al.*, 1998). Unequal sister chromatid exchange in male meiosis is the major mechanism leading to duplication of the *PLP* gene (Inoue *et al.*, 1999a; Mimault *et al.*, 1999). Additional mechanisms of genomic rearrangements operate at the *PLP* locus, as indicated by several families in which the duplicated copy invades another spot on the X chromosome (Hodes *et al.*, 2000).

Despite the large number of duplications arising from sister chromatid exchange, the expected reciprocal recombination event, namely deletion of the *PLP* locus, rarely occurs (Inoue and Lupski, 2002; Raskind *et al.*, 1991). Deletion of the *PLP* gene encompasses a much smaller segment of the X chromosome, with only two neighboring genes (Inoue and Lupski, 2002). Probably the deletion of larger sections of the X chromosome, which would comprise the majority of reciprocal recombination events arising from duplications of PLP, would cause lethality or infertility. By examining the deletion breakpoints in the three identified families, Lupski and coworkers discovered several different modes of genome rearrangement (Inoue *et al.*, 2002). This study reinforces the complexities of recombination involving the *PLP* locus that were initially observed with the PLP duplications and suggests that nonhomologous joining of ends causes *PLP* deletions (Inoue *et al.*, 2002). In addition to the loss-of-function mutations arising from deletion events, two point mutations in the *PLP* coding region at the initiation codon (Sistermans *et al.*, 1996) or the second codon (Garbern *et al.*, 1997) are null for PLP expression. Unlike the *PLP* deletions characterized to date, these null point mutations allow for a direct examination of PLP loss without complicating considerations from deletion of those genes neighboring PLP, namely the RAS superfamily member RAB9L and the thymosin β family member TMSNB (Inoue *et al.*, 2002).

About 20% of PMD patients have point mutations (single base changes or small deletions or insertions) at the *PLP* locus that alter the amino acid sequence of the PLP/

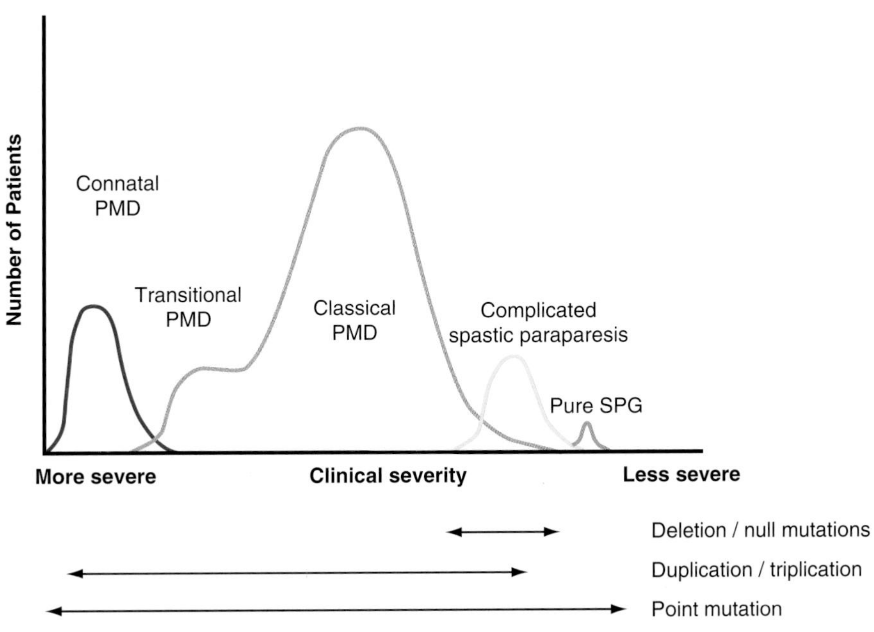


FIGURE 37.1
The clinical spectrum and relative frequency of *PLP1* mutations. The range of clinical syndromes caused by *PLP1* mutations is a set of overlapping distributions rather than a linear gradation from very severe to mild disease. The areas under the curves approximate the observed frequencies of clinical subtypes.

DM20 proteins. These include missense, nonsense, frameshift, and splicing mutations (Fig. 37.2), all of which produce abnormal PLP/DM20 proteins. Of the abnormal PLP/DM20 proteins, a majority result in severely affected patients through a toxic gain-of-function (discussed later), while the remainder create a milder form of the disease that may be categorized as loss-of-function. The loss-of-function class of abnormal proteins cannot fully perform the roles of PLP or DM20, but they do not take on new roles in oligodendrocytes. Approximately 100 distinct mutations have been discovered to date (for an up-to-date accounting of the various point mutations, refer to www.med.wayne.edu/Neurology/plp.html). An extensive collection of missense mutations (those mutations that result in amino acid substitution) in the PLP/DM20 gene exist. Certain amino acid codons have a particularly rich array of changes that offer an opportunity to investigate the consequences of a specific protein alteration on myelination and the clinical manifestations of PMD/SPG2 (Cailloux *et al.*, 2000; Hodes *et al.*, 1999). Three codons were mutated in two missense versions (V165E, V165G; L223I, L223P; Q233Z, Q233P), and one codon was subjected to five different missense mutations: the aspartate at position 202 was changed to an asparagine, histidine, valine, glycine, or glutamate residue in different PMD patients. Codon 202, located in the large external loop of PLP/DM20 (Fig. 37.2), represents a mutational "hot spot." Indeed, the entire external loop has an excessive number of mutations. While mutations are distributed throughout the PLP/DM20 coding sequence, appearing in both the transmembrane and extra-membrane domains, half of the missense mutations occur within the large external loop. The susceptibility of this region hints at conformational cues that may be important in maintaining the intraperiod line in compact myelin. A significant number of mutations are also available in the intracellular domain that is specific for PLP, including a nonsense mutation in exon3B, that enable a comparison of the roles of DM20 and PLP in the myelin sheath of man (Tab. 37.1/Fig. 37.2).

A number of splice site mutations have been uncovered in PMD patients. Of most interest are the splicing mutations that are not located at the strictly conserved positions in the donor and acceptor splice sites, including a deletion of 19 bp within intron 3 and 26 bp in intron 5 (Cailloux *et al.*, 2000; Hobson *et al.*, 2000). Although the spliced products have not been characterized in these families, splicing mutations would most likely result in

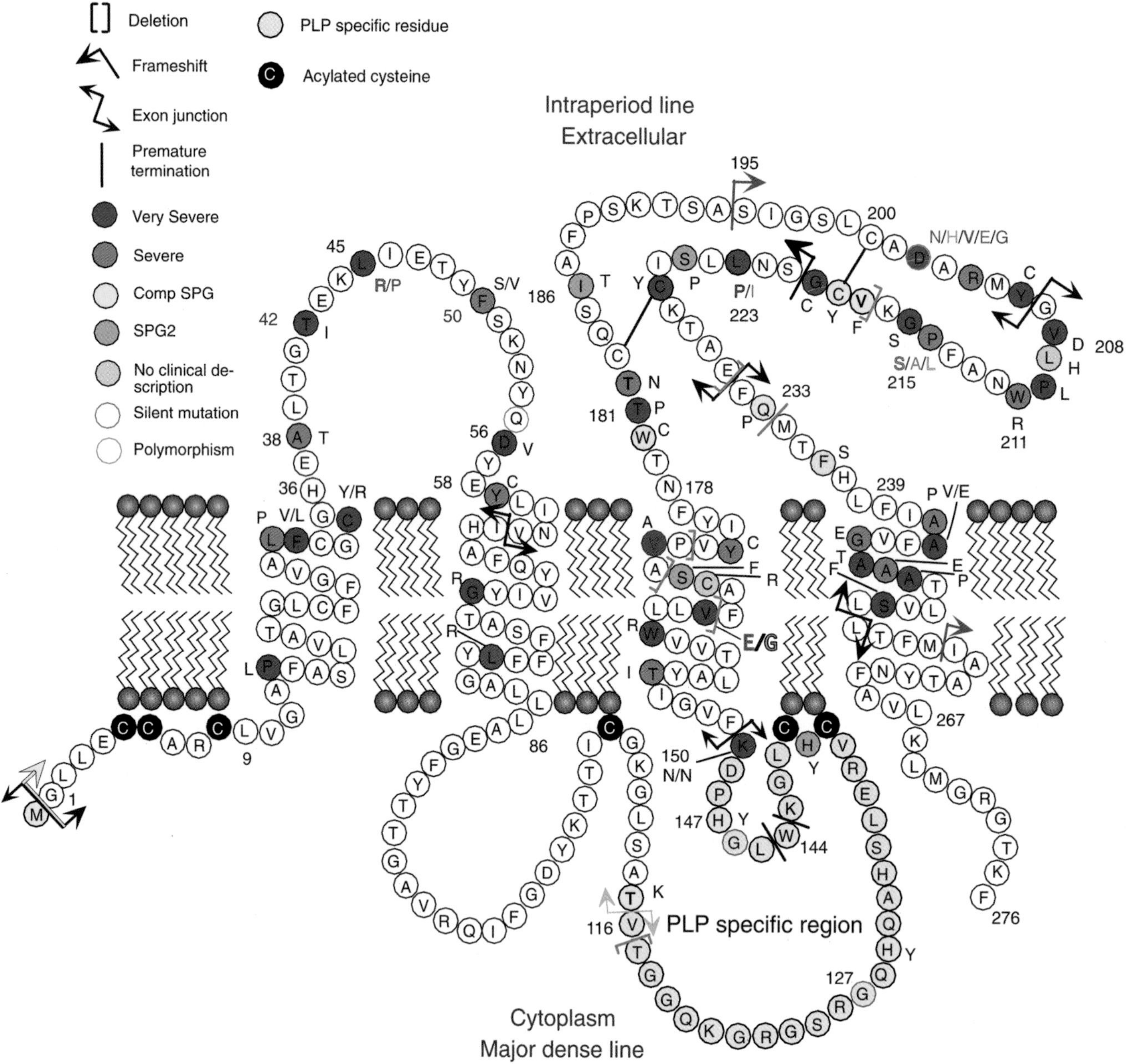


FIGURE 37.2
Point mutations of the *PLP1* gene. The orientation of the tetraspan PLP and DM20 proteins in the plasma membrane and myelin sheath is depicted together with the acylation sites (cysteine residues #5,6,8,108,138, and 140) and the disulfide bridges in the large extracellular loop. Citations for the mutations described in this figure can be found at www.med.wayne.edu/Neurology/ClinicalPrograms/PelizaeusMerzbacher/plp.html. When more than one mutation occurs at a single position, the most severe phenotype is indicated. For completeness, some mutations are presented that have been described without clinical information. When limited clinical information was available, the disease severity was assigned as follows: very severe (equivalent to "connatal") syndrome was ascribed if the patient was explicitly described as connatal, neurologic signs were present at birth or death occurred before 20 years of age; severe: neurologic signs were present in first few months of life, patient was described explicitly as intermediate or classical PMD or death occurred after 20 years of age; complicated SPG: patient was able to walk effectively for at least a few years and had CNS signs in addition to spastic paraparesis; SPG2: "pure" spastic paraparesis not associated with other CNS signs.

skipping of an exon, an event that would create an internally deleted and possibly a frameshifted abnormal PLP protein. However, mutations within intron 3 that eliminate the donor splice site have the potential of leaving the DM20 transcript and protein unscathed. The atypical splicing mutations at the *PLP* locus (Cailloux *et al.*, 2000; Hobson *et al.*, 2000) suggest that even more splicing mutations may be found in PMD/SPG2 patients, mutations that have eluded detection because sequencing efforts usually concentrate on coding regions and intron/exon junctions.

Another category of point mutations is the regulatory mutations that alter the expression of the PLP gene without affecting the protein sequence. A putative promoter mutation has been reported in a PMD family at −34 of the *PLP1* gene (Kawanishi *et al.*, 1996). Whether this is the causative change that alters PLP/DM20 expression in the reported family is not known. Additional changes may occur within regulatory elements of the *PLP* gene, which are not yet fully defined, or splice sites that affect *PLP* gene expression. Nonetheless, the C to T transition at −34 is of interest as it is within the area bound by the RNA polymerase complex prior to the commencement of transcription at the upstream initiation site (reviewed in Chapter 16). A second class of regulatory mutations that create a PMD-like disorder may arise in genes encoding transcription factors that recognize the *PLP* promoter. The transcription factors that directly bind to the *PLP* promoter are candidates (reviewed in Chapter 16), as are factors known to affect PLP expression, such as the homeodomain protein Nkx2.2 (Fu *et al.*, 2002; Qi *et al.*, 2001) or the high-mobility-group regulator Sox10 (Stolt *et al.*, 2002). One Sox10 mutation has been described that combines features of PMD, Charcot-Marie-Tooth disease type 1, and Waardenburg-Hirschsprung syndrome (Inoue *et al.*, 1999b). The occurrence of such mutations is rare, as no additional Sox10 mutations were found when screening 56 patients with Charcot-Marie-Tooth disease or 88 leukodystrophies, all patients previously sequenced for the usual candidate genes (Pingault *et al.*, 2002). Nonethess, this cohort of patients may be affected in Nkx2.2 (Fu *et al.*, 2002; Qi *et al.*, 2001) or one of the other transcription factors that influence PLP expression. Apart from the broader phenotypes expected from the mutation of a transcription factor that acts on multiple target genes, the absence of X-linkage in disorders caused by mutated transcription factors would genotypically distinguish them from PMD patients with mutations in the *PLP1* gene.

## DIAGNOSIS, PRESENTATION AND CLINICAL COURSE OF PMD/SPG2

The nomenclature of clinical syndromes arising from *PLP1* mutations has generated confusion and some controversy, and stems from the variability of syndromes caused by different mutations and from the variable expressivity of an individual mutation among family members (see Fig. 37.1 and Tab. 37.1). The most consistent features of PMD include spasticity, a lack of evidence of male-to-male transmission in the family, and generalized leukodystrophy on magnetic resonance imaging scans. However, even these relaxed criteria, applied too strictly, might exclude some patients who have only ataxia and tremor, or those infants with severe mutations who have hypotonia at onset. The diagnosis of Pelizaeus-Merzbacher disease (PMD) is thus suggested in affected individuals by the presence of a characteristic set of neurological signs and symptoms, including nystagmus, spastic paraparesis, and limb ataxia, a family history of disease consistent with an X-linked recessive pattern of inheritance, and an MRI scan demonstrating diffuse central nervous system abnormalities of myelination. The diagnosis can be unequivocally established in about 80% of patients by molecular genetic testing to identify a *PLP1* gene duplication or *PLP1* gene mutation, as discussed in the previous section on genetic mechanisms and in the discussion that follows.

Although the clinical presentation and course of PMD varies depending upon the nature of the *PLP1* mutation, the disease usually presents in one of three typical patterns. The most severe form of disease, *connatal PMD*, begins during the first weeks of life, and is associated with hypotonia, respiratory distress, stridor, nystagmus, and sometimes seizures. Because of the prominence of hypotonia and respiratory symptoms, connatal PMD can be confused with motor neuron disease or spinal muscular atrophy (Kaye *et al.*, 1994). Individuals with connatal PMD go on to develop severe spasticity with little voluntary movement, and never ambulate. In addition, they have very poor head control and cannot sit unsupported. Growth is poor, and they develop very limited language skills. These individuals usually die before the third decade of life. The most common form of disease, in contrast, *classic PMD*, begins during the neonatal period, usually within the first year of life and is associated with nystagmus, lower extremity weakness, and head titubation. Respiration is normal. Muscle tone is often reduced during infancy, but progresses to spasticity later during childhood. Motor milestones are also usually delayed in classic PMD, and most individuals never walk independently. Patients with this disease go on to develop a spastic quadraparesis, worse in the lower than in the upper extremities. Ataxia of trunk and limb movements is also a prominent feature of classic PMD, and dystonic posturing and movements also occur. Most individuals acquire some degree of language skill, which may even approach normal levels, but the speech is dysarthric and the speed of language output is usually slow. In addition, patients with the classic form of PMD also have some degree of cognitive disability. These patients can survive until the sixth decade of life. The mildest form of PMD merges clinically with syndromes of *X-linked spastic paraparesis* (SPG2). This disease begins during childhood, usually within the first 5 years of life and is associated with a mild to severe spastic paraplegia, although there may also be limb and gait ataxia. Patients with SPG2 may have nystagmus as an early sign (Bonneau *et al.*, 1993; Saugier-Veber *et al.*, 1994) but others may not develop this, or it may occur as a late sign and manifest as end-gaze rather than primary position nystagmus (Garbern *et al.*, 1997; Johnston and McKusick, 1962). Motor milestones are usually delayed, but most individuals learn to walk independently during childhood, although this ability may be lost later in life. Language skills and intelligence can be normal, although there also may be mild cognitive impairment. Individuals with this form of PMD usually have a normal life span. MRI scans are usually abnormal, but the findings can be regional or very subtle in comparison to those of patients with the more severe forms of PMD (see Fig. 37.3). Table 37.1 summarizes these three typical patterns of PMD, based on our own clinical observations as well as those of Boulloche and Aicardi (1986), Hodes *et al.* (1993), and Cailloux *et al.* (2000).

Magnetic resonance imaging (MRI) analysis of the brain is essential in the evaluation of individuals with clinical signs and symptoms of PMD/SPG2 (Ono *et al.*, 1994; Nezu *et al.*, 1998). Virtually all patients with PMD eventually have MRI findings consistent with a leukodystrophy, including diffusely increased signal intensity within the central white matter of the cerebral hemispheres, cerebellum, and brain stem, best seen on either T2-weighted or fluid attenuated inversion recovery (FLAIR) sequences, as shown in Figure 37.3. Although the relative white matter volume can be reduced and the corpus callosum thinned, brain structure is otherwise normal, including the ventricular system, basal ganglia, and cortical surface. Because myelination is an ongoing process during postnatal development, the signal intensity of myelinated tracks is not constant during this time. For this reason, the T2-weighted or FLAIR images may not be unequivocally abnormal in PMD until a child is older than 2 years of age. Patients with the more mild spastic paraplegia phenotype have similar MRI changes, but these may be less pronounced or more patchy in nature (Cambi *et al.*, 1995; Hodes *et al.*, 1999) (Fig. 37.3).

Other diagnostic considerations for individuals with the clinical features of PMD include metachromatic leukodystrophy, adrenoleukodystrophy, Krabbe disease, Cockayne disease, and Canavan disease. None of these diseases, however, are associated with nystagmus, which is common in PMD, and their diagnosis can usually be made by analysis of the appropriate lysosomal enzyme. In addition, the white matter abnormalities in these conditions are often regional rather than diffuse: The occipital white matter is most affected in adrenoleukodystrophy, while the frontal white matter is most affected in metachromatic leukodystrophy. Infants with merosin deficiency can also have dramatically increased T2 signal in the cerebral white matter, but the presence of severe weakness and hypotonia and the absence of nystagmus should direct the clinician toward consideration of myopathy. A fatal X-linked syndrome of ataxia, blindness, deafness, and mental retardation has been described and is linked to Xq21-24, but the MRI does not show a pattern of leukodystrophy, and mutations in the *PLP* coding regions have been excluded. Finally, mutations in the cell adhesion molecule gene *L1CAM* cause X-linked spastic paraplegia type 1 (SPG1), a disorder associated with mental retardation and adducted thumbs, which is allelic to the MASA syndrome (mental retardation, aphasia, shuffling gait, adducted thumbs) and X-linked hydrocephalus. MRIs of these disorders may show

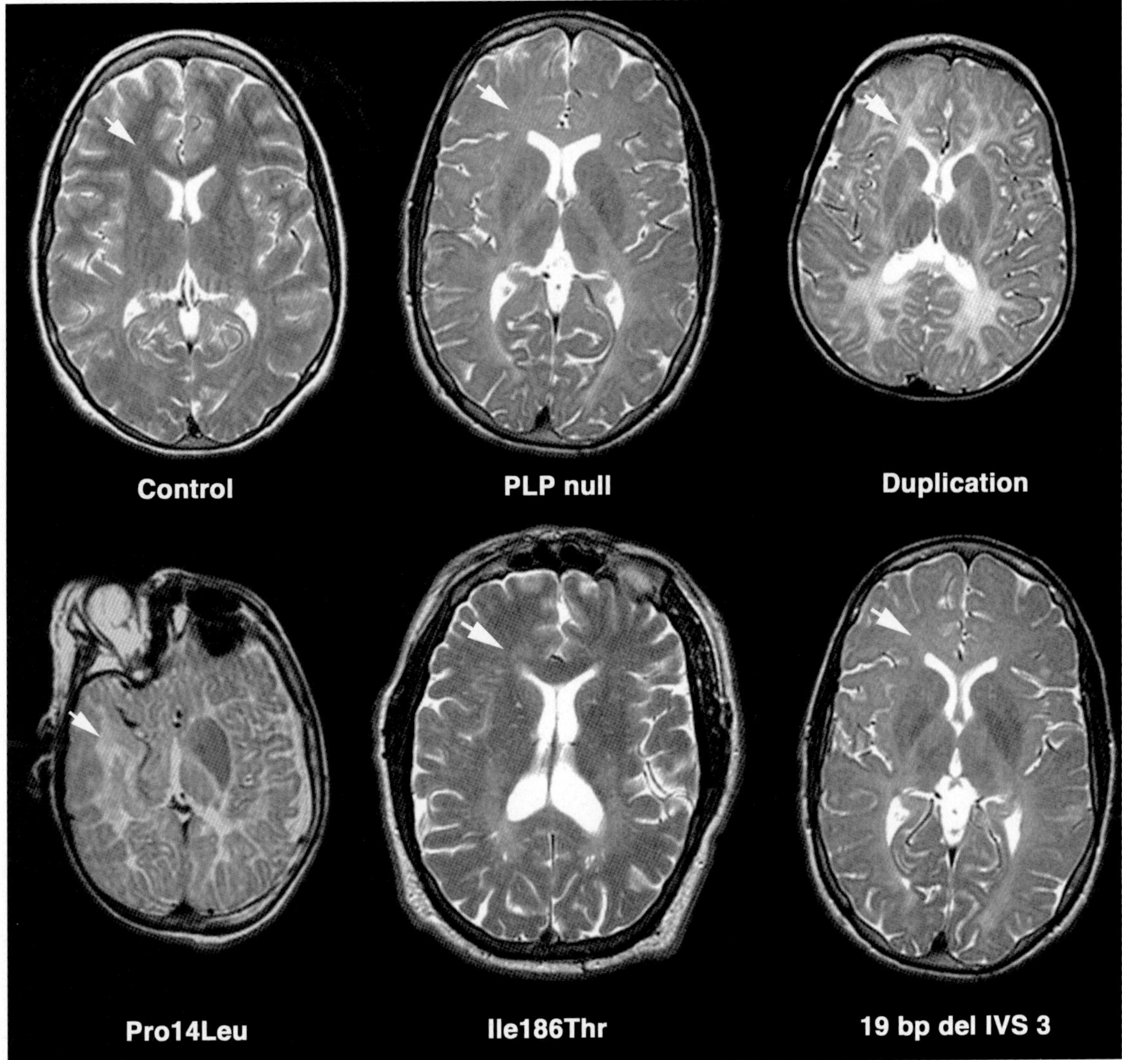


FIGURE 37.3
MRI of *PLP1* mutations with a spectrum of severity. All images are T2 weighted scans of affected males, with the exception of the control. Ages of the patients are control, 17 year old female; PLP1 null, 17 years; duplication, 12 years; Pro14Leu, 20 years; Ile186Thr, 45 years; and IVS3 deletion, 9 years. The Pro14Leu mutation represents the severely affected, connatal form of the disease, the duplication corresponds to the intermediate classical form, and the remaining images represent the mild SPG2 syndrome (PLP null, Ile186Thr and the splicing defect marked 19bp del IVS 3). The arrowhead points to areas of frontal lobe white matter and illustrates the difference in signal abnormality among this group of patients (on T2 weighted scans signal brightness increases with myelin abnormality). Note that the SPG2 patients have normal to subtle signal abnormalities compared to the duplication and connatal PMD patients.

enlarged ventricles or agenesis of the corpus callosum, but not the diffuse abnormalities of white matter consistent with a leukodystrophy.

Women with a *PLP1* gene mutation may have neurological signs and symptoms, but are not usually index cases. Several investigators have observed that, in families with severely affected males, the heterozygous women are unlikely to have clinical manifestations of PMD/SPG2, whereas in families with mildly affected males, the heterozygous women are more likely to have symptoms (Bond *et al.*, 1997; Sivakumar *et al.*, 1999). In a family with a particularly mild syndrome characterized by ataxia and mild spastic paraplegia, all three heterozygous females had neurologic signs (Hodes *et al.*, 1997). Animals with mutations of *PLP1* also exist in which severe alleles may cause transient neurologic signs in heterozygotes (Cuddon *et al.*, 1998) and mild alleles cause persistent neurologic signs in heterozygotes (Fanarraga *et al.*, 1991). These interesting phenomena will be discussed further in a subsequent section, and in Chapter 47.

### *Peripheral Neuropathy in PMD*

Some patients with PMD have a demyelinating peripheral neuropathy (Garbern *et al.*, 1997). The neuropathy in these patients is mild, however, and not usually clinically significant. Electrophysiological studies demonstrate areas of modestly slowed nerve conduction velocities distributed nonuniformly along the nerve (Garbern *et al.*, 1999).

### *Genetic Testing in PMD*

Approximately 80% of patients with clinical, genetic, and MRI features consistent with PMD have been found to have *PLP1* mutations. The genetic etiology for the other 20% of patients is not known but may be due either to mutations in areas of the PLP1 gene not routinely analyzed, such as introns and regulatory regions, or the presence of an additional autosomal or X-linked mutation that can cause the same phenotype (Osaka *et al.*, 1999). Duplication of the region surrounding the *PLP1* gene at Xq22 accounts for the majority of mutations in patients with PMD (Mimault *et al.*, 1999), perhaps up to 70%, while point mutations, small deletions, or insertions make up the rest. Deletion of the entire *PLP1* gene has been identified in a small number of patients with PMD (Boespflug-Tanguy *et al.*, 1999; Raskind *et al.*, 1991), and interstitial duplications or more complex rearrangements of the X chromosome visible on routine cytogenetic studies have been found in several others (Carrozzo *et al.*, 1997; Cremers *et al.*, 1987; Zackai *et al.*, 1997).

Because duplication of the *PLP1* region is the most common cause of PMD, identification of a *PLP1* gene duplication is the most efficient initial genetic screening test for diagnosing PMD. The duplications are of variable size, but they are usually found within an 800-kb region of the X chromosome including the *PLP1* gene (Inoue *et al.*, 1996; Inoue *et al.*, 1999a; Sistermans *et al.*, 1998; Woodward *et al.*, 1998). The duplicated region can also be found, however, at some distance from Xq22. One *PLP1* duplication has been identified at Xp22 and a second at Xq28 (Hodes *et al.*, 2000; Woodward *et al.*, 1998). Both interphase fluorescent *in situ* hybridization (FISH) and quantitative polymerase chain reaction (QPCR) have been used to detect *PLP1* duplications (Hobson *et al.*, 2000; Inoue *et al.*, 1996; Inoue *et al.*, 1999a; Shaffer *et al.*, 1997). Duplications smaller than 50 kb, however, may not be resolved by FISH, while QPCR does not provide important cytogenetic information on the location of the duplication (Shaffer *et al.*, 1997). For these reasons, both methods, interphase FISH and QPCR, should be routinely employed for the molecular genetic diagnosis of PMD.

If neither interphase FISH nor QPCR demonstrates a *PLP1* duplication, direct sequence analysis of the PLP1 gene should be performed. The *PLP1* gene encodes a relatively small protein of 277 amino acids (831 bp of DNA) and the coding sequences are contained within only seven exons. Using automated sequencing methods, therefore, it is cost-effective as well as technically straightforward to obtain the DNA sequence of the *PLP1* exons and portions of their surrounding introns. When a small mutation is found, it is sometimes possible to design an allele-specific oligonucleotide hybridization test or a simple PCR/restriction digestion assay to detect the mutation (Hobson *et al.*, 2000), which can be particularly helpful for confirmation of carrier status in females.

Prenatal DNA diagnosis of PMD in affected males at risk for the disease has been accomplished by several groups of investigators but is not routinely available. A *PLP1* duplication in an at-risk male fetus has been identified using both interphase FISH (Inoue *et al.*, 2001a) and QPCR (Regis *et al.*, 2001). A *PLP1* point mutation in an at-risk male fetus, however, has not been reported, although prenatal testing has successfully excluded such mutations (Maenpaa *et al.*, 1990; Strautnieks *et al.*, 1992). Preimplantation genetic diagnosis for PMD is possible but has not been reported. Identification of a *PLP1* duplication in single cells is also possible, although technical difficulties currently preclude its use as a diagnostic tool in patients.

### *Genotype-Phenotype Correlations*

No simple correlation has been found between a particular *PLP1* mutation or genotype, and the clinical manifestation of the disease or phenotype. Although most patients with duplications have the classic form of PMD (Inoue *et al.*, 1999a), some have the more severe connatal form (Ellis and Malcolm, 1994), while others have a milder spastic paraparesis. Inoue and coworkers recently analyzed the duplication size and structure in 20 families with PMD and suggested that the size of the PLP1 duplication correlated with the clinical phenotype (Inoue *et al.*, 1999a), so that patients with larger duplications, had more severe disease. In a similar study of 16 families with PLP duplications, however, Hobson and coworkers did not confirm this finding (Hobson, unpublished), suggesting that other structural features of the duplication, such as the location, breakpoint, or orientation, may also play a role.

Callioux and colleagues recently compared the clinical phenotype and genotype in 33 families with *PLP1* point mutations (Cailloux *et al.*, 2000). They found that single amino acid changes within evolutionarily conserved regions of the protein produced the most severe disease, while substitutions of less conserved amino acids, protein truncations, null mutations, and mutations within the *PLP1*-specific region (amino acids 116–150) produced a milder form of disease. Although exceptions to this rule occur, more severe forms of disease are likely to be associated with missense mutations within highly conserved regions of the protein.

Garbern and coworkers analyzed several families with PLP1 mutations in which no protein product was produced, so-called null mutations (Garbern *et al.*, 1997; Garbern *et al.*, 2002). These patients all had a relatively mild spastic paraparesis, which progressed during adolescence as well as an associated demyelinating peripheral neuropathy identified during electrophysiological testing. The neuropathy was not correlated with disease severity and was not found in patients with either duplications or point mutations in which protein was produced. Taken together, these data suggest that individuals with a relatively mild form of disease and peripheral neuropathy are likely to have a null mutation.

## MOLECULAR PATHOGENESIS OF PMD

Gow and Lazzarini proposed that differences in clinical severity in patients with *PLP1* coding region mutations can be accounted for by a differential effect of the specific mutation on the folding and intracellular trafficking of the protein (reviewed in Southwood and Gow, 2001). Mutations that affect the folding and transport to the cell surface of both PLP and DM20 are associated with the most severe PMD phenotypes and also cause increased oligodendrocyte cell death, while mutations that impair transport of PLP but not DM20 produce a less severe PMD phenotype that is not associated with oligodendrocyte cell death (Gow and Lazzarini, 1996; Gow *et al.*, 1998). Since mutations in which no mutant protein is synthesized cause the mildest disease, the predominant effect of *PLP1* coding region mutations is probably due to misfolded *PLP1* gene products. The cellular and molecular effects of the accumulation of misfolded PLP1 and DM20 in the RER of oligodendrocytes, rather than the absence of these proteins in the myelin sheath, are thus the cause of the clinical signs and symptoms of PMD.

Not only does the protein-misfolding hypothesis explain the differential clinical effect of *PLP* mutations, it also explains the effect of these mutations on female carriers. Female dogs that are heterozygous for a severe mutation in the canine *PLP*, for example, have neurological abnormalities early in life, but by adulthood are clinically normal, have normal numbers of oligodendrocytes, and express very little mutant *PLP* messenger RNA (Cuddon *et al.*, 1998). Female PMD carriers are also usually clinically unaffected, although some may have transient neurological abnormalities as children (Hodes *et al.*, 1995). In some PMD families, however, female heterozygotes are clinically affected, as in the family described by Pelizaeus and Merzbacher (Pelizaeus, 1885). Because of random inactivation of the X chromosome on which the *PLP* gene is located, females who are heterozygous for *PLP* mutations should express the abnormal protein in approximately 50% of their oligodendrocytes. Oligodendrocytes expressing a more severe *PLP* mutation, however, in which both PLP and DM20 are affected, undergo increased cell death and are eliminated during myelination and replaced by normal oligodendrocytes. In contrast, oligodendrocytes expressing a less severe *PLP* mutation, which does not cause cell death, are not eliminated, thus producing abnormal myelin and neurological dysfunction. Paradoxically then, females who are heterozygous for the less severe *PLP* mutations are more likely to experience neurological difficulties as adults than are females who are heterozygous for the more severe *PLP* alleles (Hodes *et al.*, 1995; Inoue *et al.*, 2001b; Sivakumar *et al.*, 1999; Sambuughin *et al.*, 1998). Similar observations have been made with experimental and naturally occurring murine *PLP* mutations (see Chapter 47).

How does accumulation of misfolded DM-20/PLP1 in the ER of oligodendrocytes affect their function? Several lines of evidence point to the involvement of the unfolded protein response (UPR), a network of genes that are induced in response to unfolded proteins and that act to regulate expression of molecular chaperones, transcription factors, caspases, and other genes (reviewed by Kaufman *et al.*, 2002). Two bZip transcription factors, CHOP (CEBPβ-homologous protein) and ATF3, are induced during the UPR and have been shown to cause apoptosis when overexpressed in transfected cells. Gow and coworkers recently found that both *CHOP* and *ATF3* expression as well as several other RER-resident molecular chaperones are similarly induced in oligodendrocytes in response to the synthesis of mutant *PLP1* gene products, implicating the UPR in the pathogenesis of oligodendrocyte cell death in PMD (Southwood *et al.*, 2002). These investigators also discovered that *rumpshaker(rsh)* mice without a functional *Chop* gene (*rsh/chop*-null double mutants) have a more severe disease than *rsh* mice, directly implicating CHOP expression in the pathogenesis of PMD. It is thus likely that the set of genes induced during the UPR plays a role in PMD pathogenesis by protecting oligodendrocytes from the toxic effects of misfolded DM-20 and PLP.

Protein misfolding has been implicated as a pathogenic mechanism in several other neurodegenerative diseases, including Alzheimer's, Parkinson's, and Huntington's diseasse (Aridor and Balch, 1999; Kopito and Ron, 2000; Taylor *et al.*, 2002). The morphological features associated with protein accumulation in these diseases include amorphous aggregates in the RER, cytoplasm or nucleus, and intermediate filament-containing aggresomes in the cytoplasm (Johnston *et al.*, 1998). Perinuclear inclusions are also observed in a variety of cell types, particularly in cultured cells treated with proteasome complex inhibitors, and are thought to form when the RER-to-cytoplasm delivery of unfolded proteins exceeds degradation by the proteasome complex. Aggresome-like inclusions are rarely found in PMD, however, because myelinating oligodendrocytes do not normally synthesize intermediate filaments. Proliferating oligodendrocyte precursor cells express vimentin and nestin in culture, but the expression of these genes is switched off as the cells differentiate (Almazan *et al.*, 2001). Although protein misfolding has been implicated in all of these diseases, the molecular mechanisms of oligodendrocyte cell death in PMD may thus be different than those in the more classic neurodegenerative diseases.

A second pathogenic mechanism in PMD is associated with the overexpression of PLP in patients with duplications of the PLP gene. Excessive amounts of normal PLP proteins have been shown to accumulate in the late endosome and lysosomal compartments of rodent cells overexpressing PLP (Simons *et al.*, 2002). Since PLP typically associates with cholesterol and other lipids to form myelin "rafts" as it trafficks through the Golgi compartment (Simons *et al.*, 2000), the shunting of excess PLP into the endosomal/lysosomal compartment effectively drains myelin lipids from the Golgi (Simons *et al.*, 2002). Presumably the transport and assembly of myelin constituents is altered in cells overexpressing PLP. Thus, while abnormal PLP proteins trigger a protein misfolding response in the rough endoplasmic reticulum, excessive PLP proteins create an imbalance in myelin constituents that adversely affects the subsequent stage of nascent myelin assembly in the Golgi network. Occasionally females with a duplication of the *PLP* gene manifest on early-onset neurological phenotype (Inoue *et al.*, 2001b). Like some carriers of *PLP* point mutations, these patients with mild PMD or spastic paraplegia show sustained clinical improvement. The recovery of these heterozygous females is probably attributable to the same mechanism favored for the point mutations, namely compensatory myelin production by the normal oligodendrocytes that contain only a single copy of the *PLP* gene.

A third mechanism of molecular pathogenesis in PMD/SPG2 occurs by loss-of-function, in patients with a deletion of the *PLP* gene (Boespflug-Tanguy *et al.*, 1999; Inoue *et al.*, 2002; Raskind *et al.*, 1991) or with point mutations at the beginning of the coding region that preclude translation (Garbern *et al.*, 1997; Sistermans *et al.*, 1996). These patients have less severe forms of the disease, with the *PLP* deletions giving rise to either a complicated form of SPG2 or a mild form of PMD (Inoue *et al.*, 2002). In mice lacking PLP, oligodendrocytes develop normally and manage to assemble a myelin sheath, yet defects in the intraperiod line of these sheaths translate into reduced conduction velocities and impaired motor coordination (Boison and Stoffel, 1994; Boison *et al.*, 1995; Klugmann *et al.*, 1997; Rosenbluth *et al.*, 1996; Yool *et al.*, 2002, reviewed in Chapter 47 by Nave). In addition, null mutations also produce axonal pathology (discussed later). These pathological changes suggest there is an absolute requirement for PLP both to maintain the structure of compact myelin and to maintain axonal integrity and function. Thus, the absence of PLP would neither trigger the unfolded protein response nor derail myelin assembly, but would instead negatively affect maintenance of the myelin sheath.

### *PLP Mutations Cause Axonal Damage*

Evidence of axonal damage has been recently found in both PMD and its animal models, a finding that is important for future understanding of the pathogenesis of demyelinating disease and its treatment. In his original description of the neuropathological features of PMD, Merzbacher noted: "*Es stellt sich nämlich heraus: daß dort, wo die Markscheiden fehlen, auch keine Achsencylinder nachweisbar sind*" (It is evident that there are no axons demonstrated where the myelin sheaths are absent) (Merzbacher, 1910). Unconvinced that axonal damage existed in PMD, Merzbacher nonetheless concluded that axons were much thinner and did not stain well with axonal stains. Definitive evidence for axonal damage in PMD was subsequently provided in several rodent models, including those caused by *PLP* point mutations (Rosenfeld and Freidrich, 1983), increased *PLP* gene dosage (Anderson *et al.*, 1998), and *PLP* null mutation (Garbern *et al.*, 2002; Griffiths *et al.*, 1998). Consistent with this interpretation, Garbern and coworkers have found evidence for axonal damage in both mice and patients with a *PLP1* null mutation by a combination of direct pathological examination of brain tissue and magnetic resonance spectroscopy (Garbern *et al.*, 2002). The axonal injury is not due to demyelination, since myelin is intact in both patients and experimental animals, or oligodendrocyte cell death, since these cells appear healthy and ensheathe axons. The extent of axonal injury increases with age and probably accounts for the progression of neurological signs and symptoms. In addition, the axonal degeneration is length dependent, suggesting that impaired axonal transport is a cause. These data suggest that progressive axonal damage is not only a common feature of the pathogenesis of PMD, it is also clinically relevant. Because axonal degeneration occurs without significant demyelination, it probably arises from the absence or perturbation of PLP-mediated oligodendrocyte-axonal interactions. Consistent with this notion, Scherer and collaborators have shown that axoglial junctions at the paranodal region are disrupted in *md* rats (Arroyo *et al.*, 2002), an animal model with a *plp* point mutation, and that these changes are probably involved in disease pathogenesis.

Interestingly, the axonal abnormalities in PMD are very similar to those described by Trapp and coworkers in multiple sclerosis (MS) (Trapp *et al.*, 1998), suggesting that the axonal abnormalities in MS, like those in PMD, may likewise result from disruption of oligodendrocyte-axonal interactions. Axonal degeneration is clinically relevant in MS, since the *N*-acetyl aspartate/creatine ratio is decreased in the brains of patients with MS, even in regions outside of MS lesions, and correlates well with clinical disability (De Stefano *et al.*, 1997; Fu *et al.*, 1998; Grossman *et al.*, 1992). Also, axonal damage in MS may underlie the secondary progressive phase of the disease, which does not respond significantly to immune modulation. Further understanding of the mechanisms of axonal degeneration in PMD will thus also be important in MS and may lead to the development of new treatment strategies for both diseases.

### *Management and Future Prospects*

Currently, there is no specific therapy for patients with PMD. The observation that most patients with PMD have a gene duplication and thus overexpress PLP or have a point mutation causing a gain-of-function precludes simple replacement gene therapy, even if appropriate delivery vehicles were to become available. In fact, for most patients, the more appropriate goal might be the *reduction* of PLP expression, such as through antisense gene therapy, since absence of PLP results in a less severe syndrome. The finding that axonal degeneration is clinically relevant in the pathogenesis of PMD also raises the possibility that therapy directed at maintaining the integrity of axons might be effective in this disorder. Cellular therapy, such as transplantation of oligodendrocyte precursors into the CNS, has shown potential in animal models of PMD (Brustle *et al.*, 1999; Duncan *et al.*, 1988; Duncan and Milward, 1995; Duncan *et al.*, 1997; Lachapelle *et al.*, 1990) and might therefore be effective in patients. Cellular therapy has not yet reversed the clinical deficits in animal models, however, and for maximum effectiveness, this therapy may need to be initiated either *in utero* or shortly after birth.

## References


Almazan, G., Vela, J. M., Molina-Holgado, E., and Guaza, C. (2001). Re-evaluation of nestin as a marker of oligodendrocyte lineage cells. *Microsc. Res. Tech.* **52**(6), 753–765.

Anderson, T. J., Montague, P., Nadon, N., Nave, K. A., and Griffiths, I. R. (1997). Modification of Schwann cell phenotype with Plp transgenes: Evidence that the PLP and DM20 isoproteins are targeted to different cellular domains. *J. Neurosci. Res.* **50**(1), 13–22.

Anderson, T. J., Schneider, A., Barrie, J. A., Klugmann, M., McCulloch, M. C., Kirkham, D., Kyriakides, E., Nave, K.-A., and Griffiths, I. R. (1998). Late-Onset Neurodegeneration in Mice with Increased Dosage of the Proteolipid Protein Gene. *J. Comp. Neurol.* **394,** 506–519.

Aridor, M., and Balch, W. E. (1999). Integration of endoplasmic reticulum signaling in health and disease. *Nat. Med.* **5,** 745–751.

Arroyo, E. J., Xu, T., Grinspan, J., Lambert, S., Levinson, S. R., Brophy, P. J., Peles, E., and Scherer, S. S. (2002). Genetic dysmyelination alters the molecular architecture of the nodal region. *J. Neurosci.* **22**(5), 1726–1737.

Bizzozero, O. A., McGarry, J. F., and Lees, M. B. (1987). Autoacylation of myelin proteolipid protein with acyl coenzyme A. *Biol Chem.* **262**(28), 13550–13557.

Boespflug-Tanguy, O., Giraud, G., Mimault, C., Isabelle, V., and Dinh, D. P. (1999). Heterogeneous rearrangements of the PLP genomic region in Pelizaeus-Merzbacher Disease: Genotype-phenotype correlation in 41 patients. *Am. J. Hum. Genet.* **65,** Program Nr: 1597.

Boison, D., Bussow, H., D'Urso, D., Muller, H. W., and Stoffel, W. (1995). Adhesive properties of proteolipid protein are responsible for the compaction of CNS myelin sheaths. *J. Neurosci.* **15**(8), 5502–5513.

Boison, D., and Stoffel, W. (1994). Disruption of the compacted myelin sheath of axons of the central nervous system in proteolipid protein-deficient mice. *Proc. Natl. Acad. Sci. U. S. A.* **91**(24), 11709–11713.

Bond, C., Si, X., Crisp, M., Wong, P., Paulson, G. W., Boesel, C. P., Dlouhy, S. R., and Hodes, M. E. (1997). Family with Pelizaeus-Merzbacher disease/X-linked spastic paraplegia and a nonsense mutation in exon 6 of the proteolipid protein gene. *Am. J. Med. Genet.* **71,** 357–360.

Bongarzone, E. R., Campagnoni, C. W., Kampf, K., Jacobs, E. C., Handley, V. W., Schonmann, V., and Campagnoni, A. T. (1999). Identification of a New Exon in the Myelin Proteolipid Protein Gene Encoding Novel Protein Isoforms That Are Restricted to the Somata of Oligodendrocytes and Neurons. *J. Neurosci.* **19**(19), 8349–8357.

Bonneau, D., Rozet, J. M., Bulteau, C., Berthier, M., Mettey, R., Gil, R., Munnich, A., and Le Merrer, M. (1993). X linked spastic paraplegia (SPG2): Clinical heterogeneity at a single gene locus. *J. Med. Genet.* **30**(5), 381–384.

Boulloche, J., and Aicardi, J. (1986). Pelizaeus-Merzbacher disease: Clinical and nosological study. *J. Child Neurol.* **1**(3), 233–239.

Brustle, O., Jones, K. N., Learish, R. D., Karram, K., Choudhary, K., Wiestler, O. D., Duncan, I. D., and McKay, R. D. (1999). Embryonic stem cell-derived glial precursors: A source of myelinating transplants *Science* **285**(5428), 754–756.

Cailloux, F., Gauthier-Barichard, F., Mimault, C., Isabelle, V., Courtois, V., Giraud, G., Dastugue, B., and Boespflug-Tanguy, O. (2000). Genotype-phenotype correlation in inherited brain myelination defects due to proteolipid protein gene mutations *Eur. J. Hum. Genet.* **8**(11), 837–845.

Cambi, F., Tang, X. M., Cordray, P., Fain, P. R., Keppen, L. D., and Barker, D. F. (1996). Refined genetic mapping and proteolipid protein mutation analysis in X-linked pure hereditary spastic paraplegia. *Neurology* **46**(4), 1112–1117.

Cambi, F., Tartaglino, L., Lublin, F., and McCarren, D. (1995). X-Linked Pure Familial Spastic Paraparesis: Characterization Of a Large Kindred With Magnetic-Resonance-Imaging Studies. *Arch. Neurol.* **52**(7), 665–669.

Campagnoni, C. W., Garbay, B., Micevych, P., Pribyl, T., Kampf, K., Handley, V. W., and Campagnoni, A. T. (1992). DM20 mRNA splice product of the myelin proteolipid protein gene is expressed in the murine heart. *J. Neurosci. Res.* **33**(1), 148–155.

Carrozzo, R., Arrigo, G., Rossi, E., Bardoni, B., Cammarata, M., Gandullia, P., Gatti, R., and Zuffardi, O. (1997). Multiple congenital anomalies, brain hypomyelination, and ocular albinism in a female with dup(X) (pter→q24::q21.32→qter) and random X inactivation. *Am. J. Med. Genet.* **72**(3), 329–334.

Cremers, F. P., Pfeiffer, R. A., van de Pol, T. J., Hofker, M. H., Kruse, T. A., Wieringa, B., and Ropers, H. H. (1987). An interstitial duplication of the X chromosome in a male allows physical fine mapping of probes from the Xq13-q22 region. *Hum. Genet.* **77**(1), 23–27.

Cuddon, P. A., Lipsitz, D., and Duncan, I. D. (1998). Myelin mosaicism and brain plasticity in heterozygous females of a canine X-linked trait *Ann. Neurol.* **44**(5), 771–779.

De Stefano, N., Matthews, P. M., Narayanan, S., Francis, G. S., Antel, J. P., and Arnold, D. L. (1997). Axonal dysfunction and disability in a relapse of multiple sclerosis: Longitudinal study of a patient. *Neurology* **49**(4), 1138–1141.

Dickinson, P. J., Griffiths, I. R., Barrie, J. M., Kyriakides, E., Pollock, G. F., and Barnett, S. C. (1997). Expression of the DM-20 isoform of the PLP gene in olfactory nerve ensheathing cells: Evidence from developmental studies. *J. Neurocytol.* **26**(3), 181–189.

Diehl, H. J., Schaich, M., Budzinski, R. M., and Stoffel, W. (1986). Individual exons encode the integral membrane domains of human myelin proteolipid protein [published erratum appears in Proc Natl Acad Sci U S A 1991 Apr;86(6), 617–8]. *Proc. Natl. Acad. Sci. U. S. A.* **83**(24), 9807–9811.

Duncan, I. D., Grever, W. E., and Zhang, S. C. (1997). Repair of myelin disease: Strategies and progress in animal models. *Mol. Med. Today* **3**(12), 554–561.

Duncan, I. D., Hammang, J. P., Jackson, K. F., Wood, P. M., Bunge, R. P., and Langford, L. (1988). Transplantation of oligodendrocytes and Schwann cells into the spinal cord of the myelin-deficient rat. *J. Neurocytol.* **17**(3), 351–360.

Duncan, I. D., and Milward, E. A. (1995). Glial cell transplants: Experimental therapies of myelin diseases.. *Brain Pathol.* **5**(3), 301–310.

Ellis, D., and Malcolm, S. (1994). Proteolipid protein gene dosage effect in Pelizaeus-Merzbacher disease *Nat. Genet.* **6**(4), 333–334.

Fanarraga, M. L., Griffiths, I. R., McCulloch, M. C., Barrie, J. A., Cattanach, B. M., Brophy, P. J., and Kennedy, P. G. (1991). Rumpshaker: An X-linked mutation affecting CNS myelination. A study of the female heterozygote. *Neuropathol. Appl. Neuro. Biol.* **17**(4), 323–334.

Fu, H., Qi, Y., Tan, M., Cai, J., Takebayashi, H., Nakafuku, M., Richardson, W., and Qiu, M. (2002). Dual origin of spinal oligodendrocyte progenitors and evidence for the cooperative role of Olig2 and Nkx2.2 in the control of oligodendrocyte differentiation. *Development* **129**(3), 681–693.

Fu, L., Matthews, P. M., De Stefano, N., Worsley, K. J., Narayanan, S., Francis, G. S., Antel, J. P., Wolfson, C., and Arnold, D. L. (1998). Imaging axonal damage of normal-appearing white matter in multiple sclerosis. *Brain* **121**(Pt 1), 103–113.

Garbern, J. Y., Cambi, F., Lewis, R., Shy, M., Sima, A., Kraft, G., Vallat, J. M., Bosch, E. P., Hodes, M. E., Dlouhy, S., Raskind, W., Bird, T., Macklin, W., and Kamholz, J. (1999). Peripheral neuropathy caused by proteolipid protein gene mutations. *Ann. N.Y. Acad. Sci* **883,** 351–365.

Garbern, J. Y., Cambi, F., Tang, X. M., Sima, A. A., Vallat, J. M., Bosch, E. P., Lewis, R., Shy, M., Sohi, J., Kraft, G., Chen, K. L., Joshi, I., Leonard, D. G., Johnson, W., Raskind, W., Dlouhy, S. R., Pratt, V., Hodes, M. E., Bird, T., and Kamholz, J. (1997). Proteolipid protein is necessary in peripheral as well as central myelin. *Neuron* **19**(1), 205–218.

Garbern, J. Y., Yool, D. A., Moore, G. J., Wilds, I. B., Faulk, M. W., Klugmann, M., Nave, K. A., Sistermans, E. A., van der Knaap, M. S., Bird, T. D., Shy, M. E., Kamholz, J. A., and Griffiths, I. R. (2002). Patients lacking the major CNS myelin protein, proteolipid protein 1, develop length-dependent axonal degeneration in the absence of demyelination and inflammation. *Brain* **125**(Pt 3), 551–561.

Gencic, S., Abuelo, D., Ambler, M., and Hudson, L. D. (1989). Pelizaeus-Merzbacher disease: An X-linked neurologic disorder of myelin metabolism with a novel mutation in the gene encoding proteolipid protein. *Am.. J. Hum. Genet.* **45**(3), 435–442.

Gow, A., Gragerov, A., Gard, A., Colman, D. R., and Lazzarini, R. A. (1997). Conservation of topology, but not conformation, of the proteolipid proteins of the myelin sheath. *J. Neurosci.* **17**(1), 181–189.

Gow, A., and Lazzarini, R. A. (1996). A cellular mechanism governing the severity of Pelizaeus-Merzbacher Disease. *Nat. Genet.* **13**(4), 422–428.

Gow, A., Southwood, C. M., and Lazzarini, R. A. (1998). Disrupted proteolipid protein trafficking results in oligodendrocyte apoptosis in an animal model of Pelizaeus-Merzbacher disease. *J. Cell Biol.* **140**(4), 925–934.

Griffiths, I., Klugmann, M., Anderson, T., Yool, D., Thomson, C., Schwab, M. H., Schneider, A., Zimmermann, F., McCulloch, M., Nadon, N., and Nave, K.-A. (1998). Axonal swellings and degeneration in mice lacking the major proteolipid of myelin. *Science* **280,** 1610–1613.

Griffiths, I. R., Dickinson, P., and Montague, P. (1995). Expression of the proteolipid protein gene in glial cells of the post-natal peripheral nervous system of rodents. *Neuropathol. Appl. Neurobiol.* **21**(2), 97–110.

Griffiths, I. R., Mitchell, L. S., McPhilemy, K., Morrison, S., Kyriakides, E., and Barrie, J. A. (1989). Expression of myelin protein genes in Schwann cells. *J. Neurocytol.* **18**(3), 345–352.

Grossman, R. I., Lenkinski, R. E., Ramer, K. N., Gonzalez-Scarano, F., and Cohen, J. A. (1992). MR proton spectroscopy in multiple sclerosis. *AJNR Am. J. Neuroradiol.* **13**(6), 1535–1543.

Gudz, T. I., Schneider, T. E., Haas, T. A., and Macklin, W. B. (2002). Myelin proteolipid protein forms a complex with integrins and may participate in integrin receptor signaling in oligodendrocytes. *J. Neurosci* **22**(17), 7398–7407.

Harding, B., Ellis, D., and Malcolm, S. (1995). A case of Pelizaeus-Merzbacher disease showing increased dosage of the proteolipid protein gene. *Neuropathol. Appl. Neurobiol.* **21**(2), 111–115.

Helynck, G., Luu, B., Nussbaum, J. L., Picken, D., Skalidis, G., Trifilieff, E., Van Dorsselaer, A., Seta, P., Sandeaux, R., Gavach, C., Heitz, F., Simon, D., and Spach, G. (1983). Brain proteolipids. Isolation, purification and effect on ionic permeability of membranes. *Eur. J. Biochem.* **133**(3), 689–695.

Hobson, G. M., Davis, A. P., Stowell, N. C., Kolodny, E. H., Sistermans, E. A., de Coo, I. F. M., Funanage, V. L., and Marks, H. G. (2000). Mutations in noncoding regions of the proteolipid protein gene in Pelizaeus-Merzbacher disease. *Neurology* **55,** 1089–1096.

Hodes, M. E., Blank, C. A., Pratt, V. M., Morales, J., Napier, J., and Dlouhy, S. R. (1997). Nonsense mutation in exon 3 of the proteolipid protein gene (PLP) in a family with an unusual form of Pelizaeus-Merzbacher disease. *Am. J. Med. Genet.* **69**(2), 121–125.

Hodes, M. E., DeMyer, W. E., Pratt, V. M., Edwards, M. K., and Dlouhy, S. R. (1995). Girl with signs of Pelizaeus-Merzbacher disease heterozygous for a mutation in exon 2 of the proteolipid protein gene. *Am. J. Med. Genet.* **55**(4), 397–401.

Hodes, M. E., Pratt, V. M., and Dlouhy, S. R. (1993). Genetics of Pelizaeus-Merzbacher disease. *Dev. Neurosci.* **15**(6), 383–394.

Hodes, M. E., Woodward, K., Spinner, N. B., Emanuel, B. S., Enrico-Simon, A., Kamholz, J., Stambolian, D., Zackai, E. H., Pratt, V. M., Thomas, I. T., Crandall, K., Dlouhy, S. R., and Malcolm, S. (2000). Additional copies of the proteolipid protein gene causing Pelizaeus-Merzbacher disease arise by separate integration into the X chromosome. *Am. J. Hum. Genet.* **67**(1), 14–22.

Hodes, M. E., Zimmerman, A. W., Aydanian, A., Naidu, S., Miller, N. R., Oller, J. L. G., Barker, B., Aleck, K. A., Hurley, T. D., and Dlouhy, S. R. (1999). Different mutations in the same codon of the proteolipid protein gene, PLP, may help in correlating genotype with phenotype in Pelizaeus-Merzbacher disease/X-linked spastic paraplegia (PMD/SPG2). *Am. J. Med. Genet.* **82**(2), 132–139.

Hudson, L. D., Puckett, C., Berndt, J., Chan, J., and Gencic, S. (1989). Mutation of the proteolipid protein gene PLP in a human X chromosome-linked myelin disorder. *Proc. Natl. Acad. Sci. USA* **86**(20), 8128–8131.

Ikenaka, K., Furuichi, T., Iwasaki, Y., Moriguchi, A., Okano, H., and Mikoshiba, K. (1988). Myelin proteolipid protein gene structure and its regulation of expression in normal and jimpy mutant mice. *J. Mol. Biol.* **199**(4), 587–596.

Ikenaka, K., Kagawa, T., and Mikoshiba, K. (1992). Selective expression of DM-20, an alternatively spliced myelin proteolipid protein gene product, in developing nervous system and in nonglial cells. *J. Neurochem.* **58**(6), 2248–2253.

Inoue, K., Kanai, M., Tanabe, Y., Kubota, T., Kashork, C. D., Wakui, K., Fukushima, Y., Lupski, J. R., and Shaffer, L. G. (2001a). Prenatal interphase FISH diagnosis of PLP1 duplication associated with Pelizaeus-Merzbacher disease. *Prenat. Diagn.* **21**(13), 1133–1136.

Inoue, K., and Lupski, J. R. (2002). Molecular mechanisms for genomic disorders. *Annu. Rev. Genomics Hum. Genet.* **3,** 199–242.

Inoue, K., Osaka, H., Imaizumi, K., Nezu, A., Takanashi, J., Arii, J., Murayama, K., Ono, J., Kikawa, Y., Mito, T., Shaffer, L. G., and Lupski, J. R. (1999a). Proteolipid protein gene duplications causing Pelizaeus-Merzbacher disease: Molecular mechanism and phenotypic manifestations. *Ann. Neurol.* **45**(5), 624–632.

Inoue, K., Osaka, H., Sugiyama, N., Kawanishi, C., Onishi, H., Nezu, A., Kimura, K., Kimura, S., Yamada, Y., and Kosaka, K. (1996). A duplicated *PLP* gene causing Pelizaeus-Merzbacher disease detected by comparative multiplex PCR. *Am. J. Hum. Genet.* **59,** 32–39.

Inoue, K., Osaka, H., Thurston, V. C., Clarke, J. T., Yoneyama, A., Rosenbarker, L., Bird, T. D., Hodes, M. E., Shaffer, L. G., and Lupski, J. R. (2002). Genomic Rearrangements Resulting in PLP1 Deletion Occur by Nonhomologous End Joining and Cause Different Dysmyelinating Phenotypes in Males and Females. *Am. J. Hum. Genet.* **71**(4), 838–853.

Inoue, K., Tanabe, Y., and Lupski, J. R. (1999b). Myelin deficiencies in both the central and the peripheral nervous systems associated with a SOX10 mutation. *Ann. Neurol.* **46**(3), 313–318.

Inoue, K., Tanaka, H., Scaglia, F., Araki, A., Shaffer, L. G., and Lupski, J. R. (2001b). Compensating for central nervous system dysmyelination: Females with a proteolipid protein gene duplication and sustained clinical improvement. *Ann. Neurol.* **50**(6), 747–754.

Johnston, A. W., and McKusick, V. A. (1962). A sex-linked recessive form of spastic paraplegia. *Am. J. Hum. Genet.* **14,** 83–94.

Johnston, J. A., Ward, C. L., and Kopito, R. R. (1998). Aggresomes: A cellular response to misfolded proteins. *J. Cell Biol.* **143**(7), 1883–1898.

Kaufman, R. J., Scheuner, D., Schroder, M., Shen, X., Lee, K., Liu, C. Y., and Arnold, S. M. (2002). The unfolded protein response in nutrient sensing and differentiation. *Nat. Rev. Mol. Cell Biol.* **3**(6), 411–421.

Kawanishi, C., Sugiyama, N., Osaka, H., Inoue, K., Suzuki, K., Onishi, H., Yamada, Y., Nezu, A., Kimura, S., and Kosaka, K. (1996). Pelizaeus-Merzbacher disease: A novel mutation in the 5′-untranslated region of the proteolipid protein gene. *Hum. Mutat.* **7**(4), 355–357.

Kaye, E. M., Doll, R. F., Natowicz, M. R., and Smith, F. I. (1994). Pelizaeus-Merzbacher disease presenting as spinal muscular atrophy: Clinical and molecular studies. *Ann. Neurol.* **36**(6), 916–919.

Klugmann, M., Schwab, M. H., Pühlhofer, A., Schneider, A., Zimmermann, F., Griffiths, I. R., and Nave, K.-A. (1997). Assembly of CNS myelin in the absence of proteolipid protein. *Neuron* **18**(1), 59–70.

Kobayashi, H., Hoffman, E. P., and Marks, H. G. (1994). The rumpshaker mutation in spastic paraplegia *Nat. Genet.* **7**(3), 351–352.

Kopito, R. R., and Ron, D. (2000). Conformational disease. *Nat. Cell Biol.* **2**(11), E207–209.

Lachapelle, F., Lapie, P., Gansmuller, A., Villarroya, H., Baumann, N., and Gumpel, M. (1990). What have we learned about the jimpy phenotype expression by intracerebral transplantations? *Ann. N.Y. Acad. Sci.* **605,** 332–345.

Macklin, W. B., Campagnoni, C. W., Deininger, P. L., and Gardinier, M. V. (1987). Structure and expression of the mouse myelin proteolipid protein gene. *J. Neurosci. Res.* **18**(3), 383–394.

Maenpaa, J., Lindahl, E., Aula, P., and Savontaus, M. L. (1990). Prenatal diagnosis in Pelizaeus-Merzbacher disease using RFLP analysis. *Clin. Genet.* **37**(2), 141–147.

McLaughlin, M., Hunter, D. J., Thomson, C. E., Yool, D., Kirkham, D., Freer, A. A., and Griffiths, I. R. (2002). Evidence for possible interactions between PLP and DM20 within the myelin sheath. *Glia* **39**(1), 31–36.

Merzbacher, L. (1910). Eine eigenarige familiär-hereditare Erkrankungsform (Aplasia axialis extra-corticalis congenita). *Z ges. Neurol. Psych.* **3,** 1–138.

Mimault, C., Giraud, G., Courtois, V., Cailloux, F., Boire, J. Y., Dastugue, B., and Boespflug-Tanguy, O. (1999). Proteolipoprotein gene analysis in 82 patients with sporadic Pelizaeus-Merzbacher Disease: Duplications, the major cause of the disease, originate more frequently in male germ cells, but point mutations do not. The Clinical European Network on Brain Dysmyelinating Disease. *Am. J. Hum. Genet.* **65**(2), 360–369.

Nave, K.-A., and Boespflug-Tanguy, O. (1996). X-linked developmental defects of myelination: From mouse mutants to human genetic diseases. *Neuroscientist* **2**(1), 33–43.

Nezu, A., Kimura, S., Takeshita, S., Osaka, H., Kimura, K., and Inoue, K. (1998). An MRI and MRS study of Pelizaeus-Merzbacher disease. *Pediatr. Neurol.* **18**(4), 334–337.

Ono, J., Harada, K., Sakurai, K., Kodaka, R., Shimidzu, N., Tanaka, J., Nagai, T., and Okada, S. (1994). MR diffusion imaging in Pelizaeus-Merzbacher disease. *Brain & Development* **16**(3), 219–223.

Osaka, H., Kawanishi, C., Inoue, K., Onishi, H., Kobayashi, T., Sugiyama, N., Kosaka, K., Nezu, A., Fujii, K., Sugita, K., Kodama, K., Murayama, K., Murayama, S., Kanazawa, I., and Kimura, S. (1999). Pelizaeus-Merzbacher disease: Three novel mutations and implication for locus heterogeneity. *Ann. Neurol.* **45**(1), 59–64.

Osaka, H., Kawanishi, C., Inoue, K., Uesugi, H., Hiroshi, K., Nishiyama, K., Yamada, Y., Suzuki, K., Kimura, S., and Kosaka, K. (1995). Novel nonsense proteolipid protein gene mutation as a cause of X-linked spastic paraplegia in twin males. *Biochem. Biophys. Res. Commun.* **215**(3), 835–841.

Pelizaeus, F. (1885). Über eine eigenthümliche Form Spastischer Lähmung mit Cerebralerschinungen auf hereditärer Grundlage (Multiple Sklerose). *Arch. Psychiatr. Nervenkr.* **16,** 698–710.

Pham-Dinh, D., Birling, M. C., Roussel, G., Dautigny, A., and Nussbaum, J. L. (1991). Proteolipid DM-20 predominates over PLP in peripheral nervous system. *Neuroreport* **2**(2), 89–92.

Pingault, V., Girard, M., Bondurand, N., Dorkins, H., Van Maldergem, L., Mowat, D., Shimotake, T., Verma, I., Baumann, C., and Goossens, M. (2002). SOX10 mutations in chronic intestinal pseudo-obstruction suggest a complex physiopathological mechanism. *Hum. Genet.* **111**(2), 198–206.

Pribyl, T. M., Campagnoni, C., Kampf, K., Handley, V. W., and Campagnoni, A. T. (1996). The major myelin protein genes are expressed in the human thymus. *J. Neurosci. Res.* **45**(6), 812–819.

Puckett, C., Hudson, L., Ono, K., Friedrich, V., Benecke, J., Dubois-Dalcq, M., and Lazzarini, R. A. (1987). Myelin-specific proteolipid protein is expressed in myelinating Schwann cells but is not incorporated into myelin sheaths. *J. Neurosci. Res.* **18**(4), 511–518.

Qi, Y., Cai, J., Wu, Y., Wu, R., Lee, J., Fu, H., Rao, M., Sussel, L., Rubenstein, J., and Qiu, M. (2001). Control of oligodendrocyte differentiation by the Nkx2.2 homeodomain transcription factor. *Development* **128**(14), 2723–2733.

Raskind, W. H., Williams, C. A., Hudson, L. D., and Bird, T. D. (1991). Complete deletion of the proteolipid protein gene (PLP) in a family with X-linked Pelizaeus-Merzbacher disease. *Am. J. Hum. Genet.* **49**(6), 1355–1360.

Regis, S., Filocamo, M., Mazzotti, R., Cusano, R., Corsolini, F., Bonuccelli, G., Stroppiano, M., and Gatti, R. (2001). Prenatal diagnosis of Pelizaeus-Merzbacher disease: Detection of proteolipid protein gene duplication by quantitative fluorescent multiplex PCR. *Prenat. Diagn.* **21**(8), 668–671.

Rosenbluth, J., Stoffel, W., and Schiff, R. (1996). Myelin structure in proteolipid protein (PLP)-null mouse spinal cord. *J. Comp. Neurol.* **371**(2), 336–344.

Rosenfeld, J., and Freidrich, V. L., Jr. (1983). Axonal swellings in jimpy mice:Does lack of myelin cause neuronal abnormalities? *Neuroscience* **10**(3), 959–966.

Ross, N. W., and Braun, P. E. (1988). Acylation in vitro of the myelin proteolipid protein and comparison with acylation in vivo: Acylation of a cysteine occurs nonenzymatically. *Neurosci Res.* **21**(1), 35–44.

Sambuughin, N., Sivakumar, K., Selenge, B., Baasanjav, D., and Goldfarb, L. G. (1998). New mutation in exon 3B of proteolipid protein gene in Mongolian family with a benign variant of X linked spastic paraplegia. *Am. J. Hum. Genet.* **63**(4), A383.

Saugier-Veber, P., Munnich, A., Bonneau, D., Rozet, J. M., Le Merrer, M., Gil, R., and Boespflug-Tanguy, O. (1994). X-linked spastic paraplegia and Pelizaeus-Merzbacher disease are allelic disorders at the proteolipid protein locus. *Nat. Genet.* **6**(3), 257–262.

Schindler, P., Luu, B., Sorokine, O., Trifilieff, E., and Van Dorsselaer, A. (1990). Developmental study of proteolipids in bovine brain: A novel proteolipid and DM-20 appear before proteolipid protein (PLP) during myelination. *J. Neurochem.* **55**(6), 2079–2085.

Seitelberger, F. (1954). Die Pelizaeus-Merzbachersche Krankheit. Klinischanatomische Untersuchungen zum Problem ihrer Stellung unter den diffusen Sklerosen. *Wien Z Nervenheilk* **9,** 228–289.

Seitelberger, F. (1970). Pelizaeus-Merzbacher disease. In "Handbook of Clinical Neurology" (P. J. Vinken and G. W. Bruyn, G., eds.), **10,** 150–220. Amsterdam, North Holland Publishing.

Shaffer, L. G., Kennedy, G. M., Spikes, A. S., and Lupski, J. R. (1997). Diagnosis of CMT1A duplications and HNPP deletions by interphase FISH: Implications for testing in the cytogenetics laboratory. *Am. J. Med. Genet.* **69**(3), 325–331.

Simons, M., Kramer, E. M., Macchi, P., Rathke-Hartlieb, S., Trotter, J., Nave, K. A., and Schulz, J. B. (2002). Overexpression of the myelin proteolipid protein leads to accumulation of cholesterol and proteolipid protein in endosomes/lysosomes: Implications for Pelizaeus-Merzbacher disease. *J. Cell Biol.* **157**(2), 327–336.

Simons, M., Kramer, E. M., Thiele, C., Stoffel, W., and Trotter, J. (2000). Assembly of Myelin by Association of Proteolipid Protein with Cholesterol- and Galactosylceramide-rich Membrane Domains. *J. Cell Biol.* **151**(1), 143–154.

Sistermans, E. A., de Coo, R. F., de Wijs, I. J., and van Oost, B. A. (1998). Duplication of the proteolipid protein gene is the major cause of Pelizaeus-Merzbacher disease. *Neurology* **50**(6), 1749–1754.

Sistermans, E. A., de Wijs, I. J., de Coo, R. F. M., Smit, L. M. E., Menko, F. H., and van Oost, B. A. (1996). A (G-to-A) mutation in the initiation codon of the proteolipid protein gene causing a relatively mild form of Pelizaeus-Merzbacher disease in a Dutch family. *Hum. Genet.* **97**(3), 337–339.

Sivakumar, K., Sambuughin, N., Selenge, B., Nagle, J. W., Baasanjav, D., Hudson, L. D., and Goldfarb, L. G. (1999). Novel exon 3B proteolipid protein gene mutation causing late-onset spastic paraplegia type 2 with variable penetrance in female family members. *Ann. Neurol.* **45**(5), 680–683.

Skalidis, G., Trifilieff, E., and Luu, B. (1986). Selective extraction of the DM-20 brain proteolipid. *J. Neurochem.* **46**(1), 297–299.

Southwood, C., and Gow, A. (2001). Molecular pathways of oligodendrocyte apoptosis revealed by mutations in the proteolipid protein gene. *Microsc. Res. Tech.* **52**(6), 700–708.

Southwood, C. M., Garbern, J., Jiang, W., Gow A. (2002). The unfolded protein response modulates diseases severity in Pelizaeus-Merzbacher disease. *Neuron.* **36**(4), 585–96.

Sporkel, O., Uschkureit, T., Bussow, H., and Stoffel, W. (2002). Oligodendrocytes expressing exclusively the DM20 isoform of the proteolipid protein gene: Myelination and development. *Glia* **37**(1), 19–30.

Stecca, B., Southwood, C. M., Gragerov, A., Kelley, K. A., Friedrich, V. L., and Gow, A. (2000). The evolution of lipophilin genes from invertebrates to tetrapods: DM-20 cannot replace proteolipid protein in CNS myelin. *J. Neurosci.* **20**(11), 4002–4010.

Stoffel, W., Hillen, H., and Giersiefen, H. (1984). Structure and molecular arrangement of proteolipid protein of central nervous system myelin. *Proc. Natl. Acad. Sci. U. S. A.* **81**(16), 5012–5016.

Stolt, C. C., Rehberg, S., Ader, M., Lommes, P., Riethmacher, D., Schachner, M., Bartsch, U., and Wegner, M. (2002). Terminal differentiation of myelin-forming oligodendrocytes depends on the transcription factor Sox10. *Genes Dev.* **16**(2), 165–170.

Strautnieks, S., Rutland, P., Winter, R. M., Baraitser, M., and Malcolm, S. (1992). Pelizaeus-Merzbacher disease: Detection of mutations Thr181—Pro and Leu223—Pro in the proteolipid protein gene, and prenatal diagnosis. *Am. J. Hum. Genet.* **51**(4), 871–878.

Taylor, J. P., Hardy, J., and Fischbeck, K. H. (2002). Toxic proteins in neurodegenerative disease. *Science* **296**(5575), 1991–1995.

Timsit, S., Martinez, S., Allinquant, B., Peyron, F., Puelles, L., and Zalc, B. (1995). Oligodendrocytes originate in a restricted zone of the embryonic ventral neural tube defined by DM-20 mRNA expression. *J. Neurosci.* **15**(2), 1012–1024.

Timsit, S. G., Bally-Cuif, L., Colman, D. R., and Zalc, B. (1992). DM-20 mRNA is expressed during the embryonic development of the nervous system of the mouse. *J. Neurochem.* **58**(3), 1172–1175.

Trapp, B. D., Peterson, J., Ransohoff, R. M., Rudick, R., Mork, S., and Bo, L. (1998). Axonal transection in the lesions of multiple sclerosis *N. Engl. J. Med.* **338**(5), 278–285.

Trofatter, J. A., Dlouhy, S. R., DeMyer, W., Conneally, P. M., and Hodes, M. E. (1989). Pelizaeus-Merzbacher disease: Tight linkage to proteolipid protein gene exon variant. *Proc. Natl. Acad. Sci. USA* **86**(23), 9427–9430.

Wahle, S., and Stoffel, W. (1998). Cotranslational integration of myelin proteolipid protein (PLP) into the membrane of endoplasmic reticulum: Analysis of topology by glycosylation scanning and protease domain protection assay. *Glia* **24**(2), 226–235.

Wang, P. J., Hwu, W. L., Lee, W. T., Wang, T. R., and Shen, Y. Z. (1997). Duplication of proteolipid protein gene: A possible major cause of Pelizaeus-Merzbacher disease. *Pediatr. Neurol.* **17**(2), 125–128.

Weimbs, T., and Stoffel, W. (1992). Proteolipid protein (PLP) of CNS myelin: Positions of free, disulfide-bonded, and fatty acid thioester-linked cysteine residues and implications for the membrane topology of PLP. *Biochemistry* **31**(49), 12289–12296.

Woodward, K., Kendall, E., Vetrie, D., and Malcolm, S. (1998). Pelizaeus-Merzbacher disease: Identification of Xq22 proteolipid-protein duplications and characterization of breakpoints by interphase FISH. *Am. J. Hum. Genet.* **63**(1), 207–217.

Yool, D., Klugmann, M., Barrie, J. A., McCulloch, M. C., Nave, K. A., and Griffiths, I. R. (2002). Observations on the structure of myelin lacking the major proteolipid protein. *Neuropathol. Appl. NeuroBiol.* **28**(1), 75–78.

Yu, W. P., Collarini, E. J., Pringle, N. P., and Richardson, W. D. (1994). Embryonic expression of myelin genes: Evidence for a focal source of oligodendrocyte precursors in the ventricular zone of the neural tube. *Neuron* **12**(6), 1353–1362.

Zackai, E. H., Stambolian, D., Enrico, A., McDonald-McGinn, D. M., Kamholz, J., Emanuel, B. S., and Spinner, N. B. (1997). Familial Pelizaeus Merzbacher disease with a pericentric inversion of the X chromosome [inv(X)(p11.4q22.1)] resulting in PLP gene duplication. *Am. J. Hum. Genet.* **61,** A144.

Zeman, W., DeMyer, W., and Falls, H. F. (1964). Pelizaeus-Merzbacher disease: A study in nosology. *J. Neuropath. Exp. Neurol.* **23,** 334–354.

Zhang, S. C., and Duncan, I. D.(2000). Remyelination and restoration of axonal function by glial cell transplantation. *Prog. Brain Res.* **127,** 515–33.

CHAPTER

# 38

# Guillain-Barre Syndrome

*John W. Griffin and Kazim Sheikh*

## INTRODUCTION

With the near eradication of polio by vaccination, Guillain-Barre syndrome (GBS) has emerged as the most frequent cause of acute flaccid paralysis worldwide. Its most frequent form, acute inflammatory demyelinating polyneuropathy (AIDP), is the prototypic acquired demyelinating disease of the peripheral nervous system. The importance of GBS in this text lies both in its own prominence as a major cause of neurologic morbidity and in the similarities and contrasts with acquired demyelinating disorders of the central nervous system.

## HISTORY

The recognition that the peripheral nervous system could be the site of involvement for paralytic diseases of the nervous system came surprisingly late. It may seem intuitive that PNS disease could lead to sensory changes and paralysis, but the publications of the work of Sir Charles Bell and Francois Magendie on the different roles of the ventral and dorsal roots emerged in the early 1820s, the definitive experiments of Johannes Muller on this topic were not published until 1831, and the consequences of nerve section awaited Augustus Waller's description in 1852 (Sanders, 1948). In any event, Robert Graves, in 1843, reviewed an epidemic outbreak of a painful paralytic disorder that occurred in Paris in 1828 and concluded that, because of the lack of documented involvement of the CNS, the disorder most likely occurred within the peripheral nervous system (Graves, 1884). The first clear description of Guillain Barre syndrome was made by the marvelously intuitive French physician Jean Baptiste Octave Landry de Thezillat in 1859 (Landry, 1859). Landry described five of his own cases and five others from the literature, including a detailed description of a woman, initially considered hysterical by her physician, who died of respiratory insufficiency. He emphasized the ascending sequence of involvement and the rapid progression. Paralysis developed within 15 days in his cases and could evolve over 2 to 3 days or "occasionally only a few hours." Of his initial 10 cases, two died of respiratory insufficiency and others had well-documented bulbar paralysis.

In the late 1890s, the degeneration of fibers in the peripheral nervous system was clear from occasional pathologic studies of acute flaccid paralysis, and one report had identified inflammatory cells around vessels and in the endoneurial space, although this feature generated little comment (Eichhorst, 1877). In 1892, Sir William Osler, the professor of medicine at Johns Hopkins Hospital, described six cases of "acute febrile polyneuritis" (Osler, 1892). These cases clinically correspond well with what we now recognize as the Guillain-Barre syndrome, although they had fever at the peak of their paralysis, a finding that remains unexplained. In 1893, Bury and Ross published an important and little known review of peripheral nerve diseases and documented more than 60 cases of acute polyneuropathies to that time (Ross and Bury, 1893). The differential diagnosis of acute flaccid paralysis 100 years ago was much longer than it is at present and included infectious and toxic disorders rarely encountered today. While it is intriguing to speculate on the diagnosis of each individual summarized by Bury and Ross, in the aggregate most of them are certainly Guillain-Barre syndrome.

Guillain-Barre syndrome was definitively described in 1916 by two French neurologists who were friends and colleagues, Georges Guillain and Jean-Alexander Barre, along with their little recognized coauthor, André Strohl (Guillain, Barre, *et al.*, 1916). Their report detailed the stories of two French soldiers in World War I who developed acute flaccid paresis. An early symptom in one was inability to stand wearing his pack and to rise after falling. Ironically, also in 1916, the first cases of epidemic polio were described from New York City, perhaps in part accounting for the fact that Guillain-Barre syndrome has been occasionally referred to as "French polio." The report by Guillain, Barre, and Strohl was a model of clinical lucidity, pointing out the depressed tendon reflexes, the rapid recovery, and the laboratory finding of elevated protein throughout cells in the spinal fluid. This final feature utilized the technique—new at that time—of lumbar puncture for diagnostic purposes and set "their" syndrome apart from poliomyelitis.

By 1948, Kernohan and Haymaker had studied 50 cases pathologically and recognized demyelination could occur in GBS (Haymaker and Kernohan, 1949). Parenthetically, the length of time required to identify the prominence of demyelination in GBS reflected the difficulty in "seeing" demyelination of individual fibers using standard paraffin sections. The best technique is teasing of nerve fibers, in which individual fibers can be followed longitudinally over multiple internodes. Teasing was utilized by Gombault in his experimental studies, in the 1880s, but was little used in subsequent pathologic studies until the 1960s.

In 1969, Asbury, Arnason, and Adams wrote their classic pathologic review of 19 Boston cases and pointed out the prominence as well as the variability of lymphocytic inflammation in these cases (Asbury, Arnason, *et al.*, 1969). Prineas in 1976 produced his classic electron micrographs of macrophage-mediated demyelination and myelin stripping (Prineas, 1981). Perhaps because of the similarities of the images in these last two reports with those of experimental allergic neuritis induced by immunization with myelin, GBS was frequently equated with EAN, and pathologic analysis of GBS largely languished for the next decade.

In 1986, Feasby and colleagues reported a patient with acute paralysis in whom physiologic and pathologic data suggested axonal degeneration without demyelination (Feasby, Gilbert, *et al.*, 1986; Feasby, Hahn, *et al.*, 1993). The possibility of "axonal GBS" was subsequently confirmed and extended by a series of studies from Northern China, conducted as collaborative studies involving Second Teaching Hospital in Shijiazhuang, Hebei Province, the Beijing Children's Hospital, the University of Pennsylvania, and the Johns Hopkins University (Griffin, Li, *et al.*, 1995; Griffin, Li, *et al.*, 1996; Siebert and Larrick, 1992). The investigators identified epidemic paralytic disease that occurred annually in the summer and had many features that were identical to AIDP in the West. However, most of the summertime cases differed from AIDP in the prominence of physiologic and pathologic features of axonal degeneration. Initially termed the "Chinese Paralytic Syndrome" to reflect its uncertain relationship to AIDP (McKhann, Cornblath, *et al.*, 1991), similar cases with prominent motor axonal involvement as a distinguishing feature were identified in many countries. For this reason, this syndrome is now termed acute motor axonal neuropathy (AMAN) (Griffin, Li, Ho, Xue, Macko, Cornblath, Gao, Yang, Tian, Mishu, McKhann, and Asbury, 1995; Griffin, Li, Macko, Ho, Hsieh, Xue, Wang, Cornblath, McKhann, and Asbury, 1996; Hafer-Macko, Hsieh, *et al.*, 1996; McKhann, Cornblath, *et al.*, 1993). In such cases, the motor system is involved exclusively or nearly exclusively (Lu, Sheikh, *et al.*, 2000). Other cases, such as those described initially by Feasby and colleagues, in which both motor involvement and sensory involvement are prominent, are designated acute motor sensory axonal neuropathy (AMSAN).

## CLINICAL MANIFESTATIONS

AIDP constitutes over 90% of GBS cases in the United States and Western Europe (Emilia-Romagna Study Group on Clinical and Epidemiological Problems in Neurology, 1998; Hadden, Cornblath, *et al.*, 1998). The dominant manifestation is usually weakness, often leading to paralysis (Asbury, Arnason, and Adams, 1969; Hughes, 1990; Ropper, Wijdicks, *et al.*, 1991). However, the initial manifestations are frequently paresthesias. In addition, there may be pain of lesser or greater severity, often vaguely localized to the back. The paresthesias may begin in the toes and "ascend" up the leg and to the hands. They occasionally involve the face or the trunk. The initial manifestations of weakness may be in the feet and ankles, but they usually come to involve proximal muscles of the arms and legs, and most ominously, the respiratory muscles. Bulbar nerves may be affected, as most often evidenced by facial weakness and difficulty with eye closure, and by dysarthria and difficulty swallowing. Hearing, vision, and smell are not affected. The involvement of extraocular movements and pupillary responses suggests elements of the Fisher syndrome described later.

The abrupt onset of weakness in GBS can cause understandable alarm to patients, but at the outset the findings on examination may be surprisingly scanty. For this reason, dating back to the original cases of Landry, hysteria has been considered a part of the initial differential diagnosis. An important clue to the neurologic nature of the underlying disease is the presence of depressed or absent tendon reflexes early. As also noted by Landry, progression can be frighteningly abrupt. In exceptional cases, patients may walk in and be in respiratory difficulties within hours. Progression may continue up to 4 weeks, with about half reaching their nadir in strength by 14 days after neurologic onset (Asbury, Arnason, *et al.*, 1978; Asbury and Cornblath, 1990; Ravn, 1967). A longer phase of initial progression suggests that the patient may have a subacute or chronic inflammatory polyneuropathy rather than GBS.

For the most part, laboratory tests served to exclude other disorders; there are no laboratory tests diagnostic of GBS. Even the "albuminocytologic dissociation" emphasized by Guillain, Barre, and Strohl (Guillain, Barré, and Strohl, 1916) is of limited diagnostic value, since the elevated spinal fluid protein often develops 2 or more weeks after onset of the disease, at a time when the diagnosis has already been established. Thus, while a markedly elevated protein at the start of the syndrome can be supportive of the diagnosis, its absence does not refute the diagnosis. Diseases that can mimic GBS necessitate, as appropriate, thorough inspection of the scalp for ticks that might cause tick paralysis, inquiry for possible exposure to botulinum toxin (for example, home canned foods), and historical inquiries for features that might suggest in intermittent porphyrias. Historical and, when relevant, serologic investigation for associated HIV or Lyme disease may be indicated.

The most valuable laboratory study is electrodiagnosis. Electrodiagnostic studies are abnormal in some fashion in most patients with GBS (Brown and Feasby, 1984; Cornblath, Mellits, *et al.*, 1988; van der Meche, Meulstee, *et al.*, 1988; van der Meché, Schmitz *et al.*, 1992b). In the uncommon instances where they are normal on the first examination, they can be expected to become abnormal on subsequent reexamination. In addition, electrodiagnostic data, as noted later, give prognostic information and help establish the class of GBS, AIDP, AMAN, or AMSAN. The findings suggestive of AIDP are those consistent with demyelination, including prolongation of F waves, prolongation of distal latencies, and reduction in motor or sensory nerve conduction velocities at the time when the action potential amplitudes are relatively preserved. Conversely, the AMAN syndrome suggested by markedly reduced compound motor action potential amplitudes with relatively normal motor conduction velocities, normal sensory nerve action potential amplitudes and velocities (McKhann, Cornblath, Griffin, Ho, Li, Jiang, Wu, Zhaori, Liu, Jou, Liu, Gao, Mao, Blaser, Mishu, and Asbury, 1993). Even this combination, however, cannot eliminate the possibility of restricted motor nerve terminal demyelination, as has been clearly demonstrated in physiologic-pathologic correlation studies in which extensive demyelination of motor nerve terminals has been demonstrated (Reisin, Cersosimo, *et al.*, 93 A.D.; Reisin, Pociecha, *et al.*).

The prognosis of AIDP is influenced by age (the older the patient, the slower the recovery), the severity at nadir, and whether or not effective immunomodulatory therapy (intravenous immunoglobulin or plasmapheresis) were used early in the treatment (Cornblath, Mellits, Griffin, McKhann, Albers, Miller, Feasby, Quaskey, and Guillain-Barre Study Group, 1988; van der Meche, Meulstee, Vermeulen, and Kievit, 1988; van der Meché, Schmitz, Meulstee, and Oomes, 1992b). In addition, the electrodiagnostic studies provide important prognostic data. Absent evoked compound motor action potentials predict a longer period to recovery (Cornblath, Mellits, Griffin, McKhann, Albers, Miller, Feasby, Quaskey, and Guillain-Barre Study Group, 1988; van der Meche, Meulstee, Vermeulen, and Kievit, 1988; van der Meché, Schmitz, Meulstee, and Oomes, 1992b). Although throughout his life Guillain emphasized the favorable outcome of patients with GBS, and the mortality in the best centers is 1 to 2.5%, 15 to 20% of patients have substantial residual weakness.

Both plasmapheresis and infusion of human immunoglobulin (HIG) improve the outcome of AIDP. Plasmapheresis, the first therapy demonstrated to benefit GBS (Consensus Conference, 1986; French Cooperative Group on Plasma Exchange in Guillain-Barre Syndrome, 1987; Guillain-Barre Study Group, 1985), has the disadvantage of the necessity for line placement in many patients and therefore is less frequently used than infusion of HIG (van der Meché, Schmitz, *et al.*, 1992a). A recent trial comparing plasmapheresis and HIG found no advantage of one over the other and no advantage to using both together (Hadden, Cornblath, Hughes, Zielasek, Hartung, Toyka, and Swan, 1998). Corticosteroids alone are of no benefit in treatment (Hughes and Swan, 1995). Ongoing trials are assessing the combination of HIG and corticosteroids.

## PATHOLOGY OF AIDP

Lymphocytic infiltration is characteristic of AIDP, but its severity can vary markedly. Typically, lymphocytes are present around endoneurial vessels, and individual lymphocytes are scattered throughout the endoneurial space (Fig. 38.1). The extensive perivascular and endoneurial cuffs of lymphocytes and the "plaque-like" demyelination seen in experimental allergic neuritis is exceptional in GBS but can occur (Fig. 38.1 A, B).

Demyelination can occur anywhere in the peripheral nervous system, from the ventral roots to the nerve terminals, but typically it clusters in the spinal roots and just distal to the spinal foramina, in the mixed spinal roots and plexuses. There can be substantial endoneurial and subperineurial edema in these sites, sufficient to lead some investigators to question if, in the unyielding space of the spinal foramina, ischemic or compressive injury to nerve could contribute to the pathogenesis of Guillain-Barre (Berciano and Garcia, 2002). In any event, extensive proximal demyelination can be associated with Wallerian-like degeneration of fibers more distally, so that many patients with absent evoked compound of motor action potential amplitudes or sensory nerve action potentials have few surviving nerve fibers in the distal regions (Haymaker and Kernohan, 1949; Honavar, Tharakan, *et al.*, 1991), yet have evidence of extensive demyelination more proximally. In other individuals, nerve terminal demyelination may be prominent (Hall, Hughes, *et al.*, 1992; Massaro, Rodriguez, *et al.*, 1998; Reisin, Cersosimo, Garcia Alvarez, Massaro, and Fejerman, 93 A.D.).

Staining for immunoglobulins in GBS nerve often shows evidence of a break in the blood nerve barrier, so that all plasma constituents, including IGM, can be found within the endoneurial space. This makes it difficult to tell with certainty whether there is binding of immunoglobulin to individual nerve fibers. In some cases, binding of complement constituents on nerve fibers has been demonstrated, and this can occur before demyelination is advanced. In three fatal cases of GBS in children, Hafer-Macko and colleagues (Hafer-Macko, Sheikh, *et al.*, 1996) found that C3d and the complement membrane attack

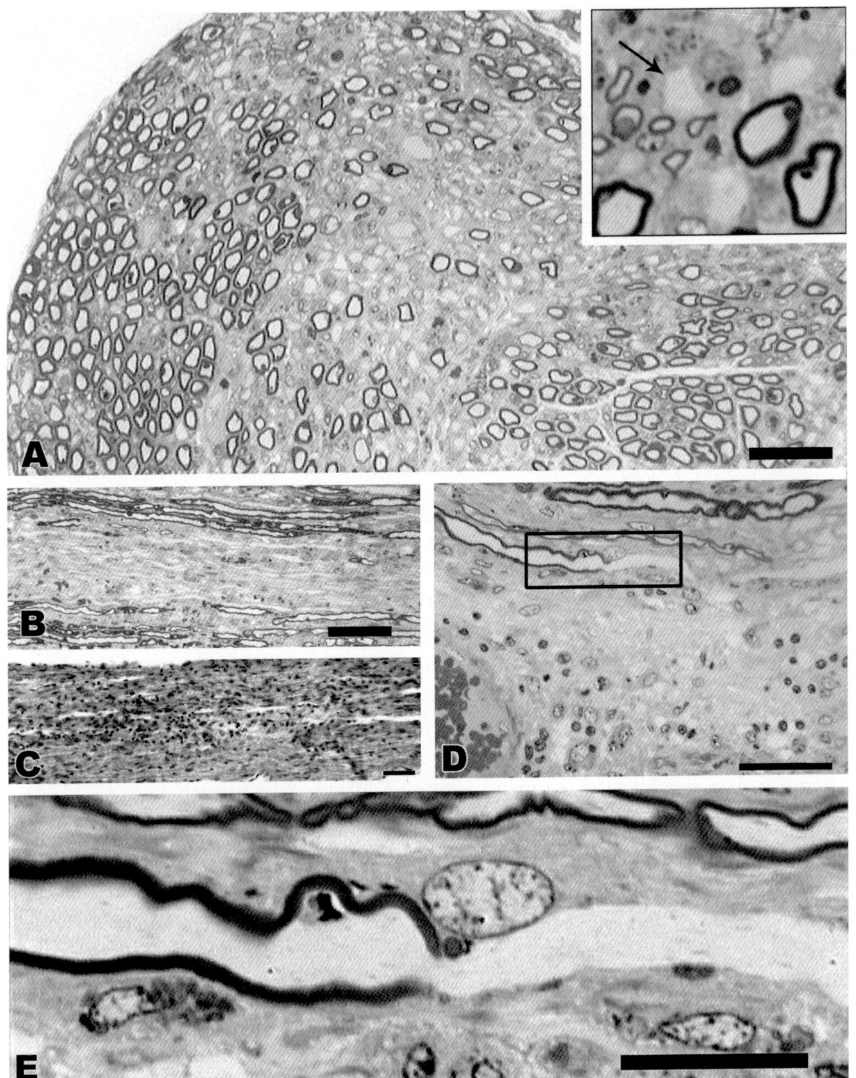

FIGURE 38.1
Pathology of AIDP. (A) This ventral rootlet from a fatal case of AIDP shows an admixture of normal myelinated nerve fibers and fully demyelinated axons, both scattered throughout the root and in the central large plaque-like zone. In the inset, a demyelinated axon is identified at higher magnification by the arrow. One micron plastic section scale bar = 50 microns. (B) A similar region in longitudinal section shows a central zone filled with demyelinated axons, flanked above and below by myelinated nerve fibers. One micron plastic section. Scale bar = 20 microns. (C) Scattered mononuclear cells in the endoneurial space in this H&E stained paraffin section of a ventral root. Scale bar = 50 microns. (D) Around the vessel to the lower left, there is extensive endoneurial edema and numerous mononuclear cells. The boxed region is seen at higher power in E. Scale bar = 50 microns. (E) A myelinated internode from the boxed region in D is seen to end abruptly at the heminode. To the right, the axon is entirely demyelinated. A large nucleus, probably of a macrophage, sits near the node. One micron plastic section. Scale bar = 20 microns.

complex neoantigen, C5b-9, affixed to the outside of nerve fibers, surrounding the abaxonal Schwann cell plasmalemma. Strikingly, these complement activation markers were not found on myelin per se. By doing light microscopic-electronmicroscopic comparisons on the same nerve fibers, such fibers were found to have early myelin vacuolization involving the outermost myelin lamellae. This vacuolization went on in other fibers to involve extensive vacuolar degeneration of myelin, and clearance of the myelin by macrophages. This sequence raises the possibility that immunoglobulin binding and complement activation lead to the formation of sublytic complement pores in the abaxonal Schwann cell cytoplasm, with entry of calcium, activation of phospholipase A and other calcium-sensitive enzymes, and consequent demyelination.

This immunopathology is not universal in AIDP; in many cases it is not possible to demonstrate complement activation markers on the surface, and macrophages invade entirely normal appearing myelin sheaths, engaging in stripping of myelin. Such cases may have different immunopathogenesis.

## ANTECEDENTS OF GBS

AIDP may follow antecedent illnesses, including infectious diseases in about two-thirds of cases and, less frequently, surgery, parturition, and other life events. Post-infectious GBS typically follows a bacterial or viral infection by 10 to 14 days. The antecedent infections that have clear links to GBS include infection with the gram-negative bacteria *Campylobacter-jejuni* (*C. jejuni*) (Jacobs, Van Doorn, *et al.*, 1996; Kaldor and Speed, 1984; Rees, Gregson, *et al.*, 1995; Walsh, Cronin, *et al.*, 1991) and the herpes virus, *Cytomegalovirus* (Dowling and Cook, 1981; Visser, van der Meché, *et al.*, 1996). *Mycoplasma pneumoniae* infection can also precede GBS (Jacobs, Rothbarth, *et al.*, 1998). A variety of disorders that alter immune function have been associated with GBS, including HIV infection (Cornblath, McArthur, *et al.*, 1987), Hodgkins disease (Lisak, Mitchell, *et al.*, 1977), and pharmacologic immunosuppression (Drachman, Patterson, *et al.*, 1970). Other antecedents include pregnancy and delivery, surgery, and an extraordinary variety of other infections. It can be associated with Lyme disease. A few vaccinations have had a suggested relationship to GBS. The Semple Rabies vaccine can clearly produce GBS, due almost certainly to the inclusion of myelin constituents in the vaccine (Hemachudha, Phanuphak, *et al.*, 1987). The 1976 influenza vaccine, the swine flu, produced a modest increase in case rate within the first weeks after immunization (Kaplan, Schonberger, *et al.*, 1983; Lasky, Terracciano, *et al.*, 1998; Schonberger, Bregman, *et al.*, 1979).

When an antecedent infection such as *Campylobacter* enteritis precedes GBS, the acute infectious manifestations and fever have generally abated before onset of the neurologic disorder. In the case of *Campylobacter*, the organism usually has been cleared by the time of neurologic presentation. Antecedent infection can be suggested by serologic studies, although *Campylobacter* serology is a specialized test and better suited to comparison of populations than individual diagnosis. In GBS, the seroprevalence of *Campylobacter* ranges from 15 to 75% in various parts of the world (Ho, Mishu, *et al.*, 1995; Kaldor and Speed, 1984; Mishu, Ilyas, *et al.*, 1993; McKhann, Cornblath, Griffin, Ho, Li, Jiang, Wu, Zhaori, Liu, Jou, Liu, Gao, Mao, Blaser, Mishu, and Asbury, 1993; Rees, Soudain, *et al.*, 1995; Speed, Kaldor, *et al.*, 1984).

Enteric infection with *Campylobacter* is the most frequent bacterial cause of diarrhea worldwide, with an estimated 2.4 million cases per year in the United States alone. Yet only about 2500 individuals develop GBS in North America annually, and only a portion of these can be ascribed to antecedent *Campylobacter* infection (Buzby, Allos, *et al.*, 1997; McCarthy, Andersson, *et al.*, 1999; Mishu and Blaser, 1993; Tauxe, 1992). Some *Campylobacter* strains are more likely to be associated with GBS than others. HS (Penner) serotyping, which detects capsular polysaccharides distinct from the lipopolysaccharide (LPS), is an important epidemiological tool in studying *C. jejuni*-associated GBS (Penner and Hennessy, 1980; Penner, Hennessy, *et al.*, 1983). Certain HS serotypes are overrepresented in GBS patients in different parts of the world. For example, HS:19, an uncommon serotype in patients with diarrhea, is isolated in up to 90% of Japanese *Campylobacter* associated GBS (Fujimoto, Yuki, *et al.*, 1992; Kuroki, Saida, *et al.*, 1993; Yuki, Takahashi, *et al.*, 1997). This serostrain is also over-represented in Chinese (Sheikh, Nachamkin, *et al.*, 1998) and Mexican (Irving Nachamkin, unpublished observations) patients with GBS, whereas HS:41 serotype is overrepresented in GBS patients from South Africa (Lastovica, Goddard, *et al.*, 1997; Prendergast, Lastovica, *et al.*, 1998). In the United Kingdom (UK), neither serotype is overrepresented (Rees, Soudain, Gregson, and Hughes, 1995). Even though the risk of GBS following *Campylobacter* is low, understanding the neuritogenic properties of the organisms has important implications for development of a *Campylobacter jejuni* vaccine, currently a priority for the military.

In general post-*Campylobacter* cases are more likely to be severe, to have prominent axonal involvement, and to have disproportionate motor involvement (Jacobs, Van Doorn, Schmitz, Tio-Gillen, Herbrink.P, Visser, Hooijkaas, and van der Meche, 1996; Rees, Gregson, and Hughes, 1995; Visser, van der Meché, *et al.*, 1995). In contrast, post-CMV cases appear are more likely to have prominent or predominant sensory involvement (Visser, van der Meché, Meulstee, Rothbarth, Jacobs, Schmitz, Van Doorn, and Dutch Guillain-Barré Study Group, 1996).

## PATHOGENETIC MECHANISMS

One of the ironies of GBS at the beginning of the 21st century is that the pathogeneses of the less frequent "variants" of GBS are better understood than that of AIDP. The model of molecular mimicry is attractive in AIDP, but the pathogenetic reconstruction of AIDP remains incomplete. The target antigens in AIDP are usually unknown and are likely to differ among different cases. The extent to which T cell-and antibody-mediation are involved is unresolved, and again may differ. These issues contrast with AMAN and with the Fisher syndrome. These variants have provided one of the most attractive examples of "molecular mimicry," in which immune attack is directed toward an antigen of an infectious agent that is similar to an antigen that is present and "seen" by the immune system on nerve fibers. These disorders are regularly associated with specific antiganglioside antibodies, and ganglioside-like moieties to be present on organisms isolated from these patients. The best-documented example is *Campylobacter jejuni*, which can have relevant ganglioside-like antigens in its lipooligo-saccharide. Among patients with *Campylobacter* infection, only those who go on to GBS have high titers of anti-ganglioside antibodies (Oomes, Jacobs, *et al.*, 1995; Rees, Gregson, and Hughes, 1995; Sheikh, Nachamkin, Ho, Willison, Veitch, Ung, Nicholson, Li, Wu, Shen, Cornblath, Asbury, McKhann, and Griffin, 1998). The recent development of successful animal models based on sensitization to these gangliosides and to the relevant *Campylobacter* antigens have substantially "closed the loop" in understanding the role of molecular mimicry in the AMAN syndrome, as described here.

The GBS variant that may bridge the way to comparable studies of AIDP is the Fisher syndrome. Described in 1956 on the basis of the triad of internal and external ophthalmoplegia, ataxia, and areflexia with little weakness, the Fisher syndrome was proposed to be a variant of GBS (Fisher, 1956). That suggestion was initially controversial, but it has subsequently been observed that many cases that present as Fisher syndrome evolve into typical AIDP. These patients may require respiratory support, ventilator assistance, and have all the other electrodiagnostic manifestations of typical AIDP. The pathology of "pure" Fisher syndrome, without more widespread weakness, is unknown because it is not a fatal disorder. However, the few cases that had gone on to death after developing a paralysis have had evidence of inflammatory demyelination.

Serologic studies established that the 90% of Fisher syndrome or Fisher-AIDP overlap cases have acute-phase serum antibodies against GQ1b gangliosides; these antibodies disappear with clinical recovery (Chiba, Kusunoki, *et al.*, 1992; Willison, Veitch, *et al.*, 1993; Yuki, Sato, *et al.*, 1993b). Fisher syndrome patients may also have antibodies that react with structurally related gangliosides containing disialosyl moieties, including GT1a, GD1b, and GT1b (Willison, Almemar, *et al.*, 1994). GQ1b is enriched in oculomotor nerves (Chiba, Kusunoki, *et al.*, 1993; Chiba, Kusunoki, *et al.*, 1997), the principal motor site affected in Fisher syndrome.

Fisher syndrome occasionally follows such antecedent infections with *Campylobacter*. *Campylobacter jejuni* lipopolysaccharides can contain ganglioside-like moieties, and several *C. jejuni* isolates from Fisher patients contain the structurally similar GQ1b-, GT1a-, and GD3-like moieties (Aspinall, McDonald, *et al.*, 1994; Jacobs, Endtz, *et al.*, 1995; Salloway, Mermel, *et al.*, 1996; Yuki, Taki, *et al.*, 1994). Rabbits immunized with *C. jejuni* LPS from patients with Fisher syndrome can produce cross-reactive antibodies recognizing

GQ1b (Goodyear, O'Hanlon, *et al.*, 1999). Willison and colleagues have undertaken a detailed analysis of the pathogenetic role of anti-GQ1b antibodies in experimental settings. They showed that anti-GQ1b antibodies stain the terminal axon at the neuromuscular junction in rat phrenic nerve-diaphragm preparations, and that anti-GQ1b antibodies could produce complement-dependent motor nerve terminal degeneration (Goodyear, O'Hanlon, Plomp, Wagner, Morrison, Veitch, Cochrane, Bullens, Molenaar, Conner, and Willison, 1999; Plomp, Molenaar, *et al.*, 1999a; Roberts, Willison, *et al.*, 1994). This degeneration was heralded by massive release of quanta from the motor nerve terminal (Goodyear, O'Hanlon, Plomp, Wagner, Morrison, Veitch, Cochrane, Bullens, Molenaar, Conner, and Willison, 1999). This effect reflected calcium entry into the terminal and preceded swelling and destruction of the terminal (Plomp, Molenaar, *et al.*, 1999b; Plomp, Molenaar, O'Hanlon, Jacobs, Veitch, Daha, Van Doorn, van der Meche, Vincent, Morgan, and Willison, 1999a). Buchwald and Toyka have found evidence of a complement-independent effect of anti-GQ1b antibodies on motor nerve terminals (Buchwald, Weishaupt, *et al.*, 1998).

Thus, an attractive reconstruction of the Fisher syndrome is that GQ1b is enriched in oculomotor nerves and that the generation of anti-GQ1b antibodies by an antecedent infection produces ophthalmoparesis because of immune-mediated injury of the oculomotor nerve terminals. Bickerstaff's brain stem encephalitis has ocular features similar to the Fisher syndrome, but associated with evidence of central nervous system involvement and T2 brightness in the brain stem on MRI studies. Such cases can also follow *Campylobacter* infection and are associated with anti-GQ1b antibodies (Yuki, Sato, *et al.*, 1993a). This suggests that antiganglioside antibodies might also be capable of producing CNS involvement when they have access.

The association of the Fisher syndrome and the axonal forms of GBS with specific antiganglioside immune responses raises the possibility that a similar association underlies AIDP. Some cases of AIDP have antiganglioside antibodies, and there have been associations of specific antiganglioside antibody patterns with specific clinical or prognostic patterns. For example, cases of AIDP with predominant motor involvement and with a poorer prognosis have been associated with IgG anti-GM1 antibodies (Jacobs, Van Doorn, Schmitz, Tio-Gillen, Herbrink.P, Visser, Hooijkaas, and van der Meche, 1996; Rees, Gregson, and Hughes, 1995; Visser, van der Meché, Van Doorn, and, *et al.*, 1995). This raises the possibility that in these cases, the poorer prognosis is associated with an increased "axonal" component, related to the anti-GM1 antibodies. One possible exception is antibody against the major PNS myelin ganglioside, LM1 (sialsylneolacto tetrasylceromide). In one thoroughly reported AIDP patient, antibody against LM1, a peripheral nerve ganglioside enriched in myelin was present in high titers at the onset of disease and fell over time (Ilyas, Willison, *et al.*, 1988). Two recent reports have identified anti-LM1 antibodies in 5 to 25% of AIDP patients (Harukawa, Utsumi, *et al.*, 2002; Yako, Kusunoki, *et al.*, 1999); in these reports they were rarely associated with axonal cases, although one other found anti-LM1 antibodies in 29% of axonal GBS.

Other candidate antigens for AIDP, including GD1b, asialo-GM1, *Gal (b1-3)GalNAc* epitope, GM2 and GT1b (Fredman, Vedeler, *et al.*, 1991; Gregson, Koblar, *et al.*, 1993; Ho, Mishu, Li, Gao, Cornblath, Griffin, Asbury, Blaser, and McKhann, 1995; Ilyas, Mithen, *et al.*, 1992; Ilyas, Willison, Quarles, Jungawala, Cornblath, Trapp, Griffin, Griffin, and McKhann, 1988; Rees, Gregson, and Hughes, 1995;), are infrequently identified. It is notable that anti-GM1 antibodies can be present in both AMAN and AIDP. The fine specificities of these antibodies or differential antibody affinity for gangliosides of neuronal and glial origin need to be explored to explain this apparent paradox. As noted, anti-galactocerebroside and anti-GM2 antibodies have been identified after antecedent infections with *Mycoplasma* and CMV, respectively. Prominent bulbar and facial involvement have been associated with anti-GT1a antibodies (Kashihara, Shiro, *et al.*, 1998; Koga, Yuki, *et al.*, 1998) and a sensory ataxic neuropathy with anti-GD1b antibodies (Miyazaki, Kusunoki, *et al.*, 2001). The latter pattern has been reproduced in a rabbit model by immunization with GD1b (Kusunoki, Hitoshi, *et al.*, 1999), in this model the target appears to be sensory ganglion cells rather than myelin.

On balance, it seems likely that relatively few cases of AIDP represent immune responses to gangliosides. The frequency of antiganglioside antibodies in AIDP, in comparison to the axonal and Fisher syndrome of patients, is low. These issues are complicated by the well-publicized difficulties in reproducibility and reliability of antiganglioside antibody assays and by the difficulties in localization in gangliosides on nerve fibers. The problem of localization of antigen with gangliosides has been improved by the availability of high titer monospecific antiganglioside antibodies, generated by immunization of genetically engineered mice deficient in gangliosides of interest. The most widely used such mice are the GD3/GD2 synthesis knockout mice, which make GD3, but no subsequent complex gangliosides (Sheikh, Sun, *et al.*, 1999). Immunization of these animals with such gangliosides as GD1a, GM1, GD1b, and GT1b have produced the high titer monospecific antibodies that can either be complement fixing (mouse IgG2a or 2b) or noncomplement fixing (mouse IgG1 or 3).

Lessons from the use of these high titer monospecific antibodies to assess ganglioside localization include the recognition that the fixation and preparation of the tissue affects the apparent localization (Gong, Tagawa, *et al.*, 2002; Lunn, Johnson, *et al.*, 2000; Sheikh, Deerinck, *et al.*, 1999). It is difficult to "see" myelin gangliosides with immunocytochemistry, except in paranodal regions, if the method of preparation does not open the myelin sheath. Thus, they may be poorly seen on fixed teased fiber preparations and yet relatively abundant in transverse fresh frozen cryostat sections. Similarly, the biochemical "surround" of gangliosides within membrane may produce crypticity of gangliosides in some settings. The abaxonal surface of Schwann cells is frequently stained by anti-ganglioside antibodies. This observation implies that if anti-glycolipid antibodies are targets in demyelination, the surface expression of glycolipid antigens on glial cells may be sufficient for antibody binding, complement activation, and calcium entry that can lead to demyelination, without a direct immune attack on myelin. Finally, there are important fine specificities of anti-gangliosides antibodies, so that some antibodies selectively stain certain neuronal and nerve fiber populations. These differences in staining patterns are not explained by ganglioside content or antibody binding to extracted gangliosides from these differentially stained neurons or nerve fibers (Fig. 38.2).

Compared to the axonal forms, AIDP has greater T-cell-mediated infiltration component (Asbury, Arnason, and Adams, 1969), the presence of T-cell activation markers in the serum and CSF of AIDP patients (Bansil, Mithen, *et al.*, 1991; Sharief, McLean, *et al.*, 1993; Sharief, Ingram, *et al.*, 1997; Sivieri, Ferrarini, *et al.*, 1997), and on the pathologic similarities to the animal model EAN (Arnason and Soliven, 1993; Hartung, Pollard, *et al.*, 1995a; Hartung, Pollard, *et al.*, 1995b). Although the trigger for T-cell activation is not clear, T cells could contribute to pathogenesis of AIDP in several ways. Activated T cells may play an important role in breakdown of the blood-nerve-barrier in recruitment of macrophages. They may also contribute to Schwann cell and myelin injury, either by direct cytotoxic mechanisms or indirectly through proinflammatory cytokines.

There is a growing interest in the role of antibody-mediated demyelination in AIDP. As noted, in some AIDP cases complement activation markers are found on the outermost Schwann cell surface and can be associated with vesicular demyelination (Hafer-Macko, Sheikh, Li, Ho, Cornblath, McKhann, Asbury, and Griffin, 1996). This pattern closely resembles the experimental nerve fiber demyelination induced by anti-galactocerebroside (GalC). GalC is a glycosphingolipid enriched in myelin (Saida, Saida, *et al.*, 1979). It is possible that in these cases the antibody and complement is more directly involved in targeting the Schwann cell and myelin, and the role of T cells may be to open the blood nerve barrier (Pollard, Westland, *et al.*, 1995; Spies, Pollard, *et al.*, 1995; Spies, Westland, *et al.*, 1995). Several clinical and experimental observations support a role for antibody-mediated mechanisms, including the response to plasmapheresis (French Cooperative Group on Plasma Exchange in Guillain-Barre Syndrome, 1987; Guillain-Barre Study Group, 1985), the presence of anti-myelin (Koski, Chou, *et al.*, 1989; Koski, Humphrey, *et al.*, 1985) and anti-glycoconjugate antibodies, and the ability of AIDP sera to induce demyelination after intraneural injection (Saida, Saida, *et al.*, 1982) or *in vitro* incubation (Birchem, Mithen, *et al.*, 1987; Koski, Chou, and Jungalwala, 1989; Mithen, Ilyas, *et al.*, 1992; Sawant-Mane, Clark, *et al.*, 1991; Sawant-Mane, Estep, *et al.*, 1994).

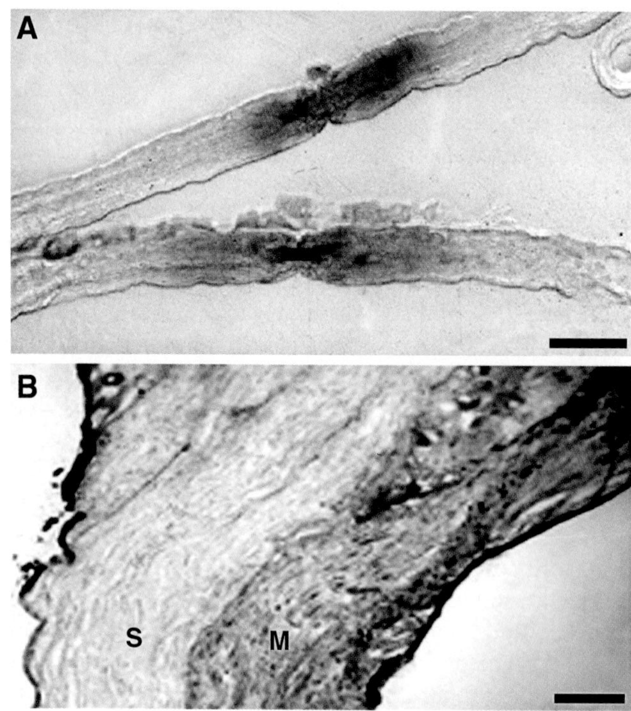


FIGURE 38.2
(A) Teased fiber preparation showing cholera toxin staining (ganglioside GM1) a node of Ranvier and paranodal Schwann cell. Scale bar = 20 microns. (B) A mixed spinal root section stained for ganglioside GD1a showing preferential staining of motor (M) compared with sensory (S) root. Scale bar = 50 microns.

## Molecular Mimicry and the AMAN Syndrome

The molecular basis for ganglioside-like mimicry is beginning to come to light following the sequencing of the *Campylobacter* genome (Parkhill, Wren, *et al.*, 2000). There are sialyltransfereases and sialic acid synthetases involved in ganglioside-like epitope expression (Gilbert, Brisson, *et al.*, 2000; Linton, Gilbert, *et al.*, 2000; Linton, Karlyshev, *et al.*, 2000). Ganglioside-like moieties have regularly been found in the GBS isolates. For example, *C. jejuni* isolates from AMAN patients with anti-GM1 antibodies patients contain GM1-like moieties (Yuki, Handa, *et al.*, 1992; Yuki, Taki, *et al.*, 1993).

The antiganglioside antibodies in AMAN are IgG species, and typically directed against GM1, GD1a, GalNac-GD1a, and occasionally GM1b (Gregson, Koblar, and Hughes, 1993; Ho, Mishu, Li, Gao, Cornblath, Griffin, Asbury, Blaser, and McKhann, 1995; Kornberg, Pestronk, *et al.*, 1994; Kuwabara, Yuki, *et al.*, 1998; Ogino, Orazio, *et al.*, 1995; Willison and Veitch, 1994; Yuki, Takahashi, Tagawa, Kashiwase, Tadokoro, and Saito, 1997; Yuki, Yoshino, Sato, and Miyatake, 1990; Yuki, Yoshino, *et al.*, 1990). Immunopathologic studies have found few lymphocytes, even in fatal cases (McKhann, Cornblath, Griffin, Ho, Li, Jiang, Wu, Zhaori, Liu, Jou, Liu, Gao, Mao, Blaser, Mishu, and Asbury, 1993), and identified binding of complement to nodes of Ranvier and the internodal axolemma (Hafer-Macko, Hsieh, Li, Ho, Sheikh, Cornblath, McKhann, Asbury, and Griffin, 1996). A characteristic feature of the axonal cases is recruitment of macrophages to the nodes and into the periaxonal space surrounding the nodes of Ranvier (Griffin, Li, Macko, Ho, Hsieh, Xue, Wang, Cornblath, McKhann, and Asbury, 1996). In the most severe cases, motor axons undergo Wallerian-like degeneration that extends from the ventral root exit zone to the motor nerve terminal (Griffin, Li, Ho, Xue, Macko, Cornblath, Gao, Yang, Tian, Mishu, McKhann, and Asbury, 1995; Griffin, Li, Macko, Ho, Hsieh, Xue, Wang, Cornblath, McKhann, and Asbury, 1996). In other cases, motor axons appear to degenerate only in their terminal regions, where the motor nerve terminal is outside the blood nerve barrier (Ho, Hsieh, *et al.*, 1997). Such cases can recover surprisingly promptly.

In northern China, the specificity of antiganglioside antibodies for the AMAN syndrome is greatest for antibodies against GD1a and the minor gangliosides, GalNAc-GD1a and GM1b. Anti-GD1a antibodies are significantly elevated in patients with AMAN (60%) compared to AIDP (4%) (Ho, Willison, *et al.*, 1999). In this group anti-GM1, anti-GM1b, and anti-GalNAc-GD1a were also more frequent in AMAN than AIDP (Yuki, Ho, *et al.*, 1999). Elevated titers of anti-GM1b and anti-GalNAc-GD1a were more commonly associated with motor-predominant variants in Japanese and Dutch patients (Ang, Yuki, *et al.*, 1999; Hao, Kaida, Kusunoki, *et al.*, 2000; Saida, *et al.*, 1999; Yuki, Ang, *et al.*, 2000). The presence of antibodies against these gangliosides is strongly related to preceding *C. jejuni* infection (Ang, Yuki, Jacobs, Koga, Van Doorn, Schmitz, and van der Meche, 1999; Chiba, *et al.*, 1994; Hao, Saida, Yoshino, Kuroki, Nukina, and Saida, 1999; Ho, Willison, Nachamkin, Li, Veitch, Ung, Wang, Liu, Cornblath, Asbury, Griffin, and McKhann, 1999; Kaida, Kusunoki, Kamakura, Motoyoshi, and Kanazawa, 2000; Kusunoki, Iwamori, *et al.*, 1996; Kusunoki, Yuki, Ho, Tagawa, Koga, Li, Hirata, and Griffin, 1999; Yuki, Ang, Koga, Jacobs, Van Doorn, Hirata, and van der Meche, 2000; Yuki, Yoshino, *et al.*, 1992), and the LPSs of *C. jejuni* carry GD1a- and GM1b-like moieties.

The correlation between AMAN, anti-GM1 antibodies and *C. jejuni* infection is not found in all patient populations (Enders, Karch, *et al.*, 1993; Vriesendorp, Mishu, *et al.*, 1993). Biochemical data and localization studies indicate that GM1-like moieties are present in both axons and myelin (O'Hanlon, Paterson, *et al.*, 1996) perhaps explaining the fact that IgG anti-GM1 antibodies are also seen in some cases of AIDP.

The basis for the motor-predominant symptoms in AMAN remains a target of investigation. The differential display of specific gangliosides on motor rather than sensory fibers is a potential explanation. GD1a localization supports this concept. GD1a has been localized by taking advantage of the ability to generate high titer monospecific antiganglioside antibodies, using mice in which the enzyme GM2/GD2 synthase was genetically targeted. These mice respond to immunization with gangliosides by raising much higher titers of monospecific antibody than seen in wild-type animals (Lunn, Johnson, Fromholt, Itonori, Huang, Vyas, Hildreth, Griffin, Schnaar, and Sheikh, 2000). The resulting anti-GD1a antibodies bind to motor axons but only a subpopulation of small sensory axons (Gong, Tagawa, Lunn, Laroy, Heffer-Lauc, Li, Griffin, Schnaar, and Sheikh, 2002). GalNAc-GD1a, a minor ganglioside in peripheral nerves, has also been associated with AMAN, and is reported to be present in human spinal motor neurons and motor nerves but not sensory nerves (Hao, Saida, Yoshino, Kuroki, Nukina, and Saida, 1999; Yoshino, 1997).

Recently Yuki *et al.* have developed a model of AMAN by immunization of rabbits with GM1 and complete Freund's adjuvant for several months (Yuki, Yamada, *et al.*, 2001). They produced Wallerian-like degeneration of motor axons without inflammation, and with evidence of IgG antibody binding to axolemma and the distinctive periaxonal macrophages seen in human AMAN. Sheikh and colleagues (unpublished) have shown that high titer monoclonal IgG anti-GD1a antibodies administered to mice produce noninflammatory axonal degeneration. Li *et al.* (Li, Xue, *et al.*, 1996) developed an animal model of AMAN by feeding a *C. jejuni* isolate from a patient with AMAN to chickens. The pathological changes in the nerves of affected chickens were similar to those seen in human cases. Unfortunately, this model has not been reproduced in other laboratories, perhaps reflecting differences in the chicken strains. Taken together, these *in vivo* models confirm that antiganglioside antibodies can produce noninflammatory axonal injury.

## RELEVANCE OF GBS TO ACQUIRED DEMYELINATING DISORDERS OF THE CNS

The Guillain Barre syndrome (GBS) and multiple sclerosis (MS) represent the major immune-mediated disorders of the PNS and the CNS, respectively. Several common themes have recently emerged. There are similarities in the immune organization of the PNS and CNS. Several recent studies have underlined the heterogeneity in the pathology and immunopathology of MS (Bruck, Lucchinetti, *et al.*, 2002; Lassmann, 1998; Lucchinetti, Bruck, *et al.*, 2000), as well as GBS. This heterogeneity includes variation in the severity of lymphocytic inflammation, in the extent to which antibody and complement appear to play roles in tissue injury, in the extent of axonal degeneration (Trapp, Bo, *et al.*, 1999).

Several conclusions from GBS might provide questions for the future in MS. First, the data for GBS suggest that the immunologic mechanism can involve molecular mimicry, at least in some GBS variants. Through this mechanism, infectious agents as diverse as CMV, EBV, *Mycoplasma*, and *Campylobacter jejuni* have been linked to GBS syndromes that appeared similar until detailed electrophysiology, pathology, and immunology were applied. Could such etiologic heterogeneity apply to MS? Second, the GBS experience suggests that the pathogenetic effector mechanisms can differ, with some disorders largely antibody-dependent, whereas the role of antibody is uncertain in others. The immunopathologic data suggest this may also apply to MS (Bruck, Lucchinetti, and Lassmann, 2002; Lassmann, 1998; Lucchinetti, Bruck, Parisi, Scheithauer, Rodriguez, and Lassmann, 2000).

Third, as the GBS experience has shown, the target antigens need not be intrinsic myelin proteins, and indeed need not be proteins. Glycolipid serology is a notoriously difficult field. Might glycolipids be antigenic in some cases of MS, or become antigenic if antigen spreading develops? The experience with Bickerstaff's brain stem encephalitis focuses this question. As noted earlier, Bickerstaff's encephalitis is an acute monophasic CNS disorder associated with eye movement abnormalities. A small number of cases have recently demonstrated that Bickerstaff's can follow *Campylobacter jejuni* infection, and can be associated with antiGQ1b antibodies, and can overlap with the Fisher syndrome (Yuki, Sato, Tsuji, Hozumi, and Miyatake, 1993a).

Finally, in both GBS and MS it is likely that multiple mechanisms render the axon vulnerable. These mechanisms include damage as a bystander to inflammatory disease, as a consequence of the intimate cell-cell interactions between the myelin-forming cell and axon, and possibly as the target of the immune attack.

## Acknowledgments

We wish to thank and acknowledge our long-term collaborators Arthur K. Asbury, David R. Cornblath, Tony W. Ho, Chung Yun Li, Guy M. McKhann, Irving Nachamkin, and Hugh J. Willison.

## References

Ang, C. W., Yuki, N., Jacobs, B. C., Koga, M., Van Doorn, P. A., Schmitz, P. I., and van der Meche, F. G. (1999). Rapidly progressive, predominantly motor Guillain-Barre syndrome with anti-GalNAc-GD1a antibodies. *Neurology* **53,** 2122–2127.

Arnason, B. G. W., and Soliven, B. (1993). Acute inflammatory demyelinating polyradiculopathy. *In* "Peripheral Neuropathy" (P. J. Dyck, P. K. Thomas, J. W. Griffin, P. A. Low, and J. F. Poduslo, eds.), pp. 1437–1497. W. B. Saunders, Philadelphia.

Asbury, A. K., Arnason, B. G., and Adams, R. D. (1969). The inflammatory lesion in idiopathic polyneuritis. *Medicine* **48,** 173–215.

Asbury, A. K., Arnason, B. G., Karp, H. R., and McFarlin, D. E. (1978). Criteria for diagnosis of Guillain-Barre syndrome. *Annals of Neurology* **3,** 565–566.

Asbury, A. K., and Cornblath, D. R. (1990). Assessment of current diagnostic criteria for Guillain-Barre syndrome. *Annals of Neurology* **27** (Supp), S21–S24.

Aspinall, G. O., McDonald, A. G., Pang, H., Kurjanczyk, L. A., and Penner, J. L. (1994). Lipopolysaccharides of *Campylobacter jejuni* serotype O:19: Structures of core oligosaccharide regions from the serostrain and two bacterial isolates from patients with the Guillain-Barré syndrome. *Biochemistry* **33,** 241–249.

Bansil, S., Mithen, F. A., Cook, S. D., Sheffet, A., and Rohowsky-Kochan, C. (1991). Clinical correlation with serum-soluble interleukin-2 receptor levels in Guillain-Barré syndrome. *Neurology* **41,** 1302–1305.

Berciano, J., and Garcia, A. (2002). Nerve ischemia in Guillain-Barre syndrome: An alternative mechanism for early conduction failure. *Rev. Neurol (Paris)* **158,** 364–365.

Birchem, R., Mithen, F. A., L'Empereur, K. M., and Wessels, M. M. (1987). Ultrastructural effects of Guillain-Barré serum in cultures containing only rat Schwann cells and dorsal root ganglion neurons. *Brain Research* **421,** 173–185.

Brown, W. F., and Feasby, T. E. (1984). Conduction block and denervation in Guillain-Barre polyneuropathy. *Brain* **107,** 219–239.

Bruck, W., Lucchinetti, C., and Lassmann, H. (2002). The pathology of primary progressive multiple sclerosis. *Mult. Scler.* **8,** 93–97.

Buchwald, B., Weishaupt, A., Toyka, K. V., and Dudel, J. (1998). Pre and postsynaptic blockade of neuromuscular transmission by MillerFishersyndrome IgG at mouse motor nerve terminals. *European Journal of Neuroscience* **10,** 281–290.

Buzby, J. C., Allos, B. M., and Roberts, T. (1997). The economic burden of Campylobacter-associated Guillain-Barre syndrome. *Journal of Infectious Disease* **176 Suppl 2,** S192-S197.

Chiba, A., Kusunoki, S., Obata, H., Machinami, R., and Kanazawa, I. (1993). Serum anti-GQ1b antibody is associated with ophthalmoplegia in Miller Fisher syndrome and Guillain-Barre syndrome: Clinical and immunohistochemical studies. *Neurology* **43,** 1911–1917.

Chiba, A., Kusunoki, S., Obata, H., Machinami, R., and Kanazawa, I. (1997). Ganglioside composition of the human cranial nerves, with special reference to pathophysiology of Miller Fisher syndrome. *Brain Research* **745,** 32–36.

Chiba, A., Kusunoki, S., Shimizu, T., and Kanazawa, I. (1992). Serum IgG antibody to ganglioside GQ1b is a possible marker of Miller Fisher syndrome. *Annals of Neurology* **31,** 677–679.

Consensus Conference (1986). Consensus Conference: The utility of therapeutic plasmapheresis for neurological disorders. *Journal of the American Medical Association* **256,** 1333–1337.

Cornblath, D. R., McArthur, J. C., Kennedy, P. G. E., Witte, A. S., and Griffin, J. W. (1987). Inflammatory demyelinating peripheral neuropathies associated with human T-cell lymphotropic virus type III infection. *Annals of Neurology* **21,** 32–40.

Cornblath, D. R., Mellits, E. D., Griffin, J. W., McKhann, G. M., Albers, J. W., Miller, R. G., Feasby, T. E., Quaskey, S. A., and Guillain-Barre Study Group (1988). Motor conduction studies in the Guillain-Barre syndrome: Description and prognostic value. *Annals of Neurology* **23,** 354–359.

Dowling, P. C., and Cook, S. D. (1981). Role of infection in Guillain-Barre syndrome: Laboratory confirmation of Herpes viruses in 41 cases. *Annals of Neurology* **9(Suppl),** 44–55.

Drachman, D. A., Patterson, P. Y., Berlin, B., and Roguska, J. (1970). Immunosuppression in the Guillain-Barre syndrome. *Archives of Neurology* **23,** 385–393.

Eichhorst, H. (1877). Neuritis acuta progressiva. *Virchow's Archiv.* 268.

Emilia-Romagna Study Group on Clinical and Epidemiological Problems in Neurology. (1998). Guillain-Barré syndrome variants in Emilia-Romagna, Italy, 1992–3: Incidence, clinical features, and prognosis. *Journal of Neurology, Neurosurgery, and Psychiatry* **65,** 218–224.

Enders, U., Karch, H., Toyka, K. V., Michels, M., Zielasek, J., Pette, M., Heesemann, J., and Hartung, H.-P. (1993). The spectrum of immune responses to *Campylobacter jejuni* and glycoconjugates in Guillain-Barre syndrome and in other neuroimmunological disorders. *Annals of Neurology* **34,** 136–144.

Feasby, T. E., Gilbert, J. J., Brown, W. F., *et al.* (1986). An acute axonal form of Guillain-Barre polyneuropathy. *Brain* **109,** 1115–1126.

Feasby, T. E., Hahn, A. F., Brown, W. F., Bolton, C. F., Gilbert, J. J., and Koopman, W. J. (1993). Severe axonal degeneration in acute Guillain-Barre syndrome: Evidence of two different mechanisms? *Journal of Neurological Science* **116,** 185–192.

Fisher, M. (1956). An unusual variant of acute idiopathic polyneuritis (syndrome of ophthalmoplegia ataxia and areflexia). *New England Journal of Medicine* **255,** 57–65.

Fredman, P., Vedeler, C. A., Nyland, H., Aarli, J. A., and Svennerholm, L. (1991). Antibodies in sera from patients with inflammatory demyelinating polyradiculoneuropathy react with ganglioside LM1 and sulphatide of peripheral nerve myelin. *Journal of Neurology* **238,** 75–79.

French Cooperative Group on Plasma Exchange in Guillain-Barre Syndrome (1987). Efficacy of plasma exchange in Guillain-Barre syndrome: Role of replacement fluids. *Annals of Neurology* **22,** 753–761.

Fujimoto, S., Yuki, N., Itoh, T., and Amako, K. (1992). Specific serotype of *Campylobacter jejuni* associated with Guillain-Barre syndrome. *Journal of Infectious Disease* **165,** 183 (letter).

Gilbert, M., Brisson, J. R., Karwaski, M. F., Michniewicz, J., Cunningham, A. M., Wu, Y., Young, N. M., and Wakarchuk, W. W. (2000). Biosynthesis of ganglioside mimics in Campylobacter jejuni OH4384. Identification of the glycosyltransferase genes, enzymatic synthesis of model compounds, and characterization of nanomole amounts by 600-mhz (1)h and (13)c NMR analysis. *Journal of Biological Chemistry* **275,** 3896–3906.

Gong, Y., Tagawa, Y., Lunn, M. P., Laroy, W., Heffer-Lauc, M., Li, C. Y., Griffin, J. W., Schnaar, R. L., and Sheikh, K. A. (2002). Localization of major gangliosides in the PNS: Implications for immune neuropathies. *Brain* **125,** 2491–2506.

Goodyear, C. S., O'Hanlon, G. M., Plomp, J. J., Wagner, E. R., Morrison, I., Veitch, J., Cochrane, L., Bullens, R. W., Molenaar, P. C., Conner, J., and Willison, H. J. (1999). Monoclonal antibodies raised against Guillain-Barre syndrome-associated Campylobacter jejuni lipopolysaccharides react with neuronal gangliosides and paralyze muscle-nerve preparations [published erratum appears in J Clin Invest 1999 Dec; 104 (12): 1771]. *J. Clin. Invest* **104,** 697–708.

Graves, R. J. (1884). Clinical Lectures on the Practice of Medicine. *New Syd. Soc.* (reprinted from the first edition, 1843)**1,** 578.

Gregson, N. A., Koblar, S., and Hughes, R. A. (1993). Antibodies to gangliosides in Guillain-Barre syndrome: Specificity and relationship to clinical features [see comments]. *Q. J. Med.* **86,** 111–117.

Griffin, J. W., Li, C. Y., Ho, T. W., Xue, P., Macko, C., Cornblath, D. R., Gao, C. Y., Yang, C., Tian, M., Mishu, B., McKhann, G. M., and Asbury, A. K. (1995). Guillain-Barre syndrome in northern China: The spectrum of neuropathologic changes in clinically defined cases. *Brain* **118,** 577–595.

Griffin, J. W., Li, C. Y., Macko, C., Ho, T. W., Hsieh, S.-T., Xue, P., Wang, F. A., Cornblath, D. R., McKhann, G. M., and Asbury, A. K. (1996). Early nodal changes in the acute motor axonal neuropathy pattern of the Guillain-Barre syndrome. *Journal of Neurocytology* **25,** 33–51.

Guillain-Barre Study Group (1985). Plasmapheresis and acute Guillain-Barre syndrome. *Neurology* **35,** 1096–1104.

Guillain, G., Barré, J. A., and Strohl, A. (1916). Sur un syndrome de radiculonebrite avec hyperalbuminose du liquide cephalo-rachidien sans reaction cellulaire. Remarques sur les caracteres cliniques et graphiques des reflexes tendineux. *Bulletin de Societe des Medicines Hopitals de Paris* **40,** 1462.

Hadden, R. D., Cornblath, D. R., Hughes, R. A., Zielasek, J., Hartung, H. P., Toyka, K. V., and Swan, A. V. (1998). Electrophysiological classification of Guillain-Barre syndrome: Clinical associations and outcome. Plasma Exchange/Sandoglobulin Guillain-Barre Syndrome Trial Group. *Annals of Neurology* **44,** 780–788.

Hafer-Macko, C., Hsieh, S.-T., Li, C. Y., Ho, T. W., Sheikh, K. A., Cornblath, D. R., McKhann, G. M., Asbury, A. K., and Griffin, J. W. (1996). Acute motor axonal neuropathy: An antibody-mediated attack on axolemma. *Annals of Neurology* **40,** 635–644.

Hafer-Macko, C., Sheikh, K. A., Li, C. Y., Ho, T. W., Cornblath, D. R., McKhann, G. M., Asbury, A. K., and Griffin, J. W. (1996). Immune attack on the Schwann cell surface in acute inflammatory demyelinating polyneuropathy. *Annals of Neurology* **39,** 625–635.

Hall, S. M., Hughes, R. A., Atkinson, P. F., McColl, I., and Gale, A. (1992). Motor nerve biopsy in severe Guillain-Barre syndrome. *Annals of Neurology* **31,** 441–444.

Hao, Q., Saida, T., Yoshino, H., Kuroki, S., Nukina, M., and Saida, K. (1999). Anti-GalNAc-GD1a antibody-associated Guillain-Barre syndrome with a predominantly distal weakness without cranial nerve impairment and sensory disturbance. *Annals of Neurology* **45,** 758–768.

Hartung, H.-P., Pollard, J. D., Harvey, G. K., and Toyka, K. V. (1995a). Immunopathogenesis and treatment of the Guillain-Barre syndrome–Part I. *Muscle & Nerve* **18,** 137–153.

Hartung, H.-P., Pollard, J. D., Harvey, G. K., and Toyka, K. V. (1995b). Immunopathogenesis and treatment of the Guillain-Barre syndrome–Part II. *Muscle & Nerve* **18,** 154–164.

Harukawa, H., Utsumi, H., Asano, A., and Yoshino, H. (2002). Anti-LM1 antibodies in the sera of patients with Guillain-Barre syndrome, Miller Fisher syndrome, and motor neuron disease. *J Peripher. Nerv. Syst.* **7,** 54–58.

Haymaker, W., and Kernohan, J. W. (1949). The Landry-Guillain-Barre syndrome. A clinicopathologic report of fifty fatal cases and a critique of the literature. *Medicine* **28,** 59–141.

Hemachudha, T., Phanuphak, P., Johnson, R. T., Griffin, D. E., Ratanavongsiri, J., and Siriprasomsup, W. (1987). Neurologic complications of Semple-type rabis vaccine: Clinical and immunologic studies. *Neurology* **37,** 550–556.

Ho, T., Hsieh, S., Nachamkin, I., Willison, H., Sheikh, K., Kiehlbauch, J., Flanigan, K., McArthur, J., Cornblath, D., McKhann, G., and Griffin, J. (1997). Motor nerve terminal degeneration provides a potential mechanism for rapid recovery in acute motor axonal neuropathy after Campylobacter infection. *Neurology* **48,** 717–724.

Ho, T. W., Mishu, B., Li, C. Y., Gao, C. Y., Cornblath, D. R., Griffin, J. W., Asbury, A. K., Blaser, M. J., and McKhann, G. M. (1995). Guillain-Barre syndrome in northern China: Relationship to *Campylobacter jejuni* infection and anti-glycolipid antibodies. *Brain* **118,** 597–605.

Ho, T. W., Willison, H. J., Nachamkin, I., Li, C. Y., Veitch, J., Ung, H., Wang, G. R., Liu, R. C., Cornblath, D. R., Asbury, A. K., Griffin, J. W., and McKhann, G. M. (1999). AntiGD1a antibody is associated with axonal but not demyelinating forms of Guillain-Barré syndrome. *Annals of Neurology* **45,** 168–173.

Honavar, M., Tharakan, J. K. J., Hughes, R. A. C., Leibowitz, S., and Winer, J. B. (1991). A clinicopathological study of the Guillain-Barre syndrome. *Brain* **114,** 1245–1269.

Hughes, R., and Swan, A. (1995). Treatment of Guillain-Barre syndrome with intravenous methylprednisolone [letter; comment]. *Annals of Neurology* **37,** 683–684.

Hughes, R. A. C. (1990). "Guillain-Barre Syndrome." Springer-Verlag, New York.

Ilyas, A. A., Mithen, F. A., Dalakas, M. C., Chen, Z.-W., and Cook, S. D. (1992). Antibodies to acidic glycolipids in Guillain-Barré syndrome and chronic inflammatory demyelinating polyneuropathy. *Journal of Neurological Science* **107,** 111–121.

Ilyas, A. A., Willison, H. J., Quarles, R. H., Jungawala, F. B., Cornblath, D. R., Trapp, B. D., Griffin, D. E., Griffin, J. W., and McKhann, G. M. (1988). Serum antibodies to gangliosides in Guillain-Barre syndrome. *Annals of Neurology* **23,** 440–447.

Jacobs, B., Van Doorn, P. A., Schmitz, P. I., Tio-Gillen, A. P., Herbrink. P, Visser, L. H., Hooijkaas, H., and van der Meche, F. G. (1996). *Campylobacter jejuni* Infections and Anti-GM1 Antibodies in Guillain-Barre Syndrome. *Annals of Neurology* **40,** 181–187.

Jacobs, B. C., Endtz, H., van der Meché, F. G. A., Hazenberg, M. P., Achtereekte, H. A., and Van Doorn, P. A. (1995). Serum anti-GQ1b IgG antibodies recognize surface epitopes on *Campylobacter jejuni* from patients with Miller Fisher syndrome. *Annals of Neurology* **37,** 260–264.

Jacobs, B. C., Rothbarth, P. H., van der Meche, F. G. A., Herbrink. P, Schmitz, P. I. M., de Klerk, M. A., and van Doorn, PA. (1998). The spectrum of antecedent infections in Guillain-Barré syndrome. *Neurology* **51,** 1110–1115.

Kaida, K., Kusunoki, S., Kamakura, K., Motoyoshi, K., and Kanazawa, I. (2000). Guillain-Barre syndrome with antibody to a ganglioside, N-acetylgalactosaminyl GD1a. *Brain* **123 (Pt 1),** 116–124.

Kaldor, J., and Speed, B. R. (1984). Guillain-Barre syndrome and *Campylobacter jejuni:* A serological study. *British Medical Journal* **288,** 1867–1870.

Kaplan, J. E., Schonberger, L. B., Hurwitz, E. S., and Katona, P. (1983). Guillain-Barre syndrome in the United States, 1978–1981: Additional observations from the national surveillance system (Letter). *Neurology* **33,** 633–636.

Kashihara, K., Shiro, Y., Koga, M., and Yuki, N. (1998). IgG Anti-GT1a antibodies which do not cross react with GQ1b ganglioside in a pharyngeal-cervical-brachial variant of Guillain-Barré syndrome. *Journal of Neurology, Neurosurgery, and Psychiatry* **65,** 799.

Koga, M., Yuki, N., Ariga, T., Morimatsu, M., and Hirata, K. (1998). Is IgG anti-GT1a antibody associated with pharyngeal-cervical-brachial weakness or oropharyngeal palsy in Guillain-Barré syndrome? *Journal of Neuroimmunology* **86,** 74–79.

Kornberg, A. J., Pestronk, A., Bieser, K., Ho, T. W., McKhann, G. M., Wu, H. S., and Jiang, Z. (1994). The clinical correlates of high-titer IgG anti-GM1 antibodies. *Annals of Neurology* **35,** 234–237.

Koski, C. L., Chou, D. K. H., and Jungalwala, F. B. (1989). Anti-peripheral nerve myelin antibodies in Guillain-Barre syndrome bind a neutral glycolipid of peripheral myelin and cross-react with Forssman antigen. *Journal of Clinical Investigation* **84,** 280–287.

Koski, C. L., Humphrey, R., and Shin, M. L. (1985). Anti-peripheral myelin antibodies in patients with demyelinating neuropathy: Quantitative and kinetic determination of serum antibody by complement component 1 fixation. *Proceedings of the National Academy of Science USA* **82,** 905–909.

Kuroki, S., Saida, T., Nukina, M., Haruta, T., Yoshioka, M., Kobayashi, Y., and Nakanishi, H. (1993). *Campylobacter jejuni* strains from patients with Guillain-Barre syndrome belong mostly to Penner serogroup 19 and contain beta-*N*-acetylglucosamine residues. *Annals of Neurology* **33,** 243–247.

Kusunoki, S., Chiba, A., Kon, K., Ando, S., Arisawa, K., Tate, A., and Kanazawa, I. (1994). N-acetylgalactosaminyl GD1a is a target molecule for serum antibody in Guillain-Barre syndrome. *Annals of Neurology* **35,** 570–576.

Kusunoki, S., Hitoshi, S., Kaida, K., Arita, M., and Kanazawa, I. (1999). Monospecific anti-GD1b IgG is required to induce rabbit ataxic neuropathy. *Ann. Neurol* **45,** 400–403.

Kusunoki, S., Iwamori, M., Chiba, A., *et al.* (1996). GM1b is a new member of antigen for serum antibody in Guillain-Barré syndrome. *Neurology* **47,** 237–242.

Kuwabara, S., Yuki, N., Koga, M., Hattori, T., Matsuura, D., Miyake, M., and Noda, M. (1998). IgG anti-GM1 antibody is associated with reversible conduction failure and axonal degeneration in Guillain-Barre syndrome. *Annals of Neurology* **44,** 202–208.

Landry, O. (1859). Note sur paralysie ascendante aigue. *Gaz. Hebdom* 472–486.

Lasky, T., Terracciano, G. J., Magder, L., Koski, C. L., Ballesteros M., Nash, D., Claek, S., Haber, P., Stolley, P. D., Schonberger, L. B., and Chen, R. T. (1998). The Guillain-Barre syndrome and the 1992–1993 and 1993–1994 influenza vaccines. *New England Journal of Medicine* **339,** 1797–1802.

Lassmann, H. (1998). Neuropathology in multiple sclerosis: New concepts. *Mult. Scler.* **4,** 93–98.

Lastovica, A. J., Goddard, E. A., and Argent, A. C. (1997). Guillain-Barre syndrome in South Africa associated with Campylobacter jejuni O:41 strains. *Journal of Infectious Disease* **176 Suppl 2,** S139-S143.

Li, C. Y., Xue, P., Gao, C. Y., Tian, W. Q., Liu, R. C., and Yang, C. (1996). Experimental *Campylobacter jejuni* infection in the chicken: An animal model of axonal Guillain-Barré syndrome. *Journal of Neurology,Neurosurgery,and Psychiatry* **61,** 279–284.

Linton, D., Gilbert, M., Hitchen, P. G., Dell, A., Morris, H. R., Wakarchuk, W. W., Gregson, N. A., and Wren, B. W. (2000). Phase variation of a beta-1,3 galactosyltransferase involved in generation of the ganglioside GM1-like lipo-oligosaccharide of campylobacter jejuni [In Process Citation]. *Molecular Microbiology* **37,** 501–514.

Linton, D., Karlyshev, A. V., Hitchen, P. G., Morris, H. R., Dell, A., Gregson, N. A., and Wren, B. W. (2000). Multiple N-acetyl neuraminic acid synthetase (neuB) genes in Campylobacter jejuni: Identification and characterization of the gene involved in sialylation of lipo-oligosaccharide. *Molecular Microbiology* **35,** 1120–1134.

Lisak, R. P., Mitchell, M., Zweiman, B., *et al.* (1977). Guillain-Barre syndrome and Hodgkin's disease: Three cases with immunological studies. *Annals of Neurology* **1,** 72–78.

Lu, J. L., Sheikh, K. A., Wu, H. S., Zhang, J., Jiang, Z. F., Cornblath, D. R., McKhann, G. M., Asbury, A. K., Griffin, J. W., and Ho, T. W. (2000). Physiological-pathological correlation in Guillain-Barre syndrome. *Neurol.* **54,** 33–39.

Lucchinetti, C., Bruck, W., Parisi, J., Scheithauer, B., Rodriguez, M., and Lassmann, H. (2000). Heterogeneity of multiple sclerosis lesions: Implications for the pathogenesis of demyelination. *Ann. Neurol* **47,** 707–717.

Lunn, M. P., Johnson, L. A., Fromholt, S. E., Itonori, S., Huang, J., Vyas, A. A., Hildreth, J. E., Griffin, J. W., Schnaar, R. L., and Sheikh, K. A. (2000). High-affinity anti-ganglioside IgG antibodies raised in complex ganglioside knockout mice: Reexamination of GD1a immunolocalization [In Process Citation]. *Journal of Neurochemistry* **75,** 404–412.

Massaro, M. E., Rodriguez, E. C., Pociecha, J., Arroyo, H. A., Sacolitti, M., Taratuto, A. L., Fejerman, N., and Reisin, R. C. (1998). Nerve biopsy in children with severe Guillain-Barre syndrome and inexcitable motor nerves. *Neurology* **51,** 394–398.

McCarthy, N., Andersson, Y., Jormanainen, V., Gustavsson, O., and Giesecke, J. (1999). The risk of Guillain-Barre syndrome following infection with Campylobacter jejuni. *Epidemiol. Infect.* **122,** 15–17.

McKhann, G. M., Cornblath, D. R., Griffin, J. W., Ho, T. W., Li, C. Y., Jiang, Z., Wu, H. S., Zhaori, G., Liu, Y., Jou, L. P., Liu, T. C., Gao, C. Y., Mao, J. Y., Blaser, M. J., Mishu, B., and Asbury, A. K. (1993). Acute motor axonal neuropathy: A frequent cause of acute flaccid paralysis in China. *Annals of Neurology* **33,** 333–342.

McKhann, G. M., Cornblath, D. R., Ho, T. W., Li, C. Y., Bai, A. Y., Wu, H. S., Yei, Q. F., Zhang, W. C., Zhaori, Z., Jiang, Z., Griffin, J. W., and Asbury, A. K. (1991). Clinical and electrophysiological aspects of acute paralytic disease of children and young adults in northern China. *The Lancet* **338,** 593–597.

Mishu, B., and Blaser, M. J. (1993). The role of *Campylobacter jejuni* infection in the initiation of Guillain-Barre syndrome. *Clinical Infectious Disease* **17,** 104–108.

Mishu, B., Ilyas, A. A., Koski, C. L., Vriesendorp, F., Cook, S. A., Mithen, F., and Blaser, M. J. (1993). Serologic evidence of previous *Campylobacter jejuni* infection in patients with the Guillain-Barre syndrome. *Annals of Internal Medicine* **118,** 947–953.

Mithen, F. A., Ilyas, A. A., Birchem, R., and Cook, S. D. (1992). Effects of Guillain-Barré sera containing antibodies against glycolipids in cultures of rat Schwann cells and sensory neurons. *Journal of Neurological Science* **112,** 223–232.

Miyazaki, T., Kusunoki, S., Kaida, K., Shiina, M., and Kanazawa, I. (2001). Guillain-Barre syndrome associated with IgG monospecific to ganglioside GD1b. *Neurology* **56,** 1227–1229.

O'Hanlon, G. M., Paterson, G. J., Wilson, G., *et al.* (1996). Anti-GM1 ganglioside antibodies cloned from autoimmune neuropathy patients show diverse binding patterns in the rodent nervous system. *J. Neuropath. Exp. Neurol.* **55,** 184–195.

Ogino, M., Orazio, N., and Latov, N. (1995). IgG anti-GM1 antibodies from patients with acute motor neuropathy are predominantly of the IgG1 and IgG3 subclasses. *Journal of Neuroimmunology* **58,** 77–80.

Oomes, P. G., Jacobs, B. C., Hazenberg, M. P. H., Banffer, J. R. J., and van der Meché, F. G. A. (1995). Anti-GM1 IgG antibodies and *Campylobacter jejuni* bacteria in Guillain-Barre syndrome: Evidence of molecular mimicry. *Annals of Neurology* **38,** 170–175.

Osler, W. (1892). "The Principles and Practice of Medicine." D. Appleton and Company, New York.

Parkhill, J., Wren, B. W., Mungall, K., Ketley, J. M., Churcher, C., Basham, D., Chillingworth, T., Davies, R. M., Feltwell, T., Holroyd, S., Jagels, K., Karlyshev, A. V., Moule, S., Pallen, M. J., Penn, C. W., Quail, M. A., Rajandream, M. A., Rutherford, K. M., van Vliet, A. H., Whitehead, S., and Barrell, B. G. (2000). The genome sequence of the food-borne pathogen Campylobacter jejuni reveals hypervariable sequences. *Nature* **403,** 665–668.

Penner, J. L., and Hennessy, J. N. (1980). Passive hemagglutination techniques for serotyping *Campylobacter fetus* subsp. *jejuni* on the basis of soluble heat-stable antigens. *Journal of Clinincal Microbiology* **12,** 732–737.

Penner, J. L., Hennessy, J. N., and Congi, A. R. V. (1983). Serotyping of *Campylobacter jejuni* and *Campylobacter coli* on the basis of thermostable antigens. *European Journal of Clinical Microbiology* **2,** 378–383.

Plomp, J. J., Molenaar, P. C., O'Hanlon, G. M., Jacobs, B. C., Veitch, J., Daha, M. R., Van Doorn, P. A., van der Meche, F. G., Vincent, A., Morgan, B. P., and Willison, H. J. (1999a). Miller Fisher anti-GQ1b antibodies: Alpha-latrotoxin-like effects on motor end plates [published erratum appears in *Ann. Neurol.* 1999;45:823]. *Annals of Neurology* **45,** 189–199.

Plomp, J. J., Molenaar, P. C., O'Hanlon, G. M., Jacobs, B. C., Veitch, J., Daha, M. R., vanDoorn, P. A., van der Meche, F. G. A., Vincent, A., Morgan, B. P., and Willison, H. J. (1999b). Miller Fisher Anti-GQ1b Antibodies: α-Latrotoxin-Like Effects on Motor End Plates. *Annals of Neurology* **45,** 189–199.

Pollard, J. D., Westland, K. W., Harvey, G. K., *et al.* (1995). Activated T cells of nonneural specificity open the blood-nerve barrier to circulating antibody. *Annals of Neurology* **37,** 467–475.

Prendergast, M. M., Lastovica, A. J., and Moran, A. P. (1998). Lipopolysaccharides from Campylobacter jejuni O:41 strains associated with Guillain-Barre syndrome exhibit mimicry of GM1 ganglioside. *Infection and Immunology* **66,** 3649–3655.

Prineas, J. W. (1981). Pathology of the Guillain-Barre syndrome. *Annals of Neurology* **9(Suppl),** 6–19.

Ravn, H. (1967). The Landry-Guillain-Barre syndrome. *Acta Neurologica Scandinavica* **30,** 8–64.

Rees, J. H., Gregson, N. A., and Hughes, R. A. C. (1995). Anti-ganglioside GM1 antibodies in Guillain-Barre syndrome and their relationship to *Campylobacter jejuni* infection. *Annals of Neurology* **38,** 809–816.

Rees, J. H., Soudain, S. E., Gregson, N. A., and Hughes, R. A. (1995). *Campylobacter jejuni* infection and Guillain-Barré syndrome. *New England Journal of Medicine* **333,** 1374–1379.

Reisin, R. C., Cersosimo, R., Garcia Alvarez, M., Massaro, M. E., and Fejerman, N. (93 A. D.). Acute "axonal" Guillain-barre syndrome in childhood. *Muscle & Nerve* **16,** 1310–1316.

Reisin, R. C., Pociecha, J., Rodriguez, E., Massaro, M. E., Arroyo, H. A., and Fejerman, N. Severe Guillain-Barre syndrome in childhood treated with human immune globulin. *Pediatric. Neurology 1996.May.* **14,** 308–312.

Roberts, M., Willison, H., Vincent, A., and Newsom-Davis, J. (1994). Serum factor in Miller-Fisher variant of Guillain-Barre syndrome and neurotransmitter release. *The Lancet* **343,** 454–455.

Ropper, A. H., Wijdicks, E. F. M., and Truax, B. T. (1991). "Guillain-Barre Syndrome." F. A. Davis Company, Philadelphia.

Ross, J., and Bury, J. S. (1893). "A Treatise on Peripheral Neuritis." Charles Griffin and Company, London.

Saida, K., Saida, T., Brown, M. J., and Silberberg, D. H. (1979). In vivo demyelination induced by intraneural injection of antigalactocerebroside serum. *American Journal of Pathology* **95,** 99–116.

Saida, T., Saida, K., Lisak, R. P., Brown, M. J., Silberberg, D. H., and Asbury, A. K. (1982). In vivo demyelinating activity of sera from patients with Guillain-Barre syndrome. *Annals of Neurology* **11,** 69–75.

Salloway, S., Mermel, L. A., Seamans, M., Aspinall, G. O., Nam Shin, J. E., Kurjanczyk, L. A., and Penner, J. L. (1996). Miller-Fisher syndrome associated with Campylobacter jejuni bearing lipopolysaccharide molecules that mimic human ganglioside GD3. *Infection and Immunology* **64,** 2945–2949.

Sanders, F. K. (1948). The thickness of myelin sheaths of normal and regenerating peripheral nerve fibers. *Proceedings of the National Academy of Science,London* **135,** 323–357.

Sawant-Mane, S., Clark, M. B., and Koski, C. L. (1991). In vitro demyelination by serum antibody from patients with Guillain-Barre syndrome requires terminal complement complexes. *Annals of Neurology* **29,** 397–404.

Sawant-Mane, S., Estep, A. 3., and Koski, C. L. (1994). Antibody of patients with Guillain-Barre syndrome mediates complement-dependent cytolysis of rat Schwann cells: Susceptibility to cytolysis reflects Schwann cell phenotype. *Journal of Neuroimmunology* **49,** 145–152.

Schonberger, L. B., Bregman, D. J., Sullivan-Bolyai, J. Z., Keenlyside, R. A., Ziegler, D. W., Retailliau, H. F., Eddins, D. L., and Bryan, J. A. (1979). Guillain-Barre syndrome following vaccination in the national influenza immunization program, United States, 1976–1977. *American Journal of Epidemiology* **110,** 105–123.

Sharief, M. K., Ingram, D. A., and Swash, M. (1997). Circulating tumor necrosis factor-alpha correlates with electrodiagnostic abnormalities in Guillain-Barre syndrome. *Annals of Neurology* **42,** 68–73.

Sharief, M. K., McLean, B., and Thompson, E. J. (1993). Elevated serum levels of tumor necrosis factor-alpha in Guillain-Barre syndrome. *Annals of Neurology* **33,** 591–596.

Sheikh, K. A., Deerinck, T. J., Ellisman, M. H., and Griffin, J. W. (1999). The distribution of ganglioside-like moieties in peripheral nerves. *Brain* **122 (Pt 3),** 449–460.

Sheikh, K. A., Nachamkin, I., Ho, T. W., Willison, H. J., Veitch, J., Ung, H., Nicholson, M., Li, C. Y., Wu, H. S., Shen, B. Q., Cornblath, D. R., Asbury, A. K., McKhann, G. M., and Griffin, J. W. (1998). Campylobacter jejuni lipopolysaccharides in Guillain-Barre syndrome: Molecular mimicry and host susceptibility. *Neurology* **51,** 371–378.

Sheikh, K. A., Sun, J. L. Y., Kawai, H., Crawford, T. O., Proia, R. L. G. J. W., and Schnaar, R. L. (1999). Mice lacking complex gangliosides develop Wallerian degeneration and myelination defects. *Proceedings of the National Academy of Science USA* **96,** 7532–7537.

Siebert, P. D., and Larrick, J. W. (1992). Competitive PCR. *Nature* **359,** 557–558.

Sivieri, S., Ferrarini, A. M., Lolli, F., Mata, S., Pinto, F., Tavolato, B., and Gallo, P. (1997). Cytokine pattern in the cerebrospinal fluid from patients with GBS and CIDP. *Journal of Neurological Science* **147,** 93–95.

Speed, B., Kaldor, J., and Cavanagh, P. (1984). Guillain-Barre syndrome associated with *Campylobacter jejuni* enteritis. *Journal of Infectious Disease* **8,** 85–86.

Spies, J. M., Pollard, J. D., Bonner, J. G., Westland, K. W., and McLeod, J. G. (1995). Synergy between antibody and P2-reactive T cells in experimental allergic neuritis. *Journal of Neuroimmunology* **57,** 77–84.

Spies, J. M., Westland, K. W., Bonner, J. G., and Pollard, J. D. (1995). Intraneural activated T cells cause focal breakdown of the blood-nerve barrier. *Brain* **118,** 857–868.

Tauxe, R. V. (1992). Epidemiology of *Campylobacter jejuni* infections in the United States and other industrialized nations. *In* "*Campylobacter jejuni:* Current Status and Future Trends" (I. Nachamkin, M. J. Blaser, and L. S. Tompkins, Eds.), pp. 9–19. American Society for Microbiology, Washington, D. C.

Trapp, B. D., Bo, L., Mork, S., and Chang, A. (1999). Pathogenesis of tissue injury in MS lesions. *Journal of Neuroimmunology* **98,** 49–56.

van der Meche, F. G. A., Meulstee, J., Vermeulen, M., and Kievit, A. (1988). Patterns of conduction failure in the Guillain-Barre syndrome. *Brain* **111,** 405–416.

van der Meché, F. G. A., Schmitz, P. I. M., and Dutch Guillain-Barre Study Group. (1992a). A randomized trial comparing intravenous immune globulin and plasma exchange in Guillain-Barre syndrome. *New England Journal of Medicine* **326,** 1123–1129.

van der Meché, F. G. A., Schmitz, P. I. M., Meulstee, J., and Oomes, P. G. (1992b). Prognostic factors in the Dutch Guillain-Barre study. Journal of Neurology 239 (suppl 2), S52. Abstract.

Visser, L. H., van der Meché, F. G. A., Meulstee, J., Rothbarth, P. Ph., Jacobs, B. C., Schmitz, P. I. M., Van Doorn, P. A., and Dutch Guillain-Barré Study Group (1996). Cytomegalovirus infection and Guillain-Barré syndrome: The clinical, electrophysiologic, and prognostic features. *Neurology* **47,** 668–673.

Visser, L. H., van der Meché, F. G. A., Van Doorn, P. A., *et al.* (1995). Guillain-Barré syndrome without sensory loss (acute motor neuropathy): A subgroup with specific clinical, electrodiagnostic and laboratory features. *Brain* **118,** 841–847.

Vriesendorp, F. J., Mishu, B., Blaser, M., and Koski, C. L. (1993). Serum antibodies to GM1, peripheral nerve myelin, and *Campylobacter jejuni* in patients with Guillain-Barre syndrome and controls: Correlation and prognosis. *Annals of Neurology* **34,** 130–135.

Walsh, F. S., Cronin, M., Koblar, S., Doherty, P., Winer, J., Leon, A., and Hughes, R. A. C. (1991). Association between glycoconjugate antibodies and Campylobacter infection in patients with Guillain-Barre syndrome. *Journal of Neuroimmunology* **34,** 43–51.

Willison, H. J., Almemar, A., Veitch, J., and Thrush, D. (1994). Acute ataxic neuropathy with cross-reactive antibodies to GD1b and GD3 gangliosides. *Neurology* **44,** 2395–2397.

Willison, H. J., and Veitch, J. (1994). Immunoglobulin subclass distribution and binding characteristics of anti-GQ1b antibodies in Miller Fisher syndrome. *Journal of Neuroimmunology* **50,** 159–165.

Willison, H. J., Veitch, J., Patterson, G., and Kennedy, P. G. E. (1993). Miller Fisher syndrome is associated with serum antibodies to GQ1b ganglioside. *Journal of Neurology,Neurosurgery,and Psychiatry* **56,** 204–206.

Yako, K., Kusunoki, S., and Kanazawa, I. (1999). Serum antibody against a peripheral nerve myelin ganglioside, LM1, in Guillain-Barre syndrome. *J Neurol Sci.* **168,** 85–89.

Yoshino, H. (1997). Distribution of gangliosides in the nervous tissues recognized by axonal form of Guillain-Barre syndrome (in Japanese). *Neuroimmunology* **5,** 174–175.

Yuki, N., Ang, C. W., Koga, M., Jacobs, B. C., Van Doorn, P. A., Hirata, K., and van der Meche, F. G. (2000). Clinical features and response to treatment in Guillain-Barre syndrome associated with antibodies to GM1b ganglioside. *Annals of Neurology* **47,** 314–321.

Yuki, N., Handa, S., Taki, T., Kasama, T., Takahashi, M., and Saito, K. (1992). Cross-reactive antigen between nervous tissue and a bacterium elicits Guillain-Barre syndrome: Molecular mimicry between gangliocide GM1 and lipopolysaccharide from Penner's serotype 19 of *Campylobacter jejuni. Biomedical Research* **13,** 451–453.

Yuki, N., Ho, T. W., Tagawa, Y., Koga, M., Li, C. Y., Hirata, K., and Griffin, J. W. (1999). Autoantibodies to GM1b and GalNAc-GD1a: Relationship to Campylobacter jejuni infection and acute motor axonal neuropathy in China. *Journal of Neurological Science* **164,** 134–138.

Yuki, N., Sato, S., Tsuji, S., Hozumi, I., and Miyatake, T. (1993a). An immunologic abnormality common to Bickerstaff's brain stem encephalitis and Fisher's syndrome. *Journal of Neurological Science* **118,** 83–87.

Yuki, N., Sato, S., Tsuji, S., Ohsawa, T., and Miyatake, T. (1993b). Frequent presence of anti-GQ1b antibody in Fisher's syndrome. *Neurology* **43,** 414–417.

Yuki, N., Takahashi, M., Tagawa, Y., Kashiwase, K., Tadokoro, K., and Saito, K. (1997). Association of Campylobacter jejuni Serotype with Antiganglioside Antibody in Guillain-Barre Syndrome and Fisher's Syndrome. *Annals of Neurology* **42,** 28–33.

Yuki, N., Taki, T., Inagaki, F., *et al.* (1993). A bacterium lipopolysaccharide that elicits Guillain-Barre syndrome has a GM1 ganglioside-like structure. *Journal of Experimental Medicine* **178,** 1771–1775.

Yuki, N., Taki, T., Takahashi, M., Saito, K., Yoshino, H., Tai, T., Handa, S., and Miyatake, T. (1994). Molecular mimicry between $GQ_{1b}$ ganglioside and lipopolysaccharides of *Campylobacter jejuni* isolated from patients with Fisher's syndrome. *Annals of Neurology* **36,** 791–793.

Yuki, N., Yamada, M., Koga, M., Odaka, M., Susuki, K., Tagawa, Y., Ueda, S., Kasama, T., Ohnishi, A., Hayashi, S., Takahashi, H., Kamijo, M., and Hirata, K. (2001). Animal model of axonal Guillain-Barre syndrome induced by sensitization with GM1 ganglioside. *Annals of Neurology* **49,** 712–720.

Yuki, N., Yoshino, H., Sato, S., and Miyatake, T. (1990). Acute axonal polyneuropathy associated with anti-$GM_1$ antibodies following *Campylobacter jejuni* enteritis. *Neurology* **40,** 1900–1902.

Yuki, N., Yoshino, H., Sato, S., Shinozawa, K., and Miyatake, T. (1992). Severe acute axonal form of Guillain-Barre syndrome associated with IgG anti-$GD_{1a}$ antibodies. *Muscle & Nerve* **15,** 899–903.

CHAPTER

# 39

# Inherited Neuropathies: Clinical, Genetic, and Biological Features

*Lawrence Wrabetz, M. Laura Feltri, Kleopas A. Kleopa, and Steven S. Scherer*

## INTRODUCTION

Neuropathy is a frequent component of numerous inherited syndromes. When it occurs in isolation, it is usually called Charcot-Marie-Tooth disease (CMT). The biology of axons and myelinating Schwann cells makes them vulnerable to the effects of mutations in a large number of genes. We emphasize the varieties of inherited demyelinating neuropathies, their clinical phenotypes, the mutations that cause these phenotypes, and update their pathogenesis gene-by-gene (for reviews, see Berger *et al.*, 2002b; Dyck *et al.*, 1993a; Harding, 1995; Kleopa and Scherer, 2002; Lupski and Garcia, 2001; Wrabetz *et al.*, 2001).

## THE CLINICAL CLASSIFICATION OF INHERITED NEUROPATHIES

Inherited neuropathies have been recognized since the late 1800s, when various forms were described by Charcot, Marie, Tooth, Herringham, Déjérine, and Sottas (Dyck *et al.*, 1993a). The dominantly inherited forms have come to be known as CMT, although an alternative designation, hereditary motor and sensory neuropathy (HMSN), has been widely used, too. CMT/HMSN was subdivided into demyelinating (CMT1) and axonal (CMT2) forms according to clinical, electrophysiological, and histological features. CMT1/HMSN I is more common and is characterized by an earlier age of onset (first or second decade of life), nerve conduction velocities (NCVs) less than 38 m/s in upper limb nerves, and segmental demyelination, remyelination, and onion bulb formations in nerve biopsies. CMT2/HMSN II has a later onset, NCVs greater than 38 m/s, and biopsies mainly show loss of myelinated axons (Dyck *et al.*, 1993a).

The terms Déjérine-Sottas syndrome (DSS), HMSN III, and CMT3 denote children who have a severe neuropathy (Dyck *et al.*, 1993a; Gabreels-Festen, 2002; Ouvrier, 1996; Ouvrier *et al.*, 1990; Plante-Bordeneuve and Said, 2002). Motor development is delayed before 3 years of age, sometimes extending to infancy. Motor abilities typically improve during the first decade, but this may be followed by progressive weakness to the point that many affected individuals use wheelchairs. Ventilatory failure (presumably caused by phrenic nerve involvement) can occur, even during infancy or childhood. Kyphoscoliosis, short stature, and foot deformities are common in older children. Sensory loss is profound, especially for modalities subserved by myelinated axons, to the point that some children have a severe sensory ataxia. Tendon reflexes are absent. Occasional patients have cranial nerve involvement—miosis, reduced pupillary responses to light, ptosis, facial weakness, nystagmus, and hearing loss. CSF protein may be elevated, and nerve roots may enhance by MRI. NCVs are very slow (<10 m/s), with marked temporal dispersion but no conduction block (Benstead *et al.*, 1990). Nerves are often enlarged, and biopsies reveal a complete absence of fibers containing normal/thick myelin sheaths and prominent "onion bulbs"; edema may be present. Axons have inappropriately thin myelin sheaths for the axonal caliber and/or are segmentally demyelinated (Fig. 39.1). Historically, DSS/CMT3/HMSN III was thought to be recessively inherited. Now it is clear that new dominant mutations in *Myelin Protein Zero* (*MPZ*), *Peripheral Myelin Protein 22 kDa* (*PMP22*), and *Early Growth Response Gene 2* (*EGR2*) are the commonest causes (Nelis *et al.*, 1999); homozygous recessive mutations of *MPZ*, *PMP22*, *EGR2*, or other genes are rarer causes (Tab. 39.1). Thus, while DSS/CMT3/HMSN III are meaningful labels of a clinical phenotype, their lack of specificity makes them difficult to use in genetic classifications. The rare recessive forms have been placed in a separate group, "CMT4" (Tab. 39.1).

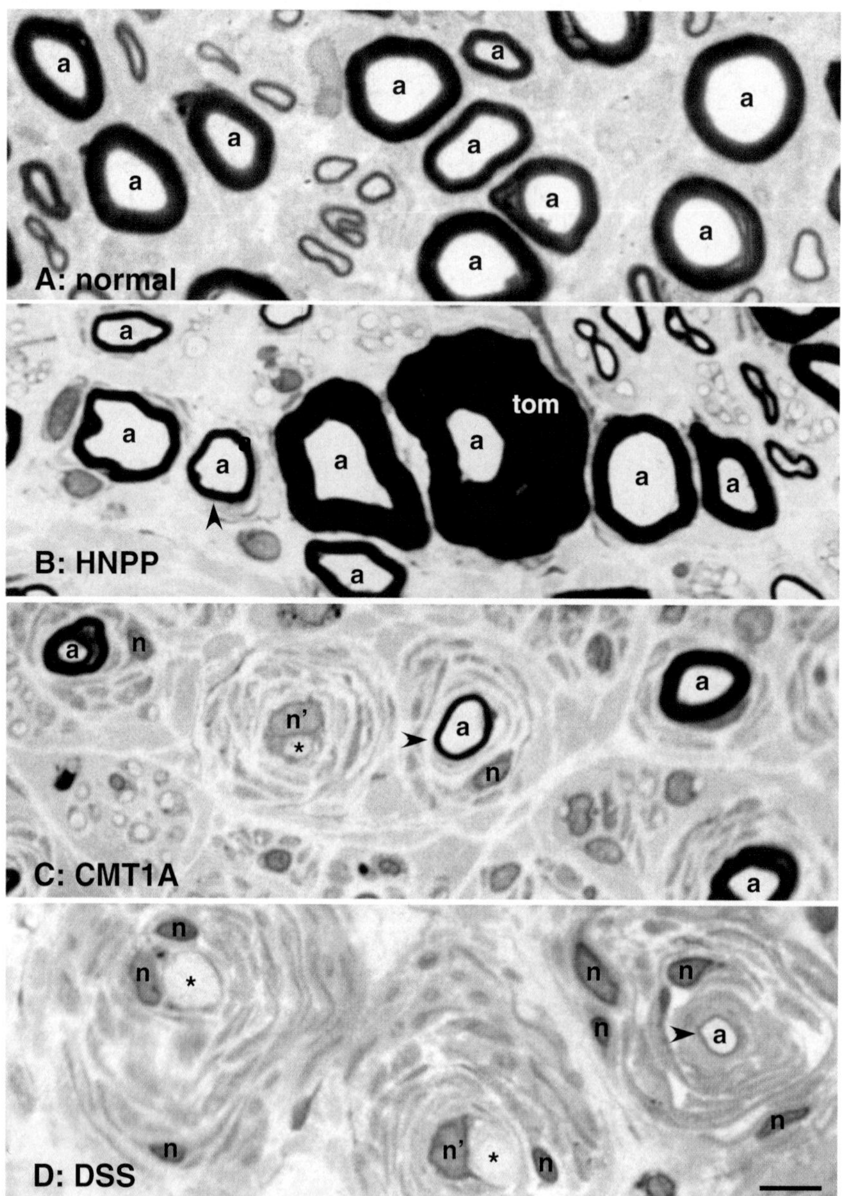


FIGURE 39.1
The pathological features of HNPP, CMT1, and DSS. These are photomicrographs of semi-thin sections of sural nerve biopsies stained with methylene blue-azure II-basic fuchsin from a 27-year-old patient with normal findings (A), a 32-year-old with HNPP (B), a 46-year-old with CMT1A (C), and a 16-year-old with dominantly inherited DSS (D), previously reported (Lynch *et al.*, 1997). Myelinated axons (a); demyelinated axons (*) and their associated Schwann cell nuclei (n); remyelinated axons (arrowheads). In B, note the tomaculum (tom). In C and D, note the supernumerary Schwann cell processes and their nuclei (n') that form "onion bulbs" around demyelinated and remyelinated axons. Scale bar 10 μm.

TABLE 39.1 Genetic Classification of the Non-syndromic Inherited Neuropathies

The table lists non-syndromic inherited neuropathies as they are classified by MIM (http://www.ncbi.nlm.nih.gov/ Omim/). Unless otherwise noted, the references are listed in the website (http://molgen-www.uia.ac.be/CMTMutations/DataSource/MutByGene.cfm). For syndromic neuropathies, see the website (http://www.neuro.wustl.edu/neuromuscular/time/hmsn.html).

| Disease (MIM) | Linkage | Affected gene | References |
|---|---|---|---|
| **CMT1 (autosomal or X-linked dominant demyelinating)** | | | |
| **HNPP** (MIM 162500) | 17p11 | *PMP22* | See text |
| **CMT1A** (MIM 118220) | 17p11 | *PMP22* (MIM 601097) | See text |
| **CMT1B** (MIM 118200) | 1q22-23 | *MPZ* (MIM 159440) | See text |
| **CMT1C** (MIM 601098) | 16p13.1.-12.3 | *LITAF/SIMPLE* | See text |
| **CMT1** | 10q21 | *EGR2* (MIM 129010) | See text |
| **CMT1X** (MIM 302800) | Xq13.1 | *GJB1* (MIM 304040) | See text |
| **Intermediate CMT (I-CMT; autosomal dominant)** | | | |
| **I-CMT1** | 10q24.1-25.1 | Outside *EGR2* and HSMN-R loci | (Verhoeven *et al.*, 2001; Villanova *et al.*, 1998) |
| **I-CMT2** | 19p12-13.2 | | (Kennerson *et al.*, 2001) |
| **CMT2 (autosomal dominant axonal/neuronal)** | | | |
| **CMT2A** (MIM 118210) | 1p35-36 | *KIF1Bβ* (MIM 605995) | See text |
| **CMT2B** (MIM 600882) | 3q13-22 | *RAB7* | (Verhoeven *et al.*, 2003) |
| **CMT2B**-not linked to 3q13-22 (no MIM) | | | (Auer-Grumbach *et al.*, 2000b) |
| **CMT2C** (with vocal cord paresis) (MIM 606071) | 12q23-24 | | Klein *et al.*, 2003 |
| **CMT2D** (MIM 601472) May be allelic to distal SMA/ HMN-V (MIM 600794) | 7p14 | *GARS* | Antonellis *et al.*, 2003 |
| **CMT2E** (MIM 162280) | 8p21 | *NEFL* | See text |
| **CMT2F** (no MIM) | 7q11-21 | | (Ismailov *et al.*, 2001) |
| **CMT2G** (MIM 604484) (proximal, Okinawa type, HSMNP or HSMNO) | 3q13.1 | | (Takashima *et al.*, 1997; Takashima *et al.*, 1999) |
| **CMT2-P$_0$** (MIM 118200) | 1q22-23 | *MPZ* | See text |
| **Severe demyelinating, autosomal dominant or recessive phenotypes ("CMT3")** | | | |
| **Dejerine-Sottas Disease/HMSN-III** (MIM 145900) | 17p11<br>1p22-23<br>Xq13.1<br>10q21<br>19q13.1<br>8p21 | *PMP22*<br>*MPZ*<br>*GJB1* (F235C)<br>*EGR2*<br>*PRX*<br>*NEFL* | See text<br>See text<br>See text<br>See text<br>See text<br>See text |
| **Congenital Hypomyelinating Neuropathy (CHN)** (MIM 605253); see also CMT4E | 10q21<br>17p11<br>1p22-23<br>11q22 | *EGR2*,<br>*PMP22*<br>*MPZ*<br>*MTMR2* | See text<br>See text<br>See text<br>See text |
| **Autosomal recessive demyelinating neuropathy ("CMT4")** | | | |
| **CMT4A** (MIM 214400) | 8q13-q21.1 | *GDAP1* | See text |
| **CMT4B-1** (MIM 601382) | 11q22 | *MTMR2* (MIM 603557) | See text |
| **CMT4B-2** (MIM 604563) | 11p15 | *MTMR13* | See text |
| **CMT4C** (MIM 601596) | 5q32 | | (Guilbot *et al.*, 1999; Le Guern *et al.*, 1996) |

(*Continues*)

TABLE 39.1 (*Continued*)

| Disease (MIM) | Linkage | Affected gene | References |
|---|---|---|---|
| **CMT4D (Lom)** (MIM 601455) | 8q24 | *NDRG1* (MIM 605626) | See text |
| **CMT4E**; same as AR CHN | | | See text |
| **CMT4F** (MIM 605260) | 19q13 | *PRX* (periaxin) (MIM 605725) | See text |
| **HMSN-R** (Russe type) (MIM 605285) | 10q23.2 | (*EGR2* excluded) | (Rogers *et al.*, 2000) |
| | **Autosomal recessive axonal neuropathy ("AR-CMT2")** | | |
| **AR-CMT2A** (CMT2B1) (MIM 605588) | 1q21.2-1q21.3 | *LMNA* | (Chaouch *et al.*, 2003; De Sandre-Giovannoli *et al.*, 2002) |
| **AR-CMT2B** (CMT2B2) (MIM 605589) | 19q13.3 | | (Leal *et al.*, 2001) |
| **Early onset AR-CMT2** | | | (Gabreels-Festen *et al.*, 1991; Ouvrier *et al.*, 1981) |
| **Congenital AR axonal neuropathy** | 5q deletion (SMA area) | | (Korinthenberg *et al.*, 1997) |
| **Lethal neonatal AR-axonal neuropathy (MIM** 604431) | | | (Vedanarayanan *et al.*, 1998; Wilmshurst *et al.*, 2001) |
| | **X-linked recessive CMT** | | |
| **CMTX2** (MIM 302801) | Xp22.2 | | (Ionasescu *et al.*, 1991, 1992) |
| **CMTX3** (MIM 302802) | Xq26 | | (Ionasescu *et al.*, 1991, 1992) |
| **Cowchock syndrome** (MIM 310490) | Xq13 | | (Cowchock *et al.*, 1985; Fischbeck *et al.*, 1986) |
| | **Hereditary sensory (and autonomic) neuropathies (HSN or HSAN)** | | |
| **HSN-1** (MIM 162400) | 9q22.1-22.3 (dominant) | *SPTLC1* | (Bejaoui *et al.*, 2001; Dawkins et al., 2001) |
| **HSN-2** | | | (Ohta *et al.*, 1973) |
| **HSN 3** (Riley-Day) (MIM 223900) | 9q31 (recessive) | *IKBKAP* | (Anderson *et al.*, 2001; Slaugenhaupt *et al.*, 2001) |
| **HSN 4** (CIPA) (MIM 256800) | 1q21-q22, recessive | *TRKA*/NGF receptor | (Indo, 2001) |
| | **Hereditary motor neuropathies (HMN or "distal SMA")** | | |
| **HMN 1** (MIM 182960) (early adulthood onset, AD or AR) | | | (Nelson and Amick, 1966) |
| **HMN 2** (MIM 158590) (also SMA-IV) | 12q24 | | (Irobi *et al.*, 2000, 2002) |
| **HMN 5** (MIM 600794) | 7p | *GARS* | Antonellis, *et al.*, 2003 |
| **HMN 7** (MIM 158580) (distal HMN with vocal paralysis-DHMNVP) | 2q14 | | (McEntagart *et al.*, 2001) |
| Distal infantile spinal muscular atrophy with diaphragm paralysis (**SMARD1**) (MIM 604320) | 11q13.2-4 | *IGHMBP2* (MIM 600502) | (Grohmann *et al.*, 1999, 2001) |
| Distal hereditary motor neuropathy, Jerash type (**HMNJ**) (MIM 605726) | 9p21.1-p12 | | (Christodoulou *et al.*, 2000) |

Please note the following: HNPP is included with CMT1; dominant *EGR2* mutations that cause a CMT1 phenotype are not given as separate name (such as CMT1D); recessive *EGR2* mutations are not listed under CMT4; CMT4E is the same as autosomal recessive CHN. For abbreviations see text.

While these clinical, electrophysiological, and pathological features distinguish DSS from CMT1 (Gabreels-Festen *et al.*, 1995; Ouvrier *et al.*, 1987), the literature contains many examples of patients who are said to have CMT (often "severe CMT") who could have just as readily been labeled DSS (see Fig. 39.2). This confusion underscores that idea that the severity of clinical findings in inherited neuropathies is a continuum; discrete subtypes are the exception, not the rule.

Congenital hypomyelinating neuropathy (CHN) is a term that should be reserved for infants who have hypotonic weakness at birth, caused by a severe neuropathy (Gabreels-Festen, 2002; Guzzetta *et al.*, 1982; Ouvrier, 1996; Ouvrier *et al.*, 1990; Phillips *et al.*, 1999; Plante-Bordeneuve and Said, 2002). Some may even have arthrogryposis caused by a prenatal onset, and swallowing or respiratory difficulties may result in death during infancy or later. NCVs are usually severely reduced (<5 m/s). Nerve biopsies reveal features that overlap with DSS, but with different predominance—greater paucity of myelin and a failure of myelinating Schwann cells to progress beyond the promyelinating stage, less frequent onion bulbs consisting of Schwann cell processes, and more redundant basal lamina ("basal lamina onion bulbs"). As in DSS, new dominant mutations, as well as recessive mutations, of *MPZ*, *PMP22*, and *EGR2*, cause CHN (Tab. 39.1). Because of their overlapping clinical and pathological features, CHN has been considered to be a more severe subtype of DSS (Guzzetta *et al.*, 1982; Tachi *et al.*, 1984). However, it is likely that the most severe cases of CHN, and those with unique pathological findings, have different genetic causes, as yet undiscovered.

The traditional approach to evaluating a neuropathy is to determine whether it is a primary "axonal" or "demyelinating" disorder. If the axon (or even the neuron) suffers the primary injury, then it is an "axonal" neuropathy; the subsequent degeneration of myelin sheaths is Wallerian degeneration and not demyelination (Griffin and Hoffman, 1993; Scherer and Salzer, 2001). Axonal neuropathies may even result in "secondary demyelination," often associated with axonal atrophy (Dyck *et al.*, 1993b). If the myelinating Schwann cells are affected first, then it is a "demyelinating" neuropathy, even though axons may degenerate subsequent to demyelination for reasons that are not well understood (Frei *et al.*, 1999; Sancho *et al.*, 1999).

For peripheral neuropathies in general, it may be difficult or even impossible, to determine whether a given neuropathy is a primary demyelinating or a primary axonal neuropathy. This is also true for inherited neuropathies, as the most widely used clinical criterion—forearm motor conduction velocities (greater or less than 38 m/s)—has turned out to be inadequate. This idea was first promulgated before the era of molecular diagnosis (Harding and Thomas, 1980) and was a heuristic criterion, as it facilitated the separation of CMT1 from CMT2. It was based on a large number of genetically heterogeneous CMT patients, whose median motor NCVs ranged from normal to very low. The distribution appeared bimodal, with one peak around 20 m/s (corresponding to CMT1), and another between 40 and 60 m/s (corresponding to CMT2). Although the two groups overlapped, they appeared to intersect at 38 m/s. This imperfect distinction between CMT1 and CMT2 has been useful, but an uncritical adherence to this criterion has contributed to the misconception that some demyelinating neuropathies are "axonal," exemplified by CMT1X. Even prior to 1980, a group of patients with "intermediate" slowing had been identified (Bradley *et al.*, 1977; Davis *et al.*, 1977; Madrid *et al.*, 1977); Figure 39 in Madrid *et al.* (1977) looks like a typical CMT1X biopsy (Sander *et al.*, 1998).

## A CELLULAR BASIS OF CLASSIFYING INHERITED NEUROPATHIES

Whereas much has been learned from comparing the genotypes and phenotypes of CMT patients, cell biological approaches have provided the key concepts of their pathogenesis. The cellular expression of the mutant protein, and the analysis of genetically authentic animal models, indicate that inherited demyelinating neuropathies are caused by the effect

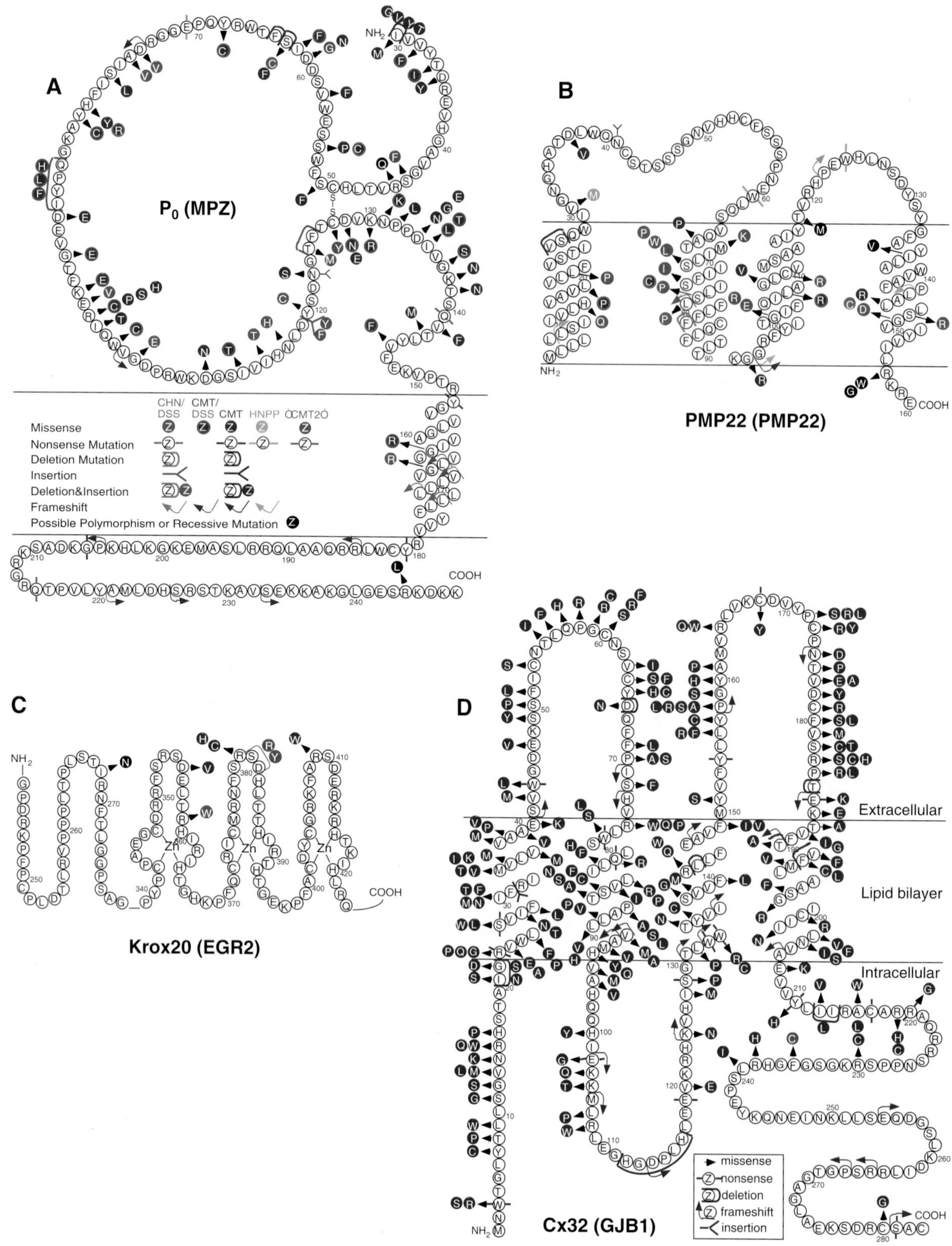


FIGURE 39.2

Schematic summary of how *MPZ*, *PMP22*, *EGR2*, and *GJB1* mutations affect $P_0$ (A), PMP22 (B), EGR2 (C), and Cx32 (D), respectively. The positions of the amino acids affected by the mutations, as well as their phenotypes, are indicated in the legend. N-linked glycosylation sites are shown for $P_0$ (amino acid 122) and PMP22 (amino acid 41). Mutations that affect the 5′ untranslated region (*GJB1*), promoter (*GJB1*), or splice sites (*MPZ* and *PMP22*) are not depicted. The patients were classified according to the published information given in the references on the website (http://molgen-www.uia.ac.be/CMTMutations/DataSource/MutByGene.cfm), but in many cases this information is insufficient to make a definitive diagnosis. Modified from (Kleopa and Scherer, 2002), with permission of Elsevier Science.

of mutations in genes that are expressed by myelinating Schwann cells and are first manifested in the myelinating Schwann cells themselves (Chapter 48 by Wrabetz *et al.*; Martini, 1997; Nave, 2001). In other words, mutations have cell autonomous effects, at least at the onset of the neuropathy. While these concepts are consistent with much of the data, there may be exceptions. For example, the clinical phenotypes of certain mutations of "myelin-related genes" indicate that their initial manifestations may be on axons (discussed later). Further, some genes that cause inherited demyelinating neuropathies may be expressed by both myelinating Schwann cells and neurons (*MTMR2*, *GDAP1*) and may have cell autonomous effects in both cell types. The analysis of animal models of these apparent exceptions should prove to be informative (Chapter 48 by Wrabetz *et al.*). Such data will likely provide new insights into how myelinating Schwann cells and axons interact to form a fundamental vertebrate adaptation—the myelinated axon.

The structure and function of myelinated axons provide many clues to understanding how mutations cause inherited demyelinating neuropathies. Because these topics are considered in detail elsewhere in this book, only a few points will be emphasized here. The myelin sheath itself can be divided into two domains, compact and noncompact myelin; each contains a nonoverlapping set of proteins. Compact myelin forms the bulk of the myelin sheath. It is largely composed of lipids, mainly cholesterol and sphingolipids, including galactocerebroside and sulfatide, and three proteins: $P_0$, PMP22, and myelin basic protein (MBP). Noncompact myelin is found in the paranodes and incisures, and it contains connexin32 (Cx32), Cx29, and myelin-associated glycoprotein (MAG). In keeping with their uniquely specialized structure, myelinating Schwann cells express high levels of myelin-related proteins and their cognate mRNAs, including $P_0$, PMP22, Cx32, Cx29, MAG, MBP, and periaxin (Scherer and Salzer, 2001).

The maintenance of a myelinating phenotype depends on the integrity of axon-Schwann cell interactions. Axonal degeneration leads to Wallerian degeneration, in which myelin sheaths are phagocytosed and previously myelinating Schwann cells dedifferentiate, expressing markers that are more characteristic of nonmyelinating Schwann cells, such as the neural cell adhesion molecule (NCAM) and the low-affinity nerve growth factor/neurotrophin receptor, $p75^{NTR}$ (Griffin and Hoffman, 1993; Scherer and Salzer, 2001). The expression of myelin-related mRNAs is down-regulated, but if axons regenerate, Schwann cells will re-ensheathe them in a manner that is highly reminiscent of development, re-express high levels of myelin-related proteins and mRNAs, and cease expressing $p75^{NTR}$ and NCAM. Nearly all myelin-related proteins and mRNAs are affected in this manner (Scherer and Salzer, 2001). It is widely believed that axons determine whether a Schwann cell will differentiate into a myelinating or nonmyelinating phenotype (Chapter 13 by Jessen and Mirsky). While the nature of the axonal signal remains to be determined, two unrelated transcription factors, POU3f1 (also known as tst-1, SCIP, and Oct-6; a POU domain family) and Egr2 (also known as Krox20, a zinc finger protein), are essential for the normal development of myelinating Schwann cells (Chapter 13 by Jessen and Mirsky). Both *Pou3f1*- and *Egr2*-null mice have drastically reduced numbers of myelinated axons, presumably because myelinating Schwann cells fail to differentiate properly (Bermingham *et al.*, 1996; Jaegle *et al.*, 1996; Topilko *et al.*, 1994). There is a surfeit of promyelinating Schwann cells—Schwann cells that associate with axons in a 1:1 manner, but lack a myelin sheath. These pathological findings resemble those found in some cases of DSS and CHN.

## CLINICAL AND MOLECULAR GENETICS OF INHERITED NEUROPATHIES

The following sections have been organized on a gene-by-gene basis. For each gene, the relevant aspects of the gene, its normal gene product, and its role in myelinating Schwann cells or neurons are mentioned to frame a discussion of how mutations affect the protein and result in neuropathy. More detailed information of each gene, the biology of its normal gene product, and relevant animal models are found in other chapters. For the original references of the mutations, see the website (http://molgen-www.uia.ac.be/CMTMutations/DataSource/MutByGene.cfm). We have focused on dysmyelinating (myelin sheaths do not form properly) and demyelinating (myelin sheaths form properly, but then breakdown) neuropathies.

## DOMINANT DYSMYELINATING AND DEMYELINATING NEUROPATHIES (CMT1, HNPP, DSS, CHN)

This is a clinically heterogenous group of disorders, spanning a wide range of disease severity, and of genetically diverse causes (Tab. 39.1).

### *PMP22* Deletions and Duplications Cause HNPP and CMT1A

#### *Genetic Aspects*

A reciprocal genetic mechanism causes the two most common inherited neuropathies, CMT1A and HNPP (Lupski and Garcia, 2001). Prior to the discovery of their genetic origins, a relationship between these two diseases had not been suspected because they are so clinically distinct. After CMT1A had been mapped to chromosome 17, it was subsequently associated with a small (1.4 megabase) internal duplication (Lupski *et al.*, 1991; Raeymaekers *et al.*, 1991). The observation that *Pmp22* mutations cause *Trembler* and *TremblerJ* (Suter *et al.*, 1992a; Suter *et al.*, 1992b)—well known mouse models of dominantly inherited demyelinating neuropathies—quickly led to the discovery that *PMP22* mapped to the duplicated segment of chromosome 17, as the region of synteny on mouse chromosome 11 containing *Pmp22* was conserved in the region of human chromosome 17 containing the duplication (Matsunami *et al.*, 1992; Patel *et al.*, 1992; Timmerman *et al.*, 1992; Valentijn *et al.*, 1992b). HNPP was subsequently mapped to the same region of chromosome 17, and the reciprocal deletion was determined to be associated with the disease (Chance *et al.*, 1993).

Two homologous DNA sequences flanking the *PMP22* gene are the molecular basis for its deletion/duplication (Lupski and Garcia, 2001). Their high degree of homology promotes unequal crossing over during meiosis, which simultaneously generates a duplicated and a deleted allele. These homologous regions are found in humans and chimpanzees, so that deletions/duplications have arisen many times during human evolution. When *de novo* deletions and duplications occur, they originate in the father. Because most cases of HNPP and CMT1A are inherited from an affected parent, their high prevalence in various ethnic groups indicates that they do not impact reproductive fitness. For example, the prevalence of HNPP in a Finnish population was 16/100,000 (Meretoja *et al.*, 1997), likely an underestimate, because many affected individuals are asymptomatic. The prevalence of CMT in various populations ranges from 4.7-41/100,000 (Dyck *et al.*, 1993a; Morocutti *et al.*, 2002; Skre, 1974), and these estimates do not include HNPP.

#### *Clinical Features of HNPP*

Episodic mononeuropathies at typical sites of nerve compression are the hallmark of HNPP (Windebank, 1993). In order of frequency, they occur in the peroneal nerve at the fibular head, the ulnar nerve at the elbow, the brachial plexus, the radial nerve at the spiral groove, and the median nerve at the wrist (Gouider *et al.*, 1995). Other nerves may be affected, and atypical presentations have been described (Mouton *et al.*, 1999; Pareyson *et al.*, 1996; Tyson *et al.*, 1996). More than half of the patients recover completely, usually within days to months, but deficits may persist. Ankle jerks may be absent in over one-third of the patients, and 12.5% are areflexic (Gouider *et al.*, 1995). Some patients with HNPP develop a progressive generalized sensory-motor neuropathy, with or without episodes of pressure palsies.

During the acute episodes of pressure palsies, electrophysiological studies may show conduction block (Sellman and Mayer, 1987). In addition to focal changes at common sites of nerve entrapment (Li *et al.*, 2002a), genetically affected individuals have a mild, sensory-motor polyneuropathy (Mouton *et al.*, 1999; Pareyson *et al.*, 1996). Sensory velocities and distal latencies are diffusely slowed, especially in the upper extremities. Motor NCVs are minimally slowed, but distal motor latencies are consistently prolonged, especially at sites prone to entrapment (Li *et al.*, 2002a). Biopsies of unpalsied nerves show focal thickenings (tomacula) caused by folding of the myelin sheath (Fig. 39.1), typically in the paranodal region, as well as segmental demyelination and remyelination (Windebank, 1993). Regions of uncompacted myelin have been noted (Jacobs and Gregory, 1991; Yoshikawa and Dyck, 1991), but this is not a specific finding (Fabrizi *et al.*, 1999; Mendell *et al.*, 1985). While it is plausible that severe focal demyelination (causing conduction block) followed by remyelination (restoring conduction) are the cellular alterations associated with the focal neuropathies, this remains to be directly demonstrated.

### *Clinical Features of* CMT1A *Caused by* PMP22 *Duplications*

CMT1A, by definition, is CMT1 linked to chromosome 17, and is almost always caused by the inheritance of the *PMP22* duplication (Lupski and Garcia, 2001). In large series, the age at onset ranges from 2 to 76 years, with most patients affected by end of the second decade (Birouk *et al.*, 1997; Harding and Thomas, 1980; Hoogendijk *et al.*, 1994; Thomas *et al.*, 1997). Neuropathy can be detected in CMT1A patients by age 5 (Berciano *et al.*, 2003), and slow nerve conduction velocities are evident even earlier (discussed later). Weakness, atrophy, and sensory loss in the lower limbs, foot deformities and areflexia are invariably present in affected patients. At a mean age of 40 years, functional disability is mild or absent in 35% of the patients, 25% are asymptomatic, 61% have difficulty walking or running but are still independent, and only one patient (less than 1%) requiring a wheelchair (Birouk *et al.*, 1997). There is considerable variability in the degree of neurological deficits within families, and even between identical twins, indicating that stochastic and environmental factors modulate disease severity (Garcia *et al.*, 1995).

In CMT1A patients with duplications, the NCVs are abnormally slowed, ranging from 5 to 35 m/s in forearm motor nerves, but most average around 20 m/s (Birouk *et al.*, 1997; Kaku *et al.*, 1993a; Lewis *et al.*, 2000; Thomas *et al.*, 1997). The lack of conduction block or temporal dispersion and the high correlation between the motor NCVs in different nerves are all hallmarks. NCVs are slow in children, even well before the clinical onset of disease. In individual patients, the motor NCVs do not change significantly even over 2 decades, whereas the motor amplitudes decrease, albeit slowly (Killian *et al.*, 1996). Conduction velocities, like clinical disability, vary widely within families (Birouk *et al.*, 1997; Kaku *et al.*, 1993b), but an early age at onset and greatly reduced median NCV are associated with a more severe course (Birouk *et al.*, 1997; Hoogendijk *et al.*, 1994). Nevertheless, motor amplitudes and the number of motor units correlate with clinical disability, indicating that axonal loss and not conduction velocity per se, cause weakness (Berciano *et al.*, 2000; Hoogendijk *et al.*, 1994; Krajewski *et al.*, 2000).

Nerve biopsies from CMT1A patients with duplications evolve during the disease (Fabrizi *et al.*, 1998; Gabreels-Festen *et al.*, 1992; Thomas *et al.*, 1997). Demyelination is more prevalent in children, and "hypomyelinated" axons (remyelinated axons with myelin sheaths that are inappropriately thin for the axonal caliber) become relatively more numerous with age (Fig. 39.1). Although some of the data were generated before genetic testing was possible, age-related axonal loss is a feature of CMT1 (Dyck *et al.*, 1989; Dyck *et al.*, 1974).

### PMP22 *Mutations Cause* CMT1A, HNPP, *and* DSS

Besides gene duplications and deletions, more than 40 different *PMP22* mutations have been identified, the majority of which lie in membrane-associated domains. These mutations are predicted to cause amino acid substitutions (missense mutations), premature stops (nonsense mutations), or frameshifts, as shown schematically in Figure 39.2, along with their associated phenotypes. Of the 38 mutations depicted, 7 cause HNPP, 6 cause

CMT1, 4 cause "severe CMT" (some of these could have been equally well called DSS), 17 cause DSS, and 4 are recessive or possible polymorphisms. Except for those with the HNPP phenotype, most patients with *PMP22* point mutations, including those with a CMT1 phenotype, are more severely affected than those harboring the duplication. They typically have an earlier age of onset, a more severe phenotype at any given age, more slowing of NCVs, and distinctive pathological changes in biopsies (Lupski and Garcia, 2001; Roa *et al.*, 1993a; Valentijn *et al.*, 1992a).

Individuals who are heterozygous for one of three *PMP22* mutations, Thr118Met, Arg157Trp, and Arg157Gly, have no discernible phenotype. Further, 1% of Europeans are heterozygous for the Thr118Met allele, which might be taken as evidence that it is a benign polymorphism (Nelis *et al.*, 1997; Young *et al.*, 2000). Homozygosity of Arg157Trp, however, causes DSS (Parman *et al.*, 1999). Further, individuals who are compound heterozygotes—a *PMP22* deletion and either Thr118Met or Arg157Gly—have a CMT1 phenotype (Numakura *et al.*, 2000; Roa *et al.*, 1993b). Thus, demyelinating neuropathy develops only when these mutant proteins are not paired with wild-type PMP22, but when it does occur, it is more severe than that caused by a null *PMP22* allele paired with wild-type PMP22 (HNPP). This confusing situation has been termed a "recessive gain of function" (Lupski, 2000).

### *How Do Loss of Function* PMP22 *Mutations Cause HNPP?*

The observation that a 1.4 megabase deletion in chromosome 17 is the common cause of HNPP immediately suggested that HNPP results from haplotype insufficiency of *PMP22*, although the potential contributions of other genes could not be excluded (Chance *et al.*, 1993). This idea was soon supported by the finding that frameshift mutations (presumed to be loss of function mutations) within *PMP22* also cause HNPP (Nicholson *et al.*, 1994; Young *et al.*, 1997), as well as the analysis of a genetically authentic animal model—*Pmp22* heterozygous null (*Pmp22*$^{+/-}$) mice (Adlkofer *et al.*, 1997a; Adlkofer *et al.*, 1995; Adlkofer *et al.*, 1997b; see also Chapter 48 by Wrabetz *et al.*). Finally, the level of PMP22 mRNA is relatively reduced in nerve biopsies from patients with HNPP, and the amount of PMP22 protein in compact myelin also appears to be reduced compared to normal nerves (Gabriel *et al.*, 1997; Schenone *et al.*, 1997; Vallat *et al.*, 1996).

PMP22 is a 160 amino acid protein with four putative transmembrane domains (Fig. 39.2). It is most abundant in peripheral nerve, mainly expressed by myelinating Schwann cells, and constitutes 2 to 5% of protein in compact myelin (Snipes *et al.*, 1992; Spreyer *et al.*, 1991; Welcher *et al.*, 1991). Although it is also expressed in a number of cell types (Baechner *et al.*, 1995; Parmantier *et al.*, 1995; Welcher *et al.*, 1991), there is no evidence that this expression plays a role in the pathogenesis of HNPP or CMT1A (Robertson *et al.*, 2002). PMP22 is synthesized in the endoplasmic reticulum (ER), where it is glycosylated, transported to the Golgi, and then to the cell membrane (Pareek *et al.*, 1993). PMP22 forms dimers, likely in the ER (D'Urso *et al.*, 1999; Tobler *et al.*, 1999). Given that reduced PMP22 expression causes HNPP, it seems paradoxical that much of it is rapidly degraded in proteasomes in normal myelinating Schwann cells (Pareek *et al.*, 1997).

The function of PMP22 is still unknown. In addition to its role in compact myelin, it was also identified as a gene (*gas3*) expressed in growth-arrested murine fibroblasts (Manfioletti *et al.*, 1990). Studies *in vitro* and in patient material further suggest that PMP22 could regulate cell proliferation (D'Urso *et al.*, 1997; Hanemann and Müller, 1998; Zoidl *et al.*, 1995), cell death (Brancolini *et al.*, 1999; Fabbretti *et al.*, 1995; Zoidl *et al.*, 1997), and differentiation (Brancolini *et al.*, 2000; Brancolini *et al.*, 1999; Hanemann *et al.*, 1996; Hanemann *et al.*, 1997). These findings have led to alternative hypotheses regarding the role of PMP22 overexpression in the pathogenesis of CMT1A, as described later.

How does a relative reduction in the amount of PMP22 produce the various features of HNPP: tomacula, uncompacted myelin, and a propensity for demyelination? One idea is that the components of compact myelin have a set stoichiometry, so that underexpression or overexpression of one component destabilizes the myelin sheath (Scherer, 1997). The evidence for this idea is still indirect. PMP22 and $P_0$ are coordinately expressed in developing and regenerating nerve (De Leon *et al.*, 1991; Notterpek *et al.*, 1999b; Snipes *et al.*, 1992; Suter *et al.*, 1994). In the interval of $P_0$ overexpression that permits normal myelination, the level of PMP22 increases proportionally to that of $P_0$, whereas those of other myelin proteins fall (Wrabetz *et al.*, 2000). An altered PMP22/$P_0$ ratio is associated with myelin pathology in CMT1A with duplicaton and HNPP (Vallat *et al.*, 1996), as well as in *Pmp22*$^{+/-}$(Adlkofer *et al.*, 1995; Gabriel *et al.*, 1997) and *Mpz*$^{+/-}$mice (Martini *et al.*, 1995b). PMP22 and $P_0$ may directly interact within compact myelin itself (D'Urso *et al.*, 1999; compare with Tobler *et al.*, 2002), and possibly in the sphingolipid/cholesterol rafts that deliver them to the myelin sheath (Erne *et al.*, 2002; Hasse *et al.*, 2002). It is conceivable that reduced PMP22/$P_0$ ratios produce a mechanical fragility in compact myelin, rendering them abnormally susceptible to compression, resulting in demyelination. Tomacula may form independently of compression, but affect paranodes, which are crucial for saltatory conduction, resulting in a mild slowing of conduction (Chapter 4 by Scherer *et al.*).

#### *What Is the Gain of Function Caused by* PMP22 *Duplication?*

Increased gene dosage of *PMP22* is the genetic basis for most patients with CMT1A; affected individuals have one extra copy of *PMP22* (three copies instead of two). Further, patients who are homozygous for the *PMP22* duplication (four copies of *PMP22*) sometimes manifest a more severe phenotype (Kaku *et al.*, 1993a; Le Guern *et al.*, 1997). The idea that gene dosage is the essential abnormality is supported by the finding that the PMP22 mRNA levels are increased in CMT1A biopsies (Hanemann *et al.*, 1994; Yoshikawa *et al.*, 1994; compare with, Kamholz *et al.*, 1994). The most direct evidence to date is that PMP22-immunoreactivity in nerve biopsies are higher in young or mildly affected patients, and return to normal in parallel with axonal loss (Gabriel *et al.*, 1997; Vallat *et al.*, 1996). It seems unlikely that the expression of PMP22 in the Schwann cells that form "onion bulbs" in CMT1A patients is related to gene dosage (Haney *et al.*, 1996; Nishimura *et al.*, 1996), as onion bulbs are PMP22-positive in nerves from patients with missense mutations (Hanemann *et al.*, 2000).

One explanation of how PMP22 overexpression results in demyelination is that PMP22 acts as a growth-arrest gene (Hanemann and Müller, 1998). In keeping with this idea, overexpressing PMP22 in cultured rat Schwann cells decreases their proliferation (Zoidl *et al.*, 1995). In addition, human Schwann cells cultured from sural nerve biopsies of CMT1A patients have decreased proliferation (Hanemann *et al.*, 1998). In other studies, the overexpression of PMP22 causes Schwann cell apoptosis (Fabbretti *et al.*, 1995; Zoidl *et al.*, 1995; Zoidl *et al.*, 1997), a feature that has been noted in inherited demyelinating neuropathies (Erdem *et al.*, 1998; Fidzianska *et al.*, 2002; Sancho *et al.*, 2001). These observations alone, however, are not definitive, as Schwann cell proliferation and even apoptosis probably occur in all neuropathies (Berciano *et al.*, 1999; Bradley and Asbury, 1972; Perkins *et al.*, 1981; Weinberg and Spencer, 1978), perhaps serving to match the number of Schwann cells and axons (Grinspan *et al.*, 1996; Trachtenberg and Thompson, 1996). Furthermore, there is no evidence for increased Schwann cell proliferation or apoptosis early in the pathogenesis in PMP22 overexpressing mice or *Pmp22*-null (*Pmp22*$^{-/-}$) mice (Sancho *et al.*, 2001).

PMP22 overexpression may perturb Schwann cell differentiation. In CMT1A biopsies, myelinating Schwann cells may express markers of nonmyelinating/denervated Schwann cells, such as p75$^{NTR}$ and NCAM, even in young patients, when most myelin sheaths look normal (Hanemann *et al.*, 1996; Hanemann *et al.*, 1997). However, this may not be a specific response to PMP22 overexpression, since these molecular changes have also been described in other myelin mutants (Giese *et al.*, 1992; Magyar *et al.*, 1996; Montag *et al.*, 1994). The PMP22 overexpressing rat ("CMT rat") provides an interesting twist on this theme (Niemann *et al.*, 2000; Sereda *et al.*, 1996). Homozygous rats have a dysmyelinating neuropathy that is much more severe than that in typical CMT1A. Nevertheless, myelin-related mRNAs are robustly expressed, but steady state levels of their cognate proteins are markedly reduced, although both PMP22 and $P_0$ reach the Golgi. As in CMT1A nerves, myelinating Schwann cells co-express p75$^{NTR}$. Thus, in the "CMT rat," myelin gene transcription appears to be uncoupled from myelin assembly, and the normal, reciprocal expression of markers of myelinating versus nonmyelinating Schwann cells is altered as described in CMT1A. Even the extreme overexpression of PMP22, however, does not prevent Schwann cells from ensheathing axons and forming at least some myelin sheaths *in vitro* (D'Urso *et al.*, 1997; Nobbio *et al.*, 2001) and *in vivo* (Robertson *et al.*, 2002; Sereda *et al.*, 1996; Chapter 48 by Wrabetz *et al.*).

Another plausible idea is that excess PMP22 arrives to and destabilizes the myelin sheath, resulting in demyelination in CMT1A (see above) (Gabriel *et al.*, 1997; Vallat *et al.*, 1996). This explanation, however, does not readily account for why even higher levels of PMP22 cause more severe dysmyelination/demyelination than in CMT1A, and that Schwann cells have altered phenotypes. Yet these more dramatic models of dysmyelination may not be relevant to the pathogenesis of CMT1A, in which the degree of overexpression is subtle.

### Most PMP22 Point Mutations Cause a Gain of Abnormal Function

Most *PMP22* point mutations cause phenotypes that are more severe than in duplication-related CMT1A or HNPP (Fig. 39.2). Since a simple loss of function of one *PMP22* allele should result in HNPP, these mutations must produce a gain of abnormal function. This idea has been directly confirmed in mice: the neuropathy in *Trembler* mice is more severe than in *TremblerJ* mice; the neuropathy in both of these mutants is much more severe than in *Pmp22* heterozygous null ($Pmp22^{+/-}$) mice (Martini, 1997). The gain of abnormal function could be either a dominant negative effect on the other wild-type *PMP22* allele, or it could be a "toxic" effect. The first clue to differentiate these possibilities is the intracellular location of mutant PMP22 in Schwann cells.

In cultured cells, dominant PMP22 mutant proteins are retained intracellularly, in the ER or the intermediate compartment (Brancolini *et al.*, 2000; Brancolini *et al.*, 1999; Colby *et al.*, 2000; D'Urso *et al.*, 1998; Dickson *et al.*, 2002; Naef *et al.*, 1997; Naef and Suter, 1999; Notterpek *et al.*, 1997; Tobler *et al.*, 1999). Thr118Met, encoded by one of the "recessive" mutations/polymorphisms (discussed earlier), in contrast, reaches the cell membrane, although not as efficiently as wild-type PMP22 (Naef and Suter, 1999), proving that this simple assay is potentially informative. In addition, the mutant proteins encoded by the *Trembler* (G150D) and *TremblerJ* alleles (L16P), aggregate abnormally in transfected cells (Tobler *et al.*, 2002). Heterologous cells, however, may be different than myelinating Schwann cells, which are highly specialized and require axonal interactions for efficient insertion of PMP22 into their cell membrane (Notterpek *et al.*, 1999b; Pareek *et al.*, 1997). Thus, it is important to confirm these findings in animal models and in patient material. To date, intracellular PMP22 has been found in nerves from both $Pmp22^{Tr/+}$ and $Pmp22^{TrJ/+}$ mice (Naef and Suter, 1999), and in rats that have been transfected with adenovirus expressing epitope-tagged versions of G150D or L16P (Colby *et al.*, 2000). Immunostaining a nerve biopsy from a "severe CMT1" patient with the same mutation that is found in *TremblerJ* mice (L16P) showed intracellular accumulation of PMP22 (wild-type and mutant protein cannot be distinguished in patients) that colocalized with an ER marker, BiP (Hanemann *et al.*, 2000). Biopsies from patients who had milder phenotypes showed different results—L105R did not show intracellular accumulation of PMP22, and G107V showed accumulation of PMP22 in supernumerary Schwann cells of onion bulbs, but not colocalized with BiP.

How can this type of intracellular retention produce gain of abnormal function? PMP22 forms dimers, so that mutant PMP22 retained in the ER or intermediate compartment could block a proportion of wild-type PMP22 from arriving to the cell membrane (a dominant-negative effect) (Naef and Suter, 1999; Tobler *et al.*, 2002; Tobler *et al.*, 1999). Such an effect could theoretically produce a phenotype somewhere between that of a heterozygous and a homozygous *PMP22*-null individual. A trans-dominant effect of PMP22 mutants on the trafficking of $P_0$ is yet another possibility. However, intracellularly retained mutant PMP22 did not alter the localization of $P_0$ in *Trembler* (G150D) and *TremblerJ* (L16P) nerves (Naef *et al.*, 1997), or in transfected, cultured Schwann cells (Tobler *et al.*, 1999). Nor can dominant-negative effects be the whole story, as $Pmp22^{Tr/-}$ mice have a worse phenotype than $Pmp22^{-/-}$ mice (Adlkofer *et al.*, 1997b). This confirms that *Pmp22*$^{Tr}$ is more deleterious than the null *Pmp22* allele, and more important, it shows that *Pmp22*$^{Tr}$ can have its effect without the presence of wild-type PMP22.

Taken together, these results suggests some *PMP22/Pmp22* alleles have a toxic gain of function deriving from an intracellular location. One possibility is that accumulation of mutant PMP22 triggers the unfolded protein response (UPR) in the ER. The UPR increases chaperone expression, attenuates protein synthesis, and increases degradation of proteins in order to eliminate abnormal proteins, which can produce cell death (reviewed in Chapter 42 by Gow; also see Mori, 2000). In *Pmp22*$^{+/+}$, *Pmp22*$^{Tr/+}$, and *Pmp22*$^{TrJ/+}$ nerves, however, PMP22 does not interact with BiP, thought to be a prerequisite for the UPR. Further, markers of the UPR, BiP, and CHOP (a transcription factor whose expression is typically induced in UPR) are not altered in mutant nerves (Dickson *et al.*, 2002). Instead, wild-type, L16P (*TremblerJ*) and G150D (*Trembler*) PMP22 complex with another ER chaperone, calnexin, both in nerves and in transfected cells, suggesting that calnexin sequestration may be deleterious (Dickson *et al.*, 2002).

The second kind of toxic gain of function could result from the rapid degradation of PMP22 from the ER (Pareek *et al.*, 1997) via the ubiquitin/proteasome pathway (Tsai *et al.*, 2002). When proteasome function is inefficient, aggresomes containing wild-type, L16P (*TremblerJ*) and G150D (*Trembler*) PMP22 form in transfected Schwann cells (Ryan *et al.*, 2002), and even in Schwann cells cultured from *TremblerJ* mice (Notterpek *et al.*, 1999a; Ryan *et al.*, 2002). L16P (*TremblerJ*) and G150D (*Trembler*) mutants aggregate more *in vitro* than does wild-type PMP22 (Tobler *et al.*, 2002). Thus, the aggregation or retention of PMP22 mutants may lead to inefficient proteasome function, which could be toxic to the cell (Bence *et al.*, 2001). However, the half-life of PMP22 mutants are only slightly increased, indicating proteasome function is only mildly impaired (Ryan *et al.*, 2002). Moreover, such toxicity usually produces increased cell death; this is not a feature of *Trembler* nerves at the onset of myelination (Sancho *et al.*, 2001).

Finally, PMP22 accumulates in lysosomes in myelinating Schwann cells of *Trembler* and *TremblerJ* mice, raising the possibility that the endosomal/lysosomal degradation pathway plays a role in the pathogenesis of demyelination (Notterpek *et al.*, 1999a; Notterpek *et al.*, 1997; Ryan *et al.*, 2002). Intracellular retention of mutant PMP22 (and, if wild-type PMP22 dimerizes with mutant PMP22, it could be retained too) could produce unstable myelin, its subsequent destruction and upregulation of the lysosomal pathway (Colby *et al.*, 2000). Alternatively, unfolded luminal protein in the ER could be delivered to lysosomes more directly, without ever passing through the myelin sheath (Dickson *et al.*, 2002; Notterpek *et al.*, 1999a; Ryan *et al.*, 2002). In *TremblerJ* nerves, there is increased degradation not only of PMP22, but also of $P_0$, which is also synthesized in the ER, and of MBP (Notterpek *et al.*, 1997), which is synthesized on free ribosomes and inserted locally into forming myelin sheaths (Colman *et al.*, 1982). This degradation of myelin components, however, could be an effect rather than a cause of demyelination.

## MPZ Mutations Cause CMT1B, DSS, CHN, and a CMT2-Like Phenotype

### *Genetic Aspects*

CMT1B was the first CMT to be mapped (Bird *et al.*, 1982), and when *MPZ* was later mapped near the *CMT1B* locus on chromosome 1 (Hayasaka *et al.*, 1993c), it was the obvious candidate gene. *MPZ* mutations were soon found to cause CMT1B, DSS, and CHN (Hayasaka *et al.*, 1993a, 1993b, 1993d; Warner *et al.*, 1996). *MPZ* mutations account for as much as 10% of CMT not due to chromosome 17 duplication (Tab. 39.2), and as ascertainment of the range of phenotypes associated with *MPZ* mutations improves, this percentage may rise. Many different *MPZ* mutations have been identified, including missense, nonsense, and frameshift mutations. Of the 84 mutations depicted in Figure 39.2, 38 cause CMT1, 22 cause "severe CMT," 13 cause DSS or CHN, 8 have been reported to cause a CMT2-like phenotype, 2 are recessive or possible polymorphisms, and 1 causes an HNPP-like phenotype. Moreover, the phenotypes of patients labeled

TABLE 39.2 The Proportion of Different CMT Mutations

| *PMP22* duplic. | *PMP22* (other) | *MPZ* | *GJB1* | Other | None | Comments |
|---|---|---|---|---|---|---|
| **52%** (79) | **7%** (5) | **3%** (5) | **8%** (11) | **2%** (3)<br>1 *EGR2*<br>1 *PRX*<br>0 *MTMR2*<br>1 *NEFL* | **33%** (50)<br>44 CMT1<br>2 CMT2<br>1 DSS<br>1 CHN<br>1 HNPP | (Boerkoel *et al.*, 2002) 153 unrelated patients with CMT1, CMT2, CMT1X, DSS, or CHN |
| **31%** (40) | **5%** (6) | **9%** (12) | **11%** (14) | N.D. | **44%** (56) (phenotypes not stated) | (Numakura *et al.*, 2002) 128 Japanese CMT patients (relatedness not stated) 74 CMT1 40 CMT2 47 unclassified |
| **58%** (98) | **1%** (2) | **2%** (4) | **7%** (12) | **0%** 0 EGR2 | **38%** (54) (phenotypes not stated) | (Mostacciuolo *et al.*, 2001) 170 unrelated Italian patients with CMT or DSS |
| **34%** (59) | **1%** (2) | **3%** (6) | **7%** (12) | N.D. | **55%** (95) (phenotypes not stated) | (Mersiyanova *et al.*, 2000a) 174 unrelated Russian patients with CMT 108 CMT1 32 CMT2 34 unclassified |
| **55%** (64) | **1%** (1) | **3%** (3) | **10%** (12) | N.D. | **31%** (36) (phenotypes not stated) | (Silander et al., 1998) 116 unrelated Finnish patients with CMT1 or DSS |
| **71%** (579) | (3/98) | (14/107) | (10/36) | N.D. | | (Nelis *et al.*, 1996) 819 unrelated CMT1 patients; *PMP22*, *MPZ*, *GJB1* mutations were looked for in some nonduplicated patients |
| **60%** (38 families) | N.D. | **2%** (1 family) | **16%** (10 families) | N.D. | **22%** (14 CMT2 families) | (Ionasescu *et al.*, 1993) 63 families (356 patients), 38 (193 patients) CMT1A, 1 (5 patients) CMT1B, 10 (110 patients) CMT1X, 14 (48 patients) CMT2 |
| **57%** (43) | N.D. | N.D. | N.D. | N.D. | **27%** (20) | (Wise *et al.*, 1993) 75 unrelated patients |

CMT1 ranges from mildly affected individuals to patients who could have equally well been called DSS.

### *Genotype-Phenotype Correlations*

How can one make sense of so many mutations and the diversity of phenotypes they cause? The lesson from *PMP22* mutations is to compare the effects of *MPZ* mutations to a null allele. Deletion of one *MPZ* allele in humans has not been described, but the comparable mutation in mice causes a late onset, demyelinating neuropathy (Martini *et al.*, 1995b; Shy *et al.*, 1997; Zielasek *et al.*, 1996). The V102 frameshift mutation, however, may be comparable to an *MPZ* deletion, as the protein would not function as a cell adhesion molecule because it lacks its transmembrane domain. It was discovered in two siblings with DSS who were both homozygous for this mutation, but their heterozygous parents and grandparents were asymptomatic (Sghirlanzoni *et al.*, 1992). Further, these heterozygous individuals had normal sensory and motor amplitudes, and their NCVs were only mildly slowed (for example, the median motor NCVs ranged from 35-42m/s). Thus, given the mild phenotypes of *MPZ* mutations with loss of function, mutations that cause DSS, severe CMT, or even CMT, must produce a gain of function, although perhaps in conjunction with a loss of function, too.

There are other mildly affected kindreds. Four siblings in their fifties were found to have the I99T mutation only after one of them appeared to develop chronic inflammatory demyelinating polyneuropathy (Donaghy *et al.*, 2000). The other three siblings had mildly reduced or even normal NCVs; one had a nerve biopsy that showed some thinly myelinated axons as well as clusters of regenerated axons. Kindreds with the D35Y, S51F, F64del, or E71x also appear to have milder neuropathies than typical CMT1B kindreds; the patient with the E71x mutation has an HNPP-like phenotype (Lagueny *et al.*, 2001).

A few *MPZ* mutations cause a CMT2-like phenotype. The best example is the S44F mutation, as clinically affected individuals have little or no slowing of NCVs despite clinically significant axonal loss (Hanemann *et al.*, 2001; Marrosu *et al.*, 1998). In contrast, clinically affected individuals with the T124M mutation have median/ulnar motor NCVs that range from "intermediate" slowing (25 to 40 m/s) to normal, whereas those in presymptomatic individuals tend to be normal (Chapon *et al.*, 1999; De Jonghe *et al.*, 1999; Misu *et al.*, 2000; Senderek *et al.*, 2000). Nerve biopsies from clinically affected patients show axonal loss, clusters of regenerated axons, and some thinly myelinated axons (Hanemann *et al.*, 2001). In spite of a late onset, many patients progress relatively rapidly to the point of using a wheelchair. In addition, abnormally reactive pupils (often the first clinical finding), dysphagia, positive sensory phenomena (including painful lacinations), and hearing loss are common. One family with the E97V mutation has a comparable phenotype, with a late onset progressive neuropathy associated with hearing loss and pupillary abnormalities (Seeman *et al.*, 2001). Two clinically affected individuals have intermediate slowing of their median motor NCVs (29 to 30 m/s), whereas a clinically unaffected boy has a nearly normal NCV (45 m/s; Seeman, personal communication). Patients with the D75V mutation have a late onset neuropathy associated with hearing loss and pupillary abnormalities, and relatively normal motor NCVs; it was not stated whether their weakness progressed rapidly (Misu *et al.*, 2000). Patients with D61G or Y119C mutations have an adult onset neuropathy (but without hearing loss or pupillary abnormalities); their NCVs were mildly slowed (median motor NCVs 39 to 43 m/s), and their biopsies showed decreased numbers of myelinated axons and clusters of regenerated axons (Senderek *et al.*, 2000). Finally, a Q141x mutation was found in two children (11 and 16 years old) who had a mild CMT phenotype and little if any slowing of motor NCVs (Young *et al.*, 2001). In sum, a few *MPZ* mutations cause a mild demyelinating neuropathy (D35Y, S51F, F64del, E71x, V102frameshift), others (D61G, I99T, Y119C) cause a late onset neuropathy that does not progress, and others (D75V, E97V, T124M) cause a complicated phenotype (rapid progression, hearing loss, or pupillary abnormalities). S44F and Q141x are the only mutations for which there is scant evidence for demyelination.

The range in clinical severity and the large number of *MPZ* mutations gives the appearance of a continuum, so that comparisons are tenuous. In addition, intrafamilial variability is notable for certain mutations (e.g., G206x; (Senderek *et al.*, 2001), but not for others (e.g., T124M; see above, or D90E; discussed later). At best, the clinical findings can be correlated with the clinical electrophysiology and nerve biopsy findings. DSS patients (described above) cannot be separated from DSS caused by mutations in other genes. Patients with "severe CMT1" overlap those with DSS, in terms of their clinical onset (often before age 3), clinical electrophysiology (forearm motor responses 8 to 15 m/s; becoming unobtainable with advanced distal muscle atrophy; absent sensory responses), and biopsy findings (severe loss of myelinated fibers, hypertrophic changes, onion bulbs, and proliferation of basal lamina). Most *MPZ* mutations appear to cause a CMT1 phenotype that is more like the one caused by *PMP22* missense mutations than by *PMP22* duplications: in the former, the age of onset is younger, atrophy appears earlier and extends to proximal muscles, and NCVs are slower (typically 10 to 20 m/s).

Nerve biopsies have revealed some possible clues. Uncompacted myelin has been reported with the S63del, E71x, R98C, R98H, C127Y mutations; other mutations have abnormally folded myelin sheaths (V32F, D61N, I62F, S78L, K96E, D109N, K130R, N131K, I135L). All of these mutations are localized in the extracellular domain, which mediates adhesion, but the phenotypes associated with both uncompacted myelin and abnormally folded myelin sheaths range from mild CMT to DSS (Gabreels-Festen *et al.*, 1996; Tachi *et al.*, 1997; Thomas *et al.*, 1994).

The report of Bird and colleagues (Bird *et al.*, 1997) of a large family with a D90E mutation is particularly instructive. The youngest members were all affected before age 10, several before age 3. Delayed walking and clumsy running were common early symptoms; absent tendon reflexes, followed by distal weakness and atrophy were early clinical findings. Proximal weakness and atrophy developed over time, and motor impairment outweighed sensory findings in most patients. The disease was insidiously progressive but did not affect longevity. The median and ulnar motor NCVs ranged from 6 to 15 m/s, changing little over time, except that distal motor responses became unobtainable, presumably due to the loss of motor axons. An autopsy of a 92-year-old affected woman revealed degeneration of fasciculus gracilis, which is consistent with severe axonal/neuronal loss caused by demyelination. In this family, an example of what is called "severe CMT1" in Figure 39.2, there was some variability in age of onset and disease severity at any given age, but the variability seems less than what has been described for CMT1A caused by *PMP22* duplications.

#### *Loss and Gain of Function Effects of* MPZ *Mutations*

$P_0$ is the most abundant protein in peripheral nerve myelin (Greenfield *et al.*, 1973). It is a single pass type I transmembrane protein with an immunoglobulin (Ig)-like fold in the extracellular domain, predicting a role in adhesion (Lemke and Axel, 1985). It has a basic/positively charged, cytoplasmic domain that likely interacts with the negatively charged phospholipids of the membrane, thereby augmenting the role of MBP in holding the apposed cytoplasmic surfaces of the membranes together (Ding and Brunden, 1995; Martini *et al.*, 1995a; Martini *et al.*, 1995b). Crystallographic analysis of the extracellular domain suggests that four $P_0$ molecules form a tetramer in *cis*, that interacts homophilically in *trans* with tetramers in apposing membrane (Shapiro *et al.*, 1996) to form the intraperiod line.

The analysis of mice that lack $P_0$ (*Mpz*$^{-/-}$ mice) confirms the importance of $P_0$, as Schwann cells form a multilamellar spiral of membrane around axons, but the myelin does not compact properly (Giese *et al.*, 1992). Mpz$^{+/-}$ mice develop a late-onset demyelinating neuropathy, indicating that halving the amount of $P_0$ destabilizes compact myelin (Martini *et al.*, 1995b; Shy *et al.*, 1997; Zielasek *et al.*, 1996). Conversely, overexpressing $P_0$ also causes dysmyelination, the severity of which is related to the level of transgene mRNA expression (Wrabetz *et al.*, 2000; Yin *et al.*, 2000). Martini (1997) has drawn a parallel between *Mpz*$^{+/-}$ mice and mild CMT and between *Mpz*$^{-/-}$ mice and DSS. This predicts that the range of severity in these human cases could represent the interval between loss of function of one and two *MPZ* alleles, consistent with a dominant-negative gain of function. That is, the mutant allele would lose adhesive function and provoke varying loss of adhesive function in the partner wild-type allele.

Aggregation assays of transfected cells show that the extracellular domain of $P_0$ can mediate homophilic intermolecular interactions (D'Urso *et al.*, 1990; Filbin *et al.*, 1990; Schneider-Schaulies *et al.*, 1990). The possibility that $P_0$ mutants have diminished adhesion has been evaluated in similar assays. Mutations in the extracellular domain that disrupt the disulfide bond (Zhang and Filbin, 1998) or N-linked glycosylation (Filbin and Tennekoon, 1993), and the I62F mutant (Matsuyama *et al.*, 2002), as well as cytoplasmic mutants that alter either an acylation site (C182A) or a PKC phosphorylation site (RSTK, residues 227 to 230) (Gao *et al.*, 2000; Wong and Filbin, 1996; Xu *et al.*, 2001) all reduced adhesion, sometimes even of a co-expressed wild-type $P_0$ (a dominant-negative effect).

Whereas the loss of adhesion alone might be expected to produce uncompacted myelin and even demyelination, as in *Mpz*$^{-/-}$ mice, what accounts for the wide range of morphological phenotypes observed in patients with *MPZ* mutations? These findings include focally-folded myelin sheaths, tomacula, axonal alterations with minimal myelin changes, and even the lack of formation of myelin. There are likely to be additional gain of function effects, stemming either from defects of the myelin sheath itself, or from another intracellular location. Comparing diverse missense mutations of the same residue raises some possibilities. For example, the S54P, S63del, S63F, R98P, R98H, and R98S mutations result in a milder phenotype (CMT1B) than the S54C, S63C, and R98C mutations, which cause severe CMT/DSS. A substitution of a cysteine generates a thiol group, which could form aberrant disulfide bonds, improperly fold, and affect trafficking.

The location or type of mutation in the $P_0$ intracellular domain is not obviously correlated with phenotype. For example, how Q215x causes CHN (Mandich *et al.*, 1999; Warner *et al.*, 1996), whereas an even longer deletion (Y181x) or a frameshift beginning after S226 causes a milder phenotype (CMT1B), remains to be determined. R228S disrupts a PKC phosphorylation site (an RSTK domain, residues 227 to 230; Brunden and Poduslo, 1987; Hilmi *et al.*, 1995; Suzuki *et al.*, 1990), and causes CMT1B (Xu *et al.*, 2001). Intracellular PKC activity modulates $P_0$ extracellular adhesion, and $P_0$ intracellular domain has been proposed to initiate signals that regulate terminal differentiation of Schwann cells (Xu *et al.*, 2001). Thus, intracellular *MPZ* mutations may provoke variable combinations of loss of extra- and intracellular adhesion, (loss of intraperiod line and major dense line compaction, respectively), together with loss of signaling function. These results further support that *MPZ* mutations act through various pathogenetic mechanisms, some mutation specific.

Unlike PMP22, there are no naturally occurring *Mpz* mutant mice, in which to analyze the effects of point mutations on trafficking. We (LW, MLF) have introduced randomly inserted copies of *Mpz*—either wild-type or mutated in the extracellular domain—that produce CHN or CMT1B-like neuropathies in transgenic mice. The nerve pathology is mutation-specific and includes either lack of myelin formation, uncompaction of myelin and tomacula, or demyelination with Schwann cell onion bulbs (Previtali *et al.*, 2000; Wrabetz *et al.*, 2000, 2002; Yin *et al.*, 2000). Since these mice also contain two normal copies of *Mpz,* the effect of the mutant alleles must include gain of function. Of note, some of the mutant proteins arrive to the myelin sheath (Previtali *et al.*, 2000), as predicted by analysis of the intraperiod line in CMT1B biopsy material (Kirschner *et al.*, 1996), whereas another (S63del) is retained intracellularly (Wrabetz *et al.*, 2002), in concordance with a study of transfected cells (Gao *et al.*, 2000). Thus, various gain of abnormal function mechanisms, originating from diverse intracellular locations are sufficient to phenocopy the variety seen in *MPZ*-related neuropathies.

## *GJB1/Cx32* Mutations Cause CMT1X

### *Genetic Aspects*

Shortly after the initial reports of autosomal dominant kindreds of CMT, Herringham (1889) reported a family in which only the males had peripheral neuropathy, many years before Morgan's description of X-linked inheritance. Although long under-recognized, CMT1X is the second most common form of CMT1, between 7 and 16% of CMT families (Tab. 39.2).

### *Clinical Features of CMT1X*

CMT1X is considered to be an X-linked dominant trait because it affects female carriers; their clinical involvement varies, likely owing to the proportion of myelinating Schwann cells that inactivate the X chromosome carrying the mutant *GJB1* allele (Scherer *et al.*, 1998). Affected women usually have a later onset (after the end of second decade) and a milder version of the same phenotype. In affected males, the clinical onset is between 5 and 20 years (Birouk *et al.*, 1998; Nicholson and Nash, 1993). Initial symptoms include difficulty running and frequent ankle sprains; foot drop and sensory loss in the legs develop later. Depending on the tempo of the disease, the distal weakness may progress to involve the gastrocnemius and soleus muscles, even to the point where assistive devices are required for ambulation. Weakness, atrophy, and sensory loss also develop in the hands, particularly in thenar muscles. These clinical manifestations are the result of a chronic, length-dependent neuropathy, and are nearly indistinguishable from those seen in patients with CMT1A or CMT1B, although atrophy, particularly of intrinsic hand muscles, positive sensory phenomena, and sensory loss may be more prominent in CMT1X patients (Hahn *et al.*, 1990).

Besides the pattern of inheritance, the degree of NCV slowing helps to distinguish CMT1A/B from CMT1X (Nicholson and Nash, 1993). In affected men, motor NCVs in the arms show "intermediate" slowing (25 to 40 m/s)—faster than in typical CMT1A (10 to 30 m/s) but slower than normal (>50 m/sec). Slowing is even evident in presymptomatic male children, prior to axonal loss (Kuntzer *et al.*, 2003). Some degree of slowing is usually found in female carriers, even asymptomatic ones. As compared to CMT1A, CMT1X patients have more heterogeneous NCVs and more distal axonal loss (Gutierrez *et al.*, 2000; Tabaraud *et al.*, 1999). The overlap in motor NCVs in CMT1X and CMT2 (discussed later) has led to the erroneous conclusion that *GJB1* mutations cause CMT1X and CMT2 (Birouk *et al.*, 1998; Boerkoel *et al.*, 2002; Silander *et al.*, 1998; Timmerman *et al.*, 1996). In all of these cases, however, CMT1X should have been considered, as there was no male-to-male transmission, and the motor NCVs of affected male patients showed intermediate slowing. In contrast to biopsies of CMT1A/B patients, there is less evidence of demyelination and remyelination and more evidence of axonal degeneration/regeneration in CMT1X (Hahn *et al.*, 2001; Sander *et al.*, 1998; Vital *et al.*, 2001).

### *Genotype-Phenotype Correlations*

CMT1X is caused by mutations in *GJB1*, the gene that encodes Cx32 (Bergoffen *et al.*, 1993). An amazing number (more than 240) and variety of mutations have been identified, affecting every domain of the Cx32 protein (Fig. 39.2), the promoter and 3′ untranslated region (Chapter 24 by Scherer and Paul), as well as deletions of the entire gene. Missense mutations alone affect 122 out of 283 amino acids, emphasizing the importance of each amino acid. Yet in spite of the large number of different mutations, the clinical severity caused by *GJB1* mutations appears to be relatively uniform in affected men, including those with a deleted gene (Dubourg *et al.*, 2001; Hahn *et al.*, 2000; Nakagawa *et al.*, 2001); *PMP22*, *MPZ*, and *EGR2* mutations clearly cause more diverse phenotypes. Only two mutations, the 265-273 deletion (Ionasescu *et al.*, 1996a) and F235C (Lin *et al.*, 1999), appear to cause "severe CMT" and/or DSS.; several others (e.g., R22x, R22Q, V163I, A147frameshift) appear to cause a more severe form of CMT1X. N175D and T191A mutations are associated with a mild phenotype. It remains to be determined whether there is a genotype-phenotype correlation in CMT1X, as most of the kindreds that have been associated with either mild or severe phenotypes are small. Genotype-phenotype correlations are being addressed in a "CMT database" led by Dr. Michael Shy at Wayne State University in collaboration with Indiana University.

Other associated manifestations of CMT1X have been reported. Hearing loss has been associated with the R142Q, T55R, and T191frameshift mutations (Lee *et al.*, 2002; Stojkovic *et al.*, 1999). This is intriguing because mutations in the genes encoding Cx43, Cx31, Cx30, and especially Cx26 are common causes of inherited hearing loss (http://www.crg.es/deafness); why these various connexins all cause hearing loss remains to be determined, but interactions between them are likely. Many mutations likely have subclinical electrophysiological evidence of slowed CNS conduction (Bähr *et al.*, 1999; Nicholson *et al.*, 1998). A few mutations (W24C, M34V, A39V, T55R, T55I, M93V, E09x, R164Q, R183S, T191frameshift; (Kleopa *et al.*, 2002; Lee *et al.*, 2002; Marques *et al.*, 1999; Panas *et al.*, 1998) have been reported to have clinical findings (such as extensor plantar responses; abnormal MRIs) that indicate CNS involvement. Two mutations (R142W and C168Y) may predispose CMT1X patients to an acute, transient CNS-related syndrome after visiting high altitudes (Paulson *et al.*, 2002).

### GJB1/Cx32 *Mutations Act Primarily through Variable Loss of Function*

Cx32 is one of about 20 connexins in mammals (Chapter 24 by Scherer and Paul). All connexins are highly homologous, with the overall structure shown in Figure 12.2—four transmembrane domain proteins, two extracellular loops, an intracellular loop, and cytoplasmic N- and C-termini. Six connexins oligomerize to form a hemichannel, or connexon; two hemichannels from apposing membranes interact to form a gap junction, a pathway that permits diffusion of ions and small molecules across membranes (Bruzzone *et al.*, 1996; White and Paul, 1999). Cx32 is localized to incisures and paranodal loops of myelinating Schwann cells and likely forms gap junctions between adjacent layers of the myelin sheath (Chapter 1 by Trapp and Kidd; Chapter 4 by Scherer *et al.*). Such a radial pathway—directly across the layers of the myelin sheath—would be advantageous as it provides a much shorter pathway (up to 1000-fold) than a circumferential route. Disruption of this radial pathway may be the reason that *GJB1/Gjb1* mutations cause demyelination in humans and in mice (Anzini *et al.*, 1997; Scherer *et al.*, 1998). However, the pathway and the rate of 5,6-carboxyfluorescein diffusion in *Gjb1*$^{-/-}$ mice did not appear to be different than in wild type mice (Balice-Gordon *et al.*, 1998), implying that another connexin also forms functional gap junctions in PNS myelin sheaths. This connexin is probably Cx29 (its human homologue is Cx31.3), which has been recently localized to the incisures (Altevogt *et al.*, 2002; Li *et al.*, 2002b). Whether another connexin, such as Cx31 (Lopez-Bigas *et al.*, 2001), is also present in incisures, remains to be determined.

The similar clinical phenotypes of most CMT1X patients suggests that most *GJB1* mutations cause a loss of function. This issue has been analyzed by expressing the mutants in heterologous cells (reviewed by Abrams *et al.*, 2000). Many mutants do not form functional channels in *Xenopus* oocytes (G12S, R15W, R22G, R22P, L90H, V95M; P172S, E208L; Y211x) or mammalian cells (C60F, V139M, R215W). Other mutants form functional channels with altered biophysical characteristics (S26L, I30N, M34T, V35M, V38M, L56F, V63I, P87A, E102G, del111-116, R220x); two of these (S26L; M34T) maintain electrical coupling, but have reduced pore diameter such that may prevent the diffusion of second messengers like IP3, cAMP, and $Ca^{2+}$ (Oh *et al.*, 1997). These studies also demonstrate that the nature of the mutation may be important, as the R15W and H94Q mutants form normal functional channels, whereas R15Q and H94Y do not (Abrams *et al.*, 2001). On the other hand, because several disease-related mutants (R15Q, H94Q, C217x, R238H, C280G, S281x) form fully functional channels (Abrams *et al.*, 2001; Castro *et al.*, 1999), these kinds of studies are limited in relation to pathogenesis of CMT1X.

Other studies have used mammalian cells to study trafficking of Cx32 mutants (reviewed in Yum *et al.*, 2002). Only one mutant is not detectably expressed in mammalian cells (e.g., 175 frameshift), but many mutants do not appear to reach the cell membrane; they appear to be retained in the ER or Golgi (G12S, R22Q, M34T, M34K, V38M, A39P, A39V, C53S, T55I, R75W, R75Q, R75P, R142W, R164Q, R164W, P172R, R183C, E186K, N205I, E208K, Y211x, C217x). Other mutants reach the cell membrane, although many of these appear to accumulate in the Golgi more than wild-type Cx32 (W3S, V13L, R15Q, S26L, M34I, M34V, V35M, V37M, C60F, V63I, M93V, del 112-117, V139M, R183H, R183S, N205S, I213V, A216W, R219C, R219H, R220x, R200G, R230C, R230L, F235C, R238H, L239I, C280G, S281x). The actual trafficking of mutants, however, may be more complex than indicated by these apparent patterns of retention (VanSlyke *et al.*, 2000; VanSlyke and Musil, 2002).

The preceding work leads to a few generalizations. Although different mutants of the same amino acid (R75P, R75Q, R75W) exhibit similar patterns of intracellular retention, this does not appear to be generally the case (Yum *et al.*, 2002). In contrast to the rest of the protein, missense mutants of intracellular carboxy terminus reach the cell membrane. Mutants that reach the cell membrane of mammalian cells usually form functional gap junctions in oocytes. Conversely, mutants that do not form functional gap junctions in oocytes do not reach the cell membrane in transfected mammalian cells. A few mutants have been expressed in cultured Schwann cells, and their localization agrees with that of transfected cell lines (Kleopa *et al.*, 2002; Yum *et al.*, 2002), but only two have been examined in myelinating Schwann cells. The 175 frameshift does not cause any discernible effects, and, as in transfected cells, no mutant protein can be detected (Abel *et al.*, 1999). The R142W mutation appears to be retained in the Golgi, and causes the retention of wild-type Cx32; it results in a mild demyelinating neuropathy (Scherer *et al.*, 1999). While much has been learned by expressing Cx32 mutants *in vitro*, the effects of these mutations are manifested in myelinating Schwann cells.

Given their overall structural similarity, it is a paradox why Cx32 mutants that accumulate in the ER do not cause as much demyelination as PMP22 mutants, which also accumulate in the ER (discussed earlier). Unlike PMP22, inhibiting proteosomes does not cause Cx32 to accumulate in aggresomes (Kleopa *et al.*, 2002; Notterpek *et al.*, 1999a; VanSlyke *et al.*, 2000). Perhaps the association between PMP22 and calnexin (Dickson *et al.*, 2002) is important in this regard. Finally, the finding that PLP mutants that cause devastating demyelination in the CNS have no known effects in myelination in the PNS may also be related to this paradox. Thus, despite their structural similarities, PMP22, Cx32, and PLP mutants have specific effects in myelinating Schwann cells.

CMT1X patients who are more severely affected, or have other manifestations such as CNS findings or hearing loss, raise the possibility that some Cx32 mutants have an additional toxic gain of function. Because connexin monomers interact, one reasonable possibility is that some Cx32 mutants have dominant-negative affects; this possibility has been shown experimentally (Bruzzone *et al.*, 1994; Omori *et al.*, 1996; Scherer *et al.*, 1999). However, Cx32 mutants cannot normally interact with themselves, as *GJB1* is subjected to X inactivation (Scherer *et al.*, 1998). Nevertheless, Cx32 mutants could have dominant-negative effects on other connexins expressed by Schwann cells or oligodendrocytes. Bruzzone *et al.* (1994) demonstrated that R142W had a dominant-negative effect on Cx26 in oocytes, but this connexin is probably not expressed by myelinating Schwann cells (Nagaoka *et al.*, 1999). In addition, channels formed by some Cx32 mutants could have a gain of function (Abrams *et al.*, 2002), although the mutant with this effect (S85C) is not associated with an unusual phenotype. Finally, expressing Cx32 "CNS mutants" (A39V, T55I, M93V, R164Q, and R183H) did not alter the distribution of Cx45 in stably transfected HeLa cells (Kleopa *et al.*, 2002). It now appears that oligodendrocytes do not express Cx45 (Kruger *et al.*, 2000); the relevant connexin may be Cx47 (Menichella *et al.*, 2003; Odermatt, 2003).

## EGR2 Mutations Cause CMT1, DSS, and CHN

*Egr2/Krox20* is a member of the early growth response gene family and encodes the zinc-finger transcription factor Krox20. As predicted by segment-specific pattern of expression of Krox20 in developing hindbrain, *Krox20/Egr2*-null mice lack rhombomeres 3 and 5 (Schneider-Maunoury *et al.*, 1993; Swiatek and Gridley, 1993). Unexpectedly, these mice were also found to have a severe dysmyelinating neuropathy (Topilko *et al.*, 1994), making *EGR2* an excellent candidate gene (Warner *et al.*, 1998), even though no CMT locus had been linked to its locus (10q21-22). To date, one recessive and six dominant *EGR2* mutations have been detected, associated with CMT1, DSS, or CHN (Fig. 39.2).

How does Krox20 function in myelination? In *Krox20/Egr2*-null mice, the development of myelinating Schwann cells appears to be "arrested" at the promyelinating stage, in which presumptive myelinating Schwann cells have formed 1:1 relationships with axons, but not yet made a myelin sheath (Topilko *et al.*, 1994). Like promyelinating Schwann cells in normal nerves, these mutant Schwann cells express early markers such as MAG, but have not up-regulated their expression of myelin-related genes. These findings suggest that axons regulate the expression of Krox20; this has been directly demonstrated (Ghazvini *et al.*, 2002; Murphy *et al.*, 1996; Zorick *et al.*, 1996, 1999). Thus, Krox20 may mediate the massive induction of myelin-related mRNAs that accompanies myelination (Stahl *et al.*, 1990), a process that has been shown to require axon-Schwann cell interactions (Scherer *et al.*, 1994). In keeping with this idea, the forced expression of EGR2 in rat Schwann cells strongly increases the expression of many myelin-related genes, including those of $P_0$, PMP22, periaxin, MAG, Cx32, MBP, choline kinase, and stearyl CoA desaturase (Nagarajan *et al.*, 2001). Whether these are direct or indirect effects remains to be determined, but Krox20 can activate the rat *Mpz* promoter 4-fold in co-transfected, cultured rat Schwann cells (Zorick *et al.*, 1999). In addition, the *GJB1/Cx32* promoter has three putative EGR2 binding sites (see Fig. 3 in Chapter 24 by Scherer and Paul), and the D355V EGR2 mutant has reduced affinity for the most 3′ EGR2 binding site (Musso *et al.*, 2001).

The one recessive mutation (I268N) falls in the R1 repressor domain (Svaren *et al.*, 1996; Svaren *et al.*, 1998); it prevents interactions with NAB co-repressors and can activate a synthetic Krox20/Egr2 target promoter *in vitro* 15-fold (Warner *et al.*, 1999). Thus, this recessive mutation may produce a gain of function by altering gene expression of myelin-related genes! In keeping with this idea, unlike *Krox20/Egr2*-null mice (Levi *et al.*, 1996; Topilko *et al.*, 1994), the three siblings who are homozygous for I268N have no brain stem or bone abnormalities and have a few myelinated axons in a sural nerve biopsy (Harati and Butler, 1985). Of the target genes that are likely to be perturbed by EGR2 overexpression in Schwann cells (Nagarajan *et al.*, 2001), *PMP22* and *MPZ* are the most likely to produce dysmyelination (Magyar *et al.*, 1996; Sereda *et al.*, 1996; Wrabetz *et al.*, 2000).

Six dominant *EGR2* mutations affect the highly conserved zinc finger DNA binding domains (Fig. 39.2). They likely act though gain of function, as heterozygous *Krox20/Egr2*-null mice appear normal. Three (R359W, S382R/D383Y, R409W) reduce DNA binding and transactivation by *in vitro* assays (Warner *et al.*, 1999), but how they function as dominants is unclear. The S382R/D383Y mutant inhibits the activation of endogenous myelin genes by wild-type EGR2 in co-transduced rat Schwann cells (Nagarajan *et al.*, 2001), but a dominant-negative effect was not found in cotransfection assays with a synthetic target promoter-reporter (Nagarajan *et al.*, 2001; Warner *et al.*, 1999). Because EGR2 is not thought to dimerize, this effect may result from a dominant effect on a partner of EGR2, such as a co-activator or adaptor. The sequestration of an EGR2 partner could explain the lack of a direct correlation between loss of DNA binding *in vitro* and the severity of the associated phenotype (Warner *et al.*, 1999). Thus, as for *PMP22* and *MPZ*, the pathogenesis of *EGR2* mutations includes components of both loss of function (reduced transactivation) and gain of abnormal function.

### Mutations in *LITAF* Cause CMT1C

Two families with dominantly inherited, typical CMT1 were mapped to 16p13.1-12.3 (Chance *et al.*, 1992b; Street *et al.*, 2002). These families, along with a new one, were found to have mutations in *LITAF* (Street *et al.*, 2003). *LITAF* (lipopolysaccharide-induced TNF-alpha factor) encodes a widely expressed transcript that is translated into a 161 amino acid protein. *LITAF* mRNA is expressed in sciatic nerve, but its level of expression is not altered in response to nerve injury, in contrast to other genes known to cause CMT1. The *LITAF* gene was originally cloned as a putative nuclear transcription factor involved in TNF$\alpha$ gene regulation, but subsequent studies indicated that the *LITAF* gene encodes a lysosomal protein (Moriwaki *et al.*, 2001). Cytoplasmic LITAF expression is found in the epidermis basal cell layer in human skin (Street *et al.*, 2003). The mutations associated with CMT1C may cluster, defining a putative domain of the LITAF protein having a critical role in peripheral nerve function. Western blot analysis suggested that the T115N and W116G mutations do not alter the level of LITAF protein in peripheral blood lymphocytes (Street *et al.*, 2003).

## RECESSIVELY INHERITED DEMYELINATING NEUROPATHIES (CMT4)

This is a heterogenous group of disorders that cause demyelinating neuropathy, although one is syndromic (Tab. 39.1). The neuropathies are usually severe, meriting the clinical diagnosis of DSS or "severe CMT" (although using the term CMT for any recessively inherited neuropathy is an expansion of its original, narrower meaning—dominantly inherited neuropathies). Each kind is rare, and tends to be more common in certain inbred populations.

### *GDAP1* Mutations Are Associated with CMT4A and AR-CMT2-Like Neuropathy

CMT4A was found in Tunisian families and mapped to the 8q13 locus (Ben Othmane *et al.*, 1993a; Ben Othmane *et al.*, 1995). Patients have a severe neuropathy that starts in the first 2 years of life, causing delayed motor development, and progressing to involve proximal muscles by the end of the first decade, to the point that many patients become wheelchair-dependent. Motor NCVs average 29 m/s in the arms, and nerve pathology includes hypomyelination, basal lamina onion bulbs, and loss of large myelinated axons. These individuals could be considered to have "severe CMT" or even DSS. These findings have been substantiated in three additional kindreds (Nelis *et al.*, 2002b).

Mutations have been identified in ganglioside-induced differentiation-associated protein-1 (*GDAP1*) in the Tunisian families (Baxter *et al.*, 2002). Surprisingly, recessive *GDAP1* mutations were found in three Spanish families manifesting a "severe CMT2" phenotype (AR-CMT2; Tab. 39.1). These patients also had a childhood onset, with distal weakness and atrophy, motor NCV of 41 m/s, and sural nerve biopsies showing loss of myelinated fibers, axonal degeneration, and no signs of demyelination (Cuesta *et al.*, 2002). Three mutations (two nonsense and one missense) were found in the Tunesian families; affected individuals were homozygous. Three alleles (one frameshift leading to premature stop and two nonsense mutations) were found in the Spanish families; affected individuals were compound heterozygous or homozygous. The affected patients described by Nelis *et al.* (2002) were homozygous for two novel mutations and one mutation previously described in compound heterozygosity. All of these mutations would be predicted to cause partial or complete loss of function. As yet, the specific mutation does not predict demyelinating CMT4A versus axonal AR-CMT2 phenotype. For example, homozygous S194x produced CMT4A in one family (Baxter *et al.*, 2002), whereas it caused AR-CMT2 in another (Nelis *et al.*, 2002b).

*GDAP1* was identified as one of several genes whose expression was induced by ganglioside synthesis in Neuro2a neuroblastoma cells (Liu *et al.*, 1999). It encodes a protein predicted to have two transmembrane domains and a glutathione S transferase domain, suggesting a role in antioxidant pathways or detoxification. It is highly expressed in brain and at lower levels in nerve and other tissues, so that it could have cell-autonomous roles in both neurons and Schwann cells (Cuesta *et al.*, 2002). Thus, specific mutations may cause cell-specific effects, producing phenotypes that suggest a neuronal (AR-CMT2) or a Schwann cell (CMT4) defect. Alternatively, a partial loss of function could have a less severe phenotype, akin to the Spanish patients, rather than a complete loss of function, akin to the Tunisian patients. Finally, GDAP1 could be involved in Schwann cell/axonal interactions, such that loss of function produces abnormalities in both (Cuesta *et al.*, 2002).

### *MTMR2* Mutations Cause CMT4B1

CMT4B has been described in Italian and Saudi Arabian families and causes a similar phenotype. Weakness was recognized between 2 and 4 years of age, progressing to wheelchair dependency by adulthhood (Houlden *et al.*, 2001; Quattrone *et al.*, 1996). Motor NCVs are uniformly slow (10 to 20 m/s in the arms), and nerve biopsies have a distinctive feature—irregular folding and redundant loops of myelin. CMT4B is caused by mutations in the myotubularin-related protein-2 gene, *MTMR2*, which belongs to the family of myotubularin-related dual specific phosphatases (Bolino *et al.*, 2000). When two Tunisian families with the same phenotype, including focally folded myelin sheaths, were linked to a different locus (11p15) named CMT4B2 (Ben Othmane *et al.*, 1999), CMT4B caused by *MTMR2* mutations was designated CMT4B1.

MTMR2 is one of 13 members of the highly conserved, 'myotubularin-related' family in humans (Laporte *et al.*, 2001). It has at least four functional domains: a GRAM domain (glucosyltransferase, Rab-like GTPase activator and myotubularin), a phosphatase domain, a SID (SET-interacting) domain, and a PDZ binding site (Laporte *et al.*, 2001). Like other members of this family, MTMR2 is widely expressed in many tissues, but is enriched in both neurons and Schwann cells from embryonic development onward (Berger *et al.*, 2002a; Bolino *et al.*, 2002). The membrane phospholipid, phosphatidylinositol-3-phosphate, PI(3)P, is a substrate of both MTMR2 and MTM1 *in vitro* (Kim *et al.*, 2002; Laporte *et al.*, 2002), although PI3,5P2 may be the preferred substrate of MTMR2 (Berger *et al.*, 2002a). *MTM1* and *MTMR2* mutations produce muscle- and nerve-specific syndromes, respectively; tissue-enriched expression, diverse substrate specificity, or differential subcellular localization could explain the lack of redundant function between family members.

The *MTMR2* mutations identified thus far predict loss of function. Five homozygous loss of function mutations in unrelated CMT4B patients, consisting of three nonsense mutations in exons 9, 11, and 12; one splice site mutation leading to the skipping of exon 13 (in-frame deletion), and one complex mutation of a 8-bp deletion combined with a 2 bp insertion, in exon 14 (Bolino *et al.*, 2000). To evaluate the frequency of *MTMR2* mutations, 183 unrelated patients with a broad spectrum of CMT and related neuropathies, were screened (Bolino *et al.*, 2000), revealing two additional heterozygous mutations in *MTMR2* associated with CHN in two unrelated patients. Heterozygous relatives were normal suggesting that these patients harbored an undetected mutation in the other *MTMR2* allele. Mutations have been subsequently reported by others in two unrelated families with CMT4B1, consisting of one base pair deletion mutation in exon 4 predicting a truncated protein, and missense mutations in exons 4 and 9 (Houlden *et al.*, 2001; Nelis *et al.*, 2002a). The majority of mutations fall in predicted functional domains.

The normal role of MTMR2 in peripheral nerve is not known; the loss of MTMR2 may have cell autonomous effects in neurons and Schwann cells. Phosphoinositides regulate intracellular membrane trafficking (Simonsen *et al.*, 2001). PI(3)P, in particular, may regulate autophagy—a transport pathway that targets cytosolic proteins and organelles to lysosomes for hydrolase-mediated degradation (Petiot *et al.*, 2000). A cell autonomous effect in myelinating Schwann cells would suggest a role for MTMR2 in the regulation of autophagy of myelin-related lipids and proteins, although why oligodendrocytes are not similarly affected is unexplained. That altered lysosomal degradation of myelin glycolipids causes PNS and CNS demyelination (the leukodystrophies) is a precedent for this idea. A cell autonomous effect in neurons would suggest that membrane recycling in axons is crucial, but a neuronal affect alone would not account for the pronounced demyelinating phenotype in these patients. Perhaps *MTMR2* mutations perturb axon-Schwann cell interactions (Berger *et al.*, 2002a). Cell-specific disruption of *Mtmr2* in mice is underway to test these ideas.

## MTMR13/*SBF2* Mutations Cause CMT4B2 with or without Glaucoma

In two large consanguineous families from Tunisia and Morocco, recessive demyelinating neuropathy associated with early onset glaucoma was mapped to 11p15, overlapping the locus for CMT4B2. Clinically, the mean age of onset was 8 years, with distal motor deficit in all four limbs, motor NCV<20m/s and myelin outfoldings on nerve biopsy. All affected family members exhibited congenital glaucoma progressing to loss of vision. An additional consanguineous Turkish family with four affected members manifested a similar neuropathy, but without glaucoma.

Two homozygous nonsense mutations in the Tunisia/Morocco families and an in frame deletion in the Turkish family were identified in *MTMR13/SBF2*, a pseudophosphatase homologue of *MTMR2*, predicting loss of function (Azzedine *et al.*, 2003; Senderek *et al.*, 2003). *MTMR13/SBF2* is expressed in multiple tissues, especially in brain, spinal cord and sciatic nerve. Its function is unknown, but by analogy to MTM1 and the pseudophosphatase MTMR9, that may form a functional pair to regulate levels of PI(3)-phosphates (Wishart and Dixon, 2002), mutations in MTMR13 may impair cooperative function with MTMR2, producing a CMT4B2 demyelinating phenotype similar to CMT4B1. The presence or absence of glaucoma in CMT4B2 may be mutation-specific.

## *NDRG1* Mutations Cause CMT4D

CMT4D is a syndromic neuropathy, with hearing loss and dysmorphic features. It was initially described in Gypsies from Lom, Bulgaria, but has been subsequently found in Gypsies in other countries (Kalaydjieva *et al.*, 1996). It has an onset in childhood, with foot deformities and abnormal gait, and progresses to severe disability by the fifth decade. Motor NCVs are severely reduced and become unobtainable after the age of 15, indicating severe axonal loss. Biopsies show demyelination, onion bulb formation, and cytoplasmic inclusions in Schwann cells (Kalaydjieva *et al.*, 1998).

CMT4D is caused by a nonsense mutation that should truncate the product of N-myc downstream-regulated gene-1 (*NDRG1*). Its function is unknown. Many cell types, including Schwann cells, express NDRG1 (Kalaydjieva *et al.*, 2000; Lachat *et al.*, 2002). It has been suggested to be associated with adherens junctions (Lachat *et al.*, 2002), which are present in myelinating Schwann cells (Fannon *et al.*, 1995; Young *et al.*, 2002). Structural prediction algorithms place NDRG1 in the $\alpha/\beta$ hydrolase superfamily, but it lacks crucial residues thought to be necessary for enzymatic activity (Shaw *et al.*, 2002). One potential clue is that its expression can be induced as part of the endoplasmic reticulum stress response (Agarwala *et al.*, 2000) perhaps CMT4D is caused by impaired endoplasmic reticulum-associated protein degradation.

## *PRX* Mutations Cause CMT4F

A large Lebanese family originally defined CMT4F (Delague *et al.*, 2000). Affected members have a DSS phenotype, with delayed motor milestones, progressing to severe distal weakness, areflexia, sensory loss, and even sensory ataxia. NCVs are severely slowed ($< 5$ m/s) or undetectable, and biopsies show thinly myelinated axons, onion bulbs, and severe axonal loss. Mutations in the periaxin gene (*PRX*) were identified in this family (Guilbot *et al.*, 2001) and in three unrelated cases (Boerkoel *et al.*, 2000). The identification of other mutations has broadened the spectrum of associated phenotypes, including patients who might have been considered to have more typical CMT1 (Takashima *et al.*, 2002).

Periaxin is a membrane-associated protein with a PDZ domain that is solely expressed in myelinating Schwann cells (Gillespie *et al.*, 1994). Its localization changes during myelination—from the adaxonal membrane (nearest the axon) to the abaxonal membrane (nearest the basal lamina) in mature myelin sheaths (Scherer *et al.*, 1995). Abaxonal periaxin interacts with the dystroglycan complex through dystrophin related protein -2 (DRP-2), thereby linking laminin-2 in the basal lamina to the actin cytoskeleton in the cytoplasm (Sherman *et al.*, 2001). This complex may also activate signal transduction from laminin to the Schwann cell (Wrabetz and Feltri, 2001).

Homozygous or compound heterozygous nonsense and frameshift mutations in *PRX* cause CMT4F. All mutations would be expected to cause loss of function; this was confirmed in one patient whose sural nerve biopsy had no periaxin (Takashima *et al.*, 2002). Myelination begins normally in *prx*-null mice; myelin outfolding develops after 6 weeks, followed by extensive demyelination by 6 months of age. In contrast to other CMT animal models, they develop a prominent allodynia and hyperalgesia (Gillespie *et al.*, 2000). Such sensory abnormalities are reminiscent of CMT4F patients.

## DEMYELINATING NEUROPATHIES AS PARTS OF OTHER SYNDROMES

Dominant demyelinating neuropathies associated with syndromes are uncommon. Patients who have large duplications of chromosome 17, including *PMP22*, are one example (Chance *et al.*, 1992a). Loss of function mutations in *PLP* cause Pelizeaus-Merzbacher disease and a mild demyelinating neuropathy (Garbern *et al.*, 1997). Dominant *SOX10* mutations cause Waardenburg-Shah/Waardenburg type IV syndrome and other "neurocristopathies." Moderate (CMT1-like) and severe (CHN-like) demyelinating neuropathies have been described, as well as CNS dysmyelination (Inoue *et al.*, 1999, 2002; Pingault *et al.*, 2000; Touraine *et al.*, 2000). Nevertheless, a screen for *SOX10* mutations in uncomplicated CMT neuropathies was unrevealing (Pingault *et al.*, 2001). SOX10 is expressed by oligodendrocytes, neural crest, and by all stages in the Schwann cell lineage (Stolt *et al.*, 2002). In keeping with its pattern of expression, SOX10 likely plays multiple roles in cellular differentiation, especially in the development of cells from the neural crest, including glial cells (Paratore *et al.*, 2001; Southard-Smith *et al.*, 1998). SOX10 may directly regulate the expression of *MPZ* and *GJB1* (Bondurand *et al.*, 2001; Peirano *et al.*, 2000). One CMT1X mutation in the *GJB1* promoter (Chapter 24 by Scherer and Paul) alters a putative SOX10 binding site and decreases the expression of the Cx32 gene in transient co-transfection assays (Bondurand *et al.*, 2001).

Demyelinating neuropathies are part of several recessive neurological syndromes, but are frequently overshadowed by other manifestations. The "classic form" of Refsum disease has a childhood onset (<20 yrs); the major clinical features are ataxia, retinitis pigmentosa, cardiomyopathy, deafness, ichthyosis, and a demyelinating neuropathy. It is caused by mutations in phytanic acid oxidase (Jansen *et al.*, 1997; Mihalik *et al.*, 1997) and is treated with a diet low in phytanic acid. Another form of this disease is caused by mutations in *PEX7*, which encodes a receptor required for importing proteins into the peroxisome (van den Brink *et al.*, 2003). A more severe variant with infantile onset is caused by mutations of *Peroxin-1*, located on chromosome 7q21-22 (Reuber *et al.*, 1997). Peroxin is required for importing peroxisomal matrix proteins. This variant is allelic to neonatal adrenoleukodystrophy and Zellweger's and their clinical features are overlapping. They include mental retardation associated with leukodystrophy, deafness, hepatomegaly, and neuropathy, although it is unclear if the neuropathy is demyelinating. Both phytanic acid and very long chain fatty acids accumulate in these patients.

Two leukodystrophies cause a recessively inherited demyelinating neuropathy. Metachromatic leukodystrophy (MIM 250100) is caused by mutations in *Arylsulfatase A* (von Figura *et al.*, 2001). Globoid cell leukodystrophy (also known as Krabbe's disease; MIM 245200) is caused by mutations in *Galactosylceramide* β*-galactosidase* (Wenger *et al.*, 2001). Both of these are lysosomal enzymes that are required for sequential steps in the degradation of sulfatide > galactocerebroside > galactose + ceramide. These glycolipids are highly enriched in oligodendrocytes and myelinating Schwann cells. In both of these disorders, the symptoms and signs referable to the CNS usually overshadow those of the PNS. At least for MLD, the severity of peripheral neuropathy seems to be related to the duration of disease, and is therefore generally inversely correlated to the severity of the CNS presentation (von Figura *et al.*, 2001). Rarely, some patients may present with a demyelinating peripheral neuropathy with little or no evident CNS findings (Comabella *et al.*, 2001; Marks *et al.*, 1997). In both disorders, peripheral nerve alterations include segmental demyelination, thin myelin sheaths, and Schwann cell inclusions.

## DOMINANT AXONAL NEUROPATHIES (CMT2)

Patients with CMT2 usually present in the second decade, but one-third of patients present up to decades later (Dyck *et al.*, 1993a). Physical findings are typically confined to the legs and progress slowly, with areflexia, distal weakness, and atrophy of both anterior and posterior calf muscles; sensory findings may be relatively mild. Sural nerve biopsies show reduced numbers of large myelinated axons, clusters of regenerated axons, and few onion bulb-like structures. CMT2 is genetically heterogeneous; kindreds have been linked to seven different loci (Tab. 39.1). The genetic abnormalities have been found in three, CMT2A, CMT2B, and CMT2E; these are discussed next.

### *KIF1B* Mutations Cause CMT2A

CMT2A patients have a typical phenotype (Ben Othmane *et al.*, 1993b; Saito *et al.*, 1997; Timmerman *et al.*, 1996). A mutation in the gene encoding kinesin1B isoforms alpha and beta (*KIF1B*), molecular motors for transporting synaptic vesicles, has been identified in one CMT2A kindred. A Q98L mutation affecting the highly conserved ATP binding region results in a loss of function (Zhao *et al.*, 2001). Haplotype insufficiency can account for the dominant phenotype in humans, as mice that are heterozygous for a null *Kif1B* allele develop neuropathy.

Kinesins are microtubule-activated ATPases—molecular "motors" that use microtubules as tracks. They form a large gene family, and each kinesin transports a specific organelle (Hirokawa, 1998). For example, in heterozygous *kifb*-null mice the levels of synaptic vesicle proteins are selectively decreased in peripheral axons. Which kinesin 1B isoform is important in the pathogenesis of CMT2A is unclear. As Mok *et al.* (2002) noted, the mutant ATP binding region is contained in both (the mutant mouse is also deficient in both by design), and cell transfection studies aimed to rescue the specific loss of $\alpha$ or $\beta$ isoform function may be flawed. This distinction is important because the cargo is isoform specific; via its carboxyl PDZ domain, KIF1B $\alpha$ may interact not only with synaptic proteins, but also Kv1.4 potassium channels, NR2 subunits of NMDA receptors, and neuronal nitric oxide synthase. Isoform-specific disruption of *KIF1B* in transgenic mice will address this question. In any case, the functions of kinesin1B isoforms explains why CMT2A is length dependent—a relative reduction in this molecular motor leads to axonal impairment starting at the most remote part of the neuron. Because axons are the longest cells in the body, they may be particularly vulnerable to defective axonal transport.

### *RAB7* Mutations Cause CMT2B

The CMT2B patients described in three reports appear to be clinically similar (Auer-Grumbach *et al.*, 2000a; De Jonghe *et al.*, 1997; Elliot *et al.*, 1997). In addition to length-dependent weakness and severe sensory loss, distal ulcerations in the feet are common, often leading to toe amputations. A similar, ulceromutilating neuropathy has been reported in an Austrian family, which did not link to the CMT2B locus (Auer-Grumbach *et al.*, 2000b), indicating further genetic heterogeneity in this phenotype. In three CMT2B families and three other unrelated CMT2B patients, two misense mutations have been described in *RAB7*, encoding a member of the Rab family of Ras-related GTPases, that are essential for proper intracellular membrane trafficking (Verhoeven *et al.*, 2003). The pathogenesis of *RAB7* mutations is unknown. *RAB7* is widely expressed, including in motor and sensory neurons, and may function in vesicle transport between late endosomes and lysosomes, or in Golgi targeting of glycosphingolipids.

### *NEFL* Mutations Cause CMT2E

Mutations in the gene that encodes the neurofilament light subunit (*NEFL)* cause CMT2E (De Jonghe *et al.*, 2001; Mersiyanova *et al.*, 2000b). In a large Russian kindred, clinical manifestations of CMT2E become apparent in the second or third decades, with difficulty walking, distal weakness, diminished sensation (including pain sensation), and absent reflexes in the legs, followed by slow progression (Mersiyanova *et al.*, 2000b). In a smaller kindred, distal weakness progressed to paresis by the fourth decade (De Jonghe *et al.*, 2001) In the Russian kindred, the median motor NCVs were mildly reduced or normal (38 to 52 m/s), whereas they were slowed well into the "demyelinating range" (median motor NCV

25 to 39 m/s; ulnar motor NCV 30 to 42 m/s) in the other kindred (De Jonghe *et al.*, 2001). Three novel mutations in Japanese patients have been reported (Yoshihara *et al.*, 2002), but the clinical description of these patients was limited to the observation that the motor NCVs were slowed (22 to 36 m/s). Finally, Jordanova *et al.* (2003) found six *NEFL* mutations (five missense and one three nucleotide deletion) in 323 unrelated patients with CMT neuropathies, some with a more severe (DSS) phenotype. A sural nerve biopsy from one patient showed both myelin outfolding, loss of myelinated fibers, and onion bulbs, as well as clusters of regenerating axons.

Neurofilaments are the main neuronal intermediate filaments and are composed of three subunits, termed heavy, medium, and light. In animal models, *Nefl* mutations have profound effects on axonal caliber (Lee *et al.*, 1994; Ohara *et al.*, 1993), potentially accounting for the slowed NCVs seen in CMT2E patients. CMT2E is autosomal dominant, suggesting that mutations produce either haploinsufficiency or gain of function. *Nefl*-null mice, however, do not appear to develop a CMT2-like neuropathy (Zhu *et al.*, 1997), whereas the L394P mutation, which is predicted to affect the coil 2B domain and thus disrupt neurofilament assembly, causes a severe peripheral neuropathy/neuronopathy in transgenic mice (Lee *et al.*, 1994). Thus, missense mutants that disorganize assembly could result in neuropathy. Consistent with this idea, several missense mutations have been reported thus far, and two of these mutant genes encode proteins that disrupt assembly and axonal transport of neurofilaments in transfected DRG neurons (Brownlees *et al.*, 2002; Perez-Olle *et al.*, 2002). In addition to axons, Schwann cells also express NEFL (Fabrizi *et al.*, 1997); whether this relates to the phenotype of CMT2E remains to be determined.

## RECESSIVELY INHERITED AXONAL NEUROPATHIES (AR-CMT2)

Axonal neuropathy is found in many recessively inherited neurological syndromes, but is rarely recognized as an isolated inherited disease. Sporadic axonal neuropathies that are presumed to be recessively inherited typically present from birth to 5 years, and progress to severe disability by the second decade or even to death during infancy (Gabreels-Festen *et al.*, 1991; Ouvrier *et al.*, 1981). NCVs and pathology are consistent with axonal degeneration, thereby distinguishing these cases from inherited demyelinating neuropathies and CMT2. We have used the term "autosomal recessive CMT2" (AR-CMT2); "CMT2B" is an alternative designation used by OMIM. Both of these terms are confusing, if not misleading, designations, as the term "CMT" was originally used to designate dominantly inherited neuropathies. The X-linked recessive CMT types listed on Table 39.1 are probably syndromic.

## MUTATIONS IN *LMNA* CAUSE AR-CMT2A/CMT2B1

In a large Moroccan family linked to 1q21.2-q21.3, the onset of symptoms in nine affected siblings was in the second decade, with severe weakness and atrophy of the distal limb muscles; proximal muscles were involved in some patients. Motor NCVs were normal or slightly slowed and biopsies showed diminished numbers of myelinated axons and clusters of regenerated axons (Bouhouche *et al.*, 1999). Two inbred Algerian families of similar phenotype were mapped to chromosome 1q21.2–21.3 and a homozygous missense mutation in *LMNA* was found to segregate with disease in both families, as well as an independent third family (Chaouch *et al.*, 2003; De Sandre-Giovannoli *et al.*, 2002).

*LMNA* encodes four isoforms of lamins A/C, all components of the nuclear envelope, and amino acid substitutions of which have already been described in limb-girdle muscular dystrophy 1B, autosomal dominant Emery-Dreifuss muscular dystrophy, dilated cardiomyopathy type 1A, autosomal dominant partial lipodystrophy, and Hutchinson–Gilford progeria syndrome. Lamins A/C are expressed in most cells. The R298C substitution in Lamin A/C affects all four isoforms and probably produces AR-CMT2A via loss of function, as *Lmna*-null mice develop a neuropathy similar to that of CMT2A patients (De Sandre-Giovannoli *et al.*, 2002; Sullivan *et al.*, 1999). In contrast, most of the other *LMNA* associated diseases occur in heterozygosity, suggesting that these diverse phenotypes arise via different gain of function effects.

## HEREDITARY SENSORY (AND AUTONOMIC) NEUROPATHIES (HSN OR HSAN)

They are grouped together for their shared characteristics—the loss of sensory (especially of small fibers) and autonomic fibers, resulting in sensory loss to the point of mutilating deformities of the hands and feet. They proved to be genetically heterogeneous (Tab. 39.1). HSN-1 is an autosomal dominant trait and manifests in adolescence with small fiber sensory loss, burning pain (distal>proximal and legs>arms), pedal deformity, acromutilation, and distal weakness. It is caused by mutations in the gene encoding serine palmitoyl transferase, long-chain base subunit 1 (*SPTLC1*) (Bejaoui *et al.*, 2001; Dawkins *et al.*, 2001). The mutations that cause HSN-1 (C133Y, C133W, V144D) reside in a conserved region, and the corresponding mutations in the yeast enzyme act as dominants because the enzyme is part of a heterodimer (Gable *et al.*, 2002). HSN-2, HSN-3, and HSN-4 are autosomal recessive. HSN-2 has its onset in early childhood with similar phenotype to HSN-1 (Dyck, 1993). HSN-3, also known as the Riley-Day syndrome or familial dysautonomia with congenital indifference to pain, is caused by mutations of *IKBKAP*, the inhibitor of κ light polypeptide gene enhancer in B cells, kinase complex-associated protein (Anderson *et al.*, 2001; Slaugenhaupt *et al.*, 2001). Onset is in infancy with absent fungiform papillae of the tongue and mainly small fiber involvement, including autonomic crises with postural hypotension and tachycardia. HSN-4 is characterized by congenital insensitivity to pain with anhydrosis (hence the alternative name, CIPA syndrome), with the associated features of small fiber sensory loss, autonomic failure, mental retardation, and acromutilation. It is caused by mutations in *TRKA*, which encodes a receptor tyrosine kinase for nerve growth factor (Indo, 2001).

## HEREDITARY MOTOR NEUROPATHIES (HMN OR "DISTAL SMA")

In these diseases, motor neurons are preferentially affected; they are also known as distal spinal muscular atrophy, "distal SMA" (Harding and Thomas, 1980). One presumes that these diseases are caused by cell autonomous effects of mutations in motor neurons, but their genetic basis is largely unknown (Tab. 39.1).

## THE PATHOGENESIS OF INHERITED AXONAL NEUROPATHIES

In many neuropathies, the clinical features tend to have a distal predilection, both in terms of first appearance and in ultimate severity. This suggests that axonal length is a factor in determining which neural elements are at risk. But distal distribution does not mean that the defect necessarily lies in the axon; it could just as well represent a primary neuron cell body abnormality. For instance, large doses of pyridoxine promptly kill large primary sensory neurons, whereas smaller doses cause only subtle shrinkage of these neurons and indolent, distal axonal degeneration (Xu *et al.*, 1989). Thus, a modest neuronal abnormality may result in distal axonopathy, but a more severe insult of the same type may cause the neuron itself to degenerate as the primary event. The inclusion of HSN-3 and HSN-4 as inherited "axonal neuropathies" is even more problematic, as they appear to result from the developmental degeneration of neurons.

In nonsyndromic neuropathies, mutations appear to act on a cell-autonomous basis, affecting either neurons or myelinating Schwann cells. The selective vulnerability of PNS neurons that leads to neuropathy may be the axons themselves—the longest cells in the body. Their prominent cytoskeleton contains intermediate filaments and microtubules, and dominant mutations in *NEFL*, the gene encoding the light subunit, cause neuropathy. Further, recessive mutations in the gigaxonin gene, which encodes a protein that likely interacts with cytoskeleton proteins, cause giant axonal neuropathy (Bomont *et al.*, 2000; Ding *et al.*, 2002; Kuhlenbaumer *et al.*, 2002). The reason for the selective vulnerability of Schwann cells (and oligodendrocytes) is less clear. Two mutations that cause dys/demyelination affect genes that are largely if not exclusively expressed in myelinating Schwann cells (*MPZ, PRX*); these mutations need not affect other cell types. However, more mutations are expressed by multiple cell types (*PMP22, GJB1, EGR2, LITAF, NDRG1, MTMR2*); why these mutations mainly affect myelinating Schwann cells remains largely a mystery.

Disability in inherited neuropathies, even demyelinating ones, correlates with axonal loss. This has been well documented in animal models (Chapter 48 by Wrabetz *et al.*) and in CMT patients (Berciano *et al.*, 2000; Dyck *et al.*, 1974, 1989; Krajewski *et al.*, 2000). The lack of a myelin sheath has pronounced effects on axonal caliber, axonal transport, and the phosphorylation and packing of neurofilaments (Chapter 1 by Trapp and Kidd). How does a myelinating Schwann cell communicate with its axon, and how is this altered by demyelination? Possibilities include trophic support from myelinating Schwann cells, the altered myelin sheath itself (Hanemann and Gabreels-Festen, 2002), signals emanating from the adaxonal Schwann cell membrane and/or cytoplasm, especially in the paranodal region, where axons and Schwann cells are intimately joined (Chapter 4 by Scherer, *et al.*). The evidence for these possibilities is provided by *Mag*-null mice, which have axonal changes that mimic those found in demyelinated axons (Yin *et al.*, 1998). Other contributing factors to demyelination or axonal loss include inflammatory changes initiated by demyelination (Maurer *et al.*, 2002) and remodeling of the extracellular matrix (Misko *et al.*, 2002; Palumbo *et al.*, 2002). In some CMT1B mutations, particularly *MPZ*T124M, axons appear to be disproportionately affected, and in a few CMT1B mutations, axonal loss is detected before altered myelin sheaths (discussed earlier). While these examples are provocative, rigorous documentation that axonal alterations preceed demyelination is still lacking.

## MAKING A MOLECULAR DIAGNOSIS

Determining the phenotypes of patients—their age of onset, historical progression, as well as their current physical findings—will usually distinguish between the CHN, DSS, CMT, and HNPP phenotypes. Other distinctive features discussed earlier, such as X-linked inheritance, may suggest a specific type of CMT, but these may not be present. Electrophysiological studies, including the median and ulnar motor NCVs, should be performed, as the degree of slowing and its uniformity should confirm or refute the clinical diagnosis and even suggest a specific subtype. In our opinion, a nerve biopsy should not be part of the initial diagnostic evaluation except in problematic cases or for research purposes.

In cases of suspected HNPP, testing for the *PMP22* deletion should be performed, as this is by far the major cause; if this is negative, then *PMP22* exons should be sequenced. In CMT patients with uniform slowing of motor NCVs between 10 and 35 m/s, testing for the *PMP22* duplication should be performed, as this is the major cause of CMT1. If the patient does not have the duplication, then *PMP22*, *MPZ*, *GJB1*, *EGR2*, and *NEFL* exons should be sequenced. In DSS with appropriately slowed NCVs, testing for the duplication will usually be negative, and sequencing of the *PMP22*, *MPZ*, *GJB1*, *EGR2*, *PRX*, and *NEFL* genes should be included in the initial evaluation. In cases where CMT1X is the most likely diagnosis (intermediate slowing of NCVs, no male-to-male transmission), sequencing *GJB1* alone is the appropriate initial test; if negative, consider sequencing *MPZ* and

*NEFL*. In cases of suspected CMT2, it is probably premature to test for *MPZ* and *NEFL* mutations alone (the only commercially available tests), but a more comprehensive battery should be available in the future as more genetic causes are found (Fig. 39.3). Discovering these causes depends on the participation of referring physicians and affected families.

## IDENTIFICATION OF OTHER CMT GENES

As summarized in Table 39.2, there are many reports regarding the proportion of different mutations that cause CMT. As noted in the table, these reports differ in the kinds of patients who were analyzed and, depending on the year of publication, whether other genes were sequenced. If one considers CMT overall, *PMP22* duplications accord for about one-half of all kindreds; the proportion goes up markedly if only CMT1 patients are considered, and even more if one only considers families with dominant inheritance. Mutations of *GJB1*, *MPZ*, and *PMP22* account for 10 to 25% of the other cases of CMT, mutations of *EGR2*, *PRX*, *MTMR2*, and *NEFL* are even rarer. A surprising finding is that no mutations have yet been identified for one-third of CMT kindreds. This issue was most elegantly illustrated in the analysis of Boerkoel *et al.* (2002), who did not identify mutations in many CMT1 kindreds.

How will we find these other CMT genes? Affected families that have no known cause of their CMT and that are large enough for linkage analysis are increasingly less common. Owing to automated sequencing, it is now possible to screen "candidate genes" as causes of CMT. To date, most of these candidates are derived from advances in the genetics and biology of myelinated axons, as described elsewhere in this book. Transcriptome analysis (Nagarajan *et al.*, 2002; Nagarajan *et al.*, 2001) and proteomics will provide even more candidates. Their sequence immediately ties them to a physical map that can be compared to mapped CMT loci.

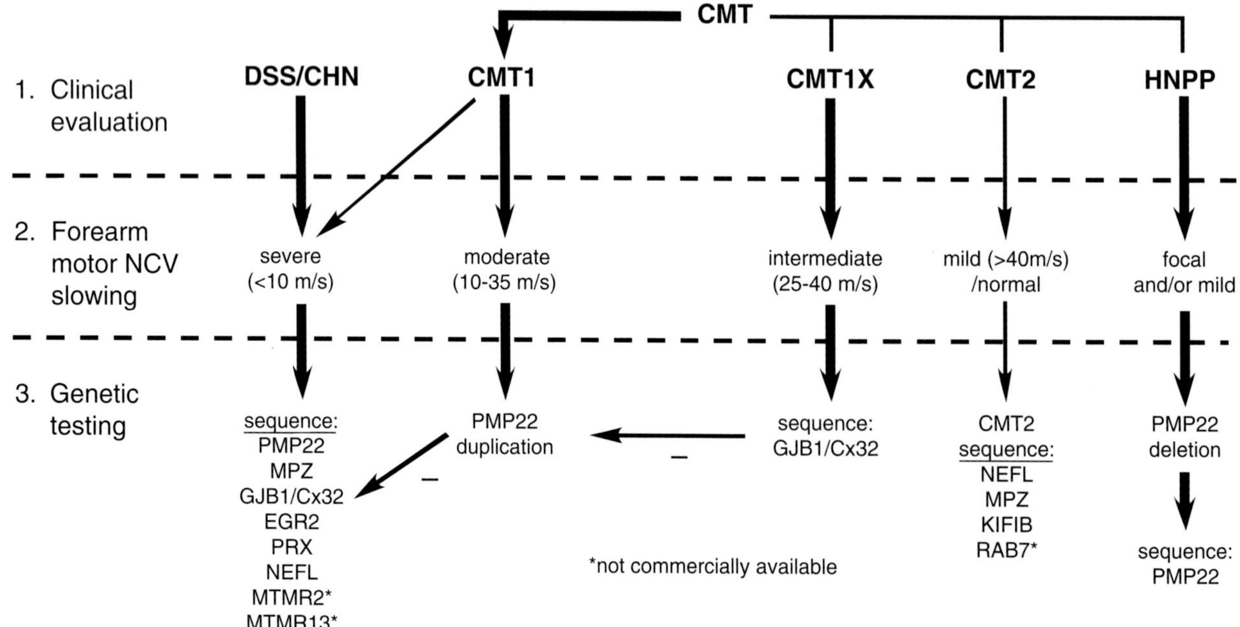


FIGURE 39.3
How to order the appropriate test in inherited neuropathies (updated information on the availability of new genetic testing can be found on the website www.genetests.org). Modified from (Kleopa and Scherer, 2002), with permission of Elsevier Science.

## SUMMARY

Inherited neuropathies are common. They are usually caused by mutations in genes that are expressed by myelinating Schwann cells or neurons, which is the biological basis for the long-standing distinction between primary "demyelinating" and "axonal" neuropathies. Neuropathies can be isolated, the primary manifestation of a more complex syndrome, or overshadowed by other aspects of the inherited disease. Increasing knowledge of the molecular genetic causes of inherited neuropathies facilitates a faster and more accurate diagnosis, setting the stage for the development of specific therapeutic interventions.

### References

Abel, A., Bone, L. J., Messing, A., Scherer, S. S., and Fischbeck, K. F. (1999). Studies in transgenic mice indicate a loss of connexin32 function in X-linked Charcot-Marie-Tooth disease. *J. Neuropathol. Exp. Neurol.* **58,** 702–710.

Abrams, C. K., Bennett, M. V. L., Verselis, V. K., and Bargiello, T. A. (2002). Voltage opens unopposed gap junction hemichannels formed by a connexin 32 mutant associated with X-linked Charcot-Marie-Tooth disease. *Proc. Natl. Acad. Sci. USA* **99,** 3980–3984.

Abrams, C. K., Freidin, M. M., Verselis, V. K., Bennett, M. V. L., and Bargiello, T. A. (2001). Functional alterations in gap junction channels formed by mutant forms of connexin 32: Evidence for loss of function as a pathogenic mechanism in the X-linked form of Charcot-Marie-Tooth disease. *Brain Res.* **900,** 9–25.

Abrams, C. K., Oh, S., Ri, Y., and Bargiello, T. A. (2000). Mutations in connexin 32: The molecular and biophysical bases for the X-linked form of Charcot-Marie-Tooth disease. *Brain Res. Rev.* **32,** 203–214.

Adlkofer, K., Frei, R., Neuberg, D. H.-H., Zielasek, J., Toyka, K. V., and Suter, U. (1997a). Heterozygous peripheral myelin protein 22-deficient mice are affected by a progressive demyelinating peripheral neuropathy. *J. Neurosci.* **17,** 4662–4671.

Adlkofer, K., Martini, R., Aguzzi, A., Zielasek, J., Toyka, K. V., and Suter, U. (1995). Hypermyelination and demyelinating peripheral neuropathy in *pmp22*-deficient mice. *Nat. Genet.* **11,** 274–280.

Adlkofer, K., Naef, R., and Suter, U. (1997b). Analysis of compound heterozygous mice reveals that the Trembler mutation can behave as a gain-of-function allele. *J. Neurosci. Res.* **49,** 671–680.

Agarwala, K. L., Kokame, K., Kato, H., and Miyata, T. (2000). Phophorylation of RTP, an ER stress-response cytoplasmic protein. *Biochem. Biophys. Res. Comm.* **272,** 641–647.

Altevogt, B. M., Kleopa, K. A., Postma, F. R., Scherer, S. S., and Paul, D. L. (2002). Cx29 is uniquely distributed within myelinating glial cells of the central and peripheral nervous systems. *J. Neurosci.* **22,** 6458–6470.

Anderson, S. L., Coli, R., Daly, I. W., Kichula, E. A., Rork, M. J., Volpi, S. A., Ekstein, J., and Rubin, B. Y. (2001). Familial dysautonomia is caused by mutations of the IKAP gene. *Amer. J. Hum. Genet.* **68,** 753–758.

Antonellis, A., Ellsworth, R. E., Sambuughin, N., Puls, I., Abel, A., Lee-Lin, S. Q., Jordanova, A., Kremensky, I., Christodoulou, K., Middleton, L. T., Sivakumar, K., Ionasescu, V., Funalot, B., Vance, J. M., Goldfarb, L. G., Fischbeck, K. H., and Green, E. D. (2003) Glycyl tRNA synthetase mutations in Charcot-Marie-Tooth disease type 2D and distal spinal muscular atrophy type V. *Amer, J. Hum. Genet.* **72,** 1293–1299.

Anzini, P., Neuberg, D. H.-H., Schachner, M., Nelles, E., Willecke, K., Zielasek, J., Toyka, K., Suter, U., and Martini, R. (1997). Structural abnormalities and deficient maintenance of peripheral nerve myelin in mice lacking the gap junction protein connexin32. *J. Neurosci.* **17,** 4545–4561.

Auer-Grumbach, M., De Jonghe, P., Wagner, K., Verhoeven, K., Hartung, H.-P., and Timmerman, V. (2000a). Phenotype-genotype correlations in a CMT2B family ith refined 3q13-q22 locus. *Neurology* **55,** 1552–1557.

Auer-Grumbach, M., Wagner, K., Timmerman, V., De Jonghe, P., and Hartung, H.-P. (2000b). Ulcero-mutilating neuropathy in an Austrian kinship without linkage to hereditary motor and sensory neuropathy IIB and hereditary sensory neuropathy I loci. *Neurology* **54,** 45–52.

Azzedine, H., Bolino, A., Taieb, T., Birouk, N., Di Duca, M., Bouhouche, A., Benamou, S., Mrabet, A., Hammadouche, T., Chkili, T., Gouider, R., Ravazzolo, R., Brice, A., Laporte, J., and Le Guern, E. (2003). Mutations in MTMR13, a new pseudo-phosphatase homologue of MTMR2 and Sbf1, are responsible for an autosomal recessive demyelinating form of Charcot-Marie-Tooth disease associated with early-onset glaucoma. *Amer. J. Hum. Genet.* **72,** 1143–1153.

Baechner, D., Liehr, T., Hameister, H., Altenberger, H., Grehl, H., Suter, U., and Rautenstrauss, B. (1995). Widespread expression of the peripheral myelin protein-22 gene (PMP22) in neural and non-neural tissues during murine development. *J. Neurosci. Res.* **42,** 733–741.

Bähr, M., Andres, F., Timmerman, V., Nelis, E., Van Broeckhoven, C., and Dichgans, J. (1999). Central visual, acoustic, and motor pathway involvement in a Charcot-Marie-Tooth family with an Asn205Ser mutation in the connexin32 gene. *J. Neurol. Neurosurg. Psychiat.* **66,** 202–206.

Balice-Gordon, R. J., Bone, L. J., and Scherer, S. S. (1998). Functional gap junctions in the Schwann cell myelin sheath. *J. Cell Biol.* **142,** 1095–1104.

Baxter, R. V., Ben Othmane, K., Rochelle, J. M., Stajich, J. E., Hulette, C., Dew-Knight, S., Hentati, F., Ben Hamida, M., Bel, S., Stenger, J. E., Gilbert, J. R., Pericak-Vance, M., and Vance, J. M. (2002). Ganglioside-induced differentiation-associated protein-1 is mutant in Charcot-Marie-Tooth disease type 4A/8q21. *Nat. Genet.* **30,** 21–22.

Bejaoui, K., Wu, C. Y., Sheffler, M. D., Haan, G., Ashby, P., Wu, L. C., De Jonghe, P., and Brown, R. H. (2001). SPTLC1 is mutated in hereditary sensory neuropathy, type 1. *Nat. Genet.* **27,** 261–262.

Ben Othmane, K., Hentati, F., Lennon, F., Hamida, C. B., Biel, S., Roses, A. D., Pericak-Vance, M. A., Hamida, M. B., and Vance, J. M. (1993a). Linkage of a locus (CMT4A) for autosomal recessive Charcot-Marie-Tooth disease to chromosome 8q. *Hum. Mol. Genet.* **2,** 1625–1628.

Ben Othmane, K., Johnson, E., Menold, M., Graham, F. L., BenHamida, M., Hasegawa, O., Rogala, A. D., Ohnishi, A., PericakVance, M., Hentati, F., and Vance, J. M. (1999). Identification of a new locus for autosomal recessive Charcot-Marie-Tooth disease with focally folded myelin on chromosome 11p15. *Genomics* **62,** 344–349.

Ben Othmane, K., Loeb, D., Hayworth-Hodgte, R., Hentati, F., Rao, N., Roses, A. D., Hamida, K. B., Pericak, M. A., and Vance, J. M. (1995). Physical and genetic mapping of the CMT4A locus and exclusion of PMP-22 as a defect in CMT4A. *Genomics* **28,** 286–290.

Ben Othmane, K., Middleton, L. T., Lopest, L. J., Wilkinson, K. M., Lennon, F., Rozear, M. P., Stajich, J. M., Gaskell, P. C., Roses, A. D., Pericak-Vance, M. A., and Vance, J. M. (1993b). Localization of a gene (CMT2A) for autosomal dominant Charcot-Marie-Tooth disease type 2 to chromosome 1p and evidence of genetic heterogeneity. *Genomics* **17,** 370–375.

Bence, N. F., Sampat, R. M., and Kopito, R. R. (2001). Impairment of the ubiquitin-proteasome system by protein aggregation. *Science* **292,** 1552–1555.

Benstead, T., Kuntz, N., Miller, R., and Daube, J. (1990). The elecrophysiologic profile of Déjérine-Sottas disease (HMSN III). *Muscle Nerve* **13,** 586–592.

Berciano, J., Garcia, A., Calleja, J., and Combarros, O. (2000). Clinico-electrophysiological correlation of extensor digitorum brevis muscle atrophy in children with Charcot-Marie-Tooth disease 1A duplication. *Neuromuscular Disord.* **10,** 419–424.

Berciano, J., Garcia, A., and Combarros, O. (2003). Initial semeiology in childrin with Charcot-Marie-Tooth disease 1A duplication. *Muscle Nerve* **27,** 34–39.

Berciano, M. T., Fernandez, R., Pena, E., Calle, E., Villagra, N. T., and Lafarga, M. (1999). Necrosis of Schwann cells during tellurium-induced primary demyelination: DNA fragmentation, reorganization of splicing machinery, and formation of intranuclear rods of actin. *J. Neuropathol. Exp. Neurol.* **58,** 1234–1243.

Berger, P., Bonneick, S., Willi, S., Wymann, M., and Suter, U. (2002a). Loss of phosphatase activity in myotubularin-related protein 2 is associated with Charcot-Marie-Tooth disease type 4B1. *Hum. Mol. Genet.* **11,** 1569–1579.

Berger, P., Young, P., and Suter, U. (2002b). Molecular cell biology of Charcot-Marie-Tooth disease. *Neurogenetics* **4,** 1–15.

Bergoffen, J., Scherer, S. S., Wang, S., Oronzi-Scott, M., Bone, L., Paul, D. L., Chen, K., Lensch, M. W., Chance, P., and Fischbeck, K. (1993). Connexin mutations in X-linked Charcot-Marie-Tooth disease. *Science* **262,** 2039–2042.

Bermingham, J. R., Jr.,, Scherer, S. S., O'Connell, S., Arroyo, E., Kalla, K., Powell, F. R., and Rosenfeld, M. G. (1996). tst-1/SCIP/Oct-6 regulates a unique step in peripheral myelination and is required for normal respiration. *Genes Dev.* **10,** 1751–1762.

Bird, T. D., Kraft, G. H., Lipe, H. P., Kenney, K. L., and Sumi, S. M. (1997). Clinical and pathological phenotype of the original family with Charcot-Marie-Tooth type 1B: A 20-year study. *Ann. Neurol.* **41,** 463–469.

Bird, T. D., Ott, J., and Giblett, E. R. (1982). Evidence for linkage of Charcot-Marie-Tooth neuropathy to the Duffy locus on chromosome 1. *Am. J. Genet.* **34,** 388–394.

Birouk, N., Gouider, R., Le Guern, E., Gugenheim, M., Tardieu, S., Maisonobe, T., Le Forestier, N., Agid, Y., Brice, A., and Bouche, P. (1997). Charcot-Marie-Tooth disease type 1A with 17p11.2 duplication—Clinical and electrophysiological phenotype study and factors influencing disease severity in 119 cases. *Brain* **120,** 813–823.

Birouk, N., Le Guern, E., Maisonobe, T., Rouger, H., Gouider, R., Gugenheim, M., Tardieu, S., Gugenheim, M., Routon, M. C., Leger, J. M., Agid, Y., Brice, A., and Bouche, P. (1998). X-linked Charcot-Marie-Tooth disease with connexin 32 mutations—clinical and electrophysiological study. *Neurology* **50,** 1074–1082.

Boerkoel, C. F., Takashima, H., Garcia, C. A., Olney, R. K., Johnson, J., Berry, K., Russo, P., Kennedy, S., Teebi, A. S., Scavina, M., Williams, L. L., Mancias, P., Butler, I. J., Krajewski, K., Shy, M., and Lupski, J. R. (2002). Charcot-Marie-Tooth disease and related neuropathies: Mutation distribution and genotype-phenotype correlation. *Ann. Neurol.* **51,** 190–201.

Boerkoel, C. F., Takashima, H., Stankiexicz, P., Garcia, C. A., Leber, S. M., Rhee-Morris, L., and Lupski, J. R. (2000). Periaxin mutations cause recessive Dejerine-Sottas neuropathy. *Amer. J. Hum. Genet.* **68,** 325–333.

Bolino, A., Marigo, V., Ferrera, F., Loader, J., Romio, L., Leoni, A., Di Duca, M., Cinti, R., Cecchi, C., Feltri, M. L., Wrabetz, L., Ravazzolo, R., and Monaco, A. P. (2002). Molecular characterization and expression analysis of Mtmr2, a mouse homologue of MTMR2, the myotubularin-related-2 gene mutated in CMT4B. *Gene* **283,** 17–26.

Bolino, A., Muglia, M., Conforti, F. L., LeGuern, E., Salih, M. A. M., Georgiou, D. M., Christodoulou, K., Hausmanowa-Petrusewicz, I., Mandich, P., Schenone, A., Gambardella, A., Bono, F., Quattrone, A., Devoto, M., and Monaco, A. P. (2000). Charcot-Marie-Tooth type 4B is caused by mutations in the gene encoding myotubularin-related protein-2. *Nat. Genet.* **25,** 17–19.

Bomont, P., Cavalier, L., Blondeau, F., Hamida, C. B., Belal, S., Tazir, M., Demir, E., Topaloglu, H., Korinthenberg, R., Tuysuz, B., Landrieu, P., Hentati, F., and Koenig, M. (2000). The gene encoding gigaxonin, a new member of the cytoskeletal BTB/kelch repeat family, is mutated in giant axonal neuropathy. *Nat Genet* **26,** 370–374.

Bondurand, N., Girard, M., Pingault, V., Lemort, N., Dubourg, O., and Goossens, M. (2001). Human connexin 32, a gap junction protein altered in the X-linked form of Charcot-Marie-Tooth disease, is directly regulated by the transcription factor SOX10. *Hum. Mol. Genet.* **10,** 2783–2795.

Bouhouche, A., Benomar, A., Birouk, N., Mularoni, A., Meggouh, F., Tassin, J., Grid, D., Vandenberghe, A., Yahyaoui, M., Chkili, T., Brice, A., and LeGuern, E. (1999). A locus for an axonal form of autosomal recessive Charcot-Marie-Tooth disease maps to chromosome 1q21.2q21.3. *Amer. J. Hum. Genet.* **65,** 722–727.

Bradley, W. G., and Asbury, A. K. (1972). Radioautographic studies of Schwann cell behavior: I. Acrylamide neuropathy in the mouse. *J. Neuropathol. Exp. Neurol.* **29,** 500–506.

Bradley, W. G., Madrid, R., and Davis, D. J. F. (1977). The peroneal muscular atrophy syndrome—clinical, genetic, electrophysiological and nerve biopsy studies. 3. Clinical, electrophysiological and pathological correlations. *J. Neurol. Sci.* **32,** 123–136.

Brancolini, C., Edomi, P., Marzinotto, S., and Schneider, C. (2000). Exposure at the cell surface is required for gas3/PMP22 to regulate both cell death and cell spreading: Implication for the Charcot-Marie-Tooth type 1A and Dejerine-Sottas diseases. *Mol. Biol. Cell.* **11,** 2901–2914.

Brancolini, C., Marzinotto, S., Edomi, P., Agostoni, E., Fiorentini, C., Müller, H. W., and Schneider, C. (1999). Rho-dependent regulation of cell spreading by the tetraspan membrane protein Gas3/PMP22. *Mol. Biol. Cell.* **10,** 2441–2459.

Brownlees, J., Ackerley, S., Grierson, A. J., Jacobsen, N. J., Shea, K., Anderton, B. H., Leigh, P. N., Shaw, C. E., and Miller, C. C. (2002). Charcot-Marie-Tooth disease neurofilament mutations disrupt neurofilament assembly and axonal transport. *Hum. Mol. Genet.* **11,** 2837–2844.

Brunden, K. R., and Poduslo, J. F. (1987). A phorbol ester-sensitive kinase catalyzes the phosphorylation of P0 glycoprotein in myelin. *J. Neurochem.* **49,** 1863–1872.

Bruzzone, R., T. W. White, S. S. Scherer, Fischbeck, K. H., and Paul, D. L. (1994). Null mutations of connexin32 in patients with X-linked Charcot-Marie-Tooth disease. *Neuron* **13,** 1253–1260.

Bruzzone, R., White, T. W., and Paul, D. L. (1996). Connections with connexins: The molecular basis of direct intercellular signaling. *Eur. J. Biochem.* **238,** 1–27.

Castro, C., Gomez-Hernandez, J. M., Silander, K., and Barrio, L. C. (1999). Altered formation of hemichannels and gap junction channels caused by C-terminal connexin-32 mutations. *J. Neurosci.* **19,** 3752–3760.

Chance, P. F., Alderson, M. K., Leppig, K. A., Lensch, M. W., Matsunami, N., Smith, B., Swanson, P. D., Odelberg, S. J., Disteche, C. M., and Bird, T. D. (1993). DNA deletion associated with hereditary neuropathy with liability to pressure palsies. *Cell* **72,** 143–151.

Chance, P. F., Bird, T. D., Matsunami, N., Lensch, M. W., Brothman, A. R., and Feldman, G. M. (1992a). Trisomy-17p associated with Charcot-Marie-Tooth neuropathy Type-1A phenotype—evidence for gene dosage as a mechanism in CMT1A. *Neurology* **42,** 2295–2299.

Chance, P. F., Matsunami, N., Lensch, W., Smith, B., and Bird, T. D. (1992b). Analysis of the DNA duplication 17p11.2 in Charcot-Marie-Tooth neuropathy type-1 pedigrees—additional evidence for a third autosomal CMT1 locus. *Neurology* **42,** 2037–2041.

Chaouch, M., Allal, Y., De Sandre-Giovannoli, A., Vallat, J. M., Amerel-Khedoud, A., Kassouri, N., Chaouch, A., Sindou, P., Hammadouche, T., Tazir, M., Levy, N., and Grid, D. (2003). The phenotypic manifestations of autosomal recessive axonal Charcot-Marie-Tooth due to a mutation in Lamin A/C gene. *Neuromuscular Disord.* **13,** 60–67.

Chapon, F., Latour, P., Diraison, P., Schaeffer, S., and Vandenberghe, A. (1999). Axonal phenotype of Charcot-Marie-Tooth disease associated with a mutation in the myelin protein zero gene. *J. Neurol. Neurosurg. Psychiat.* **66,** 779–782.

Christodoulou, K., Zamba, E., Tsingis, M., Mubaidin, A., Horani, K., AbuSheik, S., El Khateeb, M., Kyriacou, K., Kyriakides, T., Al Qudah, A. K., and Middleton, L. (2000). A novel form of distal hereditary motor neuronopathy maps to chromosome 9p21.1-p12. *Ann. Neurol.* **48,** 877–884.

Colby, J., Nicholson, R., Dickson, K. M., Orfali, W., Naef, R., Suter, U., and Snipes, G. J. (2000). PMP22 carrying the Trembler or Trembler-J mutation is intracellularly retained in myelinating Schwann cells. *Neurobiol. Dis.* **7,** 561–573.

Colman, D. R., Kreibich, G., Frey, A. B., and Sabatini, D. D. (1982). Synthesis and incorporation of myelin polypeptides into CNS myelin. *J. Cell Biol.* **95,** 598–608.

Comabella, M., Waye, J. S., Raguer, N., Eng, B., Dominguez, C., Navarro, C., Borras, C., Krivit, W., and Montalban, X. (2001). Late-onset metachromatic leukodystrophy clinically presenting as isolated peripheral neuropathy: Compound heterozygosity for the IVS2+1G -> A mutation and a newly identified missense mutation (Thr408Ile) in a Spanish family. *Ann. Neurol.* **50,** 108–112.

Cowchock, R. S., Duckett, S. W., Streletz, L. J., Graziani, L. J., and Jackson, L. G. (1985). X-linked sensory-motor neuropathy type II with deafness and mental retardation: A new disorder. *Am. J. Hum. Genet.* **20,** 307–315.

Cuesta, A., Pedrola, L., Sevilla, T., Garcia-Planells, J., Chumillas, M. J., Mayordomo, F., Le Guern, E., Marin, I., Vilchez, J. J., and Palau, F. (2002). The gene encoding ganglioside-induced differentiation-associated protein 1 is mutated in axonal Charcot-Marie-Tooth type 4A disease. *Nat. Genet.* **30,** 22–25.

D'Urso, D., Brophy, P. J., Staugaitis, S. M., Gillespie, C. S., Frey, A. B., Stempak, J. G., and Colman, D. R. (1990). Protein zero of peripheral nerve myelin: Biosynthesis, membrane insertion, and evidence for homotypic interaction. *Neuron* **4,** 449–460.

D'Urso, D., Ehrhardt, P., and Müller, H. W. (1999). Peripheral myelin protein 22 and protein zero: A novel association in peripheral nervous system myelin. *J. Neurosci.* **19,** 3396–3403.

D'Urso, D., Prior, R., Greiner-Petter, R., Gabreels-Festen, A. A. W. M., and Müller, H. W. (1998). Overloaded endoplasmic reticulum-Golgi compartments, a possible pathomechanism of peripheral neuropathies caused by mutations of the peripheral myelin protein PMP22. *J. Neurosci.* **18,** 731–740.

D'Urso, D., Schmalenbach, C., Zoidl, G., Prior, R., and Müller, H. W. (1997). Studies on the effects of altered PMP22 expression during myelination in vitro. *J. Neurosci. Res.* **48,** 31–42.

Davis, D. J. F., Bradley, W. G., and Madrid, R. (1977). The peroneal muscular atrophy syndrome—clinical, genetic, electrophysiological and nerve biopsy studies. 1. Clinical, genetic, and electrophysiological findings and classification. *J. Génét. Hum.* **26,** 311–349.

Dawkins, J. L., Hulme, D. J., Brahmbhatt, S. B., Auer-Grumbach, M., and Nicholson, G. A. (2001). Mutations in SPTLC1, encoding serine palmitoyltransferase, long chain base subunit-1, cause hereditary sensory neuropathy type I. *Nat. Genet.* **27,** 309–312.

De Jonghe, P., Mersivanova, I., Nelis, E., Del Favero, J., Martin, J. J., Van Broeckhoven, C., Evgrafov, O. C., and Timmerman, V. (2001). Further evidence that neurofilament light chain gene mutations can cause Charcot-Marie-Tooth disease type 2E. *Ann. Neurol.* **49,** 245–249.

De Jonghe, P., Timmerman, V., Ceuterick, C., Nelis, E., De Vriendt, E., Lofgren, A., Vercruyssen, A., Verellen, C., Van Maldergem, L., Martin, J. J., and Van Broeckhoven, C. (1999). The Thr124Met mutation in the peripheral myelin protein zero (MPZ) gene is associated with a clinically distinct Charcot-Marie-Tooth phenotype. *Brain* **122,** 281–290.

De Jonghe, P., Timmerman, V., Nelis, E., Martin, J.-J., and Van Broeckhoven, C. (1997). Charcot-Marie-Tooth disease and related peripheral neuropathies. *J. Peripher. Nerv. Syst.* **2,** 370–387.

De Leon, M., Welcher, A. A., Suter, U., and Shooter, E. M. (1991). Identification of transcriptionally regulated genes after sciatic nerve injury. *J. Neurosci. Res.* **29,** 437–448.

De Sandre-Giovannoli, A., Chaouch, M., Kozlov, S., Vallat, J. M., Tazir, M., Kassouri, N., Szepetowski, P., Hammadouche, T., Vandenberghe, A., Stewart, C. L., Grid, D., and Levy, N. (2002). Homozygous defects in LMNA, encoding lamin A/C nuclear-envelope proteins, cause autosomal recessive axonal neuropathy in human (Charcot-Marie-Tooth disorder type 2) and mouse. *Amer. J. Hum. Genet.* **70,** 726–736.

Delague, V., Bareil, C., Tuffery, S., Bouvagnet, P., Chouery, E., Koussa, S., Maisonobe, T., Loiselet, J., Megarbane, A., and Claustres, M. (2000). Mapping of a new locus for autosomal recessive demyelinating Charcot-Marie-Tooth disease to 19q13.1–13.3 in a large consanguineous Lebanese family: Exclusion of MAG as a candidate gene. *Amer. J. Hum. Genet.* **67,** 236–243.

Dickson, K. M., Bergeron, J. J. M., Shames, I., Colby, J., Nguyen, D. T., Chevet, E., Thomas, D. Y., and Snipes, G. J. (2002). Association of calnexin with mutant peripheral myelin protein-22 ex vivo: A basis for gain-of-function ER diseases. *Proc. Natl. Acad. Sci. USA* **99,** 9852–9857.

Ding, J. Q., Liu, J. J., Kowal, A. S., Nardine, T., Bhattacharya, P., Lee, A., and Yang, Y. M. (2002). Microtubule-associated protein 1B: A neuronal binding partner for gigaxonin. *J. Cell Biol.* **158,** 427–433.

Ding, Y., and Brunden, K. R. (1995). The cytoplasmic domain of myelin glycoprotein $P_0$ interacts with negatively charged phospholipid bilayers. *J. Biol. Chem.* **269,** 10764–10770.

Donaghy, M., Sisodiya, S. M., Kennett, R., McDonald, B., Haites, N., and Bell, C. (2000). Steroid responsive polyneuropathy in a family with a novel myelin protein zero mutation. *J. Neurol. Neurosurg. Psychiat.* **69,** 799–805.

Dubourg, O., Tardieu, S., Birouk, N., Gouider, R., Leger, J. M., Maisonobe, T., Brice, A., Bouche, P., and LeGuern, E. (2001). Clinical, electrophysiological and molecular genetic characteristics of 93 patients with X-linked Charcot-Marie-Tooth disease. *Brain* **124,** 1958–1967.

Dyck, P. J. (1993). Neuronal atrophy and degeneration predominantly affecting peripheral sensory and autonomic neurons. *In* "Peripheral Neuropathy" 3rd ed., vol.2 (P. J. Dyck, P. K. Thomas, J. W. Griffin, P. A. Low and J. F. Poduslo, eds.), 1065–1093. W. B. Saunders, Philadelphia.

Dyck, P. J., Chance, P., Lebo, R., and Carney, J. A. (1993a). Hereditary motor and sensory neuropathies. *In* "Peripheral Neuropathy" 3rd ed., vol.2 (P. J. Dyck, P. K. Thomas, J. W. Griffin, P. A. Low, and J. F. Poduslo, eds.), 1094–1136. W. B. Saunders,, Philadelphia.

Dyck, P. J., Giannini, D., and Lais, A. (1993b). Pathologic alterations of nerves. *In* "Peripheral Neuropathy " 3rd ed., vol.1 (P. J. Dyck, P. K. Thomas, J. W. Griffin, P. A. Low, and J. F. Poduslo, eds.),3rd ed., 514–595. W. B. Saunders, Philadelphia.

Dyck, P. J., Karnes, J. L., and Lambert, E. H. (1989). Longitudinal study of neuropathic deficits and nerve conduction abnormalities in hereditary motor and sensory neuropathy type 1. *Neurology* **39,** 1302–1308.

Dyck, P. J., Lais, A. C., and Offord, K. P. (1974). The nature of myelinated nerve fiber degeneration in dominately inherited hypertrophic neuropathy. *Mayo Clinic Proc.* **49,** 34–39.

Elliot, J. L., Kwon, J. M., Goodfellow, P. J., and Yee, W.-C. (1997). Hereditary motor and sensory neuropathy IIB: Clinical and electrophysiological characteristics. *Neurology* **48,** 23–28.

Erdem, S., Mendell, J. R., and Sahenk, Z. (1998). Fate of Schwann cell in CMT1A and HNPP: Evidence for apoptosis. *J. Neuropathol. Exp. Neurol.* **57,** 635–642.

Erne, B., Sansano, S., Frank, M., and Schaeren-Wiemers, N. (2002). Rafts in adult peripheral nerve myelin contain major structural myelin proteins and myelin and lymphocyte protein (MAL) and CD59 as specific markers. *J. Neurochem.* **82,** 550–562.

Fabbretti, E., Edomi, P., Brancolini, C., and Schneider, C. (1995). Apoptotic phenotype induced by overexpression of wild-type *gas3/PMP22:* Its relation to the demyelinating peripheral neuropathy CMT1A. *Genes Dev.* **9,** 1846–1856.

Fabrizi, C., Kelly, B. M., Gillespie, C. S., Schlaepfer, W. W., Scherer, S. S., and Brophy, P. J. (1997). Transient expression of the neurofilament proteins NF-L and NF-M by Schwann cells is regulated by axonal contact. *J. Neurosci. Res.* **50,** 291–299.

Fabrizi, G. M., Cavallaro, T., Taioli, F., Orrico, D., Morbin, M., Simonati, A., and Rizzuto, N. (1999). Myelin uncompaction in Charcot-Marie-Tooth neuropathy type 1A with a point mutation of peripheral myelin protein-22. *Neurology* **53,** 846–851.

Fabrizi, G. M., Simonati, A., Morbin, M., Cavallaro, T., Taioli, F., Benedetti, M. D., Edomi, P., and Rizzuto, N. (1998). Clinical and pathological correlations in Charcot-Marie-Tooth neuropathy type 1A with the 17p11.2p12 duplication: A cross-sectional morphometric and immunohistochemical study in twenty cases. *Muscle Nerve* **21,** 869–877.

Fannon, A. M., Sherman, D. L., Ilyina-Gragerova, G., Brophy, P. J., Friedrich, V. L., and Colman, D. R. (1995). Novel E-cadherin mediated adhesion in peripheral nerve: Schwann cell architecture is stabilized by autotypic adherens junctions. *J. Cell Biol.* **129,** 189–202.

Fidzianska, A., Drac, H., and Rafalowska, J. (2002). Phenomenon of Schwann cell apoptosis in a case of congenital hypomyelinating neuropathy with basal lamina onion bulb formation. *Brain Develop.* **24,** 727–731.

Filbin, M. T., and Tennekoon, G. I. (1993). Homophilic adhesion of the myelin P0 protein requires glycosylation of both molecules in the homophilic pair. *J. Cell Biol.* **122,** 451–459.

Filbin, M. T., Walsh, F. S., Trapp, B. D., Pizzey, J. A., and Tennekoon, G. I. (1990). Role of P0 protein as a homophilic adhesion molecule. *Nature* **344,** 871–872.

Fischbeck, K. H., ar-Rushdi, N., Pericak-Vance, M., Rozear, M., Roses, A. D., and Fryns, J. P. (1986). X-linked neuropathy: Gene localization with DNA probes. *Ann. Neurol.* **20,** 527–532.

Frei, R., Motzing, S., Kinkelin, I., Schachner, M., Koltzenburg, M., and Martini, R. (1999). Loss of distal axons and sensory Merkel cells and features indicative of muscle denervation in hindlimbs of P0-deficient mice. *J. Neurosci.* **19,** 6058–6067.

Gable, K., Han, G., Monaghan, E., Bacikova, D., Natarajan, M., Williams, R., and Dunn, T. M. (2002). Mutations in the yeast LCB1 and LCB2 genes, including those corresponding to the hereditary sensory neuropathy type I mutations, dominantly inactivate serine palmitoyltransferase. *J. Biol. Chem.* **277,** 10194–10200.

Gabreels-Festen, A. (2002). Dejerine-Sottas syndrome grown to maturity: Overview of genetic and morphological heterogeneity and follow-up of 25 patients. *J. Anat.* **200,** 341–356.

Gabreels-Festen, A. A. W. M., Bolhuis, P. A., Hoogendijk, J. E., Valentijn, L. J., Eshuis, E. J. H. M., and Gabreels, F. J. M. (1995). Charcot-Marie-Tooth disease type 1A: Morphological phenotype of the 17p duplication versus PMP22 point mutations. *Acta Neuropathol.* **90,** 645–649.

Gabreels-Festen, A. A. W. M., Hoogendijk, J. E., Meijerink, P. H. S., Gabreels, F. J. M., Bolhuis, P. A., Vanbeersum, S., Kulkens, T., Nelis, E., Jennekens, F. G. I., Devisser, M., Vanengelen, B. G. M., Van Broeckhoven, C., and Mariman, E. C. M. (1996). Two divergent types of nerve pathology in patients with different P0 mutations in Charcot-Marie-Tooth disease. *Neurology* **47,** 761–765.

Gabreels-Festen, A. A. W. M., Joosten, E. M. G., Gabreels, F. J. M., Jennekens, F. G. I., Gooskens, R. H. J. M., and Stegeman, D. F. (1991). Hereditary motor and sensory neuropathy of neuronal type with onset in early childhood. *Brain* **114,** 1855–1870.

Gabreels-Festen, A. A. W. M., Joosten, E. M. G., Gabreels, F. J. M., Jennekens, F. G. I., and Kempen, T. W. J. (1992). Early morphological features in dominantly inherited demyelinating motor and sensory neuropathy (HMSN Type-I). *J. Neurol. Sci.* **107,** 145–154.

Gabriel, J. M., Erne, B., Pareyson, D., Sghirlanzoni, A., Taroni, F., and Steck, A. J. (1997). Gene dosage effects in hereditary peripheral neuropathy—Expression of peripheral myelin protein 22 in Charcot-Marie-Tooth disease type 1A and hereditary neuropathy with liability to pressure palsies nerve biopsies. *Neurology* **49,** 1635–1640.

Gao, Y., Li, W., and Filbin, M. T. (2000). Acylation of myelin P0 protein is required for adhesion. *J. Neurosci. Res.* **60,** 704–713.

Garbern, J. Y., Cambi, F., Tang, X. M., Sima, A. A. F., Vallat, J. M., Bosch, E. P., Lewis, R., Shy, M., Sohi, J., Kraft, G., Chen, K. L., Joshi, I., Leonard, D. G. B., Johnson, W., Raskind, W., Dlouhy, S. R., Pratt, V., Hodes, M. E., Bird, T., and Kamholz, J. (1997). Proteolipid protein is necessary in peripheral as well as central myelin. *Neuron* **19,** 205–218.

Garcia, C. A., Malamut, R. E., Englnad, J. D., Parry, G. S., Liu, P., and Lupski, J. R. (1995). Clinical variability in two pairs of identical twins with the Charcot-Marie-Tooth disease type 1A duplication. *Neurology* **45,** 2090–2093.

Ghazvini, M., Mandemakers, W., Jaegle, M., Piirsoo, M., Driegen, S., Koutsourakis, M., Smit, X., Grosveld, F., and Meijer, D. (2002). A cell type-specific allele of the POU gene Oct-6 reveals Schwann cell autonomous function in nerve development and regeneration. *EMBO J.* **21,** 4612–4620.

Giese, K. P., Martini, R., Lemke, G., Soriano, P., and Schachner, M. (1992). Mouse $P_0$ gene disruption leads to hypomyelination, abnormal expression of recognition molecules, and degeneration of myelin and axons. *Cell* **71,** 565–576.

Gillespie, C. S., Sherman, D. L., Blair, G. E., and Brophy, P. J. (1994). Periaxin, a novel protein of myelinating Schwann cells with a possible role in axonal ensheathment. *Neuron* **12,** 497–508.

Gillespie, C. S., Sherman, D. L., Fleetwood-Walker, S. M., Cottrell, D. F., Tait, S., Garry, E. M., Wallace, V. C. J., Ure, J., Griffiths, I. R., Smith, A., and Brophy, P. J. (2000). Peripheral demyelination and neuropathic pain behavior in periaxin-deficient mice. *Neuron* **26,** 523–531.

Gouider, R., Le Guern, E., Gugenheim, M., Tardieu, S., Maisonobe, T., Leger, J. M., Vallat, J. M., Agid, Y., Bouche, P., and Brice, A. (1995). Clinical, electrophysiologic, and molecular correlations in 13 families with hereditary neuropathy with liability to pressure palsies and a chromosome 17p11.2 deletion. *Neurology* **45,** 2018–2023.

Greenfield, S., Brostoff, S., Eylar, E. H., and Morell, P. (1973). Protein composition of myelin of the peripheral nervous system. *J. Neurochem.* **20,** 1207–1216.

Griffin, J. W., and Hoffman, P. N. (1993). Degeneration and regeneration in the peripheral nervous system. *In* "Peripheral Neuropathy" 3rd ed., vol.1 (P. J. Dyck, P. K. Thomas, P. A. Low, and J. F. Poduslo, eds.), 361–376. W. B. Saunders, Philadelphia.

Grinspan, J. B., Marchionni, M., Reeves, M., Coulaloglou, M., and Scherer, S. S. (1996). Axonal interactions regulate Schwann cell apoptosis in developing peripheral nerve: Neuregulin receptors and the role of neuregulins. *J. Neurosci.* **16,** 6107–6118.

Grohmann, K., Schuelke, M., Diers, A., Hoffmann, K., Lucke, B., Adams, C., Bertini, E., Leonhardt-Horti, H., Muntoni, F., Ouvrier, R., Pfeufer, A., Rossi, R. N., Van Maldergem, L., Wilmshurst, J. M., Wienker, T. F., Sendtner, M., Rudnik-Schöneborn, S., Zerres, K., and Hübner, C. (2001). Mutations in the gene encoding immunoglobulin mu-binding protein 2 cause spinal muscular atrophy with respiratory distress type 1. *Nat. Genet.* **29,** 75–77.

Grohmann, K., Wienker, T. F., Saar, K., Rudnik-Schöneborn, S., Stoltenburg-Didinger, G., Rossi, R. N., Nürnberg, G., Pfeufer, A., Wirth, B., Reis, A., Zerres, K., and Hübner, C. (1999). Diaphragmatic spinal muscular atrophy with respiratory distress is heterogeneous, and one form is linked to chromosome 11q13-q21. *Amer. J. Hum. Genet.* **65,** 1459–1462.

Guilbot, A., Kessali, M., Ravise, N., Hammadouche, T., Bouhouche, A., Maisonobe, T., Grid, D., Brice, A., and Guern, E. L. (1999). The autosomal recessive form of CMT disease linked to 5q31-q33. *Ann. N. Y. Acad. Sci.* **883,** 56–59.

Guilbot, A., Williams, A., Ravise, N., Verny, C., Brice, A., Sherman, D. L., Brophy, P. J., Le Guern, E., Delague, V., Bareil, C., Megarbane, A., and Claustres, M. (2001). A mutation in periaxin is responsible for CMT4F, an autosomal recessive form of Charcot-Marie-Tooth disease. *Hum. Mol. Genet.* **10,** 415–421.

Gutierrez, A., England, J. D., Sumner, A. J., Ferer, S., Warner, L. E., Lupski, J. R., and Garcia, C. A. (2000). Unusual electrophysiological findings in X-linked dominant Charcot-Marie-Tooth disease. *Muscle Nerve* **23,** 182–188.

Guzzetta, F., Ferriere, G., and Lyon, G. (1982). Congenital demyelinating neuropathy. Pathological findings compared with polyneuropathies starting later in life. *Brain* **105,** 395–416.

Hahn, A., Ainsworth, P. J., Bolton, C. F., Bilbao, J. M., and Vallat, J.-M. (2001). Pathological findings in the X-linked form of Charcot-Marie-Tooth disease: A morphometric and ultrastructural analysis. *Acta Neuropathol.* **101,** 129–139.

Hahn, A. F., Ainsworth, P. J., Naus, C. C. G., Mao, J., and Bolton, C. F. (2000). Clinical and pathological observations in men lacking the gap junction protein connexin 32. *Muscle Nerve,* S39-S48.

Hahn, A. F., Brown, W. F., Koopman, W. J., and Feasby, T. E. (1990). X-linked dominant hereditary motor and sensory neuropathy. *Brain* **113,** 1511–1525.

Hanemann, C. O., D'Urso, D., Gabreels-Festen, A. A. W. M., and Müller, H. W. (2000). Mutation-dependent alteration in cellular distribution of peripheral myelin protein 22 in nerve biopsies from Charcot-Marie-Tooth type 1A. *Brain* **123,** 1001–1006.

Hanemann, C. O., and Gabreels-Festen, A. A. (2002). Secondary axon atrophy and neurological dysfunction in demyelinating neuropathies. *Curr. Opin. Neurol.* **15,** 611–615.

Hanemann, C. O., Gabreels-Festen, A. A. W. M., and De Jonghe, P. (2001). Axon damage in CMT due to mutation in myelin protein P0. *Neuromuscular Disord.* **11,** 753–756.

Hanemann, C. O., Gabreels-Festen, A. A. W. M., Müller, H. W., and Stoll, G. (1996). Low affinity NGF receptor expression in CMT1A nerve biopsies of different disease stages. *Brain* **119,** 1461–1469.

Hanemann, C. O., Gabreels-Festen, A. A. W. M., Stoll, G., and Müller, H. W. (1997). Schwann cell differentiation in Charcot-Marie-Tooth disease type 1A (CMT1A): Normal number of myelinating Schwann cells in young CMT1A patients and neural cell adhesion molecule expression in onion bulbs. *Acta Neuropathol.* **94,** 310–315.

Hanemann, C. O., and Müller, H. W. (1998). Pathogenesis of Charcot-Marie-Tooth IA (CMTIA) neuropathy. *Trends Neurosci.* **21,** 282–286.

Hanemann, C. O., Rosenbaum, C., Kupfer, S., Wosch, S., Stoegbauer, F., and Müller, H. W. (1998). Improved culture methods to expand Schwann cells with altered growth behaviour from CMT1A patients. *Glia* **23,** 89–98.

Hanemann, C. O., Stoll, G., D'Urso, D., Fricke, W., Martin, J. J., Van Broeckhoven, C., Mancardi, G. L., Bratke, I., and Müller, H. W. (1994). Peripheral myelin protein-22 expression in Charcot-Marie-Tooth disease type Ia sural nerve biopsies. *J. Neurosci. Res.* **37,** 654–659.

Haney, C., Snipes, G. J., Shooter, E. M., Suter, U., Garcia, C., Griffin, J. W., and Trapp, B. D. (1996). Ultrastructural distribution of PMP22 in Charcot-Marie-Tooth disease type 1A. *J. Neuropathol. Exp. Neurol.* **55,** 290–299.

Harati, Y., and Butler, I. J. (1985). Congenital hypomyelinating neuropathy. *J. Neurol. Neurosurg. Psychiat.* **48,** 1269–1276.

Harding, A. E. (1995). From the syndrome of Charcot, Marie and Tooth to disorders of peripheral myelin proteins. *Brain* **118,** 809–818.

Harding, A. E., and Thomas, P. K. (1980). The clinical features of hereditary motor and sensory neuropathy types I and II. *Brain* **103,** 259–280.

Hasse, B., Bosse, F., and Müller, H. W. (2002). Proteins of peripheral myelin are associated with glycosphingolipid/cholesterol-enriched membranes. *J. Neurosci. Res.* **69,** 227–232.

Hayasaka, K., Himoro, M., Sato, W., Takada, G., Uyemura, K., Shimizu, N., Bird, T. D., Conneally, P. M., and Chance, P. F. (1993a). Charcot-Marie-Tooth neuropathy type 1B is associated with mutations of the myelin P0 gene. *Nat. Genet.* **5,** 31–34.

Hayasaka, K., Himoro, M., Sawaishi, Y., Nanao, K., Takahashi, T., Takada, G., Nicholson, G. A., Ouvrier, R. A., and Tachi, N. (1993b). De novo mutation of the myelin Po gene in Dejerine-Sottas disease (hereditary motor and sensory neuropathy type III). *Nat. Genet.* **5,** 266–268.

Hayasaka, K., Himoro, M., Wang, Y. M., Takata, M., Minoshima, S., Shimizu, N., Miura, M., Uyemura, K., and Takada, G. (1993c). Structure and chromosomal localization of the gene encoding the human myelin protein zero (MPZ). *Genomics* **17,** 755–758.

Hayasaka, K., Takada, G., and Ionasescu, V. V. (1993d). Mutation of the myelin $P_0$ gene in Charcot-Marie-Tooth neuropathy type-1B. *Hum. Mol. Genet.* **2,** 1369–1372.

Herringham, W. P. (1889). Muscular atrophy of the peroneal type affecting many members of a family. *Brain* **11,** 230–236.

Hilmi, S., Fournier, M., Valeins, H., Gandar, J. C., and Bonnet, J. (1995). Myelin P0 glycoprotein: Identification of the site phosphorylated in vitro and in vivo by endogenous protein kinases. *J. Neurochem.* **64,** 902–907.

Hirokawa, N. (1998). Kinesin and dynein superfamily proteins and the mechanism of organelle transport. *Science* **279,** 519–526.

Hoogendijk, J. E., de Visser, M., Bolhuis, P. A., Hart, A. A. M., and de Visser, B. W. O. (1994). Hereditary motor and sensory neuropathy type I—clinical and neurographical features of the 17p duplication subtype. *Muscle Nerve* **17,** 85–90.

Houlden, H., King, R. H. M., Wood, N. W., Thomas, P. K., and Reilly, M. M. (2001). Mutations in the 5' region of the myotubularin-related protein 2 (MTMR2) gene in autosomal recessive hereditary neuropathy with focally folded myelin. *Brain* **124,** 907–915.

Indo, Y. (2001). Molecular basis of congenital insensitivity to pain with anhidrosis (CIPA): Mutations and polymorphisms in TRKA (NTRK1) gene encoding the receptor tyrosine kinase for nerve growth factor. *Hum. Mutat.* **18,** 462–471.

Inoue, K., Shilo, K., Boerkoel, C. F., Crowe, C., Sawady, J., Lupski, J. R., and Agamanolis, D. P. (2002). Congenital hypomyelinating neuropathy, central dysmyelination, and Waardenburg-Hirschsprung disease: Phenotypes linked by SOX10 mutation. *Ann Neurol* **52,** 836–842.

Inoue, K., Tanabe, Y., and Lupski, J. R. (1999). Myelin deficiencies in both the central and the peripheral nervous systems associated with a SOX10 mutation. *Ann. Neurol.* **46,** 313–318.

Ionasescu, V., Ionasescu, R., and Searby, C. (1996a). Correlation between connexin 32 gene mutations and clinical phenotype in X-linked dominant Charcot-Marie-Tooth neuropathy. *Am. J. Med. Genet.* **63,** 486–491.

Ionasescu, V. V., Ionasescu, R., and Searby, C. (1993). Screening of dominantly inherited Charcot-Marie-Tooth neuropathies. *Muscle Nerve* **16,** 1232–1238.

Ionasescu, V. V., Trofatter, J., and Haines, J. L. (1991). Heterogeneity in X-linked recessive Charcot-Marie-Tooth neuropathy. *Amer. J. Hum. Genet.* **48,** 1075–1083.

Ionasescu, V. V., Trofatter, J., Haines, J. L., Summers, A. M., Ionasescu, R., and Searby, C. (1992). X-linked recessive Charcot-Marie-Tooth neuropathy—clinical and genetic study. *Muscle Nerve* **15,** 368–373.

Irobi, J., Nelis, E., Verhoeven, K., DeVriendt, E., Dierick, I., DeJonghe, P., VanBroeckhoven, C., and Timmerman, V. (2002). Mutation analysis of 12 candidate genes for distal hereditary motor neuropathy type II (Distal HMN II) linked to 12q24.3. *J. Peripher. Nerv. Syst.* **7,** 87–95.

Irobi, J., Tissir, F., De Jonghe, P., De Vriendt, E., Van Broeckhoven, C., Timmerman, V., and Beuten, J. (2000). A clone contig of 12q24.3 encompassing the distal hereditary motor neuropathy type II gene. *Genomics* **65,** 34–43.

Ismailov, S. M., Fedotov, V. P., Dadali, E. L., Polyakov, A. V., Van Broeckhoven, C., Ivanov, V. I., De Jonghe, P., Timmerman, V., and Evgrafov, O. V. (2001). A new locus for autosomal dominant Charcot-Marie-Tooth disease type 2 (CMT2F) maps to chromosome 7q11-q21. *Eur. J. Human Genet.* **9,** 646–650.

Jacobs, J. M., and Gregory, R. (1991). Uncompacted lamellae as a feature of tomaculous neuropathy. *Acta Neuropathol.* **83,** 87–91.

Jaegle, M., Mandemakers, W., Broos, L., Zwart, R., Karis, A., Visser, P., Grosveld, F., and Meijer, D. (1996). The POU factor Oct-6 and Schwann cell differentiation. *Science* **273,** 507–510.

Jansen, G. A., Hogenhout, E. M., Ferdinandusse, S., Waterham, H. R., Ofman, R., Jakobs, C., Skjeldal, O. H., and Wanders, R. J. A. (1997). Human phytanoyl-CoA hydroxylase: Resolution of the gene structure and the molecular basis of Refsum's disease. *Nat. Genet.* **17,** 190–193.

Jordanova, A., De Jonghe, P., Boerkoel, C. F., Takashima, H., De Vriendt, E., Ceuterick, C., Martin, J.-J., Butler, I. J., Mancias, P., Papasozomenos, S. C., Terespolsky, D., Potochi, L., Brown, C. W., Shy, M., Rita, D. A., Tournev, I., Kremensky, I., Lupski, J. R., and Timmerman, V. (2003). Mutations in the neurofilament light chain geen (*NEFL*) cause early onset severe Charcot-Marie-Tooh disease. *Brain* **126,** 590–597.

Kaku, D. A., Parry, G. J., Malamut, R., Lupski, J. R., and Garcia, C. A. (1993a). Nerve conduction studies in Charcot-Marie-Tooth polyneuropathy associated with a segmental duplication of chromosome 17. *Neurology* **43,** 1806–1808.

Kaku, D. A., Parry, G. J., Malamut, R., Lupski, J. R., and Garcia, C. A. (1993b). Uniform slowing of conduction velocities in Charcot-Marie-Tooth disease polyneuropathy type 1. *Neurology* **43,** 2664–2667.

Kalaydjieva, L., Gresham, D., Gooding, R., Heather, L., Baas, F., de Jonge, R., Blechschmidt, K., Angelicheva, D., Chandler, D., Worsley, P., Rosenthal, A., King, R. H. M., and Thomas, P. K. (2000). *N-myc downstream-regulated gene 1* is mutated in hereditary motor and sensory neuropathy-Lom. *Amer. J. Hum. Genet.* **67,** 47–58.

Kalaydjieva, L., Hallmayer, J., Chandler, D., Savov, A., Nikolova, A., Angelicheva, D., King, R. H. H., Ishpekova, B., Honeyman, K., Calafell, F., Shmarov, A., Petrova, J., Turnev, I., Hristova, A., Moskov, M., Stancheva, S., Petkova, I., Bittles, A. H., Georgieva, V., Middleton, L., and Thomas, P. K. (1996). Gene mapping in Gypsies identifies a novel demyelinating neuropathy on chromosome 8q24. *Nat. Genet.* **14,** 214–217.

Kalaydjieva, L., Nikolova, A., Turnev, I., Petrova, J., Hristova, A., Ishpekova, B., Petkova, I., Shmarov, A., Stancheva, S., Middleton, L., Merlini, L., Trogu, A., Muddle, J. R., King, R. H. M., and Thomas, P. K. (1998). Hereditary motor and sensory neuropathy—LOM, a novel demyelinating neuropathy associated with deafness in gypsies—Clinical, electrophysiological and nerve biopsy findings. *Brain* **121,** 399–408.

Kamholz, J., Shy, M., and Scherer, S. S. (1994). Elevated expression of messenger RNA for peripheral myelin protein 22 in biopsied peripheral nerves of patients with Charcot-Marie-Tooth disease type IA. *Ann. Neurol.* **36,** 451–452.

Kennerson, M. L., Zhu, D., Gardner, R. J. M., Storey, E., Merory, J., Robertson, S. P., and Nicholson, G. A. (2001). Dominant intermediate Charcot-Marie-Tooth neuropathy maps to chromosome 19p12-p13.2. *Amer. J. Hum. Genet.* **69,** 883–888.

Killian, J. M., Tiwari, P. S., Jacobson, S., Jackson, R. D., and Lupski, J. R. (1996). Longitudinal studies of the duplication form of Charcot-Marie-Tooth polyneuropathy. *Muscle Nerve* **19,** 74–78.

Kim, S. A., Taylor, G. S., Torgersen, K. M., and Dixon, J. E. (2002). Myotubularin and MTMR2, phosphatidylinositol 3-phosphatases mutated in myotubular myopathy and type 4B Charcot-Marie-Tooth disease. *J. Biol. Chem.* **277,** 4526–4531.

Kirschner, D. A., Szumowski, K., Gabreels-Festen, A. A. W. M., Hoogendijk, J. E., and Bolhuis, P. A. (1996). Inherited demyelinating peripheral neuropathies: Relating myelin packing abnormalities to P0 molecular defects. *J. Neurosci. Res.* **46,** 502–508.

Klein, C. J., Cunningham, I. M., Atkinson, E. J., Schaid, D. J., Hebbring, S. J., Anderson, S. A., Klein, D. M., Dyck, P. J. B., Litchy, W. J., Thibodeau, S. N. (2003). The gene for HMSN2C maps to 12q23-24 - A region of neuromuscular disorders. *Neurology* **60,** 1151–1156.

Kleopa, K. A., and Scherer, S. S. (2002). Inherited Neuropathies. *Neurol. Clin. N. Am.* **20,** 679–709.

Kleopa, K. A., Yum, S. W., and Scherer, S. S. (2002). Cellular mechanisms of connexin32 mutations associated with CNS manifestations. *J. Neurosci. Res.* **68,** 522–534.

Korinthenberg, R., Sauer, M., Ketelsen, U. P., Hanemann, C. O., Stoll, G., Graf, M., Baborie, A., Volk, B., Wirth, B., Rudnik-Schoneborn, S., and Zerres, K. (1997). Congenital axonal neuropathy caused by deletions in the spinal muscular atrophy region. *Ann. Neurol.* **42,** 364–368.

Krajewski, K. M., Lewis, R. A., Fuerst, D. R., Turansky, C., Hinderer, S. R., Garbern, J., Kamholz, J., and Shy, M. E. (2000). Neurological dysfunction and axonal degeneration in Charcot-Marie-Tooth disease. *Brain* **123,** 1516–1527.

Kruger, O., Plum, A., Kim, J. S., Winterhager, E., Maxeiner, S., Hallas, G., Kirchhoff, S., Traub, O., Lamers, W. H., and Willecke, K. (2000). Defective vascular development in connexin 45-deficient mice. *Development* **127,** 4179–4193.

Kuhlenbaumer, G., Young, P., Oberwittler, C., Hunermund, G., Schirmacher, A., Domschke, K., Ringelstein, B., and Stogbauer, F. (2002). Giant axonal neuropathy (GAN): Case report and two novel mutations in the gigaxonin gene. *Neurology* **58,** 1273–1276.

Kuntzer, T., Dunarnd, M., Schorderet, D. F., Vallat, J.-M., Hahn, A. F., and Bogousslavsky, J. (2003). Phenotypic expresssion of a Pro 87 to Leu mutatin in the connexin 32 gene in a large Swiss family with Charcot-Marie-Tooth neuropathy. *J. Neurol. Sci.*, **87,** 77–86.

Lachat, P., Shaw, P., Gebhard, S., Van Belzen, N., Chaubert, P., and Bosman, F. T. (2002). Expression of NDRG1, a differentiation-related gene, in human tissues. *Histochem. Cell. Biol.* **118,** 399–408.

Lagueny, A., Latour, P., Vital, G., LeMasson, G., Rouanet, M., Ferrer, X., Vital, C., and Vandenberghe, A. (2001). Mild recurrent neuropathy in CMT1B with a novel nonsense mutation in the extracellular domain of the MPZ gene. *J Neurol Neurosurg Psychiat* **70,** 232–235.

Laporte, J., Blondeau, F., Buj-Bello, A., and Mandel, J. L. (2001). The myotubularin family: From genetic disease to phosphoinositide metabolism. *Trends Genet* **17,** 221–228.

Laporte, J., Liaubet, L., Blondeau, F., Tronchere, H., Mandel, J. L., and Payrastre, B. (2002). Functional redundancy in the myotubularin family. *Biochem Biophys Res Commun* **291,** 305–312.

Le Guern, E., Gouider, R., Mabin, D., Tardieu, S., Birouk, N., Parent, P., Bouche, P., and Brice, A. (1997). Patients homozygous for the 17p11.2 duplication in Charcot-Marie-Tooth type 1A disease. *Ann. Neurol.* **41,** 104–108.

Le Guern, E., Guilbot, A., Kessali, M., Ravise, N., Tassin, J., Maisonobe, T., Grid, D., and Brice, A. (1996). Homozygosity mapping of an autosomal recessive form of demyelinating Charcot-Marie-Tooth disease to chromosome 5q23-q33. *Hum. Mol. Genet.* **5,** 1685–1688.

Leal, A., Morera, B., DelValle, G., Heuss, D., Kayser, C., Berghoff, M., Villegas, R., Hernandez, E., Mendez, M., Hennies, H. C., Neundorfer, B., Barrantes, R., Reis, A., and Rautenstrauss, B. (2001). A second locus for an axonal form of autosomal recessive Charcot-Marie-Tooth disease maps to chromosome 19q13.3. *Amer. J. Hum. Genet.* **68,** 269–274.

Lee, M. J., Nelson, I., Houlden, H., Sweeney, M. G., Hilton-Jones, D., Blake, J., Wood, N. W., and Reilly, M. M. (2002). Six novel connexin32 (GJB1) mutations in X-linked Charcot-Marie-Tooth disease. *J. Neurol. Neurosurg. Psychiat.* **73,** 304–306.

Lee, M. K., Marzalek, J. R., and Cleveland, D. W. (1994). A mutant neurofilament subunit causes massive, selective motor neuron death: Implications for the pathogenesis of human motor neuron disease. *Neuron* **13,** 975–988.

Lemke, G., and Axel, R. (1985). Isolation and sequence of a cDNA encoding the major structural protein of peripheral myelin. *Cell* **40,** 501–508.

Levi, G., Topilko, P., Schneider-Maunoury, S., Lasagna, M., Mantero, S., Cancedda, R., and Charnay, P. (1996). Defective bone formation in Krox-20 mutant mice. *Development* **122,** 113–120.

Lewis, R. A., Sumner, A. J., and Shy, M. E. (2000). Electrophysiological features of inherited demyelinating neuropathies: A reappraisal in the era of molecular diagnosis. *Muscle Nerve* **23,** 1472–1487.

Li, J., Krajewski, K., Shy, M. E., and Lewis, R. A. (2002a). Hereditary neuropathy with liability to pressure palsy—The electrophysiology fits the name. *Neurology* **58,** 1769–1773.

Li, X., Lynn, B. D., Olson, C., Meier, C., Davidson, K. G. V., Yasumura, T., Rash, J. E., and Nagy, J. L. (2002b). Connexin29 expression, immunocytochemistry and freeze-fracture replica immunogold labelling (FRIL) in sciatic nerve. *Eur. J. Neurosci.* **16,** 795–806.

Lin, G. S., Glass, J. D., Shumas, S., Scherer, S. S., and Fischbeck, K. H. (1999). A unique mutation in connexin32 associated with severe, early onset CMTX in a heterozygous female. *Ann. N. Y. Acad. Sci.* **883,** 481–485.

Liu, H., Nakagawa, T., Kanematsu, T., Uchida, T., and Tsuji, S. (1999). Isolation of 10 differentially expressed cDNAs in differentiated Neuro2a cells induced through controlled expression of the GD3 synthase gene. *J. Neurochem.* **72,** 1781–1790.

Lopez-Bigas, N., Olive, M., Rabionet, R., Ben-David, O., Martinez-Matos, J. A., Bravo, O., Bachs, I., Volpini, V., Gasparini, P., Avraham, K. B., Ferrer, I., Arbones, M. L., and Estivill, X. (2001). Connexin 31 (GJB3) is expressed in the peripheral and auditory nerves and causes neuropathy and hearing impairment. *Hum. Mol. Genet.* **10,** 947–952.

Lupski, J. R. (2000). Recessive Charcot-Marie-Tooth disease. *Ann. Neurol.* **47,** 6–8.

Lupski, J. R., and Garcia, C. A. (2001). Charcot-Marie-Tooth peripheral neuropathies and related disorders. *In* "The Metabolic & Molecular Basis of Inherited Disease" vol.4 (C. R. Scriver, A. L. Beaudet, W. S. Sly, D. Valle, B. Childs, and K. W. Kinzler, eds.), 5759–5788. McGraw-Hill, New York.

Lupski, J. R., Montes de Oca-Luna, R., Slaugenhaupt, S., Pentao, L., Guzzetta, V., Trask, B. J., Saucedo-Cardenas, O., Barker, D. F., Chakravarti, A., and Patel, P. I. (1991). DNA duplication associated with Charcot-Marie-Tooth disease type IA. *Cell* **66,** 219–232.

Lynch, D. R., Hara, H., Yum, S., Chance, P. J., Scherer, S. S., Bird, S. J., and Fischbeck, K. H. (1997). Autosomal dominant transmission of Dejerine-Sottas disease (HMSN III). *Neurology* **49,** 601–603.

Madrid, R., Bradley, W. G., and Davis, D. J. F. (1977). The peroneal muscular atrophy syndrome—clinical, genetic, electrophysiological and nerve biopsy studies. 2. Observations on pathological changes in sural nerve biopsies. *J. Neurol. Sci.* **32,** 91–122.

Magyar, J. P., Martini, R., Ruelicke, T., Aguzzi, A., Adlkofer, K., Dembic, Z., Zielasek, J., Toyka, K. V., and Suter, U. (1996). Impaired differentiation of Schwann cells in transgenic mice with increased *PMP22* gene dosage. *J. Neurosci.* **16,** 5351–5360.

Mandich, P., Mancardi, G. L., Varese, A., Soriani, S., DiMaria, E., Bellone, E., Bado, M., Gross, L., Windebank, A. J., Ajmar, F., and Schenone, A. (1999). Congenital hypomyelination due to myelin protein zero Q215X mutation. *Ann. Neurol.* **45,** 676–678.

Manfioletti, G., Ruaro, M. E., Del Sal, G., Philipson, L., and Schneider, C. (1990). A growth arrest-specific (*gas*) gene codes for a membrane protein. *Mol. Cell. Biol.* **10,** 2914–2930.

Marks, H. G., Scavina, M. T., Kolodny, E. H., Palmieri, M., and Childs, J. (1997). Krabbe's disease presenting as a peripheral neuropathy. *Muscle Nerve* **20,** 1024–1028.

Marques, W., Sweeney, M. G., Wood, N. W., and Wroe, S. J. (1999). Central nervous system involvement in a novel connexin 32 mutation affecting identical twins. *J. Neurol. Neurosurg. Psychiat.* **66,** 803–804.

Marrosu, M. G., Vaccargiu, S., Marrosu, G., Vannelli, A., Cianchetti, C., and Muntoni, F. (1998). Charcot-Marie-Tooth disease type 2 associated with mutation of the myelin protein zero gene. *Neurology* **50,** 1397–1401.

Martini, R. (1997). Animal models for inherited peripheral neuropathies. *J. Anat.* **191,** 321–336.

Martini, R., Mohajeri, M. H., Kasper, S., Giese, K. P., and Schachner, M. (1995a). Mice doubly deficient in the genes for P0 and myelin basic protein show that both proteins contribute to the formation of the major dense line in peripheral nerve myelin. *J. Neurosci.* **15,** 4488–4495.

Martini, R., Zielasek, J., Toyka, K. V., Giese, K. P., and Schachner, M. (1995b). Protein zero (P0)-deficient mice show myelin degeneration in peripheral nerves characteristic of inherited human neuropathies. *Nat. Genet.* **11,** 281–285.

Matsunami, N., Smith, B., Ballard, L., Lensch, M. W., Robertson, M., Albertsen, H., Hanemann, C. O., Muller, H. W., Bird, T. D., White, R., and Chance, P. F. (1992). Peripheral myelin protein-22 gene maps in the duplication in chromosome-17p11.2 associated with Charcot-Marie-Tooth-1A. *Nat. Genet.* **1,** 176–179.

Matsuyama, W., Nakagawa, M., Takashima, H., and Osame, M. (2002). Altered trafficking and adhesion function of MPZ mutations and phenotypes of Charcot-Marie-Tooth disease 1B. *Acta Neuropathol.* **103,** 501–508.

Maurer, M., Kobsar, I., Berghoff, M., Schmid, C. D., Carenini, S., and Martini, R. (2002). Role of immune cells in animal models for inherited neuropathies: Facts and visions. *J. Anat.* **200,** 405–414.

McEntagart, M., Norton, N., Williams, H., Teare, M. D., Dunstan, M., Baker, P., Houlden, H., Reilly, M., Wood, N., Harper, P. S., Futreal, P. A., Williams, N., and Rahman, N. (2001). Localization of the gene for distal hereditary motor neuronopathy VII (DHMN-VII) to chromosome 2q14. *Amer. J. Hum. Genet.* **68,** 1270–1276.

Mendell, J. R., Sahenk, Z., Whitaker, J. N., Trapp, B. D., Yates, A. J., Griggs, R. C., and Quarles, R. H. (1985). Polyneuropathy and IgM monoclonal gammopathy: Studies on the pathogenetic role of anti-myelin-associated glycoprotein antibody. *Ann. Neurol.* **17,** 243–254.

Menichella, D. M., Goodenough, D. A., Sirkowski, E., Scherer, S. S., Paul, D. L., (2003). Connexins are critical for normal myelination in the central nervous system. *J. Neurosci.* **23**, 5963–5973.

Meretoja, P., Silander, K., Kamino, H., Aula, P., Meretoja, A., and Savontaus, M.-L. (1997). Epidemiology of herediatry neuropathy with liability to pressure palises (HNPP) in southwestern Finland. *Neuromusc. Disord.* **7,** 529–532.

Mersiyanova, I. V., Ismailov, S. M., Polyakov, A. V., Dadali, E. L., Fedotov, V. P., Nelis, E., Lofgren, A., Timmerman, V., Van Broeckhoven, C., and Evgrafov, O. V. (2000a). Screening for mutations in the peripheral myelin genes PMP22, MPZ and Cx32 (GJB1) in Russian Charcot-Marie-Tooth neuropathy patients. *Hum. Mutat.* **15,** 340–347.

Mersiyanova, I. V., Perepelov, A. V., Polyakov, A. V., Sitnikov, V. F., Dadali, E. L., Oparin, R. B., Petrin, A. N., and Evgrafov, O. V. (2000b). A new variant of Charcot-Marie-Tooth disease type 2 is probably the result of a mutation in the neurofilament-light gene. *Amer. J. Hum. Genet.* **67,** 37–46.

Mihalik, S. J., Morrell, J. C. D., Sacksteder, K. A., Watkins, P. A., and Gould, S. J. (1997). Identification of PAHX, a Refsum disease gene. *Nat. Genet.* **17,** 185–189.

Misko, A., Ferguson, T., and Notterpek, L. (2002). Matrix metalloproteinase mediated degradation of basement membrane proteins in Trembler J neuropathy nerves. *J. Neurochem.* **83,** 885–894.

Misu, K., Yoshihara, T., Shikama, Y., Awaki, E., Yamamoto, M., Hattori, N., Hirayama, M., Takegami, T., Nakashima, K., and Sobue, G. (2000). An axonal form of Charcot-Marie-Tooth disease showing distinctive features in association with mutations in the peripheral myelin protein zero gene (Thr124Met or Asp75Val). *J. Neurol. Neurosurg. Psychiat.* **69,** 806–811.

Mok, H., Shin, H., Kim, S., Lee, J. R., Yoon, J., and Kim, E. (2002). Association of the kinesin superfamily motor protein KIF1Balpha with postsynaptic density-95 (PSD-95), synapse-associated protein-97, and synaptic scaffolding molecule PSD-95/discs large/zona occludens-1 proteins. *J. Neurosci.* **22,** 5253–5258.

Montag, D., Giese, K. P., Bartsch, U., Martini, R., Lang, Y., Bluthmann, H., Karthigasan, J., Kirschner, D. A., Wintergerst, E. S., Nave, K.-A., Zielasek, J., Toyka, K. V., Lipp, H.-P., and Schachner, M. (1994). Mice deficient for the myelin-associated glycoprotein show subtle abnormalities in myelin. *Neuron* **13,** 229–246.

Mori, K. (2000). Tripartite management of unfolded proteins in the endoplasmic reticulum. *Cell* **101,** 451–454.

Moriwaki, Y., Begum, N. A., Kobayashi, M., Matsumoto, M., Toyoshima, K., and Seya, T. (2001). *Mycobacterium bovis* bacillus Calmette-Guerin and its cell wall complex induce a novel lysosomal membrane protein, SIMPLE, that bridges the missing link between lipopolysaccharide and p53-inducible gene, LITAF (PIG7) and estrogen-inducible gene, EET-1. *J. Biol. Chem.* **276,** 23065–23076.

Morocutti, C., Colazza, G. B., Soldati, G., DAlessio, C., Damiano, M., Casali, C., and Pierelli, F. (2002). Charcot-Marie-Tooth disease in Molise, a central-southern region of Italy: An epidemiological study. *Neuroepidemiology* **21,** 241–245.

Mostacciuolo, M. L., Righetti, E., Zortea, M., Bosello, V., Schiavon, F., Vallo, L., Merlini, L., Siciliano, G., Fabrizi, G. M., Rizzuto, N., Milani, M., Baratta, S., and Taroni, F. (2001). Charcot-Marie-Tooth disease type I and related demyelinating neuropathies: Mutation analysis in a large cohort of Italian families. *Hum. Mutat.* **18,** 32–41.

Mouton, P., Tardieu, S., Gouider, R., Birouk, N., Maisonobe, T., Dubourg, O., Brice, A., Le Guern, E., and Bouche, P. (1999). Spectrum of clinical and electrophysiological features in HNPP patients with the 17p11.2 deletion. *Neurology* **52,** 1440–1446.

Murphy, P., Topilko, P., Schneider-Maunoury, S., Seitanidou, T., Baron-Van Evercooren, A., and Charnay, P. (1996). The regulation of *Krox*-20 expression reveals important steps in the control of peripheral glial cell development. *Development* **122,** 2847–2857.

Musso, M., Balestra, P., Bellone, E., Cassandrini, D., Di Maria, E., Doria, L. L., Grandis, M., Mancardi, G., Schenone, A., Levi, G., Ajmar, F., and Mandar, P. (2001). The D355V mutation decreases EGR2 binding to an element within the Cx32 promoter. *Neurobiol. Dis.* **8,** 700–706.

Naef, R., Adlkofer, K., Lescher, B., and Suter, U. (1997). Aberrant protein trafficking in *Trembler* suggests a disease mechanism for hereditary human peripheral neuropathies. *Mol. Cell. Neurosci.* **9,** 13–25.

Naef, R., and Suter, U. (1999). Impaired intracellular trafficking is a common disease mechanism of PMP22 point mutations in peripheral neuropathies. *Neurobiol. Dis.* **6,** 1–14.

Nagaoka, T., Oyamada, M., Okajima, S., and Takamatsu, T. (1999). Differential expression of gap junction proteins connexin26, 32, and 43 in normal and crush-injured rat sciatic nerves: Close relationship between connexin43 and occludin in the perineurium. *J. Histochem. Cytochem.* **47,** 937–948.

Nagarajan, R., Le, N., Mahoney, H., Araki, T., and Milbrandt, J. (2002). Deciphering peripheral nerve myelination by using Schwann cell expression profiling. *Proc Nat Acad Sci USA* **99,** 8998–9003.

Nagarajan, R., Svaren, J., Le, N., Araki, T., Watson, M., and Milbrandt, J. (2001). EGR2 mutations in inherited neuropathies dominant-negatively inhibit myelin gene expression. *Neuron* **30,** 355–368.

Nakagawa, M., Takashima, H., Umehara, F., Arimura, K., Miyashita, F., Takenouchi, N., Matsuyama, W., and Osame, M. (2001). Clinical phentoype in X-linked Charcot-Marie-Tooth disease with an entire deletion of the connexin 32 coding sequence. *J. Neurol. Sci.* **185,** 31–36.

Nave, K.-A. (2001). Myelin-specific genes and their mutations in the mouse. *In* "Glial Cell Development" (K. R. Jessen and W. D. Richardson, eds.), 177–208. Oxford University Press, Oxford.

Nelis, E., Erdem, S., Tan, E., Lofgren, A., Ceuterick, C., De Jonghe, P., Van Broeckhoven, C., Timmerman, V., and Topaloglu, H. (2002a). A novel homozygous missense mutation in the myotubularin-related protein 2 gene associated with recessive Charcot-Marie-Tooth disease with irregularly folded myelin sheaths. *Neuromuscul Disord* **12,** 869–873.

Nelis, E., Erdem, S., Van den Bergh, P. Y. K., Belpaire-Dethiou, M.-C., Ceuterick, C., Van Gerwen, V., Cuesta, A., Pedrola, L., Palau, F., Gabreels-Festen, A. A. W. M., Verellen, C., Tan, E., Demirci, M., Van Broeckhoven, C., De Jonghe, P., Topaloglu, H., and Timmerman, V. (2002b). Mutations in GDAP1. Autosomal recessive CMT with demyelination and axonopathy. *Neurology* **59,** 1865–1872.

Nelis, E., Haites, N., and Van Broeckhoven, C. (1999). Mutations in the peripheral myelin genes and associated genes in inherited peripheral neuropathies. *Hum. Mutat.* **13,** 11–28.

Nelis, E., Holmberg, B., Adolfsson, R., Holmgren, G., and VanBroeckhoven, C. (1997). PMP22 Thr(118)Met: Recessive CMT1 mutation or polymorphism? *Nat. Genet.* **15,** 13–14.

Nelis, E., Van Broeckhoven, C., and co-authors (1996). Estimation of the mutation frequencies in Charcot-Marie-Tooth disease type 1 and hereditary neuropathy with liability to pressure palsies: A European collaborative study. *Eur. J. Human Genet.* **4,** 25–33.

Nelson, J. W., and Amick, L. D. (1966). Heredofamilial progressive spinal muscular atrophy: A clinical and electromyographic study of a kinship. *Neurology* **16,** 306.

Nicholson, G., and Nash, J. (1993). Intermediate nerve conduction velocities define X-linked Charcot-Marie-Tooth neuropathy families. *Neurology* **43,** 2558–2564.

Nicholson, G., Valentijn, L. J., Cherryson, A. K., Kennerson, M. L., Bragg, T. L., DeKroon, R. M., Ross, D. A., Pollard, J. D., McLeod, J. G., Bolhuis, P. A., and Baas, F. (1994). A frame shift mutation in the PMP22 gene in hereditary neuropathy with liability to pressure palsies. *Nat. Genet.* **6,** 263–266.

Nicholson, G. A., Yeung, L., and Corbett, A. (1998). Efficient neurophysiological selection of X-linked Charcot-Marie-Tooth families. *Neurology* **51,** 1412–1416.

Niemann, S., Sereda, M. W., Suter, U., Griffiths, I. R., and Nave, K. A. (2000). Uncoupling of myelin assembly and Schwann cell differentiation by transgenic overexpression of peripheral myelin protein 22. *J. Neurosci.* **20,** 4120–4128.

Nishimura, T., Yoshikawa, H., Fujimura, H., Sakoda, S., and Yanagihara, T. (1996). Accumulation of peripheral myelin protein 22 in onion bulbs and Schwann cells of biopsied nerves from patients with Charcot-Marie-Tooth disease type 1A. *Acta Neuropathol.* **92,** 454–460.

Nobbio, L., Mancardi, G., Grandis, M., Levi, G., Surer, U., Nave, K. A., Windebank, A. J., Abbruzzese, M., and Schenone, A. (2001). PMP22 transgenic dorsal root ganglia cultures show myelin abnormalities similar to those of human CMT1A. *Ann. Neurol.* **50,** 47–55.

Notterpek, L., Ryan, M. C., Tobler, A. R., and Shooter, E. M. (1999a). PMP22 accumulation in aggresomes: Implications for CMT1A pathology. *Neurobiol. Dis.* **6,** 450–460.

Notterpek, L., Shooter, E. M., and Snipes, G. J. (1997). Upregulation of the endosomal-lysosomal pathway in the *Trembler-J* neuropathy. *J. Neurosci.* **17,** 4190–4200.

Notterpek, L., Snipes, G. J., and Shooter, E. M. (1999b). Temporal expression pattern of peripheral myelin protein 22 during in vivo and in vitro myelination. *Glia* **25,** 358–369.

Numakura, C., Lin, C. Q., Ikegami, T., Guldberg, P., and Hayasaka, K. (2002). Molecular analysis in Japanese patients with Charcot-Marie-Tooth disease: DGGE analysis for PMP22, MPZ, and Cx32/GJB1 mutations. *Hum. Mut.* **20,** 392–398.

Numakura, C., Lin, C. Q., Oka, N., Akiguchi, I., and Hayasaka, K. (2000). Hemizygous mutation of the peripheral myelin protein 22 gene associated with Charcot-Marie-Tooth disease type 1. *Ann. Neurol.* **47,** 101–103.

Odermatt, B., Wellershaus, K., Wallraff, A., Seifert, G., Degen, G., Euwens, C., Fuss, B., Bussow, H., Schilling, K., Stenhauser, C., Willecke, K. (2003). Connexin 47 (Cx47)-deficient mice with enhanced green fluorescent protein reporter gene reveal predominant oligodendrocytic expression of Cx47 and display vacuolized myelin in the CNS. *J. Neurosci.* **23,** 4549–4559.

Oh, S., Ri, Y., Bennett, M. V. L., Trexler, E. B., Verselis, V. K., and Bargiello, T. A. (1997). Changes in permeability caused by connexin 32 mutations underlie X-linked Charcot-Marie-Tooth disease. *Neuron* **19,** 927–938.

Ohara, O., Gahara, Y., Miyake, T., Teraoka, H., and Kitamura, T. (1993). Neurofilament deficiency in quail caused by nonsense mutation in neurofilament-L gene. *J. Cell Biol.* **121,** 387–395.

Ohta, M., Ellefson, R. D., Lambert, E. H., and Dyck, P. J. (1973). Hereditary sensory neuropathy, type II. Clinical, electrophysiologic, histologic, and biochemical studies of a Quebec kinship. *Arch. Neurol.* **29,** 23–37.

Omori, Y., Mesnil, M., and Yamasaki, H. (1996). Connexin 32 mutations from X-linked Charcot-Marie-Tooth disease patients: Functional defects and dominant negative effects. *Mol. Biol. Cell* **7,** 907–916.

Ouvrier, R. (1996). Correlation between the histopathologic, genotypic, and phenotypic features of hereditary peripheral neuropathies in childhood. *J. Child Neurol.* **11,** 133–146.

Ouvrier, R. A., McLeod, J. G., and Conchin, T. E. (1987). The hypertrophic forms of hereditary motor and sensory neuropathy. A study of hypertrophic Charcot-Marie-Tooth disease (HMSN type I) and Dejerine-Sottas disease (HMSN type III) in childhood. *Brain* **110,** 121–148.

Ouvrier, R. A., McLeod, J. G., Morgan, G. J., Wise, G. A., and Conchin, T. E. (1981). Hereditary motor and sensory neuropathy of neuronal type with onset in early childhood. *J. Neurol. Sci.* **51,** 181–197.

Ouvrier, R. A., McLeod, J. G., and Pollard, J. D. (1990). "Peripheral Neuropathy in Childhood." Raven Press, New York.

Palumbo, C., Massa, R., Panico, M. B., DiMuzio, A., Sinibaldi, P., Bernardi, G., and Modesti, A. (2002). Peripheral nerve extracellular matrix remodeling in Charcot-Marie-Tooth type 1 disease. *Acta Neuropathol.* **104,** 287–296.

Panas, M., Karadimas, C., Avramopoulos, D., and Vassilopoulos, D. (1998). Central nervous system involvement in four patients with Charcot-Marie-Tooth disease with connexin 32 extracellular mutations. *J. Neurol. Neurosurg. Psychiat.* **65,** 947–948.

Paratore, C., Goerich, D. E., Suter, U., Wegner, M., and Sommer, L. (2001). Survival and glial fate acquisition of neural crest cells are regulated by an interplay between the transcription factor Sox10 and extrinsic combinatorial signaling. *Development* **128,** 3949–3961.

Pareek, S., Notterpek, L., Snipes, G. J., Naef, R., Sossin, W., Laliberte, J., Iacampo, S., Suter, U., Shooter, E. M., and Murphy, R. A. (1997). Neurons promote the translocation of peripheral myelin protein 22 into myelin. *J. Neurosci.* **17,** 7754–7762.

Pareek, S., Suter, U., Snipes, G. J., Welcher, A. A., Shooter, E. M., and Murphy, R. A. (1993). Detection and processing of peripheral myelin protein PMP22 in cultured Schwann cells. *J. Biol. Chem.* **268,** 10372–10379.

Pareyson, D., Scaioli, V., Taroni, F., Botti, S., Lorenzetti, D., Solari, A., Ciano, C., and Sghirlanzoni, A. (1996). Phenotypic heterogeneity in hereditary neuropathy with liability to pressure palsies associated with chromosome 17p11.2–12 deletion. *Neurology* **46,** 1133–1137.

Parman, Y., Plante-Bordeneuve, V., Guiochon-Mantel, A., Eraksoy, M., and Said, G. (1999). Recessive inheritance of a new point mutation of the PMP22 gene in Dejerine-Sottas disease. *Ann. Neurol.* **45,** 518–522.

Parmantier, E., Cabon, F., Braun, C., Durso, D., Müller, H. W., and Zalc, B. (1995). Peripheral myelin protein-22 is expressed in rat and mouse brain and spinal cord motoneurons. *Eur. J. Neurosci.* **7,** 1080–1088.

Patel, P. I., Roa, B. B., Welcher, A. A., Schoenerscott, R., Trask, B. J., Pentao, L., Snipes, G. J., Garcia, C. A., Francke, U., Shooter, E. M., Lupski, J. R., and Suter, U. (1992). The gene for the peripheral myelin protein-PMP-22 is a candidate for Charcot-Marie-Tooth disease type-1A. *Nat. Genet.* **1,** 159–165.

Paulson, H., Garbern, J. Y., Hoban, T. F., Krajewski, K. M., Lewis, R. A., Fischbeck, K. H., Grossman, R. I., Lenkiski, R., Kamholz, J. A., and Shy, M. E. (2002). Transient CNS white matter abnormality in X-linked Charcot-Marie-Tooth disease. *Ann. Neurol.* **52,** 429–434.

Peirano, R. I., Goerich, D. E., Riethmacher, D., and Wegner, M. (2000). Protein zero gene expression is regulated by the glial transcription factor Sox10. *Mol. Cell. Biol.* **20,** 3198–3209.

Perez-Olle, R., Leung, C. L., and Liem, R. K. H. (2002). Effects of Charcot-Marie-Tooth-linked mutations of the neurofilament light subunit on intermediate filament formation. *J. Cell Sci.* **115,** 4937–4946.

Perkins, C. S., Aguayo, A. J., and Bray, G. M. (1981). Schwann cell multiplication in trembler mice. *Neuropathol. Appl. Neurobiol.* **7,** 115–126.

Petiot, A., Ogier-Denis, E., Blommaart, E. F., Meijer, A. J., and Codogno, P. (2000). Distinct classes of phosphatidylinositol 3′-kinases are involved in signaling pathways that control macroautophagy in HT-29 cells. *J. Biol. Chem.* **275,** 992–998.

Phillips, J. P., Warner, L. E., Lupski, J. R., and Garg, B. P. (1999). Congenital hypomyelinating neuropathy: Two patients with long-term follow-up. *Pediat. Neurol.* **20,** 226–232.

Pingault, V., Bondurand, N., LeCaignec, C., Tardieu, S., Lemort, N., Dubourg, O., Le Guern, E., Goossens, M., and Boespflug-Tanguy, O. (2001). The SOX10 transcription factor: Evaluation as a candidate gene for central and peripheral hereditary myelin disorders. *J. Neurol.* **248,** 496–499.

Pingault, V., Guiochon-Mantel, A., Bondurand, N., Faure, C., Lacroix, C., Lyonnet, S., Goosens, M., and Landrieu, P. (2000). Peripheral neuropathy with hypomyelination, chronic intestinal pseudo-obstruction and deafness: A developmental neural crest syndrome related to a SOX10 mutation. *Ann. Neurol.* **48,** 671–676.

Plante-Bordeneuve, V., and Said, G. (2002). Dejerine-Sottas disease and hereditary demyelinating neuropathy of infancy. *Muscle Nerve* **26,** 608–621.

Previtali, S. C., Quattrini, A., Fasolini, M., Panzeri, M. C., Villa, A., Filbin, M. T., Li, W. H., Chiu, S. Y., Messing, A., Wrabetz, L., and Feltri, M. L. (2000). Epitope-tagged $P_0$ glycoprotein causes Charcot-Marie-Tooth-like neuropathy in transgenic mice. *J. Cell Biol.* **151,** 1035–1045.

Quattrone, A., Gambardella, A., Bono, F., Aguglia, U., Bolino, A., Bruni, A. C., Montesi, M. P., Oliveri, R. L., Sabatelli, M., Tamburrini, O., Valentino, P., Van Broeckhoven, C., and Zappia, M. (1996). Autosomal recessive hereditary motor and sensory neuropathy with focally folded myelin sheaths: Clinical, electrophysiologic, and genetic aspects of a large family. *Neurology* **46,** 1318–1324.

Raeymaekers, P., Timmerman, V., Nelis, E., De Jonghe, P., Hoogendijk, J., Baas, F., Barker, D. F., Martin, J. J., De Visser, M., Bolhius, P. A., and Van Broeckhoven, C. (1991). Duplication in chromosome 17p11.2 in Charcot-Marie-Tooth neuropathy type 1a (CMT1a). *Neuromusc. Disord.* **1,** 93–97.

Tachi, N., Kozuka, N., Ohya, K., Chiba, S., and Sasaki, K. (1997). Tomaculous neuropathy in Charcot-Marie-Tooth disease with myelin protein zero gene mutation. *J. Neurol. Sci.* **153,** 106–109.

Takashima, H., Boerkoel, D. F., De Jonghe, P., Ceuterick, C., Martin, J.-J., Voit, T., Schroder, J.-M., Williams, A., Brophy, P. J., Timmerman, V., and Lupski, J. R. (2002). Periaxin mutations cause a broad spectrum of demyelinating neuropathies. *Ann. Neurol.* **51,** 709–715.

Takashima, H., Nakagawa, M., Nakahara, K., Suehara, M., Matsuzaki, T., Higuchi, I., Higa, H., Arimura, K., Iwamasa, T., Izumo, S., and Osame, M. (1997). A new type of hereditary motor and sensory neuropathy linked to chromosome 3. *Ann. Neurol.* **41,** 771–780.

Takashima, H., Nakagawa, M., Suehara, M., Saito, M., Saito, A., Kanzato, N., Matsuzaki, T., Hirata, K., Terwilliger, J. D., and Osame, M. (1999). Gene for hereditary motor and sensory neuropathy (Proximal dominant form) mapped to 3q13.1. *Neuromuscular Disord.* **9,** 368–371.

Thomas, F. P., Lebo, R. V., Rosoklija, G., Ding, X. S., Lovelace, R. E., Latov, N., and Hays, A. P. (1994). Tomaculous neuropathy in chromosome 1 Charcot-Marie-Tooth syndrome. *Acta Neuropathol.* **87,** 91–97.

Thomas, P. K., Marques, W., Davis, M. B., Sweeney, M. G., King, R. H. M., Bradley, J. L., Muddle, J. R., Tyson, J., Malcolm, S., and Harding, A. E. (1997). The phenotypic manifestations of chromosome 17p11.2 duplication. *Brain* **120,** 465–478.

Timmerman, V., De Jonghe, P., Spoelders, P., Simokovic, S., Lofgren, A., Nelis, E., Vance, J., Martin, J.-J., and Van Broeckhoven, C. (1996). Linkage and mutation analysis of Charcot-Marie-Tooth neuropathy type 2 families with chromosomes 1p35-p36 and Xq13. *Neurology* **46,** 1311–1318.

Timmerman, V., Nelis, E., Vanhul, W., Nieuwenhuijsen, B. W., Chen, K. L., Wang, S., Othman, K. B., Cullen, B., Leach, R. J., Hanemann, C. O., De Jonghe, P., Raeymaekers, P., van Ommen, G.-J. B., Martin, J.-J., Müller, H. W., Vance, J. M., Fischbeck, K. H., and Van Broeckhoven, C. (1992). The peripheral myelin protein gene PMP-22 is contained within the Charcot-Marie-Tooth disease Type-1A duplication. *Nat. Genet.* **1,** 171–175.

Tobler, A. R., Liu, N., Mueller, L., and Shooter, E. M. (2002). Differential aggregation of the Trembler and TremblerJ mutants of peripheral myelin protein 22. *Proc. Natl. Acad Sci. USA* **99,** 483–488.

Tobler, A. R., Notterpek, L., Naef, R., Taylor, V., Suter, U., and Shooter, E. M. (1999). Transport of *Trembler-J* mutant peripheral myelin protein 22 is blocked in the intermediate compartment and affects the transport of the wild-type protein by direct interaction. *J. Neurosci.* **19,** 2027–2036.

Topilko, P., Schneider-Maunoury, S., Levi, G., Baron-Van Evercooren, A., Ben Younes Chennoufi, A., Seitanidou, T., Babinet, C., and Charnay, P. (1994). Krox-20 controls myelination in the peripheral nervous system. *Nature* **371,** 796–799.

Touraine, R. L., Attie-Bitach, T., Manceau, E., Korsch, E., Sarda, P., Pingault, V., EnchaRazavi, F., Pelet, A., Auge, J., Nivelon-Chevallier, A., Holschneider, A. M., Munnes, M., Doerfler, W., Goossens, M., Munnich, A., Vekemans, M., and Lyonnet, S. (2000). Neurological phenotype in Waardenburg syndrome type 4 correlates with novel SOX10 truncating mutations and expression in developing brain. *Amer. J. Hum. Genet.* **66,** 1496–1503.

Trachtenberg, J. T., and Thompson, W. J. (1996). Schwann cell apoptosis and its regulation at the developing neuromuscular junction. *Nature* **379,** 174–177.

Tsai, B., Ye, Y., and Rapoport, T. A. (2002). Retro-translocation of proteins from the endoplasmic reticulum into the cytosol. *Nat. Rev. Mol. Cell. Biol.* **3,** 246–255.

Tyson, J., Malcolm, S., Thomas, P. K., and Harding, A. E. (1996). Deletions of chromosome 17p11.2 in multifocal neuropathies. *Ann. Neurol.* **39,** 180–186.

Valentijn, L. J., Baas, F., Wolterman, R. A., Hoogendijk, J. E., van den Bosch, N. H. A., Zorn, I., Gabreels-Festen, A. W. M., de Visser, M., and Bolhuis, P. A. (1992a). Identical point mutations of PMP-22 in Trembler-J mouse and Charcot-Marie-Tooth disease Type-1A. *Nat. Genet.* **2,** 288–291.

Valentijn, L. J., Bolhuis, P. A., Zorn, I., Hoogendijk, J. E., Vandenbosch, N., Hensels, G. W., Stanton, V. P., Housman, D. E., Fischbeck, K. H., Ross, D. A., Nicholson, G. A., Meershoek, E. J., Dauwerse, H. G., Vanommen, G. J. B., and Baas, F. (1992b). The peripheral myelin gene PMP-22/GAS-3 is duplicated in Charcot-Marie-Tooth disease type-1A. *Nat. Genet.* **1,** 166–170.

Vallat, J. M., Sindou, P., Preux, P. M., Tabaraud, F., Milor, A. M., Couratier, P., Le Guern, E., and Brice, A. (1996). Ultrastructural PMP22 expression in inherited demyelinating neuropathies. *Ann. Neurol.* **39,** 813–817.

van den Brink, D. M., Brites, P., Haasjes, J., Wierzbicki, A. S., Mitchell, J., Lambert-Hamill, M., de Belleroche, J., Jansen, G. A., Waterham, H. R., and Wanders, R. J. A. (2003). Identification of *PEX7* as the second gene involved in Refsum disease. *Amer. J. Hum. Genet.* **72,** 471–477.

VanSlyke, J. K., Deschênes, S. M., and Musil, L. S. (2000). Intracellular transport, assembly, and degradation of wild-type and disease-linked mutant gap junction proteins. *Mol. Biol. Cell.* **11,** 1933–1946.

VanSlyke, J. K., and Musil, L. S. (2002). Dislocation and degradation from the ER are regulated by cytosolic stress. *J. Cell Biol.* **157,** 381–394.

Vedanarayanan, V. V., Smith, S., Subramony, S. H., Bock, G. O., and Evans, O. B. (1998). Lethal neonatal autosomal recessive axonal sensorimotor polyneuropathy. *Muscle Nerve* **21,** 1473–1477.

Verhoeven, K., De Jonghe, P., Coen, K., Verpoorten, N., Auer-Grumbach, M., Kwon, J. M., FitzPatrick, D., Schmedding, E., De Vriendt, E., Jacobs, A., Van Gerwen, V., Wagner, K., Hartung, H.-P., and Timmerman, V. (2003). Mutations in the small GTP-ase late endosomal protein RAB7 cause Charcot-Marie-Tooth disease type 2B neuropathy. *Amer. J. Hum. Genet.* **72,.**

Verhoeven, K., Villanova, M., Rossi, A., Malandrini, A., DeJonghe, P., and Timmerman, V. (2001). Localization of the gene for the intermediate form of Charcot-Marie-Tooth to chromosome 10q24.1-q25.1. *Amer J Hum Genet* **69,** 889–894.

Villanova, M., Timmerman, V., De Jonghe, P., Malandrini, A., Rizzuto, N., Van Broeckhoven, C., Guazzi, G. C., and Rossi, A. (1998). Charcot-Marie-Tooth disease: An intermediate form. *Neuromuscular Disord.* **8,** 392–393.

Vital, A., Ferrer, X., Lagueny, A., Vandenberghe, A., Latour, P., Goizet, C., Canron, M. H., Louiset, P., Petry, K. G., and Vital, C. (2001). Histopathological features of X-linked Charcot-Marie-Tooth disease in 8 patients from 6 families with different connexin32 mutations. *J. Peripher. Nerv. Syst.* **6,** 79–84.

von Figura, K., Gieselmann, V., and Jaeken, J. (2001). Metachromatic leukodystrophy. *In* "The Metabolic & Molecular Basis of Inherited Disease," vol.3 (C. R. Scriver, A. L. Beaudet, W. S. Sly, D. Valle, B. Childs, and K. W. Kinzler, eds.), 3695–3724. McGraw-Hill, New York.

Warner, L. E., Hilz, M. J., Appel, S. H., Killian, J. M., Watters, G. V., Wheeler, C., Witt, D., Bodell, A., Nelis, E., Van Broeckhoven, C., and Lupski, J. R. (1996). Clinical phenotypes of different MPZ ($P_0$) mutations may include Charcot-Marie-Tooth type 1B, Dejerine-Sottas, and congenital hypomyelination. *Neuron* **17,** 451–460.

Warner, L. E., Mancias, P., Butler, I. J., McDonald, C. M., Keppen, L., Koob, K. G., and Lupski, J. R. (1998). Mutations in the early growth response 2 (EGR2) gene are associated with hereditary myelinopathies. *Nat. Genet.* **18,** 382–384.

Warner, L. E., Svaren, J., Milbrandt, J., and Lupski, J. R. (1999). Functional consequences of mutations in the early growth response 2 gene (EGR2) correlate with severity of human myelinopathies. *Hum. Mol. Genet.* **8,** 1245–1251.

Weinberg, H. J., and Spencer, P. S. (1978). The fate of Schwann cells isolated from axonal contact. *J. Neurocytol.* **7,** 555–569.

Welcher, A. A., Suter, U., DeLeon, M., Snipes, G. J., and Shooter, E. M. (1991). A myelin protein is encoded by the homologue of a growth arrest-specific gene. *Proc. Natl. Acad. Sci. USA* **88,** 7195–7199.

Wenger, D. A., Suzuki, K., Suzuki, Y., and Suzuki, K. (2001). Galactosyl ceramide lipidosis: Globoid cell leukodystrophy (Krabbe disease). *In* "The Metabolic & Molecular Basis of Inherited Disease" vol.3 (C. R. Scriver, A. L. Beaudet, W. S. Sly, D. Valle, B. Childs, and K. W. Kinzler, eds.), 3669–3694. McGraw-Hill, New York.

White, T. W., and Paul, D. L. (1999). Genetic diseases and gene knockouts reveal diverse connexin functions. *Annu. Rev. Physiol.* **61,** 283–310.

Wilmshurst, J. M., Bye, A., Rittey, C., Adams, C., Hahn, A. F., Ramsay, D., Pamphlett, R., Pollard, J. D., and Ouvrier, R. (2001). Severe infantile axonal neuropathy with respiratory failure. *Muscle Nerve* **24,** 760–768.

Windebank, T. (1993). Inherited recurrent focal neuropathies. *In* "Peripheral Neuropathy" vol.2 (P. J. Dyck, P. K. Thomas, J. W. Griffin, P. A. Low, and J. F. Poduslo, eds.), 1137–1148. W. B. Saunders, Philadelphia.

Wise, C. A., Garcia, C. A., Davis, S. N., Zhang, H. J., Liu, P. T., Patel, P. I., and Lupski, J. R. (1993). Molecular analyses of unrelated Charcot-Marie-Tooth (CMT) disease patients suggest a high frequency of the CMTIA duplication. *Amer. J. Hum. Genet.* **53,** 853–863.

Wishart, M. J., and Dixon, J. E. (2002). PTEN and myotubularin phosphatases: From 3-phosphoinositide dephosphorylation to disease. Phosphatase and tensin homolog deleted on chromosome ten. *Trends Cell Biol.* **12,** 579–585.

Wong, M. H., and Filbin, M. T. (1996). Dominant-negative effect on adhesion by myelin $P_0$ protein truncated in its cytoplasmic domain. *J. Cell Biol.* **134,** 1531–1541.

Wrabetz, L., D'Antonio, M., Dati, G., Fratta, P., Previtali, S., Imperiale, D., Zielasek, J., Toyka, K., Messing, A., Feltri, M.-L., and Quattrini, A. (2002). Transgenic mice expressing the CMT1B mutant *Mpz*(delser63) develop demyelinating neuropathy. *2002 Abstract Viewer/Itinerary Planner. Washington, DC: Society for Neuroscience* **(Online),** Program No. 523.527.

Wrabetz, L., and Feltri, M. L. (2001). Do Schwann cells stop, Dr(o)P2, and roll? *Neuron* **30,** 642–644.

Wrabetz, L., Feltri, M. L., Hanemann, C. O., and Müller, H. W. (2001). The molecular genetics of hereditary demyelinating neuropathies. *In* "Glial Cell Development" (K. R. Jessen and W. D. Richardson, eds.), 331–354. Oxford University Press, Oxford.

Wrabetz, L., Feltri, M. L., Quattrini, A., Imperiale, D., Previtali, S., DAntonio, M., Martini, R., Yin, X. H., Trapp, B. D., Zhou, L., Chiu, S. Y., and Messing, A. (2000). P0 glycoprotein overexpression causes congenital hypomyelination of peripheral nerves. *J Cell Biol* **148,** 1021–1033.

Xu, W. B., Shy, M., Kamholz, J., Elferink, L., Xu, G., Lilien, J., and Balsamo, J. (2001). Mutations in the cytoplasmic domain of P0 reveal a role for PKC-mediated phosphorylation in adhesion and myelination. *J Cell Biol* **155,** 439–445.

Xu, Y., Sladky, J. T., and Brown, M. J. (1989). Dose-dependent expression of neuronopathy after experimental pyridoxine intoxication. *Neurology* **39,** 1077–1083.

Yin, X., Kidd, G. J., Wrabetz, L., Feltri, M. L., Messing, A., and Trapp, B. D. (2000). Schwann cell myelination requires timely and precise targeting of P0 protein. *J. Cell Biol.* **148,** 1009–1020.

Yin, X. H., Crawford, T. O., Griffin, J. W., Tu, P. H., Lee, V. M. Y., Li, C. M., Roder, J., and Trapp, B. D. (1998). Myelin-associated glycoprotein is a myelin signal that modulates the caliber of myelinated axons. *J. Neurosci.* **18,** 1953–1962.

Yoshihara, T., Yamamoto, M., Hattori, N., Misu, K., Mori, K., Koike, H., and Sobue, G. (2002). Identification of novel sequence variants in the neurofilament-light gene in a Japanese population: Analysis of Charcot-Marie-Tooth disease patients and normal individuals. *J. Peripher. Nerv. Syst.* **7,** 221–224.

Yoshikawa, H., and Dyck, P. J. (1991). Uncompacted inner myelin lamellae in inherited tendency to pressure palsy. *J. Neuropathol. Exp. Neurol.* **50,** 649–657.

Yoshikawa, H., Nishimura, T., Nakatsuji, Y., Fujimura, H., Himoro, M., Hayasaka, K., Kakoda, S., and Yanagihara, T. (1994). Elevated expression of messenger RNA for peripheral myelin protein 22 in biopsied peripheral nerves of patients with Charcot-Marie-Tooth disease type 1A. *Ann. Neurol.* **35,** 445–450.

Young, P., Boussadia, O., Berger, P., Leone, D. P., Charnay, P., Kemler, R., and Suter, U. (2002). E-cadherin is required for the correct formation of autotypic adherens junctions of the outer mesaxon but not for the integrity of myelinated fibers of peripheral nerves. *Mol. Cell. Neurosci.* **21,** 341–351.

Young, P., Grote, K., Kuhlenbaumer, G., Debus, O., Kurlemann, H., Halfter, H., Funke, H., Ringelstein, E. B., and Stogbauer, E. (2001). Mutation analysis in Charcot-Marie Tooth disease type 1: Point mutations in the MPZ gene and the GJB1 gene cause comparable phenotypic heterogeneity. *J. Neurol.* **248,** 410–415.

Young, P., Stogbauer, F., Eller, B., deJonghe, P., Lofgren, A., Timmerman, V., Rautenstrauss, B., Oexle, K., Grehl, H., Kuhlenbaumer, G., VanBroeckhoven, C., Ringelstein, E. B., and Funke, H. (2000). PMP22 Thr118Met is not a clinically relevant CMT1 marker. *J. Neurol.* **247,** 696–700.

Young, P., Wiebusch, H., Stogbauer, F., Ringelstein, B., Assmann, G., and Funke, H. (1997). A novel frameshift mutation in PMP22 accounts for hereditary neuropathy with liability to pressure palsies. *Neurology* **48,** 450–452.

Yum, S. W., Kleopa, K. A., Shumas, S., and Scherer, S. S. (2002). Diverse trafficking abnormalities for connexin32 mutants causing CMTX. *Neurobiol. Dis.* **11,** 43–52.

Zhang, K., and Filbin, M. T. (1998). Myelin P0 protein mutated at Cys21 has a dominant-negative effect on adhesion of wild type P0. *J. Neurosci. Res.* **53,** 1–6.

Zhao, C., Takita, J., Tanaka, Y., Setou, M., Nakagawa, T., Takeda, S., Yang, H. W., Terada, S., Nakata, T., Takei, Y., Saito, M., Tsuji, S., Hayashi, Y., and Hirokawa, N. (2001). Charcot-Marie-Tooth disease type 2A caused by mutation in a microtubule motor KIF1Bβ. *Cell* **105,** 587–597.

Zhu, Q., Couillard-Despres, S., and Julien, J. P. (1997). Delayed maturation of regenerating myelinated axons in mice lacking neurofilaments. *Exp. Neurol.* **148,** 299–316.

Zielasek, J., Martini, R., and Toyka, K. V. (1996). Functional abnormalities in $P_0$-deficient mice resemble human hereditary neuropathies linked to $P_0$ gene mutations. *Muscle Nerve* **19,** 946–952.

Zoidl, G., Blass-Kampmann, S., D'Urso, D., Schmalenback, C., and Müller, H. W. (1995). Retroviral-mediated gene transfer of the peripheral myelin protein PMP22 in Schwann cells: Modulation of cell growth. *EMBO J.* **14,** 1122–1128.

Zoidl, G., D'Urso, D., Blass-Kampmann, S., Schmalenbach, C., Kuhn, R., and Muller, H. W. (1997). Influence of elevated expression of rat wild-type PMP22 and its mutant PMP22Trembler on cell growth of NIH3T3 fibroblasts. *Cell Tiss. Res.* **287,** 459–470.

Zorick, T. S., Syroid, D. E., Arroyo, E., Scherer, S. S., and Lemke, G. (1996). The transcription factors SCIP and Krox-20 mark distinct stages and cell fates in Schwann cell differentiation. *Mol. Cell. Neurosci.* **8,** 129–145.

Zorick, T. S., Syroid, D. E., Brown, A., Gridley, T., and Lemke, G. (1999). Krox-20 controls SCIP expression, cell cycle exit and susceptibility to apoptosis in developing myelinating Schwann cells. *Development* **126,** 1397–1406.

CHAPTER

# 40

# Infectious Demyelinating Diseases

*Richard T. Johnson and Eugene O. Major*

## INTRODUCTION

Viral infections can lead to acute or chronic demyelinating diseases of the central or peripheral nervous systems in animals and humans. These diseases can be acute or chronic with progressive or relapsing-remitting courses. The loss of myelin with *relative* sparing of axons may or may not be associated with inflammation or gliosis, and oligodendrocytes or Schwann cells may or may not be altered. The mechanisms of demyelination are varied.

Natural infections of rodents (mouse hepatitis and Theiler's viruses), canines (canine distemper virus), and ruminants (visna of sheep and caprine arthritis-encephalitis viruses) have been associated with central nervous system (CNS) demyelination; see Chapter 44. This chapter focuses on three human CNS demyelinating diseases: acute disseminated encephalomyelitis (ADEM), also known as post-infectious encephalomyelitis, progressive multifocal leukoencephalopathy (PML), and multiple sclerosis (MS).

These three diseases have very different clinical courses and distinctive pathological features, although all share the essential element of demyelination. ADEM and PML have antithetic modes of pathogenesis; the former is a predominantly extraneural infection resulting in a virus-induced host autoimmune response, and the latter is a direct lytic infection of oligodendrocytes in an immunocompromised host. The role of infections in MS is unclear; epidemiological studies implicate an early life exposure in the genesis of the disease that could represent an infection. Exacerbations of disease more often follow viral-like illnesses and patients with MS have abnormal immune responses to viruses, including the intrathecal generation of antibodies to measles and a variety of other agents.

## PROPOSED MECHANISMS OF VIRUS-INDUCED DEMYELINATION

Several mechanisms have been proposed to explain the demyelination seen with viral infections, and in MS when an infectious etiology has been postulated (Tab. 40.1). The most straightforward mechanism to explain CNS myelin loss is the selective destruction of the myelin maintaining cells, oligodendrocytes. This mechanism is responsible for the loss of myelin in PML, a disease characterized by infection and lysis of oligodendrocytes (discussed later).

In the immunocompetent host, immune responses are often proposed to explain myelin destruction. Most agents associated with CNS demyelination are enveloped viruses. Viral envelopes are formed by insertion of virus-coded proteins into the lipid bilayer of the cell membrane. The core or nucleocapsid of the virus then acquires the envelope by budding through the modified membrane. Hypothetically, immune responses against viral proteins within the membrane could caused myelin membrane damage *in situ*. Alternatively, virus

TABLE 40.1 **Proposed Mechanisms of Virus-Induced CNS Demyelination**

| **CNS infection** |
|---|
| Infection of oligodendrocytes |
| Direct destruction |
| Pathogenic immune response to viral antigens on cell membranes |
| Introduction of cell membranes into systematic circulation |
| Infection of other CNS cells |
| Release of cytokines or viral proteins toxic to myelin supporting cells or myelin membranes |
| ***Extraneural infection*** |
| Molecular mimicry (virus proteins and myelin proteins) |
| Disruption of immune responses |

replicating in oligodendrocytes could transport sequestered myelin antigens into the systemic circulation.

Infection of macrophages, microglia or astrocytes may release soluble cytokines, chemokines or viral proteins, which are toxic to other uninfected CNS cells. Visna virus infections of sheep have a long incubation period followed by either a progressive or remitting and relapsing course, accompanied by patchy demyelinated lesions simulating MS. However, infection is limited to cells of macrophage origin. In the brain, macrophages and microglia appear to release a cytokine or similar soluble substance that results in demyelination (Kennedy *et al.*, 1985). A related lentivirus, human immunodeficiency virus (HIV), has subsequently been shown to infect the same restricted cell population in the human brain. Viral proteins as well as cytokines released from infected macrophages and microglia have also been implicated in the pathogenesis of HIV encephalopathy (Power and Johnson, 2001).

Demyelination can also result from immune responses against myelin in the absence of nervous system infection. Molecular mimicry, in which an immune response to an environmental agent cross-reacts with a host antigen, has been a popular postulated mechanism. A similar amino acid sequence contained in both viral protein and myelin proteins might allow systemic virus replication to induce an immune response against an epitope on the CNS myelin. Searching sequence databases for commonality of encephalitogenic sequences of myelin basic protein and viral proteins turned up a sequence within the P protein of hepatitis B virus. Inoculation of this synthesized viral sequence into rabbits resulted in an inflammatory response in the brain (Fujinami and Oldstone, 1985). In natural infections, *Camphylobactor* infections followed by the axonal form of Guillian-Barre syndrome are probably due to similarities between bacterial and axonal proteins (Moran and Prendergast, 2001), and cellular damage in HTLV-1-associated myelopathy (tropical spastic paraparesis) appears related, in part, to homology between nuclear ribonuclear neuronal protein and the tax protein of HTLV-1 (Levin *et al.*, 2002).

Finally, infection of lymphoid cells may disrupt normal cellular immune responses. Activated T cells normally traffic through the CNS, but only those recognizing an antigen remain (Irani and Griffin, 1996). Thus, in systemic infections causing lymphocyte activation, CNS traffic of T cells is increased. If normally suppressed responses to self-antigens are disrupted by the infection, autoimmune disease can occur such as ADEM associated with measles virus infections (discussed later).

For over half a century, the focus on experimental autoimmune (allergic) encephalomyelitis (EAE) as the prototype autoimmune disease biased thought on virus-induced demyelination. In recent years, studies of humoral immune responses in the pathogenesis of Guillian-Barre syndrome and focus on toxic effects of cytokines and viral proteins in studies of neurological complications of HIV infections have provided a more balanced perspective.

# ACUTE DISSEMINATED ENCEPHALOMYELITIS

## Definition

ADEM is an acute, inflammatory, demyelinating disease of the brain and spinal cord. In most patients it has an abrupt onset days to several weeks after a viral exanthem or virus-like illness. But the disease is not specific to viruses and has been reported after several bacterial illnesses, immunizations, and drug and serum administration.

The nosology is confusing, since the disease has been described under a remarkable variety of names. Post-infectious, parainfectious, post-exanthematous, post-vaccinal, post-measles, and post-influenzal encephalomyelitis have been applied to describe the clinical settings. Acute disseminated encephalomyelitis, perivascular myclinoclasis, perivenous encephalitis, and acute demyelinating encephalomyelitis have been coined to describe the pathological features. Allergic encephalomyelitis, immune-mediated encephalomyelitis, hyperergic encephalomyelitis, and disseminated vasculomyelinopathy imply knowledge of pathogenetic mechanisms (Johnson *et al.*, 1985). Since the essential features for diagnosis are the neuropathological changes, ADEM will be used here except in specific cases such as post-measles and post-vaccinal encephalomyelitis.

Acute hemorrhagic necrotizing leukoencephalits is generally regarded as a more intense, "hyperacute" form of ADEM. However, this rare acute demyelinating disease has distinct clinical and pathological features and is associated with a different spectrum of antecedent infections.

## Epidemiology

ADEM was a common disease in the mid-20th century, representing about one-third of all cases of encephalitis. The most common cause of ADEM was measles, which, along with ADEM cases following rubella and mumps, has been largely eliminated in regions of the world that have adequately protected children with the measles-mumps-rubella (MMR) vaccine. The second major cause of ADEM was a vaccine, vaccinia virus, which was discontinued after the worldwide eradication of natural smallpox in 1977. More recently, the varicella vaccine has further reduced the risk of ADEM. Now in countries with active childhood vaccination programs, ADEM makes up less than 10% of the cases of encephalitis, and the most common antecedent illnesses are nonspecific respiratory infections (Johnson, 1998).

The incidence of ADEM after clinically distinctive virus illnesses is highly variable (Tab. 40.2); the incidence after Epstein-Barr (EB) virus, *Mycoplasma pneumoniae*, influenza, and nonspecific upper respiratory infections are uncertain. The clinical findings after specific infections show some distinctive features, and the mortality and morbidity rates are quite different. Despite the common pathology, the pathogenesis may vary. Most data on pathogenesis relate to post-measles encephalomyelitis.

## Pathology

In acute fatal cases the brain may be congested and swollen. On gross sections, vessels are prominent in white matter with discoloration along the veins.

TABLE 40.2 Postinfectious Encephalomyelitis with Perivenular Demyelination Associated with Exanthematous Viral Infections

| | Case rate | Fatality rate | Sequelae rate |
|---|---|---|---|
| Vaccinia | 1:63 to 1:250,000 | 10% | Rare |
| Measles | 1:1000 | 25% | Frequent |
| Varicella[a] | 1:10,000 | 5% | 10% |
| Rubella[a] | 1:20,000 | 20% | Very rare |

[a]Estimates difficult to determine because of frequency of toxic encephalopathy or Reye's syndrome (different pathology) and acute cerebellar ataxia (unknown pathology) and the rare documentation of perivenular demyelinating disease.

On microscopic examination mononuclear cells are prominent along the small veins. In intense acute cases, polymorphonuclear cells may also be present. Pallor and loss of myelin staining is seen along the vessels; its perivenular localization often produces flame shaped lesions. In the spinal cord, this causes a characteristic radial pattern (Fig. 40.1), a pattern distinctive from the plaques of demyelination seen in PML or MS. Patients dying later in disease show even more sharply demarcated lesions and lipid-laden macrophages (Johnson *et al.*, 1985).

Immunocytochemical staining of myelin proteins also distinguishes ADEM from PML and MS. In ADEM, as in EAE, areas demonstrating loss of myelin basic protein and myelin-associated glycoprotein are concordant (Gendelman *et al.*, 1984). In PML, the area of myelin-associated glycoprotein loss is distinctly larger than the area of myelin basic protein loss in demyelinated lesions. Presumably this reflects a direct attack on the myelin membranes in ADEM and EAE; whereas in PML, where disease results from oligodendrocyte infection, the myelin-associated glycoprotein, concentrated in the periaxonal, most distal extensions of the myelin membrane, is lost first. Thus, in PML lesions, areas of decreased myelin-associated glycoprotein staining are two to three times larger than areas of myelin basic protein loss. Demyelinated plaques in MS show a mixture of patterns, suggesting different pathogenic mechanisms accounting for myelin loss (Gendelman *et al.*, 1985).

In acute hemorrhagic necrotizing leukoencephalitis, the brain is usually strikingly swollen with evidence of herniation. Gross hemorrhages are evident. Microscopically both veins and arterioles show fibrinoid necrosis. This vascular necrosis is associated with transudates of fibrin into the tissue, extravasation of red blood cells, and tissue

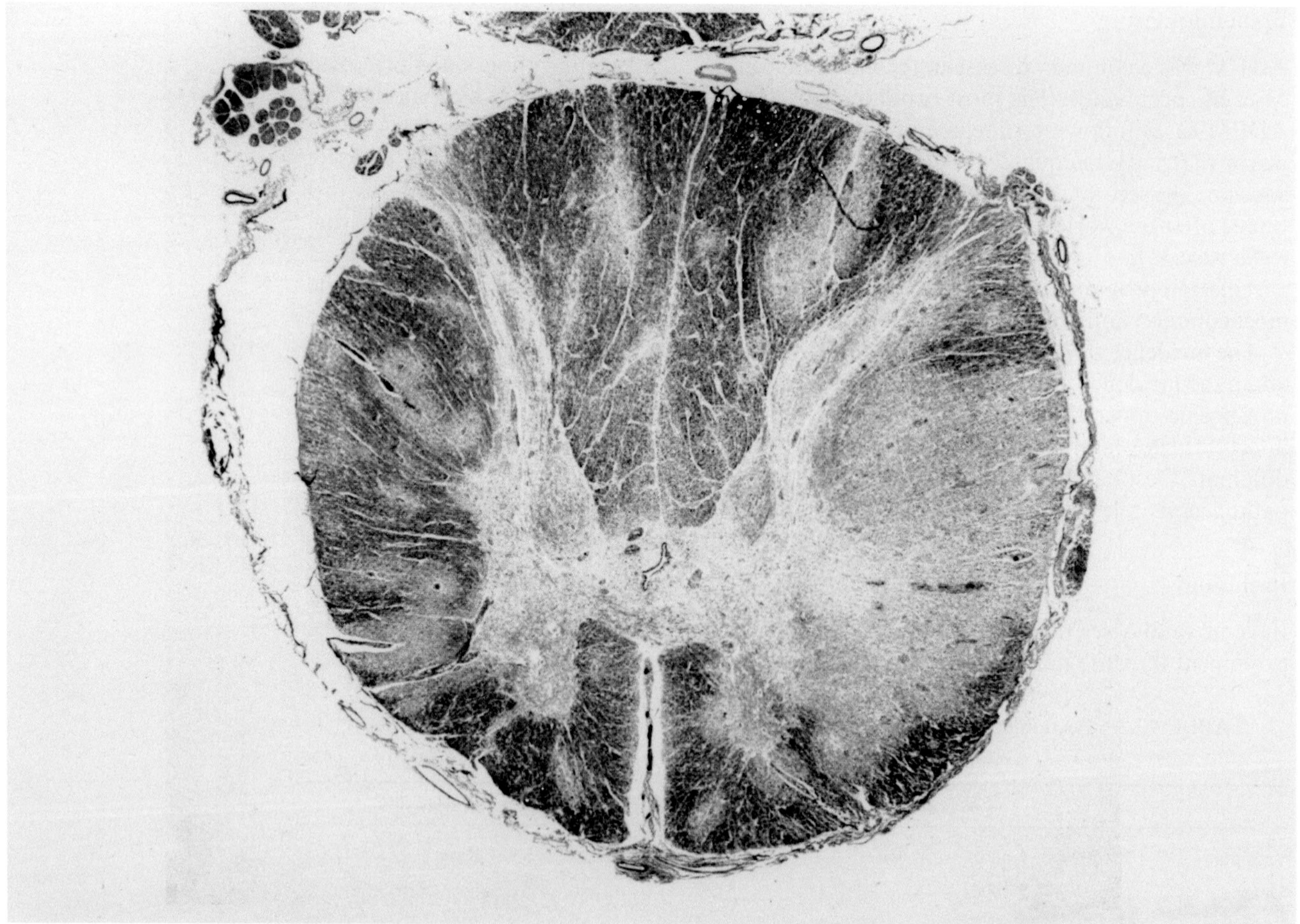

**FIGURE 40.1**
ADEM following varicella. This 12-year-old girl developed paraparesis abruptly 2 weeks after the onset of uncomplicated chickenpox. Over the next 3 days the disease evolved with arm weakness, blindness, respiratory distress, seizures, and death. Section of spinal cord shows the characteristic pattern of perivenular demyelination.

necrosis. The inflammatory infiltrate is predominantly polymorphonuclear. These findings are most intense in the white matter; and despite the large necrotic areas, there are regions where myelin loss with relative sparing of axons is evident.

## Pathogenesis

The pathological changes in ADEM resemble those seen in the "neuroparalytic accidents" reported after post-exposure vaccination for rabies using killed virus prepared in animal brain and spinal cord. Indeed, the similarity between the demyelinating encephalomyelitis after vaccination with vaccinia virus to prevent smallpox and the complications of rabies vaccine led Rivers and Schwentker (1935) to studies in monkeys. Animals repeatedly inoculated with emulsions of normal brain developed neurological signs and had perivenular demyelination. This was the discovery of EAE. Subsequently Kabat and colleagues (1947) found that in some species, a single injection of brain could induce the disease if brain inoculum was emulsified in adjuvant. Others showed that specific sequences of myelin basic protein and proteolipid protein could cause disease, and that disease could be passively transferred with sensitized lymphocytes (Paterson, 1960) (see Chapter 43).

EAE mimics ADEM and post-rabies vaccine encephalitis (Tab. 40.3). Lymphocytes from patients with post-rabies vaccine encephalomyelitis (Hemachudha *et al.*, 1988), post-measles encephalitis, post-varicella cerebellar ataxia, and encephalomyelitis following respiratory infections have been shown to proliferate when cultured in the presence of myelin basic protein. The gap in these parallels is that patients with ADEM have not been injected with myelin proteins.

Studies of the pathogenesis of ADEM have focused primarily on measles because the clinical diagnosis is easy, the incidence of ADEM is high compared to other infections, and the neurological complications of measles are homogeneous. Generalization of these studies to ADEM and other post-infectious complications of other viruses is cautioned, since the systemic pathogenesis and effects on the immune system by the other agents are variable.

**TABLE 40.3 Comparisons of Experimental Allergic Encephalomyelitis with Encephalomyelitis after Rabies Vaccine and Viral Infections**

| | Experimental allergic encephalomyelitis | Post-rabies vaccine encephalomyelitis | Postinfectious encephalomyelitis |
|---|---|---|---|
| Inducing event | Inoculation with CNS tissue or myelin basic Protein | Inoculation with CNS tissue | Infection with enveloped viruses |
| Latent period | 10–21 days | 7–42 days | 10–40 days[a] |
| Clinical forms | | | |
| Acute onset | + | + | + |
| Monophasic disease | + | + | + |
| Occasional chronic or relapsing forms | + | + | + |
| Pathologic findings | | | |
| Perivenular lymphocytes | | | |
| Perivenular demyelination | + | + | + |
| Immunological studies | | | |
| Lymphocytes stimulated *in vitro* by myelin basic protein | + | + | + |
| *In vitro* demyelination by lymphocytes | + | ? | + |
| Anti-myelin protein antibodies | + | + | − |

[a]From beginning of incubation periods.
From Johnson (1998).

Measles was the first virus shown to cause immunosuppression. von Pirquet (1908) demonstrated that children had a conversion of positive tuberculin reactions during measles, and for weeks thereafter. Subsequent studies showed inhibition of lymphocyte responses to mitogens for up to 4 weeks after uncomplicated measles virus infection. The magnitude of inhibition of lymphocyte proliferation was the same in children with uncomplicated measles, in those with pneumonitis related to immunodeficiency, and in those with ADEM thought to be due to an autoimmune response (Hirsch *et al.*, 1984). In contrast, spontaneous proliferation of CD4, CD8, and B lymphocytes was found, as well as signs of immune activation, which included lymphoproliferation of lymphocytes in the presence of myelin basic protein in 15% of cases of uncomplicated measles and in 47% of those with ADEM (Johnson *et al.*, 1984).

The mechanisms underlying the profound suppression of cell-mediated immunity accompanying measles is still not fully understood. *In vitro* infection of human monocytes specifically down-regulates IL-12 production, a cytokine critical in cell-mediated immunity (Karp *et al.*, 1996), however disruption at other sites in the complex cytokine network is likely.

In a subsequent study of ADEM after varied infections, T-cell lines were established from patients. The frequency of cell lines reactive to myelin basic protein was ten times higher in patients with ADEM than patients with encephalitis or controls. IL-4 was the prominent cytokine secreted by T-cell lines from patients with ADEM during the recovery phase (Pohl-Koppe *et al.*, 1998). This finding supports a more general relevance of T-cell responses to myelin proteins in the pathogenesis of ADEM.

## Clinical Features

ADEM is best defined by its unique pathology, because many of the causative agents are associated with multiple post-infectious syndromes and many of the clinical syndromes and imaging studies overlap with other disease processes. The two most clearly defined cases of ADEM are those following vaccinia and measles virus infections. Each follows a clinically distinct exanthem and presents a similar clinical course and consistent pathology. In contrast, neurological syndromes associated with rubella, varicella, mumps, and influenza may include direct encephalitis, Reye's syndrome, and acute cerebellar ataxia—all of which may have different mechanisms of pathogenesis not characterized by demyelination (Tab. 40.2).

The common clinical features are a lag of 3 days to 3 weeks after the exanthem or respiratory disease, an abrupt onset of headache, fever, and impaired consciousness, and the finding of focal neurological signs. The disease reaches a nadir within days, and recovery is variable, depending, in large part, on the causative agent. The spinal fluid usually shows a modest pleocytosis and mild protein elevation, but can also appear normal. The myelin basic protein content may be elevated, particularly early in disease. In some cases, magnetic resonance imaging has proved an effective method of differentiation from acute encephalitis or Reye's syndrome. Multifocal white matter lesions of similar age are found, which may or may not enhance. When enhancement is seen in all lesions simultaneously (Fig. 40.2), the image is characteristic of ADEM.

Acute ADEM not associated with viral exanthems can be difficult to differentiate from acute viral encephalitis or, in some cases, the initial attack of MS. A viral prodrome, high lesion load on magnetic resonance imaging involving deep gray matter, and the absence of oligoclonal bands in the spinal fluid favor a diagnosis of ADEM (Hynson *et al.*, 2001). Followup studies of patients diagnosed with ADEM have shown a subsequent diagnosis of MS in some patients, raising the question of whether ADEM might be a part of an "MS spectrum" (Hartung and Grossman, 2001). MS is not, however, an outcome of classical ADEM following measles or vaccinia infections, and ADEM has a very distinctive neuropathology.

### *Measles*

Measles probably remains the most common cause of ADEM worldwide. Although indigenous measles has been eliminated from the Western Hemisphere and Western

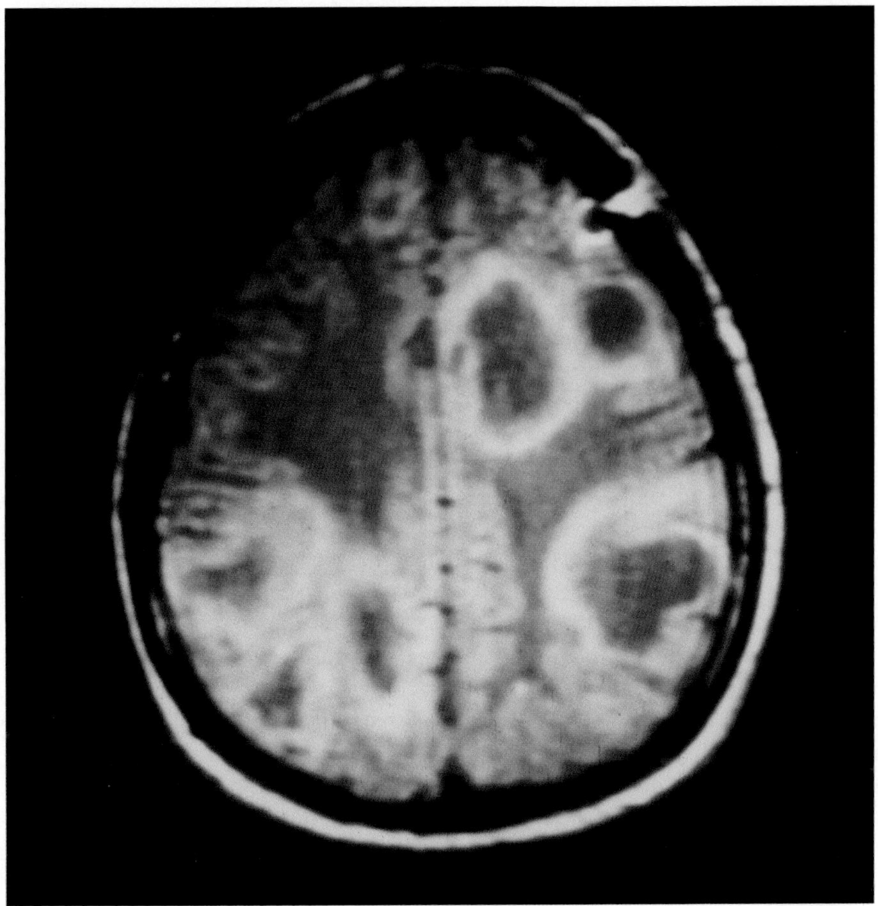

**FIGURE 40.2**
ADEM after primary Epstein-Barr virus infection. This college student had classical monospot positive infectious mononucleosis. Two weeks after onset, she developed multifocal neurological signs and coma. The enhanced MRI at that time shows widespread white mater lesions with intense enhancement. She subsequently recovered and returned to school with minimal sequelae.

Europe, it still causes over 1 million childhood deaths each year, largely in developing countries. Measles continues to rank as the third most common infectious cause of childhood death worldwide, following diarrheal illnesses and malaria. The most frequent fatal complications of measles, pneumonitis, gastroenteritis, and secondary bacterial infections, result from a depression of cell-mediated immune responses extending for 1 to 4 weeks after the rash. Prior to the emergence of HIV, measles virus was the most important and lethal causes of a virus-induced immunodeficiency syndrome. However, the major neurological complication of measles infection, ADEM, was assumed to be an allergic or autoimmune disease. Although this initially appeared to be a paradox, studies of measles and HIV have shown that immune activation can suppress immune responses as well as release autoimmune responses.

The incidence of post-measles encephalitis is reasonably constant, at about 1 per 1000 cases, and is age dependent, since children under 2 years of age seldom develop encephalitis. It does not appear to be nutritionally dependent, as are some opportunistic infections. Thus, populations such as those of West Africa tend to suffer high rates of measles mortality from opportunistic infections and infant deaths. On the other hand, more affluent countries without adequate immunization programs have greater mortality and morbidity from post-measles encephalitis, because older children become infected. Although polyneuritis, toxic encephalopathy and acute hemiplegia of possible vascular etiology have been reported with measles, over 95% of the neurological illnesses are represented by ADEM.

The incubation period of measles is 10 to 14 days. The prodrome and period of infectivity is marked by coryza, conjunctivitis, cough, and the pathognomonic Koplik spots on the buccal mucosa. Coincident with the antibody response and the end of infectivity, a maculopapular rash develops on the face and trunk, later spreading to the extremities. Virus can be recovered from the rash, and for up to 5 days after the appearance of the rash, viral antigen or RNA can be found in epithelioid cells of the lung, gut, bladder, and lymphoid organs (Moench *et al.*, 1988). On rare occasions, viral antigen and RNA can also be detected in cerebrovascular endothelial cells (Esolen *et al.*, 1995). Although there is no evidence of infection of neural cells, approximately 50% of children have an abnormal electroencephalogram during the rash (Gibbs *et al.*, 1959), and approximately 30% have a pleocytosis (Ojala, 1947).

Post-measles encephalitis typically develops 4 to 5 days after the onset of the rash, but may precede the rash or be delayed until 3 weeks after. Typically the child is afebrile, the rash is fading and the child is returning to normal activities, when fever returns with headache. Obtundation is frequent and may progress to coma. Generalized or focal seizures occur in about half of the children. Multifocal neurological signs may include cranial nerve abnormalities, pyramidal tract signs, abnormal movements, and ataxia. Sensory deficits are infrequent. The spinal fluid may show a modest mononuclear cell pleocytosis but is acellular in about one-third of the patients. Protein elevations are variable, but many have high levels of myelin basic protein in spinal fluid, particularly early in the course of the encephalitis. Elevated IgG synthesis and oligoclonal bands are usually absent (Johnson *et al.*, 1984). Mortality and morbidity are high. Between 10 and 40% mortality are reported, and neurological sequellae are found in the majority of survivors. Prognosis has been linked to length of stupor or coma (Tyler, 1957), but remarkable recoveries can be seen after prolonged coma (Johnson *et al.*, 1984).

The measles vaccine is an attenuated live virus, which has led to the question of whether or not the vaccine may, on rare occasions, cause ADEM. The vaccine virus can produce fever, but in early tests of the vaccine, no abnormalities were found on electroencephalograms that are common with wild-type virus infections. Post-liscencing studies reported one case of encephalitis per million children following vaccination, a number lower than the observed background of two per million cases of encephalitis or encephalopathy per month, suggesting a coincidental relationship between vaccine and disease. Further analysis, however, showed some clustering of cases during the 6 to 15 days after immunization, suggesting a possible relationship (Landrigan and Witte, 1973). Since no histopathological studies have been reported in post-vaccine illnesses, whether or not a few of these cases represent rare cases of ADEM remains unknown.

### *Vaccinia*

Until recently, the neurological complications of smallpox and vaccinia were of only historical interest; the last case of natural smallpox was observed in 1977, and within a few years vaccinia inoculation had been abandoned worldwide. Recent threats of bioterrorism have led to consideration of renewed vaccinia virus inoculation, and the risks of ADEM must be reconsidered.

In retrospect, ADEM accompanied smallpox but was hidden under the devastating systemic disease (Marsden and Hurst, 1932). In the 1920s, ADEM became appreciated as a complication of immunization with vaccinia virus. The incidence of complications after vaccination is extraordinarily variable; an incidence of 1 in 63 is cited for one Dutch vaccine program (but a variety of types of illness were included) (DeVries, 1960). During World War II, an incidence of post-vaccinal encephalomyelitis in England was estimated 1 per 175,000 (Miller, 1953), a subsequent retrospective analysis in the United States estimated 1 per 200,000; during the sidewalk vaccination of 5 million people in New York in 1947 a similar incidence of about 1 per 100,000 was estimated, and during the more recent mass vaccination during the smallpox outbreak in the United Kingdom in 1962, passive reporting estimated neurological complications in 1 per 20,000 (Spillane and Wells, 1964). The variation in incidence may be due to different ethnic populations, different patches of virus, and certainly variable and often poor data collection. ADEM is clearly more common with primary immunization, and some data suggest that incidence increases with age.

At the time of maximal cutaneous reaction or shortly thereafter, patients with ADEM develop fever, nuchal rigidity and obtundation, Movement disorders including tremor, ataxia, trismus, and myoclonus are specifically mentioned in several reports (Miller and Stanton, 1954; Spillane and Wells, 1964). Fatality rates are as varied as incidence rates, but are generally lower than those for post-measles encephalomyelitis, and sequellae are less frequent.

The pathogenesis is assumed to resemble that of measles, but vaccinia virus usually replicates only in the dermis. In some patients a viremia is found, and this is more prolonged in patients with ADEM. Virus has been recovered from brains and spinal fluids of patients with ADEM (Brooks, 1979). Which hematogenous cells are infected and the effect on immune responses has not been studied.

In considering the resumption of vaccination some have recommended (1) vaccination of those likely to encounter victims (first-responders, family health care providers, and clinic and emergency room personnel), (2) vaccination of all who request vaccine, or (3) mandatory universal vaccination. In any of these scenarios, most of those receiving vaccine would be over age 2 and a majority would be receiving primary vaccinations, two factors that presumably increase the risk of ADEM. If the incidence of ADEM were 1 per 20,000 vaccinees (some would consider that figure high; others low) in the United States, we might anticipate 10,000 cases of ADEM with 1000 deaths if universal immunization were the option chosen.

### *Varicella*

Of the neurological complications accompanying chickenpox, fully 50% are acute cerebellar ataxia, which complicates 1 in 4000 chickenpox cases. Typical ADEM is quite rare but does occur (Fig. 40.1). The most dreaded complication is Reye's syndrome, in which fatty degeneration of the liver is accompanied by life threatening brain edema, but in this disease both inflammation and demyelination are absent.

Post-varicella cerebellar ataxia has a good prognosis and the absence of fatalities leave the histopathology undefined. In several cases of acute ataxia with chickenpox, lymphoproliferative responses in the presence of myelin basic protein have been reported, suggesting a pathogenesis similar to post-measles encephalomyelitis (Johnson *et al.*, 1984; Lisak *et al.*, 1977). Antibodies reacting with sections of cerebrum and cerebellum were reported in 3 of 8 children with post-varicella cerebellar ataxia, suggesting that humoral immune responses may also be involved (Adams *et al.*, 2000).

The typical ADEM resembles post-measles ADEM; disease onset is abrupt at 4 to 15 days after the onset of rash. Fever, headache, obtundation, seizures, and focal neurological signs are common (Gollomp and Fahn, 1987). Neuropathological studies are similar.

### *Rubella*

Rubella is the fourth exanthem classically associated with ADEM. It is estimated that an incidence of 1 per 20,000 cases develop ADEM. The onset is typical; during the week after the rash, fever, headache, and obtundation develop often with seizures. Focal neurological signs are usually not found, but a pleocytosis is. Fatalities do occur, but most have failed to show the typical hallmarks of ADEM; a minority has shown characteristic perivenular inflammation and demyelination suggesting varied types of post-rubella encephalopathies. In a single child, a lymphoproliferative response to myelin basic protein was documented (Johnson *et al.*, 1985).

### *Human Immunodeficiency Virus*

HIV has been associated with a remarkable spectrum of neurological diseases. Acute meningitis and acute demyelinating polyneuritis (Guillian-Barre syndrome) have often been seen about the time of initial seroconversion. These are assumed to be autoimmune disorders associated with the initial activation of CD4 cells. A small number of newly infected individuals have developed a fatal encephalomyelitis, and pathological studies have shown ADEM (Narciso *et al.*, 2001; Silver *et al.*, 1997).

Years later with onset of AIDS different central and peripheral nervous system diseases are prominent associated with intense immunodeficiency. HIV dementia, which develops in 20 to 40% of AIDS patients, can be characterized by "diffuse myelin pallor," visualized on magnetic resonance imaging as a hypodense lesion of white matter, primarily in the cerebral hemispheres, and in pathological sections by a pallor of myelin staining. Initially thought to represent demyelination, immunocytochemical staining for myelin proteins has failed to show myelin loss. The abnormal signal on imaging and pallor of staining seem to reflect a breakdown of the blood-brain barrier (Power *et al.*, 1993). In addition to the prominent diffuse pallor of myelin, small flame-shaped areas of demyelination without inflammation are occasionally seen along vessels; these may represent the residua of minor or subclinical demyelinating encephalitis that occurred at the time of seroconversion.

### *Other Agents*

Several viruses have been associated with ADEM that are also associated with apparent acute encephalitis or meningitis. In neurological complications of mumps virus, EB virus, and influenza A and B virus infections, virus has been recovered from brain or spinal fluid and pathological findings have been varied; some suggest direct effects of virus replication in neural cells and some histopathologically are ADEM (Hart and Earle, 1975).

Mumps was the single most common viral cause of viral meningitis, but over 90% of these illnesses are now prevented in countries with adequate MMR vaccine administration. Indeed, mumps may be the most neuroinvasive virus, since examination of spinal fluid in patients with uncomplicated parotitis showed that fully 50% had a pleocytosis. Fortunately, mumps is not highly neurovirulent, and the common neurological complication is benign meningitis. In patients with mumps meningitis, virus can readily be isolated from spinal fluid, and viral nucleocapsids can be visualized by electron microscopy within ependymal cells found in spinal fluid (Herndon *et al.*, 1974). This suggests a similar pathogenesis of CNS invasion in humans as seen in hamsters, where mumps virus selectively infects ependymal cells (Johnson, 1968). Serious CNS complications of mumps virus infections are rare. Even prior to immunization, when mumps virus infection was universal, only four to five deaths from mumps encephalitis were reported to the Centers for Disease Control each year. Of those cases, about half showed the histological findings of perivenular demyelination (Schwarz *et al.*, 1968).

The neurological complications of EB virus infections pose an even more confusing spectrum of disease. Typically these disorders arise 1 to 2 weeks after the onset of clinical infectious mononucleosis. About 1% of patients have neurological complications, but these vary from Guillian-Barre syndrome and acute cerebellar ataxia (usually associated with autoimmune responses) to meningitis, encephalitis, and myelitis typical of direct infections (Gautier-Smith, 1965). The finding of viral DNA by PCR is not meaningful, since EB virus is latent in B lymphocytes and a single B cell traversing through cerebral circulation or drifting into spinal fluid could give a positive signal. As with mumps virus infections, intrathecal antibody synthesis and oligoclonal bands of IgG in the spinal fluid may be found; this is in contrast to post-measles encephalomyelitis but does not exclude an immunopathological mechanism. Again, the diagnosis of ADEM is pathology-based. In the rare fatal cases of encephalitis, a necrotizing polioencephalitis is found; but in others perivenular demyelination has been reported (Paskavitz *et al.*, 1995).

Both influenza A and B have been, on rare occasions, related to Reye's syndrome, acute transverse myelitis, and Guillian-Barre syndrome. The association with pathologically verified ADEM is very rare (Hoult and Flewett, 1960). *Mycoplasma pneumonia* is also associated with a variety of neurological complications including the occasional case of ADEM (Riedel *et al.*, 2001). A diagnosis of ADEM is often entertained clinically, but autopsy studies of fatal cases have generally shown brain edema or perivascular inflammation without convincing demyelination. Recent anecdotal reports of probable ADEM associated with hepatitis C virus (Sacconi *et al.*, 2001), attenuated polio vaccine virus (Ozawa *et al.*, 2000), and acute herpetic gingivostomatitis (Ito *et al.*, 2000) may be coincidental.

### Acute Hemorrhagic Necrotizing Leukoencephalopathy

This acute hemorrhagic disease has been regarded as a more intense form of ADEM and as a distinct entity. The clinical setting is similar. Usually 1 to 20 days following a virus-like illness, the disease develops with fever, obtundation, seizures, and focal neurological signs. Although reported in individual cases after measles and chickenpox, most follow a non-specific upper respiratory infection. In Asia, a number of cases have been associated with influenza virus infections (Voudris *et al.*, 2001); recently several cases were reported with *Mycoplasma pneumoniae* infections (Pfausler *et al.*, 2002). In contrast to ADEM, the illness is fulminant with signs suggesting an expanding mass lesion, and the majority of patients die within 5 days. The spinal fluid shows polymorphonuclear cells and red cells; in addition, a peripheral leukocytosis and proteinuria are usually found.

The arguments linking acute hemorrhagic necrotizing leukoencephalitis to ADEM are (1) the similar clinical setting despite a distinct spectrum of precipitating illnesses, (2) an apparent continuum of pathology with cases clearly showing features of both diseases, and (3) the animal model of hyperacute EAE that resembles hemorrhagic necrotizing leukoencephalitis (Levine and Wenk, 1965). In a single case, a proliferative response of the patient's lymphocytes was demonstrated when cultured with myelin basic protein (Behan *et al.*, 1968).

### Prevention and Treatment

Few arenas of medicine have celebrated the extraordinary success in disease prevention at as an astonishing cost-benefit ratio as in the prevention of infections with vaccines. The measles vaccine alone prevents between 2 million and 3 million deaths each year, reduces the burden of permanently neurologically impaired by even greater numbers, has reduced childhood deafness by 10%, and has virtually eliminated subacute sclerosing panencephalitis from countries with sustained vaccine programs. The cessation of vaccination to prevent smallpox and the introduction of vaccine programs to prevent mumps, rubella, and chickenpox have decreased the incidence of ADEM dramatically.

Treatment is less effective. Although the literature abounds with anecdotal claims of the benefits of corticosteroids, no randomized placebo-controlled study supports their value. Several studies of sequential patients with measles encephalitis who did or did not receive steroids or ACTH showed no difference in mortality or morbidity (Ziegra, 1961). These studies may be applicable only to measles, and empiric treatment with steroids remains common in ADEM, particularly when there is any evidence of increased intracranial pressure. One retrospective study of post-infectious encephalomyelitis showed higher mortality and morbidity rates among those who had received corticosteroids. On the assumption that the more seriously ill would tend to be treated, the data were reanalyzed to include only patients admitted in coma. Even in this reevaluation the mortality was higher in treated patients (Boe *et al.*, 1965).

Supportive treatment is important since children can have remarkable recoveries after prolonged coma. Therefore lowering of fever, management of seizures, careful management of fluids, reducing increased intracranial pressure, and prevention of urinary and respiratory tract and skin infections are paramount. Mechanical ventilation is often necessary.

## PROGRESSIVE MULTIFOCAL LEUKOENCEPHALOPATHY

### Definition

#### *PML*

In the 1950s, a rapidly progressing neurologic syndrome was observed in a patient suffering from chronic lymphatic leukemia (CLL). Although the cause was ruled to be a result of leukemic cells that had infiltrated the brain, post-mortem examination revealed bizarre, enlarged nuclei and demyelination, which was not consistent with the diagnosis. A few years later, another patient with CLL developed similar neurologic symptoms. Again, autopsy revealed demyelinated plaques populated by cells with enlarged, dense nuclei, which were hypothesized to be oligodendrocytes with an unusual, undescribed pathology. The results were published in 1958 as the first clinical and neuropathological description of a new disease, progressive multifocal leukoencephalopathy (PML), also known as Richardson's disease after E. P. Richarson, who was responsible for the initial description (Astrom *et al.*, 1958). There were early suspicions that PML was caused by a virus; however, the etiologic agent was not identified until 1971 as the human polyomavirus, JC Virus. Like other polyomaviruses, JCV was named after the initials of the patient from whom virus was first isolated (Padgett *et al.*, 1971)

Initially the disease was mainly associated with patients suffering from lymphoproliferative and myeloproliferative diseases such as CLL, Hodgkin's disease, and sarcoidosis (Richardson, 1974). Following the description of PML, retrospective review of the literature uncovered several similar accounts in patients with dementia suffering from a variety of underlying immunosuppressive disorders. The accounts dated back as far as 1930 with pathologic features consistent with PML (Hallervorden, 1930). PML is almost exclusively associated with an underlying cellular immunodeficiency. Prior to the AIDS epidemic, the association was most frequently observed in patients with Hodgkin's disease and CLL. In the decades following, the exponential rise in the incidence of AIDS resulted in a much larger and rapidly growing population of immunosuppressed individuals. Presently, PML has become an increasingly common complication in AIDS patients, and has been the AIDS defining illness in approximately 1% of the cases. It is expected that approximately 4 to 5% of all AIDS patients will eventually develop this disease (Berger and Major, 1999).

### *JC Virus*

JCV is a small, noneneveloped virus, approximately 45 nm in diameter. The viral capsid is icosahedral in symmetry, and made up of the 3 viral capsid proteins encoded by the late region of the JCV genome. After translation and transcription in the cytoplasm, nuclear localization signals located on the amino terminal region transport the proteins to the nucleus, where the virion particles are assembled (Moreland and Garcea, 1991). Capsid assembly is governed by the major structural protein, Vp1, which accounts for more than 70% of the entire viral protein content. Vp1 also contains the antigenic epitopes to which a specific antibody response is mounted, and it is responsible for the ability of JCV to agglutinate human type O erythrocytes (Shah *et al.*, 1977; Wang *et al.*, 1999).

Located inside the viral capsid are the JCV minchromosomes, each of which is a single molecule of viral DNA complexed with cellular and nuclear histones. The complete genome is a closed, circular supercoiled structure, approximately 5.13 kb in length (Frisque *et al.*, 1984). Transcription occurs in both directions starting from the highly conserved origin of replication, marked by a single EcoR1 restriction site. Extensive sequencing data has revealed that the genome can be functionally divided into three regions: the early region, encoding two nonstructural proteins; the late region, encoding three capsid proteins; and the regulatory region. The early region, located on the proximal side of the origin, is transcribed and expressed early after viral entry. Counterclockwise transcription of this region starting from the EcoR1 site, followed by differential splicing, produces two major mRNA species encoding the Large T and small t antigens. It is known that Large T is a nonstructural, DNA binding protein with multiple functions (Fanning, 1992), one of which is the initiation of JC viral DNA replication by the unwinding and separation of the two strands of DNA so that the polymerases can function. Furthermore, it autoregulates to prevent transcription of the early genes during the later stages of infection, when the structural genes are being produced. Large T also plays a part in the malignant transformation of cells by binding to cell cycle regulatory proteins as well as tumor suppressors such as p53 and pRB, resulting in cellular malignant transformation.

The late region, located on the distal side of the origin, is encoded in the strand of DNA complementary to the strand that encodes the early genes. Clockwise transcription from the origin of replication yields the capsid proteins VP1, VP2, and VP3, as well as the Agnoprotein. VP1, VP2, and VP3, as discussed earlier, are the structural proteins that make up the viral capsid. Agnoprotein in related viruses has been implicated in DNA binding and localization of VP1 to the nucleus (Cole, 1996, Carswell and Alwine, 1986). A recent report describing the presence of JCV agnoprotein in the cytoplasm of infected cells, suggests that protein shuttles freely between the cytoplasm and the nucleus and is important for JCV proliferation (Okada *et al.*, 2001). Early gene expression must take place before viral DNA replication can proceed, since the early products, Large T and small t, are necessary for the expression of the late gene products. Thus, efficient expression of those late structural proteins occurs only after viral transcription and translation have taken place. The noncoding sequences located between the early and late genes contain the origin of replication, the JCV promoter, and enhancer sequences. Collectively, this area is also known as the viral regulatory region (RR), thought to control host range for lytic infection.

Studies of JCV infection in various cell types have demonstrated the extremely narrow host range of this virus. It has been shown that in cell culture systems, human glial cells are the most susceptible to infection as well as the most conducive to virion production (Wroblewska *et al.*, 1980). It was originally hypothesized that the Large T viral protein defined the neurotropism of JCV, since the virus was shown to be able to replicate in nonglial cell types only in the presence of JCV or SV40 Large T protein, both of which share significant homology (Feigenbaum *et al.*, 1987). Subsequent studies interchanged the JCV promoter with other viral promoters and used the constructs to infect various cell types. The results have suggested that the cell type specificity of JCV may also be a function of the viral promoter (Feigenbaum *et al.*, 1992). The restricted growth in cell types from extra neural tissue such as kidney and tonsil has led to questions regarding the nature of JCV susceptibility. Is JCV host cell restriction at the level of binding and entry or is it at the molecular level? The recent identification of the specific cell surface receptor for JCV has provided some answers to these questions (Liu *et al.*, 1998). The receptor, an $\alpha$ 2-6 linked sialic acid, is a commonly expressed ganglioside found on the surface of various cells. Indeed, binding studies of JCV have shown that the virus can bind to and enter numerous cell types via this receptor, both susceptible and nonsusceptible.

Thus, unlike other viruses, viral susceptibility to JCV is not a function of specific receptor binding and entry. The focus has now shifted to intracellular factors that may contribute to the specificity of this virus. The regulatory region of JCV has several binding sites for the NF1 family of transcription factors. A comparison of relative NF1 expression between highly susceptible cells from the human fetal brain (HFB) and a nonsusceptible epithelial cell line (HeLa), demonstrated that one class in particular, NF1-D, was elevated in the HFB cells (Sumner *et al.*, 1996). Further studies have shown that overexpression of NF1-D in a normally nonpermissive cell line can render the cells susceptible to JCV infection, as determined by early and late gene production (Monaco *et al.*, 2001). The regulatory region of this virus has been of much interest, because it is becoming increasingly clear that despite effective virus binding or the presence of viral DNA in the cells, productive infection only occurs in the cell types that express the appropriate transcriptional factors. The very narrow host range and the cell type specificity of JCV are unique properties of this virus.

## Epidemiology

It would be expected that the incidence of PML would be higher in the geographic areas coinciding with a large HIV infected population. However, since the technology required to make a definitive diagnosis of PML may not readily be available in such areas, the actual incidence of this disease may be masked to some extent. As such, the entire worldwide incidence of PML has not yet been determined. However, serological studies of human polyomaviruses in geographically isolated regions have yielded much information on the natural distribution of JCV in human populations. The first study published in 1973 described a random sampling of 406 individuals from the state of Wisconsin, screened for the presence of JCV antibodies. The results showed that approximately 70% of assayed individuals had significant antibody titers to JCV in their blood. However, the percentage dropped dramatically in very young children, suggesting that initial infection and seroconversion most likely occurs during early childhood (Padgett and Walker, 1973). Much larger studies were conducted shortly thereafter to study the worldwide distribution of human polyomaviruses. Again, JCV infection was prevalent worldwide, as demonstrated by the presence of antibodies in infected individuals. The majority of adolescents and a much higher percentage of adults (80%) showed elevated levels of JCV-specific antibodies (Brown *et al.*, 1975,Walker and Padgett, 1983).

A more recent epidemiological study of the incidence of PML in the United States was conducted from 1979 to 1994. The survey reported the incidence of PML among HIV infected individuals as 1.6%. However, since the data only included PML cases that were diagnosed ante mortem, and not new cases discovered at autopsy, the authors felt that the numbers were an under-representation of the actual prevalence of the disease. It was also reported that 89% of the PML cases were attributed to HIV infection during this time period (Holman *et al.*, 1991). A recently concluded seroepidemiological study examining the circulation of human polyomaviruses in the population determined that 80% of the population exhibited antibodies to JCV (Maher, D. *et al.*, in press).

## Pathogenesis

The exact route of JCV transmission, initial infection and pathogenesis continues to be investigated. Seroepidemiologial studies have proven that the majority of the healthy, human population has antibodies against the virus, although the percentage drops in very young children. Thus, it is postulated that initial infection and seroconversion occurs within the first 6 years of life with no associated clinical symptoms. The initial route of infection remains elusive, although one study has reported JCV replication in human tonsillar tissue, implicating a site of latency and also a primary infection route via inhalation (Monaco *et al.*, 1998). Trafficking B lymphocytes (Tornatore *et al.*, 1992) may then carry the virus from the tonsillar and stromal tissue to other latent sites, including the bone marrow, tonsils, colon epithelial cells, and kidney (Jensen and Major, 1999; Laghi *et al.*, 1999) (Fig. 40.3). It is well documented that the virus is excreted in the urine of healthy individuals as well as patients with PML (Agostini *et al.*, 1996). Transmission via this route is unlikely, however, because the predominant genotype found in urine isolates has not be shown to be able to cause a robust infection in any type of human cell (Ault, 1997). Systemic circulation of the virus to these different compartments is thought to be via a hematogenous route, most likely involving infected B lymphocytes. Lymphocytes may shuttle the virus across the blood brain barrier during a period of severe immune deficiency, which sets the stage for the onset of PML when JCV infection is passed from the lymphocytes to the highly susceptible glial cell population.

## Pathology

The initial descriptions of PML were focused on the histopathological features associated with the disease, such as the enlarged oligodendroglial nuclei and bizarre, giant astrocytes. The swollen nuclei of infected oligodendrocytes usually display a change in chromatin pattern. They often appear more homogenous or will have the chromatin concentrated at the periphery, near the nuclear membrane. The nuclei have also been described as having "ground glass" appearance, which is due to the presence of numerous inclusion bodies. Electron microscopy has revealed that these inclusion bodies are actually a dense, crystalline, or filamentous array of JC virion particles (Aksamit, 1995).

Upon gross examination, demyelinated plaques and lesions can be visible to the naked eye. The foci of demyelination are initially few and randomly distributed. They can range in size from millimeters to centimeters in diameter, occasionally coalescing to form even larger lesions. The lesions have been identified throughout the white matter of the brain, including the cerebral hemispheres, cerebellum, medulla, and even spinal cord. However, lesions are most commonly located in the subcortical white matter, near the gray-white matter junction, which is an area of increased cerebral blood flow. This lends support to the hypothesis of viral entry into the CNS via hematogenous dissemination. However,

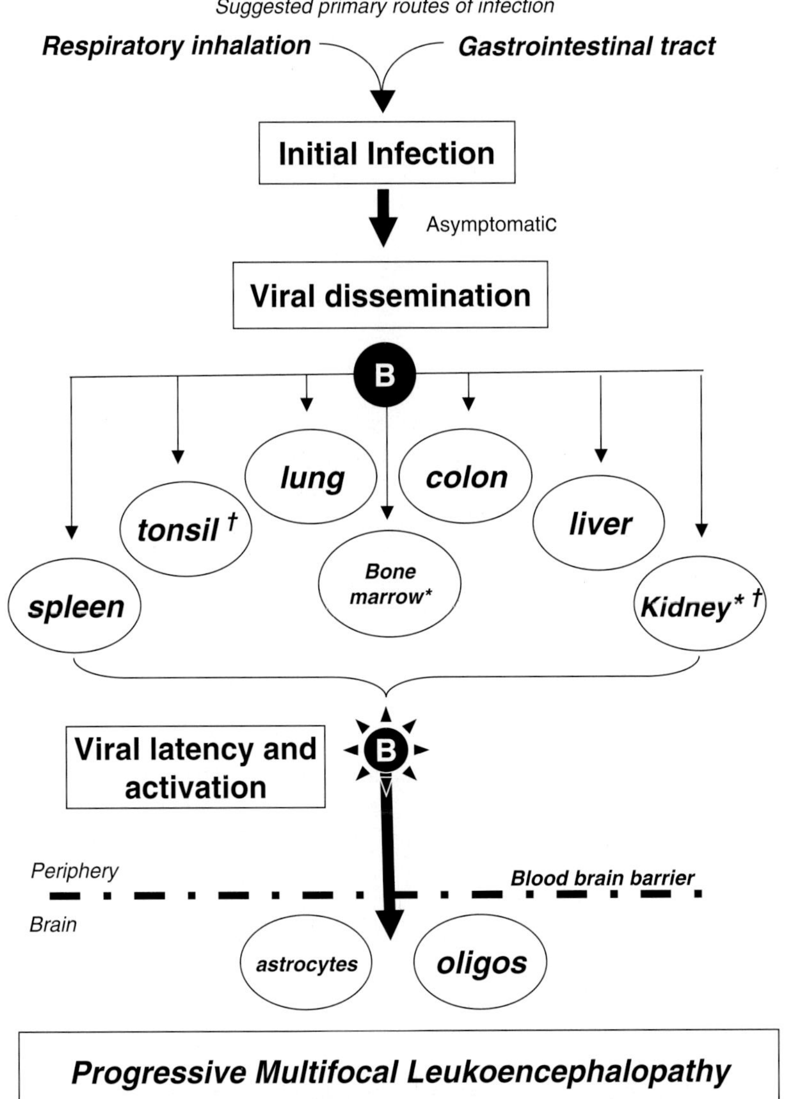


**FIGURE 40.3**
Pathogenesis of progressive multifocal leukoencephalopathy. Primary infection is followed by an extended period of latency in several anatomical compartments. Current data implicate the kidneys and bone marrow as potential sites for JCV latency (*). Active JCV replication has been demonstrated in tonsillar tissue as well as in kidney (†). Following viral activation, infected B lymphocytes may traffic the virus across the blood brain barrier and into the parenchyma of the brain, where the infection is then passed to the highly susceptible glial cell population, ultimately resulting in the pathological and clinical symptoms associated with PML.

lesions do not follow the cerebral vasculature of the brain. Microscopic examination of the plaques shows lytic destruction of oligodendrocytes, myelin degradation, but sparing of the associated axons. Active viral replication and capsid formation in infected oligodendrocytes is followed by cytolysis and viral release to surrounding cells. Susceptible cell types will follow the same pattern, resulting in a lesion where infected oligodendrocytes are concentrated at the periphery, encroaching outwards as the lesion grows. Thus, JCV is disseminated by cell-to-cell contact. Oligodendrocytes can be found throughout the lesion, often with enlarged, basophilic nuclei. Astrocytes found in this area may be hypertrophied and severely enlarged, while neurons are typically spared. In some cases, lipid-laden macrophages have been identified in the center of the lesions as well, evidence of active myelin degradation.

The mechanism behind JCV induced demyelination is primarily through the lytic infection of oligodendrocytes. However, there is some evidence that JCV large T protein may interfere with the production of myelin. Inflammatory infiltrates are rare in PML, although there is a pronounced active astrocytosis in the lesions.

## Radiographic Findings

Besides the onset of clinical symptoms, one of the first indicators of PML is a lesion visualized by CT or MRI. Lesions are often difficult to attribute to a specific disease because, radiologically, they can appear very similar. As a general rule, PML lesions are multifocal and noncontrast enhancing. The location and extent of lesioning can vary, however. As such, radiographic imaging cannot be used alone to diagnose PML.

Neuroimaging has remained one of the most important tools in studying the PML patient (Thurnher *et al.*, 1997). The noninvasive visualization of lesions is helpful for a preliminary diagnosis, especially in cases where suspected lesions are in areas where the risk of biopsy is too high. By computerized tomography (CT) scan, the demyelinated lesions appear as asymmetrically distributed subcortical areas of decreased signaling intensity. Contrast enhancement is very rarely seen, indicating an intact blood brain barrier. CT scans are limited in detecting the extent of lesions occurring deeper in the brain, such as in the cerebellum or brainstem.

Magnetic resonance imaging (MRI) is extremely sensitive in determining not only the number of lesions, but the extent as well. In fact, MRI has been shown to be more sensitive than CT in both aspects, often revealing lesions where the CT scan previously appeared normal. As such, MRI is the preferred diagnostic technique for the evaluation of potential PML cases. In contrast to the hypodense lesions seen in CT scans, demyelinated lesions appear as patchy areas of increased signal intensity by T2 weighted MRI. T1 weighted images exhibit a decrease in signal intensity, as opposed to the hyperintense T2 weighted images. T1 related decrease in signal intensity is consistent with demyelination.

Metabolic assays generally have not been of much use in studying PML because lesions tend to occur either in the myelinated white matter or at the gray white matter junction.

## Clinical Features

Viral reactivation and lytic JCV infection of oligodendrocytes can cause demyelination in any white matter tract located throughout the brain. The clinical symptoms seen in PML patients are consistent with the extent and location of subcortical white matter destruction, with no inflammatory changes in the CSF. Furthermore, the spectrum of symptoms in HIV-associated PML patients is nearly identical to that of PML associated with other underlying immune deficiencies. The most common presenting symptoms are known collectively as the "triad," which include a progressive deterioration of visual, motor, and cognitive functions. In HIV associated PML cases, the onset of neurological signs and symptoms may actually precede a diagnosis of AIDS in HIV infected patients and has been added to the list of AIDS defining illnesses.

The most common presenting ailments are motor abnormalities. By the time of diagnosis, the majority of patients will exhibit signs of moderate to severe weakness, which typically affects limbs on one side of the body (hemiparesis). Gait abnormalities (Berger and Major, 1999) or difficulty performing routine motor tasks are often accompanied by complaints of lethargy or impaired movement of the arms and legs. Visual deficits also account for a significant percentage of presenting symptoms. The severity of the symptoms often correlate with the extent of lesioning. Hemianopsia, or blindness in one-half the visual field in each eye is common.

Predictors of longer survival time with PML include lack of clinical progression during the first 2 months of treatment (De Luca *et al.*, 2001), contrast enhancement and mass effect (Berger, 2000) in HIV patients, concomitant treatment with HAART and importantly, low JCV virus levels in the CSF (Yiannoutsos *et al.*, 1999).

## Treatment and Immune Deficiency

There is no established therapy, as yet, for the effective treatment of PML. Although there have been isolated reports in individual patients, large-scale studies have been difficult to conduct, due to the limited number of possible test subjects. Attempts to treat the disease have traditionally been aimed at curing the underlying immune deficit, thereby alleviating symptoms of opportunistic infections. Therapies aimed specifically against JCV have also been investigated, but with mixed results. Such antiviral therapies are difficult due to the fact that the drugs not only interfere with the virus but also with the normal functioning of the host cell.

Cytarabine, or Ara-C, is a nucleoside, well established as a chemotherapeutic agent to treat various malignant disorders, but has also been reported to be beneficial in the treatment of PML patients. Positive case reports, in addition to preliminary results suggesting that the drug may have some activity against JCV in primary human cells *in vitro* (Hou and Major, 1998), prompted the undertaking of ACTG 243, the largest clinical trial, as yet, for any opportunistic infection associated with AIDS. HIV infected, biopsy proven PML patients were administered Ara-C, either intravenously or intrathecally, with or without concomitant antiretroviral therapy. Patients were monitored for clinical signs and viral load during treatment. The results from this trial showed that the administration of Ara-C resulted in no statistical difference between the outcome of treated patients to untreated controls (Hall *et al.*, 1998). However, this and other trials investigating Ara-C resulted in data showing the prognostic value of JC viral load in the CSF. Patients with a reduction in the levels of virus present in the CSF had a significant increase in survival time (De Luca *et al.*, 1999; Yiannoutsos *et al.*, 1999).

Cidofovir is an antiviral agent that is active against a broad spectrum of human DNA viruses, best documented in the treatment of cytomegalovirus (CMV) retinitis, a significant complication in AIDS patients, or genital herpes. There have been several reports of success in treating AIDS-related PML with the drug, particulary in European countries. Although failures have been reported, the addition of cidofovir to preexisting antiretroviral therapy in AIDS patients seemed to have improved the symptoms of PML, even in cases where the course of the disease worsened despite highly active antiretroviral therapy (Portilla *et al.*, 2000). Significant radiological improvements, marked by decreases in the extent of lesions, have also been reported in response to cidofovir therapy (Cardenas *et al.*, 2001). In contrast, the results from the only clinical trial specifically using cidofovir in relation to PML, ACTG protocol 363, were far less encouraging. Reported at the $8^{th}$ Conference on Retroviruses and Opportunistic Infections, the preliminary statistical analysis revealed no difference in prognosis between patients receiving cidofovir and those without (Marra *et al.*, 2002).

Since the beginning of the AIDS pandemic, the most common underlying immune deficit resulting in PML has been HIV infection. Combination retroviral therapy also known as highly active anti-retroviral therapy or HAART has been frequently reported to increase the immune status, clinical and radiological symptoms, and survival times in some PML patients (Inui *et al.*, 1999). The presence of JCV in the CSF or the initiation of a JCV-specific humoral intrathecal response have been used as markers for viral replication and immune status, both of which may possess prognostic value for the progression of PML. This is particularly true with the advent of HAART therapy, which in multicenter analyses has been successfully correlated with longer survival.

However, despite prolonged survival, HAART did not always halt the rapid neurological deterioration of PML, suggesting that early intervention with a drug specific for JCV will be necessary to stabilize the destruction of the white matter (Gasnault *et al.*, 1999). Similar case reports have also shown that patients can develop PML while on HAART therapy, and that a decrease in HIV viral load and increase in CD4+ cell counts does not always correlate with resolution of neurological symptoms, again emphasizing the need for a definitive antiviral treatment (Tantisiriwat *et al.*, 1999). It also appears that the initiation of HAART therapy in patients with a high JC viral load at the time of diagnosis does not have a significant effect on the surival of the patients following treatment, whereas patients with median or low viral loads at diagnosis do have prolonged survival on HAART (Taoufik *et al.*, 2000).

One recently completed study retrospectively analyzed a series of PML patients being treated with HAART in three northern Italian neurological clinics. The trial revealed that although approximately 50 percent of the patients did show disease stabilization and longer survival in response to HAART, the rapid immune reconstitution could speed the progression of PML as a result of the circulation of lymphocytes that are actively infected by JCV (Cinque *et al.*, 2001).

### Conclusions

PML is the only human demyelinating disease with a known direct viral infection of oligodendrocytes. It remains a challenge to understand how a virus with such a widespread presence in the normal human population can be targeted so specifically to oligodendrocytic destruction in the brain of immune compromised individuals. Once considered exceedingly rare, PML has been given much attention recently due to the continual rise in the incidence of AIDS and other immunosuppressive disorders due to chemotherapy in cancer patients and preventative measures against graft rejection in transplant recipients. Since the majority of the population has already been infected with JCV, and a significant percentage of AIDS patients will develop the disease, it is critically important to establish an effective treatment regimen and develop methods to screen severely immunocompromised patients for the potential risk of developing PML.

## MULTIPLE SCLEROSIS

### Definition

Although the plaques of MS on gross brain and spinal cord specimens had been previously described, the clinical complex of multifocal remitting and relapsing disease and pathological correlation with plaques of sclerosis was made by Charcot in 1868. In keeping with his times, he postulated that exposure to cold, physical injury or emotional stress caused the disease. Over the next 15 years, Koch and Pasteur laid the foundations of microbiology and immunology, so it is not surprising that in 1884 Pierre Marie, a student and successor of Charcot as Professor of Neurology in Paris, proposed a microbial cause of MS. Indeed, in the afterglow of Pasteur's discovery of a post-exposure vaccine to protect against rabies, Marie prematurely predicted that a vaccine would soon be available for MS.

Speculation concerning an infectious agent as a cause of MS has recurred over the past century but has gained greater credence over the past 50 years because of three areas of investigation: (1) epidemiologic studies have suggested that MS results, in part, from a childhood environmental exposure followed by a long latency; (2) studies of viral diseases of animals and humans have documented that infections can have long incubation periods, give rise to relapsing and remitting courses, and cause demyelination; (3) studies of patients with MS have consistently shown abnormal immune responses to viral antigens, particularly the intrathecal synthesis of antibodies to viral antigens.

MS is defined as a demyelinating disease of the CNS with lesions separated in space and time and *in which other diagnoses have been ruled out*. Before the recovery of *Borellia burgdorferi* or the human T-cell lymphotropic virus, some cases of Lyme disease and tropical spastic paraparesis fell within the definition of MS. We may view these observations from two perspectives: (1) in the past we made erroneous diagnoses now corrected by greater knowledge or (2) what we define as MS may have multiple causes and manifestations, and with more specific diagnoses the syndrome will become better and more narrowly defined.

The epidemiology, pathology, and clinical features of MS are comprehensively covered in other chapters. Discussion in this chapter will focus on features suggesting possible infectious causes.

## Epidemiology

### *Geographic and Ethnic Distribution*

The prevalence of MS is highly variable, dependent on geography and ethnicity. The prevalence of over 200 per 100,000 in the Shetland and Orkney Islands of the North Atlantic contrasts with prevalences approaching 1 per 100,000 in areas of Africa. This variance is not explained by clinical sophistication or quality of health care as once believed. Even within Europe and North America a north/south gradient or zones exist with higher incidence related to higher latitude. This appears to be reflected in the Southern Hemisphere, where the incidence of MS is higher in southern than northern areas of Australia and higher on the south than the north island of New Zealand (Kurtzke, 1993).

In Northern Europe, Canada, and the Northern United States, prevalence rates are high and range from 30 to 80 cases per 100,000. In Southern Europe and the Southern United States, moderate rates of 6 to 29 are usual. Low prevalence rates are defined as those below 5 per 100,000 and prevail in Northern South America and all known areas of Africa and Asia. Remarkable exceptions to the general correlation of latitude to prevalence are exemplified by the absence of MS in Eskimos, and a prevalence in excess of 150 per 100,000 in Sardinia (Montomoli *et al.*, 2002). The incidence of MS is clearly tied to geography, but whether this reflects immigration routes of Northern Europeans carrying susceptibility genes, or whether it reflects regional exposure still provokes controversy.

MS is more common in women than men in all regions, which supports the postulated immune-mediated pathogenesis. Distribution among racial groups is also unequal; it is more common in whites than Asians, and more common in Asians than African Americans. This supports genetic factors in causation, but it is difficult to accredit this solely to genetic factors since the prevalence in non-whites in the United States increases with increasing latitude, implicating the importance of environmental agents (Lowis, 1988). MS prevalence also correlates to a lesser extent with higher socioeconomic class and urbanization.

Little data are available to determine whether the prevalence of MS has increased over time. The increasing identification of occasional cases in those ethnic group previously thought to be spared from the disease (native-born Andeans residents, black South Africans, Eastern European gypsies, etc.) may represent better medical care and availability of imaging or may represent a genuine spread of MS to previously unaffected populations. In Rochester, Minnesota, a stable rate was noted for many years and a more recent survey showed a striking rise (Wynn *et al.*, 1990). Prevalence data are hard to compare, since the earlier diagnosis and longer survival increase prevalence rates and incidence rates are less accessible

### *Familial Aggregation and Genetics*

The risk of MS is significantly increased in the siblings and progeny of MS patients. This is striking in twins where the Canadian study has shown monozygotic twins had a concordance rate of 30.8% and dizygotic sex-alike twins had a concordance rate of 4.7% (Sadovnick *et al.*, 1993). This strengthens the long recognized genetic component of causation; however, 70% of the monozygotic twins were discordant suggesting important nongenetic factors. The Canadian study subsequently evaluated adopted, nonbiological relatives and could find little effect of shared environment (Ebers *et al.*, 1995).

### *Migration Studies*

Studies of populations migrating from high-risk regions to low-risk regions and studies of patterns of disease on North Atlantic islands have provided the strongest support for the role of a childhood exposure followed by a long incubation period. These investigations began after World War II when Dean (1970) observed that the majority of patients with MS in South Africa were immigrants from the United Kingdom or Northern Europe, even though they made up less that 10% of the population. He determined a prevalence of 50 per 100,000 in this population, compared with 11 per 100,000 in native born English-speaking South Africans, 3 per 100,000 in white Africaans speaking natives, and absence of MS in black, native-born South Africans. Further analysis showed that migration prior to age 15 years led to a risk similar to that of native born English South Africans; and migration as an adult resulted in a risk similar to that of the country of origin (Dean and Kurtzke, 1971). Similar risk of early life exposure for migrants have been reported from Israel, Australia, Hawaii, and the Antilles. Recent studies of migrants from the United Kingdom and Ireland to varied latitudes in Australia showed prevalence in migrants was considerably less than their country of origin, but did not show a shift at age 15, suggesting that environmental factors may operate over a period of many years and not only in childhood (Hammond *et al.*, 2000). Studies of migrants from low risk regions to high risk regions suggest a similar phenomenon but are less complete.

Similar evidence of early life exposure is provided by studies of World War II veterans. In the United States, residence at birth and military induction showed a sharp north to south differential in risk for MS. Residence after induction and at the onset of disease showed no geographic correlation indicating that risk was acquired prior to conscription (Beebe *et al.*, 1967).

### *Apparent Epidemics*

Continental incidence rates appear rather stable, but studies of island populations of Norse ancestry in the North Atlantic have shown fluctuations suggesting epidemics. Prevalence rates on the Shetland and Orkney Islands repeatedly showed the highest rates worldwide, but the breakdown of incidences of new cases per year show an abrupt upsurge in the late 1930s, and an equally sudden decline in new cases in 1971, suggesting an epidemic during the intervening 3 decades (Kurtzke, 2000)

The data from the Faeroe Islands are even more dramatic. No cases of MS were documented prior to 1943; then 16 patients had onsets between 1943 and 1949 with three subsequent waves of cases. The onset of the initial outbreak coincided with the British occupation of the islands from 1940 to 1945, and detailed analysis showed a spatial relationship between villages where MS patients lived and where British troops had been quartered. The studies in the Faeroes have concluded that MS is not only an acquired disease but that it is a transmissible disease (Kurtzke, 2000).

MS has long been recognized in Iceland, but a reexamination of their rates show a rise in incidence in 1922, which plateaued until 1945 when a rise in incidence occurred over the subsequent decade. Again this followed the occupation by American, Canadian, and British military forces.

### *Epidemiological Evidence of a Specific Virus*

Although late childhood or adolescent infection with a virus, followed by a long incubation has been suggested by epidemiological investigations, very little data implicate a specific agent. A number of reports confirm that measles and other common childhood infections occur at a more advanced age in MS patients than in controls (Bachmann and Kesselring, 1998). A history of infectious mononucleosis is more frequent in MS patients, indicating later infection, since infections with the ubiquitous EB virus are generally asymptomatic in children and manifest with mononucleosis only when infections is delayed until adolescence and young adult life. These findings favoring late acquisition of common infections simply may reflect that persons who develop MS may have had more sheltered childhoods.

An unexplained north to south gradient of varicella-zoster virus infection occurs with chickenpox being an almost universal disease of elementary school children in temperate zones and an infrequent disease of children in the tropics. In the tropics more adult cases, and even adult epidemics, occur (Ross, 1998). An excess of spring births of persons who develop MS has been cited to implicate an infectious etiology, but this correlation would implicate maternal or neonatal infection, which is not consistent with the migration studies.

Animal exposures have been investigated extensively. Initially, the Faeroe Island outbreak was postulated to be related to canine distemper virus, a viral infection thought to have been imported by the British officers' dogs. Subsequently a cluster of MS cases in

Sitka, Alaska, was noted to have followed a canine distemper outbreak 4 to 5 years previously (Cook and Dowling, 1982). Studies of MS patients have not confirmed antibody responses to canine distemper specific polypeptides.

### *Viral Infections and Exacerbations*

Patients often relate exacerbations of MS to psychological stress, physical trauma or physical fatigue, but prospective studies quite consistently show a relationship only with symptoms of respiratory infections (Casetta and Granieri, 2000; Marrie *et al.*, 2000). A recent study extended the findings to show that exacerbations in the contest of a systemic infections lead to more sustained damage (Buljevac et al., 2002).

A number of studies have also examined activation of human herpesviruses with exacerbations, particularly EB virus and human herpesvirus 6 (HHV6), but also active replication of herpes simplex type 1 has been associated with exacerbations (Ferrante *et al.*, 2000). The obvious dilemma in these studies is the precise timing of the onset of the exacerbation and the activation of the latent virus—that is, determining which came first.

## Pathology

Electron microscopic studies in 1964 identified papovavirus particles in inclusion bodies of PML and in 1965 identified structures resembling morbillivirus nucleocapsids in the inclusions in subacute sclerosing panencephalitis. Amid the exuberance over finding viruses by electron microscopy of poorly fixed autopsy and biopsy tissues, a number of studies reported "viruslike" particles in MS brains. The ovoid membrane bodies of 30 to 200 nm in diameter are now thought to represent myelin breakdown products, the dense intracytoplasmic granules of 60 to 80 nm diameter probably represent nonspecific changes in reactive astrocytes, and the intranuclear structures in inflammatory cells originally identified as myxovirus nucleocapsids are now believed to be nonspecific alterations in nuclear chromatin. None of these or other structures have been definitively identified as viral in nature (Johnson and Herndon, 1974).

Although the neuropathology of MS in covered in Chapter 31, one perspective of the pathology that may be relevant to causation is the heterogeneity of lesions in MS. Lucchinetti, *et al.* (2000) analyzed acute demyelinating lesions in 51 biopsies and 32 autopsies from MS patients. All cases contained at least one active lesion with inflammation, macrophages with myelin debris, and demyelination. CD3 T cells, macrophages, and occasional plasma cells characterized all patterns, but in some cases the demyelination was perivenular and in others not. Some had plaques with sharp margins, others were ill-defined. In some, oligodendrocytes persisted in demyelinated foci and remyelination was evident, in others apoptosis of oligodendrocytes was associated with wider loss of myelin associated glycoprotein. Despite this heterogeneity there was homogeneity among active lesions in the same patient. They divided the cases into four patterns, but the parallels of some to ADEM and others to PML are very suggestive of different modes of pathogenesis.

In viral diseases, consistency of a clinical-pathological syndrome does not imply a single causative agent. When lymphocytic choriomeningitis virus was recovered from spinal fluid it was regarded as *the* cause of benign aseptic meningitis, yet subsequent studies have implicated more than 100 different viruses in that syndrome. Conversely a single virus can evoke varied clinical-pathological responses such a varicella-zoster virus which can cause ADEM, Reye's disease, acute myelitis, vasculitis, and postherpetic neuralgia.

Among clinical laboratory tests, the intrathecal synthesis of IgG and the presence of spinal fluid oligoclonal bands are hallmarks of MS. Other diseases that consistently show these abnormalities are infectious processes—neurosyphilis, neuroborreliosis, subacute sclerosing panencephalitis, HTLV-1 associated myelitis, and other chronic infections. In these diseases, intrathecal antibodies can be shown to react with viral antigens; the antigen(s) in MS are unknown but the analysis of IgG heavy chain sequences in MS brains suggest an antigen driven response rather than a nonspecific B-cell activation (Smith-Jensen *et al.*, 2000).

## Virological Studies

Studies of patients with MS have implicated poxviruses, herpesviruses, rhabdoviruses, orthomyxoviruses, paramyxoviruses, coronaviruses, flaviviruses, picornaviruses, retroviruses, and a variety of unclassified or mythical agents. Several parasites and bacteria have also been implicated. Assays of antibodies in serum and in spinal fluid have consistently shown higher titers of various antibodies in MS patients than in controls, inoculations of patient fluids or tissues into cell cultures or laboratory animals have shown changes interpreted as evidence of virus replication, or finally the change in quantity or topography of an agent known to persist in humans has been interpreted as suggesting a causal relationship to MS.

### *Serological Studies*

In 1962, the first report appeared that titers of antibodies to measles virus were higher in the serum of MS patients than controls. The same antibodies were detectable in the spinal fluids of 75% of MS patients and not in spinal fluids of controls (Adams and Imagawa, 1962). Initially, these findings were regarded with skepticism, but study after study confirmed these odd findings; more than 30 confirmations have been published. Subsequently other studies showed higher titers and intrathecal synthesis of antibodies to a variety of other viruses, but never with the magnitude or consistency of measles antibodies (Tab. 40.4). In one study, 23% of patients with MS had disproportionately high antibodies to 2 or more viruses in the spinal fluid (Norrby *et al.*, 1974); in another study one patient was reported who had evidence of intrathecal synthesis of antibody to 11 different viruses (Salmi *et al.*, 1983). In general, twin studies have shown higher levels in antibody in the serum or spinal fluid of the affected twin than of the healthy twin (Kinnunen *et al.*, 1990).

The range of responses has suggested a nonspecific activation of B cells, but responses against one protein of a virus and not another (Nath and Wolinsky, 1990), and studies of the antibody variable regions suggest a more specific response. The finding of higher serum antibody titers to measles is not specific to MS. Similar higher titers have been reported in systemic lupus erythematosus, chronic hepatitis, and Reiter syndrome. In MS, as in these other diseases, individual levels of antimeasles antibody are not remarkable, as they are in subacute sclerosing panencephalitis, but the mean titer of large group of patients is consistently higher than the mean of a group of matched controls. Furthermore, measles infection is not a prerequisite to MS, since cases of MS have been observed, presenting prior to the acquisition of measles.

**TABLE 40.4 Higher Antiviral Antibodies in Multiple Sclerosis Than in Controls**

| Serum | CSF |
|---|---|
| *Measles* | *Measles* |
| Parainfluenza 3 | Parainfluenza 1, 2, 3 |
| Influenza C | Influenza A, B |
| Varicella | Varicella |
| Herpes simplex | Herpes simplex |
| Human herpes virus—6 | Human herpes virus 6 |
| Epstein-Barr | Epstein-Barr |
| Rubella | Rubella |
| | Mumps |
| | Respiratory syncytial |
| | Coronaviruses |
| | Adenoviruses |
| Borna disease virus | Borna disease virus |
| HTLV-I (gag) | HTLV-I (gag) |
| HTLV-II | Simian Virus-5 |

Modified from Johnson (1998).

### *Isolation Reports*

Recovery of agents from MS has a colorful history. During the first half of the 20th century extensive interest was given a putative spirochete. In 1917, the agent was claimed to have been recovered from the spinal fluid of patients with MS inoculated into guinea pigs and rabbits. In 1952, direct staining of the agent in brain and spinal cord led to its naming as *Spirochaeta myelophthora* (Steiner, 1952). Interest was rekindled in 1957 with further claims of cultivation of spirochetes from spinal fluids (Ichelson, 1957), claims that later reports failed to confirm. This controversy was finally settled by extensive negative results using the precise methods recommended for cultivation but substituting autoclaved water (Kurtzke *et al.*, 1962).

In the 1930s in England, an organism tentatively named *Spherula insularis*, possibly a Mycoplasma, was reported to have been isolated from spinal fluid of 176 of 189 patients with MS (Chevassut, 1930). A vaccine was made, and more than 100 patients were given the vaccine prior to an abrupt retraction (Purves-Stewart, 1931). In 1956, *Toxoplasma gondii* was alleged to have been isolated from spinal fluid and blood of MS patients, but that too went unconfirmed. A number of claims of transmission to primates and other animals were made, but agents were not characterized and results remained unconfirmed (Johnson, 1985).

The first recovery of a virus that evoked serious consideration was the 1946 Soviet claim of recovery of a virus in mice inoculated with spinal fluid and brain tissue of two patients with MS (Margulis *et al.*, 1946). The virus was shown independently to be rabies virus; whether the patient diagnosis was wrong or the agents were laboratory contaminants was unknown. No laboratories confirmed the isolations, although the original laboratory reported subsequent similar isolations.

In 1964, herpes simplex virus was recovered from the spinal fluid of a patient with MS (Gudnadottir *et al.*, 1964). This virus subsequently was shown to be a type 2 herpes simplex strain; the type that has subsequently be isolated frequently from spinal fluid in recurrent meningitis. This may also represent the first isolation of "normal flora" from MS specimens and the beginning of the persistent question of cause or effect.

Some of the viruses on Table 40.5 have subsequently been retracted as laboratory contaminants (scrapie and measles), some are thought to represent animal viruses recovered from inoculated laboratory animals (chimpanzee cytomegalovirus and corona-

**TABLE 40.5 Viruses Recovered from Patients with Multiple Sclerosis (MS)**

| | |
|---|---|
| Rabies virus | 1946<br>1964 |
| Herpes simplex virus, type 2 | 1964 |
| Scrapie agent | 1965 |
| MS-associated agent | 1972 |
| Parainfluenza virus 1 | 1972 |
| Measles virus | 1972 |
| Simian virus 5 | 1978 |
| Chimpanzee cytomegalovirus | 1979 |
| Coronavirus | 1980 |
| SMON-like virus | 1982 |
| Tick-borne encephalitis flavivirus | 1982 |
| HTLV-I | 1985 |
| LM7 (retrovirus) | 1989 |
| Herpes simplex virus, type 1 | 1989 |
| Human herpesvirus 6 | 1994 |
| Endogenous retroviruses | 1998 |

HTLV, human T-cell lymphotrophic virus, SMON, subacute myelo-optico-neuropathy.

virus), and some probably do not represent viruses but only laboratory observations interpreted as representing viral activity not verified in independent laboratories (MS-associated agent and SMON virus). A critique of these reported isolations previously has been published (Johnson, 1998).

During the National Institutes of Health studies of slow infections, tissues from MS patients were inoculated into chimpanzees. No evidence of transmission has been observed over the subsequent 30 years. This is not definitive evidence against a viral cause, however. During those studies tissue from PML and subacute sclerosing panencephalitis, diseases now known to be caused by viruses, were similarly inoculated into chimpanzees with negative long-term observations.

### *Agents of Current Interest*

Over the past 5 years the literature on infectious agents and MS has been dominated by studies of the herpesviruses, EB and human herpesvirus 6 (HHV6), endogenous retroviruses, and a bacterium, *Chlamydia pneumoniae*. In contrast to prior attempts to recover a unique MS virus, these all represent ubiquitous agents that persist in humans, and studies have focused on quantitation and cellular sites of infection. In each case the difficult question is whether changes are related to causation or whether replication and host cells changes are secondary to the immunological changes in MS.

***Epstein Barr virus*** Interest continues in the long postulated role of EB virus in MS. As mentioned earlier, the age of acquisition determines disease in this infection. Early life infections, as occur in tropical climes and impoverished communities, lead to immunity but no clinical illness; delayed infections in adolescence and young adult life often lead to the syndrome of infectious mononucleosis. Furthermore, even in case-controlled studies MS patients report a greater frequency of preceding infectious mononucleosis. Prevalence of antibodies to EB virus in MS patients is greater than in controls, and in most studies 100% have antibodies against EB, an extent of seropositivity unique to EB virus. A number of authors have suggested that EB infection is a prerequisite to development of MS (Ascherio and Munch, 2000; Munch *et al.*, 1998; Myhr *et al.*, 1998) Longitudinal studies have also found an association between EB virus activation and disease activity in MS patients (Wandinger *et al.*, 2000)).

There have been several reports of patients with neurological complications of primary EB virus infections who went on to develop progressive or relapsing disease subsequently diagnosed as MS (Bray *et al.*, 1992; Shaw and Alvord, 1987). One 6-year-old had 11 episodes of relapsing disease with high titers of EB antibodies. At death, the neuropathological diagnosis was typical MS, and PCR of the brain showed EB virus sequences (Pedneault *et al.*, 1992).

EB virus maintains latency in B cells, which are not present, or at least very rare, in normal nervous tissue. B cells are a feature of the inflammatory response in MS and other inflammatory and infectious diseases. Therefore, the presence of EB DNA determined by PCR may only reflect the presence of B cells; detection of viral proteins in cells or infectious virus in brain or spinal fluid are evidence of active infection, but again this could represent nonspecific activation during the attack of MS.

***Human herpesvirus 6*** HHV6 is a recently recovered human herpesvirus. The virus is ubiquitous with a 70 to 100% seroprevalence in adult populations worldwide. Two variants have been distinguished, and the B variant is the predominant cause of exanthem subitum in childhood. Encephalitis has long been a recognized complication of exanthem subitum. After primary infection, HHV6 remains latent primarily in T cells, but the virus is pleiotropic, with latency in B cells and CNS glial cells having been reported (Soldan *et al.*, 2001).

Similar with many other viruses, higher levels of serum antibodies and presence of spinal fluid antibodies to HHV6 were reported in many MS patients. In addition, HHV6 DNA was detected in spinal fluid by PCR (Wilborn *et al.*, 1994). The report by Challoner and colleagues in 1995 made HHV6 a serious candidate as the cause of MS. They found

HHV6 DNA in the majority of MS and control brains, but protein expression was primarily in MS brains. Furthermore, immunocytochemical staining showed positive meningeal cells in both groups, but in MS lesions there was staining of cells adjacent to the plaques thought to be neurons and oligodendrocytes. Many conflicting publications have followed. HHV6 IgM in serum and spinal fluid, higher titers of antibodies in serum, and higher frequency of antibody in spinal fluid have all been reported in MS patients compared to controls; and all of these findings have been refuted in other studies. More frequent detection of HHV6 DNA in peripheral blood mononuclear cells, serum, spinal fluid, and brain of MS patients have been reported; and again others have failed to confirm the claims. In one study of lymphoproliferative responses to HHV6 antigens by MS patients, more frequent responses of patients was found to the A variant, although most data has implicated the B variant (Soldan *et al.*, 2000).

Several reported results raise a need for confirmation or extension. One group reported immunocytochemical staining in 90% of sections showing active demyelinating lesions and only 13% in tissue sections free of active disease (Knox *et al.*, 2000); this level of sensitivity and specificity is unique among reports. Recently elevated serum and spinal fluid levels of membrane cofactor protein CD46 were reported in MS patients; this is important because CD46 is a receptor for HHV6 (as well as measles, the traditionally most implicated virus) and is a regulator of the complement cascade involved in antibody mediated immunopathology (Soldan *et al.*, 2001). This provocative finding may lead to new mechanisms by which viruses might evoke in immune-mediated diseases.

*Endogenous retroviruses* Human endogenous retroviruses (HERVs) are DNA sequences present within human chromosomes and make up about 2% of the human genome. The characteristic presence of long terminal repeats followed by *gag, pol, and env* genes identify their retroviral origins; they are thought to represent ancestral infections in which integrated DNA is now passed on in Mendelian fashion. Comparisons to ERVs of apes and old world monkeys suggest that some entered our genome 25 million years ago (Voisset *et al.*, 1999). HERVs are defective in that they do not code infectious particles or transmit horizontally. Some do encode functional proteins, and complementation may result in virion formation.

No endogenous retroviruses have been convincingly associated with human disease. The potential to enhance downstream cellular genes has led to speculation that they might be involved in autoimmune disease. They have been proposed as factors in the pathogenesis of MS, systemic lupus erythematosus, Sjogren's disease, and type 1 diabetes (Perron and Seigneurin, 1999).

In 1991 a retrovirus was reported budding from a cell line of meningeal cells established from the spinal fluid of a patient with MS (Perron *et al.*, 1991). Subsequently, C-type retrovirus particles were found in peripheral blood mononuclear cells cultured from several patients with MS, but this proved to be a different HERV (Christensen *et al.*, 1998).

Several recent studies suggest that increased expression of these viruses is a consequence of immune activity rather than the cause. Johnston *et al.* (2001) showed that levels of HERV RNA increased in cultured macrophages nonspecifically stimulated *in vitro*; several HERVs were also expressed in brain tissue of patients with human immunodeficiency virus infections and with MS, correlating with tumor necrosis factor expression and macrophage activation. In another study (Dolei *et al.*, 2002), analysis of blood for HERV reported detection in all MS patients, most patients with other inflammatory neurological disease and rarely in healthy donors. The role of these viruses as cofactors rather than simply secondary responders remains unclear.

*Chlamydia pneumoniae* *C. pneumoniae* is an obligate intracellular Gram-negative bacterium. It is a common respiratory pathogen causing pharyngitis, bronchitis and atypical pneumonia. Seroprevalence is 40 to 70% in adults, with most seroconversions occurring during adolescence. Numerous attempts to relate *C. pneumoniae* to chronic disease have been made, most notably coronary artery disease and atherosclerosis. Because the bacteria persist in human macrophages, PCR studies of tissues with macrophage infiltrates often are positive.

After observing a single patient with apparent acute MS from whom *C. pneumonia* was recovered from spinal fluid and who improved with antibiotic therapy, the Vanderbilt group undertook an extensive study. From spinal fluid of MS patients, they cultured *C. pneumoniae* from 64% but recovered bacteria from only 11% of spinal fluids from patients with other diseases. PCR was positive in 97% compared to 18% in control patients. Spinal fluid IgG directed against the bacterium was found in 97%, compared to 18% with other neurological diseases (Sriram *et al.*, 1999). Subsequently they reported that oligoclonal bands in spinal fluids of patients with MS not only reacted with *C. pneumoniae* antigens (116 of 17 patients) but could be partially or completely adsorbed by antigens (Yao *et al.*, 2001). A large number of contradictory reports have followed. Some have been confirmatory to some facets, but none with the high percentages of the initial report; the majority have been negative A recent report, for example, using PCR detected *C. pneumoniae* in spinal fluid of 21% of MS patients, in 43% of patients with other neurological diseases, and in no healthy controls (Gieffers *et al.*, 2001). This would suggest that inflammatory responses that recruit macrophages into the spinal fluid, where under normal circumstances they are not found, can carry in C. *pneumonia*. Better standardization of both cultivation and PCR methods are needed before fair comparisons of studies can be made.

## SUMMARY

It is clear that a diverse array of viruses can infect the human central nervous system. The resulting viral infections can result in a wide variety of clinical and pathological symptoms. While some viruses may cause widespread inflammation and neurodegeneration, other viruses may remain latent in the CNS and only produce pathological changes during reactivation. Viral induced demyelination can occur both from direct infection of the myelin-producing oligodendrocytes, as in PML, or by indirect mechanisms that have yet to be determined. The final outcome of a viral CNS infection will depend not only on viral characteristics, but also the interaction between virus and host cell. Understanding factors such as immune modulation and host cell regulation of viral gene expression could improve current methods of diagnosis or even lead to innovative methods for therapeutic intervention.

### References


Adams C, Diadori P, *et al.* (2000). Autoantibodies in childhood post-varicella acute cerebellar ataxia. *Can J Neurol Sci* **27,** 316–320.

Adams JM, Imagawa DT (1962). Measles antibodies in multiple sclerosis. *Proc Soc Exp Biol Med* **111.**

Agostini HT, Ryschkewitsch CF, *et al.* (1996). Genotype profile of human polyomavirus JC excreted in urine of immunocompetent individuals. *J Clin Microbiol* **34,** 159–164.

Aksamit AJ, Jr. (1995). Progressive multifocal leukoencephalopathy: A review of the pathology and pathogenesis. *Microsc Res Tech* **32,** 302–311.

Ascherio A, Munch M (2000). Epstein-Barr virus and multiple sclerosis. *Epidemiology* **11,** 220–224.

Astrom KE, Mancall EL, *et al.* (1958). Progressive Multifocal Leukoencephalopathy. *Brain* **81,** 93–127.

Ault GS (1997). Activity of JC virus archetype and PML-type regulatory regions in glial cells. *J Gen Virol* **78 (Pt 1),** 163–169.

Bachmann S, Kesselring J (1998). Multiple sclerosis and infectious childhood diseases. *Neuroepidemiology* **17,** 154–160.

Beebe GW, Kurtzke JF, *et al.* (1967). Studies on the natural history of multiple sclerosis. 3. Epidemiologic analysis of the army experience in World War II. *Neurology* **17,** 1–17.

Behan PO, Geschwind N, *et al.* (1968). Delayed hypersensitivity to encephalitogenic protein in disseminated encephalomyelitis. *Lancet* **2,** 1009–1012.

Berger JR (2000). Progressive Multifocal Leukoencephalopathy. *Curr Treat Options Neurol* **2,** 361–368.

Berger JR, Major EO (1999). Progressive Multifocal Leukoencephalopathy. *In* "Textbook of AIDS Medicine" (T.C. Merigan, J. G. Bartlett, and D. Bolognesi, eds.), pp. 403–419. Williams and Wilkins, Baltimore.

Boe J, Solberg CO, *et al.* (1965). Corticosteroid treatment of acute meningoencephalitis: A retrospective study of 346 cases. *Br Med J* **1,** 1094–1095.

Bray PF, Culp KW, *et al.* (1992). Demyelinating disease after neurologically complicated primary Epstein-Barr virus infection. *Neurology* **42,** 278–282.

Brooks BR (1979). Virus-associated neurological syndromes. *In* "Diagnosis of Viral Infections" (D. Lennette, S. Spector, and K. Thompson, eds.), pp. 183–203. University Park Press. Baltimore, Maryland.

Brown P, Tsai T, *et al.* (1975). Seroepidemiology of human papovaviruses. Discovery of virgin populations and some unusual patterns of antibody prevalence among remote peoples of the world. *Am J Epidemiol* **102,** 331–340.

Buljevac, D., Flach, H. Z., Hop, W. C., Hijdra, D., Laman, J. D., Savelkoul, H. F., van Der Meche, F. G., van Doorn, P. A., Hintzen, R. O. (2002). Prospective study on the relationship between infections and multiple sclerosis exacerbations. *Brain* **125**, 952–960.

Cardenas RL, Cheng KH, *et al.* (2001). The effects of cidofovir on progressive multifocal leukoencephalopathy: An MRI case study. *Neuroradiology* **43,** 379–382.

Carswell S, Alwine JC (1986). Simian virus 40 agnoprotein facilitates perinuclear-nuclear localization of VP1, the major capsid protein. *J Virol* **60,** 1055–1061.

Casetta I, Granieri E (2000). Clinical infections and multiple sclerosis: Contribution from analytical epidemiology. *J Neurovirol* **6 Suppl 2,** S147–151.

Chevassut K (1930). The etiology of disseminated sclerosis. *Lancet* **1,** 552–560.

Christensen T, Dissing Sorensen P, *et al.* (1998). Expression of sequence variants of endogenous retrovirus RGH in particle form in multiple sclerosis. *Lancet* **352,** 1033.

Cinque P, Pierotti C, *et al.* (2001). The good and evil of HAART in HIV-related progressive multifocal leukoencephalopathy. *J Neurovirol* **7,** 358–363.

Cole CN (1996). Polyomavirinae: The viruses and their replication. *In "Fields Virolog"* (B. N. Fields, D. M. Knipe, and P. M. Howley, eds.), pp 1997–2025. Lippincott-Raven, Philadelphia.

Cook SD, Dowling PC (1982). Distemper and multiple sclerosis in Sitka, Alaska. *Ann Neurol* **11,** 192–194.

De Luca A, Giancola ML, *et al.* (1999). Clinical and virological monitoring during treatment with intrathecal cytarabine in patients with AIDS-associated progressive multifocal leukoencephalopathy. *Clin Infect Dis* **28,** 624–628.

De Luca A, Giancola ML, *et al.* (2001). Potent anti-retroviral therapy with or without cidofovir for AIDS-associated progressive multifocal leukoencephalopathy: Extended follow-up of an observational study. *J Neurovirol* **7,** 364–368.

Dean G (1970). The multiple sclerosis problem. *Sci Am* **223,** 40–46.

Dean G, Kurtzke JF (1971). On the risk of multiple sclerosis according to age at immigration to South Africa. *Br Med J* **3,** 725–729.

DeVries E (1960). "Postvaccinal Perivenous Encephalitis." Elsevier Science, Amsterdam.

Dolei A, Serra C, *et al.* (2002). Multiple sclerosis-associated retrovirus (MSRV) in Sardinian MS patients. *Neurology* **58,** 471–473.

Ebers GC, Sadovnick AD, *et al.* (1995). A genetic basis for familial aggregation in multiple sclerosis. Canadian Collaborative Study Group. *Nature* **377,** 150–151.

Esolen LM, Takahashi K, *et al.* (1995). Brain endothelial cell infection in children with acute fatal measles. *J Clin Invest* **96,** 2478–2481.

Fanning E (1992). Simian virus 40 large T antigen: The puzzle, the pieces, and the emerging picture. *J Virol* **66,** 1289–1293.

Feigenbaum L, Hinrichs SH, *et al.* (1992). JC virus and simian virus 40 enhancers and transforming proteins: Role in determining tissue specificity and pathogenicity in transgenic mice. *J Virol* **66,** 1176–1182.

Feigenbaum L, Khalili K, *et al.* (1987). Regulation of the host range of human papovavirus JCV. *Proc Natl Acad Sci U S A* **84,** 3695–3698.

Ferrante P, Mancuso R, *et al.* (2000). Molecular evidences for a role of HSV-1 in multiple sclerosis clinical acute attack. *J Neurovirol* **6 Suppl 2,** S109–114.

Frisque RJ, Bream GL, *et al.* (1984). Human polyomavirus JC virus genome. *J Virol* **51,** 458–469.

Fujinami RS, Oldstone MB (1985). Amino acid homology between the encephalitogenic site of myelin basic protein and virus: Mechanism for autoimmunity. *Science* **230,** 1043–1045.

Gasnault J, Taoufik Y, *et al.* (1999). Prolonged survival without neurological improvement in patients with AIDS-related progressive multifocal leukoencephalopathy on potent combined antiretroviral therapy. *J Neurovirol* **5,** 421–429.

Gautier-Smith PC (1965). Neurological complications of glandular fever (infectious mononucleosis). *Brain* **88,** 323–334.

Gendelman HE, Pezeshkpour GH, *et al.* (1985). A quantitation of myelin-associated glycoprotein and myelin basic protein loss in different demyelinating diseases. *Ann Neurol* **18,** 324–328.

Gendelman HE, Wolinsky JS, *et al.* (1984). Measles encephalomyelitis: Lack of evidence of viral invasion of the central nervous system and quantitative study of the nature of demyelination. *Ann Neurol* **15,** 353–360.

Gibbs FA, Gibbs EL, *et al.* (1959). Electroencephalographic abnormality i "uncomplicated" childhood diseases. *JAMA* **171,** 1050–1055.

Gieffers J, Pohl D, *et al.* (2001). Presence of Chlamydia pneumoniae DNA in the cerebral spinal fluid is a common phenomenon in a variety of neurological diseases and not restricted to multiple sclerosis. *Ann Neurol* **49,** 585–589.

Gollomp SM, Fahn S (1987). Transient dystonia as a complication of varicella. *J Neurol Neurosurg Psychiatry* **50,** 1228–1229.

Gudnadottir M, Helgadottir H, *et al.* (1964). Virus isolated from the brain of a patient with multiple sclerosis. *Exp Neurol* **9,** 85–95.

Hall CD, Dafni U, *et al.* (1998). Failure of cytarabine in progressive multifocal leukoencephalopathy associated with human immunodeficiency virus infection. AIDS Clinical Trials Group 243 Team. *N Engl J Med* **338,** 1345–1351.

Hallervorden J (1930). Eigennartige und nicht rubriziebare Prozesse. *In* "Hadbuch der Geiteskranheiten" (O. Bumke, ed.), pp 1063–1107. Springer, Berlin.

Hammond SR, English DR, *et al.* (2000). The age-range of risk of developing multiple sclerosis: Evidence from a migrant population in Australia. *Brain* **123 (Pt 5),** 968–974.

Hart MN, Earle KM (1975). Haemorrhagic and perivenous encephalitis: A clinical-pathological review of 38 cases. *J Neurol Neurosurg Psychiatry* **38,** 585–591.

Hartung HP, Grossman RI (2001). ADEM: Distinct disease or part of the MS spectrum? *Neurology* **56,** 1257–1260.

Hemachudha T, Griffin DE, *et al.* (1988). Immunologic studies of patients with chronic encephalitis induced by post-exposure Semple rabies vaccine. *Neurology* **38,** 42–44.

Herndon RM, Johnson RT, *et al.* (1974). Ependymitis in mumps virus meningitis. Electron microscopical studies of cerebrospinal fluid. *Arch Neurol* **30,** 475–479.

Hirsch RL, Griffin DE, *et al.* (1984). Cellular immune responses during complicated and uncomplicated measles virus infections of man. *Clin Immunol Immunopathol* **31,** 1–12.

Holman RC, Janssen RS, *et al.* (1991). Epidemiology of progressive multifocal leukoencephalopathy in the United States: Analysis of national mortality and AIDS surveillance data. *Neurology* **41,** 1733–1736.

Hou J, Major EO (1998). The efficacy of nucleoside analogs against JC virus multiplication in a persistently infected human fetal brain cell line. *J Neurovirol* **4,** 451–456.

Hoult JG, Flewett TH (1960). Influenza encephalopathy and post-influenzal encephalitis: Histological and other observations. *BMG* **1,** 1847–1850.

Hynson JL, Kornberg AJ, *et al.* (2001). Clinical and neuroradiologic features of acute disseminated encephalomyelitis in children. *Neurology* **56,** 1308–1312.

Ichelson RR (1957). Cultivation of spirochaetes from spinal fluids of multiple sclerosis cases and engative controls. *Proc Soc Exp Biol Med* **95,** 57–58.

Inui K, Miyagawa H, *et al.* (1999). Remission of progressive multifocal leukoencephalopathy following highly active antiretroviral therapy in a patient with HIV infection. *Brain Dev* **21,** 416–419.

Irani DN, Griffin DE (1996). Regulation of lymphocyte homing into the brain during viral encephalitis at various stages of infection. *J Immunol* **156,** 3850–3857.

Ito T, Watanabe A, *et al.* (2000). Acute disseminated encephalomyelitis developed after acute herpetic gingivostomatitis. *Tohoku J Exp Med* **192,** 151–155.

Jensen PN, Major EO (1999). Viral variant nucleotide sequences help expose leukocytic positioning in the JC virus pathway to the CNS. *J Leukoc Biol* **65,** 428–438.

Johnson RT (1968). Mumps virus encephalitis in the hamster. Studies of the inflammatory response and noncytopathic infection of neurons. *J Neuropathol Exp Neurol* **27,** 80–95.

Johnson RT (1985). Viral aspects of multiple sclerosis. *In* "Handbook of Clinical Neurology" (P. J. Vinken, G. W. Bruyn, and H. L. Klawans, eds.), pp 319–336. Elsevier Science, Amsterdam.

Johnson RT (1998). Postinfectious demyleinating diseases. *In* "Viral Infections of the Nervous System" (R. T. Johnson , ed.), pp 181–210. Lippincott-Raven, Philadelphia.

Johnson RT, Griffin DE, *et al.* (1984). Measles encephalomyelitis–clinical and immunologic studies. *N Engl J Med* **310,** 137–141.

Johnson RT, Griffin DE, *et al.* (1985). Postinfectious encephalomyelitis. *Semin Neurol* **5,** 180–190.

Johnson RT, Herndon RM (1974). Virologic studies of multiple sclerosis and other chronic and relapsing neurological diseases. *Prog Med Virol* **18,** 214–228.

Johnston JB, Silva C, *et al.* (2001). Monocyte activation and differentiation augment human endogenous retrovirus expression: Implications for inflammatory brain diseases. *Ann Neurol* **50,** 434–442.

Kabat EA, Wolfe A, *et al.* (1947). The rapid production of acute disseminated encephalomyelitis in rhesus monkey by injection of heterologous and homologous brain tissue with adjuvants. *J Exp Med* **85,** 117–130.

Karp CL, Wysocka M, *et al.* (1996). Mechanism of suppression of cell-mediated immunity by measles virus. *Science* **273,** 228–231.

Kennedy PG, Narayan O, *et al.* (1985). Persistent expression of Ia antigen and viral genome in visna-maedi virus-induced inflammatory cells. Possible role of lentivirus-induced interferon. *J Exp Med* **162,** 1970–1982.

Kinnunen E, Valle M, *et al.* (1990). Viral antibodies in multiple sclerosis. A nationwide co-twin study. *Arch Neurol* **47,** 743–746.

Knox KK, Brewer JH, *et al.* (2000). Human herpesvirus 6 and multiple sclerosis: Systemic active infections in patients with early disease. *Clin Infect Dis* **31,** 894–903.

Kurtzke JF (1993). Epidemiologic evidence for multiple sclerosis as an infection. *Clin Microbiol Rev* **6,** 382–427.

Kurtzke JF (2000). Multiple sclerosis in time and space-geographic clues to cause. *J Neurovirol* **6 Suppl 2,** S134–140.

Kurtzke JF, Martin A, *et al.* (1962). Microbiology in multiple sclerosis-evaluation of Ichelson's organism. *neurology* **12,** 915–922.

Laghi L, Randolph AE, *et al.* (1999). JC virus DNA is present in the mucosa of the human colon and in colorectal cancers. *Proc Natl Acad Sci U S A* **96,** 7484–7489.

Landrigan PJ, Witte JJ (1973). Neurologic disorders following live measles-virus vaccination. *Jama* **223,** 1459–1462.

Levin MC, Lee SM, *et al.* (2002). Autoimmunity due to molecular mimicry as a cause of neurological disease. *Nat Med* **8,** 509–513.

Levine S, Wenk EJ (1965). A hyperacute form of allergic encephalomyelitis. *Am J Pathol* **47,** 61–88.

Lisak RP, Mitchell M, *et al.* (1977). Guillain-Barre syndrome and Hodgkin's disease: Three cases with immunological studies. *Ann Neurol* **1,** 72–78.

Liu CK, Wei G, *et al.* (1998). Infection of glial cells by the human polyomavirus JC is mediated by an N-linked glycoprotein containing terminal alpha(2–6)-linked sialic acids. *J Virol* **72,** 4643–4649.

Lowis GW (1988). Ethnic factors in multiple sclerosis: A review and critique of the epidemiological literature. *Int J Epidemiol* **17,** 14–20.

Lucchinetti C, Bruck W, *et al.* (2000). Heterogeneity of multiple sclerosis lesions: Implications for the pathogenesis of demyelination. *Ann Neurol* **47,** 707–717.

Margulis MS, Soloviev VD, *et al.* (1946). Aetiology and pathogenesis of acute sporadic disseminated encephalomyelitis and multiple sclerosis. *J Neurol Neurosurg Psychiatry.*

Marra CM, Rajicic N, *et al.* (2002). A pilot study of cidofovir for progressive multifocal leukoencephalopathy in AIDS. *Aids* **16,** 1791–1797.

Marrie RA, Wolfson C, *et al.* (2000). Multiple sclerosis and antecedent infections: A case-control study. *Neurology* **54,** 2307–2310.

Marsden JP, Hurst EW (1932). Acute perivascular myelinoclasis ("acute disssemination encephalopmyelitis") in smallpox. *Brain* **55,** 181–225.

Miller HG (1953). Prognosis of neurologic illness following vaccination against smallpox. *Arch Neurol* **69,** 695–706.

Miller HG, Stanton JB (1954). Neurological sequelae of prophylactic inoculation. *Q J Med* **23,** 1–27.

Moench TR, Griffin DE, *et al.* (1988). Acute measles in patients with and without neurological involvement: Distribution of measles virus antigen and RNA. *J Infect Dis* **158,** 433–442.

Monaco MC, Jensen PN, *et al.* (1998). Detection of JC virus DNA in human tonsil tissue: Evidence for site of initial viral infection. *J Virol* **72,** 9918–9923.

Monaco MC, Sabath BF, *et al.* (2001). JC virus multiplication in human hematopoietic progenitor cells requires the NF-1 class D transcription factor. *J Virol* **75,** 9687–9695.

Montomoli C, Allemani C, *et al.* (2002). An ecologic study of geographical variation in multiple sclerosis risk in central Sardinia, Italy. *Neuroepidemiology* **21,** 187–193.

Moran AP, Prendergast MM (2001). Molecular mimicry in Campylobacter jejuni and Helicobacter pylori lipopolysaccharides: Contribution of gastrointestinal infections to autoimmunity. *J Autoimmun* **16,** 241–256.

Moreland RB, Garcea RL (1991). Characterization of a nuclear localization sequence in the polyomavirus capsid protein VP1. *Virology* **185,** 513–518.

Munch M, Riisom K, *et al.* (1998). The significance of Epstein-Barr virus seropositivity in multiple sclerosis patients? *Acta Neurol Scand* **97,** 171–174.

Myhr KM, Riise T, *et al.* (1998). Altered antibody pattern to Epstein-Barr virus but not to other herpesviruses in multiple sclerosis: A population based case-control study from western Norway. *J Neurol Neurosurg Psychiatry* **64,** 539–542.

Narciso P, Galgani S, *et al.* (2001). Acute disseminated encephalomyelitis as manifestation of primary HIV infection. *Neurology* **57,** 1493–1496.

Nath A, Wolinsky JS (1990). Antibody response to rubella virus structural proteins in multiple sclerosis. *Ann Neurol* **27,** 533–536.

Norrby E, Link H, *et al.* (1974). Comparison of antibodies against different viruses in cerebrospinal fluid and serum samples from patients with multiple sclerosis. *Infect Immun* **10,** 688–694.

Ojala A (1947). On changes in the cerebrospinal fluid during measles. *Ann Med Intern Fenn* **36,** 321–331.

Okada Y, Endo S, *et al.* (2001). Distribution and function of JCV agnoprotein. *J Neurovirol* **7,** 302–306.

Ozawa H, Noma S, *et al.* (2000). Acute disseminated encephalomyelitis associated with poliomyelitis vaccine. *Pediatr Neurol* **23,** 177–179.

Padgett BL, Walker DL (1973). Prevalence of antibodies in human sera against JC virus, an isolate from a case of progressive multifocal leukoencephalopathy. *J Infect Dis* **127,** 467–470.

Padgett BL, Walker DL, *et al.* (1971). Cultivation of papova-like virus from human brain with progressive multifocal leucoencephalopathy. *Lancet* **1,** 1257–1260.

Paskavitz JF, Anderson CA, *et al.* (1995). Acute arcuate fiber demyelinating encephalopathy following Epstein-Barr virus infection. *Ann Neurol* **38,** 127–131.

Paterson PY (1960). Transfer of allergic encephalomyelitis in rats by means of lymph node cells. *J Exp Med* **111,** 119–136.

Pedneault L, Katz BZ, *et al.* (1992). Detection of Epstein-Barr virus in the brain by the polymerase chain reaction. *Ann Neurol* **32,** 184–192.

Perron H, Lalande B, *et al.* (1991). Isolation of retrovirus from patients with multiple sclerosis. *Lancet* **337,** 862–863.

Perron H, Seigneurin JM (1999). Human retroviral sequences associated with extracellular particles in autoimmune diseases: Epiphenomenon or possible role in aetiopathogenesis? *Microbes Infect* **1,** 309–322.

Pfausler B, Engelhardt K, *et al.* (2002). Post-infectious central and peripheral nervous system diseases complicating Mycoplasma pneumoniae infection. Report of three cases and review of the literature. *Eur J Neurol* **9,** 93–96.

Pohl-Koppe A, Burchett SK, *et al.* (1998). Myelin basic protein reactive Th2 T cells are found in acute disseminated encephalomyelitis. *J Neuroimmunol* **91,** 19–27.

Portilla J, Boix V, *et al.* (2000). Progressive multifocal leukoencephalopathy treated with cidofovir in HIV-infected patients receiving highly active anti-retroviral therapy. *J Infect* **41,** 182–184.

Power C, Johnson RT (2001). Neuroimmune and neurovirological aspects of human immunodeficiency virus infection. *Adv Virus Res* **56,** 389–433.

Power C, Kong PA, *et al.* (1993). Cerebral white matter changes in acquired immunodeficiency syndrome dementia: Alterations of the blood-brain barrier. *Ann Neurol* **34,** 339–350.

Purves-Stewart J (1931). Disseminated sclerosis-experimental vaccine treatment. *Lancet* **1,** 440–441.

Richardson EP, Jr. (1974). Our evolving understanding of progressive multifocal leukoencephalopathy. *Ann N Y Acad Sci* **230,** 358–364.

Riedel K, Kempf VA, *et al.* (2001). Acute disseminated encephalomyelitis (ADEM) due to Mycoplasma pneumoniae infection in an adolescent. *Infection* **29,** 240–242.

Rivers TM, Schwentker FF (1935). Encephalomyelitis accompanied by myelin destruction experimentally produced in monkeys. *J Exp Med* **61,** 689–702.

Ross RT (1998). The varicella-zoster virus and multiple sclerosis. *J Clin Epidemiol* **51,** 533–535.

Sacconi S, Salviati L, *et al.* (2001). Acute disseminated encephalomyelitis associated with hepatitis C virus infection. *Arch Neurol* **58,** 1679–1681.

Sadovnick AD, Armstrong H, *et al.* (1993). A population-based study of multiple sclerosis in twins: Update. *Ann Neurol* **33,** 281–285.

Salmi A, Reunanen M, *et al.* (1983). Intrathecal antibody synthesis to virus antigens in multiple sclerosis. *Clin Exp Immunol* **52,** 241–249.

Schwarz GA, Yang DC, *et al.* (1968). Meningoencephalomyelitis with epidemic parotitis. *Arch Neurol* **11,** 453–462.

Shah KV, Ozer HL, *et al.* (1977). Common structural antigen of papovaviruses of the simian virus 40-polyoma subgroup. *J Virol* **21,** 179–186.

Shaw CM, Alvord EC, Jr. (1987). Multiple sclerosis beginning in infancy. *J Child Neurol* **2,** 252–256.

Silver B, McAvoy K, *et al.* (1997). Fulminating encephalopathy with perivenular demyelination and vacuolar myelopathy as the initial presentation of human immunodeficiency virus infection. *Arch Neurol* **54,** 647–650.

Smith-Jensen T, Burgoon MP, *et al.* (2000). Comparison of immunoglobulin G heavy-chain sequences in MS and SSPE brains reveals an antigen-driven response. *Neurology* **54,** 1227–1232.

Soldan SS, Fogdell-Hahn A, *et al.* (2001). Elevated serum and cerebrospinal fluid levels of soluble human herpesvirus type 6 cellular receptor, membrane cofactor protein, in patients with multiple sclerosis. *Ann Neurol* **50,** 486–493.

Soldan SS, Leist TP, *et al.* (2000). Increased lymphoproliferative response to human herpesvirus type 6A variant in multiple sclerosis patients. *Ann Neurol* **47,** 306–313.

Spillane JD, Wells CEC (1964). The neurology of Jennerian vaccination: A clinical account of the neurological complications which occurred during the smallpox epidemic in South Wales in 1962. *Brain* **87,** 1–44.

Sriram S, Stratton CW, *et al.* (1999). Chlamydia pneumoniae infection of the central nervous system in multiple sclerosis. *Ann Neurol* **46,** 6–14.

Steiner G (1952). Acute plaques in multiple sclerosis, their pathogenetic significance and role of spirochaetes as etiological factor. *J Neuropathol Exp Neurol* **11,** 343–372.

Sumner C, Shinohara T, *et al.* (1996). Expression of multiple classes of the nuclear factor-1 family in the developing human brain: Differential expression of two classes of NF-1 genes. *J Neurovirol* **2,** 87–100.

Tantisiriwat W, Tebas P, *et al.* (1999). Progressive multifocal leukoencephalopathy in patients with AIDS receiving highly active antiretroviral therapy. *Clin Infect Dis* **28,** 1152–1154.

Taoufik Y, Delfraissy JF, *et al.* (2000). Highly active antiretroviral therapy does not improve survival of patients with high JC virus load in the cerebrospinal fluid at progressive multifocal leukoencephalopathy diagnosis. *Aids* **14,** 758–759.

Thurnher MM, Thurnher SA, *et al.* (1997). Progressive multifocal leukoencephalopathy in AIDS: Initial and follow-up CT and MRI. *Neuroradiology* **39,** 611–618.

Tornatore C, Berger JR, *et al.* (1992). Detection of JC virus DNA in peripheral lymphocytes from patients with and without progressive multifocal leukoencephalopathy. *Ann Neurol* **31,** 454–462.

Tyler HR (1957). Nuerological complications of rubeola (measles). *Medicine (Baltimore)* **36,** 147–167.

Voisset C, Blancher A, *et al.* (1999). Phylogeny of a novel family of human endogenous retrovirus sequences, HERV-W, in humans and other primates. *AIDS Res Hum Retroviruses* **15,** 1529–1533.

von Pirquet C (1908). Das Verhalten der kutanen Tuberkulin-reaktion wahrend der Masern. *Dtsch Med Wochenschr* **34,** 1297–1300.

Voudris KA, Skaardoutsou A, *et al.* (2001). Brain MRI findings in influenza A-associated acute necrotizing encephalopathy of childhood. *Eur J Paediatr Neurol* **5,** 199–202.

Walker DL, Padgett BL (1983). The epidemiology of human polyomaviruses. *Prog Clin Biol Res* **105,** 99–106.

Wandinger K, Jabs W, *et al.* (2000). Association between clinical disease activity and Epstein-Barr virus reactivation in MS. *Neurology* **55,** 178–184.

Wang M, Tzeng TY, *et al.* (1999). Human anti-JC virus serum reacts with native but not denatured JC virus major capsid protein VP1. *J Virol Methods* **78,** 171–176.

Wilborn F, Schmidt CA, *et al.* (1994). A potential role for human herpesvirus type 6 in nervous system disease. *J Neuroimmunol* **49,** 213–214.

Wroblewska Z, Wellish M, *et al.* (1980). Growth of JC virus in adult human brain cell cultures. *Arch Virol* **65,** 141–148.

Wynn DR, Rodriguez M, *et al.* (1990). A reappraisal of the epidemiology of multiple sclerosis in Olmsted County, Minnesota. *Neurology* **40,** 780–786.

Yao SY, Stratton CW, *et al.* (2001). CSF oligoclonal bands in MS include antibodies against Chlamydophila antigens. *Neurology* **56,** 1168–1176.

Yiannoutsos CT, Major EO, *et al.* (1999). Relation of JC virus DNA in the cerebrospinal fluid to survival in acquired immunodeficiency syndrome patients with biopsy-proven progressive multifocal leukoencephalopathy. *Ann Neurol* **45,** 816–821.

Ziegra SR (1961). Corticosteroid treatment for measles encephalitis. *J Pediatr* **59,** 322–323.

CHAPTER

# 41

# Ischemic White Matter Damage

*Peter K. Stys and Stephen G. Waxman*

Central nervous system axons play the critical role of transmitting electrical impulses within the central nervous system (CNS) with high fidelity and reliability. The unique architecture of myelinated axons allows these structures to conduct action potentials rapidly in an energy efficient manner. A coordinated organization of axonal ion channels is required to effect this, in addition to a highly specialized myelin sheath. Together, the axonal ion channels conduct the necessary ionic currents, while the myelin sheath provides a capacitative shield that greatly reduces stray trans-axolemmal current leaks, thereby ensuring rapid, reliable, and efficient saltatory conduction (Waxman *et al.*, 1995). The highly specialized architecture of myelinated fibers renders them prone to functional disruption when any of the critical components are deranged. A variety of axonal disorders is characterized by irreversible compromise of conduction through central tracts, resulting in varying degrees of clinical disability, which depends on the severity of damage and location of the affected pathways. Common examples include acute stroke, hypoxic/ischemic white matter injury that can result in periventricular leukomalacia and cause cerebral palsy, and more chronic states such as vascular dementia from long-standing microangiopathic pathology, trauma (for example, in closed head and spinal cord injuries), and a variety of demyelinating disorders such as multiple sclerosis. Together, these disorders represent a huge personal and socio-economic burden on Western populations. We believe that a key to devising successful therapies for these disorders lies in a thorough understanding of the fundamental mechanisms of ischemic CNS injury. While white matter injury mechanisms share a number of common steps with those seen in gray matter (for an excellent review, see Lipton, 1999), there are also unique features. This chapter summarizes our current knowledge of the deleterious events triggered to induce anoxic/ischemic damage in mammalian white matter.

## THE SCOPE OF WHITE MATTER INJURY

Cerebrovascular disease is a leading cause of death and disability, with close to 600,000 new cases each year in Canada and the United States alone. While much work has focused on gray matter injury mechanisms, white matter tracts are also damaged in the vast majority of strokes. Up to one-quarter of all strokes are lacunar in nature, involving predominantly white matter tracts in the brain (Fisher, 1982). Indeed, ~ 50% of the adult human CNS is composed of white matter (Zhang and Sejnowski, 2000), yet we know far less about this tissue than gray matter regions. Traumatic spinal cord injury is another example of a devastating condition affecting mainly young adults, with more than 10,000 new cases per year in the United States (Gibson, 1992); the yearly cost of care for the estimated 250,000 individuals living with spinal cord injuries exceeds $10 billion per year. In the United States alone, it is estimated that nearly 2 million people suffered a head injury in 1990 (Collins, 1990). Recent data suggest that the majority of these (~ 1.5 million) suffered some form of *brain* injury as a result (Sosin *et al.*, 1996). Diffuse axonal injury is a central feature of brain trauma. Microscopically, this type of injury is characterized by the appearance of numerous swollen axonal "retraction balls" separated from the distal fiber, mainly due to "secondary axotomy," whereby axons are biochemically (rather than mechanically) transected in the first hours after mild to moderate injury (Povlishock and Christman, 1995). The mechanisms of this axotomy are not well understood but seem to be accompanied by mitochondrial swelling, nodal "blebs," focal loosening of the myelin sheath, disorganization of neurofilaments, localized disruption of axoplasmic transport, and finally axonal disconnection (Maxwell *et al.*, 1997). A recent study suggests focal accumulation of Ca with activation of calpain may be responsible (Buki *et al.*, 1998), and we have recently shown that "controlled" Ca influx (rather than nonspecific Ca overload through disrupted axolemma) via reverse Na-Ca exchange and voltage-gated Ca channels plays a key role (Wolf *et al.*, 2001).

Finally, lessons learned about ischemic injury to white matter may be very relevant to multiple sclerosis, afflicting an estimated 350,000 people in Europe and North America alone (Weinshenker, 1996). Recent work has made it clear that this disease causes irreversible disability partly, if not mainly, because of axonal degeneration, rather than demyelination (Bjartmar and Trapp, 2001; Ferguson *et al.*, 1997; Kornek and Lassmann, 1999; Rieckmann and Smith, 2001; Trapp *et al.*, 1998; Waxman, 2000). Although the mechanisms responsible for this axonal loss are not yet fully understood, there are indications that some mechanisms that have been elucidated from studies of ischemic white matter injury may play a role, and this may open up therapeutic opportunities.

## CNS ENERGY METABOLISM

Cells of the mammalian CNS require a continuous supply of oxygen and glucose to support normal metabolism and uninterrupted signaling. Indeed, it is estimated that over 50% of resting ATP consumption is accounted for by ion pumping, with the Na-K-ATPase being by far the greatest consumer (Erecinska and Dagani, 1990; Erecinska and Silver, 1989), operating to maintain normal Na and K gradients across cell membranes. While glucose consumption is two to three times greater in gray than in white matter (Clarke and Sokoloff, 1994), white matter is nevertheless heavily dependent on a continuous supply of energy: optic nerves maintained *in vitro* quickly depolarize within minutes of the onset of anoxia, with only a small fraction of resting membrane potential supported by glycolysis (Leppanen and Stys, 1997). Conversely, blocking glycolysis either pharmacologically—for example, using iodoacetate, an irreversible blocker of glyceraldehyde 3-phosphate dehydrogenase (Devlin, 1992, p. 308) or by removing glucose—also causes a marked depolarization of central axons; however, the onset of membrane potential failure is delayed compared to anoxia, with the compound action and resting membrane potentials being well preserved for 20 minutes or more (Brown *et al.*, 2001a; Stys, 1998; Stys *et al.*, 1998) (Fig. 41.1).

In the case of pharmacological inhibition of glycolysis, this delay is thought to be due residual consumption of energy substrates (e.g., amino acids) by the Krebs cycle and ATP generation by oxidative metabolism (Leppanen and Stys, 1997; Stryer, 1988). Removing glucose also has a delayed effect on membrane potential and the disappearance of the compound action potential, which begin to decay after only 40 minutes of aglycemia (Brown *et al.*, 2001a; Wender *et al.*, 2000). In this case, with the glycolytic pathways unblocked, it is likely that once residual substrates that fuel the Krebs cycle are depleted, energy is supplied to axons by catabolism of glycogen (Wender *et al.*, 2000). Because astrocytes contain the only substantial source of glycogen in the CNS (Koizumi, 1974; Sorg and Magistretti, 1991; Swanson *et al.*, 1989), it is thought that these cells generate lactate through glycolysis, which is exported to, then taken up by, axons via specific monocarboxylate transporters (Wender *et al.*, 2000). Although there are suggestions that neurons use lactate preferentially, especially during activation (Tsacopoulos and Magistretti, 1996), the issue of whether neurons and axons utilize glucose directly is still

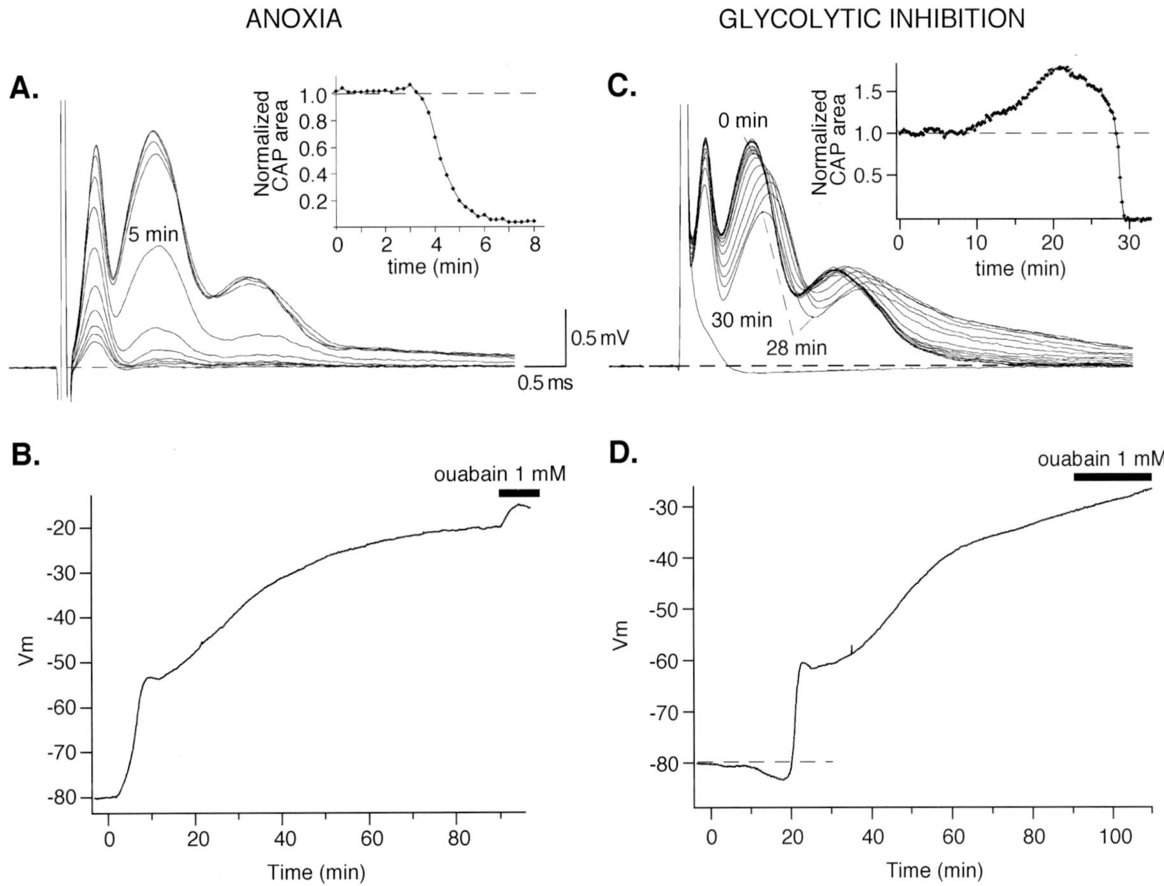


FIGURE 41.1
(A, B) Representative compound action and resting membrane potentials from rat optic nerve exposed to *in vitro* anoxia (beginning at time 0). Compound action potentials are abolished within minutes of anoxia, paralleling the quick depolarization of resting potential. Blocking the Na-K-ATPase with ouabain (B) reveals that a small component of resting membrane potential is supported by glycolytic ATP even after 1 hr of anoxia. (C, D) Similar records from optic nerves this time exposed to *in vitro* glycolytic inhibition using iodoacetate (a paradigm that is independent of residual traces of glucose or glycogen availability). In contrast to anoxia, during glycolytic block excitability and resting membrane potential are maintained for at least 20 minutes before rapidly collapsing, probably at the time of exhaustion of alternate substrates being metabolized by the Krebs cycle (see text). Reproduced from Stys, 1998, with permission.

unsettled. Recent evidence suggests that neuronal elements will use both substrates if available (Chih *et al.*, 2001). Figure 41.2 summarizes the presumed modes of energy substrate utilization in white matter of the mammalian CNS.

## EARLY CONSEQUENCES OF ENERGY DEPRIVATION

The heavy reliance of white matter on a continuous supply of energy substrates implies that transmembrane ionic gradients and membrane polarization will be rapidly compromised when ATP levels fall. Using ion-sensitive microelectrodes, Ransom and colleagues demonstrated a quick rise of $[K]_o$ in optic nerve within 5 minutes of anoxia onset, from a baseline of 3 mM to ~15 mM, coupled with an acidification of the extracellular space by 0.3 pH units (Ransom *et al.*, 1992). The rise in $[K]_o$ closely parallels the rapid anoxic depolarization of optic nerves and loss of excitability (which may be reversible depending on the duration of anoxia, see below). Using Ca-sensitive microelectrodes, Brown *et al.* (1998) observed a fall in $[Ca]_o$, presumably reflecting accumulation into an intracellular compartment. What these studies do not reveal is which cellular elements

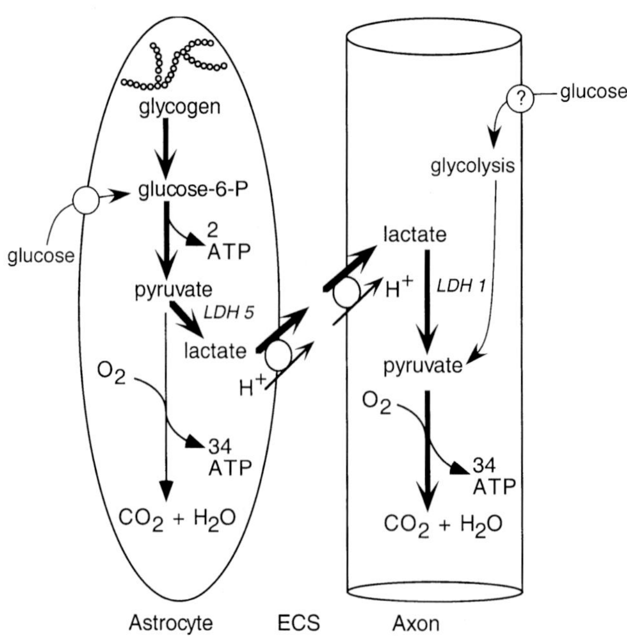


FIGURE 41.2
Simplified model depicting utilization of energy substrates in white matter. Astrocytes are known to take up glucose and metabolize it to lactate through glycolytic pathways. Under substrate-limited conditions, glial-derived lactate can support axonal function. Although not firmly established, under energy-replete conditions it is likely that both glia and axons can take up and metabolize glucose directly. Modified from Wender *et al.*, 2000, with permission, and B. R. Ransom, personal communication.

(e.g., axons or glia) are sourcing or accumulating ions. It is well known that astrocytes are able to survive on glycolysis alone for prolonged periods of time (Callahan *et al.*, 1990; Yu *et al.*, 1989). Hypoxia alone causes little change in astrocytic [Na] and only a modest increase of free $[Ca]_i$ from ~150 to ~280 nM (Rose *et al.*, 1998; Silver *et al.*, 1997). Even ischemic astrocytes do not accumulate substantial Na acutely, but cytosolic [Ca] rises more than with hypoxia alone, to ~600 nM (Rose *et al.*, 1998; Silver *et al.*, 1997). Central axons however behave more like neuronal elements, being much more sensitive even to anoxia alone. Figure 41.3 shows a plot of axoplasmic Na, K and Ca changes in large optic nerve axons subjected to *in vitro* anoxia. Axoplasmic [K] falls from a resting level of ~150 mM to less than 10% after 1h of anoxia, while [Na] rises from ~20 to ~100 mM. Because Ca is largely bound in the cytosol, the concentrations of this ion are shown in mmol/kg dry weight because the electron probe microanalysis technique used to measure these ions (more accurately, elements) reports *total* (free + bound) amounts. Total axonal Ca rises by approximately five-fold during 60 minutes of *in vitro* anoxia, but the ionized [Ca], most relevant to biological (including pathological) processes, may increase much more. Using guinea pig spinal cord slices subjected to focal compression injury *in vitro*, LoPachin and colleagues (LoPachin *et al.*, 1999) observed elemental changes similar to those seen during anoxia. Thus, a rise in axoplasmic Na and Ca, and a loss of K seem to be a general feature of the response of injured nerve fibers.

We have recent evidence of a very substantial rise in axoplasmic free [Ca] using confocal microscopy and Ca-sensitive dyes. During *in vitro* ischemia, we observed a substantial fluorescence increase, indicating a rise in free [Ca] into the micromolar range, possibly exceeding 10 μM or more, though accurate calibrations in myelinated fibers are difficult to perform (Nikolaeva and Stys, 2002; Ren *et al.*, 2000). Figure 41.4 shows confocal images of optic nerve subjected to *in vitro* ischemia in perfusate containing normal [Ca] (2 mM) and in zero-Ca/EGTA bath. Surprisingly, there was a substantial increase in ionized axoplasmic Ca in the absence of bath Ca, implying release of this ion from an intracellular pool. Recent experiments from our lab indicate that endoplasmic reticulum Ca stores, controlled by ryanodine and IP3 receptors, play a major role in injury to certain white matter tracts such

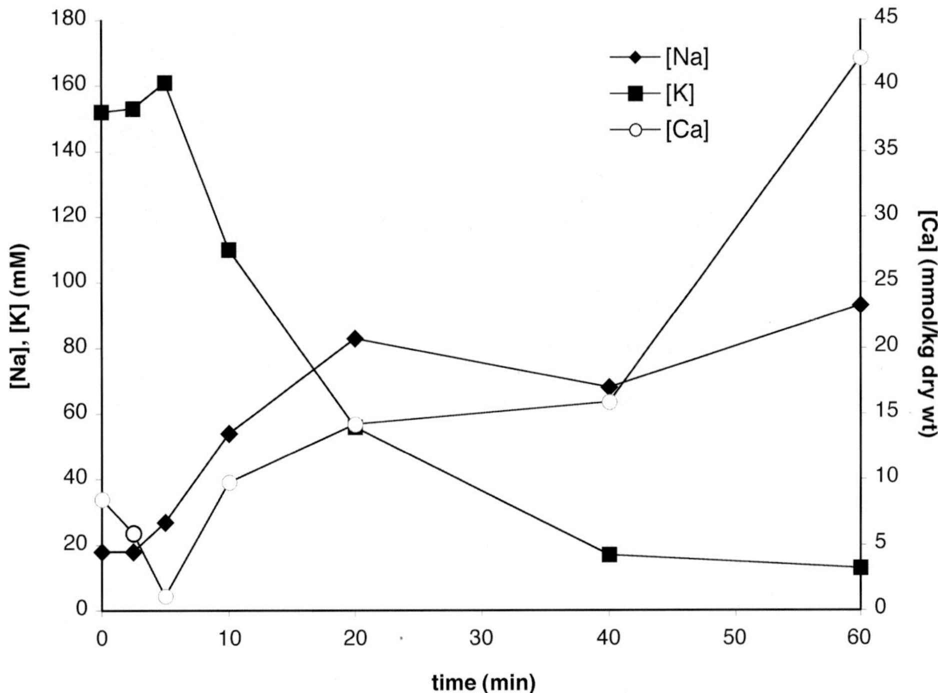


FIGURE 41.3
Graph of changes in axoplasmic [Na], [K] and [Ca] in large optic nerve axons subjected to *in vitro* anoxia (beginning at time 0). [Na] and [K] are shown as free, ionized fractions in mM (see Stys *et al.*, 1997, for details), whereas Ca, which is almost totally bound in cells, is reported in mmol/kg dry weight. During 1 hour of anoxic exposure, axoplasmic Na increases about five-fold from a baseline of ~ 20 mM. There is a parallel severe loss of K. Total Ca content (including axoplasm and ER, but excluding mitochondria) increases gradually about five-fold over baseline. Note that normal baseline Ca content in axons approaches 1 mM as an equivalent concentration, indicating substantial intracellular sources of Ca that likely contribute to white matter injury when released during ischemia (see text).

as dorsal columns of the spinal cord. While dorsal columns respond to *anoxia* in a manner that is similar to optic nerves (degree of functional injury, rescue by zero-Ca perfusate) (Imaizumi *et al.*, 1997, 1999; Li *et al.*, 1999, 2000), ischemia (oxygen and glucose deprivation) causes far greater injury that cannot be prevented by removal of Ca from the bath (Ouardouz *et al.*, 2003). More detailed investigation revealed that L-type Ca channel blockers are robustly protective in ischemic dorsal columns, but *only* in Ca-free perfusate. This apparent paradox can be explained by the fact that dihydropyridine Ca channel blockers inhibit the voltage sensor on L-type Ca channels (Rios and Brum, 1987), which is crucial for depolarization-mediated activation of ryanodine receptors and Ca release from the endoplasmic reticulum, a mechanism identical to "excitation-contraction coupling" in skeletal muscle. Taken together, it is very likely that perhaps the most proximal source of deleterious Ca increase during ischemia is release of this ion from "axoplasmic reticulum" (see Fig. 41.5), both via ryanodine receptor activation by axonal depolarization sensed by L-type Ca channels, and by activation of IP3 receptors by second messengers (Ouardouz *et al.*, 2003; Thorell *et al.*, 2002). In addition to release of internal Ca stores into the cytosol, there is also a net accumulation of Ca originating from the extracellular space inferred by $[Ca]_o$ measurements (Brown *et al.*, 1998) and demonstrated directly by electron probe microanalysis (Fig. 41.3) (LoPachin and Stys, 1995; Stys and LoPachin, 1998).

## INJURY MECHANISMS TRIGGERED BY ENERGY FAILURE

As mentioned in the previous section, excitability of white matter tracts is abolished within minutes of the onset of anoxia or ischemia, but this does not imply an irreversible loss of

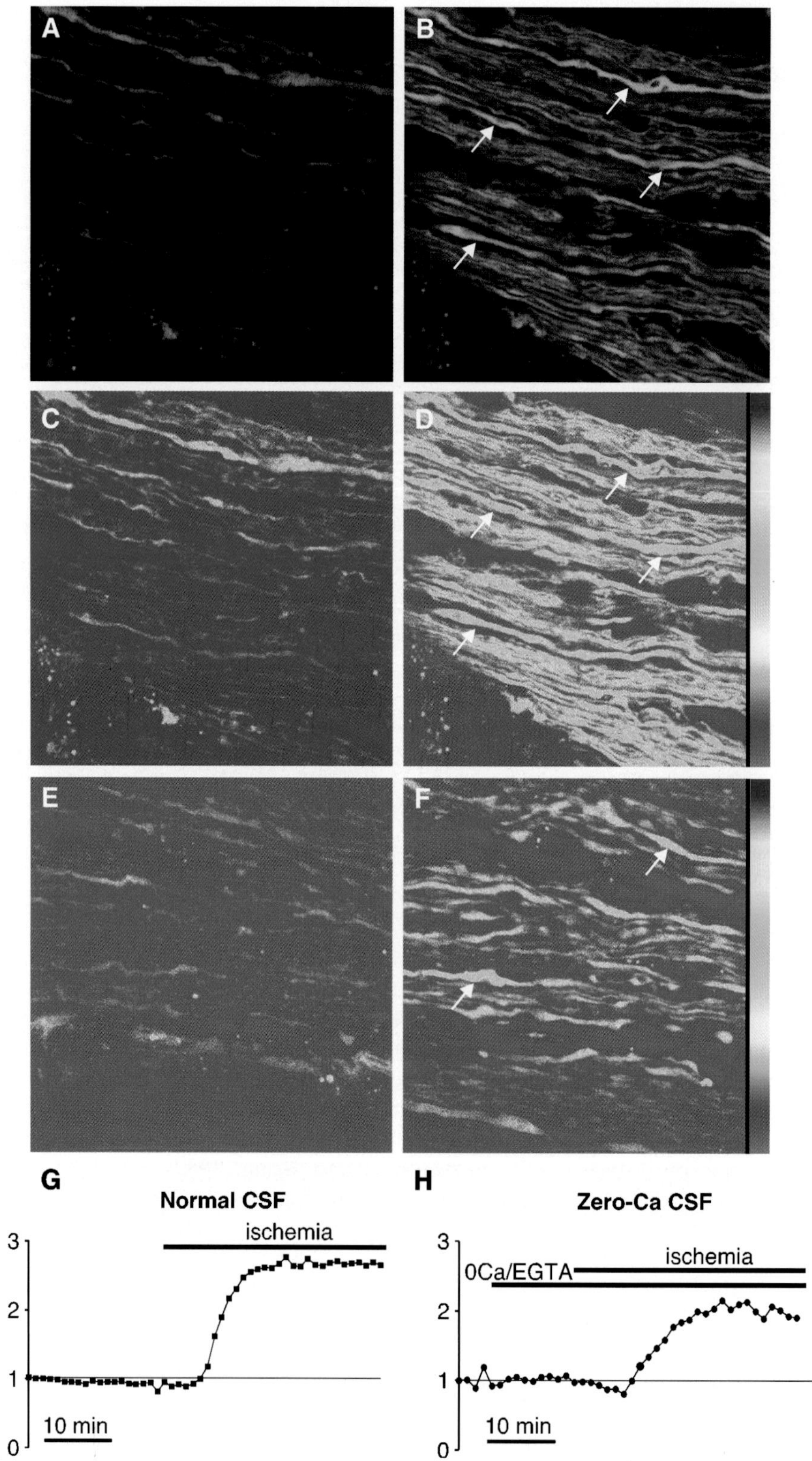


FIGURE 41.4

Confocal images of rat optic nerve axons (arrows) loaded with the Ca-sensitive dye Oregon Green 488 BAPTA-1 dextran. The Ca-sensitive green signal is weak in control nerves (A) because of the normally low resting [Ca] in healthy fibers. *In vitro* ischemia in normal CSF (containing 2 mM Ca) causes axoplasmic [Ca] to rise (B). Panels C and D are the same fields as in A and B but in pseudocolor to better illustrate the changes in [Ca]. A different experiment shows control nerve (E) and a substantial Ca increase in axons bathed in Ca-free perfusate during ischemia (F), indicating release of Ca from intracellular stores. Quantitative changes in Ca-sensitive fluorescence are shown for optic nerves subjected to *in vitro* ischemia in normal Ca-replete CSF (G) and Ca-free bath (H).

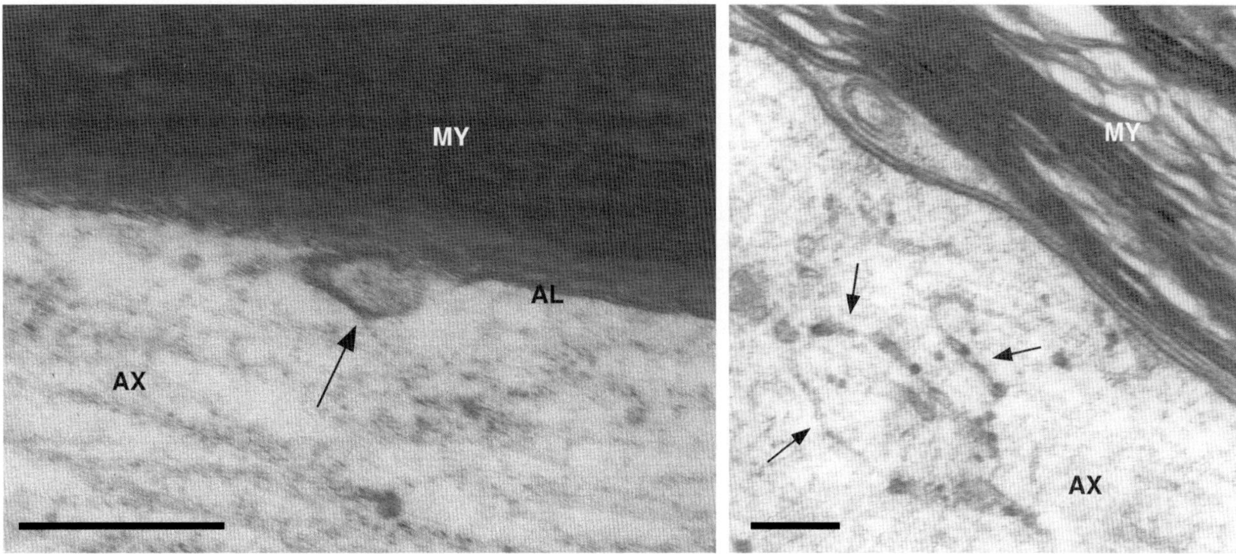


FIGURE 41.5
Electron micrographs of rat dorsal column axons reveal endoplasmic reticulum profiles in the cortical as well as the central axoplasm. Circular, elongated, or irregular cisternae frequently abutted the axolemma. It is hypothesized that this "axoplasmic reticulum" represents internal Ca storage compartments that can be released by depolarization-induced activation of ryanodine receptors (analogous to excitation-contraction coupling in skeletal muscle) or chemically by receptor-controlled synthesis of IP3. MY: myelin; AX: axoplasm; AL: axolemma. Scale bars 200 nm. Modified from Ouardouz *et al.*, 2003 with permission.

function. For instance in adult optic nerve, if anoxia is maintained for only 10 to 15 minutes *in vitro*, although electrogenesis is completely abolished, re-oxygenation allows complete functional recovery; the longer anoxia is applied, the worse the post-anoxic recovery, so that after 90 minutes of anoxic exposure at 37°C, no return of function is observed (Fern *et al.*, 1998). Predictably, *in vitro* ischemia produces greater injury compared to anoxia alone (Ouardouz *et al.*, 2003; Stys and Jiang, 2002; Stys and Ouardouz, 2002; Tekkok and Goldberg, 2001). The key role of cellular Ca overload in anoxic white matter damage was demonstrated in 1990 by Stys and colleagues: removal of bath Ca (with the addition of the Ca chelator EGTA) allowed complete functional (Stys *et al.*, 1990) and structural (Waxman *et al.*, 1993) recovery, despite a more rapid acute loss of excitability (Stys, Ransom, and Waxman, unpublished; Tekkok and Goldberg, 2001). Indeed, Ca depletion allowed substantial functional recovery of optic nerve function even after 3 hours of continuous *in vitro* ischemia, whereas with Ca-replete perfusate, such an insult causes liquefaction and complete destruction of the tissue (Sim and Stys, unpublished).

The central role of Ca in white matter injury was subsequently confirmed in a number of other tracts such as spinal cord dorsal columns and corpus callosum, using various paradigms including anoxia, simulated ischemia, and traumatic injury (Agrawal and Fehlings, 1996; Brown *et al.*, 2001a; Imaizumi *et al.*, 1997; Li *et al.*, 2000; Tekkok and Goldberg, 2001). Thus, it appears that excess accumulation of Ca ions in the cytosol is a central event. The key question then is, what are the mechanisms promoting Ca overload in axons and glia during injury? In a series of experiments in 1992 on anoxic optic nerve, we showed that functional injury (and presumably Ca overload, a prediction which was later confirmed directly by electron probe x-ray microanalysis; see Stys and LoPachin, 1998) was almost completely dependent on Na influx through Na channels which could be blocked by micromolar TTX (Stys *et al.*, 1992a). This Na- and depolarization-dependent Ca overload was found be mediated in large part by reverse Na-Ca exchange. The Na-Ca exchanger is a key player in maintaining Ca homeostasis in all excitable cells, utilizing the transmembrane Na gradient to export one Ca ion from the cytosol for three or four Na ions flowing in (Blaustein and Lederer, 1999; Dong *et al.*, 2002) (although recent work indicates that a 4Na-1Ca:1K exchanger exists in the brain as well; see Dong *et al.*, 2001; Kiedrowski *et al.*, 2002). The electrogenic nature and reversibility of this transport system implies that collapse of the Na

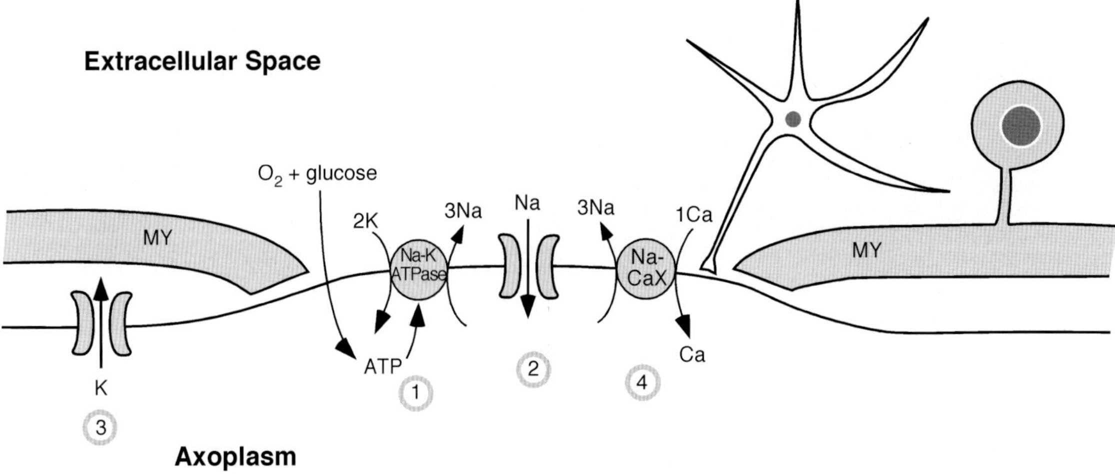


FIGURE 41.6
Simplified diagram illustrating sequence of interrelated events leading to anoxic injury of a central myelinated axon. Interruption of energy supply leads to failure of ATP-dependent pumps such as axolemmal Na-K-ATPase (1). Reduction of Na pumping across the axolemma leads to accumulation of axoplasmic Na mainly through noninactivating Na channels (2). The rise in $[Na]_i$, coupled with depolarization caused by K efflux through a variety of K channels (3) stimulates the Na-Ca exchanger to operate in the Ca import mode, overloading the axon with damaging amounts of this cation (4).

gradient or membrane depolarization (two invariable consequences of compromised white matter tracts) will bias the exchanger toward the Ca import mode, potentially culminating in Ca overload and irreversible cellular injury. From these studies emerged a simple model of white matter anoxic injury summarized in Figure 41.6. Subsequent experiments confirmed that this mechanism operates in many other axonal tracts as well, in response to anoxia, ischemia and various traumatic models (Imaizumi *et al.*, 1997; Li *et al.*, 2000; Kapoor *et al.*, 2003; Tekkok *et al.*, 2000; Wolf *et al.*, 2001).

Careful inspection of the time course of axonal Na accumulation (see Fig. 41.3) reveals a continuous rise in [Na] over tens of minutes, suggesting that a substantial axolemmal Na conductance persists throughout most of the anoxic period, even at a time when axons are strongly depolarized (compare with Fig. 41.1B). Classical Hodgkin-Huxley kinetics imply inactivation of Na channels in depolarized axonal membranes, yet the preceding results suggest that a finite Na permeability persists even in depolarized axons. Such "noninactivating" Na conductance has been demonstrated in many types of neurons (for a review, see Taylor, 1993) and was confirmed directly in optic nerve (Stys *et al.*, 1993) axons as well. This route of pathological Na flux in injured axons may have important implications for the design of therapeutic agents, with several classes of Na channel blockers having preferential selectivity at open, noninactivating Na channels.

More recent studies indicate that reverse Na-Ca exchange may not be the only route of extracellular Ca influx. Several groups found that a variety of voltage-gated channel subtypes contribute to white matter injury. Antagonists of L-type Ca channels were found to be partially protective against optic nerve anoxic injury, with the $Ca_V1.2$ and 1.3 isoforms demonstrated immunohistochemically in axons and astrocytes (Brown *et al.*, 2001b; Fern *et al.*, 1995a). Curiously, the dihydropyridines nifedipine and nimodipine failed to reduce accumulation of total axoplasmic Ca induced by anoxia (Stys and LoPachin, 1998). The reason for this discrepancy is not clear, but in light of recent data (Ouardouz *et al.*, 2003), perhaps these Ca channel blockers are protective because they reduce depolarization-induced release from ryanodine-sensitive stores (see previous section), which would explain the improved physiological outcome with no difference in *total* axonal Ca accumulation. In addition to L-type, N-type Ca channels have also been implicated in anoxic and traumatic white matter injury (Agrawal *et al.*, 2000; Fern *et al.*, 1995a; Wolf *et al.*, 2001).

Interestingly, while the mechanisms of axonal injury in MS are poorly understood, its pathophysiology may include some features in common with ischemia and trauma, in that an important role of Ca is suggested by several lines of evidence (for a review see Rieckmann and Maurer, 2002): glutamate, released by activated macrophages/microglia, has deleterious effects on CNS white matter, in part through activation of glial AMPA/kainate receptors (Li and Stys, 2000; Pitt *et al.*, 2000; Stys and Li, 2000). We have evidence that group I metabotropic glutamate receptors may be involved in the release of toxic amounts of Ca from IP3-dependent stores in white matter (Stys and Ouardouz, 2002). Moreover, a very interesting recent study by Goldberg and colleagues suggests that AMPA/kainate receptor-mediated damage to oligodendrocytes *in vitro* induces release of reactive oxygen species that secondarily injure axons (Underhill and Goldberg, 2002). From these studies, it is very likely that the toxic amounts of glutamate known to be released in inflammatory areas of MS plaques may promote Ca-dependent damage not only to glia but to axons as well, ultimately causing axonal degeneration. Nitric oxide (NO) is another factor that is produced in relatively high concentrations by macrophages (and other cells) at sites of inflammation (Bo *et al.*, 1994; Cross *et al.*, 1998). NO causes axonal dysfunction probably because of an interaction with mitochondrial cytochrome c oxidase, leading to a competitive inhibition of $O_2$ utilization (Bolanos *et al.*, 1997; Cooper, 2002; Garthwaite *et al.*, 2002; Smith *et al.*, 2001); thus, it is possible that tissue in the vicinity of an inflammatory lesion remains "chemically hypoxic." Such a state could in turn invoke the Ca-dependent injury processes that have been described in anoxic/ischemic white matter. Such mechanistic overlap might allow us to capitalize on knowledge gained from work on white matter anoxia/ischemia to devise successful protective strategies for inflammatory white matter disorders.

Complicating the issue of white matter damage in inflammatory disorders further, recent studies indicate that, in addition to demyelination and axon degeneration, dysregulated expression of ion channels (an "acquired channelopathy") occurs in experimental allergic encephalomyelitis (EAE) and MS (Black *et al.*, 2000; Waxman, 2001). An interesting recent report indicates that $Ca_v2.2$, the pore-forming subunit of N-type Ca channels, not only accumulates within axonal spheroids of actively demyelinating lesions in MS and EAE but is also inserted into the axolemma, suggesting that injured axons may be preferentially susceptible to Ca-mediated injury by ion entering through ectopically targeted channels (Kornek *et al.*, 2001).

As in many other cell types (Orrenius and Nicotera, 1996; Schanne *et al.*, 1979), Ca is thought to represent the "final common pathway" of cell injury in white matter as well. It is highly likely that once cytosolic [Ca] rises excessively, a large number of Ca-dependent pathways are stimulated culminating in irreversible tissue destruction. Many crucial biochemical pathways are modulated by Ca ions including calpains, phospholipases, endonucleases, NO synthase, mitochondrial free radical generation, protein kinase C, and others. Experiments in both traumatic, anoxic/ischemic and immune-mediated demyelinating paradigms clearly indicate the important role of calpain overactivation in producing breakdown of key structural proteins including spectrin, neurofilament, and myelin basic protein (Buki *et al.*, 1999; Jiang and Stys, 2000; McCracken *et al.*, 2001; Schumacher *et al.*, 2000, 2001; Stys and Jiang, 2002). Calpain substrates are not limited to just these proteins, with additional relevant targets for possible proteolysis including the Ca-ATPase (Salamino *et al.*, 1994); tau, tubulin, ankyrin (Rami *et al.*, 1997); the myelin proteins MAG and PLP (Deshpande *et al.*, 1995; Schaecher *et al.*, 2001; Shields *et al.*, 1999); calmodulin-binding proteins (e.g., G-proteins), protein kinase C, calcineurin, phospholipase C (Kampfl *et al.*, 1997); NMDA and AMPA receptors (Bi *et al.*, 1998a, 1998b, 1998c; Gellerman *et al.*, 1997); L-type Ca channels (Hell *et al.*, 1996); NCAM and N-cadherin (Covault *et al.*, 1991); and calpain also appears to play an important role in the induction of apoptosis and the mitochondrial permeability transition (Lipton, 1999) (discussed later). In all likelihood, many if not most of the other Ca-dependent pathways are also overdriven in injured white matter, conspiring to cause irreversible damage to this tissue. The corollary is that blocking only one (e.g., calpain) or even a few of the Ca-stimulated pathways would not improve functional outcome, as has been shown in optic nerve: predictably, direct pharmacological calpain inhibition was very effective at reducing calpain-dependent spectrin degradation (and by inference calpain activation in general), but did not at all improve physiological outcome (Jiang and Stys, 2000; Stys and Jiang, 2002).

Although white matter is structurally and functionally simpler than gray matter, recent data indicate that many more signaling pathways may be involved in the genesis of white matter ischemic injury than was previously appreciated (e.g., Fig. 41.6). A thorough discussion of each is beyond the scope of this chapter, and the reader is referred to the cited references for more details. In addition to "direct" Ca sourcing pathways such as Na-Ca exchange, voltage-gated Ca channels and intracellular Ca release channels, other pathways modulate the degree of injury, including somewhat surprisingly, several neurotransmitters. For instance, both endogenously released GABA and adenosine are protective against anoxia in the optic nerve: application of exogenous GABA or adenosine, or blocking reuptake of GABA or adenosine with nipecotic acid or propentofylline, respectively, are protective, whereas blocking GABA-B (phaclofen) or adenosine receptors (theophylline) worsens outcome (Fern *et al.*, 1994, 1995b, 1996b). Release of both adenosine and GABA in white matter regions was confirmed in an *in vivo* cat model of global cerebral ischemia (Dohmen *et al.*, 2001), lending further support to the "autoprotective" role of these substances proposed by Fern *et al.* (1996a). These two neurotransmitter receptors appear to modulate a convergent pathway involving a G-protein/protein kinase C cascade, although which molecular complex is then targeted and which cellular elements are protected by this mechanism (i.e., axon cylinder versus glia) is unknown. Most investigations on white matter injury have been focused on aberrant cation flux, but Malek and Stys (2002) have data indicating that anion transporters may also contribute to damage. Evidence from the anoxic optic nerve model suggests that Cl channels attempt to normalize a Cl dysequilibrium mediated by the K-Cl co-transporter, itself driven to accumulate abnormal amounts of Cl because of the collapse of the K gradient. Thus, blocking certain Cl channels with niflumic acid worsens injury, but blocking the K-Cl co-transporter with furosemide is partially protective. Analysis of waveshapes suggests that these effects may be mediated in large part at the myelin sheath, so that pathological Cl-dependent volume changes might be disrupting axo-glial architecture leading to slowing and failure of action potential propagation (Malek *et al.*, 2002).

Reperfusion injury has been implicated in many tissues including brain, heart, and even in spinal cord white matter directly (Darley *et al.*, 1991; Jalc *et al.*, 1995; White *et al.*, 2000). As if starvation of the CNS of energy substrates is not bad enough, ironically, restoring oxygen and glucose supply can be additionally injurious. Free radical and NO production are both stimulated during the reperfusion period, and mitochondrial matrix Ca rises to an extreme degree, exceeding its baseline level by ~30 to 100-fold; this is true for organelles in both hippocampal neurons (Taylor *et al.*, 1999) and white matter axons (LoPachin and Stys, 1995; Stys and LoPachin, 1996). Such a large Ca accumulation will not only damage mitochondria, as these quantities of ion precipitate out of the aqueous phase, but the accumulating electrical charge carried by a rapid influx of Ca ions will also severely hamper attempts by a rejuvenated electron transport chain to restore the negative matrix potential; this potential is essential for the resumption of ATP synthesis, rather than *consumption* of precious glycolytically-derived ATP, which occurs when mitochondria are depolarized (Nicholls and Budd, 2000). Moreover, high mitochondrial Ca loads will also promote opening of the mitochondrial permeability transition, further accelerating the rundown of any remaining electrochemical gradients across the inner membrane. Therefore, paradoxically, these events may induce a permanent state of "chemical hypoxia" and a worsening energy deficit at a time when cellular energy metabolism should be restarting. A recent report demonstrated an apoptotic mode of cell death, particularly involving oligodentrocytes in traumatically injured spinal cord white matter (Casha *et al.*, 2001). It is interesting to speculate on the link between the mitochondrial permeability transition (promoted by excessive Ca levels), release of cytochrome c, and the induction of apoptosis by activation of caspases (Lipton, 1999; MacManus and Buchan, 2000), perhaps reflecting an additional, more delayed, deleterious effect of mitochondrial Ca overload that occurs during, and especially after, the termination of ischemia and other insults.

## WHITE MATTER EXCITOTOXICITY

White matter is a tissue devoid of chemical synapses in the traditional sense, but this does not preclude the possibility of physiological and pathological signaling between elements involving traditional neurotransmitters. Indeed, the previous section describes experiments clearly demonstrating a role of endogenously released GABA and adenosine in white matter anoxic injury. While gray matter "excitotoxicity" has been the subject of intense study for several decades, the effect of glutamate on white matter has received attention only in recent years, with this excitotoxin implicated in all modes of white matter injury examined so far. Numerous studies have shown that both oligodendrocytes and astrocytes possess glutamate receptors of the AMPA and kainate (but not NMDA) subtypes (Agrawal and Fehlings, 1997b; Garcia-Barcina and Matute, 1996; Jensen and Chiu, 1993; Matute *et al.*, 1997; for reviews see Matute *et al.*, 2002; Steinhauser and Gallo, 1996). White matter astrocytes express all AMPA and kainate receptor subunits except GluR4. In contrast, oligodendrocytes express only GluR3 and GluR4 AMPA receptor subunits (notably lacking GluR2), as well as all kainate subunits except GluR5 (Garcia-Barcina and Matute, 1996, 1998; Matute *et al.*, 2002). The absence of GluR2 in oligodendrocytes may render them particularly susceptible to Ca flux through these Ca-permeable receptors. Persistent activation of these non-NMDA ionotropic receptors causes injury to oligodendrocytes both in cell culture and *in vivo* (Matute *et al.*, 1997, 1998; McDonald *et al.*, 1998; Yoshioka *et al.*, 1995, 1996). Astrocytes are more resistant to excitotoxicity, but can be severely injured when exposed to AMPA receptor agonists particularly when desensitization is blocked (David *et al.*, 1996). As an extension to these findings, a number of investigators have shown that glutamate receptor antagonism is protective against a number of insults affecting white matter. Spinal cord injury examined using both an *in vitro* clip compression model (Agrawal and Fehlings, 1997b) and an *in vivo* contusion model (Rosenberg *et al.*, 1999a; Wrathall *et al.*, 1997) was ameliorated in the presence of 2,3-dihydro-6-nitro-7-sulfamoyl-benzo(f)quinoxaline (NBQX), a selective antagonist of AMPA/kainate receptors. More recent work has confirmed that AMPA/kainate receptors play an important role in hypoxic/ischemic white matter injury as shown by *in vitro* models, for example, corpus callosum (Tekkok and Goldberg, 2001) and spinal dorsal column (Li *et al.*, 1999). This mechanism was confirmed *in vivo* both in the adult brain (McCracken *et al.*, 2002) and in the immature animal, with oligodendrocytes being particularly vulnerable (Follett *et al.*, 2000). Predictably, NMDA receptor antagonists are ineffective at protecting white matter from ischemic injury (Yam *et al.*, 2000), in line with the known lack of effects of NMDA receptor activation (or inhibition) in this tissue (Agrawal and Fehlings, 1997b; Li and Stys, 2000). Interestingly, two recent studies using a model of EAE reported a beneficial effect of systemically administered NBQX, with reduction of oligodendroglial and axonal damage, along with a parallel improvement in clinical scores (Pitt *et al.*, 2000; Smith *et al.*, 2000). Finally, a role for metabotropic glutamate receptors in ischemic and traumatic white matter injury has been proposed, which may actually couple back to the potentially very important mechanism of release of internal Ca stores, via a phospholipase C-dependent mechanism acting on IP3 receptors (Agrawal *et al.*, 1998; Stys and Ouardouz, 2002).

Taken together, these data strongly suggest that as in gray matter, a variety of disorders damage white matter via excitotoxic mechanisms. Important questions that arise include which white matter elements are injured by excessive glutamate release? And how is this excitotoxin released in a tissue without synaptic machinery? Using an isolated spinal white matter preparation, Li and Stys (2000) showed that activation of AMPA receptors caused significant functional injury to dorsal columns measured electrophysiologically. Immunohistochemistry revealed that oligodendrocytes and astrocytes were damaged, revealed by an increase in calpain-mediated breakdown of the cytoskeletal protein spectrin (Fig. 41.7). In addition, using a marker for degenerated myelin basic protein (Matsuo *et al.*, 1998), it

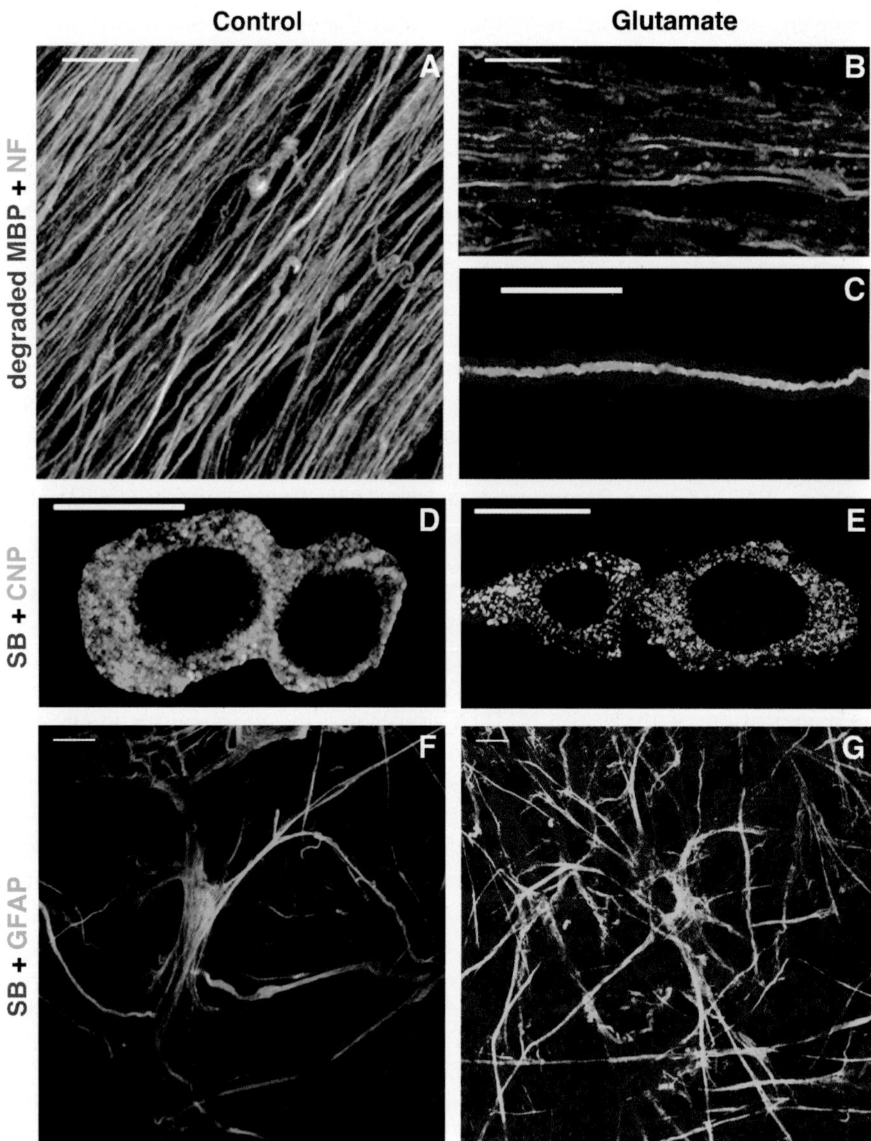


FIGURE 41.7
Confocal microscopic images of dorsal columns stained with standard markers (neurofilament, CNPase, GFAP to identify axon cylinders, oligodendrocytes, and astrocytes, respectively) and markers of cellular injury after 3 hour in normal CSF or CSF containing 1 mM glutamate. Panels A, B, and C show tissue double stained for neurofilament (green) and degenerated myelin basic protein (red). Control images show no myelin damage, whereas exposure to glutamate caused marked injury to myelin (arrowheads). Panels D and E identify oligodendrocytes using CNPase (green), showing cytoskeletal damage revealed by spectrin breakdown ("SBP," red) in glutamate-treated versus control tissue. GFAP (green in panels F and G) identifies astrocytes that also sustained cytoskeletal damage. In contrast, axon cylinders showed no appreciable increase in spectrin breakdown after an equivalent treatment (not shown). Scale bars 10 μm. Modified from Li and Stys, 2000, with permission.

was shown that the myelin sheath itself is damaged by AMPA receptor stimulation (Figs. 41.7B and 41.7C) (Li and Stys, 2000). While it is not yet clear whether myelin damage results primarily from overactivation of Ca-permeable AMPA receptors, or whether the sheath degenerated secondarily as a result of injury to the cell body of the oligodendrocyte, immunohistochemistry suggests that GluR4 (but not GluR2) subunits may be located on the myelin sheath itself (Li and Stys, 2000), raising the possibility that this structure may be directly vulnerable to elevated ambient glutamate levels. Whether or not axons *per se* are vulnerable to glutamate exposure is less certain. In contrast to glia, axons did not exhibit any discernible breakdown of spectrin in response to an excitotoxic insult (Li and Stys, 2000). On the other hand, Tekkök and Goldberg (2001) presented evidence of *axonal* protection by NBQX in an *in vitro* model of central white matter ischemic injury. However, recent evidence suggests that axonal degeneration in response to an excitotoxic challenge occurs secondarily to oligodendroglial injury, mediated by generation of free radicals (Underhill and Goldberg, 2002).

How glutamate effects injury is poorly understood, but several mechanisms are possible. The first is simple Ca overload mediated by Ca-permeable AMPA receptors. During periods of energy depletion such as hypoxia/ischemia, what might normally be a manageable Ca load could now become a toxic accumulation leading to over-activation of the many Ca-dependent systems discussed earlier. A second mechanism that is perhaps important during lower intensity but more chronic exposures to glutamate does not involve not a receptor-dependent pathway, but the uptake of glutamate by oligodendrocytes via a glutamate-cystine exchange mechanism. This in turn depletes cystine and thereby glutathione, rendering the cells vulnerable to oxidative stress (Oka *et al.*, 1993). A similar mechanism has also been proposed for astrocytes (Chen *et al.*, 2000). This mechanism may represent a component of the free radical-mediated axonal damage originating from oligodendrocytes challenged with glutamate (Underhill and Goldberg, 2002).

There is now little doubt that many white matter tracts are vulnerable to excitotoxins, whether applied exogenously or released endogenously in the setting of an insult such as ischemia, trauma, or immune-mediated demyelination. In general, glutamate can be released (1) in a vesicular manner (i.e., Ca-dependent synaptic release), (2) in a nonvesicular manner by reversal of the Na-dependent glutamate transporters (Attwell *et al.*, 1993), (3) through volume-sensitive anion channels (Rutledge *et al.*, 1998), or (4) by exocytosis from astrocytes (Pasti *et al.*, 2001). As noted in previous sections, anoxia, ischemia, and trauma all result in marked ionic deregulation mainly in axons, causing depolarization, loss of K and a rise in Na. A major mechanism for terminating excitatory synaptic transmission is uptake of glutamate by Na-dependent glutamate transporters. This transport system couples the movement of glutamate or aspartate with Na and H in exchange for K in an electrogenic manner, with a typical stoichiometry of 3 Na, 1 H, 1 glutamate: 1 K (Levy *et al.*, 1998; Zerangue and Kavanaugh, 1996). This ratio of ion coupling implies electrogenic transport, indicating that collapse of Na and K gradients, together with depolarization, will drive this transporter in the reverse, glutamate export mode, in a manner similar to that proposed for physiological release of glutamate in immature optic nerve (Kriegler and Chiu, 1993). Cytoplasm, including axoplasm, is known to contain millimolar concentrations of glutamate that far exceed the low micromolar levels in brain extracellular space (Attwell *et al.*, 1993; Fonnum, 1984). Calculations suggest that extracellular glutamate concentrations may reach hundreds of micromolar in response to an anoxic/ischemic insult in white matter (Li *et al.*, 1999), supported by direct measurements of elevated extracellular glutamate levels using microdialysis *in vivo* (Graf *et al.*, 1998). Further evidence for a major role of reverse Na-dependent glutamate transport was provided by the significant protection against both anoxia and trauma in spinal cord white matter, afforded by dihydrokainate and L-trans-pyrrolidine-2,4-dicarboxylic acid (Li *et al.*, 1999), specific inhibitors of Na-dependent glutamate transport (Arriza *et al.*, 1994; Griffiths *et al.*, 1994). Using a semi-quantitative immunohistochemical technique, these authors went on to show that it is mainly axon cylinders, and to a lesser extent oligodendrocytes, that source glutamate during an anoxic challenge (Li *et al.*, 1999), in keeping with the proposed order of ischemic vulnerability of these elements in adult white matter (axons > oligodendrocytes >> astrocytes). During *ischemia* (versus anoxia as in the above study), however, immature oligodendrocytes release substantial quantities of glutamate that in turn activates receptors on these same cells to cause death, in effect creating a "fatal glutamate release feedback loop" (Fern and Moller, 2000). Other modes of glutamate release have not been investigated in injured white matter, but may also include anion channel mediated release, or exocytotic release during more severe injury where astrocytic [Ca] would be expected to rise.

## RATIONAL NEUROPROTECTIVE STRATEGIES

In the past 10 years, our knowledge of the basic mechanisms of white matter injury has progressed significantly from the relatively simple three-step model shown in Figure 41.6 to a much more comprehensive and complex picture summarized in Figure 41.8. The most effective therapeutic strategies can now be rationally proposed by carefully observing the interdependencies of the various steps in the injury cascade. One can see that, for example, a noninactivating voltage gated Na conductance (probably due, at least in part in mature axons, to $Na_v1.6$, which displays a prominent persistent conductance; see Smith *et al.*, 1998) occupies a central location in the injury process for the following reasons: (1) during Na pump failure, this conductance will provide a pathway for influx of Na into the axoplasm, in turn promoting K efflux through a variety of K channels, resulting in axonal depolarization and axoplasmic Na accumulation. (2) The depolarization will in turn gate $Ca_v1.2$, which will activate ryanodine receptors and release Ca from intracellular stores.

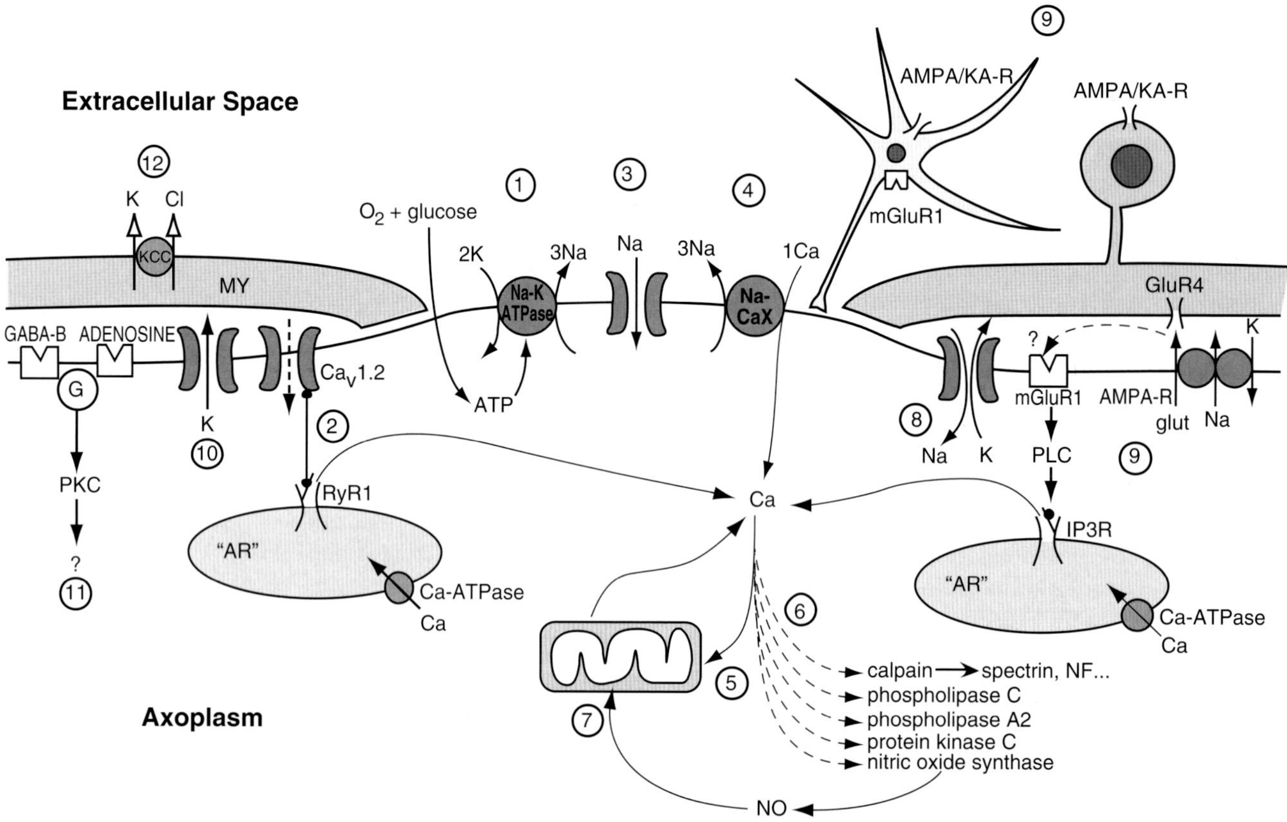


FIGURE 41.8
Diagram illustrating interrelated events leading to injury of a central myelinated axon. Interruption of energy supply leads to failure of ATP-dependent pumps (1). Perhaps the first source of raised axonal [Ca] is from internal stores, which may be released by an "excitation-contraction coupling"-like mechanism and by generation of IP3 from activation of mGluR1 (2). Reduction of Na pumping across the axolemma leads to accumulation of axoplasmic Na via a noninactivating Na conductance (3). The rise in $[Na]_i$, coupled with depolarization caused by K efflux through a variety of K channels (10) stimulates the Na-Ca exchanger to operate in the Ca import mode (4). The accumulation of axonal Ca in turn leads to mitochondrial injury, especially during reoxygenation (5), and to activation of a number of Ca-dependent enzyme systems that damage the fiber (6). One of these is nitric oxide synthase, which may generate sufficient quantities of NO to further inhibit mitochondrial respiration (7). Some Na influx may occur through Na/K permeable inward rectifier channels (8) (Eng *et al.*, 1990; Stys *et al.*, 1998). Glial injury, especially oligodendrocytes and myelin (MY) damage, is exacerbated by excess glutamate release by the Na-K-glutamate transporter, which releases this transmitter under conditions of axoplasmic Na loading and depolarization. AMPA receptors on astrocytes, oligodendrocytes, and even myelin mediate direct damage to these structures (9). Endogenously released transmitters such as GABA and adenosine appear to play an "autoprotective" role (11). Recent evidence also suggest anion transporters such as the K-Cl co-transporter participate in volume dysregulation in glia and the myelin sheath, contributing to conduction abnormalities (12). The locations of the various channels and transporters are drawn for convenience and do not necessarily reflect their real distributions in axons.

(3) Depolarization and increased $[Na]_i$ will together drive the reversal of the Na-Ca exchanger leading to axonal Ca overload and reverse Na-dependent glutamate transport, which will cause release of toxic amounts of glutamate, leading to activation of AMPA/kainate and metabotropic glutamate receptors. For these reasons, targeting Na channels is an attractive option.

A major problem with such a strategy is that Na channels also play a key physiological role: the genesis of action potentials. While TTX, a specific, state-independent blocker of voltage-gated Na channels (Catterall, 1980), is very protective in a variety of white matter injury paradigms both *in vitro* and *in vivo* (Imaizumi *et al.*, 1997; Rosenberg *et al.*, 1999b; Stys *et al.*, 1992a; Tekkok and Goldberg, 2001; Teng and Wrathall, 1997), it is not a viable therapeutic option in the clinical setting because of the potency of the Na channel blocking effect. Certain agents from the local anesthetic and anti-arrhythmic classes are preferentially active at the open conformation of the voltage-gated Na channel (Khodorov, 1991; Wang *et al.*, 1987; Yeh and Tanguy, 1985) and should therefore be relatively selective for the noninactivating Na channel subtype implicated in axonal injury. These "use-dependent" or "phasic" Na channel blockers have the potential of allowing normal signaling to proceed unhindered along axons (because the time a rapidly inactivating Na channel spends in the open conformation during an action potential is very brief, therefore the agent will have little opportunity to access its binding site on the channel protein), yet effectively block a persistently open state that occurs during pathological conditions with prolonged depolarization. This hypothesis was tested using analogs of local anesthetics and anti-arrhythmics known to preferentially block open, noninactivation Na channels, in the *in vitro* anoxic optic nerve model (Stys *et al.*, 1992b; Stys, 1995). Examples are shown in Figure 41.9. While the prototypical local anesthetic lidocaine is an effective neuroprotective agent, it exerts its actions at the expense of severe depression of preinjury action potentials. In contrast, the permanently charged quaternary lidocaine analog QX-314 was very effective

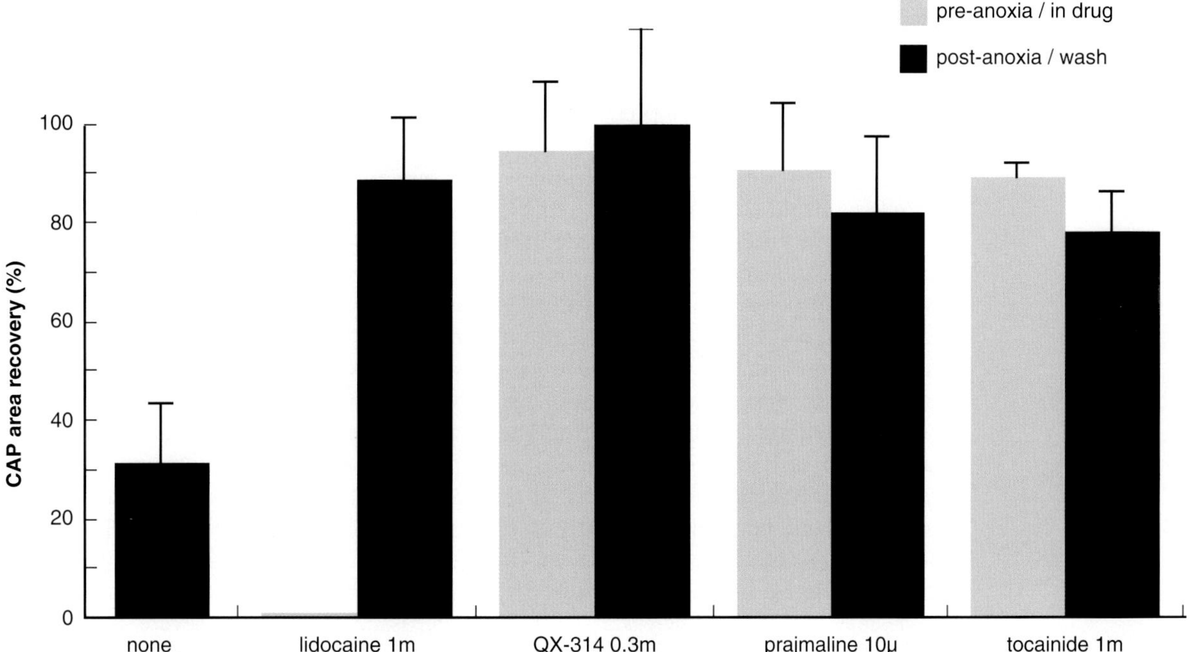


FIGURE 41.9
Bar graph showing examples of effects of various Na channel blockers on pre-anoxic and post-anoxic optic nerve compound action potential (CAP). Gray bars show the degree of depression of excitability in optic nerve before anoxia is applied. Black bars show CAP recovery after anoxia and wash of drug. Control recovery without blockers is about 20 to 30% of pre-anoxic CAP area. Lidocaine (1 mM) is a very effective neuroprotectant, but at the expense of severe depression of electrogenesis. In contrast, "use-dependent" Na channel blockers, particularly the permanently charged analogs such as QX-314 and prajmaline that are thought to be more selective for the open conformation of the Na channel, are highly neuroprotective with minimal anesthetic effect. Data from Stys, 1995.

at a concentration that showed little inhibition of normal electrogenesis. Charged molecules such as QX-314 are thought to be more selective for the open conformation of Na channels (Khodorov, 1991; Wang *et al.*, 1987; Yeh and Tanguy, 1985), which is likely the main reason for its favorable profile.

A serious practical problem with charged compounds is their poor penetration across the blood-brain barrier. QX-314, for instance, although it is a very effective neuroprotectant *in vitro*, fails to enter into the rat CNS to any measurable degree after systemic administration (Stys, unpublished observations). We are then faced with the paradoxical requirement of a charged species for maximal open Na channel blockade versus neutrality to allow CNS penetration. A compromise can be reached by selecting an ionizable compound with a pKa near physiological pH that will exist in both neutral and charged forms. Studies with the antiarrhythmic mexiletine, a primary amine with a pKa of 8.4, showed that this drug is not only effective *in vitro* against optic nerve anoxia but also penetrates into the CNS reaching neuroprotective concentrations after intraperitoneal injection (Hewitt *et al.*, 2001; Stys and Lesiuk, 1996). Moreover, the intracellular acidosis that occurs during anoxia/ischemia will increase the proportion of the protonated form, trapping more drug in the cytosol, further raising the concentration of charged drug where it is most needed. This rationale was confirmed with other Na channel blocking agents including anticonvulsants and a number of other antiarrhythmics and local anesthetics (Fern *et al.*, 1993; Stys *et al.*, 1992b; Stys, 1995). The *in vivo* situation is likely far more complex (discussed later), which may be why these agents confer only modest protection in the whole animal subjected, for example, to an *in vivo* spinal cord injury (Agrawal and Fehlings, 1997a). Moreover, in the clinical setting, systemic side effects of drugs need to be considered. Na channel blockers may have potent adverse effects on peripheral organs such as the cardiovascular system. Nevertheless, proof of principle in an *in vivo* model of axonal degeneration is provided by the observation by Lo *et al.* (2002) of robust protection of white matter axons in EAE with phenytoin at serum levels within the range used in the clinical setting (Fig. 41.10) and by Bechtold and colleagues (2002) using the antiarrhythmic flecainide at doses that had very few adverse clinical effects. Recent advances in our molecular understanding of Na channel subtype distributions in various organs and different parts of the CNS raises the potential for the design of agents that will specifically target a certain Na channel isoform and even a specific conformational state using knowledge of molecular pharmacology. In the case of white matter, mature myelinated fibers are endowed mainly with $Na_v1.6$ at nodes of Ranvier (Caldwell *et al.*, 2000), so targeting these channels with selective agents may minimize peripheral cardiovascular side effects while maximizing the desired blocking action.

Anoxic *in vitro* models of white matter injury have been very useful for dissecting out injury mechanisms, but may display only a subset of the steps unleashed during more severe (and perhaps more clinically realistic) injury *in vivo*. For instance, as effective as TTX is at protecting white matter against anoxia *in vitro* (Imaizumi *et al.*, 1997; Stys *et al.*, 1992a), this agent is ineffective during more severe insults including more prolonged simulated *in vitro* ischemia using oxygen-glucose deprivation (Stys and Ouardouz, 2002), where previously dormant pathways may now be recruited. In ischemic (as opposed to anoxic) dorsal columns, protection is only apparent if Ca is removed from the bath and Na channels are blocked (Ouardouz *et al.*, 2003), suggesting that during ischemia internal Ca stores are unloaded independently of Ca entry across cell membranes, with both sources needing to be blocked for protection. If this observation is confirmed, it would suggest that neuroprotective strategies designed to control Ca influx across plasma membranes are necessary but not sufficient to fully protect tissue after more severe insults; optimal protection against ischemia will likely need to simultaneously address the release of internal Ca stores.

Another target apparent from Figure 41.8 is the glutamate receptor, particularly the AMPA/kainate class. This receptor appears to be primarily involved in damage to glia and myelin. A number of studies have confirmed the efficacy of AMPA receptor antagonists such as NBQX and GYKI52466 in *in vitro* anoxic, ischemic and traumatic white matter injury models (Agrawal and Fehlings, 1997b; Li *et al.*, 1999; Stys and Ouardouz, 2002).

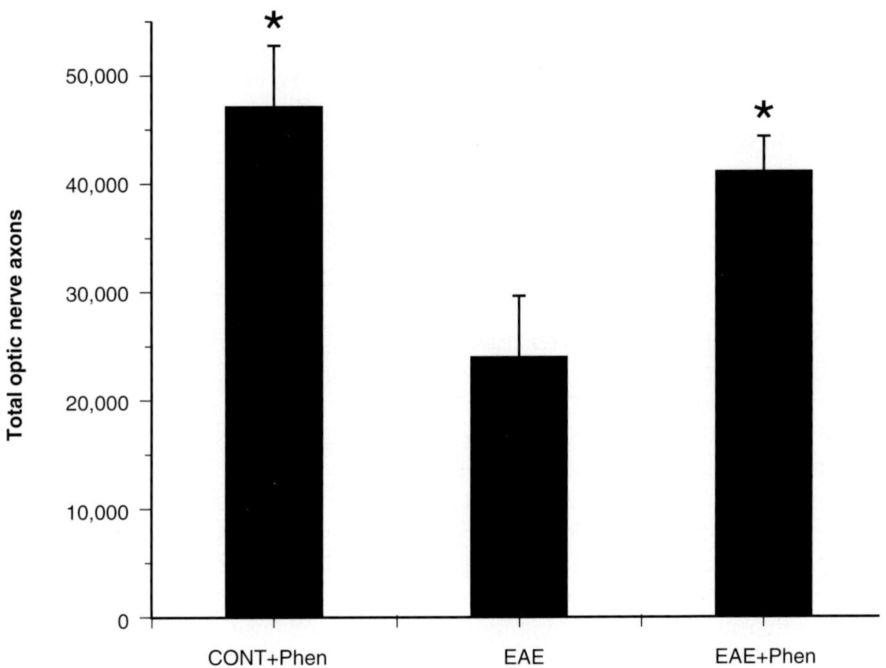


FIGURE 41.10
Total number of axons within optic nerves of control (no EAE, treated with phenytoin), EAE, and phenytoin treated EAE mice. There is a significant decrease in number of optic nerve axons in EAE. Phenytoin has a protective effect and produces a significant increase in the number of axons, compared to untreated EAE. Bars, means ± SD, * $p < 0.001$ compared to EAE. Reproduced from Lo *et al.*, 2002, with permission.

Equally important is the recent observation of white matter protection by AMPA receptor blockers in several *in vivo* models of ischemia, spinal cord injury, and auto-immune demyelination (Kanellopoulos *et al.*, 2000; McCracken *et al.*, 2002; Pitt *et al.*, 2000; Rosenberg *et al.*, 1999a; Smith *et al.*, 2000; Wrathall *et al.*, 1994, 1997). Coupled with the known beneficial effects of these agents against gray matter injury (Akins and Atkinson, 2002), this class of drug represents an attractive option and deserves further study.

While much of our understanding of white matter injury mechanisms has been obtained from *in vitro* models of anoxia or ischemia, emerging evidence suggests an unexpected degree of overlap with other white matter disorders, including trauma and immune-mediated demyelination. In the latter case, NO produced in inflammatory lesions may play a key role. Kapoor *et al.* (2003) have hypothesized that NO acts by impeding mitochondrial respiration. Drawing parallels from work on white matter anoxic injury, they have shown that partial blockade of Na channels with low doses of flecainide or lidocaine, or of the Na-Ca exchanger with bepridil, have a protective effect on axons exposed to NO. Extending these predictions to *in vivo* models of demyelination, two groups have recently demonstrated the utility of state-dependent Na channel blockers in ameliorating histological damage and clinical disability in an animal model of MS, experimental allergic encephalomyelitis (EAE). Bechtold *et al.* (2002) showed that flecainide, a class I anti-arrhythmic that blocks open Na channels preferentially (Ragsdale *et al.*, 1996), and which reduces NO-mediated axonal injury (discussed earlier), was significantly neuroprotective in a model of chronic relapsing EAE. Using a different class of Na channel blocking agent, Lo *et al.* (2002) have demonstrated that the anticonvulsant phenytoin (which is partially protective in an anoxic white matter model; see Fern *et al.*, 1993), can ameliorate clinical progression and prevent axonal degeneration in a similar model.

Finally, with the recent advent of reperfusion strategies in stroke using intravenous or intra-arterial thrombolysis (Meschia *et al.*, 2002) we are now faced with the potential of inducing reperfusion injury when ischemic regions have their blood flow restored. Mitochondria appear particularly vulnerable to reperfusion injury as described previously. Therefore strategies aimed at limiting mitochondrial Ca overload, perhaps by timed inhibition of the Ca uniporter, or the mitochondrial permeability transition or introduction of free radical scavengers, may reduce injury during the reperfusion phase. This has not been tested in white matter injury models.

## CONCLUSION

Given the key role that white matter tracts play in the overall operation of the CNS, it is essential that any protective or restorative strategies consider this tissue on a footing equal to its gray matter counterpart. Over the past decade, the many neuroprotective trials in stroke and traumatic brain injury were designed mainly if not exclusively with the goal of rescuing the neuron and the synapse, exhibiting a naïve inattention to the importance of axonal connections. We would argue that one of the main reasons for the failure of so many (indeed all!) acute neuroprotective trials (DeGraba and Pettigrew, 2000; Lees, 2000; Maas, 2001) is the fact that white matter pathophysiology was neglected in the design of these strategies. Over the past 10 years we have learned a great deal about how this tissue is damaged by ischemia, trauma, and immune attack, which positions the research community to now rationally devise the "next phase" of neuroprotective studies on the CNS, tailored to the protection of both gray and white matter regions.

### Acknowledgments

Work in the laboratory of PKS supported in part by grants from the Heart and Stroke Foundation of Ontario, National Institute of Neurological Disorders and Stroke, Canadian Institutes of Health Research, Ontario Neurotrauma Foundation, Canadian Stroke Network, Premier's Research Excellence Award from the Province of Ontario, Canadian MS Society, and the generosity of private donors.

Work in the laboratory of SGW supported in part by grants from the Rehabilitation Research Service and Medical Research Service, VA, and the National Multiple Sclerosis Society, and by gifts from the PVA and EPVA.

### References

Agrawal S. K., Fehlings M. G. (1996). Mechanisms of secondary injury to spinal cord axons in vitro–role of Na+, Na+-K+-ATPase, the Na+-H+ exchanger, and the Na+-Ca2+ exchanger. *J. Neurosci.* 16:545–552.

Agrawal S. K., Fehlings M. G. (1997a). The effect of the sodium channel blocker QX-314 on recovery after acute spinal cord injury. *J Neurotrauma* 14:81–88.

Agrawal S. K., Fehlings M. G. (1997b). Role of NMDA and non-NMDA ionotropic glutamate receptors in traumatic spinal cord axonal injury. *J. Neurosci.* 17:1055–1063.

Agrawal S. K., Theriault E., Fehlings M. G. (1998). Role of group I metabotropic glutamate receptors in traumatic spinal cord white matter injury. *J Neurotrauma* 15:929–941.

Agrawal S. K., Nashmi R., Fehlings M. G. (2000). Role of L- and N-type calcium channels in the pathophysiology of traumatic spinal cord white matter injury. *Neuroscience* 99:179–188.

Akins P. T., Atkinson R. P. (2002). Glutamate AMPA receptor antagonist treatment for ischaemic stroke. *Curr Med Res Opin* 18 Suppl 2:s9–13.

Arriza J. L., Fairman W. A., Wadiche J. I., Murdoch G. H., Kavanaugh M. P., Amara S. G. (1994). Functional comparisons of three glutamate transporter subtypes cloned from human motor cortex. *J. Neurosci.* 14:5559–5569.

Attwell D., Barbour B., Szatkowski M. (1993). Nonvesicular release of neurotransmitter. *Neuron* 11:401–407.

Bechtold D. A., Kapoor R., Smith K. J. (2002). Axonal protection in experimental inflammatory demyelinating disease achieved by flecainide therapy. *Soc. Neurosci. Abstr.* 93.7.

Bi R., Bi X., Baudry M. (1998a). Phosphorylation regulates calpain-mediated truncation of glutamate ionotropic receptors. *Brain Res* 797:154–158.

Bi X., Chen J., Baudry M. (1998b). Calpain-mediated proteolysis of GluR1 subunits in organotypic hippocampal cultures following kainic acid treatment. *Brain Res* 781:355–357.

Bi X., Rong Y., Chen J., Dang S., Wang Z., Baudry M. (1998c). Calpain-mediated regulation of NMDA receptor structure and function. *Brain Res* 790:245–253.

Bjartmar C., Trapp B. D. (2001). Axonal and neuronal degeneration in multiple sclerosis: Mechanisms and functional consequences. *Curr. Opin. Neurol.* 14:271–278.

Black J. A., Dib-Hajj S., Baker D., Newcombe J., Cuzner M. L., Waxman S. G. (2000). Sensory neuron -specific sodium channel SNS is abnormally expressed in the brains of mice with experimental allergic encephalomyelitis and humans with multiple sclerosis. *Proc. Natl. Acad. Sci. U.S.A.* 97:11598–11602.

Blaustein M. P., Lederer W. J. (1999). Sodium/calcium exchange: Its physiological implications. *Physiol. Rev.* 79:763–854.

Bo L., Dawson T. M., Wesselingh S., Mork S., Choi S., Kong P. A., Hanley D., Trapp B. D. (1994). Induction of nitric oxide synthase in demyelinating regions of multiple sclerosis brains. *Ann Neurol* 36:778–786.

Bolanos J. P., Almeida A., Stewart V., Peuchen S., Land J. M., Clark J. B., Heales S. J. (1997). Nitric oxide - mediated mitochondrial damage in the brain: Mechanisms and implications for neurodegenerative diseases. *J Neurochem* 68:2227–2240.

Brown A. M., Fern R., Jarvinen J. P., Kaila K., Ransom B. R. (1998). Changes in $[Ca^{2+}]_o$ during anoxia in CNS white matter. *Neuroreport* 9:1997–2000.

Brown A. M., Wender R., Ransom B. R. (2001a). Ionic mechanisms of aglycemic axon injury in mammalian central white matter. *J. Cereb. Blood Flow Metab.* 21:385–395.

Brown A. M., Westenbroek R. E., Catterall W. A., Ransom B. R. (2001b). Axonal L-type Ca(2+) channels and anoxic injury in rat CNS white matter. *J. Neurophysiol.* 85:900–911.

Buki A., Povlishock J. T., Siman R., Christman C. W. (1998). the role of calpain-mediated spectrin proteolysis (CMSP) in traumatically induced axonal injury (AI). *Soc. Neurosci. Abstr.* 24:252.

Buki A., Siman R., Trojanowski J. Q., Povlishock J. T. (1999). The role of calpain-mediated spectrin proteolysis in traumatically induced axonal injury. *J. Neuropathol. Exp. Neurol.* 58:365–375.

Caldwell J. H., Schaller K. L., Lasher R. S., Peles E., Levinson S. R. (2000). Sodium channel Nav1.6 is localized at nodes of Ranvier, dendrites, and synapses. *Proc. Natl. Acad. Sci. U.S.A.*

Callahan D. J., Engle M. J., Volpe J. J. (1990). Hypoxic injury to developing glial cells: Protective effect of high glucose. *Pediatr Res* 27:186–190.

Casha S., Yu W. R., Fehlings M. G. (2001). Oligodendroglial apoptosis occurs along degenerating axons and is associated with FAS and p75 expression following spinal cord injury in the rat. *Neuroscience* 103:203–218.

Catterall W. A. (1980). Neurotoxins that act on voltage-sensitive sodium channels in excitable membranes. *Annu. Rev. Pharmacol. Toxicol.* 20:15–43.

Chen C. J., Liao S. L., Kuo J. S. (2000). Gliotoxic action of glutamate on cultured astrocytes. *J Neurochem* 75:1557–1565.

Chih C. P., Lipton P., Roberts E. L., Jr. (2001). Do active cerebral neurons really use lactate rather than glucose? *Trends Neurosci.* 24:573–578.

Clarke D. D., Sokoloff L. (1994). Circulation and energy metabolism of the brain. *In* "Basic Neurochemistry" (G. J. Siegel, B. W. Agranoff, R. W., Albers, and P. B. Molinoff, eds.), 5th ed., pp. 645–680. Raven Press, New York.

Collins J. G. (1990). Types of injuries by selected characteristics. *Vital Health Stat.*:1–68.

Cooper C. E. (2002). Nitric oxide and cytochrome oxidase: Substrate, inhibitor or effector? *Trends Biochem. Sci.* 27:33–39.

Covault J., Liu Q. Y., el-Deeb S. (1991). Calcium-activated proteolysis of intracellular domains in the cell adhesion molecules NCAM and N-cadherin. *Brain Res Mol Brain Res* 11:11–16.

Cross A. H., Manning P. T., Keeling R. M., Schmidt R. E., Misko T. P. (1998). Peroxynitrite formation within the central nervous system in active multiple sclerosis. *J Neuroimmunol* 88:45–56.

Darley U. V., Stone D., Smith D., Martin J. F. (1991). Mitochondria, oxygen and reperfusion damage. *Ann. Med.* 23:583–588.

David J. C., Yamada K. A., Bagwe M. R., Goldberg M. P. (1996). AMPA receptor activation is rapidly toxic to cortical astrocytes when desensitization is blocked. *J. Neurosci.* 16:200–209.

DeGraba T. J., Pettigrew L. C. (2000). Why do neuroprotective drugs work in animals but not humans? *Neurol Clin* 18:475–493.

Deshpande R. V., Goust J. M., Hogan E. L., Banik N. L. (1995). Calpain secreted by activated human lymphoid cells degrades myelin. *J. Neurosci. Res.* 42:259–265.

Devlin T. M. (Ed.). (1992). "Textbook of Biochemistry," 3rd ed. Wiley-Liss, New York.

Dohmen C., Kumura E., Rosner G., Heiss W. D., Graf R. (2001). Adenosine in relation to calcium homeostasis: Comparison between gray and white matter ischemia. *J Cereb Blood Flow Metab* 21:503–510.

Dong H., Dunn J., Lytton J. (2002). Stoichiometry of the Cardiac Na+/Ca2+ exchanger NCX1.1 measured in transfected HEK cells. *Biophys J* 82:1943–1952.

Dong H., Light P. E., French R. J., Lytton J. (2001). Electrophysiological characterization and ionic stoichiometry of the rat brain K(+)-dependent NA(+)/CA(2+) exchanger, NCKX2. *J Biol Chem* 276:25919–25928.

Eng D. L., Gordon T. R., Kocsis J. D., Waxman S. G. (1990). Current-clamp analysis of a time-dependent rectification in rat optic nerve. *J. Physiol. (Lond.)* 421:185–202.

Erecinska M., Dagani F. (1990). Relationships between the neuronal sodium/potassium pump and energy metabolism. Effects of K+, Na+, and adenosine triphosphate in isolated brain synaptosomes. *J. Gen. Physiol.* 95:591–616.

Erecinska M., Silver I. A. (1989). ATP and brain function. *J. Cereb. Blood Flow Metab.* 9:2–19.

Ferguson B., Matyszak M. K., Esiri M. M., Perry V. H. (1997). Axonal damage in acute multiple sclerosis lesions. *Brain* 120:393–399.

Fern R., Davis P., Waxman S. G., Ransom B. R. (1998). Axon conduction and survival in CNS white matter during energy deprivation: A developmental study. *J. Neurophysiol.* 79:95–105.

Fern R., Moller T. (2000). Rapid ischemic cell death in immature oligodendrocytes: A fatal glutamate release feedback loop. *J Neurosci* 20:34–42.

Fern R., Ransom B. R., Waxman S. G. (1995a). Voltage-gated calcium channels in CNS white matter: Role in anoxic injury. *J. Neurophysiol.* 74:369–377.

Fern R., Ransom B. R., Waxman S. G. (1996a). Autoprotective mechanisms in the CNS: Some new lessons from white matter. *Mol. Chem. Neuropathol.* 27:107–129.

Fern R., Ransom B. R., Waxman S. G. (1996b). White matter stroke: Autoprotective mechanisms with therapeutic implications. *Cerebrovasc. Dis.* 6:59–65.

Fern R., Ransom B., Stys P. K., Waxman S. G. (1993). Pharmacological protection of CNS white matter during anoxia: Actions of phenytoin, carbamazepine and diazepam. *J. Pharmacol. Exp. Ther.* 266:1549–1555.

Fern R., Waxman S. G., Ransom B. R. (1994). Modulation of anoxic injury in CNS white matter by adenosine and interaction between adenosine and GABA. *J. Neurophysiol.* 72:2609–2616.

Fern R., Waxman S. G., Ransom B. R. (1995b). Endogenous GABA attenuates CNS white matter dysfunction following anoxia. *J. Neurosci.* 15:699–708.

Fisher C. M. (1982). Lacunar strokes and infarcts: A review. *Neurology* 32:871–876.

Follett P. L., Rosenberg P. A., Volpe J. J., Jensen F. E. (2000). NBQX attenuates excitotoxic injury in developing white matter. *J. Neurosci.* 20:9235–9241.

Fonnum F. (1984). Glutamate: A neurotransmitter in mammalian brain. *J. Neurochem.* 42:1–11.

Garcia-Barcina J. M., Matute C. (1996). Expression of kainate-selective glutamate receptor subunits in glial cells of the adult bovine white matter. *Eur. J. Neurosci.* 8:2379–2387.

Garcia-Barcina J. M., Matute C. (1998). AMPA-selective glutamate receptor subunits in glial cells of the adult bovine white matter. *Brain Res. Mol. Brain Res.* 53:270–276.

Garthwaite G., Goodwin D. A., Batchelor A. M., Leeming K., Garthwaite J. (2002). Nitric oxide toxicity in CNS white matter: An in vitro study using rat optic nerve. *Neuroscience* 109:145–155.

Gellerman D. M., Bi X., Baudry M. (1997). NMDA receptor-mediated regulation of AMPA receptor properties in organotypic hippocampal slice cultures. *J Neurochem* 69:131–136.

Gibson C. J. (1992). Overview of spinal cord injury. *Phys. Med. Rehab. Clin. North Am.* 3:699–709.

Graf R., Dohmen C., Kumura E., Rosner G., Heiss W.-D. (1998). Extracellular shifts of GABA, adenosine and ion activities in cortical gray and subcortical white matter during global ischemia in cats. *Soc. Neurosci. Abstr.* 24:983.

Griffiths R., Dunlop J., Gorman A., Senior J., Grieve A. (1994). L-trans-pyrrolidine-2,4-dicarboxylate and cis-1-aminocyclobutane-1,3-dicarboxylate behave as transportable, competitive inhibitors of the high-affinity glutamate transporters. *Biochem. Pharmacol.* 47:267–274.

Hell J. W., Westenbroek R. E., Breeze L. J., Wang K. K., Chavkin C., Catterall W. A. (1996). N-methyl-D-aspartate receptor-induced proteolytic conversion of postsynaptic class C L-type calcium channels in hippocampal neurons. *Proc Natl Acad Sci U S A* 93:3362–3367.

Hewitt K. E., Stys P. K., Lesiuk H. J. (2001). The use-dependent sodium channel blocker mexiletine is neuroprotective against global ischemic injury. *Brain Res.* 898:281–287.

Imaizumi T., Kocsis J. D., Waxman S. G. (1997). Anoxic injury in the rat spinal cord-pharmacological evidence for multiple steps in Ca2+-dependent injury of the dorsal columns. *J. Neurotrauma* 14:299–311.

Imaizumi T., Kocsis J. D., Waxman S. G. (1999). The role of voltage-gated Ca2+ channels in anoxic injury of spinal cord white matter. *Brain Res.* 817:84–92.

Jalc P., Marsala J., Jalcova H. (1995). Postischemic reperfusion causes a massive calcium overload in the myelinated spinal cord fibers. *Mol. Chem. Neuropathol.* 25:143–153.

Jensen A. M., Chiu S. Y. (1993). Expression of glutamate receptor genes in white matter: Developing and adult rat optic nerve. *J. Neurosci.* 13:1664–1675.

Jiang Q., Stys P. K. (2000). Calpain inhibitors confer biochemical, but not electrophysiological, protection against anoxia in rat optic nerves. *J. Neurochem.* 74:2101–2107.

Kampfl A., Posmantur R. M., Zhao X., Schmutzhard E., Clifton G. L., Hayes R. L. (1997). Mechanisms of calpain proteolysis following traumatic brain injury: Implications for pathology and therapy. A review and update. *J. Neurotrauma* 14:121–134.

Kanellopoulos G. K., Xu X. M., Hsu C. Y., Lu X., Sundt T. M., Kouchoukos N. T. (2000). White matter injury in spinal cord ischemia: Protection by AMPA/kainate glutamate receptor antagonism. *Stroke* 31:1945–1952.

Kapoor R., Davies M., Blaker P. A., et al (2003). Protection of axons from degeneration caused by nitric oxide can be achieved using blockers of the sodium channel and sodium-calcium exchanger. *Ann. Neurol.* in press.

Khodorov B. I. (1991). Role of inactivation in local anesthetic action. *Ann. N. Y. Acad. Sci.* 625:224–248.

Kiedrowski L., Czyz A., Li X. F., Lytton J. (2002). Preferential expression of plasmalemmal K-dependent Na+/Ca2+ exchangers in neurons versus astrocytes. *Neuroreport* 13:1529–1532.

Koizumi J. (1974). Glycogen in the central nervous system. *Prog. Histochem. Cytochem.* 6:1–37.

Kornek B., Lassmann H. (1999). Axonal pathology in multiple sclerosis. A historical note. *Brain Pathol.* 9:651–656.

Kornek B., Storch M. K., Bauer J., Djamshidian A., Weissert R., Wallstroem E., Stefferl A., Zimprich F., Olsson T., Linington C., Schmidbauer M., Lassmann H. (2001). Distribution of a calcium channel subunit in dystrophic axons in multiple sclerosis and experimental autoimmune encephalomyelitis. *Brain* 124:1114–1124.

Kriegler S., Chiu S. Y. (1993). Calcium signaling of glial cells along mammalian axons. *J. Neurosci.* 13:4229–4245.

Lees K. R. (2000). Neuroprotection. *Br Med Bull* 56:401–412.

Leppanen L. L., Stys P. K. (1997). Ion transport and membrane potential in CNS myelinated axons. II: Effects of metabolic inhibition. *J. Neurophysiol.* 78:2095–2107.

Levy L. M., Warr O., Attwell D. (1998). Stoichiometry of the glial glutamate transporter GLT-1 expressed inducibly in a chinese hamster ovary cell line selected for low endogenous Na+-dependent glutamate uptake. *J. Neurosci.* 18:9620–9628.

Li S., Jiang Q., Stys P. K. (2000). Important role of reverse Na(+)-Ca(2+) exchange in spinal cord white matter injury at physiological temperature. *J. Neurophysiol.* 84:1116–1119.

Li S., Mealing G. A., Morley P., Stys P. K. (1999). Novel injury mechanism in anoxia and trauma of spinal cord white matter: Glutamate release via reverse Na+-dependent glutamate transport. *J. Neurosci.* 19:RC16.

Li S., Stys P. K. (2000). Mechanisms of ionotropic glutamate receptor-mediated excitotoxicity in isolated spinal cord white matter. *J. Neurosci.* 20:1190–1198.

Lipton P. (1999). Ischemic cell death in brain neurons. *Physiol. Rev.* 79:1431–1568.

Lo A. C., Black J. A., Waxman S. G. (2002). Neuroprotection of axons with phenytoin in experimental allergic encephalomyelitis. *Neuroreport* 13:1909–1912.

LoPachin R. M., Gaughan C. L., Lehning E. J., Kaneko Y., Kelly T. M., Blight A. (1999). Experimental spinal cord injury: Spatiotemporal characterization of elemental concentrations and water contents in axons and neuroglia. *J. Neurophysiol.* 82:2143–2153.

LoPachin R. M., Stys P. K. (1995). Elemental composition and water content of rat optic nerve myelinated axons and glial cells: Effects of in vitro anoxia and reoxygenation. *J. Neurosci.* 15:6735–6746.

Maas A. I. (2001). Neuroprotective agents in traumatic brain injury. *Expert Opin Investig Drugs* 10:753–767.

MacManus J. P., Buchan A. M. (2000). Apoptosis after experimental stroke: Fact or fashion? *J Neurotrauma* 17:899–914.

Malek S., Coderre E., Stys P. K. (2002). K-Cl cotransporter mediates injurious Cl flux in anoxic/ischemic CNS white matter. *J. Neurosci.*:in prep.

Malek S., Stys P. K. (2002). Effects of Na and Cl fluxes during anoxia on the compound action potential of rat optic nerve. *Soc. Neurosci. Abstr.* 95.9.

Matsuo A., Akiguchi I., Lee G. C., McGeer E. G., McGeer P. L., Kimura J. (1998). Myelin degeneration in multiple system atrophy detected by unique antibodies. *Am J Pathol* 153:735–744.

Matute C. (1998). Characteristics of acute and chronic kainate excitotoxic damage to the optic nerve. *Proc. Natl. Acad. Sci. U.S.A.* 95:10229–10234.

Matute C., Alberdi E., Ibarretxe G., Sanchez-Gomez M. V. (2002). Excitotoxicity in glial cells. *Eur J Pharmacol* 447:239–246.

Matute C., Sanchez-Gomez M. V., Martinez-Millan L., Miledi R. (1997). Glutamate receptor-mediated toxicity in optic nerve oligodendrocytes. *Proc. Natl. Acad. Sci. U.S.A.* 94:8830–8835.

Maxwell W. L., Povlishock J. T., Graham D. L. (1997). A mechanistic analysis of nondisruptive axonal injury: A review. *J. Neurotrauma* 14:419–440.

McCracken E., Dewar D., Hunter A. J. (2001). White matter damage following systemic injection of the mitochondrial inhibitor 3-nitropropionic acid in rat. *Brain Res* 892:329–335.

McCracken E., Fowler J. H., Dewar D., Morrison S., McCulloch J. (2002). Grey matter and white matter ischemic damage is reduced by the competitive AMPA receptor antagonist, SPD 502. *J Cereb Blood Flow Metab* 22:1090–1097.

McDonald J. W., Althomsons S. P., Hyrc K. L., Choi D. W., Goldberg M. P. (1998). Oligodendrocytes from forebrain are highly vulnerable to AMPA/kainate receptor-mediated excitotoxicity. *Nat. Med.* 4:291–297.

Meschia J. F., Miller D. A., Brott T. G. (2002). Thrombolytic treatment of acute ischemic stroke. *Mayo Clin Proc* 77:542–551.

Nicholls D. G., Budd S. L. (2000). Mitochondria and neuronal survival. *Physiol. Rev.* 80:315–360.

Nikolaeva M. A., Stys P. K. (2002). Calcium changes in ischemic rat optic nerve axons studied by confocal microscopy. *Soc. Neurosci. Abstr.* 299.6.

Oka A., Belliveau M. J., Rosenberg P. A., Volpe J. J. (1993). Vulnerability of oligodendroglia to glutamate: Pharmacology, mechanisms, and prevention. *J. Neurosci.* 13:1441–1453.

Orrenius S., Nicotera P. (1996). Mechanisms of calcium-related cell death. *In* "Cellular and Molecular Mechanisms of Ischemic Brain Damage" (B. K. Siesjo and T. Wieloch, eds.), pp. 137–152. Raven Press, New York.

Ouardouz, M., Nikolaeva, M., Coderre, E., Zamponi, G. W., McRory, J. E., Trapp, B. D., Yin, X., Wang, W., Woulfe, J., Stys, P. K. (2003). Depolarization-induced $Ca^{2+}$release in ischemic spinal cord white matter involves L-type $Ca^{2+}$ channel activation of ryanodine receptors. *Neuron* **40**, 53–63.

Pasti L., Zonta M., Pozzan T., Vicini S., Carmignoto G. (2001). Cytosolic calcium oscillations in astrocytes may regulate exocytotic release of glutamate. *J. Neurosci.* 21:477–484.

Pitt D., Werner P., Raine C. S. (2000). Glutamate excitotoxicity in a model of multiple sclerosis. *Nat. Med.* 6:67–70.

Povlishock J. T., Christman C. W. (1995). Diffuse axonal injury. *In* "The Axon: Structure, Function and Pathophysiology" (S. G. Waxman, J. D. Kocsis, and P. K. Stys, eds.), pp. 504–529. Oxford University Press, New York.

Ragsdale D. S., McPhee J. C., Scheuer T., Catterall W. A. (1996). Common molecular determinants of local anesthetic, antiarrhythmic, and anticonvulsant block of voltage-gated Na+ channels. *Proc Natl Acad Sci U S A* 93:9270–9275.

Rami A., Ferger D., Krieglstein J. (1997). Blockade of calpain proteolytic activity rescues neurons from glutamate excitotoxicity. *Neurosci. Res.* 27:93–97.

Ransom B. R., Walz W., Davis P. K., Carlini W. G. (1992). Anoxia-induced changes in extracellular $K^+$ and pH in mammalian central white matter. *J. Cereb. Blood Flow Metab.* 12:593–602.

Ren Y., Ridsdale A., Coderre E., Stys P. K. (2000). Calcium imaging in live rat optic nerve myelinated axons in vitro using confocal laser microscopy. *J. Neurosci. Meth.* 102:165–176.

Rieckmann P., Maurer M. (2002). Anti-inflammatory strategies to prevent axonal injury in multiple sclerosis. *Curr Opin Neurol* 15:361–370.

Rieckmann P., Smith K. J. (2001). Multiple sclerosis: More than inflammation and demyelination. *Trends Neurosci* 24:435–437.

Rios E., Brum G. (1987). Involvement of dihydropyridine receptors in excitation-contraction coupling in skeletal muscle. *Nature* 325:717–720.

Rose C. R., Waxman S. G., Ransom B. R. (1998). Effects of glucose deprivation, chemical hypoxia, and simulated ischemia on $Na^+$ homeostasis in rat spinal cord astrocytes. *J. Neurosci.* 18:3554–3562.

Rosenberg L. J., Teng Y. D., Wrathall J. R. (1999a). 2,3-dihydroxy-6-nitro-7-sulfamoyl-benzo(*f*)quinoxaline reduces glial loss and acute white matter pathology after experimental spinal cord contusion. *J. Neurosci.* 19:464–475.

Rosenberg L. J., Teng Y. D., Wrathall J. R. (1999b). Effects of the sodium channel blocker tetrodotoxin on acute white matter pathology after experimental contusive spinal cord injury. *J. Neurosci.* 19:6122–6133.

Rutledge E. M., Aschner M., Kimelberg H. K. (1998). Pharmacological characterization of swelling-induced D-[3H]aspartate release from primary astrocyte cultures. *Am. J. Physiol.* 274:C1511–1520.

Salamino F., Sparatore B., Melloni E., Michetti M., Viotti P. L., Pontremoli S., Carafoli E. (1994). The plasma membrane calcium pump is the preferred calpain substrate within the erythrocyte. *Cell Calcium* 15:28–35.

Schaecher K. E., Shields D. C., Banik N. L. (2001). Mechanism of myelin breakdown in experimental demyelination: A putative role for calpain. *Neurochem Res* 26:731–737.

Schanne F. A., Kane A. B., Young E. E., Farber J. L. (1979). Calcium-dependence of toxic cell death: A final common pathway. *Science* 206:700–702.

Schumacher P. A., Siman R. G., Fehlings M. G. (2000). Pretreatment with calpain inhibitor CEP-4143 inhibits calpain I activation and cytoskeletal degradation, improves neurological function, and enhances axonal survival after traumatic spinal cord injury. *J. Neurochem.* 74:1646–1655.

Shields D. C., Schaecher K. E., Saido T. C., Banik N. L. (1999). A putative mechanism of demyelination in multiple sclerosis by a proteolytic enzyme, calpain. *Proc. Natl. Acad. Sci. U.S.A.* 96:11486–11491.

Silver I. A., Deas J., Erecinska M. (1997). Ion homeostasis in brain cells: Differences in intracellular ion responses to energy limitation between cultured neurons and glial cells. *Neuroscience* 78:589–601.

Smith K. J., Kapoor R., Hall S. M., Davies M. (2001). Electrically active axons degenerate when exposed to nitric oxide. *Ann. Neurol.* 49:470–476.

Smith M. R., Smith R. D., Plummer N. W., Meisler M. H., Goldin A. L. (1998). Functional analysis of the mouse Scn8a sodium channel. *J. Neurosci.* 18:6093–6102.

Smith T., Groom A., Zhu B., Turski L. (2000). Autoimmune encephalomyelitis ameliorated by AMPA antagonists. *Nat Med* 6:62–66.

Sorg O., Magistretti P. J. (1991). Characterization of the glycogenolysis elicited by vasoactive intestinal peptide, noradrenaline and adenosine in primary cultures of mouse cerebral cortical astrocytes. *Brain Res* 563:227–233.

Sosin D. M., Sniezek J. E., Thurman D. J. (1996). Incidence of mild and moderate brain injury in the United States, 1991. *Brain Inj.* 10:47–54.

Steinhauser C., Gallo V. (1996). News on glutamate receptors in glial cells. *Trends Neurosci* 19:339–345.

Stryer L. (1988). "Biochemistry." W. H. Freeman, New York.

Stys P. K. (1995). Protective effects of antiarrhythmic agents against anoxic injury in CNS white matter. *J. Cereb. Blood Flow Metab.* 15:425–432.

Stys P. K. (1998). Anoxic and ischemic injury of myelinated axons in CNS white matter: From mechanistic concepts to therapeutics. *J. Cereb. Blood Flow Metab.* 18:2–25.

Stys P. K., Hubatsch D. A., Leppanen L. L. (1998). Effects of K+ channel blockers on the anoxic response of central myelinated axons. *NeuroReport* 9:447–453.

Stys P. K., Jiang Q. (2002). Ca2+-mediated calpain-dependent neurofilament breakdown in anoxic and ischemic central white matter axons. *Neurosci. Lett.* 328:150–154.

Stys P. K., Lehning E. J., Sauberman A. J., LoPachin R. M. (1997). Intracellular concentrations of major ions in rat myelinated axons and glia: Calculations based on electron probe X-ray microanalyses. *J. Neurochem.* 68:1920–1928.

Stys P. K., Lesiuk H. (1996). Correlation between electrophysiological effects of mexiletine and ischemic

Stys P. K., Li S. (2000). Glutamate-induced white matter injury: Excitotoxicity without synapses. *The Neuroscientist* 6:230–233.

Stys P. K., LoPachin R. M. (1996). Elemental composition and water content of rat optic nerve myelinated axons during in vitro post-anoxia reoxygenation. *Neuroscience* 73:1081–1090.

protection of CNS white matter. *Neuroscience* 71:27–36.

Stys P. K., LoPachin R. M. (1998). Mechanisms of ion flux in anoxic myelinated CNS axons. *Neuroscience* 82:21–32.

Stys P. K., Ouardouz M. (2002). Role of glutamate receptors in spinal cord dorsal column ischemia. *Soc. Neurosci. Abstr.*:298.298.

Stys P. K., Ransom B. R., Waxman S. G. (1992b). Tertiary and quaternary local anesthetics protect CNS white matter from anoxic injury at concentrations that do not block excitability. *J. Neurophysiol.* 67:236–240.

Stys P. K., Ransom B. R., Waxman S. G., Davis P. K. (1990). Role of extracellular calcium in anoxic injury of mammalian central white matter. *Proc. Natl. Acad. Sci. USA*. 87:4212–4216.

Stys P. K., Sontheimer H., Ransom B. R., Waxman S. G. (1993). Non-inactivating, TTX-sensitive $Na^+$ conductance in rat optic nerve axons. *Proc. Natl. Acad. Sci. USA*. 90:6976–6980.

Stys P. K., Waxman S. G., Ransom B. R. (1992a). Ionic mechanisms of anoxic injury in mammalian CNS white matter: Role of $Na^+$ channels and $Na^+$ -$Ca^{2+}$ exchanger. *J. Neurosci.* 12:430–439.

Swanson R. A., Yu A. C., Sharp F. R., Chan P. H. (1989). Regulation of glycogen content in primary astrocyte culture: Effects of glucose analogues, phenobarbital, and methionine sulfoximine. *J. Neurochem.* 52:1359–1365.

Taylor C. P. (1993). Na+ currents that fail to inactivate. *Trends Neurosci.* 16:455–460.

Taylor C. P., Weber M. L., Gaughan C. L., Lehning E. J., LoPachin R. M. (1999). Oxygen/glucose deprivation in hippocampal slices: Altered intraneuronal elemental composition predicts structural and functional damage. *J. Neurosci.* 19:619–629.

Tekkok S. B., Goldberg M. P. (2001). AMPA/kainate receptor activation mediates hypoxic oligodendrocyte death and axonal injury in cerebral white matter. *J. Neurosci.* 21:4237–4248.

Tekkok S. B., Hyrc K. L., Underhill S. M., Goldberg M. P. (2000). Na+/Ca2+ exchange blocker KB-R7943 protects axons and oligodendrocytes during oxygen glucose deprivation. *Soc. Neurosci. Abstr.* 26:2065.

Teng Y. D., Wrathall J. R. (1997). Local blockade of sodium channels by tetrodotoxin ameliorates tissue loss and long -term functional deficits resulting from experimental spinal cord injury. *J. Neurosci.* 17:4359–4366.

Thorell W. E., Leibrock L. G., Agrawal S. K. (2002). Role of RyRs and IP3 receptors after traumatic injury to spinal cord white matter. *J. Neurotrauma* 19:335–342.

Trapp B. D., Peterson J., Ransohoff R. M., Rudick R., Mork S., Bo L. (1998). Axonal transection in the lesions of multiple sclerosis. *N. Engl. J. Med.* 338:278–285.

Tsacopoulos M., Magistretti P. J. (1996). Metabolic coupling between glia and neurons. *J. Neurosci.* 16:877–885.

Underhill S. M., Goldberg M. P. (2002). Axons potentiate oligodendrocyte vulernability to excitotoxicity. *Soc. Neurosci. Abstr.* 299.7.

Wang G. K., Brodwick M. S., Eaton D. C., Strichartz G. R. (1987). Inhibition of sodium currents by local anesthetics in chloramine-T-treated squid axons. The role of channel activation. *J. Gen. Physiol.* 89:645–667.

Waxman S. G. (2000). Multiple sclerosis as a neuronal disease. *Arch Neurol* 57:22–24.

Waxman S. G. (2001). Transcriptional channelopathies: an emerging class of disorders. *Nat. Rev. Neurosci.* 2:652–659.

Waxman S. G., Black J. A., Ransom B. R., Stys P. K. (1993). Protection of the axonal cytoskeleton in anoxic optic nerve by decreased extracellular calcium. *Brain Res.* 614:137–145.

Waxman S. G., Kocsis J. D., Stys P. K., (Eds.). (1995). "The Axon: Structure, Function and Pathophysiology." Oxford University Press, New York.

Weinshenker B. G. (1996). Epidemiology of multiple sclerosis. *Neurol Clin* 14:291–308.

Wender R., Brown A. M., Fern R., Swanson R. A., Farrell K., Ransom B. R. (2000). Astrocytic glycogen influences axon function and survival during glucose deprivation in central white matter. *J Neurosci* 20:6804–6810.

White B. C., Sullivan J. M., DeGracia D. J., O'Neil B. J., Neumar R. W., Grossman L. I., Rafols J. A., Krause G. S. (2000). Brain ischemia and reperfusion: Molecular mechanisms of neuronal injury. *J Neurol Sci* 179:1–33.

Wolf J. A., Stys P. K., Lusardi T., Meaney D., Smith D. H. (2001). Traumatic axonal injury induces calcium influx modulated by tetrodotoxin-sensitive sodium channels. *J. Neurosci.* 21:1923–1930.

Wrathall J. R., Choiniere D., Teng Y. D. (1994). Dose-dependent reduction of tissue loss and functional impairment after spinal cord trauma with the AMPA/kainate antagonist NBQX. *J. Neurosci.* 14:6598–6607.

Wrathall J. R., Teng Y. D., Marriott R. (1997). Delayed antagonism of AMPA/kainate receptors reduces long-term functional deficits resulting from spinal cord trauma. *Exp. Neurol.* 145:565–573.

Yam P. S., Dunn L. T., Graham D. I., Dewar D., McCulloch J. (2000). NMDA receptor blockade fails to alter axonal injury in focal cerebral ischemia. *J Cereb Blood Flow Metab* 20:772–779.

Yeh J. Z., Tanguy J. (1985). Na channel activation gate modulates slow recovery from use-dependent block by local anesthetics in squid giant axons. *Biophys. J.* 47:685–694.

Yoshioka A., Bacskai B., Pleasure D. (1996). Pathophysiology of oligodendroglial excitotoxicity. *J. Neurosci. Res.* 46:427–437.

Yoshioka A., Hardy M., Younkin D. P., Grinspan J. B., Stern J. L., Pleasure D. (1995). Alpha-amino-3 -hydroxy-5-methyl-4-isoxazolepropionate (AMPA) receptors mediate excitotoxicity in the oligodendroglial lineage. *J. Neurochem.* 64:2442–2448.

Yu, A. C. H., Gregory G. A., Chan P. H. (1989). Hypoxia-induced dysfunctions and injury of astrocytes in primary cell cultures. *J. Cereb. Blood Flow Metab.* 9:20–28.

Zerangue N., Kavanaugh M. P. (1996). Flux coupling in a neuronal glutamate transporter. *Nature* 383:634–637.

Zhang K., Sejnowski T. J. (2000). A universal scaling law between gray matter and white matter of cerebral cortex. *Proc Natl Acad Sci U S A* 97:5621–5626.

CHAPTER

# 42

# Protein Misfolding as a Disease Determinant

*Alexander Gow*

## INTRODUCTION

"Conformational diseases" is the term used increasingly to refer to a large eclectic group of degenerative disorders with far greater similarities in pathophysiology than is apparent clinically. As this umbrella term suggests, conformational diseases arise at least in part from perturbations to three-dimensional structure in one or more cellular proteins stemming from genetic missense or nonsense mutations or from unclear etiology. At least some of these diseases can be loosely regarded as evolutionarily conserved in the sense that molecular mechanisms underlying pathogenesis in mammals are known to operate in and modify the behavior of yeast and fungi and, perhaps, organisms in many phyla (Prusiner, 1998; Uptain and Lindquist, 2002).

In humans, the deposition of abnormally folded proteins have been found in most organs including CNS, kidney, liver, heart, bones, and joints. Curiously, deposits typically occur in CNS but not other organs or vice versa, but the etiology of this apparent arbitrary division is currently unknown (Pepys, 2001). The amyloidosis group of conformational diseases comprises systemic degenerative disorders that mainly involve the peripheral organs. As the name indicates, these diseases arise from the deposition of amyloid in tissue that is extracellular and is composed of any one of approximately 20 proteins having little in common except for a capacity to generate insoluble fibrillar deposits with a stable β-sheet structure. This common secondary structure motif, which involves interactions between the amino acid main chain atoms, is a generic property of polypeptides that can be generated using purified proteins *in vitro* (reviewed by Dobson, 2001). Nevertheless, specific diseases with distinct clinical phenotypes result from the accumulation of particular proteins, which suggests that unique properties of the misfolded polypeptide chains drive the pathophysiology.

An important aspect of pathogenesis in systemic amyloidoses is the dependence on abnormally high concentrations of major components of the amyloid fibrils. For example, chronic infections and inflammation cause sustained overproduction of acute phase proteins such as serum amyloid A protein, which is the apolipoprotein component of high density lipoprotein. Processed forms of this protein are most commonly deposited in kidney leading to renal failure. $A\beta_2M$ amyloidosis is a complication of long-term hemodialysis, for which the $\beta_2$-microglobulin component of HLA class I molecules accumulates in the bones and joints. $\beta_2$-microglobulin is normally exclusively removed from blood by the proximal tubules of the kidney; however, this clearance is inefficient after kidney failure and cannot be effected by hemodialysis, which leads to chronic elevation of $\beta_2$-microglobulin levels in plasma.

The major focus of this review is the group of conformational diseases that stem from aberrant protein folding in the central nervous system (CNS). The number of disorders included in this group has been growing rapidly and includes several well-known diseases—Alzheimer's disease, Parkinson's disease, prion protein diseases, Huntington's disease and frontotemporal dementias—for which important findings have been reported in recent years.

## PROTEIN INCLUSION DISEASES

A major focus of a large number of studies appearing in the literature in recent years has been to identify cellular conditions leading to the generation of altered protein conformations as well as changes in protein processing and aggregation. Such pathology is commonplace in neurodegenerative diseases and stems from increased β-sheet secondary structure and aggregation of one or more of several proteins that lead to formation of the amyloid-like deposits and inclusion bodies observed in Alzheimer's disease, Parkinson's disease, advanced Down's syndrome, and frontotemporal dementia and Parkinsonism linked to chromosome 17 (FTDP-17). The proteins involved in this pathology include amyloid precursor protein-derived peptides (e.g., Aβ), α-synuclein and the microtubule-associated protein, tau (Trojanowski, 2002). However, amyloid deposits and inclusions are also found in other diseases including prion diseases, Huntington's disease, most spinocerebellar ataxias, and serpinopathies (reviewed in Cummings and Zoghbi, 2000; Lomas and Carrell, 2002).

The degree to which amyloid deposits and inclusions contribute to neurodegenerative pathophysiology is currently unclear and, in some if not most cases, their presence may reflect secondary processes stemming from upstream events (Cummings and Zoghbi, 2000; Trojanowski, 2002). Despite the persistence of these protein aggregates in the parenchyma as prominent features or hallmarks of specific disorders, deposits and inclusions are increasingly thought to be nontoxic. Indeed, for several spinocerebellar ataxias inclusions are not detected in neuronal populations that are primarily affected but rather are observed in nontarget neurons from brain regions exhibiting little to no other pathology or clinical involvement (Cummings and Zoghbi, 2000). On the other hand, proteins that comprise the protein aggregates are directly implicated in pathogenesis of several diseases. For example, amyloid fibrils composed of the Aβ peptide are prominent features of sporadic Alzheimer's disease and mutations in the amyloid precursor protein lead to increased deposition of Aβ amyloid in familial Alzheimer's disease. In similar fashion, sporadic and familial forms of Parkinson's disease involve α-synuclein in Lewy bodies while FTDP-17 involves tau in neurofibrillary tangles and prion disease involves PrP protein in inclusions. Thus, the genes that are mutated in familial forms of these diseases encode proteins, which are major components of the inclusions observed in sporadic forms of the same diseases.

A relatively simple explanation to accommodate apparently opposing views about the relevance of amyloid and inclusions in neurodegenerative disease is that the monomeric or oligomeric forms of the proteins are the toxic species and cells attempt to neutralize this toxicity by sequestering the protein into large aggregates. Indeed, recent *in vivo* data indicate as much for neurodegenerative changes associated with alternatively folded forms of the prion protein in scrapie and Creutzfeldt-Jakob disease (CJD) and β-amyloid protein in Alzheimer's disease (Ma and Lindquist, 2002; Ma *et al.*, 2002a; Walsh *et al.*, 2002). Accordingly, several factors—the level of expression of amyloidogenic or inclusion-forming protein, a cell's capacity to form nontoxic deposits, and the sequence of events leading to altered protein conformation or oligomerization (genetic mutation or upstream pathologic processes)—are thought to influence the susceptibility of any given cell to alternatively folded forms of proteins that give rise to a particular disease. In the discussion that follows, we consider data for a number of degenerative diseases in the context of protein misfolding.

## Prion Diseases

Prion-related disorders in mammals are perhaps the archival class of conformational diseases and have been identified in various mammalian species including scrapie in sheep and goats, bovine spongioform encephalitis, chronic wasting disease in deer and elk, as well as Creutzfeldt-Jakob disease (CJD) and Kuru in humans (Prusiner, 1998). These diseases involve a cellular prion protein, $PrP^{C}$, which is encoded by the evolutionarily conserved *PRNP* gene. The function of $PrP^{C}$ is poorly defined and can adopt an abnormal higher-ordered conformation under certain conditions to generate the $PrP^{Sc}$ isoform (Wechselberger *et al.*, 2002). This alternative conformation exhibits unusual properties because it propagates by converting other $PrP^{C}$ molecules to the $PrP^{Sc}$ form. An important aspect of pathogenesis, and ultimately therapy, is that continued expression of *PRNP* is necessary for development of disease, which has been demonstrated by the complete resistance of *Prnp*-null mice to high titer infection with infective prion particles (Bueler *et al.*, 1993). Thus, prions are infectious particles and, when transferred between organisms, elicit degenerative disease through subversion of normal protein folding.

Details of the mechanism underlying conversion of $PrP^{C}$ to $PrP^{Sc}$ or $PrP^{Sc}$–like structural isoforms have come to light and can be divided into two major stages (Hegde *et al.*, 1998, 1999; Ma and Lindquist, 2002; Ma *et al.*, 2002a). The first stage involves a byproduct of $PrP^{C}$ synthesis and folding in the endoplasmic reticulum (ER) prior to trafficking through the secretory pathway to the cell surface. A significant proportion of nascent PrP polypeptide chains either fail to adopt appropriate higher-ordered structures or adopt alternate transmembrane topologies (CtmPrP), and these unstable intermediates are retrotranslocated from the ER to the cytosol for rapid degradation by the ubiquitin-proteasome complex. Missense mutations in PrP identified from CJD patients generate these intermediates at higher frequencies than those observed for either wild-type PrP or for amino acid changes that are not associated with CJD, resulting in retrotranslocation of a greater proportion of nascent PrP polypeptides.

The second stage of PrP conversion is thought to occur stochastically at low frequency and involves adoption of $PrP^{Sc}$-like conformations by retrotranslocated polypeptides in the cytosol. Such structural changes serve as molecular templates for the structural conversion of additional $PrP^{C}$ molecules, which homopolymerize and are extremely resistant to degradation by the cell. Furthermore, polymer formation is dependent on monomer concentration in the cytosol; thus, the higher likelihood for misfolding of familial CJD variant PrP accounts for the greater efficiency of $PrP^{Sc}$ conversion and self-association. In this light, the mechanism through which prions contribute to pathogenesis appears to involve a toxic gain-of-function of misfolded PrP rather than a loss of function for the cell. In strong support of this notion, *Prnp*-null mice exhibit no observable neurologic phenotype (Bueler *et al.*, 1993).

## Serpinopathies

One of the clearest examples of diseases that stem from a toxic gain-of-function associated with altered protein conformation involves mutations in $\alpha_1$-ANTITRYPSIN ($\alpha_1$-AT) and related genes that encode serine protease inhibitors (reviewed in Carrell and Lomas, 2002; Lomas and Carrell, 2002). $\alpha_1$-AT is secreted into the bloodstream by the liver and functions primarily to protect connective tissue by irreversibly inhibiting elastase that is secreted by leukocytes in the lungs. Patients harboring mutations in the coding region of $\alpha_1$-AT exhibit reduced serpin activity in the blood and are at risk for developing emphysema in adulthood. Patients that are homozygous for mutations causing the most severe form of disease, so-called *PiZZ* alleles, show virtually no serpin activity or protein in the blood. Rather, nascent polypeptides homopolymerize to form linear chains that are visible using electron microscopy and accumulate in the ER of hepatocytes.

Approximately 10 to 15% of *PiZZ* patients develop neonatal cirrhosis. Because $\alpha_1$-AT has no known function in liver, this additional hepatic phenotype likely represents an acquired toxic property of the mutant protein related to its accumulation in the ER.

Major factors contributing to liver damage involve those that cause inflammatory responses that raise body temperature and induce the expression of acute phase genes such as $\alpha_1$-AT (Crowther, 2002). Furthermore, those patients that develop severe liver pathology exhibit other abnormalities in skin fibroblasts. Specifically, the fibroblasts exhibit reduced capacity to degrade misfolded polypeptides through the ubiquitin-proteasome pathway following retrotranslocated from the ER (Wu *et al.*, 1994). Currently, the relevance to disease severity of these lower-than-normal rates of ER-associated protein degradation (ERAD) is unknown. However, it is conceivable that hepatocytes in most *PiZZ* patients are resistant to damage because the ERAD pathway is sufficiently active to minimize the accumulation of polymerized mutant $\alpha_1$-AT that would otherwise lead to cell dysfunction or death.

More recently, one form of autosomal-dominant familial encephalopathy with inclusion bodies (FEN1B) has been linked to mutations in the *PI12* gene, which encodes the neurally restricted neuroserpin protein. A hallmark of this neurodegenerative disease is the presence of eosinophilic Collins bodies in neurons of the substantia nigra and deeper layers of cerebral cortex, which bear striking resemblance to the periodic-acid-Schiff positive inclusions in hepatocytes of *PiZZ* patients. Indeed, in one pedigree with a particularly severe form of this dementia, life span is reduced to 2 decades and inclusions develop in essentially all neurons (Davis *et al.*, 1999a, 1999b). Currently, the aggregation state of the mutant serpins that mediate the toxic effects in neurons and hepatocytes—monomers, small aggregates, or large polymers—has not been determined; however, these mutant proteins adopt stable higher-ordered structures within the ER and, at least for $\alpha_1$-AT, do not induce expression of the molecular chaperone, BiP (Graham *et al.*, 1990). Nevertheless, a substantial proportion of these serpin polymers are stably associated with the ER-localized calcium binding-protein, calnexin (Le *et al.*, 1994).

## Cytoplasmic Inclusion Diseases

A conformational disease for which defective ERAD in neurons of the substantia nigra plays a critical role in pathogenesis is Parkinson's disease (reviewed in Crowther, 2002; Kruger *et al.*, 2002). To date, mutations in two genes, *PARKIN* and *α-SYNUCLEIN*, have been clearly linked to familial disease. *PARKIN* encodes an E3 ubiquitin ligase, which normally polyubiquitinates proteins that are destined for proteasomal degradation (Shimura *et al.*, 2000). Furthermore, considerable evidence links another locus containing the *UCH-L1* gene to familial Parkinson's disease, the gene product of which encodes a ubiquitin hydrolase that serves to recycle ubiquitin monomers during ubiquitinated substrate degradation by the proteasome. The fact that an O-glycosylated form of α-synuclein is a major component of cytoplasmic inclusions, called Lewy bodies, in nigral neurons from most Parkinson's patients provides a compelling link between the rare familial forms and sporadic forms of disease. In addition, α-synuclein that is present in Lewy bodies is typically ubiquitinated (by the *PARKIN* gene product), which suggests that perturbed or defective proteasome function is a major mechanism underlying Lewy body formation and pathogenesis in most patients. However, Lewy bodies are rarely observed in patients harboring *PARKIN* mutations, which indicates that the pathophysiology of Parkinson's disease is independent of these inclusions; thus, Lewy bodies probably are not toxic to neurons and may be secondary aspects of the disease phenotype. Rather, oligomers of at least some of the components of inclusions are currently thought to be the active species for cell dysfunction or death.

Parkinson's disease is a member of a diverse group of cytoplasmic inclusion disorders known collectively as tauopathies (reviewed in Lee *et al.*, 2001). Other well-known members include Alzheimer's disease, amyotrophic lateral sclerosis, Creutzfeldt-Jakob disease, Down's syndrome, FTDP-17, and Pick's disease. The hallmark pathological features of tauopathies are the appearance of filaments in the parenchyma, called neuropil threads, and filamentous inclusions composed of paired-helical and straight filaments. These protein aggregates are labeled by antibodies raised against phosphorylated tau protein. Other pathology may also accompany the tau-positive filament tangles, including: β-amyloid deposits observed in Alzheimer's disease and Lewy bodies found in Parkinson's disease.

Clear evidence that tau plays an important role in the pathophysiology of tauopathies comes from mapping of mutations in many FTDP-17 kindreds to the *TAU* gene. These mutations appear to alter splicing of *TAU* primary transcripts or induce hyperphosphorylation of tau and reduce its affinity for microtubules, which leads to tau aggregation and neurofibrillary tangle formation. Furthermore, several sporadic disorders known as frontotemporal dementias cause clinical symptoms that are similar to FTDP-17 and appear to perturb *TAU* gene expression in several ways, including modifying the splicing of primary transcripts, increasing gene expression, or increasing tau phosphorylation. On the other hand, pathogenesis in sporadic Alzheimer disease is widely thought to involve an amyloid cascade with Aβ peptide as the building block and tau pathology as a secondary event (Hardy and Allsop, 1991).

## Expanded Trinucleotide-Repeat Diseases

The spinocerebellar ataxia (SCA) group of neurological diseases are autosomal-dominant neurodegenerative disorders characterized by progressive motor symptoms, with a particularly severe impact on hypoglossal nuclei, in the absence of cognitive impairment (Orr and Zoghbi, 2001). Trinucleotide expansions in some of these diseases occur in the untranslated regions of unrelated genes and appear to cause disease through disparate mechanisms. On the other hand, expanded repeats also occur in coding regions to form large polyglutamine tracts (encoded by the trinucleotide, CAG) beyond a threshold size of 20 to 40 residues. Additional diseases known to be caused by trinucleotide repeat expansions in protein coding regions include dentatorubropallidoluysian atrophy, Huntington and Kennedy diseases (reviewed in Cummings and Zoghbi, 2000).

Studies in transgenic mice have revealed a number of important principles governing pathogenesis in the trinucleotide expansion diseases, some of which are known to be relevant to other conformational diseases. Working with pathogenic forms of *SCA1* containing arrays of 77 to 82 CAG repeats (corresponding to a glutamine tract, 77 to 82Q), which encode ataxin-1 and aggregate to form nuclear inclusions, Orr and colleagues first determined that nuclear localization of this protein is required for aggregation and subsequent neurodegeneration (Klement *et al.*, 1998). Second, ataxin-1 self-association/aggregation and inclusion body formation are not required for pathogenesis, which suggests that nuclear-localized, monomeric ataxin-1 is the primary toxic species once the glutamine domain is sufficiently large (Klement *et al.*, 1998). Third, the ubiquitin-proteasome pathway directly modulates disease severity by serving to ubiquitinate pathogenic forms of ataxin-1 and promote incorporation into inclusion bodies. Indeed, this pathway normally serves to ameliorate disease as demonstrated by an exacerbation of the phenotype of ataxin-1(82Q) transgenic mice that harbor two null alleles of the E3 ubiquitin ligase gene, *Ube3a* (Cummings *et al.*, 1999). Finally, the presence of small chaperones in ataxin-1 inclusion bodies, and the mitigating effects of overexpressing inducible hsp70 in ataxin-1(82Q) transgenic mice, indicate that inappropriate or incomplete protein folding may be an important mediator of pathophysiology (Cummings *et al.*, 1998, 2001). Notably, overexpression of hsp70 does not influence formation of inclusions but may reduce the toxicity of ataxin-1 monomers by sequestration to form nontoxic complexes.

An important aspect of pathology in trinucleotide repeat diseases is reflected by the observation that the polyglutamine tract may be sufficient for pathogenesis. For example, widespread expression of a polyglutamine tract under transcriptional control of the human cytomegalovirus immediate-early promoter in transgenic mice conferred progressive behavioral abnormalities but only localized neuronal loss (Reddy *et al.*, 1998). Furthermore, addition of 146 CAG repeats into the coding region of the *Hprt* gene, which encodes a ubiquitously expressed cytoplasmic protein that does not normally contain a glutamine-rich domain, causes Huntington's disease–like symptoms and premature death of mice (Ordway *et al.*, 1997). However, the absence of cell death in these animals indicates that the neuronal loss observed in Huntington's disease may arise from a loss of function of the huntingtin protein. Thus, these data indicate that although polyglutamine tracts are likely to be intrinsically toxic, disease-specific phenotypes, and the loss of particular neuronal subtypes are likely to stem from loss- or gain-of-function associated with the mutant protein harboring the polyglutamine domain.

## DISEASES FOR WHICH DEPOSITS OR INCLUSIONS ARE NOT PROMINENT FEATURES OF PATHOLOGY

In contrast to the diseases discussed previously, a number of familial degenerative disorders are not associated with protein deposits or inclusion bodies despite the fact that changes in protein conformation are known to arise from the associated genetic lesions. Presumably, either these proteins are toxic at far lower concentrations than proteins causing inclusion diseases or the primary structures of these proteins do not comprise amino acid domains that are amyloidogenic if improperly folded. One of the best characterized of these noninclusion diseases is the leukodystrophy, Pelizaeus-Merzbacher disease (PMD). Clinical symptoms associated with mutations causing PMD are apparent at birth or within the first year of life, which is consistent with the notion that the mutant gene products are extremely toxic to cells and cause apoptosis long before they accumulate in amounts necessary to form inclusion bodies. In comparison, ages of onset of even juvenile forms of inclusion body diseases are rarely less than the first decade of life. A major focus of studies aimed at characterizing the molecular mechanisms underlying pathogenesis of PMD has been to identify signaling pathways downstream of the synthesis of the mutant proteins that lead to cell dysfunction or apoptosis. These pathways are discussed in detail in this chapter because of their growing relevance to the pathogenesis of inclusion body diseases.

### The *PLP1* gene and Pelizaeus-Merzbacher disease

The leukodystrophies are a diverse group of rare central nervous system (CNS) disorders that arise from a variety of neurodegenerative processes in the white matter. Genetic lesions and biochemical defects underlying pathogenesis of several of these diseases have been described over the past 15 years (Berger *et al.*, 2001; Schiffmann and Boespflug-Tanguy, 2001). Pelizaeus-Merzbacher disease (PMD) is one example for which mutations were identified in the *proteolipid protein 1* gene (*PLP1*) in the late 1980s (Gencic *et al.*, 1989; Hudson *et al.*, 1989) but for which the molecular mechanisms are only now coming to light. Thus, a novel mechanism involving a recently elucidated signaling cascade that is activated by the accumulation of mutant proteins in the secretory pathway appears to play a direct role in pathogenesis. This mechanism could account for 20 to 25% of PMD cases and may be causative for many degenerative diseases involving protein misfolding.

PMD is an *X*-chromosome linked hypomyelinating disease caused by mutations in the *PLP1* gene, which encodes a major CNS myelin protein. The *PLP1* gene is comprised of 7 exons, all of which contribute to the open reading frame, and exon 3 contains a central cryptic splice-site that is utilized to generate two protein isoforms, PLP1 and DM-20. Thus, the smaller DM-20 protein lacks a 35 amino acid polypeptide encoded by exon 3B, which, in PLP1, contributes to a hydrophilic domain in the middle of the protein. This domain is exposed to the cytoplasm and is known as the PLP1-specific peptide. Absence of the PLP1-specific peptide has no effect on overall membrane topology, and both protein isoforms span the bilayer four times with the amino- and carboxyl-termini exposed to the cytoplasm (Gow *et al.*, 1997). However, topography of the second extracellular loop of DM-20 may differ from that of PLP1, which may serve to regulate myelin membrane compaction and lamellar spacing in a manner slightly different to that of PLP1 (Stecca *et al.*, 2000).

### Three Genetic Lesions Confer Pelizaeus-Merzbacher Disease

The clinical spectrum of PMD is very broad and ranges from severe forms associated with a phenotype at birth, quadriparesis and dramatically reduced life span, to milder forms associated only with spastic paraparesis. Three types of genetic lesions associated with PMD account for 80 to 90% of diagnoses and are characterized by gene deletions, gene duplications and coding region mutations (Garbern *et al.*, 1999).

### PLP1 *Gene Null Alleles*

*PLP1*-null mutations have been identified in several patients, including a complete deletion of the gene and an in-frame stop codon after the first amino acid (Garbern *et al.*, 1997), and all exhibit a similar mild clinical phenotype characterized by moderate spastic quadriparesis, mild cognitive delay, ataxia, and a demyelinating peripheral neuropathy (Garbern *et al.*, 1997; Nave and Boespflug-Tanguy, 1996; Raskind *et al.*, 1991; Sistermans *et al.*, 1996). In contrast to this Schwann cell pathology, demyelination in the CNS is virtually absent although neurons undergo progressive length-dependent axonal degeneration principally in cervical and thoracic regions of the ascending and descending corticospinal tracts (Garbern *et al.*, 2002). These data demonstrate the importance of *PLP1* gene products for long term maintenance of oligodendrocyte-axon interactions even in the PNS where this gene is expressed at very low levels by Schwann cells.

#### *Supernumerary Copies of the* PLP1 *gene*

The second and most common cause of PMD is the duplication within an approximately 800 kb region of the *X*-chromosome flanking the *PLP1* gene. Studies in animal models show that overexpression of PLP1 and/or DM-20 is sufficient to cause CNS hypomyelination in transgenic mice (Gow *et al.*, 1998; Kagawa *et al.*, 1994; Macklin *et al.*, 1995; Mastronardi *et al.*, 1993; Readhead *et al.*, 1994); thus, gene duplications in humans likely cause PMD in similar fashion. The molecular mechanism responsible for generating this genetic lesion is currently unknown, but may involve extensive DNA repeat regions that predispose the *X*-chromosome to nonreciprocal homologous recombination as is known for duplications in Charcot-Marie-Tooth 1A (Reiter *et al.*, 1996) and Smith-Magenis syndrome (Chen *et al.*, 1997). Clinical phenotypes associated with duplications are variable and have not been characterized in detail; however, data from transgenic mice suggest a direct relationship between the level of overexpression and disease severity (Inoue *et al.*, 1996).

#### *Missense and Nonsense Mutations in the* PLP1 *Gene*

The third major genetic defect in PMD involves coding region mutations in the *PLP1* gene, which arise from missense, nonsense, and splice-site mutations that either preserve the reading frame or cause frame-shifted and truncated proteins. More than 50 distinct mutations have been described worldwide and the clinical phenotypes associated with these mutations span the severity spectrum. Most coding region mutations identified to date affect the primary structure of both DM-20 and PLP1, and the majority of these mutations confer severe disease. On the other hand, perhaps the only region of the open reading frame where different missense mutations confer milder phenotypes encodes the PLP1-specific peptide.

## Animal Models of Pelizaeus-Merzbacher Disease

An important tool set that has contributed significantly to the current level of understanding about the pathogenesis of PMD is the large number of spontaneously occurring animal models from several species that are available for study. The best characterized models in older literature are the canine *shaking* pup (*shp*), *myelin-deficient* rat (*md*) and *jimpy* mouse (*jp*). Mouse mutants have received considerable attention in recent years because of the identification of patients with the same mutations (Kobayashi *et al.*, 1994; Yamamoto *et al.*, 1998), including the *rumpshaker* mouse (*rsh*) and the *myelin synthesis-deficient* mouse (*msd*), and perhaps more importantly because of the application of genetic manipulations to generate wild-type *Plp1* overexpressing transgenic mice—strains designated *4e-Plp*, *#72* and *#66*—and homologous recombinant null alleles (Boison and Stoffel, 1994; Hudson and Nadon, 1992; Kagawa *et al.*, 1994; Klugmann *et al.*, 1997; Readhead *et al.*, 1994; Stecca *et al.*, 2000).

A useful aspect of pathophysiology associated with *Plp1* coding region mutations in the mouse models is a relatively reliable association between disease severity and life span. Mutations causing severe disease such as *jp*, *msd* and the recently described *4J* mutation (Pearsall *et al.*, 1997), shorten life span to less than 4 weeks while mild phenotypes are generally associated with normal life spans. This correlation is not clear-cut in PMD patients, and mutations causing severe disease do so through greater functional disability. Together, the mouse mutants comprise the full spectrum of genetic lesions and disease severities found in patients, including mild and severe forms of disease arising from overexpression and coding region mutations. Moreover, a number of the clinical symptoms as well as hypomyelination and oligodendrocyte cell death observed in patients are recapitulated in these animals.

## Evidence for Three Distinct Pathogenic Mechanisms for Pelizaeus-Merzbacher Disease

Although PMD is found to be a monogenic disease in the majority of patients, considerable evidence indicates that each of the three types of genetic lesions in the *PLP1* gene causes disease by distinct mechanisms. Early data from *Plp1* overexpressing transgenic mice show that morphological abnormalities in oligodendrocyte cell bodies from these animals are confined to Golgi profiles, which become distended during myelinogenesis (Kagawa *et al.*, 1994; Readhead *et al.*, 1994).

Immunocytochemical evidence indicates that oligodendrocytes in these animals appear to function relatively normally at early ages; however, the processes from these cells eventually lose contact with axons leading to demyelination (Gow *et al.*, 1998). Recent *in vitro* studies have now shed light on a cellular mechanism that underlies pathophysiology, which revolves around inappropriate trafficking and accumulation of cholesterol and lipid raft components into lysosomes (Simons *et al.*, 2002).

There are good reasons to suspect that disease associated with coding region mutations arises from gain-of-function effects rather than the loss of function observed for gene deletions. First, coding region mutations cause a broad spectrum of disease severities, while null alleles consistently yield mild disease (Garbern *et al.*, 1999). Second, peripheral neuropathy is associated with null alleles but not with the vast majority of coding region mutations. Third, the degree of myelination in null patients and transgenic mice is close to normal whereas most coding region mutations are associated with a significant loss to virtual absence of myelin. Finally, gene expression profiles between null alleles and coding region mutations are distinct (see Figures 42.3B and 42.4B).

## Molecular Pathogenesis of Missense Mutations Causing Pelizaeus-Merzbacher Disease

The availability of naturally occurring, noncomplimenting myelin mutant rodents such as the *jp* and *msd* mouse strains as well as mutations in other species enabled detailed analyses of the biochemical and cellular phenotypes associated with mutations in the *PLP1* gene long before identification of the genetic lesions.

### *Early Observations*

Characterization of the molecular mechanism underlying coding region mutations in PMD has been greatly assisted by the availability of animal models; biopsy procedures in PMD patients were discontinued in the 1950s and this disease is rare enough so that autopsy material is not forthcoming. Early studies in animals such as the *jp* mouse, *md* rat and canine *shp* predate identification of the genetic lesions in these animals; however, *X*-chromosome linkage and similarities in phenotype, morphology and biochemical analyses of white matter suggested that the affected loci in these animals might be allelic (for reviews see Hudson and Nadon, 1992; Skoff and Knapp, 1992). In these early studies, several observations have been key to the development of current hypotheses to account for pathogenesis in PMD (Gow *et al.*, 1998). First, immunoelectron microscopy studies looking at *Plp1* gene products in wild-type and *jp* mice revealed striking differences in the intracellular localization of these proteins in the secretory pathway of oligodendrocytes (Nussbaum and Roussel, 1983; Roussel *et al.*, 1987; Schwob *et al.*, 1985). Furthermore, transmission electron microscopy of oligodendrocytes revealed amorphous precipitates in the ER of some *Plp1* mutant animals, including *shp* and *jp* mice (reviewed in Duncan, 1990). Such precipitates are relatively common in a number of cell types in which mutant proteins accumulate in the ER (Rutishauser and Spiess, 2002).

Another series of watershed morphometric observations in *jp* mice laid out the consequences for oligodendrocytes expressing many mutant forms of *Plp1* gene products (Ghandour and Skoff, 1988; Knapp *et al.*, 1986). Although not fully appreciated at the time, *jp* oligodendrocytes exhibit the canonical morphological features of apoptosis (Gow *et al.*, 1998; Grinspan *et al.*, 1998; Lipsitz *et al.*, 1998) but decreases in the size of the oligodendrocyte population in the first 14 days after birth is not a feature of disease (Ghandour and Skoff, 1988). Presumably, the rate of differentiation of oligodendrocyte progenitors in these mutants at early ages is roughly equivalent to cell death. However, whether this population receives environmental signals at later times to shut down proliferation and differentiation, or whether the progenitor population becomes depleted, remains an open question.

A common interpretation of the phenotypes of *Plp1* mutant animals at one time was that the oligodendrocytes failed to differentiate to the point that they would express high levels of *Plp1* gene products. Findings from embryos showing *Plp1* gene expression in the CNS from mid-gestation further fueled this view (Timsit *et al.*, 1992); however, ablation of the *Plp1* gene in mice by homologous recombination reveal no apparent consequence for oligodendrocyte differentiation and has effectively put such a notion to rest (Boison and Stoffel, 1994; Klugmann *et al.*, 1997; Stecca *et al.*, 2000). A more likely interpretation of pathology in the mouse mutants is that as oligodendrocyte progenitors differentiate and express *Plp1* gene products, they undergo apoptosis, which effectively eliminates the differentiated cell pool. The fact that progenitors continue to divide and replenish this cell population provides a plausible explanation for the apparent differentiation defect. An effective demonstration of the presence of differentiated oligodendrocytes in *msd* brain is shown in Figure 42.1. Myelin basic protein (MBP) immunofluorescence staining of cerebellum from a P18 *msd* mouse shows an abundance of this protein in the white matter, which is similar to littermate controls (Fig. 42.1A). Such staining would not be detected in the absence of differentiated, myelin membrane-synthesizing oligodendrocytes, and previous studies have reached similar conclusions (Ghandour and Skoff, 1988). Indeed, staining of cortex in P18 *msd* mice using antibodies against MBP and PLP1/DM-20 (top row, Fig. 42.1B) clearly demonstrates the presence of oligodendrocyte membrane around nearby axons with a morphological appearance similar to myelin sheaths in wild-type and *rsh* mice (Gow *et al.*, 1998). In contrast, PLP1/DM-20 is confined to oligodendrocyte cell bodies in *msd* and *rsh* mice (bottom row, Fig. 42.1B). Together, these data lend strong support to the view that the oligodendrocyte cell lineage differentiates normally before undergoing apoptosis in response to the expression of mutant *Plp1* gene products.

### *Recent Data and the Protein Misfolding Hypothesis*

The search for molecular mechanisms underlying pathogenesis of PMD led to a series of *in vitro* experiments by several groups where wild-type and mutant forms of PLP1 and DM-20 were expressed in transfected or transduced cells in culture (Gow *et al.*, 1994a, 1997; Gow and Lazzarini, 1996; Jung *et al.*, 1996; Kalwy *et al.*, 1997; Sinoway *et al.*, 1994; Thomson *et al.*, 1997; Yamada *et al.*, 1999, 2001). Together, these data demonstrate that normal intracellular trafficking of *PLP1* gene products through the secretory pathway to the cell surface and into the endocytic pathway to lysosomes is perturbed by single amino acid changes throughout the coding region. An essentially invariant consequence of missense mutations is defective trafficking of PLP1. However, mutations fall into two classes based on whether they block trafficking of PLP1 and DM-20 (class I mutations) or PLP1 but not DM-20 (class II mutations). Interestingly, a strong correlation is apparent between

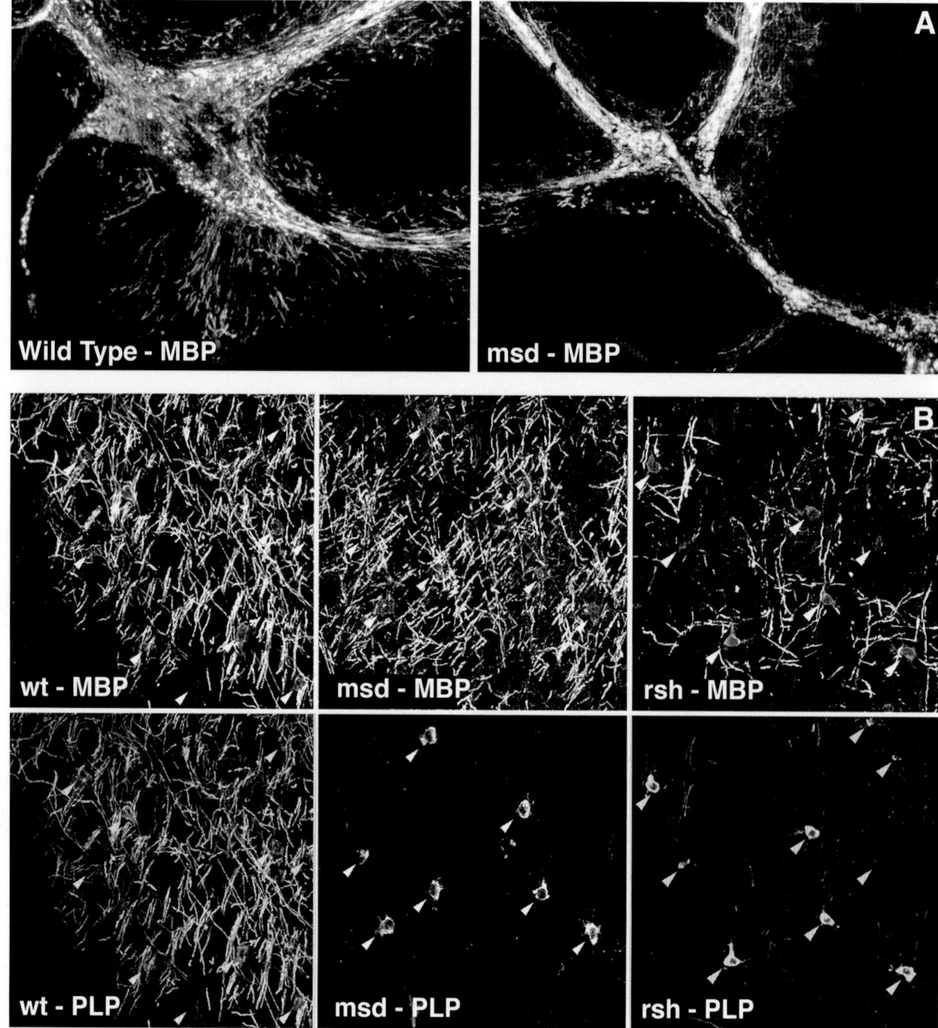


FIGURE 42.1
MBP and PLP1/DM-20 immunocytochemistry in *msd* and *rsh* mouse brains. (A) The intensities of MBP staining in wild-type and *msd* cerebella are similar. (B) MBP staining in the cortex shows many myelin sheath profiles in wild-type as well as *msd* and *rsh* mice. Although PLP1/DM-20 colocalizes with MBP in wild-type tissue, this protein is largely confined to the cell bodies of oligodendrocytes in the mutant animals.

class II mutations and mild forms of disease in patients (Tab. 42.1) and a simple interpretation of these data is that disease severity correlates with the amount of protein that is retained in the perinuclear regions of the cells (Gow and Lazzarini, 1996).

A hallmark of interrupted trafficking of these proteins is their accumulation in the ER, which is often seen as perinuclear localization in tubulovesicular profiles that colocalize with ER markers such as the molecular chaperone, BiP, as well as their absence on the cell surface and in lysosomes (Gow *et al.*, 1994b). Importantly, observations from *in vitro* paradigms using transfected fibroblasts are similar to those observed for mutant forms of PLP1/DM-20 *in vivo* (Gow *et al.*, 1998; Roussel *et al.*, 1987) and suggests that disruption to PLP1/DM-20 trafficking is not an artifact or a consequence of cell type-specific processes but rather is a general phenomenon in cell biology. Indeed, interrupted trafficking and ER accumulation of dozens of secretory pathway proteins with missense mutations have been reported and a number have been shown to be stably associated with molecular chaperones such as BiP. Unfortunately, the propensity for PLP1 and DM-20 to aggregate in solution renders similar experiments technically challenging.

The intracellular trafficking defects that are observed for most mutant forms of PLP1 and DM-20 suggest that these proteins do not adopt stable higher-ordered structures after

TABLE 42.1 Intracellular Trafficking of PLP1 and DM-20 for Mutations Identified in PMD Patients and Animal Models

| Class | Disease Severity | Missense Mutation | Intracellular Accumulation in Transfected COS-7 Cells | | | |
|---|---|---|---|---|---|---|
| | | | PLP1 | | DM-20 | |
| | | | Endoplasmic Reticulum | Cell Surface | Endoplasmic Reticulum | Cell Surface |
| Wild type | - | - | | x | | x |
| I | Severe | L14P | x | | x | |
| | | H36P (*shp*) | x | | x | |
| | | A38S (*4J*) | x | | x | |
| | | T74P (*md*) | x | | x | |
| | | W162R | x | | x | |
| | | T181P | x | | x | |
| | | L223P | x | | x | |
| | | A242V (*msd*) | x | | x | |
| II | Mild | H36Q (*pt*) | x | | | x |
| | | T155I | x | | | x |
| | | I186T (*rsh*) | x | | | x |
| | | D202H | x | | | x |
| | | D202E | x | | | x |
| | | P215S | x | | | x |
| | | V218F | x | | | x |
| | | V218I | x | | | x |
| | | L223I | x | | | x |

synthesis in the ER. In such cases, proteins generally remain in this compartment until they are hydrolyzed via the ubiquitin/proteasome pathway. This pathway is known as ER-associated degradation (ERAD), which operates constitutively in most cell types and involves: retrotranslocation of defective or excess wild-type polypeptides through the ER membrane into the cytoplasm, polyubiquitination, and proteolysis in the proteasome (reviewed in Brodsky and McCracken, 1999). In light of the facts that ERAD is evolutionarily conserved in eukaryotes and that secretory pathway proteins are constantly flowing through this pathway, it is reasonable to expect that cells should cope efficiently with mutant proteins in the ER. However, conceivably, the rates of synthesis of some mutant proteins could be so great as to overwhelm the cells capacity to degrade them. In such cases, misfolded proteins would accumulate in the ER and eventually threaten cell viability (reflecting a loss of homeostasis), and the cell might be expected to react to this metabolic stress by suppressing protein synthesis and activating genetic programs to alleviate the toxic effects of protein accumulation. One such signaling pathway that serves to reestablish homeostasis in cells in response to misfolded protein accumulation in the ER is called the unfolded protein response (UPR).

## The UPR Signaling Cascade

Early awareness of the UPR at the cellular level dates back to the 1970s and 1980s as a result of examining the intracellular trafficking of wild-type and mutant forms of transmembrane proteins through the secretory pathway (reviewed by Garoff, 1985; Kozutsumi *et al.*, 1988). Retention of mutants in the ER, which could also be effected by drugs such as tunicamycin to block N-glycosylation of glycoproteins, led to the notion that the ER serves as a quality control organelle in which individual proteins must adopt stable three-dimensional structures before gaining entry into the remaining membrane compartments of the cell (Bonifacino and Lippincott-Schwartz, 1991; Gething and Sambrook, 1992; Hammond and Helenius, 1995; Klausner and Sitia, 1990; Rose and Doms, 1988). A number of "UPR-effector" proteins, such as molecular chaperones like BiP that belong to the hsp70 family, had been identified by the late 1980s, but the bulk of the characterization and integration of UPR components into a cohesive signaling pathway has been achieved over the past 10 years.

### *Components of the UPR*

Although our knowledge about the complexity and function of the UPR is still evolving, a number of central players have been defined (for recent reviews, Harding *et al.*, 2002; Kaufman *et al.*, 2002; Ma and Hendershot, 2001). The UPR can be broadly divided into two components; one that modulates homeostasis at the level of transcription while the other component modulates homeostasis through translational repression. Table 42.2 lists well characterized upstream components of the UPR in mammals as well as their major functions and targets and Figure 42.2 shows the flow of information in this signaling cascade from activation in the ER to the nucleus.

Three proteins that have been characterized to date, which we refer to as "UPR-initiator" proteins, serve as direct monitors of protein flux through the ER. A fourth protein, ATF4, which may be activated by signals outside of the UPR, regulates the expression of important UPR target genes. These initiators activate a number of "UPR-effector" proteins that assist cells in adapting to imposed stress to establish homeostasis, as well as to participate negative feedback loops that deactivate UPR signaling. Thus, Ire1 (Fig. 42.2A) and PERK (Fig. 42.2B) are ER-resident receptor kinases, each with a luminal domain that associates with the molecular chaperone, BiP. In the event of an increase in the level of unstable nascent polypeptide intermediates in the ER, BiP dissociates from BiP-Ire1 and/or BiP-PERK complexes, which frees up these initiator proteins for dimerization, autotransphosphorylation, and signaling to the nucleus (Bertolotti *et al.*, 2000). Activated Ire1 and PERK also exhibit additional properties—endoribonuclease activity for Ire1 and an eIF2α kinase activity for PERK—and effect transcriptional modulation and global translational repression, respectively (Harding *et al.*, 2002). Ire1 catalyzes processing of an mRNA that encodes the XBP-1 transcription factor, which in turn induces expression of molecular chaperone genes (reviewed in Ma and Hendershot, 2001). On the other hand, PERK-mediated phosphorylation of the alpha subunit of eIF2 (eIF2α) inhibits GDP/GTP exchange on this factor by the guanine nucleotide exchange factor (GEF), eIF2B, and blocks binding of Met-tRNA$_f^{met}$ to eIF2. Consequently, blocking formation of the eIF2•GTP•Met-tRNA$_f^{met}$ ternary complex ensures that

TABLE 42.2 Summary of the Functions and Targets of UPR Associated Proteins

| Protein | Group | Function | Targets | Reference |
|---|---|---|---|---|
| Ire1 | Initiator | Kinase/ endonuclease | *Xbp-1 mRNA splicing* | (Mori *et al.*, 1993)<br>(Cox and Walter, 1996)<br>(Wang *et al.*, 1998a) |
| PERK | | eIF2α-kinase | eIF2 | (Harding *et al.*, 1999) |
| ATF4 | | Transcription factor | *CHOP* gene | (Fawcett *et al.*, 1999) |
| ATF6 | | Transcription factor | *XBP-1* gene | (Yoshida *et al.*, 2000) |
| Xbp-1 | Effector | Transcription factor | Molecular Chaperone expression | (Yoshida *et al.*, 2001)<br>(Calfon *et al.*, 2002) |
| CHOP | | Transcription factor | ATF3, apoptosis-related genes | (Ubeda *et al.*, 1996) |
| ATF3 | | Transcription factor | *CHOP* gene repressor | (Wolfgang *et al.*, 1997)<br>(Bole *et al.*, 1986) |
| BiP | | Molecular chaperone | Unfolded protein binding | (Kozutsumi *et al.*, 1988) |
| ERp59 | | Disulfide bond formation | Nascent ER polypeptides | (Ferrari and Soling, 1999) |
| ERp72 | | Disulfide bond formation | Nascent ER polypeptides | (Ferrari and Soling, 1999) |
| eIF2 | | Ribosome assembly | Met-tRNAi | (Harding *et al.*, 2000) |
| Gadd34 | | Phosphatase binding | PP1 | (Novoa *et al.*, 2001) |

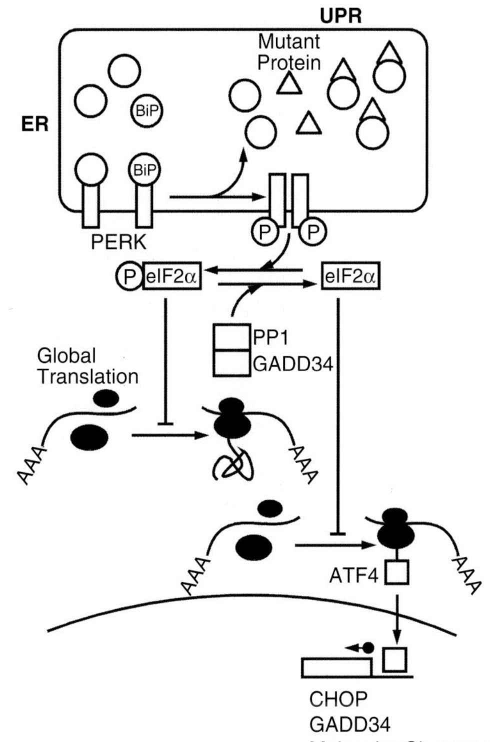


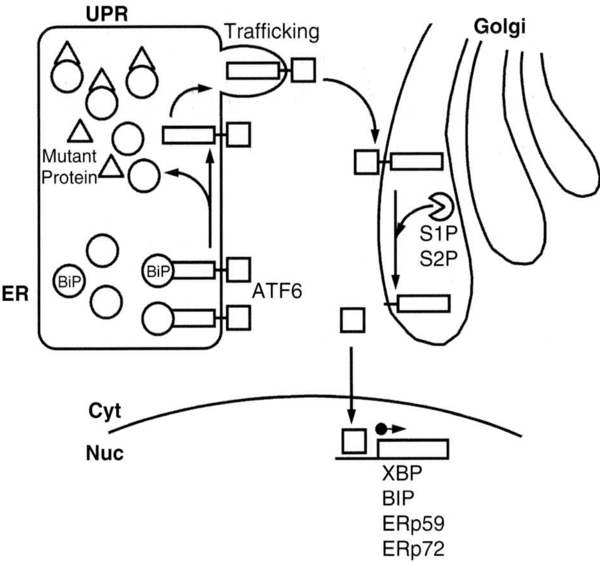


FIGURE 42.2
UPR signaling is initiated through three proteins and regulates transcription and translation.(A) The Ire1 receptor is localized to the ER and modulates transcription through XBP-1. (B) The PERK receptor is localized to the ER and represses global translation through phosphorylation of eIF2α. ATF4 is encoded by a cytoplasmic mRNA that is translated in response to changes in the rate of protein synthesis and regulates transcription. (C) ATF6 is a membrane-tethered protein that is localized in the ER but is released to the Golgi during a UPR and regulates transcription after cleavage by proteases.

recruitment of initiator tRNA to the 40S ribosome preinitiation complex cannot occur (reviewed in Kimball, 1999). Furthermore, phosphorylated eIF2 competitively inhibits the GEF activity of eIF2B and leads to rapid repression of all translation in the cell.

Under cellular conditions where the eIF2 is partially phosphorylated and global protein synthesis is only partially inhibited, the translation of specific classes of mRNAs yield proteins that serve to propagate UPR signaling into the nucleus. One such class of mRNAs is constitutively present in most cell types and a representative example of this class is an mRNA that encodes the transcription factor, ATF4. Importantly, the 5′ region of this mRNA includes a short open reading frame (called a 5′ ORF) that, under normal conditions, is translated to yield an inactive protein. However, when the available pool of eIF2 becomes partially phosphorylated, translation initiation on this mRNA switches to a downstream open reading frame (ORF) that encodes the active transcription factor. Apparently, as ribosomal scanning positions the 40S ribosomal subunit at the initiation codon of the 5′ ORF under normal cellular conditions, the abundance of ternary complexes ensures rapid binding and prompt 80S ribosome assembly. However, eIF2$\alpha$ phosphorylation drives down the level of ternary complexes, which delays formation of the pre-initiation complex and increases the probability that the small ribosomal subunit will move beyond the AUG of the 5′ UTR. This process is known as bypass scanning. In such cases, the 40S ribosome continues along the mRNA to find the downstream ORF where ternary complex binding enables ribosome assembly and translation to generate ATF4 (DeGracia *et al.*, 2002; Harding *et al.*, 2000).

One of the consequences of bypass scanning is induction of ATF4 target genes that encode: several molecular chaperones including BiP, which help to alleviate ER stress and negatively regulate the initiation of UPR signaling (Bertolotti *et al.*, 2000); GADD34 protein, which negatively regulates translational repression by recruiting the protein phosphatase PP1 to dephosphorylate eIF2 and reestablish ribosome assembly; and the transcription factor CHOP, which plays a pivotal role in UPR signaling and has been shown to induce apoptosis in several cell types (Harding *et al.*, 2000). Similar to *ATF4*, *CHOP* mRNA contains a 5′ ORF (Jousse *et al.*, 2001), which suggests that CHOP function is likely to be important under conditions where eIF2 is phosphorylated. Furthermore, accumulation of GADD34 in the cytoplasm likely ensures that translational repression triggered by PERK is temporary and that CHOP is only transiently translated (Novoa *et al.*, 2001). A further requirement for CHOP to function as a transcription factor is phosphorylation by p38 kinase, which imparts additional constraints on CHOP function (Wang and Ron, 1996).

ATF6 is a third UPR-initiator protein and is an ER membrane-tethered transcription factor that is released into the cytosol by S1P/S2P proteases in response to the accumulation of unfolded proteins. These proteases are unlikely to be specific activators for the UPR signaling pathway because they also process another well-characterized membrane-tethered transcription factor, SREBP, which plays a central role in cholesterol biosynthesis (Lee *et al.*, 2002; Ye *et al.*, 2000). Interestingly, tethered-ATF6 is retained in the ER in a complex with BiP under normal conditions but is released for trafficking to the Golgi apparatus in response to ER stress where it is proteolytically cleaved (Shen *et al.*, 2002). Targets of ATF6 include *XBP-1*, genes encoding molecular chaperones and the protein disulfide isomerases, ERp59, and ERp72 (Okada *et al.*, 2002).

### *Many UPR-Effector Proteins Are Constitutively Expressed*

During the course of normal development and maintenance, individual cells continually synthesize membrane components in the ER for delivery to other compartments, including the Golgi apparatus, cell surface, endosomes, and lysosomes. In addition to general transcriptional regulation of individual components by cell-type specific factors, membrane biogenesis through the secretory pathway is regulated at the level of bulk flow, or flux, by several components of the UPR. For example, molecular chaperones such as BiP are normally present in the ER of most cells under physiological conditions, which suggests that XBP-1 and ATF6 are continually processed at low levels. Transcription factors such as CHOP and ATF3 are also expressed at low levels, thereby implying PERK activation and ATF4 translation. However, the limited studies of UPR-effector genes carried using normal cells at cellular homeostasis suggests that such low level expression reflects the activity of UPR signaling-independent mechanisms (Brewer *et al.*, 1997). Nevertheless, the fact that UPR-effectors are present in cells under normal conditions and are strongly induced by the UPR suggests that these proteins, and by direct extension the UPR, operate to protect cells against metabolic stress involving the ER and to preserve or re-establish cellular homeostasis. The consequence for cells in which homeostasis cannot be regained is often apoptosis by activation of caspase cascades. These cascades may involve the initiator-caspase 12 in mice but not in humans (Fischer *et al.*, 2002) where, presumably, another caspase family member is activated.

In light of the constitutive activity of UPR-effectors, how is the normal expression of genes encoding these proteins distinguished from cell stress-related expression? One possibility may be through the utilization of conserved cis-elements in the proximal promoters of UPR-effector genes to induce transcription (Lee, 2001; Ma *et al.*, 2002b; Yoshida *et al.*, 1998). Indeed, two such elements have been well-characterized in mammalian cells, namely the unfolded protein response element (UPRE) and the endoplasmic reticulum stress element (ERSE), which are found in the promoters of many molecular chaperones. A third element, called the C/EBP-ATF composite element, has recently been identified in the *CHOP* promoter and is critical for induction of this gene by UPR signaling. A number of transcription factors activated by the UPR are known to bind to the UPRE, ERSE and C/EBP-ATF motifs, including XBP-1, ATF3, ATF4, ATF6, C/EBP, NF-Y and YY1, and TFII-I.

## Involvement of the UPR in Pelizaeus-Merzbacher Disease and Animal Models

The first indication that activation of the UPR is a feature of disease in *Plp1* mutant animals came from a demonstration that the *Bip* gene is induced in the brains of *jp* and *msd* mice although, curiously, *Bip* gene induction is not observed in *md* rats or the canine *shp* model (Hudson and Nadon, 1992). More recent experiments focused exclusively on the mouse mutants demonstrate induction of a number of molecular chaperones, but the magnitudes of these increases are relatively modest (Southwood and Gow, 2001). Nevertheless, these observations have prompted a detailed examination of UPR activation in *Plp1* mutant mice (Southwood *et al.*, 2002).

### *The UPR Is Activated in Pelizaeus-Merzbacher Disease*

Northern blots in Figure 42.3A reveal induced expression of six UPR-effector genes in the spinal cords of *msd*, *jp* and *rsh* mice. The *Chop* gene is genetically downstream of PERK and ATF4 and *Atf3* is regulated by CHOP (Chen *et al.*, 1996). On the other hand, *Bip*, *ERp59* and *ERp72* are downstream of Ire1 and ATF6. Importantly, northern blots in Figure 42.3B demonstrate that the same set of UPR-effector proteins are induced in subcortical white matter compared with occipital gray matter from a PMD patient (Δ*exon6*). This patient harbors a splice-site mutation at the splice donor site of exon 6 that causes skipping of this exon (Hobson *et al.*, 2000; Southwood *et al.*, 2002). These data contrast with the results obtained from the nonplaque region of a patient with multiple sclerosis (MS). In this case, the *BIP* gene is the only gene for which expression is significantly different between white and gray matter, and is actually increased in gray matter. The significance of these data for MS is presently unclear and is under further investigation. Importantly, characterization of UPR-effector genes inside active plaques and adjacent gray and white matter regions may reveal important aspects of the pathophysiology as has been alluded to in previous studies.

Induced expression of UPR-effector genes in *msd* and *rsh* mice has been confirmed with immunocytochemical data, which show not only that CHOP is localized to the nuclei of *Plp1*-positive oligodendrocytes, but also ATF3. Both of these bZip transcription factors are thought to remain cytoplasmic until their activation through phosphorylation by MAP kinases p38 and JNK, respectively (Wang and Ron, 1996). It is not currently known if CHOP and ATF3 are present in the same oligodendrocytes at the same time or whether there is a temporal expression pattern; however, developmental northern analyses in spinal cords of *msd* mice indicate that *Chop* induction precedes that of *Atf3*, possibly by as much as 5 days (Southwood *et al.*, 2002). Studies of liver regeneration in rat indicate that these two transcription factors are not normally colocalized in the same cells and may antagonize each others expression (Chen *et al.*, 1996; Wolfgang *et al.*, 1997).

A significant distinction between CHOP and ATF3 expression in *msd* mice is the expression of ATF3 by microglia in addition to oligodendrocytes, while CHOP

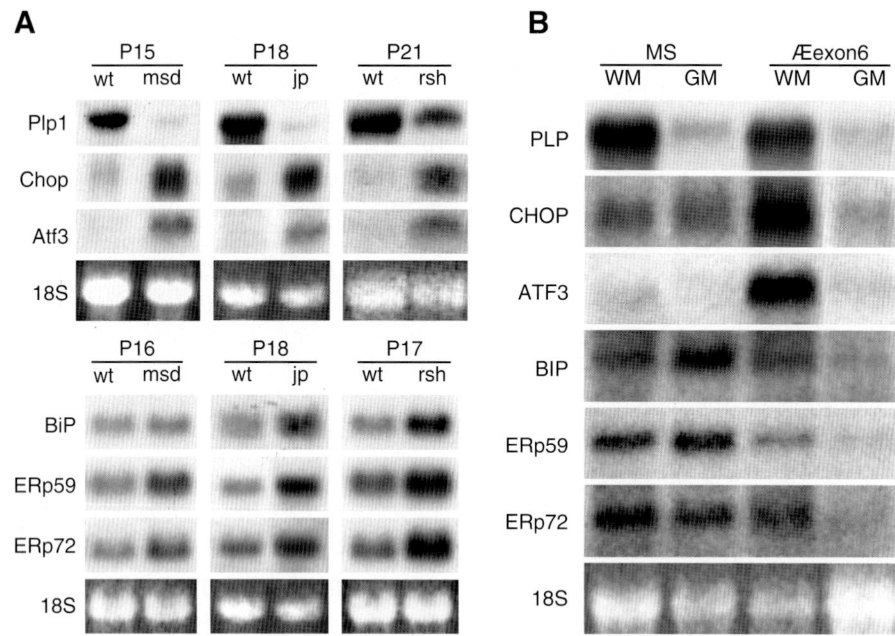


FIGURE 42.3
Northern blotting shows the induction of six genes encoding UPR-effector proteins. (A) Induction of genes in *msd*, *jp*, and *rsh* mice. (B) Induction of genes in PMD but not an MS patient.

is expressed only in oligodendrocytes. Although morphology, proliferation, and gene expression of microglia are altered in response to mutant *Plp1* expression (reviewed by Vela *et al.*, 1998), the signals that induce these changes remain unclear. However, there is no evidence for *Plp1* expression and activation of the UPR in this cell type, which indicates that *Atf3* expression is induced by a broader range of signals than is *Chop* and that ATF3 may have additional functions outside of the UPR.

### *The UPR Modulates Disease Severity in Animal Models of Pelizaeus-Merzbacher Disease*

Considering changes in cell behavior at the level of transcription in response to UPR signaling, the greatest attention has been focused on the transcription factors that effect these changes and to gain insight into the compensatory mechanisms that cells employ to establish or maintain homeostasis. CHOP has been particularly well studied in this regard, partly because it was one of the first UPR-induced transcription factors identified and because of the important role this protein plays in initiating apoptosis in at least some cell types (Ubeda *et al.*, 1996; Wang *et al.*, 1996; Zinszner *et al.*, 1998). From these studies, CHOP is widely believed to be a pro-apoptotic transcription factor (reviewed in Harding *et al.*, 2002).

The central role proposed for CHOP in the UPR, as well as its strong induction in oligodendrocytes of *Plp1* mutant mice, suggests that this transcription factor might be a critical modulator of disease severity in PMD patients. Indeed, previous studies in animal models have suggested that severe disease correlates with abnormally high levels of oligodendrocyte death (Gow *et al.*, 1998; Schneider *et al.*, 1992). To explore the potential involvement of CHOP in modulating disease severity, *rsh* mice were crossed with *Chop*-null mice (Zinszner *et al.*, 1998) and examined using a Kaplan-Meier analysis (Southwood *et al.*, 2002).

Changes in life span for *rsh* mice in the absence of CHOP is dramatic. While *rsh* mice live approximately 2 years, *Chop*-null/*rsh* double-mutant mice die as early as 5 weeks of age and have an average life span of less than 10 weeks. Furthermore, these animals exhibit seizures not unlike that of *jp* and *msd* mice, which is a more severe form of disease than is usually observed for *rsh* mice, and indicates that CHOP serves as an anti-apoptotic transcription factor in PMD. Although the mechanism underlying the functional switch between pro-apoptotic and anti-apoptotic properties is unknown, it is likely that the fate of cells after UPR activation is determined by the downstream target genes of CHOP as well as other UPR-induced transcription factors. In this regard, CHOP appears to regulate overlapping but distinct targets in oligodendrocytes compared to other cell types (Southwood *et al.*, 2002; Wang *et al.*, 1998b).

A similar heterogeneity in CHOP target genes has also been observed in transfected COS-7 cells expressing a mutant form of the mitochondrial protein, OTC, that misfolds in the mitochondrial matrix. Under these conditions, expression of *Chop* and four nuclear-encoded mitochondrial molecular chaperones is induced but not the expression of five ER-localized molecular chaperones. Furthermore, promoters regulating expression of the mitochondrial chaperones contain *cis*-elements that bind the CHOP/C/EBPβ heterodimer *in vitro*. Conversely, induction of a UPR using tunicamycin or thapsigargin induces expression of ER-localized molecular chaperones but not those localized to mitochondria (Zhao *et al.*, 2002). A simple interpretation of these data is that CHOP is expressed in response to the accumulation of unfolded proteins in at least two organelles and CHOP target gene selection is regulated in conjunction with unknown organelle-specific factors.

#### *Activation of the UPR Is Specific for Coding Region Mutations in PLP1*

In the light of data from early immunoelectron microscopy studies in *jp* mice, which showed that mutant PLP1/DM-20 were largely localized to the ER of oligodendrocytes (Roussel *et al.*, 1987), the demonstration that the UPR is activated in PMD tissue and *Plp1* mutant animals is a consistent and satisfying outcome. But is the UPR activated when the *PLP1* gene is overexpressed in duplication patients or transgenic mice? Immunoelectron microscopy and immunocytochemical studies show that most wild-type PLP1/DM-20 accumulates in the myelin sheaths. Nonetheless, these proteins are detectable in oligodendrocyte cell bodies and are localized largely to the Golgi apparatus (Nussbaum *et al.*, 1985; Schwob *et al.*, 1985). Interestingly, morphological evidence from *Plp1* overexpressor transgenic mice suggests that the products from this gene also accumulate in the Golgi apparatus and may perturb the function of this organelle. If so, the levels of PLP1/DM-20 in the ER should be relatively normal and the UPR would not be expected to be induced. Indeed, the data in Figure 42.4 suggest that this is the case. Immunocytochemical staining of wild-type cerebellum shows strong anti-PLP1/DM-20 reactivity in white matter tracts (Fig. 42.4Aa). CHOP is not expressed (Fig. 42.4Ab) by any of the cells in this field, the positions of which are revealed by the nuclear DAPI stain (Fig. 42.4Ac). White matter tracts in the cerebellum are weakly labeled with anti-PLP1/DM-20 antibodies in transgenic *4e-Plp* overexpressor mice and several oligodendrocyte cell bodies are heavily labeled (arrowheads, Fig. 42.4Ad). Nevertheless, CHOP is not induced in these cells. Staining of cerebellum with antibodies against ATF3 also fails to label oligodendrocytes (data not shown). Consistent with these findings, northern blots of autopsy material from a PMD duplication patient (Fig. 42.4B) show that neither *CHOP* nor *ATF3* are induced in white matter compared to gray matter. Together, these data support the contention that the UPR is an important feature of the pathophysiology in PMD caused by coding region mutations.

### Other Noninclusion Diseases Associated with Activation of the UPR

With a great deal of attention focused on the delineation of UPR signaling pathways in the basic science and clinical arenas, a growing number of diseases that stem from mutations in proteins that may activate a UPR are coming to light. For example, patients with Wolcott-Rallison syndrome disease harbor mutations in the *PERK* gene and clinical symptoms such as neonatal type I diabetes, mental retardation, cardiovascular abnormalities, hepatic and renal dysfunction and other multisystemic manifestations (Delepine *et al.*, 2000). The most likely cause of disease in these patients is the failure of cells to repress protein translation in response to metabolic or heat-induced stress, which places homeostasis at risk and leads to cell death. Currently, it is unclear why many of these diseases do not appear to be associated with intracellular inclusion bodies.

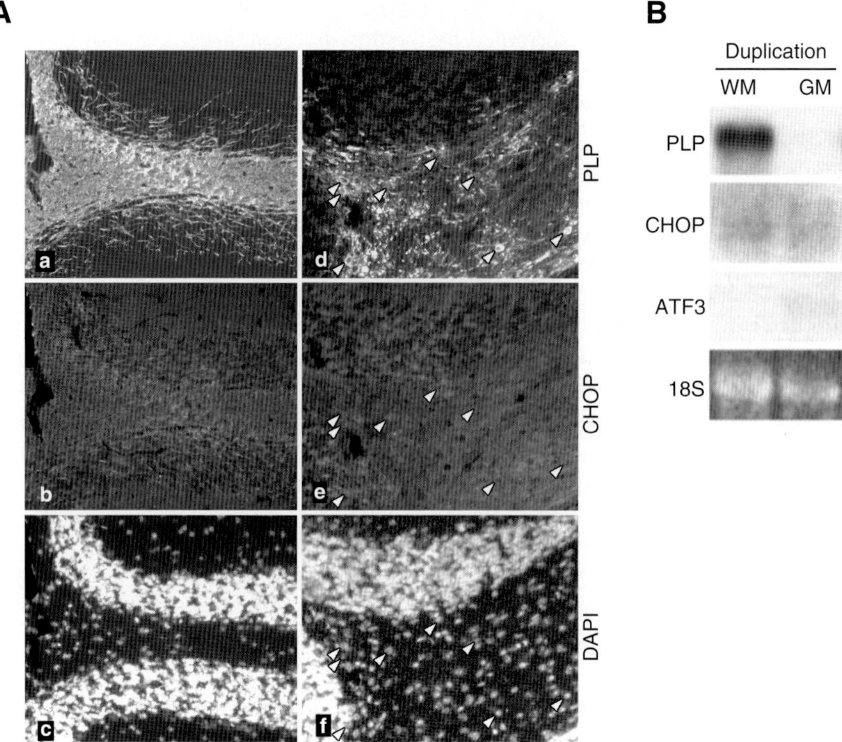


FIGURE 42.4
UPR induction is not a feature of disease in PLP1 overexpressors. (A) CHOP is not expressed by wild-type oligodendrocytes or oligodendrocytes overexpressing a wild-type *Plp1* transgene. (B) Northern blotting shows that neither CHOP nor ATF3 are induced in white matter of a PMD patient with a duplicated wild-type *PLP1* gene.

Missense mutations in several genes cause the group of peripheral neuropathies known collectively as Charcot-Marie-Tooth disease and involve the *PMP22*, *MPZ*, and *CONNEXIN 32* genes. Heterologous expression, in transfected fibroblasts, of mutant forms of PMP-22 identified from patients have been examined in greatest detail. In similar fashion to *PLP1*, missense mutations disrupt the normal intracellular trafficking of PMP-22 through the secretory pathway to the cell surface and the mutant proteins accumulate in the ER (D'Urso *et al.*, 1998; Naef *et al.*, 1997; Sanders *et al.*, 2001; Tobler *et al.*, 1999). Such accumulation has been demonstrated in PNS-myelinating Schwann cells from patient biopsy specimens and is associated with increased expression of molecular chaperones. These data suggest that the UPR is activated in CMT; however, widespread apoptosis is not a feature of even the most severe forms of CMT, which may mean that misfolded PNS myelin-specific proteins are more easily degraded than those in the CNS or that Schwann cells and oligodendrocytes differ in their sensitivity to UPR inducing metabolic stress.

Cystic fibrosis stems from genetic mutations that perturb normal function of the chloride transporter protein, CFTR (recently reviewed by Gelman and Kopito, 2002). Although this disease affects several cell types in patients, the most prominent pathology is observed in lung. Extensive analysis of *CFTR* mutations from the 1200 or so mutations and polymorphisms that have been described for this gene indicate that four or more distinct mechanisms may account for pathophysiology: class I mutations are null or functionally null; class II mutations are associated with interrupted intracellular trafficking in the ER; class III mutations arise from abnormal plasma membrane recycling, endocytosis, or lysosomal transport; and class IV mutations stem from defects in channel activation and regulation by interacting proteins. By far the most common mutation in the *CFTR* gene (> 90% of patients of Northern European descent) involves an in-frame deletion of three nucleotides that encode phenylalanine at position 508 (ΔF508) of this

1480 amino acid protein. The ΔF508 mutation is commonly designated as a class II mutation from both *in vitro* and *in vivo* studies (Denning *et al.*, 1992; Kartner *et al.*, 1992), although the extent of the intracellular trafficking defect exhibits cell type dependence (Kalin *et al.*, 1999). The ΔF508 mutation is also noteworthy from the perspective of pharmacological strategies for ameliorating disease. Thus, this mutation can form functional chloride channels in cells if it reaches the plasma membrane, which can be accomplished by reducing the growth temperature or by treating cells with protein stabilizing agents such as glycerol and sorbitol (Colledge *et al.*, 1995; Gelman and Kopito, 2002; Sato *et al.*, 1996).

Despite the fact that mutant CFTR does not form inclusions in patients, *in vitro* paradigms can be manipulated to yield perinuclear inclusions of polyubiquitylated protein (Johnston *et al.*, 1998). Intermolecular folding of wild-type CFTR does not appear to proceed efficiently in the ER because >75% of nascent chains are degraded by the proteasome complex under normal physiological conditions (Jensen *et al.*, 1995). Inhibition of this ERAD pathway leads to accumulation of wild-type or mutant CFTR in the cytosol in the form of large perinuclear aggregates called aggresomes (Johnston *et al.*, 1998). In fibroblasts, aggresomes are bordered by intermediate filaments such as vimentin and it is possible that these structures serve to sequester the mutant protein aggregates until such times as they can be degraded by the proteasome complex. Aggresome formation is not restricted to CTFR accumulation; presenilin I also forms these complexes (Johnston *et al.*, 1998), and we have also observed these structures in transfected cells overexpressing wild-type PLP1 in the presence or absence of the proteasome inhibitor MG132 (unpublished observations, and Gow *et al.*, 1994a). The morphological and biochemical characterization of aggresomes by Kopito and colleagues, as well as the demonstration that misfolded protein aggregates impair the function of the ERAD pathway (Bence *et al.*, 2001; Johnston *et al.*, 1998; Kopito and Sitia, 2000) provide an important interpretation of inclusion pathology that is observed in many neurodegenerative diseases.

Another example of a disease that may involve the UPR is a cell-type specific disease, called leukoencephalopathy with vanishing white matter (VWM). VWM is associated with mutations in any of the subunits of the ubiquitously expressed GEF protein, eukaryotic initiation factor 2B (eIF2B). eIF2B catalyzes the GDP-GTP exchange on eIF2 to enable binding of Met-tRNA$_f^{met}$ and its subsequent recruitment to the ribosome preinitiation complex. Furthermore, eIF2 is the central regulator of global protein translation in the cell and, in particular, the phosphorylation status of the eIF2α subunit determines whether-or-not eIF2B GEF activity is induced or inhibited by eIF2•GDP (Kimball, 1999). Mutations that modify the interaction between eIF2B and eIF2 or alter the activities of these initiation factors, as is likely to be the case in VWM, diminish the ability of cells to regulate protein synthesis in response to cell stress and even under normal physiological conditions. For unknown reasons in VWM disease, oligodendrocytes and neurons appear to be selectively sensitive compared to other cell types following transient core temperature elevations such as those experienced during infections (Leegwater *et al.*, 2001; van der Knaap *et al.*, 1997; van der Knaap *et al.*, 2002).

Evidence that is now beginning to emerge from several groups implicates the UPR in familial forms of Parkinson's disease, in particular those associated with mutations in the *PARKIN* gene. Although Parkinson's disease is considered here and elsewhere as an inclusion disorder, patients with *PARKIN* mutations rarely exhibit inclusion pathology. One of the substrates of parkin E3 ligase is the parkin-associated endothelin receptor-like receptor, Pael-R, which has been shown to accumulate with α-synuclein in Lewy bodies from sporadic Parkinson's patients (Imai *et al.*, 2001). Pael-R is a transmembrane protein that is expressed by oligodendrocyte lineage cells and dopamine neurons and is most abundant in corpus callosum and substantia nigra. A substantial portion of this receptor is normally conjugated to ubiquitin, suggesting either that the protein is synthesized in excess and residual polypeptide chains are subsequently degraded by the ERAD pathway, or that the protein does not readily adopt a stable higher-ordered conformation and many of the nascent chains are targeted to the ERAD pathway. When overexpressed in transfected cells, Pael-R is also polyubiquitinated and induces robust apoptosis that is enhanced by concomitant inhibition of proteasome function and diminished by coexpression of wild-type parkin. These data indicate that Pael-R expression induces an unfolded protein response, which leads to apoptosis of these cells (Imai *et al.*, 2001). Consistent with this notion, analysis of autopsied frontal lobes from autosomal-recessive juvenile Parkinson's patients (AR-JP, associated with mutations in the *PARKIN* gene) reveals substantial accumulation of detergent-insoluble Pael-R compared to control tissue. Importantly, the absence of Lewy bodies in the parenchyma of AR-JP patients indicates that Pael-R may accumulate in the ER and may kill the nigral neurons through activation of the unfolded protein response pathway in similar fashion to that observed in cell culture experiments (Imai *et al.*, 2001).

Unexpectedly, the pathophysiology of several experimental models of Parkinson's disease also involves activation of the UPR, at least for *in vitro* systems (Ryu *et al.*, 2002). As determined by SAGE analysis and northern blotting, PC12 cell-derived dopamine neurons grown in the presence of 6-hydroxydopamine, $MPP^+$ or rotenone induce a number of UPR target genes encoding: heat shock proteins and molecular chaperones; CHOP and one of its DNA-binding partners, C/EBPβ ubiquitin and ubiquitin-conjugating enzymes and proteasome subunits. Furthermore, western blotting reveals that two of the UPR-initiator proteins, PERK and Ire1, are phosphorylated, that eIF2α is phosphorylated and that the mRNA encoding ATF4 is translated in the presence of these Parkinson's mimetic agents.

Several recent studies also suggest that familial Alzheimer's disease may involve activation of the UPR although some of these data are currently conflicting. While investigating the proteolytic cleavage and nuclear localization of the cytoplasmic tail of Ire1 in response to UPR activation, two groups have demonstrated that the polytopic presenilin (PS) protein and Ire1 physically interact and that proteolytic processing of Ire1 is defective in cells derived from *PS I*-null mice or transfected neurons expressing mutant forms of PS I identified in patients (Katayama *et al.*, 1999; Niwa *et al.*, 1999); two related *PRESENILIN* genes are known in mammals and their encoded products are believed to exhibit γ-secretase activity or are closely associated with γ-secretase. Moreover, these groups find that tunicamycin-induced signal transduction from the ER to the nucleus is attenuated in cells from *PS I*-null mice, which results in blunted induction of the molecular chaperone, BiP, in response to tunicamycin treatment. On the other hand, a third group (Sato *et al.*, 2000) has demonstrated in *PS I*/*PS II*-double null cells that Ire1 and PERK activation and signaling are not compromised after indution of the UPR. Furthermore, induction of *Bip* and *Chop* expression occur normally in the absence of PS or the presence of mutant forms of PS I identified in familial Alzheimer's patients or in autopsied brains from sporadic Alzheimer's patients.

## Toward a Set of Criteria to Identify Novel UPR-Associated Diseases

To recognize additional degenerative diseases that may involve mutations in secretory pathway proteins that activate the UPR, it is important to develop a set of criteria that may be used to screen out diseases for which other mechanisms underlie pathogenesis. Toward this end, three factors are worthy of consideration.

### Null Alleles

Complete gene deletions or nonsense mutations at the 5′ end of the open reading frame represent the strongest cases for loss-of-function disease and particular care should be taken to characterize the phenotype from these genetic lesions for comparison with phenotypes arising from other mechanisms. Although these null alleles could yield recessive or semi-dominant phenotypes, they would be expected to confer disease that is significantly more mild than, or clinically distinct from, at least a portion of allelic mutations. With this criterion, it is possible to eliminate diseases for which mutations simply abolish protein function even in the event that those mutations disrupt protein trafficking.

For example, mutations in the immunoglobulin superfamily neural cell adhesion molecule, L1, underlie a variety of clinical symptoms collectively referred to as CRASH

(Fransen *et al.*, 1995). Heterologous expression of missense mutations in transfected fibroblasts reveals that most fail to traverse the secretory pathway but rather are retained in the ER (De Angelis *et al.*, 2002; Moulding *et al.*, 2000). However, available evidence suggests that the clinical symptoms are probably not associated with activation of the UPR. In particular, expression of mutant L1 under transcriptional control of the L1 promoter in transgenic mice yields a phenotype that is indistinguishable from the null allele using several criteria (Runker *et al.*, 2003). These data indicate that mutant forms of L1 are nonfunctional and that the disease symptoms are consistent with a loss-of-function phenotype. A second example of a disease where missense mutations cause protein accumulation in the ER, but where clinical symptoms more likely arise from loss of function is autosomal dominant retinitis pigmentosa (ADRP). In this case, *Rhodopsin*-null mice exhibit very similar retinal degeneration as do transgenic mice expressing mutant forms of rhodopsin identified in ADRP patients (Humphries *et al.*, 1997; Olsson *et al.*, 1992). In contrast, *PLP1*-null alleles identified in PMD patients consistently yield more mild forms of disease than most missense mutations. In addition, null patients exhibit peripheral neuropathy, which is a feature of disease distinct from that observed in patients with coding region mutations (Shy *et al.*, 2003).

### *Dominant and Semi-Dominant Alleles*

Accumulation of mutant proteins in the ER frequently occurs at the level of nascent polypeptide synthesis and prior to the integration of these protein monomers into multimeric complexes in the ER. Accordingly, a single mutant copy of a gene encoding an abundant secretory pathway protein may be sufficient to induce the clinical symptoms of a UPR-associated disease. Moreover, addition of wild-type copies of this gene (e.g., by gene therapy) would not be expected to ameliorate the phenotype because toxicity of the mutant protein would not be associated with a loss of function. In fact, such a strategy may exacerbate disease by increasing flux through the secretory pathway and placing heavier demands on the ER. In this regard, the introduction of supernumerary copies of a wild-type *Plp1* gene into mice harboring the $Plp1^{jp}$ allele fails to ameliorate the severe disease conferred by the *jp* allele even though transgene-derived wild-type PLP1 and DM-20 in these animals can traverse the secretory pathway to the myelin sheath (Schneider *et al.*, 1995). Clearly, disease in this case is not a consequence of the absence of *Plp1* gene products in the myelin but rather is a consequence of mutant protein accumulation in the secretory pathway (Gow *et al.*, 1998; Nussbaum and Roussel, 1983; Roussel *et al.*, 1987).

### *Recessive Alleles*

In general, it is likely to be difficult to identify UPR-associated diseases exhibiting recessive phenotypes without the aid of biopsy or autopsy material to demonstrate perinuclear accumulation of mutant proteins or without using *in vitro* approaches to examine intracellular trafficking of the mutant proteins in transfected cells in culture. For genes expressed at relatively low levels, it is reasonable to expect that a coding region mutation in one allele might not yield a sufficient amount of protein accumulation to overwhelm the UPR and cause disease. However, such mutations may do so if both gene copies are mutated. This case has clearly been shown by several groups in mice (Power *et al.*, 1996; Turnley *et al.*, 1991; Yoshioka *et al.*, 1991). For example, transgene-derived expression of the H-2K$^b$ protein in oligodendrocytes using the cell type-specific MBP promoter/enhancer causes a dysmyelinating phenotype in some hemizygous lines while others are asymptomatic. Although this MHC molecule has a wild-type sequence, it normally resides in the ER until forming a ternary complex with $\beta_2$-microglobulin and a polypeptide supplied by a TAP tansporter. Because oligodendrocytes usually express neither $\beta_2$-microglobulin nor the transporter, H-2K$^b$ accumulates in the ER of these cells. Importantly, the disease phenotype is dependent on transgene expression above a threshold, which can be breached in high expressing hemizygous lines, by breeding an asymptomatic line to homozygosity or by increasing gene dosage through the breeding of two asymptomatic hemizygous lines.

## SUMMARY

Although involvement of the UPR is suspected in a number of common degenerative disorders, until recently too little has been known or understood about this signaling cascade for any meaningful exploration of human disease. However, rapid progress over the past 2 years by several prominent laboratories has yielded an important framework of information with which to assess the role of this signaling pathway in many degenerative diseases. In this regard, coding region mutations in the *PLP1* gene are associated with induction of the UPR *in vitro*, in the CNS of animal models of PMD, and in a PMD patient. The activation of this signaling cascade occurs in animals with severe and mild forms of disease and does not determine disease severity per se. However, UPR activation is directly involved in modulating disease severity in the sense that interfering with the function of this pathway negatively affects cell survival. Thus, PMD is the first example of a degenerative disease in which the UPR is not only activated but also modulates disease severity.

### Acknowledgments

My warm thanks to Cherie Southwood for her critical review of this work and comments. This work is supported by grants from NINDS (RO1 NS43783), the National Multiple Sclerosis Society (RG 2891-B-2), and the Childrens Research Center of Michigan.

### References

Bence, N. F., Sampat, R. M., and Kopito, R. R. (2001). Impairment of the ubiquitin-proteasome system by protein aggregation. *Science* **292,** 1552–15525.

Berger, J., Moser, H. W., and Forss-Petter, S. (2001). Leukodystrophies: Recent developments in genetics, molecular biology, pathogenesis and treatment. *Curr Opin Neurol* **14,** 305–312.

Bertolotti, A., Zhang, Y., Hendershot, L. M., Harding, H. P., and Ron, D. (2000). Dynamic interaction of BiP and ER stress transducers in the unfolded-protein response. *Nat. Cell Biol.* **2,** 326–332.

Boison, D., and Stoffel, W. (1994). Disruption of the compacted myelin sheath of axons of the central nervous system in proteolipid protein-deficient mice. *Proc. Natl. Acad. Sci. USA* **91,** 11709–11713.

Bole, D., Hendershot, L. M., and Kearney, J. (1986). Posttranslational association of immunoglobulin heavy chain binding protein with nascent heavy chains in nonsecreting and secreting hybridomas. *J. Cell Biol.* **102,** 1558–1566.

Bonifacino, J. S., and Lippincott-Schwartz, J. (1991). Degradation of proteins within the endoplasmic reticulum. *Curr. Opin. Cell Biol.* **3,** 592–600.

Brewer, J. W., Cleveland, J. L., and Hendershot, L. M. (1997). A pathway distinct from the mammalian unfolded protein response regulates expression of endoplasmic reticulum chaperones in non-stressed cells. *EMBO J.* **16,** 7207–7216.

Brodsky, J. L., and McCracken, A. A. (1999). ER protein quality control and proteasome-mediated protein degradation. *Semin. Cell Dev. Biol.* **10,** 507–513.

Bueler, H., Aguzzi, A., Sailer, A., Greiner, R. A., Autenried, P., Aguet, M., and Weissmann, C. (1993). Mice devoid of PrP are resistant to scrapie. *Cell* **73,** 1339–1347.

Calfon, M., Zeng, H., Urano, F., Till, J. H., Hubbard, S. R., Harding, H. P., Clark, S. G., and Ron, D. (2002). IRE1 couples endoplasmic reticulum load to secretory capacity by processing the XBP-1 mRNA. *Nature* **415,** 92–96.

Carrell, R. W., and Lomas, D. A. (2002). Alpha1-antitrypsin deficiency—a model for conformational diseases. *N Engl J Med* **346,** 45–53.

Chen, B. P., Wolfgang, C. D., and Hai, T. (1996). Analysis of ATF3, a transcription factor induced by physiological stresses and modulated by gadd153/Chop10. *Mol. Cell. Biol.* **16,** 1157–1168.

Chen, K. S., Manian, P., Koeuth, T., Potocki, L., Zhao, Q., Chinault, A. C., Lee, C. C., and Lupski, J. R. (1997). Homologous recombination of a flanking repeat gene cluster is a mechanism for a common contiguous gene deletion syndrome. *Nat. Genet.* **17,** 154–163.

Colledge, W. H., Abella, B. S., Southern, K. W., Ratcliff, R., Jiang, C., Cheng, S. H., MacVinish, L. J., Anderson, J. R., Cuthbert, A. W., and Evans, M. J. (1995). Generation and characterization of a delta F508 cystic fibrosis mouse model. *Nat Genet* **10,** 445–452.

Cox, J. S., and Walter, P. (1996). A novel mechanism for regulating activity of a transcription factor that controls the unfolded protein response. *Cell* **87,** 391–404.

Crowther, D. C. (2002). Familial conformational diseases and dementias. *Hum Mutat* **20,** 1–14.

Cummings, C. J., Mancini, M. A., Antalffy, B., DeFranco, D. B., Orr, H. T., and Zoghbi, H. Y. (1998). Chaperone suppression of aggregation and altered subcellular proteasome localization imply protein misfolding in SCA1. *Nat Genet* **19,** 148–154.

Cummings, C. J., Reinstein, E., Sun, Y., Antalffy, B., Jiang, Y., Ciechanover, A., Orr, H. T., Beaudet, A. L., and Zoghbi, H. Y. (1999). Mutation of the E6-AP ubiquitin ligase reduces nuclear inclusion frequency while accelerating polyglutamine-induced pathology in SCA1 mice. *Neuron* **24,** 879–692.

Cummings, C. J., Sun, Y., Opal, P., Antalffy, B., Mestril, R., Orr, H. T., Dillmann, W. H., and Zoghbi, H. Y. (2001). Over-expression of inducible HSP70 chaperone suppresses neuropathology and improves motor function in SCA1 mice. *Hum Mol Genet* **10,** 1511–1518.

Cummings, C. J., and Zoghbi, H. Y. (2000). Trinucleotide repeats: Mechanisms and pathophysiology. *Annu Rev Genomics Hum Genet* **1,** 281–328.

D'Urso, D., Prior, R., Greiner-Petter, R., Gabreels-Festen, A. A., and Muller, H. W. (1998). Overloaded endoplasmic reticulum-Golgi compartments, a possible pathomechanism of peripheral neuropathies caused by mutations of the peripheral myelin protein PMP22. *J. Neurosci.* **18,** 731–740.

Davis, R. L., Holohan, P. D., Shrimpton, A. E., Tatum, A. H., Daucher, J., Collins, G. H., Todd, R., Bradshaw, C., Kent, P., Feiglin, D., Rosenbaum, A., Yerby, M. S., Shaw, C. M., Lacbawan, F., and Lawrence, D. A. (1999a). Familial encephalopathy with neuroserpin inclusion bodies. *Am J Pathol* **155,** 1901–1913.

Davis, R. L., Shrimpton, A. E., Holohan, P. D., Bradshaw, C., Feiglin, D., Collins, G. H., Sonderegger, P., Kinter, J., Becker, L. M., Lacbawan, F., Krasnewich, D., Maenke, M., Lawrence, D. A., Yerby, M. S., Shaw, C. M., Gooptu, B., Elliot, P. R., Finch, J. T., Carrell, R. W., and Lomas, D. A. (1999b). Familial dementia caused by polymerization of mutant neuroserpin. *Nature* **401,** 376–379.

De Angelis, E., Watkins, A., Schafer, M., Brummendorf, T., and Kenwrick, S. (2002). Disease-associated mutations in L1 CAM interfere with ligand interactions and cell-surface expression. *Hum Mol Genet* **11,** 1–12.

DeGracia, D. J., Kumar, R., Owen, C. R., Krause, G. S., and White, B. C. (2002). Molecular pathways of protein synthesis inhibition during brain reperfusion: Implications for neuronal survival or death. *J Cereb Blood Flow Metab* **22,** 127–141.

Delepine, M., Nicolino, M., Barrett, T., Golamaully, M., Lathrop, G. M., and Julier, C. (2000). EIF2AK3, encoding translation initiation factor 2-alpha kinase 3, is mutated in patients with Wolcott-Rallison syndrome. *Nat Genet* **25,** 406–409.

Denning, G. M., Anderson, M. P., Amara, J. F., Marshall, J., Smith, A. E., and Welsh, M. J. (1992). Processing of mutant cystic fibrosis transmembrane conductance regulator is temperature-sensitive. *Nature* **358,** 761–764.

Dobson, C. M. (2001). The structural basis of protein folding and its links with human disease. *Philos Trans R Soc Lond B Biol Sci* **356,** 133–145.

Duncan, I. D. (1990). Dissection of the phenotype and genotype of the X-linked myelin mutants. *In* "Myelination and Dysmyelination" (I. D. Duncan, R. P. Skoff, and D. R. Colman, eds.), Vol. 605 , pp. 110–121. New York Academy of Sciences, New York.

Fawcett, T. W., Martindale, J. L., Guyton, K. Z., Hai, T., and Holbrook, N. J. (1999). Complexes containing activating transcription factor (ATF)/cAMP-responsive-element-binding protein (CREB) interact with the CCAAT/enhancer-binding protein (C/EBP)-ATF composite site to regulate Gadd153 expression during the stress response. *Biochem J* **339,** 135–141.

Ferrari, D. M., and Soling, H. D. (1999). The protein disulphide-isomerase family: Unravelling a string of folds. *Biochem J* **339,** 1–10.

Fischer, H., Koenig, U., Eckhart, L., and Tschachler, E. (2002). Human caspase 12 has acquired deleterious mutations. *Biochem Biophys Res Commun* **293,** 722–726.

Fransen, E., Lemmon, V., Van Camp, G., Vits, L., Coucke, P., and Willems, P. J. (1995). CRASH syndrome: Clinical spectrum of corpus callosum hypoplasia, retardation, adducted thumbs, spastic paraparesis and hydrocephalus due to mutations in one single gene, L1. *Eur J Hum Genet* **3,** 273–284.

Garbern, J., Cambi, F., Shy, M., and Kamholz, J. (1999). The molecular pathogenesis of Pelizaeus-Merzbacher disease. *Arch. Neurol.* **56,** 1210–1214.

Garbern, J. Y., Cambi, F., Tang, X. M., Sima, A. A., Vallat, J. M., Bosch, E. P., Lewis, R., Shy, M., Sohi, J., Kraft, G., Chen, K. L., Joshi, I., Leonard, D. G., Johnson, W., Raskind, W., Dlouhy, S.R., Pratt, V., Hodes, M.E., Bird, T., and Kamholz, J. (1997). Proteolipid protein is necessary in peripheral as well as central myelin. *Neuron* **19,** 205–218.

Garbern, J. Y., Yool, D. A., Moore, G. J., Wilds, I. B., Faulk, M. W., Klugmann, M., Nave, K. A., Sistermans, E. A., van der Knaap, M. S., Bird, T. D., Shy, M. E., Kamholz, J. A., and Griffiths, I. R. (2002). Patients lacking the major CNS myelin protein, proteolipid protein 1, develop length-dependent axonal degeneration in the absence of demyelination and inflammation. *Brain* **125,** 551–561.

Garoff, H. (1985). Using recombinant DNA techniques to study protein targeting in the eukaryotic cell. *Annu. Rev. Cell Biol.* **1,** 403–445.

Gelman, M. S., and Kopito, R. R. (2002). Rescuing protein conformation: Prospects for pharmacological therapy in cystic fibrosis. *J Clin Invest* **110,** 1591–1597.

Gencic, S., Abuelo, D., Ambler, M., and Hudson, L. D. (1989). Pelizaeus-Merzbacher disease: An X-linked neurologic disorder of myelin metabolism with a novel mutation in the gene encoding proteolipid protein. *Am. J. Hum. Genet.* **45,** 435–442.

Gething, M.-J., and Sambrook, J. (1992). Protein folding in the cell. *Nature* **355,** 33–45.

Ghandour, M., and Skoff, R. (1988). Expression of galactocerebroside in developing normal and jimpy oligodendrocytes *in situ. J. Neurocytol.* **17,** 485–498.

Gow, A., Friedrich, V. L., and Lazzarini, R. A. (1994a). Intracellular transport and sorting of the oligodendrocyte transmembrane proteolipid protein. *J. Neurosci. Res.* **37,** 563–573.

Gow, A., Friedrich, V. L., and Lazzarini, R. A. (1994b). Many naturally occurring mutations of myelin proteolipid protein impair its intracellular transport. *J. Neurosci. Res.* **37,** 574–583.

Gow, A., Gragerov, A., Gard, A., Colman, D. R., and Lazzarini, R. A. (1997). Conservation of topology, but not conformation, of the proteolipid proteins of the myelin sheath. *J. Neurosci.* **17,** 181–189.

Gow, A., and Lazzarini, R. A. (1996). A cellular mechanism governing the severity of Pelizaeus-Merzbacher disease. *Nat. Genet.* **13,** 422–428.

Gow, A., Southwood, C. M., and Lazzarini, R. A. (1998). Disrupted proteolipid protein trafficking results in oligodendrocyte apoptosis in an animal model of Pelizaeus-Merzbacher disease. *J. Cell Biol.* **140,** 925–934.

Graham, K., Le, A., and Sifers, R. (1990). Accumulation of the insoluble PiZ variant of human $\alpha_1$-antitrypsin within the hepatic endoplasmic reticulum does not elevate the steady-state level of grp78/BiP. *J. Biol. Chem.* **265,** 20463–20468.

Grinspan, J. B., Coulalaglou, M., Beesley, J. S., Carpio, D. F., and Scherer, S. S. (1998). Maturation-dependent apoptotic cell death of oligodendrocytes in myelin-deficient rats. *J. Neurosci. Res.* **54,** 623–634.

Hammond, C., and Helenius, A. (1995). Quality control in the secretory pathway. *Curr. Op. Cell Biol.* **7,** 523–529.

Harding, H. P., Calfon, M., Urano, F., Novoa, I., and Ron, D. (2002). Transcriptional and Translational Control in the Mammalian Unfolded Protein Response. *Annu Rev Cell Dev Biol* **18,** 18.

Harding, H. P., Novoa, I., Zhang, Y., Zeng, H., Wek, R., Schapira, M., and Ron, D. (2000). Regulated translation initiation controls stress-induced gene expression in mammalian cells. *Mol. Cell* **6,** 1099–1108.

Harding, H. P., Zhang, Y., and Ron, D. (1999). Protein translation and folding are coupled by an endoplasmic reticulum-resident kinase. *Nature* **397,** 271–274.

Hardy, J., and Allsop, D. (1991). Amyloid deposition as the central event in the aetiology of Alzheimer's disease. *Trends Pharmacol Sci* **12,** 383–388.

Hegde, R. S., Mastrianni, J. A., Scott, M. R., DeFea, K. A., Tremblay, P., Torchia, M., DeArmond, S. J., Prusiner, S. B., and Lingappa, V. R. (1998). A transmembrane form of the prion protein in neurodegenerative disease. *Science* **279,** 827–834.

Hegde, R. S., Tremblay, P., Groth, D., DeArmond, S. J., Prusiner, S. B., and Lingappa, V. R. (1999). Transmissible and genetic prion diseases share a common pathway of neurodegeneration. *Nature* **402,** 822–826.

Hobson, G. M., Davis, A. P., Stowell, N. C., Kolodny, E. H., Sistermans, E. A., de Coo, I. F., Funanage, V. L., and Marks, H. G. (2000). Mutations in noncoding regions of the proteolipid protein gene in Pelizaeus-Merzbacher disease. *Neurology* **55,** 1089–96.

Hudson, L. D., and Nadon, N. L. (1992). Amino acid substitutions in proteolipid protein that cause dysmyelination. *In* "Myelin: Biology and Chemistry" (R. E. Martenson, ed.), pp. 677–702. CRC Press, Boca Raton, FL.

Hudson, L. D., Puckett, C., Berndt, J., Chan, J., and Gencic, S. (1989). Mutation of the proteolipid protein gene PLP in a human X chromosome-linked myelin disorder. *Proc. Natl. Acad. Sci. U. S. A.* **86,** 8128–8131.

Humphries, M. M., Rancourt, D., Farrar, G. J., Kenna, P., Hazel, M., Bush, R. A., Sieving, P. A., Sheils, D. M., McNally, N., Creighton, P., Erven, A., Boros, A., Gulya, K., Capecchi, M. R., and Humphries, P. (1997). Retinopathy induced in mice by targeted disruption of the rhodopsin gene. *Nat. Genet.* **15.**

Imai, Y., Soda, M., Inoue, H., Hattori, N., Mizuno, Y., and Takahashi, R. (2001). An unfolded putative transmembrane polypeptide, which can lead to endoplasmic reticulum stress, is a substrate of Parkin. *Cell* **105,** 891–902.

Inoue, Y., Kagawa, T., Matsumura, Y., Ikenaka, K., and Mikoshiba, K. (1996). Cell death of oligodendrocytes or demyelination induced by overexpression of proteolipid protein depending on expressed gene dosage. *Neurosci. Res.* **25,** 161–172.

Jensen, T. J., Loo, M. A., Pind, S., Williams, D. B., Goldberg, A. L., and Riordan, J. R. (1995). Multiple proteolytic systems, including the proteasome, contribute to CFTR processing. *Cell* **83,** 129–135.

Johnston, J. A., Ward, C. L., and Kopito, R. R. (1998). Aggresomes: A cellular response to misfolded proteins. *J. Cell Biol.* **143,** 1883–1898.

Jousse, C., Bruhat, A., Carraro, V., Urano, F., Ferrara, M., Ron, D., and Fafournoux, P. (2001). Inhibition of CHOP translation by a peptide encoded by an open reading frame localized in the chop 5′UTR. *Nucleic Acids Res* **29,** 4341–4351.

Jung, M., Sommer, I., Schachner, M., and Nave, K. A. (1996). Monoclonal antibody O10 defines a conformationally sensitive cell-surface epitope of proteolipid protein (PLP): Evidence that PLP misfolding underlies dysmyelination in mutant mice. *J. Neurosci.* **16,** 7920–7929.

Kagawa, T., Ikenaka, K., Inoue, Y., Kuriyama, S., Tsujii, T., Nakao, J., Nakajima, K., Aruga, J., Okano, H., and Mikoshiba, K. (1994). Glial cell degeneration and hypomyelination caused by overexpression of myelin proteolipid protein gene. *Neuron* **13,** 427–442.

Kalin, N., Claass, A., Sommer, M., Puchelle, E., and Tummler, B. (1999). DeltaF508 CFTR protein expression in tissues from patients with cystic fibrosis. *J Clin Invest* **103,** 1379–1389.

Kalwy, S. A., Smith, R., and Kidd, G. J. (1997). Myelin proteolipid protein expressed in COS-1 cells is targeted to actin-associated surfaces. *J Neurosci Res* **48,** 201–211.

Kartner, N., Augustinas, O., Jensen, T. J., Naismith, A. L., and Riordan, J. R. (1992). Mislocalization of delta F508 CFTR in cystic fibrosis sweat gland. *Nat Genet* **1,** 321–327.

Katayama, T., Imaizumi, K., Sato, N., Miyoshi, K., Kudo, T., Hitomi, J., Morihara, T., Yoneda, T., Gomi, F., Mori, Y., Nakane, Y., Takeda, J., Tsuda, T., Itoyama, Y., Murayama, O., Takashima, A., St. George-Hyslop, P., Takeda, M., and Tohyama, M. (1999). Presenilin-1 mutations downregulate the signalling pathway of the unfolded-protein response. *Nat Cell Biol* **1,** 479–485.

Kaufman, R. J., Scheuner, D., Schroder, M., Shen, X., Lee, K., Liu, C. Y., and Arnold, S. M. (2002). The unfolded protein response in nutrient sensing and differentiation. *Nat Rev Mol Cell Biol* **3,** 411–421.

Kimball, S. R. (1999). Eukaryotic initiation factor eIF2. *Int. J. Biochem. Cell Biol.* **31,** 25–29.

Klausner, R. D., and Sitia, R. (1990). Protein degradation in the endoplasmic reticulum. *Cell* **62,** 611–614.

Klement, I. A., Skinner, P. J., Kaytor, M. D., Yi, H., Hersch, S. M., Clark, H. B., Zoghbi, H. Y., and Orr, H. T. (1998). Ataxin-1 nuclear localization and aggregation: Role in polyglutamine-induced disease in SCA1 transgenic mice. *Cell* **95,** 41–53.

Klugmann, M., Schwab, M. H., Puhlhofer, A., Schneider, A., Zimmermann, F., Griffiths, I. R., and Nave, K.-A. (1997). Assembly of CNS myelin in the absence of proteolipid protein. *Neuron* **18,** 59–70.

Knapp, P., Skoff, R., and Redstone, D. (1986). Oligodendroglial cell death in jimpy mice: An explanation for the myelin deficit. *J. Neurosci.* **6,** 2813–2822.

Kobayashi, H., Hoffman, E. P., and Marks, H. G. (1994). The *rumpshaker* mutation in spastic paraplegia. *Nat. Genet.* **7,** 351–352.

Kopito, R. R., and Sitia, R. (2000). Aggresomes and Russell bodies. Symptoms of cellular indigestion? *EMBO Rep* **1,** 225–231.

Kozutsumi, Y., Segal, M., Normington, K., Gething, M. J., and Sambrook, J. (1988). The presence of malfolded proteins in the endoplasmic reticulum signals the induction of glucose-regulated proteins. *Nature* **332,** 462–464.

Kruger, R., Eberhardt, O., Riess, O., and Schulz, J. B. (2002). Parkinson's disease: One biochemical pathway to fit all genes? *Trends Mol Med* **8,** 236–240.

Le, A., Steiners, J. L., Ferrell, G. A., Shaker, J. C., and Sifers, R. N. (1994). Association between calnexin and a secretion-incompetent variant of human $\alpha_1$-antitrypsin. *J. Biol. Chem.* **269,** 7514–7519.

Lee, A. S. (2001). The glucose-regulated proteins: Stress induction and clinical applications. *Trends Biochem Sci* **26,** 504–510.

Lee, K., Tirasophon, W., Shen, X., Michalak, M., Prywes, R., Okada, T., Yoshida, H., Mori, K., and Kaufman, R. J. (2002). IRE1-mediated unconventional mRNA splicing and S2P-mediated ATF6 cleavage merge to regulate XBP1 in signaling the unfolded protein response. *Genes Dev* **16,** 452–466.

Lee, V. M., Goedert, M., and Trojanowski, J. Q. (2001). Neurodegenerative tauopathies. *Annu Rev Neurosci* **24,** 1121–1159.

Leegwater, P. A., Vermeulen, G., Konst, A. A., Naidu, S., Mulders, J., Visser, A., Kersbergen, P., Mobach, D., Fonds, D., van Berkel, C. G., Lemmers, R. J., Frants, R. R., Oudejans, C. B., Schutgens, R. B., Prank, J. C., and vander Knapp, M. S. (2001). Subunits of the translation initiation factor eIF2B are mutant in leukoencephalopathy with vanishing white matter. *Nat Genet* **29,** 383–388.

Lipsitz, D., Goetz, B. D., and Duncan, I. D. (1998). Apoptotic glial cell death and kinetics in the spinal cord of the myelin-deficient rat. *J. Neurosci. Res.* **51,** 497–507.

Lomas, D. A., and Carrell, R. W. (2002). Serpinopathies and the conformational dementias. *Nat Rev Genet* **3,** 759–768.

Ma, J., and Lindquist, S. (2002). Conversion of PrP to a Self-Perpetuating PrPSc-like Conformation in the Cytosol. *Science* **298,** 1785–1788.

Ma, J., Wollmann, R., and Lindquist, S. (2002a). Neurotoxicity and Neurodegeneration When PrP Accumulates in the Cytosol. *Science* **298,** 1781–1785.

Ma, Y., Brewer, J. W., Diehl, J. A., and Hendershot, L. M. (2002b). Two distinct stress signaling pathways converge upon the CHOP promoter during the mammalian unfolded protein response. *J Mol Biol* **318,** 1351–1365.

Ma, Y., and Hendershot, L. M. (2001). The unfolding tale of the unfolded protein response. *Cell* **107,** 827–30.

Macklin, W. B., Trapp, B. D., Kagawa, T., and Ikenaka, K. (1995). Hypomyelination in transgenic mice with multiple copies of the myelin proteolipid protein gene. *J. Neurochem.* **64,** S86.

Mastronardi, F. G., Ackerley, C. A., Arsenault, L., Roots, B. I., and Moscarello, M. A. (1993). Demyelination in a transgenic mouse: A model for multiple sclerosis. *J. Neurosci. Res.* **36,** 315–324.

Mori, K., Ma, W., Gething, M.-J., and Sambrook, J. (1993). A transmembrane protein with a cdc2+/CDC28-related kinase activity is required for signalling from the ER to the nucleus. *Cell* **74,** 743–756.

Moulding, H. D., Martuza, R. L., and Rabkin, S. D. (2000). Clinical mutations in the L1 neural cell adhesion molecule affect cell-surface expression. *J Neurosci* **20,** 5696–5702.

Naef, R., Adlkofer, K., Lescher, B., and Suter, U. (1997). Aberrant protein trafficking in Trembler suggests a disease mechanism for hereditary human peripheral neuropathies. *Mol. Cell. Neurosci.* **9,** 13–25.

Nave, K.-A., and Boespflug-Tanguy, O. (1996). X-linked developmental defects of myelination: From mouse mutants to human genetic diseases. *The Neuroscientist* **2,** 33–43.

Niwa, M., Sidrauski, C., Kaufman, R. J., and Walter, P. (1999). A role for presenilin-1 in nuclear accumulation of Ire1 fragments and induction of the mammalian unfolded protein response. *Cell* **99,** 691–702.

Novoa, I., Zeng, H., Harding, H. P., and Ron, D. (2001). Feedback inhibition of the unfolded protein response by GADD34-mediated dephosphorylation of eIF2alpha. *J Cell Biol* **153,** 1011–1022.

Nussbaum, J. L., and Roussel, G. (1983). Immunocytochemical demonstration of the transport of myelin proteins through the Golgi apparatus. *Cell Tissue Res.* **234,** 547–559.

Nussbaum, J.-L., Roussel, G., Wunsch, E., and Jolles, P. (1985). Site-specific antibodies to rat myelin proteolipids directed against the C-terminal hexapeptide. *J. Neurol. Sci.* **68,** 89–100.

Okada, T., Yoshida, H., Akazawa, R., Negishi, M., and Mori, K. (2002). Distinct Roles of ATF6 and PERK in Transcription during the Mammalian Unfolded Protein Response. *Biochem J* **16.**

Olsson, J. E., Gordon, J. W., Pawlyk, B. S., Roof, D., Hayes, A., Molday, R. S., Mukai, S., Cowley, G. S., Berson, E. L., and Dryja, T. P. (1992). Transgenic mice with a rhodopsin mutation (pro23his): A mouse model of autosomal dominant retinitis pigmentosa. *Neuron* **9,** 815–830.

Ordway, J. M., Tallaksen-Greene, S., Gutekunst, C. A., Bernstein, E. M., Cearley, J. A., Wiener, H. W., Dure, L. S. t., Lindsey, R., Hersch, S. M., Jope, R. S., Albin, R. L., and Detloff, P. J. (1997). Ectopically expressed CAG repeats cause intranuclear inclusions and a progressive late onset neurological phenotype in the mouse. *Cell* **91,** 753–763.

Orr, H. T., and Zoghbi, H. Y. (2001). SCA1 molecular genetics: A history of a 13 year collaboration against glutamines. *Hum Mol Genet* **10,** 2307–2311.

Pearsall, G. B., Nadon, N. L., Wolf, M. K., and Billings-Gagliardi, S. (1997). Jimpy-4J mouse has a missense mutation in exon 2 of the Plp gene. *Dev. Neurosci.* **19,** 337–341.

Pepys, M. B. (2001). Pathogenesis, diagnosis and treatment of systemic amyloidosis. *Philos Trans R Soc Lond B Biol Sci* **356,** 203–10; discussion 210–211.

Power, C., Kong, P., and Trapp, B. (1996). Major histocompatibility class I expression in oligodendrocytes induces hypomyelination in transgenic mice. *J. Neurosci. Res.* **44,** 165–173.

Prusiner, S. B. (1998). Prions. *Proc Natl Acad Sci U S A* **95,** 13363–13383.

Raskind, W. H., Williams, C. A., Hudson, L. D., and Bird, T. D. (1991). Complete deletion of the proteolipid protein gene (PLP) in a family with X-linked Pelizaeus-Merzbacher disease. *Am. J. Hum. Genet.* **49,** 1355–1360.

Readhead, C., Schneider, A., Griffiths, I. R., and Nave, K.-A. (1994). Premature arrest of myelin formation in transgenic mice with increased proteolipid protein gene dosage. *Neuron* **12,** 583–595.

Reddy, P. H., Williams, M., Charles, V., Garrett, L., Pike-Buchanan, L., Whetsell, W. O., Jr., Miller, G., and Tagle, D. A. (1998). Behavioural abnormalities and selective neuronal loss in HD transgenic mice expressing mutated full-length HD cDNA. *Nat Genet* **20,** 198–202.

Reiter, L. T., Murakami, T., Koeuth, T., Pentao, L., Muzny, D. M., Gibbs, R. A., and Lupski, J. R. (1996). A recombination hotspot responsible for two inherited peripheral neuropathies is located near a mariner transposon-like element. *Nat. Genet.* **12,** 288–297.

Rose, J. K., and Doms, R. W. (1988). Regulation of protein export from the endoplasmic reticulum. *Annu. Rev. Cell Biol.* **4,** 257–288.

Roussel, G., Meskovic, N. M., Trifilieff, E., Artault, J.-C., and Nussbaum, J.-L. (1987). Arrest of proteolipid transport through the Golgi apparatus in Jimpy brain. *J. Neurocytol.* **16,** 195–204.

Runker, A. E., Bartsch, U., Nave, K. A., and Schachner, M. (2003). The C264Y missense mutation in the extracellular domain of L1 impairs protein trafficking in vitro and in vivo. *J Neurosci* **23,** 277–286.

Rutishauser, J., and Spiess, M. (2002). Endoplasmic reticulum storage diseases. *Swiss Med Wkly* **132,** 211–222.

Ryu, E. J., Harding, H. P., Angelastro, J. M., Vitolo, O. V., Ron, D., and Greene, L. A. (2002). Endoplasmic reticulum stress and the unfolded protein response in cellular models of Parkinson's disease. *J Neurosci* **22,** 10690–10698.

Sanders, C. R., Ismail-Beigi, F., and McEnery, M. W. (2001). Mutations of peripheral myelin protein 22 result in defective trafficking through mechanisms which may be common to diseases involving tetraspan membrane proteins. *Biochemistry* **40,** 9453–9459.

Sato, N., Urano, F., Yoon Leem, J., Kim, S. H., Li, M., Donoviel, D., Bernstein, A., Lee, A. S., Ron, D., Veselits, M. L., Sisoda, S. S., and Thinakaran, G. (2000). Upregulation of BiP and CHOP by the unfolded-protein response is independent of presenilin expression. *Nat. Cell Biol.* **2,** 863–870.

Sato, S., Ward, C. L., Krouse, M. E., Wine, J. J., and Kopito, R. R. (1996). Glycerol reverses the misfolding phenotype of the most common cystic fibrosis mutation. *J Biol Chem* **271,** 635–638.

Schiffmann, R., and Boespflug-Tanguy, O. (2001). An update on the leukodsytrophies. *Curr Opin Neurol* **14,** 789–794.

Schneider, A., Griffiths, I., Readhead, C., and Nave, K.-A. (1995). Dominant-negative action of the jimpy mutation in mice complemented with an autosomal transgene for myelin proteolipid protein. *Proc. Natl. Acad. Sci.* **92,** 4447–4451.

Schneider, A., Montague, P., Griffiths, I., Fanarraga, M., Kennedy, P., Brophy, P., and Nave, K.-A. (1992). Uncoupling of hypomyelination and glial cell death by a mutation in the proteolipid protein gene. *Nature* **358,** 758–761.

Schwob, V. S., Clark, H. B., Agrawal, D., and Agrawal, H. C. (1985). Electron microscopic immunocytochemical localization of myelin proteolipid protein and myelin basic protein to oligodendrocytes in rat brain during myelination. *J. Neurochem.* **45,** 559–571.

Shen, J., Chen, X., Hendershot, L., and Prywes, R. (2002). ER stress regulation of ATF6 localization by dissociation of BiP/GRP78 binding and unmasking of Golgi localization signals. *Dev Cell* **3,** 99–111.

Shimura, H., Hattori, N., Kubo, S., Mizuno, Y., Asakawa, S., Minoshima, S., Shimizu, N., Iwai, K., Chiba, T., Tanaka, K., and Suzuki, T. (2000). Familial Parkinson disease gene product, parkin, is a ubiquitin-protein ligase. *Nat Genet* **25,** 302–305.

Shy, M., Hobson, G., Boespflug-Tanguy, O., Garbern, J., Sperle, K., Jain, M., Li, W., Gow, A., Rodriguez, D., Bertini, E., Mancias, P., Krajewski, K., Lewis, R. A., Kamholz, J., and members of the ENEDD (2003). Schwann cell expression of PLP1 but not its alternatively spliced isoform DM20 is necessary to prevent demyelinating peripheral neuropathy. *Ann Neurol* (in press).

Simons, M., Kramer, E. M., Macchi, P., Rathke-Hartlieb, S., Trotter, J., Nave, K. A., and Schulz, J. B. (2002). Overexpression of the myelin proteolipid protein leads to accumulation of cholesterol and proteolipid protein in endosomes/lysosomes: Implications for Pelizaeus-Merzbacher disease. *J Cell Biol* **157,** 327–336.

Sinoway, M. P., Kitagawa, K., Timsit, S., Hashim, G. A., and Colman, D. R. (1994). Proteolipid protein interactions in transfectants: Implications for myelin assembly. *J. Neurosci. Res.* **37,** 551–562.

Sistermans, E. A., de Wijs, I. J., de Coo, R. F. M., Smit, L. M. E., Menko, F. H., and van Oost, B. A. (1996). A (G-to-A) mutation in the initiation codon of the proteolipid protein gene causing a relatively mild form of Pelizaeus-Merzbacher disease in a Dutch family. *Hum. Genet.* **97,** 337–339.

Skoff, R. P., and Knapp, P. E. (1992). Phenotypic expression of X-linked genetic defects affecting myelination. *In* "Myelin: Biology and Chemistry" (R. E. Martenson, ed.), pp. 653–676. CRC Press, Boca Raton, FL.

Southwood, C. M., Garbern, J., Jiang, W., and Gow, A. (2002). The unfolded protein response modulates disease severity in Pelizaeus-Merzbacher disease. *Neuron* **36,** 585–596.

Southwood, C. M., and Gow, A. (2001). Molecular mechanisms of disease stemming from mutations in the proteolipid protein gene. *Micros. Res. Tech.* **52,** 700–708.

Stecca, B., Southwood, C. M., Gragerov, A., Kelley, K. A., Friedrich, V. L. J., and Gow, A. (2000). The evolution of lipophilin genes from invertebrates to tetrapods: DM-20 cannot replace PLP in CNS myelin. *J. Neurosci.* **20,** 4002–4010.

Thomson, C. E., Montague, P., Jung, M., Nave, K.-A., and Griffiths, I. R. (1997). Phenotypic severity of murine Plp mutants reflects in vivo and in vitro variations in transport of PLP isoproteins. *Glia* **20,** 322–332.

Timsit, S. G., Bally-Cuif, L., Colman, D. R., and Zalc, B. (1992). DM-20 mRNA is expressed during the embryonic development of the nervous system of the mouse. *J. Neurochem.* **58,** 1172–1175.

Tobler, A. R., Notterpek, L., Naef, R., Taylor, V., Suter, U., and Shooter, E. M. (1999). Transport of Trembler-J mutant peripheral myelin protein 22 is blocked in the intermediate compartment and affects the transport of the wild-type protein by direct interaction. *J. Neurosci.* **19,** 2027–2036.

Trojanowski, J. Q. (2002). Tauists, Baptists, Syners, Apostates, and new data. *Ann Neurol* **52,** 263–265.

Turnley, A. M., Morahan, G., Okano, H., Bernard, O., Mikoshiba, K., Allison, J., Bartlett, P. F., and Miller, J. A. F. P. (1991). Dysmyelination in transgenic mice resulting from expression of class I histocompatibility molecules in oligodendrocytes. *Nature* **353,** 566–569.

Ubeda, M., Wang, X.-Z., Zinszner, H., Wu, I., Habener, J., and Ron, D. (1996). Stress-induced binding of transcription factor CHOP to a novel DNA-control element. *Mol. Cell. Biol.* **16,** 1479–1489.

Uptain, S. M., and Lindquist, S. (2002). Prions as protein-based genetic elements. *Annu Rev Microbiol* **56,** 703–41.

van der Knaap, M. S., Barth, P. G., Gabreels, F. J., Franzoni, E., Begeer, J. H., Stroink, H., Rotteveel, J. J., and Valk, J. (1997). A new leukoencephalopathy with vanishing white matter. *Neurology* **48,** 845–855.

van der Knaap, M. S., Leegwater, P. A., Konst, A. A., Visser, A., Naidu, S., Oudejans, C. B., Schutgens, R. B., and Pronk, J. C. (2002). Mutations in each of the five subunits of translation initiation factor eIF2B can cause leukoencephalopathy with vanishing white matter. *Ann Neurol* **51,** 264–270.

Vela, J. M., Gonzalez, B., and Castellano, B. (1998). Understanding glial abnormalities associated with myelin deficiency in the jimpy mutant mouse. *Brain Res Brain Res Rev* **26,** 29–42.

Walsh, D. M., Klyubin, I., Fadeeva, J. V., Cullen, W. K., Anwyl, R., Wolfe, M. S., Rowan, M. J., and Selkoe, D. J. (2002). Naturally secreted oligomers of amyloid beta protein potently inhibit hippocampal long-term potentiation in vivo. *Nature* **416,** 535–539.

Wang, X.-Z., Harding, H. P., Zhang, Y., Jolicoeur, E. M., Kuroda, M., and Ron, D. (1998a). Cloning of mammalian Ire1 reveals diversity in the ER stress responses. *EMBO J.* **17,** 5708–5717.

Wang, X.-Z., Kuroda, M., Sok, J., Batchvarova, N., Kimmel, R., Chung, P., Zinszner, H., and Ron, D. (1998b). Identification of novel stress-induced genes downstream of *chop*. *EMBO J.* **17,** 3619–3630.

Wang, X.-Z., Lawson, B., Brewer, J. W., Zinszner, H., Sanjay, A., Mi, L.-J., Boorstein, R., Kreibich, G., Hendershot, L. M., and Ron, D. (1996). Signals from the stressed endoplasmic reticulum induce C/EBP-homologous protein (CHOP/GADD153). *Mol. Cell. Biol.* **16,** 4273–4280.

Wang, X.-Z., and Ron, D. (1996). Stress-induced phosphorylation and activation of the transcription factor CHOP (GADD153) by p38 MAP Kinase. *Science* **272,** 1347–1349.

Wechselberger, C., Wurm, S., Pfarr, W., and Hoglinger, O. (2002). The physiological functions of prion protein. *Exp Cell Res* **281,** 1–8.

Wolfgang, C. D., Chen, B. P., Martindale, J. L., Holbrook, N. J., and Hai, T. (1997). gadd153/Chop10, a potential target gene of the transcriptional repressor ATF3. *Mol. Cell. Biol.* **17,** 6700–6707.

Wu, Y., Whitman, I., Molmenti, E., Moore, K., Hippenmeyer, P., and Perlmutter, D. H. (1994). A lag in intracellular degradation of mutant $\alpha_1$-antitrypsin correlates with the liver disease phenotype in homozygous PiZZ $\alpha_1$-antitrypsin deficiency. *Proc. Natl. Acad. Sci. USA* **91,** 9014–9018.

Yamada, M., Ivanova, A., Yamaguchi, Y., Lees, M. B., and Ikenaka, K. (1999). Proteolipid protein gene product can be secreted and exhibit biological activity during early development. *J. Neurosci.* **19,** 2143–2151.

Yamada, M., Jung, M., Tetsushi, K., Ivanova, A., Nave, K. A., and Ikenaka, K. (2001). Mutant Plp/DM20 cannot be processed to secrete PLP-related oligodendrocyte differentiation/survival factor. *Neurochem Res* **26,** 639–645.

Yamamoto, T., Nanba, E., Zhang, H., Sasaki, M., Komaki, H., and Takeshita, K. (1998). Jimpy(msd) mouse mutation and connatal Pelizaeus-Merzbacher disease. *Am. J. Med. Genet.* **75,** 439–440.

Ye, J., Rawson, R. B., Komuro, R., Chen, X., Dave, U. P., Prywes, R., Brown, M. S., and Goldstein, J. L. (2000). ER stress induces cleavage of membrane-bound ATF6 by the same proteases that process SREBPs. *Mol Cell* **6,** 1355–1364.

Yoshida, H., Haze, K., Yanagi, H., Yura, T., and Mori, K. (1998). Identification of the cis-acting endoplasmic reticulum stress response element responsible for transcriptional induction of mammalian glucose-regulated proteins. Involvement of basic leucine zipper transcription factors. *J. Biol. Chem.* **273,** 33741–33749.

Yoshida, H., Matsui, T., Yamamoto, A., Okada, T., and Mori, K. (2001). XBP1 mRNA Is Induced by ATF6 and Spliced by IRE1 in Response to ER Stress to Produce a Highly Active Transcription Factor. *Cell* **107,** 881–891.

Yoshida, H., Okada, T., Haze, K., Yanagi, H., Yura, T., Negishi, M., and Mori, K. (2000). ATF6 activated by proteolysis binds in the presence of NF-Y (CBF) directly to the cis-acting element responsible for the mammalian unfolded protein response. *Mol Cell Biol* **20,** 6755–6767.

Yoshioka, T., Feigenbaum, L., and Jay, G. (1991). Transgenic mouse model for central nervous system demyelination. *Mol. Cell. Biol.* **11,** 5479–5486.

Zhao, Q., Wang, J., Levichkin, I. V., Stasinopoulos, S., Ryan, M. T., and Hoogenraad, N. J. (2002). A mitochondrial specific stress response in mammalian cells. *Embo J* **21,** 4411–4419.

Zinszner, H., Kuroda, M., Wang, X., Batchvarova, N., Lightfoot, R. T., Remotti, H., Stevens, J. L., and Ron, D. (1998). CHOP is implicated in programmed cell death in response to impaired function of the endoplasmic reticulum. *Genes Dev.* **12,** 982–995.

SECTION V

# ANIMAL MODELS OF HUMAN DISEASE

CHAPTER

# 43

# Experimental Autoimmune Encephalomyelitis

*Hans Lassmann*

## INTRODUCTION

The concept that brain inflammation can be induced by an autoimmune reaction against the central nervous system was born from clinical observations made at the turn of the 20th century in the course of testing the safety and efficacy of different vaccinations (Remlinger, 1928). Immunization with certain vaccines, in particular with rabies vaccines, which were produced by the propagation of the infectious agents in nervous tissue, in rare instances were associated with an acute inflammatory central nervous system (CNS) disease—postvaccinal leucoencephalomyelitis. Based on these observations, Rivers *et al.* (1933) immunized monkeys by repeated intramuscular injections of sterile extracts of normal rabbit brain tissue. They observed after 46 to 85 such injections the development of a chronic inflammatory demyelinating diseases of the central nervous system, which in its essential features resembled the lesions present in multiple sclerosis.

Although these studies established the concept of autoimmunity as a mechanism to induce inflammatory demyelinating brain disease, the practical use of this experimental model was limited due to species restrictions and poor reproducibility. This problem was overcome by the introduction of potent immune stimulating adjuvants, such as Freund's complete adjuvans (Freund *et al.*, 1950). With these tools the disease could be induced in nearly all vertebrate species in a highly reproducible manner. These models, which were then denominated "experimental autoimmune encephalomyelitis (EAE)," became the most important tools to study brain inflammation in general or the immunological mechanisms of organ-specific autoimmunity. They further were instrumental to unravel the mechanisms, leading to immune-mediated tissue damage in the central nervous system.

The pathology in the central nervous system in autoimmune encephalomyelitis reflects an inflammatory demyelinating disease, which in many respects is similar to its human counterparts, such as acute disseminated leucoencephalomyelitis, acute haemorhagic leucoencephalomyelitis, and multiple sclerosis (Alvord, 1970; Lassmann, 1983; Raine *et al.*, 1974). The inflammatory reaction is dominated by a mononuclear cell infiltrate, mainly consisting of T lymphocytes and macrophages accompanied by microglia activation. Pathological alterations are concentrated in the white matter (leucoencephalitis), although gray matter areas can be involved too. The essential structural lesions in the CNS are confluent areas (plaques) of primary demyelination with partial axonal preservation. However, axonal injury and destruction is regularly found in all areas of demyelination. The lesions are further characterized by the formation of a dense astrocytic scar, called reactive gliosis. Parallel to demyelination a variable degree of remyelination can be found, which can lead to complete restoration of the demyelinated tissue. A detailed comparison of such EAE lesions with those found in acute disseminated leucoencephalitis, and multiple sclerosis revealed that most essential pathological features of human inflammatory demyelinating disease are closely reflected in these EAE models (Lassmann, 1983).

## BASIC MECHANISMS OF AUTOIMMUNE-MEDIATED INFLAMMATORY BRAIN DISEASE

Since sensitization with nervous system tissue leads to an autoimmune disease, which is restricted to the central or the peripheral nervous system, it became clear already at an early stage that specific immune reactions, either mediated by T lymphocytes or antibodies, have to be involved in its pathogenesis. Classical work by Philip Paterson (1960) provided first clear evidence that the disease is basically mediated by T lymphocytes. T cells, isolated from actively sensitized animals with autoimmune encephalomyelitis, induced a similar disease, when passively transferred to normal naïve recipients, provided the donor cells and recipient animals are matched by their histocompatibility antigens. In contrast, intravenous transfer of serum or purified antibodies, derived from sensitized and diseased animals, did not induce disease (Chase, 1959).

A major breakthrough in the study of T-cell immunology in EAE was the development of a technique, which allowed to isolate and propagate monospecific T-cell lines or clones, which were able to transfer inflammatory brain disease to naïve recipients, which was first established in rats (Ben Nun *et al.*, 1981) and later in mice (Zamvil *et al.*, 1985). This allowed for the first time an in depth analysis of the antigen-specificity and the immunological properties of T cells, responsible for the initiation and propagation of autoimmune CNS inflammation.

There is, however, a major difference in the pathology of the CNS lesions between EAE, induced by passive transfer of T lymphocytes and that present in animals, which have been actively sensitized with whole CNS tissue or myelin. While in the latter the inflammatory process is associated with widespread primary demyelination or tissue damage, passive transfer of autoreactive T cells in general leads to an inflammatory brain disease with little or absent demyelination (Fig. 43.1). Thus, in actively induced EAE additional immune responses seem to be involved which modify the basic T-cell-mediated inflammatory process.

A major component, which is involved in this modification, are antibodies, directed against antigens, which are exposed in the extracellular space and are thus accessible for antibodies *in vivo*. Active sensitization of animals with whole CNS tissue or myelin may give rise to antibodies, which are able to induce demyelination *in vitro* in organotypic myelinating tissue culture (Bornstein and Appel, 1961). Intravenous injections of such antibodies fails to induce disease, because their entry into the CNS is restricted by the intact blood brain barrier. However, when directly injected into the cerebrospinal fluid or the CNS tissue with either complement or cytokines, which activate macrophages, they induce primary demyelination (Lassmann *et al.*; 1981; Vass *et al.*, 1992). Furthermore, when such antibodies are injected intravenously into animals with EAE, induced by transfer of auto-reactive T lymphocytes, they may effectively transform the pure T-cell-mediated inflammation into an inflammatory demyelinating type of pathology, which is similar to that observed after active sensitization of the animals with brain tissue (Linington *et al.*, 1988; Schlüsener *et al.*, 1987).

Thus, on this basis three different disease models are available, which can be used to address fundamentally different questions regarding the pathogenesis of inflammatory demyelinating diseases.

### 1. EAE Induced by Passive Transfer of Autoreactive T-Lymphocytes (PT-EAE)

In this model memory T lymphocytes, directed against antigens of the CNS, are isolated from sensitized donors and are transferred into naïve histocompatible recipients (Ben Nun

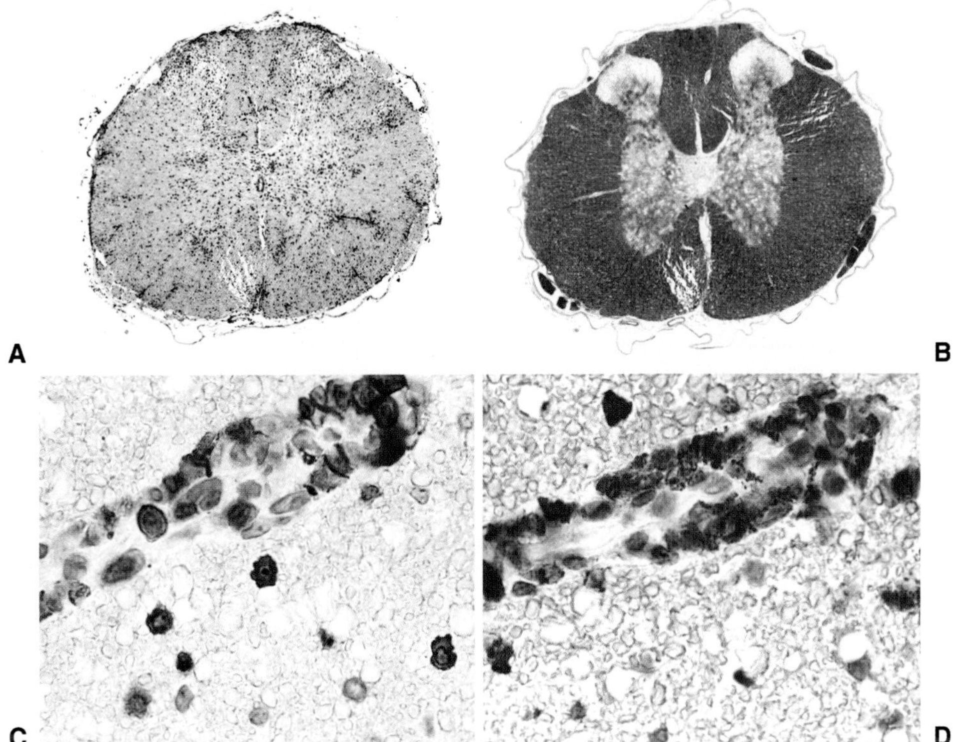


FIGURE 43.1
Brain inflammation induced by passive transfer of MBP-reactive Th1 cells; perivascular inflammatory infiltrates in the spinal cord (A) with minimal or absent demyelination or tissue injury (B). The infiltrates are composed of T lymphocytes (C) and macrophages (D). (A) immunocytochemistry for ED1 (macrophages); ×: 100. (B) Luxol fast blue myelin stain; ×: 100. (C) immunocytochemistry for W 3/13 (T cells); × 500. (D) Immunocytochemistry for ED1 (macrophages); × 500.

*et al.*, 1981). Thus, this model is induced by T cells, which are already immunologically primed and it is not complicated by the immunological processes, which occur during the sensitization in the peripheral immune system. It is thus an ideal model to study the mechanisms, how T cells start the inflammatory process in the CNS, and to analyze the effects on the target tissue, which they exert either alone or in cooperation with activated macrophages or microglia cells. Specific questions that have been addressed in these models include those that involve the mechanisms of immune surveillance of the CNS, the interaction of T cells and macrophages with the blood brain barrier and the analysis, how inflammatory cells—and in particular T cells—are cleared from established inflammatory brain lesions.

When monospecific T-cell lines or clones are used, the disease of PT-EAE follows a very reproducible course. Disease and brain inflammation starts between 3 and 5 days after transfer, reaches its clinical peak between days 5 to 8, and declines thereafter (Ben Nun *et al.*, 1981; Wekerle *et al.*, 1986). In general, the inflammatory process in the CNS is cleared after 15 days, leaving the CNS tissue either unaffected or in the case of severe encephalitis with some degree of perivascular astrocytic scaring. In rare instances, in particular in mouse models, a single passive transfer of autoreactive T cells may lead to a chronic disease (Mokhtarian *et al.*, 1984; Zamvil *et al.*, 1985), which is associated with more widespread demyelination and tissue damage (Fig. 43.2).

## 2. Co-transfer EAE (CoT-EAE)

In this model disease is induced, as in classical PT-EAE, by the passive transfer of encephalitogenic T lymphocytes (Linington *et al.*, 1988). At the onset of brain inflammation and disease (3 to 4 days after T-cell transfer) antibodies, soluble inflammatory

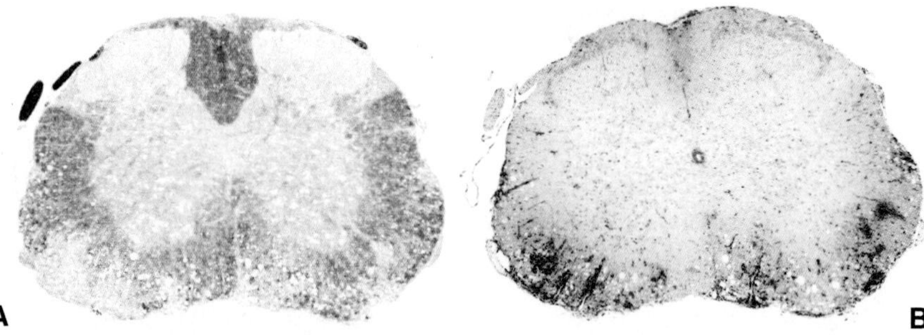


FIGURE 43.2
Chronic T-cell-mediated EAE in the mouse following sensitization with MOG peptide 35–55. The inflammatory process is associated with demyelination and tissue damage. (A) Luxol fast blue myelin stain, sowing areas of myelin loss in the ventral portions of the white matter; ×: 50. (B) Adjacent section stained with the macrophage marker Mac 3 reveals massive macrophage infiltration in the areas of demyelination; ×: 50.

mediators or other cells of the immune system are transferred intravenously. This allows to study, whether inflammatory mediators or immune cells, which by themselves are unable to induce brain inflammation, may modulate disease and pathology of T-cell-mediated disease.

Co-transfer EAE has been extensively analyzed to define the pathogenic role of demyelinating antibodies *in vivo* (Linington *et al.*, 1988). When such antibodies are transferred at the onset of T-cell-mediated brain inflammation the severity of clinical disease is massively augmented and the pathological alterations in the CNS are transformed from a pure inflammatory to an inflammatory demyelinating phenotype. The pathological outcome is determined by the balance between the encephalitogenic T-cell response and the concentration of circulating demyelinating antibodies (Lassmann *et al.*, 1988). This model allows to evaluate the pathogenic potential of CNS directed autoantibodies (Weerth *et al.*, 1999) and to study the immunological mechanisms of antibody-mediated brain tissue damage *in vivo* (Litzenburger *et al.*, 1998). Furthermore, it is also useful to address more general questions on the cell biology and functional consequences of de- and remyelination, in particular, when an exactly timed model of de and remyelination is required (Di Bello *et al.*, 1999).

Co-transfer EAE is, however, not restricted to the study of antibodies. It further allows to test immunomodulatory effects of cytokines or the functional role of regulatory T-cell populations in acute T-cell-mediated brain inflammation.

## 3. EAE, Induced by Active Sensitization (A-EAE)

This is the most complex model of EAE, since it covers not only the effector stage of brain inflammation, as it is done in PT-EAE and CoT-EAE, but also includes the induction phase of the immune response, such as the sensitization of naïve T cells and B cells as well as their propagation and polarization into different effector and regulatory T-cell populations.

Active immunization of susceptible animals in general induces an acute neurological disease, which starts between 10 and 20 days after sensitization (Alvord, 1970). Depending on the mode of sensitization, the nature of the sensitizing antigen, and the genetic background of the animals, a chronic relapsing or chronic progressive disease may develop (Lassmann, 1983, Raine, 1985). The pathology of the acute phase of the disease (10 to 20 days after sensitization) is dominated by the inflammatory reaction and mainly mediated through the T-cell response. Chronic disease is generally associated with severe demyelination or tissue damage and involves in addition to T cells other immunological mechanisms, such as for instance pathogenic antibodies (Fig. 43.3). In comparison to models of transfer EAE, A-EAE has several advantages. It can easily be induced even in laboratories, where the complex T-cell line technology is not established and, if properly handled, chronic inflammatory demyelinating disease can be induced for studies of basic cell biological

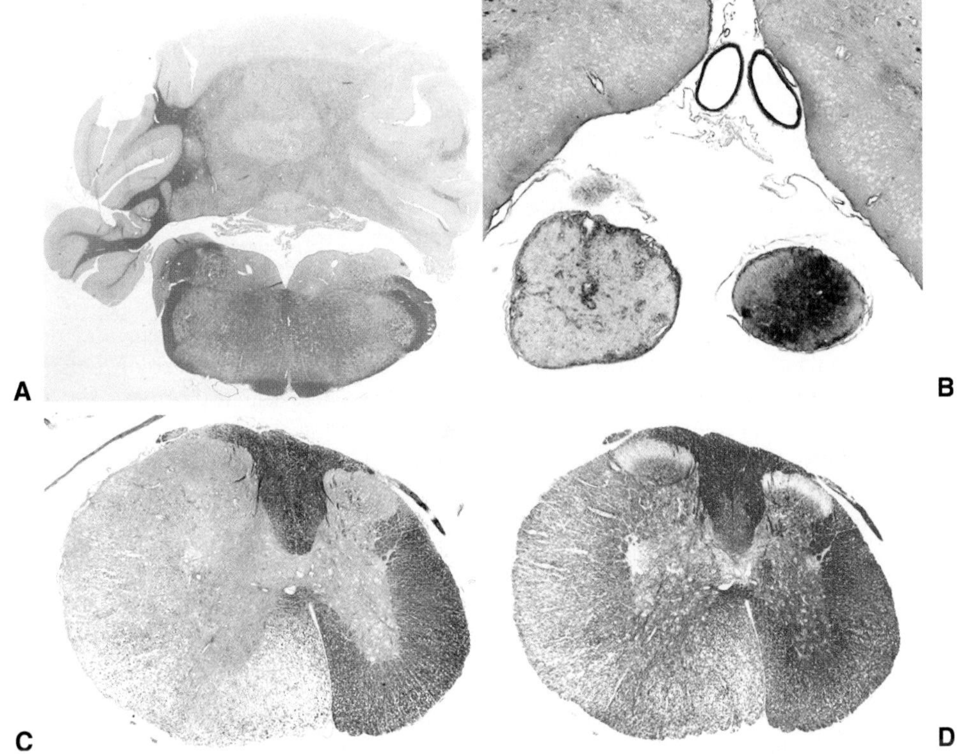


FIGURE 43.3
Inflammatory demyelinating disease induced in rats by active sensitization with MOG. In this case, the lesions are induced by a cooperation of encephalitogenic T cells and demyelinating antibodies. Large plaques of demyelination are present in the cerebellar white matter (A), the optic nerve (B) and the spinal cord (C). The axonal density within the lesion is reduced, in part by edema and tissue swelling and in part by axonal injury (D). (A–C) Luxol fast blue myelin stain. (D) Bielschowsky silver impregnation for axons. (A) × 15. (B) 100. (C, D) × 40.

aspects of demyelination, remyelination, and tissue injury. It furthermore allows the study of basic mechanisms of the induction of autoimmunity and of immune regulation. Its disadvantage lies in its complexity, which makes it difficult to clearly spot the individual immunopathogenetic mechanisms involved in its pathogenesis.

## TARGET ANTIGENS IN THE CENTRAL NERVOUS SYSTEM FOR AUTOIMMUNITY

T lymphocytes and antibodies recognize their antigen in different ways (for review, see Wekerle, 1998). T cells recognize small peptides, bound to molecules of the major histocompatibility complex (MHC) on the surface of antigen presenting cells. $CD8^+$ T cells use class I MHC and $CD4^+$ T cells class II MHC molecules for antigen recognition. In the normal central nervous system, the expression of both classes of MHC molecules is restricted to some perivascular macrophages and microglia cells, class I molecules being additionally present on endothelial cells (Traugott *et al.*, 1983, Matsumoto and Fujiwara, 1986). While class I MHC can be expressed on all cell types of the nervous system under inflammatory conditions, the expression of class II molecules is more restricted and predominantly found on leukocytes and microglia cells (Vass and Lassmann, 1990).

For T-cell antigen recognition, proteins have to be cleaved into small peptides in intracellular compartments of the antigen presenting cells; they have then to be attached to respective MHC molecule and transported to the surface of the antigen presenting cell, where they are recognized by the T cell through their specific T-cell receptor. This antigen recognition requires additional co-ligation between T cells and antigen presenting cells through adhesion molecules and co-stimulatory molecules. The selection of the proper peptide not only depends on the T-cell receptor, but also on its binding abilities to the MHC molecule and its proteolytic cleavage sites. In an outbred population or in different inbred strains, which have different MHC haplotypes, the antigenic peptides will be different. Thus, the antigenic peptide, which drives an autoimmune disease, may be the same in different animals from the same inbred strain, but in general will differ between different individuals of an outbred population. It has, however, to be noted that both extracellular as well as intracellular proteins may be presented in this way and may thus be targets for the cell-mediated immunity.

In contrast, antibodies recognize their antigen within the intact protein and do not require specific antigen presentation. Thus, a pathogenic antibody will recognize its target across histocompatibility barriers, provided the antigen has the respective interspecies homology in protein sequence and structure. The limitation of antibodies to be pathogenic is its accessibility of the target epitope *in vivo*. This implies that the antigen (epitope) has to be either located on the cell surface or in the extracellular space and the epitope recognized by the antibody must not be hidden within the tertiary structure of the protein. Due to these major differences in epitope recognition between T cells and antibodies, their roles in CNS autoimmunity have to be discussed separately.

### T-Cell-mediated Autoimmunity

For a long time myelin basic protein, one of the major myelin proteins, was believed to be the only brain antigen responsible for the induction of EAE. It was the first that had been identified and chemically characterized (Kies *et al.*, 1960). The reason for this was that it is relatively easy to purify and due to its hydrophilic nature it is readily available for use in immunological test systems. Myelin basic protein is highly encephalitogenic, which means that it is able to induce EAE even in minute concentrations (Alvord, 1970).

MBP induces a strong encephalitogenic T-cell response in all vertebrate species tested so far. However, the peptide epitopes of the MBP molecule, which are recognized by encephalitogenic T cells, differ between different species and between different strains of the same species (Alvord, 1984; Swanborg, 2001). Furthermore, even within a given inbred strain frequently more than one peptide epitopes of the MBP molecule can drive a T-cell response, which each may differ in their encephalitogenic potential. This complex situation makes it difficult or even impossible to prove the pathogenetic potential of a T-cell response against MBP in humans.

This problem is further complicated by the fact that MBP is only one candidate antigen for an encephalitogenic T-cell response. Another antigen, which can drive an encephalitogenic T-cell response, is proteolipid protein (PLP; Sobel and Kuchroo, 1992). Similar to the situation with MBP the peptide epitopes within the PLP molecule, which are responsible for the induction of T-cell-mediated encephalitis, vary between animal species and strains.

In recent years encephalitogenic T-cell responses were identified, directed against a variety of other myelin and oligodendrocyte proteins, such as myelin oligodendrocyte glycoprotein (Linington *et al.*, 1993), myelin associated glycoprotein (Morris-Downes *et al.*, 2002; Weerth *et al.*, 1999), cyclic nucleotide phosphodieserase (Morris-Downes *et al.*, 2002; Rosener *et al.*, 1997), and oligodendrocytic basic protein (Maatta *et al.*, 1998; Morris-Downes *et al.*, 2002), as well as against proteins expressed in other glial cells, such as for instance S-100 protein (Kojima *et al.*, 1994). These data suggest that any CNS protein, which is able to stimulate a T-cell response (and this probably applies to most of them), is a possible candidate for a T-cell-mediated encephalomyelitis. The spectrum of possible target auto-antigens for an encephalitogenic T-cell response in humans is thus very broad.

In addition, brain inflammation was also induced by T cells, which react through molecular mimicry with brain proteins as well as proteins from infectious agents (Bhardwaj *et al.*, 1993; Moktharian *et al.*, 1999; Wucherpfennig and Strominger, 1995). This does not require complete sequence identity between the respective peptides, but just a peptide structure, which in its motive is similar in the essential anchor sequences that mediate the binding to the MHC molecule and the T-cell receptor (Wucherpfennig and Strominger, 1995). This further increases the possible number of peptide sequences, which may give rise for an encephalitogenic T-cell response.

T-cell autoimmunity can also be induced against other molecules than peptides, such as for instance glycolipids and complex carbohydrates. In this situation antigen presentation is different, since these molecules are not presented by classical MHC molecules but by molecules of the CD1 complex (Moody *et al.*, 1999; Moody and Besra, 2001). CD1 molecules are nonpolymorphic and thus do not differ between different outbred members of the same species. Some of the CD1 molecules have a deep hydrophobic grove, which allows the binding of glycolipid molecules. The specific T-cell response is directed against the complex carbohydrate structure of the respective glycolpipds.

Specific T-cell reactions against a variety of glycolipids in the central nervous system, such as gangliosides or sulfatides have been identified in humans, in particular in multiple sclerosis patients and such molecules are, thus, potential targets for T-cell-mediated autoimmunity (Shamshiev *et al.*, 1999, 2002). Due to species differences in the structure and function of CD1 molecules and the anti-lipid T-cell response, experimental evidence for the encephalitogenic potential of such T cells so far is indirect.

## Target Antigens for Antibody-Mediated Demyelination and Tissue Destruction

As mentioned earlier, the basic requirement for an antibody to be pathogenic is the accessibility of the target antigen in the intact tissue. Thus, the target antigen has either to be present in the extracellular space or expressed on the extracellular surface of cells. This to a large extent reduces the number of potentially pathogenic target antigens, since it excludes all those epitopes which are exclusively present in the cell cytoplasm or in other compartments, which are not accessible from the extracellular space. The pathogenic potential of antibodies can be tested when they are directly applied together with either activated macrophages or complement to organotypic cultures of CNS tissue (Bornstein and Appel, 1961). Alternatively, such antibodies can be directly injected into the cerebrospinal fluid or the CNS tissue (Jankovic *et al.*, 1965, Lassmann *et al.*, 1981). Furthermore, their pathogenic potential *in vivo* can be tested in models of co-transfer EAE (Linington *et al.*, 1988).

This basic principle has been extensively studies for antibodies against myelin components. Thus, antibodies against MBP, which is located at the cytoplasmic face of the cell membrane in compact myelin sheaths, do not induce demyelination *in vitro* or *in vivo*. In contrast, MOG, which is located on the extracellular surface of oligodendrocytes and myelin sheaths, is a target for antibody-mediated demyelination (Linington *et al.*, 1988). The situation is more complex for antigens, such as PLP or MAG, which at least contain epitopes, which are located on the extracellular face of the myelin membrane. Nevertheless, antibodies against these antigens did not induce demyelination *in vitro* (Seil *et al.*, 1980,, 1981). This could be explained by the complex architecture of the myelin sheath. The extracellular compartment within the compact myelin sheath (interperiod line) is secluded from the brain extracellular space by tight junctions, which prohibit the entry of serum proteins into the compact myelin. Similarly, diffusion of extracellular proteins is restricted into the periaxonal space where MAG is located.

In addition, the epitope recognized by the antibody has to be accessible *in vivo* within the complex tertiary structure of the molecule. As an example, most antibodies, which were directed against linear peptide epitopes of MOG, even against those which are contained in the extracellular domain of the molecule, did not bind to native MOG on the surface of transfected cells (Haase *et al.*, 2001).

Thus, so far only a small number of molecules has been identified as targets for demyelinating antibodies. They include MOG as well as certain glycolipids, which are exposed on the myelin surface, such as galactocerebroside (Dubois-Dalcq *et al.*, 1970). In principle, however, also antibodies against other cellular targets of the CNS, such as astrocytes or neurons, could be pathogenic and could modulate the pathology of T-cell-mediated encephalitis. Interestingly, in some multiple sclerosis patients, antibodies have been detected, which are directed against progenitor cells of oligodendrocytes (Niehaus *et al.*, 2000). It has to be determined in the future whether such antibodies can impair remyelination in inflammatory demyelinating lesions of the CNS.

## WHAT T-CELL POPULATIONS ARE RESPONSIBLE FOR THE INDUCTION OF BRAIN INFLAMMATION?

The immune system is controlled by different T lymphocyte populations. Helper T cells (Th-cells), by their production of cytokines may either recruit and activate effector cells, such as macrophages or granulocytes or may stimulate B-cell differentiation and antibody production. Cytotoxic T lymphocytes (Tc-cells) destroy in an antigen-specific manner specific target cells through their cytotoxic machinery. Regulatory T cells (Tr-cells), again through cytokine production, modulate or down-regulate immune reactions. Furthermore, antigen recognition differs between T-cell subsets. $CD4^+$ T cells recognize antigenic peptides in the context of class II MHC molecules, $CD8^+$ T cells use class I MHC molecules and T cells directed against complex carbohydrates or glycolipis require CD1 molecules for antigen presentation. Finally, the first antigen contact of naïve T cells may polarize T cells toward the production of Th/Tc1 cytokines such as interferon-gamma (IFN-$\gamma$) or tumor necrosis factor alpha (TNF-$\alpha$), of Th/Tc2 cytokines, such as interleukin 4, 5, and 10 or of immunoregulatory cytokines, such as transforming growth factor beta (TGF-$\beta$). Thus, many different T-cell populations with fundamentally different function may be involved in the initiation and regulation of T-cell-mediated brain inflammation.

### Th-1 Cells in EAE

EAE has for long been regarded as the paradigmatic model of an autoimmune disease mediated by Th-1 cells (for review see Lafaille, 1998; Owens *et al.*, 2001). This assumption is mainly based on studies of EAE models, induced by sensitization with MBP. The disease can be transferred by intravenous injection of monospecific autoreactive Th-1 polarized T-cell lines and clones. The initial stage of brain inflammation is dominated by local production of Th-1 cytokines, while during the recovery phase of the disease Th-2 cytokines become more prominent in the lesions (Issazadeh *et al.*, 1995a, 1995b). The disease, induced by active sensitization can be inhibited by deletion of $CD4^+$ T cells and by blockade of class II MHC molecules and inhibition or genetic deletion of Th-1-related cytokines, in particular interleukin 12 may ameliorate disease. In addition, disease susceptibility of different animal strains is to a large extent controlled by the MHC class II complex (Olsson *et al.*, 2000). These data clearly document the ability and importance of Th-1 cells for disease induction in EAE, but they do not rule out possible additional pathogenetic roles of other T-cell populations.

### Th-2 Cells in EAE

Th-2 cells are generally believed to be protective in EAE (Lafaille, 1998). They dominate in lesions of animals, which recover from disease (Issazadeh *et al.*, 1995a, 1995b). Sensitization strategies, which favor a Th-2 response, are in general protective against brain inflammation in this model (Wekerle, 1998). Thus, immune deviation from Th-1 to Th-2 responses is proposed as a valid therapeutic option for T-cell-mediated brain diseases, such as multiple sclerosis and this notion is supported by a large number of experimental studies, showing such effects in MBP-induced EAE (Hohlfeld, 1997).

There are, however, a variety of new data that indicate that the situation is more complicated. It was shown that Th-2 polarized T cells against myelin basic protein can induce brain inflammation following passive transfer, although profound immunosuppression of recipient animals was required (Laffaille *et al.*, 1997). The pathology of the brain lesions in this model was different from that induced by Th-1 cells, the lesions being associated with profound tissue destruction, and the inflammatory infiltrates dominated by granulocytes. Thus, in principle, Th-2 cells are able to directly induce brain inflammation and cerebral tissue damage. A possible role of Th-2 immune responses is also suggested from studies in EAE, induced by sensitization with MOG. With this antigen the disease is driven by a synergy of pathogenic T-cell and antibody responses. Furthermore, in the chronic stage of the disease its severity is determined rather by the antibody than the T-cell response (Stefferl *et al.*, 1999). Thus, in such a situation any stimulation of the antibody response may be detrimental. In this model, sensitization procedures or therapeutic strategies, which stimulate Th-2 responses may be associated with more severe disease as well as more demyelination and tissue damage compared to that in a classical Th-1-mediated autoimmune encephalomyelitis (Genain *et al.*, 1996). This may also be associated with a Th-2 driven antibody response (Tsunoda *et al.*, 2000) and an inflammatory pathology, dominated by the infiltration of granulocytes and eosinophils (Storch *et al.*, 1998).

## Class I MHC restricted Cytotoxic T cells

Similar to that of Th-2 cells, the role of class I restricted CD8+ T lymphocytes has for long been regarded as inhibitory or regulatory. This again is mainly based on data, obtained in EAE models, induced with myelin basic protein. Blockade of antigen presentation by the class II pathway, either through antibodies or by genetic deletion of CD4 or MHC class II molecules in general prevents EAE. In contrast, blockade of $CD8^+$ lymphocytes through antibodies or genetic deletion resulted in increased disease severity and, in chronic models, in increased numbers of relapses (Jiang *et al.*, 1992; Koh *et al.*, 1992). In addition, cytotoxic class I MHC restricted T cells were shown to destroy encephalitogenic Th-1 cells in an antigen specific manner through recognition of peptides of the respective T-cell receptor (Sun *et al.*, 1988). Thus, these data taken together suggest that class I restricted T cells in EAE may function as regulatory T cells instrumental in suppression of acute disease and relapses.

This concept was challenged by the observation that passive transfer of a T-cell population, which was enriched with MOG reactive, class I restricted $CD8^+$ cells can induce brain inflammation in normal recipient mice. In addition, these T cells induced more severe tissue damage than Th-1 cells alone (Sun *et al.*, 2001). In another experiment, myelin basic protein reactive CD8+ T cells were raised from animals, which were genetically deficient for MBP. Such T cells, when passively transferred into recipients, which did express MBP in the CNS, induced brain inflammation (Huseby *et al.*, 2001). Disease, however, was only seen when the recipients were immunosuppressed and treated with Il-2 before transfer. The lesions in the brain showed T-cell and macrophage infiltrates, like in classical PT-EAE; brain tissue damage, however, when present resembled the pathology of brain ischemia. Whether this was due to a vasculitic reaction, induced by class I restricted T cells or by other mechanisms is so far unclear.

To avoid the problem of tolerance for class I–restricted T cells against autoantigens, their possible pathogenicity has also been tested in transgenic models. The strategy in these experiments was to express a foreign antigen under a CNS specific promotor. Upon peripheral immunization with the respective antigen, the animals develop an inflammatory disease of the central nervous system, associated with destruction of the cells, expressing the transgene, which was mainly mediated by class I restricted T cells (Evans *et al.*, 1996). This was also achieved following passive transfer of cytotoxic T cells (Oldstone *et al.*, 1993). We recently used a similar model (Cornet *et al.*, 2001), in which influenza haemagglutinin is expressed under the GFAP promotor. We then transferred class I restricted cytotoxic T cells, derived from a T-cell receptor transgenic animal, in which the T-cell repertoire entirely consists of HA reactive class I MHC restricted T cells (Lassmann *et al.* unpublished). These studies showed that such T cells can induce brain inflammation in normal transgenic recipients. Similar as in PT-EAE with Th-1 cells, antigen specific activation of the T cells is required to allow them to home in the CNS. The pathological alterations in the CNS in this model were characterized by inflammatory infiltrates, mainly composed by activated T lymphocyte. The lesions showed little recruitment of haematogenous macrophages but were associated with profound microglia activation, selective loss, and apoptotic destruction of antigen-containing astrocytes without bystander damage of other CNS elements, such as myelin, oligodendrocytes, neurons, or axons (Fig. 43.4). Thus, the pathology of these lesions was much more selective compared to that found after transfer of Th-1 cells. These data together with recent *in vitro* studies suggest a major pathogenic role of cytotoxic, class I MHC restricted T cells in inflammatory brain diseases (Neumann *et al.*, 2002).

These studies clearly show that not only Th-1 cells, but also class I restricted cytotoxic T cells and, under certain conditions also Th-2 cells, can induce or contribute to T-cell-mediated autoimmune inflammation in the CNS. The question is why this was overlooked during many years of EAE research. The reason for this may be twofold. First, most studies on the immunology of EAE concentrated on the T-cell response against myelin basic protein. This antigen induces a disease which is purely T-cell mediated. Antibodies against MBP do not recognize their target antigen *in vivo* and thus are not pathogenic. When, however, like in MOG-induced EAE antibodies play a major role in the pathogenesis of brain disease, a stimulation of Th-2 responses may play a role in augmentation and

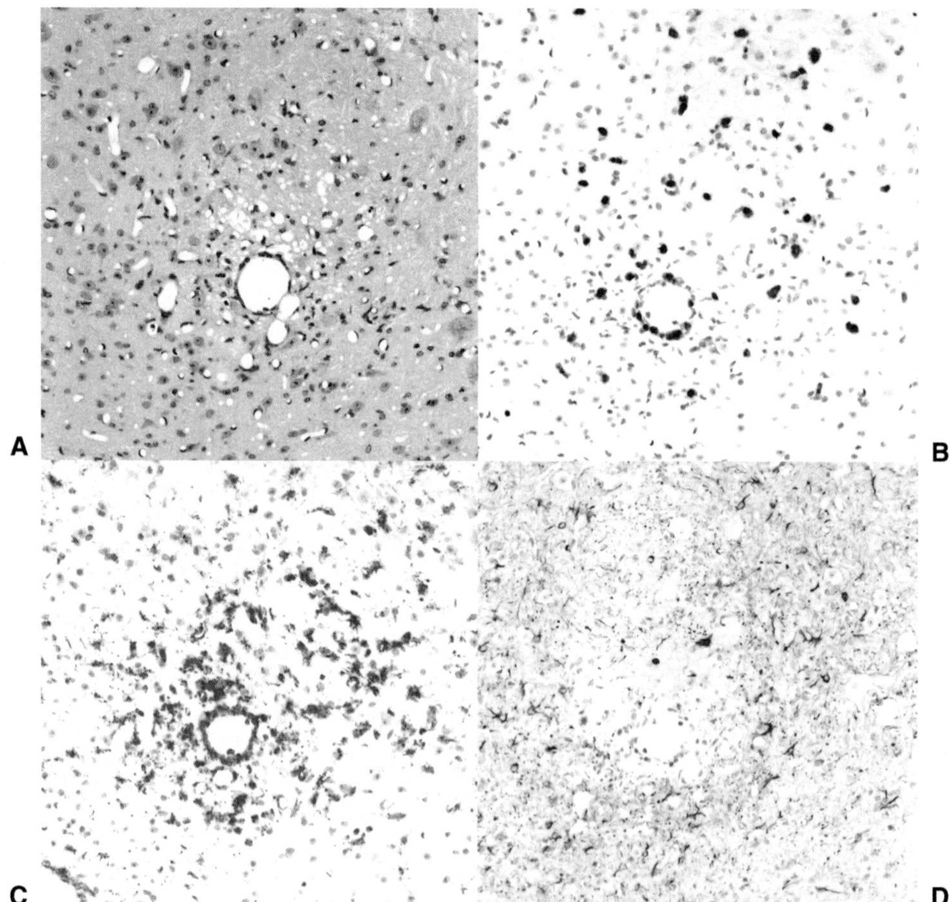


FIGURE 43.4
Brain inflammation induced by class I MHC restricted cytotoxic T cells; passive transfer of haemaglutinin reactive $CD8^+$ T cells in recipient animals, which express haemaglutinin under the GFAP promotor in astrocytes. Perivascular inflammation with vacuolization of the tissue (A) is associated with a difuse infiltration of T lymphocytes in the tissue (B) and an activation of local microglia cells (C). This process leads to degenerative changes and loss of astrocytes in the inflamed areas (D). (A) Haematoxylin/eosin stain. (B) Immunocytochemistry for CD3. (C) Immunocytochemistry for Mac-3. (D) Immunocytochemistry for GFAP. All figures ×: 300.

modification of the disease. Second, thymic deletion and peripheral tolerization may be more efficient for class I restricted cytotoxic T cells than for Th-1 cells. This may account for many classical EAE antigens, such as MBP or PLP, since they are expressed not only in the nervous system, but also in peripheral tissues, including the thymus (Voskuhl, 1998). A strong encephalitogenic class I restricted T-cell response has, thus, so far only been achieved by sensitization with either a foreign antigen or with an autoantigen, which is not expressed at all in peripheral tissues, such as MOG (Sun *et al.*, 2001) or MBP in MBP-deficient animals (Huseby *et al.*, 2001). This, however, does not rule out that a pathogenic class I restricted autoimmune response could be induced by molecular mimicry between infectious agents and autoantigens in the CNS (Evans *et al.*, 1996; Wucherpfennig and Strominger, 1995).

## IMMUNE SURVEILLANCE OF THE CNS AND THE INDUCTION OF INFLAMMATION

The models of PT-EAE and in particular the introduction of monospecific autoreactive T-cell lines and clones (Ben Nun *et al.*, 1981) paved the way for detailed studies on the mechanisms of immune surveillance of the brain and on the molecular requirements for the induction of brain inflammation. As mentioned earlier, intravenous injection of activated autoreactive Th-1 cells leads to an inflammatory brain disease (Fig. 43.5), which starts 3 to 4 days after transfer. Inflammation reaches its peak around day 5 to 7 and then declines. The time of disease onset in part depends upon the number of T cells, which are transferred, with lower numbers leading to a delay of a few days. However, even with transfer of

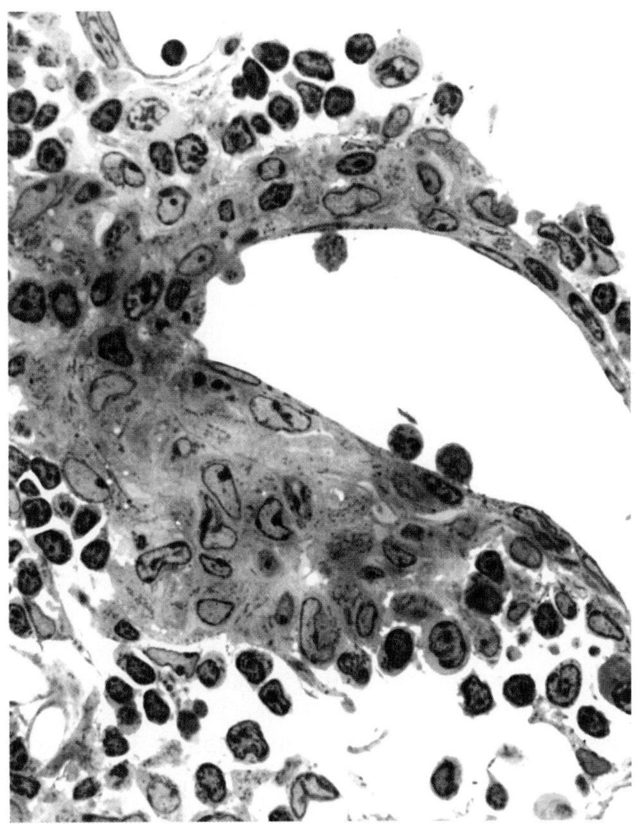

FIGURE 43.5
Inflammatory infiltrate in T-cell-mediated EAE; massive perivascular accumulation of Lymphocytes and macrophages. Toluidine blue stained plastic section; × 2000.

very high cell numbers, an incubation period of at least 72 hours remains (Flügel *et al.*, 2001). Detailed quantitative studies on T-cell infiltration in the CNS revealed that within the first hours after intravenous transfer some T cells enter the CNS. This early wave of T cells is antigen independent, being similar after transfer of autoreactive MBP-specific cells or T lymphocytes directed against an irrelevant antigen, which is not present in the CNS (Hickey *et al.*, 1991; Wekerle *et al.*, 1986). However, only CNS-specific T cells induce an inflammatory CNS disease. During the initial phase of CNS inflammation, 3 to 4 days after transfer, antigen specific T cells dominate in the lesions (Bauer *et al.*, 1998; Flügel *et al.*, 2001). Thereafter, additional T cells and macrophages from the host are recruited into the lesion, which at the peak of clinical disease and brain inflammation dominate the inflammatory infiltrates (Bauer *et al.*, 1998). This is associated with local up-regulation of class I and class II MHC molecules, both on inflammatory cells and local glia cells and by profound activation of local microglia. Both the antigen specific as well as the secondarily recruited T cells are rapidly cleared from the lesions by apoptotic destruction (Bauer *et al.*, 1998).

These data suggest that the normal blood brain barrier does restrict the entry of most circulating leukocytes into the CNS. This, however, is not the case for T lymphocytes, which have been activated by their specific antigen in the periphery. A peripheral activation of these cells, for instance, in the course of an infection, will start the process of immune surveillance of the brain. In the absence of the specific antigen, the T cells will either be locally destroyed by apoptosis or possibly also leave the brain through lymphatic drainage. In case they encounter their specific antigen in the CNS, they will be reactivated, start to produce pro-inflammatory cytokines, such as gamma-interferon or TNF-$\alpha$, and initiate the local inflammatory response.

It is, however, important to note that freshly *in vitro* activated T cells have only a limited capability to reach the CNS and their direct injection into the cerebrospinal fluid does not induce inflammation and disease. Instead these cells have after their transfer to migrate in a predictable way through the peripheral lymphatic system, where they obtain specific phenotypic and functional characteristics that allow them to migrate to and home in the CNS and mediate the inflammatory response (Flügel *et al.*, 2001).

### Leukocyte Entry into the CNS Is Controlled by Adhesion Molecules and Chemokines

The process of leukocyte migration through vascular barriers is controlled by adhesion molecules and chemokines and occurs in several consecutive steps (Luster, 1998; Springer, 1994). The first step is characterized by loose attachment of the cells to the endothelial surface. It leads to rolling of leukocytes along the luminal surface of the vessels and is mainly mediated by the interaction between selectins and carbohydrates. Then the leukocytes firmly attach to the endothelial surface by the interaction of adhesion molecules of the intergrin and immunoglobulin family. This firm attachment initiates transmigration, which either may occur in a trans-endothelial route through endothelial channels or in a paracellular route. Migration of inflammatory cells through the vessel wall requires the activation of proteases, which dissolve the inter-endothelial junctions and/or the basement membrane.

This process of trans-endothelial migration of leukocytes is further regulated by the interaction between chemokines and their receptors (reviewed by Luster, 1998). Chemokines are a family of small proteins which are produced and secreted both, by leukocytes and by cells of the target tissue. They diffuse toward the vessel wall and may become attached to the luminal surface of endothelial cells. There they are recognized by leukocytes, which express the respective receptors. In addition, leukocytes are attracted by soluble chemokines and migrate along their concentration gradient. Chemokines may either activate leukocyte adhesion molecules and thus support the firm attachment of the cells to the endothelial surface. In addition, through different members of the chemokine family and their interaction with specific receptors, which are expressed on different leukocyte subsets, they determine which leukocytes (T cells, B cells, macrophages, or granulocytes) are attracted to the inflammatory focus. Thus, chemokines determine the quality of the inflammatory reaction.

Adhesion molecules and chemokines play a major role in controlling brain inflammation (for review see Lee and Benveniste, 1999; Huang *et al.*, 2000; Ransohoff, 1999). Endothelial cells of the normal blood brain barrier show only a low basal level of adhesion molecule expression (Lee and Benveniste, 1999), and there is only a minor synthesis of chemokines in the normal brain (Huang *et al.*, 2000). This may explain, why it is permissive for transmigration only of activated T cells with high levels of adhesion molecule and chemokine receptor expression (Flügel *et al.*, 2001). When inflammation, however, is initiated cerebral endothelial cells become activated and express high levels of adhesion molecules. Furthermore local synthesis of chemokines in perivascular macrophages and astrocytes create a pro-inflammatory environment, which attracts more T cells and macrophages into the lesions.

In line with this concept a variety of adhesion molecules have been detected on brain endothelia within EAE lesions and this is associated with increased binding of leukocytes to the inflamed vessels in *in vitro* assays (Engelhardt *et al.*, 1994). Vascular cell adhesion molecule (VCAM) seems to be particularly important, since blockade of the interaction with its binding partner on leukocytes consistently reduces the severity of brain inflammation in EAE *in vivo* (Yednock *et al.*, 1992).

The spectrum of chemokines, present in classical EAE lesions is broad and includes mainly chemokines, which are associated with the recruitment of T lymphocytes and monocytes/macrophages (Godiska *et al.*, 1995) and it appears to differ depending upon the stage of the disease. Thus, in the acute phase of EAE different chemokines may be involved than in chronic lesions (Kennedy *et al.*, 1998) Their respective receptors are expressed on leukocytes within the lesions (Fife *et al.*, 2001; Izikson *et al.*, 2000; Jee *et al.*, 2002; Matsui *et al.*, 2002,). Blockade of certain chemokine receptors, such as for instance CCR2 through antibodies or through genetic deletion is a potent anti-inflammatory therapy in EAE (Fife *et al.*, 2000; Izikson *et al.*, 2000). To what extent other chemokines are present in atypical EAE lesions, such as those with profound granulocyte infiltration, is so far undetermined.

Besides classical chemokines there are other molecules with similar pro-inflammatory function. One of those are components of the complement system, such as C3 or C5, which interact with the respective complement receptors on leukocytes. Thus, complement inactivation or blockade of complement receptors may not only inhibit tissue damage but in addition has a profound anti-inflammatory effect (Huitinga *et al.*, 1993). Chemokine function may however also be mediated through certain neuropeptides (Numao and Agrawal, 1992; Ruff *et al.*, 1985), and in EAE the neuropeptide secretoneurin appears to attract macrophages into sites of brain inflammation (Storch *et al.*, 1996).

## MHC-Expression and T-cell Activation in the CNS

As discussed earlier in detail, T lymphocytes recognize their antigen only, when it is presented in the context of MHC molecules. Thus, MHC expression in the CNS is the prerequisite that T cells in the inflammatory focus get activated through specific recognition of their antigen, liberated within the tissue. MHC expression in the normal CNS tissue is strictly controlled (Matsumoto and Fujiwara, 1986) and only present on perivascular and meningeal macrophages and few microglia cells. In addition, MHC class I molecules are present on the luminal surface of cerebral endothelial cells. The suppression of MHC antigen expression is an active process and depends on the electrical activity of the neurons (Neumann *et al.*, 1996, 1997). Blockade of electrical activity by tetrodotoxin in brain slices leads to rapid up-regulation of MHC expression not only in the neurons themselves but also in glia cells, which are located in their vicinity. The active suppression of MHC expression by electrically active neurons is at least in part mediated by neurotrophic factors, signaled through the p75 neurotrophin receptor (Neumann *et al.*, 1998).

In EAE, irrespective of the mode of disease induction, MHC molecules are up-regulated within the inflammatory CNS lesions (Hickey *et al.*, 1985; Matsumoto and Fujiwara, 1986;

Sobel and Colvin, 1985). The extent of up-regulation reflects the severity of the inflammatory process. Most extensive expression is found on invading leukocytes and on microglia. In case of intense inflammation, class I molecules can also be found on other cells, such as astrocytes and some oligodendrocytes or neurons. In contrast, class II molecules can be found on microglia and only rarely on some astrocytes and ependymal cells. This graded response of MHC molecule up-regulation in the CNS is also seen after direct injection of gamma-interferon into the cerebrospinal fluid or the CNS tissue (Vass and Lassmann, 1990). Also in this situation microglia respond most prominently, while expression on other glial cells is only found after application of rather high concentrations of this cytokine.

These data suggest that antigen recognition by T cells in the CNS occurs in different steps. In the normal CNS tissue in the course of immune surveillance, antigen presentation occurs on meningeal and perivascular macrophages. This implies that an autoantigen, which may be recognized by T cells in the normal brain, has to be liberated into the brain's extracellular space and has to diffuse to the perivascular or menigeal compartment, where it is presented by cells, constitutively expressing MHC molecules. When inflammation is started, MHC antigens are up-regulated in a graded manner, first on microglia and only in conditions with intense inflammation also on other cells of the CNS. Thus, during the development of inflammatory brain lesions and in particular in chronic inflammatory processes more and additional antigen presenting cells are recruited, which may amplify the T-cell-mediated inflammatory reaction.

This concept is supported also by data, obtained in the model of EAE induced in radiation bone marrow chimeras. In this model, bone marrow transplantation is performed, using cells with a partially different MHC haplotype. These new bone marrow cells, at least in this particular rat model, replace the population of meningeal and perivascular macrophages, but not the parenchymal cells in the CNS tissue such as neurons, oligodendrocytes, astrocytes, and microglia (Hickey *et al.*, 1992). PT-EAE induced by T cells with an MHC haplotype, corresponding to that of the transplanted bone marrow cells, results in brain inflammation, similar to that present in fully histocompatible animals (Hickey and Kimura, 1988). These data show that antigen presentation by the population of meningeal and perivascular macrophages alone is sufficient to induce the basic inflammatory reaction of autoimmune encephalomyelitis. It is, however, expected, but so far not formally proven that this basic inflammatory reaction may be amplified by antigen presentation through additional cells of the CNS tissue.

Direct antigen presentation by cells of the CNS is required for cytotoxicity mediated by class I MHC restricted T cells. Thus, when EAE is induced by transfer of class I restricted cytotoxic T cells the apoptotic destruction of the specific target cells is associated with profound class I expression in the respective cells (Lassmann unpublished). Not surprisingly no disease and CNS lesions are found when such T cells are transferred into ß-2 microglobulin deficient mice (Sun *et al.*, 2001).

## CLEARANCE OF BRAIN INFLAMMATION IN AUTOIMMUNE ENCEPHALOMYELITIS

The CNS is different from other organs, since it lacks classical lymphatic vessels. Yet in acute autoimmune encephalomyelitis the inflammatory lesions subside within five to ten days after the peak of inflammation and clinical disease. Thus, there must be ways and mechanisms, how inflammatory cells, which have entered the CNS in the course of immune surveillance or inflammation, are cleared from the tissue.

An important observation was reported by Pender (Pender *et al.*, 1991), who draw the attention to the fact that numerous cells within EAE lesions are destroyed by apoptosis. A more detailed analysis of the cell types undergoing apoptosis in the lesions revealed that they were predominantly T lymphocytes. Furthermore, since programmed cell death is a rapid procedure, the quantitative data suggested that within a 24-hour time period more than twice the number of cells present in the lesions are removed by apoptosis (Schmied *et al.*, 1993). Thus, T-cell-mediated inflammation in acute EAE can only be maintained as long as there is a continuous supply of new T cells entering the CNS from the peripheral circulation. Using prelabeled T lymphocytes for PT-EAE it became clear that not only those T cells that recognize the specific antigen in the CNS, but also all other secondarily recruited T cells are eliminated from the lesions through programmed cell death (Bauer *et al.*, 1998). Besides T cells, B lymphocytes also have been shown to undergo apoptosis in inflammatory CNS lesions (White *et al.*, 2000), while plasma cells seem to be resistant. Detailed quantitative data on the elimination of B cells are, however, so far not available.

The immunological mechanisms that are responsible for this efficient destruction of T cells in the CNS are so far not clear and several different pathways may be involved (Gold *et al.*, 1997; Pender and Rist, 2001). Antigen specific T cells may be driven into apoptosis by contact with excess of soluble antigen, liberated in the CNS in the course of tissue damage, and TNF signaling through the TNF-receptor I seems to be involved in this process (Bachmann *et al.*, 1999). In addition, astrocytes express Fas-ligand, which may induce cell death through activation of the Fas-receptor, which is expressed on activated T lymphocytes (Bechmann *et al.*, 2000). This may explain why in the CNS apoptotic destruction of T cells is mainly found within the CNS parenchyme and not in the meningeal and perivascular space. These data, however, do not exclude that other, so far unknown CNS-specific mechanisms play and additional role.

This efficient local destruction of lymphocytes within inflamed brain tissue has several important consequences. It suggests that apoptotic destruction of the specific cells of the immune system is the major mechanism to terminate T-cell-mediated inflammation in the CNS. It may further explain why after acute EAE the original encephalitogenic T-cell population may be clonaly deleted from the immune repertoire. Finally, an impairment of this clearance process may be involved in the pathogenesis of chronic inflammatory diseases of the CNS. The lack of apoptotic destruction of fully differentiated plasma cells may explain the long lasting intrathecal immunoglobulin synthesis following cerebral inflammation.

While it is clear now that the vast majority of lymphocytes do not leave the CNS but are locally destroyed within the tissue, the situation seems to be different for macrophages. Although some of these cells within the lesions can be found, which show morphological changes of apoptosis, their number is very low (White *et al.*, 1998). Whether macrophages leave the CNS through lymphatic drainage pathways has to be determined.

## DETERMINANT-SPREADING AS A MECHANISM TO PROPAGATE AUTOIMMUNITY

In some animal species and strains, EAE induced by a single antigenic peptide may develop into a chronic inflammatory disease of the nervous system. When the T-cell immune response in such animals is followed over time, a broadening of the immune response to different peptide epitopes of the same protein or even to peptides of different proteins can be seen (Mc Rae *et al.*, 1995; Yu *et al.*, 1996). This process has been defined as determinant- or epitope-spreading and it is believed to be a major mechanism, responsible for chronification of an autoimmune disease. This cannot only be observed in primary autoimmune diseases, such as EAE, but may also happen as a consequence of virus-induced inflammation in the brain and may be one possible mechanism, how virus infections can trigger a neurological autoimmune disease (Miller and Eagar, 2001).

The basis for the induction of antigen-spreading is the liberation of brain antigens in an inflammatory environment and the genetic susceptibility of the organism to mount a respective autoimmune response. The question of where the autoimmune response is triggered is still unresolved. This is not trivial, since the induction of a new T-cell response requires the stimulation of naïve, unprimed T cells by professional antigen presenting cells, such as dendritic cells. The normal brain does not contain dendritic cells and they are also not induced in or recruited into the CNS by simple tissue injury. However, in chronic inflammatory lesions, in particular also in chronic EAE lesions, cells can be found, which phenotypically resemble dendritic cells and express the costimulatory molecules, necessary to stimulate naïve T cells (Serafini *et al.*, 2000). The source of these dendritic like cells is still controversial. They may either be recruited from the circulation by specific chemokines. Alternatively, some data suggest that microglia are undifferentiated haematopoetic progenitor cells, which have the potential to differentiate either into tissue macrophages or dendritic cells, depending on the cytokine milieu in the lesions (Fischer and Reichmann, 2001). It is thus feasible that naïve T cells, which are nonspecifically recruited into the inflammatory focus, are then locally primed with CNS antigen, presented by local dendritic cells and locally differentiate into autoimmune memory cells (Miller *et al.*, 1995; Vanderlugt *et al.*, 1998). The alternative mechanism for the induction of antigen-spreading is that brain antigens are either de novo expressed in or reach the lymphatic tissues, after being liberated in the lesions (Voskuhl, 1998).

## MECHANISMS OF TISSUE DAMAGE IN INFLAMMATORY LESIONS OF THE CNS

Brain inflammation in EAE is associated with damage and destruction of CNS tissue. Different forms of tissue damage may occur in the white matter. Primary demyelination is defined as a process, which leads to destruction of myelin sheaths with relative preservation of axons. Although all primary demyelinating lesions show some degree of axonal injury and loss, the characteristic feature of such lesions is that within the areas of complete loss of myelin preserved axons are still present in high density. Such primary demyelinating lesions have to be distinguished from lesions with unselective tissue damage In this situation, axons are affected to a similar extent compared to myelin and the degeneration of myelin occurs in parallel or secondary to axonal loss (secondary demyelination). In both situations, astrocytes built up a dense scar tissue (Fig. 7). Finally, in most severe lesions, all tissue elements can be destroyed, leading to cytstic necrosis. All three different forms of tissue injury can be found in EAE lesions (Lassmann, 1983), the quality and quantity of tissue damage is highly variable between different models and depends on the genetic background of the animals, the mode of sensitization, the nature of the sensitizing antigen, and the chronicity of the disease. Overall in acute EAE the pathology is dominated by inflammation and tissue damage or demyelination is sparse. In contrast, chronic models of EAE are generally associated with extensive demyelination or tissue damage. In addition, EAE models that are exclusively mediated by Th1 cells show less pronounced tissue injury than those in which the immune response is directed against multiple antigens and inflammation is mediated by multiple different immune mechanisms (Lassmann, 1983).

In immunological terms tissue destruction can occur by specific immune reactions, either through antigen recognition by cytotoxic T cells or by specific antibodies. This is generally associated with a high degree of selectivity of the cellular injury. In contrast, tissue may be destroyed by activated effector cells, such as macrophages, microglia, or granulocytes, independently of specific antigen recognition on the target cells. This type of damage is called "bystander damage" (Wisniweski and Bloom, 1975). Such bystander damage may show a certain degree of specificity, since for instance myelin sheaths or oligodendrocytes are in general more susceptible to toxic macrophage products than neurons or astrocytes. In more severe lesions, bystander damage, however, is always associated with profound unselective tissue injury.

A variety of different immunological mechanisms appear to be involved in the induction of tissue injury in EAE and their relative importance for disease outcome varies between species and strains of animals. These mechanisms include direct T-cell-mediated cytotoxicity, tissue injury induced by toxic products of activated effector cells, such as macrophages, microglia, or granulocytes, specific antibodies that can damage tissue either

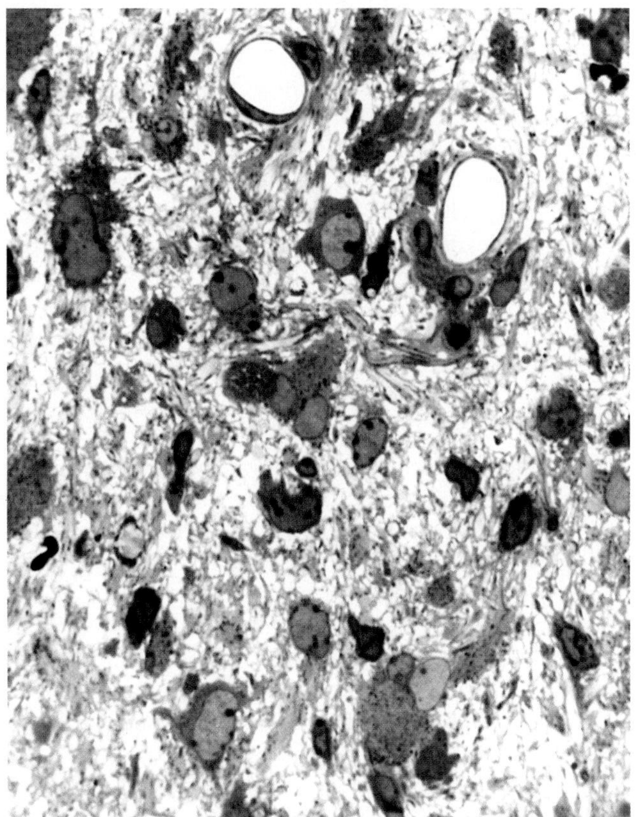

FIGURE 43.7
Glial scar formation in chronic EAE lesions; numerous reactive astrocytes are present within the lesion, forming the scar with a dense network of cell processes. Toluidine blue-stained plastic section; × 2000.

through complement activation or the interaction with activated macrophages, or, in very severe lesions, hypoxic or ischemic metabolic disturbances.

## Direct T-cell-mediated Cytotoxicity

In principle, both class I and class II–restricted T lymphocytes have a cytotoxic potential. $CD8^+$ T cells, however, are more effective in tissue destruction, since class I MHC expression is less restricted in comparison to class II. Thus, *in vitro*, all cells of the nervous system, including neurons, axons, oligodendrocytes, astrocytes, or microglia can be destroyed by cytotoxic T cells in an antigen-specific class I MHC restricted way (Neumann *et al.*, 2002). This is different for CD4+T lymphocytes, which can only lyse antigen presenting macrophages or microglia and astrocytes (Sun and Wekerle, 1986).

As discussed earlier, passive transfer of autoreactive $CD8^+$ T lymphocytes can lead to brain inflammation with very selective destruction of the respective antigen-containing target cells. The immunological requirements for such a direct T-cell-mediated killing is the expression of MHC class I molecules on the surface of the target cells, allowing specific antigen presentation and the interaction with T cells via an "immunological synapse" (Grakoui *et al.*, 1999). T cells can kill their targets either through their cytotoxic granules, which mainly contain perforin and granzymes. Perforin impairs the membrane stability of the target cells, while granzymes, getting access to the cell cytoplasm, start the apoptotic cascade. This is a rapid process, leading to cell destruction within less than 1 hour. In addition, T cells can destroy their targets also through the activation of death receptors, belonging to the Fas- or TNF receptor family. This death pathway is more protracted, the target cells being destroyed within several hours after the insult (for review, see Neumann *et al.*, 2002).

EAE is generally regarded as a disease mediated by class II restricted Th2 cells. Most of the immunological data in this respect, however, were obtained from EAE models induced by sensitization with myelin basic protein. Since MBP is at least in part expressed in peripheral lymphatic tissue (Voskuhl, 1998), immune control of class I restricted T-cell reactions against this antigen may be under strict regulation. In line with this concept, a significant immune response of $CD8^+$ T cells can be induced only in MBP-deficient animals (Huseby *et al.*, 2001). However, sensitization with MOG, which is not expressed in peripheral tissues of mice, leads to a profound class I MHC restricted immune response, which was shown to be encephalitogenic after passive transfer of the respective T cells. Thus, these data suggest that cytotoxic T lymphocytes may play a major pathogenic role in chronic MOG-induced EAE in mice, while in other EAE models their role may be limited.

### Antibody-Mediated Tissue Injury

As mentioned earlier, antibodies directed against target antigens, which are accessible from the extracellular space *in vivo*, may modulate clinical disease and pathology in T-cell-mediated EAE. This process has most intensively been investigated for demyelinating antibodies, which have been recognized already in early studies of EAE (Bornstein and Appel, 1961). Antibody-mediated tissue injury in the course of T-cell-mediated EAE leads to a very selective destruction of the target structures and plays a key role in the pathogenesis of the extensive and widespread demyelination, present in MOG induced EAE in rats (Storch *et al.*, 1998) or primates (Genain *et al.*, 1999) and in guinea pigs after sensitization with whole CNS tissue or myelin (Lebar *et al.*, 1986, Linington and Lassmann, 1987, Figs. 43.3 and 43.6).

Although mice with chronic EAE may too develop a potential demyelinating antibody response, its role in the pathogenesis of the lesions is less evident. This is best exemplified in anti-MOG B-cell transgenic animals (Litzenburger *et al.*, 1998). These animals develop a massive antibody response against MOG, which recognizes a surface determinant of the molecule and is thus potentially pathogenic. In spite of this, these animals only show a moderate increase in demyelination in comparison to wild-type animals with the same T-cell-mediated EAE. The reason for this rather poor antibody-mediated demyelinating response may reside in the relative inefficacy of most mouse strains in the antibody-mediated activation of the complement system.

Tissue damage through antibodies may be accomplished by two different ways. Complement is activated by the immune complexes, leading to accumulation of the terminal lytic complement complex on the surface of the target cells. This will lead to disturbance of membrane homeostasis and lysis of the respective cells. Thus, blockade of the complement system is an effective way to prevent antibody-mediated demyelination in EAE (Piddlesden *et al.*, 1994). In addition, macrophages or microglia express Fc- and complement-receptors, which allow them to attach to antibody targeted myelin and initiate its destruction (Brosnan *et al.*, 1977).

### Tissue Injury through Activated Macrophages or Microglia Cells

Macrophages or activated microglia cells play a central role in EAE. The severity of clinical disease as well as the amount of tissue damage within the CNS correlates significantly with the extent of macrophage, but not of T-cell infiltration in the lesions (Berger *et al.*, 1997). In addition, deletion of macrophages or blockade of macrophage function ameliorate disease and tissue damage (Huitinga *et al.*, 1990). As shown by studies performed *in vitro* and *in vivo*, activated macrophages produce a variety of different toxic mediators, which are not only instrumental in the defense against foreign pathogens but can also destroy local tissue in the course of an inflammatory reaction.

#### *Proteases*

Therapeutic intervention in EAE with protease inhibitors ameliorates clinical disease and tissue damage in the CNS (Brosnan *et al.*, 1980). Based on these findings the role of

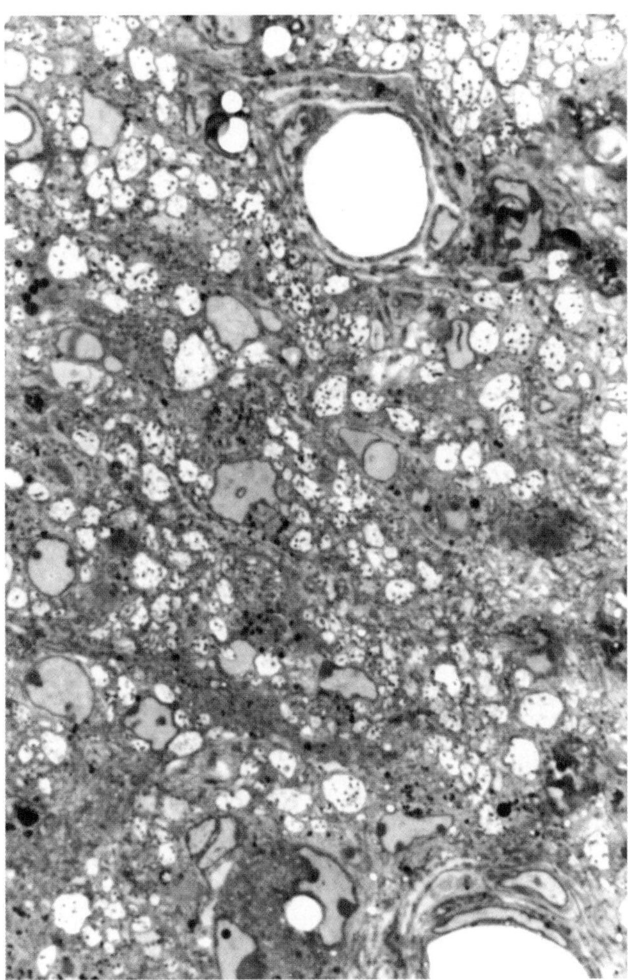

FIGURE 43.6
Primary demyelination in EAE, induced by a cooperation of encephalitogenic T cells and demyelinating antibodies in a guinea pig, sensitized with whole CNS tissue. Numerous demyelinated axons are embedded in a dense glial scar tissue. Toluidine blue stained plastic section; × 2000.

proteases in the pathogenesis of this disease and as possible targets for therapy has been extensively studied (reviewed in Cuzner and Opdenakker, 1999). Various different proteases are produced and expressed within the lesions, predominantly within activated inflammatory cells such as T cells, macrophages or, when present, granulocytes (Clements *et al.*, 1997; Teesalu *et al.*, 2001), as well as in astrocytes (Teesalu *et al.*, 2001), and can also be detected in the cerebrospinal fluid (Gijbels *et al.*, 1993). Their biological activity in the lesions was shown by in situ zymography (Teesalu *et al.*, 2001). They are in general secreted as inactive precursor and have to be cleaved to become biologically active (Cuzner and Opdenakker, 1999). Furthermore, their activity within the lesions is strictly controlled by specific inhibitors, such as tissue inhibitors of metalloproteases (TIMPs; Cuzner and Opdenakker, 1999), which are also expressed within the lesions, in particular in astrocytes (Teesalu *et al.*, 2001). Thus, their biological activity in the lesions depends on the balance between the active enzyme and its inhibitor.

Proteases are involved in several essentially different steps in the development of EAE lesions. First, they are required for the migration of inflammatory cells through the blood brain barrier. Second, they may cleave extracellularely liberated CNS proteins, such as for instance MBP, and thus increase the amount of peptides, which may be presented to T cells (Fabry *et al.*, 1994; Opdenakker and Van Damme, 1994). Both effects will potentiate the inflammatory reaction and a blockade of proteases will have an anti-inflammatory effect. Third, proteases liberated in the lesions may directly be involved in tissue destruction.

Direct intracerebral injection of proteases in concentrations, similar to those present in inflammatory lesions, induce myelin and axonal damage (Anthony *et al.*, 1998).

Protease inhibition may thus be a valuable target for anti-inflammatory therapy. This has been established in different EAE models *in vivo*, in which treatment with various protease inhibitors has a beneficial effect on clinical disease and tissue damage (Clements *et al.*, 1997; Gijbels *et al.*, 1994). Interestingly, some of the effects of β-interferon on brain inflammation may also be mediated through its inhibition of matrix metalloprotease activity (Leppert *et al.*, 1996).

### *Tumor Necrosis Factor-Alpha (TNF-α)*

TNF-α is a key cytokine, regulating inflammation and tissue damage in brain inflammation (for review, see Probert *et al.*, 2000). It is highly expressed in the lesions of EAE, in particular in the early stages of their evolution (Issazadeh *et al.*, 1995a). The cellular sources of TNF-α in inflammatory brain lesions are lymphocytes and macrophages as well as activated microglia (Frei *et al.*, 1987) and astrocytes (Liebermann *et al.*, 1989). TNF-α exerts serveral pro-inflammatory actions, such as the induction of adhesion molecules and chemokines (Butcher and Picker, 1996), and may induce macrophage activation. In addition, TNF-α and lymphotoxin-alpha (LT-α) may directly induce cell damage by the activation of the death domain of the TNF-receptor-1. This may occur in oligodendrocytes *in vitro* (D'Souza *et al.*, 1995; Selmaj and Raine, 1988) and may lead to primary demyelination (Selmaj and Raine, 1988).

Over-expression of TNF-α *in vivo* in transgenic animals leads to demyelination and apoptosis of oligodendrocytes (Akassoglou *et al.*, 1998) or when expressed only at low levels in the CNS may, although not being pathogenic by itself, aggravate demyelination in EAE (Taupin *et al.*, 1997). For these reasons, TNF-α has long been regarded as a prime candidate for therapeutic intervention in inflammatory demyelinating diseases. However, treatment of EAE animals with antibodies against TNF-α or TNF-R1 blocking agents revealed conflicting results (for review, see Probert *et al.*, 2000). While most studies showed a beneficial effect some studies revealed the opposite (Willenborg *et al.*, 1995). The situation may be in part explained by results obtained in transgenic models with a deletion of TNF/LT or the TNF-R1. When EAE is induced in these animals, demyelination and tissue destruction are reduced by 80% in comparison to that in wild-type controls. On the other hand, the degree of brain inflammation is significantly increased (Eugster *et al.*, 1999), and local destruction of T cells in the lesions by apoptosis is reduced (Bachmann *et al.*, 1999). Thus, as recently reviewed by Probert *et al.* (2000), signaling through the TNF-R1 pathway in EAE may have a dual function. It may thus be pro-inflammatory and may induce selective tissue damage, but simultaneously it may have an anti-inflammatory effect, possibly being involved in the control of T-cell autoimmunity. Importantly, these TNF-R1-mediated effects on EAE differ between animal strains (Kassiotis *et al.*, 1999; Körner *et al.*, 1997; Liu *et al.*, 1998), underlining the genetic influence on the mechanisms of inflammation and tissue damage in EAE.

### *Reactive Oxygen and Nitrogen Species*

Reactive oxygen and nitrogen species (ROS and RNI) are important toxic mediators produced mainly by activated leukocytes. They may play a major role in the pathogenesis of inflammatory demyelinating diseases, both in humans and experimental models (for review, see Smith *et al.*, 1999; Smith and Lassmann, 2002; Willenborg *et al.*, 1999). ROS may directly destroy target cells through direct membrane damage by lipid peroxidation and the induction of apoptosis. Oligodendrocytes and myelin are particularly vulnerable to their action, possible due to the elaborate cell processes built by these cells (Kim and Kim, 1991; Noble *et al.*, 1994). Thus, therapies that limit superoxide production show consistent beneficial effects in EAE (Smith *et al.*, 1999).

The situation with reactive nitrogen intermediates is more complex. They may either alone or in combination with ROS interfere with the pathogenesis of EAE lesions at a variety of different levels. Similar as ROS nitric oxide radicals induce oligodendrocyte death *in vitro*, these cells being much more sensitive compared to astrocytes and microglia

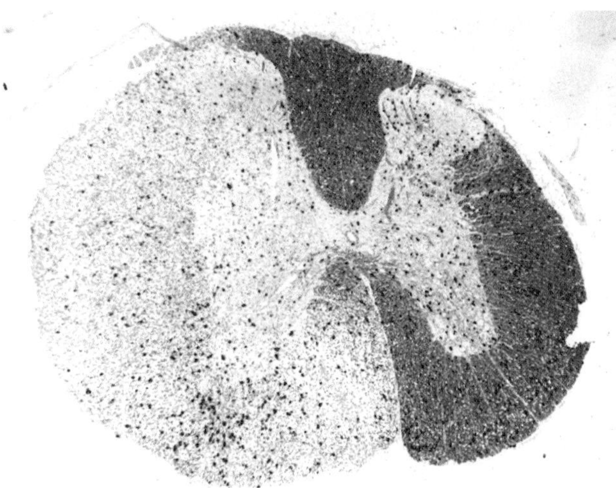

FIGURE 43.9
Oligodendrocytes in an actively demyelinating EAE lesions stained by in situ hybridization for PLP mRNA (black cells). In comparison to the normal white matter, the density of oligodendrocytes is reduced in the lesions. However, even during the process of active demyelination, there are oligodendrocytes present, which contain myelin protein mRNAs and in some areas they form clusters of high density. *In situ* hybridization for PLP mRNA (black) and immunocytochemistry for PLP protein (red); × 60.

may interfere with the development of the disease. Thus, an effect of the treatment on clinical disease or lesion volume in the CNS does not necessarily imply that this is due to remyelination.

There are only few instances where remyelination is impaired in EAE lesions. Obviously in very destructive EAE lesions, remyelination is limited by axonal loss. In addition, repeated demyelinating episodes within the same area of the CNS reduces the remyelinating capacity of the tissue. This is best exemplified in the model of repeated co-transfer EAE with encephalitogenic T cells and demyelinating anti-MOG antibodies. While after the first co-transfer remyelination occurs rapidly and completely, after each subsequent co-transfer of T cells and antibodies, the remyelinating capacity of the tissue declines (Linington *et al.*, 1992). Although not formally proven, these data suggest that the pool of progenitor cells that may accomplish remyelination is limited and gradually becomes used up in the course of repeated demyelinating episodes.

Another model that shows impaired remyelination is MOG-induced EAE in the Brown Norway (BN) rat. These rats differ from other rat strains in two ways. First, immunization with MOG in this strain results in a vigorous demyelinating antibody response, which is more severe compared to other rat strains (Stefferl *et al.*, 1999). Second, these animals express MOG at an earlier stage of myelination and remyelination in comparison to other rat strains. The consequence of these two factors is that MOG is expressed in remyelinating lesions already at a time when the blood brain barrier is still impaired and anti-MOG antibodies can reach the lesions in high concentration. These remyelinating oligodendrocytes are then rapidly destroyed by antibodies and complement (Storch *et al.*, unpublished).

Although these data give some insights as to how remyelination can be impaired in inflammatory demyelinating lesions, there must be additional other mechanisms that are responsible for the low degree of remyelination in chronic MS plaques, which so far are not reproduced in EAE.

## THE GOOD SIDE OF INFLAMMATION: PROTECTIVE AUTOIMMUNITY

For many years, inflammation has been considered to inevitably be harmful for the central nervous system. On the other hand, it was difficult to explain why nature permitted brain autoimmunity to occur with relative ease. In other words, liberation of antigen in the central nervous system can induce autoimmune reactions on the T-cell as well as antibody level. The reason for this apparent discrepancy may be found in recent immunological studies, which show that inflammatory cells can produce a variety of cytokines or growth factors that help to repair damaged tissue (Schwartz, 2001).

Cells of the immune system, including T cells, B cells, and macrophages, in particular when they are activated, can produce neurotrophic factors (Besser and Wank, 1999; Kerschensteiner *et al.*, 1999; Moalem *et al.*, 2000). These neurotrophic factors may exert their action not only on the nervous tissue, but also on the immune system. Within the nervous system, activated leukocytes within an inflammatory focus may be the major source of neurotrophins, being more important than resident neurons or glia cells, and leukocyte-derived neurotrophins are biologically active and can rescue neurons *in vitro* (Kerschensteiner *et al.*, 1999). In addition, neurotrophins may directly act on cells of the immune system, mainly having anti-inflammatory functions. As an example, nerve growth factor can modulate EAE by its direct action on macrophages through the p75 NT-receptor (Flügel *et al.*, 2001). It inhibits MHC-expression and impairs immigration of inflammatory cells into the brain, possibly by down-regulating adhesion molecule expression.

Recent studies suggest that inflammatory reactions in the brain may stimulate regeneration and repair of CNS lesions. In experimental models of brain or spinal cord trauma, clinical deficit is less pronounced in animals with mild T-cell-mediated autoimmune inflammation (Hamarberg *et al.*, 2000; Moalem *et al.*, 1999). This is associated with significantly less tissue damage and attempts of axonal regeneration and sprouting. The mechanisms behind these effects are apparently mediated by neurotrophins, produced by inflammatory cells in these conditions. Functional blockade of neurotrophins with sepcific antibodies abolishes the beneficial effect of inflammation.

Inflammation apparently has a major effect on remyelination in demyelinating lesions. Remyelination is stimulated by macrophages *in vitro* (Diemel *et al.*, 1998), and macrophage depletion blocks remyelination in a model of toxic demyelination (Kotter *et al.*, 2001). Interestingly, this effect may in part be due to the action of TNF-$\alpha$, which may promote the proliferation of oligodendrocyte progenitors as well as remyelination (Arnett *et al.*, 2001). Thus, the same cytokine may be cytotoxic in mature oligodendrocyte but stimulate the recruitment of new oligodendrocytes from progenitors.

Although the concept that inflammation may promote tissue repair is not new and has been recognized for long time as a mechanism of wound healing, its importance in inflammatory CNS diseases has only recently received attention. This has major consequences. In a disease like multiple sclerosis, remyelination is extensive in acute and in active lesions of chronic disease, but is sparse in chronic inactive demyelinated plaques. Active remyelination thus occurs on a background of profound inflammation. This is similar in EAE models, where remyelination is present and extensive in lesions that contain profound inflammatory infiltrates. In the light of these findings, it may turn out that complete blockade of inflammation in multiple sclerosis patients by extensive immunosuppression may be counterproductive. Thus, changing the quality of inflammation by immune modulation may be the better therapeutic strategy than complete immunosuppression.

## EAE IS AN ENVIRONMENTALLY INDUCED DISEASE WITH POLYGENIC BACKGROUND

Although T-cell or antibody-mediated autoimmune reactions have been described to occur following trauma or viral infections of the CNS, so far no spontaneous form of autoimmune encephalomyelitis has been described in any animal species. Active immunization with nervous system antigens is therefore essential for the induction of autoimmune encephalomyelitis. In addition, however, the incidence, severity and phenotypic manifestation of disease is highly influenced by the genetic background of the animal. The genetic regulation of EAE is very complex and its complete review would go beyond the scope of this chapter. Thus, only some principal aspects will be discussed (for more detailed review, see Olsson *et al.*, 2000, and Sundvall *et al.*, 1995).

The gene region with the most prominent effect on disease susceptibility in EAE is the MHC region (Encinas *et al.*, 1996; Olsson *et al.*, 2000). Within the MHC complex, class II genes have the strongest effect and MHC-controlled high disease susceptibility is associated with increased production of pro-inflammatory Th1 cytokines by encephalitogenic T cells. Thus, a major influence of the MHC region is due to its qualitative and quantitative control of T-cell antigen recognition (Weissert *et al.*, 1998). A detailed analysis of intra-MHC recombinant rat strains, however, revealed additional effects, mediated by genes in the class I and class III region (Weissert *et al.*, 1998). Whether these effects reflect a pathogenic contribution of class I MHC restricted T cells is so far undetermined, since the MHC complex contains numerous other genes, which are involved in the control of immune function.

Besides the control by the MHC, complex EAE is regulated by many other, non-MHC genes (Dahlmann *et al.*, 1999). Genome wide screening of EAE animals revealed more than 10 additional susceptibility loci with influence on disease incidence, chronicity, or severity. Interestingly, many of these gene regions are not specific for EAE, but are additionally associated with other autoimmune diseases, such as autoimmune neurits or uveitis, adjuvant or collagen-induced arthritis, or insulin-dependent diabetes melitus, and synthenic regions appeared in the genomic screen of multiple sclerosis patients (Olsson *et al.*, 2000). The individual genes and their possible function are so far undetermined but may be involved in general immune regulation, in the mechanisms of immune-mediated tissue damage, or may determine the susceptibility of the nervous tissue for inflammation-induced damage.

There are several possible examples for such effects. The major differences in the extent of antibody-mediated demyelination in MOG-EAE between different species and strains may be due to the genetically determined ability of antibodies to activate complement and by polymorphisms in the MOG gene itself (Stefferl *et al.*, 1999). In addition, the type and activation stage of effector cells within EAE lesions seems to be genetically controlled. While classical EAE in rats is associated with massive recruitment of haematogenous macrophages, in Wistar rats lesions are characterized by massive T-cell infiltration, microglia activation but nearly complete absence of macrophage recruitment (Storch *et al.*, 2002). Detailed genetic mapping revealed that this effect is associated with genes in the class II and the nonclassical class I region of the MHC complex. This difference in effector cells in the lesions has a major influence on the type of immune-mediated tissue damage. In spite of a similar extent of demyelination, axonal injury is much more severe in animals with macrophage-dominated lesions, compared to those where microglia prevail (Storch *et al.*, 2002).

Susceptibility of the target tissue may also be controlled by neurotrophic factors. As an example, the extent of oligodendrocyte damage and demyelination in EAE is much more severe in animals with a deficiency for ciliary neurotrophic factor compared to intact controls (Linker *et al.*, 2002).

## CONCLUSIONS

EAE research was started with the naïve approach to develop a simple model for multiple sclerosis that allows to unravel its pathogenesis and evaluate preclinically new therapeutic strategies. After nearly 70 years of EAE research, we have learned a lot about basic immunology, the mechanisms of autoimmunity, and the pathogenesis of brain inflammation. It, however, also became clear that EAE is a very complex disease with a broad spectrum of different immunological mechanisms, their pathogenic contribution being determined by the genetic background of the animal and the mode of disease induction. Thus, there is no single EAE. Instead there are multiple different models, each of which allows us to study only certain specific aspects of brain inflammation or inflammation-induced tissue damage. This is extremely useful for elucidating basic pathogenetic mechanisms involved in inflammatory brain diseases and can also be utilized to test the principal feasibility of therapeutic approaches. However, since human inflammatory brain diseases and in particular multiple sclerosis are similarly complex, its use for screening of new MS therapies deserves a critical and cautious approach.

## References

Akassoglou, K., Bauer, J., Kassiotis, G., Pasparakis, M., Lassmann, H., Kollias, G., and Probert, L. (1998). Oligodendrocyte apoptosis and primary demyelination induced by local TNF/p55TNF receptor signaling in the central nervous system of transgenic mice: Models for multiple sclerosis with primary oligodendrogliopathy. *Amer. J. Pathol.* **153,** 801–813.

Albina, J. E., Henry, W. L Jr. (1991). Suppression of lymphocyte proliferation through the nitric oxide synthesizing pathway. *J Surg Res.* **50,** 403–409.

Alvord, E. C. Jr. (1970). Acute disseminated encephalomyelitis and "allergic" encephalopathies. *In* "Handbook of Clinical Neurology" (P. I. Vinken and G. W. Bruyn, eds.), Vol. 9, pp. 500–571. Elsevier, New York.

Alvord, E. C. Jr. (1984). Species restricted encephalitogenic determinants. *In* "Experomental Allergic Encephalomyelitis: A Useful Model for Multiple Sclerosis" (E. C. Alvord, M. W. Kies, A. J. Suckling, eds.), pp. 523–537, Alan R. Liss, New York.

Anthony, D. C., Miller, K. M., Fearn, S., Townsend, M. J., Opdenakker, G., Wells, G. M., Clements, J. M., Chandler, S., Gearing, A. J., and Perry, V. H. (1998). Matrix metalloproteinase expression in an experimentally-induced DTH model of multiple sclerosis in the rat CNS. *J Neuroimmunol.* **87,** 62–72.

Arnett, H. A., Mason, J., Marino, M., Suzuki, K., Matsushima, G. K., and Ting, J. P. (2001). TNF alpha promotes proliferation of oligodendrocyte progenitors and remyelination. *Nat Neurosci.* **4,** 1116–1122.

Bachmann, R., Eugster, H. P., Frei, K., Fontana, A., and Lassmann, H. (1999). Impaiment of TNF-receptor 1 signalling but not Fas-signalling diminishes T-cell apoptosis in MOG-peptide induced chronic demyelinating autoimmune encephalomyelitis in mice. *Amer J Pathol* **154,** 1417–1422.

Bauer, J., Bradl, M., Hickey, W. F., Forss-Petter, S., Breitschopf, H., Linington, C., Wekerle, H., and Lassmann, H. (1998). T cell apoptosis in inflammatory brain lesions. Destruction of T cells does not depend on antigen recognition. *Am J Pathol* **153,** 715–724.

Bechmann, I.; Lossau, S., Steiner, B., Mor, G., Gimsa, U., and Nitsch, R. (2000). Reactive astrocytes upregulate Fas (CD95) and Fas ligand (CD95L) expression but do not undergo programmed cell death during the course of anterograde degeneration. *Glia.* **32,** 25–41.

Ben Nun, A., Wekele H., and Cohen, I. R. (1981). The rapis isolation of clonable antigen-specific T lymphocyte lines capable of mediating autoimmune encephalomyelitis. *Eur. J. Immunol.* **11,** 195–199.

Berger, T., Weerth, S., Kojima, K., Linington, C., Wekerle, H., and Lassmann, H. (1997). Experimental autoimmune encephalomyelitis: The antigen specificity of T-lymphocytes determines the topography of lesions in the central and peripheral nervous system. *Lab Invest* **76,** 355–364.

Besser, M., and Wank, R. (1999). Cutting edge: Clonally restricted production of the neurotrophins brain-derived neurotrophic factor and neurotrophin-3 mRNA by human immune cells and Th1/Th2-polarized expression of their receptors. *J Immunol.* **162,** 6303–6306.

Bhardwaj, V., Kumar, V., Geysen, H. M., and Sercarz, E. E. (1993). Degenerate recognition of a dissimilar antigenic peptide by myelin basic protein-reactive T cells. Implications for thymic education and autoimmunity. J *Immunol.* **151,** 5000–5010.

Bielefeldt, K., Whiteis, C. A., Chapleau, M. W., and Abboud, F. M. (1999). Nitric oxide enhances slow inactivation of voltage-dependent sodium currents in rat nodose neurons. *Neurosci Lett.* **271,** 159–162.

Blakemore, W. F., and Keirstead, H. S. (1999). The origin of remyelinating cells in the central nervous system. *J Neuroimmunol.* **98,** 69–76.

Bolanos, J. P., Almeida, A., Stewart, V., Peuchen, S., Land, J. M., Clark, J. B., and Heales, S. J. (1997). Nitric oxide-mediated mitochondrial damage in the brain: Mechanisms and implications for neurodegenerative diseases. *J Neurochem.* **68,** 2227–2240.

Bornstein, M. B., and Appel S. H. (1961). The application of tissue culture to the study of experimental "allergic" encephalomyelitis. I. Patterns of demyelination. *J. Neuropathol. Exp. Neurol.* **20,** 141–147.

Brosnan, C. F., Cammer, W., Norton, W. T., and Bloom, B. R. (1980). Proteinase inhibitors suppress the development of experimental allergic encephalomyelitis. *Nature.* **285,** 235–237.

Brosnan, C. F., Stoner, G. L., Bloom, B. R., and Wisniewski, H. M. (1977). Studies on demyelination by activated lymphocytes in the rabbit eye. II. Antibody dependent cell mediated demyelination. *J. Immunol.* **118,** 2103–2111.

Butcher, E. C., and Picker, L. J. (1996). Lymphocyte homing and homeostasis. *Science* **272,** 60–66.

Cannella, B., Hoban, C. J., Gao, Y. L., Garcia-Arenas, R., Lawson, D., Marchionni, M., Gwynne, D., and Raine, C. S. (1998). The neuregulin, glial growth factor 2, diminishes autoimmune demyelination and enhances remyelination in a chronic relapsing model for multiple sclerosis. *Proc Natl Acad Sci US* **95,** 10100–10105.

Chase, W. M. A. (1959). A critique of attempts at passive transfer of sensitivity to nervous tissue. *In* "Allergic Encephalomyelitis" (M. vW. Kies and E. vC. Alvord, eds.), pp. 348–374. Thomas, Springfield, IL.

Clements, J. M., Cossins, J. A., Wells, G. M., Corkill, D. J., Helfrich, K., Wood, L. M., Pigott, R., Stabler, G., Ward, G. A., Gearing, A. J., and Miller, K. M. (1997). Matrix metalloproteinase expression during experimental autoimmune encephalomyelitis and effects of a combined matrix metalloproteinase and tumour necrosis factor-alpha inhibitor. *J Neuroimmunol.* **74,** 85–94.

Cornet, A., Savidge, T. C., Cabarrocas, J., Dend, W. L., Colombel, J. F., Lassmann, H., Desreumaux, P., and Liblau, R. S. (2001). Enterocolitis induced by autoimmune targeting of enteric glia cells: A possible mechanism in Crohn's disease? *Proc Natl Acad Sci* (USA) **98,** 13306–13311.

Cuzner, M. L., and Opdenakker, G. (1999). Plasminogen activators and matrix metalloproteinases, mediators of extracellular proteolysis in inflammatory demyelination of the central nervous system. *J. Neuroimmunol.* **94,** 1–14.

Dahlmann, I., Wallstrom E., Weissert, R., Storch, M., Kornek, B., Jacobsson, L., Linington, C., Luthman, H., Lassmann, H., and Olsson, T. (1999). Linkage analysis of myelin oligodendrocyte glycoprotein-induced experimental autoimmune encephalomyelitis in the rat identifies a locus controlling demyelination on chromosome 18. *Hum Mol Genet* **8,** 2183–2190.

DiBello, I. C., Dawson, M. R., Levine, J. M., and Reynolds, R. (1999). Generation of oligodendroglial progenitors in acute inflammatory demyelinating lesions of the rat brain stem is associated with demyelination rather than inflammation. *J. Neurocytol.* **28,** 365–381.

Diemel, L. T., Copelman, C. A., and Cuzner, M. L. (1998). Macrophages in CNS remyelination: Friend or foe? *Neurochem-Res.* **23,** 341–347.

D'Souza, S., Alinauskas, K., McCrea, E., Goodyer, C., and Antel, J. P. (1995). Differential susceptibility of human CNS-derived cell populations to TNF-dependent and independent immune-mediated injury. *J Neurosci.* **15,** 7293–7300.

Dubois-Dalcq, M., Niedieck, B., and Buyse, M. (1970)/ Action of anti-cerebroside sera on myelinated nervous tissue cultures. *Pathologica Europea* **5,** 331–347.

Encinas, J. A., Weiner, H. L., and Kuchroo, V. K. (1996). Inheritance of susceptibility to experimental autoimmune encephalomyelitis. *J Neurosci Res.* **45,** 655–669.

Engelhardt, B., Conley, F. K., and Butcher, E. C. (1994). Cell adhesion molecules on vessels during inflammation in the mouse central nervous system. *J Neuroimmunol.* **51,** 199–208.

Eugster, H. P., Frei, K., Bachmann, R., Bluethmann, H., Lassmann, H., and Fontana, A. (1999). Severity of symptoms and demyelination in MOG-induced EAE depends on TNFR1. *Eur. J. Immunol.* **29,** 626–632.

Evans, C. F., Horwitz, M. S., Hobbs, M. V., and Oldstone, M. B. (1996). Viral infection of transgenic mice expressing a viral protein in oligodendrocytes leads to chronic central nervous system autoimmune disease. *J Exp Med.* **184,** 2371–2384.

Fabry, Z., Raine, C. S., and Hart, M. N. (1994). Nervous tissue as an immune compartment: The dialect of the immune response in the CNS. *Immunol Today.* **15,** 218–224.

Fife, B. T., Huffnagle, G. B., Kuziel, W. A., and Karpus, W. J. (2000). CC chemokine receptor 2 is critical for induction of experiemntal autoimmune encephalomyelitis. *J. Exp. Med.* **192,** 899–905.

Fife, B. T., Paniagua, M. C., Lukcs, N. W., Kunkel, S. L., and Karpus, W. J. (2001). Selective CC chemokine receptor expression by central nervous system-infiltrating encephalitogenic T cells during experimental autoimmune encephalomyelitis. *J. Neurosci. Res.* **66,** 705–714.

Fischer, H. G., and Reichmann, G. (2001). Brain dendritic cells and macrophages/microglia in central nervous system inflammation. *J Immunol* **166,** 2717–2726.

Flugel, A., Berkowicz, T., Ritter, T., Labeur, M., Jenne, D. E., Li, Z., Ellwart, J. W., Willem, M., Lassmann, H., and Wekerle, H (2001). Migratory activity and functional changes of green fluorescent effector cells before and during experiemntal autoimmune encephalomyelitis. *Immunity* **14,** 547–560.

Flugel, A., Matsumoro, K., Neumann, H., Klinkert, W. E., Birnbacher, R., Lassmann, H., Otten, U., and Wekerle, H (2001). Anti inflammatory activity of nerve growth factor in experimental autoimmune encephalomyelitis: Inhibition of monocyte transendeothelial migration. *Eur J Immunol* **13,** 11–22.

Frei, K., Siepl, C., Groscurth, P., Bodmer, S., Schwerdel, C., and Fontana, A. (1987). Antigen presentation and tumor cytotoxicity by interferon-gamma-treated microglial cells. *Eur J Immunol.* **17,** 1271–1278.

Freund, J., Lipton, M. M., and Morrison, L. R. (1950). Demyelination in the guinea pig chronic allergic encephalomyelitis produced by injecting guinea pig brain in oil emulsion containing a variant of mycobacterium butyricum. *Arch. Pathol.* **50,** 108–121.

Genain, C. P., Abel, K., Belmar, N., Villinger, F., Rosenberg, D. P., Linington, C., Raine, C. S., and Hauser, S. L. (1996). Late complications of immune deviation therapy in a non-human primate. Science **274,** 2054–2057.

Genain, C. P., Cannella, B., Hauser, S. L., and Raine, C. S. (1999). Autoantibodies to MOG mediate myelin damage in MS. *Nat. Med.* **5,** 170–175.

Gijbels, K., Galardy, R. E., and Steinman, L. (1994). Reversal of experimental autoimmune encephalomyelitis with a hydroxamate inhibitor of matrix metalloproteases. *J Clin Invest.* **94,** 2177–2182.

Gijbels, K., Proost, P., Masure, S., Carton, H., Billiau, A., and Opdenakker, G. (1993). Gelatinase B is present in the cerebrospinal fluid during experimental autoimmune encephalomyelitis and cleaves myelin basic protein. *J Neurosci Res.* **36,** 432–440.

Godiska, R., Chantry, D., Dietsch, G. N., and Gray, P. W. (1995) Chemokine expression in murine experimental allergic encephalomyelitis. *J. Neuroimmunol.* **58,** 167–176.

Gold, R., Hartung, H. P., and Lassmann, H. (1997). T-cell apoptosis in autoimmune diseases: Termination of inflammation in the nervous system and other sites with specialized immune-defense mechanisms. *Trends Neurosci* **20,** 399–404.

Grakoui, A., Bromley, S. K., Sumen, C., Davis, M. M., Shaw, A. S., Allen, P. M., and Dustin, M. L. (1999). The immunological synapse: A molecular machine controlling T cell activation. *Science* **285,** 221–227.

Haase, C. G., Guggenmos, -J., Brehm, U., Andersson, M., Olsson, T., Reindl, M., Schneidewind, J. M., Zettl, U. K., Heidenreich, F., Berger, T., Wekerle, H., Hohlfeld, R., and Linington, C. (2001). The fine specificity of the myelin oligodendrocyte glycoprotein autoantibody response in patients with multiple sclerosis and normal healthy controls. *J Neuroimmunol.* **114,** 220–225.

Hammarberg, H., Lidman, O., Lundberg, C., Eltayeb, S. Y., Gielen, A. W., Muhallab, S., Svenningsson, A., Linda, H., van-Der-Meide, P. H., Cullheim, S., Olsson, T., and Piehl, F. (2000). Neuroprotection by encephalomyelitis: Rescue of mechanically injured neurons and neurotrophin production by CNS-infiltrating T and natural killer cells. *J Neurosci.* **20,** 5283–5291.

Hickey, W. F., Hsu, B. L., and Kimura, H. (1991). T lymphocyte entry into the central nervous system. *J Neurosci Res* **28,** 254–260.

Hickey, W. F., and Kimura, H. (1988). Perivascular microglia cells of the CNS are bone marrow derived and present antigen in vivo. *Science* **239,** 290–293.

Hickey, W. F., Osborn, J. F., and Kirby, W. W. (1985) Expression of Ia molecules by astrocytes during acute experiemntal allergic encephalomyelitis. *Cell. Immunol.* **91,** 528–535.

Hickey, W. F., Vass, K., and Lassmann, H. (1992). Bone marrow derived elements in the central nervous system: An immunohistochemical and ultrastructural survey of rat chimeras. *J Neuropath Exp Neurol* **51,** 246–256.

Hohlfeld, R. (1997). Biotechnological agents for the immunotherapy of multiple sclerosis. Principles, problems and persectives, *Brain* **120,** 865–916.

Huang, D., Han, Y., Rani, M. R., Glabinski, A., Trebst, C., Sorensen, T., Tani, M., Wang, J., Chien, P., O'Bryan, S., Bielecki, B., Zhou, Z. L., Majumder, S., and Ransohoff, R. M. (2000). Chemokines and chemokine receptors in inflammation of the nervous system: Manifold roles and exquisite regulation. *Immunol Rev.* **177,** 52–67.

Huitinga, I., Damoiseaux, J. G., Dopp, E. A., and Dijkstra, C. D. (1993). Treatment with anti-CR3 antibodies ED7 and ED8 suppresses experimental allergic encephalomyelitis in Lewis rats. *Eur J Immunol.* **23,** 709–715.

Huitinga. I., Rooijen, N., deGroot, C. J. A., Uitdehaag, B. M. J., and Dijkstra, C. D. (1990). Suppression of experiemntal allergic encephalomyelitis after elimination of macrophages. *J. Exp. Med.***172,** 1025–1033.

Huseby, E. S., Liggitt, D., Brabb, T., Schnabel, B., Ohlen, C., and Goverman, J. (2001). A pathogenic role for myelin-specific CD8 (+) T cells in a model for multiple sclerosis. *J Exp Med* **194,** 669–676.

Issazadeh, S., Ljungdahl, A., Höjeberg, B., Mustafa, M., and Olsson, T. (1995a). Cytokine production in the central nervous system of Lewis rats with experimental autoimmune encephalomyelitis: Dynamics of mRNA expression for interleukin 10, interleukin 12, cytolysin, tumor necrosis factor a and tumor necrosis factor ß. *J Neuroimmunol.* **61,** 205–212.

Issazadeh, S., Mustafa, M., Ljungdahl, A., Hojeberg, B., Dagerlind, A., Elde, R., and Olsson, T. (1995b). Interferon gamma, interleukin 4 and transforming growth factor beta in experimental autoimmune encephalomyelitis in Lewis rats: Dynamics of cellular mRNA expression in the central nervous system and lymphoid cells. *J Neurosci Res.* 1995 **40,** 579–590.

Izikson, L., Klein, R. S., Charo, I. F., Weiner, H. L., and luster, A. D. (2000). Resistance to experimental autoimmune encephalomyelitis in mice lacking the CC chemokine receptor (CCR) 2. *J. Exp. Med.* **192,** 1075–1080..

Jankovic, B., Draskoci, M., and Janjic, M. (1965). Passive transfer of "allergic" encephalomyelitis with anti-brain serum, injected into the lateral ventricle of the brain. *Nature* **207,** 428–429.

Jee, Y., Yoon, W. K., Okura, Y., Tanuma, N., and Matsumoto, Y. (2002). Upregulation of monocyte chemotactic protein-1 and CC chemokine receptor 2 in the central nervous system is closely associated with relapse of autoimmune encephalomyelitis in Lewis rats. *J. Neuroimmunol.* **128,** 49–57.

Jiang, H., Zhang, S. L., and Pernis, B. (1992). Role of $CD8^+$ T cells in murine experimental allergic encephalomyelitis. *Science* **256,** 1213–1215.

Kapoor, R., Davies, M., and Smith, K. J. (1999). Temporary axonal conduction block and axonal loss in inflammatory neurological disease. A potential role for nitric oxide? *Ann N Y Acad Sci.* **893,** 304–308.

Kassiotis, G., Pasparakis, M., Kollias, G., and Probert, L. (1999). TNF accelerates the onset but does not alter the incidence and severity of myelin basic protein-induced experimental autoimmune encephalomyelitis. *Eur J Immunol.* **29,** 774–780.

Kennedy, K. J., Strieter, R. M., Kunkel, S. L., Lucas, N. W., and Karpus, W. J. (1998). Acute and relapsing experimental autoimmune encephalomyelitis are regulated by differential expression of the CC chemokines macrophage inflammatory protein-1alpha and monocyte chemotactic protein-1. *J. Neuroimmunol.* **92,** 98–108.

Kerschensteiner, M., Gallmeier, E., Behrens, L., Leal, V. V., Misgeld, T., Klinkert, W. E., Kolbeck, R., Hoppe, E., Oropeza-Wekerle, R. L., Bartke, I., Stadelmann, C., Lassmann, H., Wekerle, H., and Hohlfeld, R. (1999). Activated human T cells, B cells, and monocytes produce brain-derived neurotrophic factor in vitro and in inflammatory brain lesions: A neuroprotective role of inflammation? *J Exp Med.* **189,** 865–870.

Kies, M. W., Murphy, J. B., and Alvord, E. C. (1960). Fractionation of guinea pig brain proteins with encephalitogenic activity. *Fed. Proc.* **19,** 207.

Kim, Y. S., and Kim, S. U. (1991). Oligodendroglial cell death induced by oxygen radicals and its protection by catalase. *J Neurosci Res.* **29,** 100–106.

Koh, D. R., Fung-Leung, W. P., Ho, A., Gray, D., Acha-Orbea, H., and Mak, T. W. (1992). Less mortality but more relapses in experimental allergic encephalomyelitis in CD8 −/− mice. *Science* **256,** 1210–1213.

Kojima, K., Berger, Th., Lassmann, H., Hinze-Selch, D., Zhang, Y., Germann, J., Reske, K., Wekerle, H., and Linington, C. (1994). Experimental autoimmune panencephalitis and uveoretinitis transfered to the Lewis rat by T-lymphocytes specific for the S100ß molecule, a calcium binding protein of astroglia. *J Exp Med* **180,** 817–829.

Korner, H., Lemckert, F. A., Chaudhri, G., Etteldorf, S., and Sedgwick, J. D. (1997). Tumor necrosis factor blockade in actively induced experimental autoimmune encephalomyelitis prevents clinical disease despite activated T cell infiltration to the central nervous system. *Eur J Immunol.* **27,** 1973–1981.

Kotter, M. R., Setzu, A., Sim, F. J., Van-Rooijen, N., and Franklin, R. J. (2001). Macrophage depletion impairs oligodendrocyte remyelination following lysolecithin-induced demyelination. *Glia.* **35,** 204–212.

Kubes, P., Suzuki, M., and Granger, D. N. (1991). Nitric oxide: An endogenous modulator of leukocyte adhesion. *Proc Natl Acad Sci USA.* **88,** 4651–4655.

Lafaille, J. (1998). The role of Helper T cell subsets in autoimmune disease. *Cytokine & Growth Factor Reviews* **9,** 139–151.

Lafaille, J. J., Keere, F. V., Hsu, A. L., Baron, J. L., Haas, W., Raine, C. S., and Tonegawa, S. (1997). Myelin basic protein-specific T helper 2 (Th2) cells cause experimental autoimmune encephalomyelitis in immunodeficient hosts rather than protect them from disease. *J. Exp. Med.* **186,** 307–312.

Lassmann, H. (1983). "Comparative Neuropathology of Chronic Experimental Allergic Encephalomyelitis and Multiple Sclerosis." Springer, Berlin, Heidelberg, New York.

Lassmann, H., Brunner, C., Bradl, M., and Linington, C. (1988). Experimental allergic encephalomyelitis: The balance between encephalitogenic T-lymphocytes and demyelinating antibodies determines size ans structure of demyelinated lesions. *Acta Neuropathol.* **75,** 566–576.

Lassmann, H., Kitz, K., and Wisniewski, H. M. (1981). In vivo effect of sera from animals with chronic relapsing experimental allergic encephalomyelitis on central and peripheral myelin. *Acta. Neuropathol.* **55,** 297–306.

Lebar, R., Lubetzki, C., Vincent, C., Lombrail, P., and Poutry, J. M. (1986). The MS autoantigen of central nervous system myelin, a glycoprotein present in oligodendrocyte membranes. *Experimental Immunol.* **66,** 423–443.

Lee, S. J., and Benveniste, E. N. (1999). Adhesion molecule expression and regulation on cells of the central nervous system. *J. Neuroimmunol.* **98,** 77–88.

Leppert, D., Waubant, E., Burk, M. R., Oksenberg, J. R., and Hauser, S L. (1996). Interferon beta-1b inhibits gelatinase secretion and in vitro migration of human T cells: A possible mechanism for treatment efficacy in multiple sclerosis. *Ann Neurol.* **40,** 846–852.

Lieberman, A. P., Pitha, P. M., Shin, H. S., Shin, M. L. (1989). Production of tumor necrosis factor and other cytokines by astrocytes stimulated with lipopolysaccharide or a neurotropic virus. *Proc Natl Acad Sci USA* **86,** 6348–6352.

Linington, C., Berger, Th., Perry, L., Weerth, S., Hinze-Selch, D., Zhang, Y., Lu, H., Lassmann, H., and Wekerle, H. (1993). T cells specific for the myelin oligodendroglia glycoprotein mediate an unusual autoimmune inflammatory response in the central nervous system. *Eur J Immunol* **23,** 1364–1372.

Linington, C., Bradl, M., Lassmann, H., Brunner, C., and Vass, K. (1988). Augmentation of demyelination in rat acute allergic encephalomyelitis by circulating antibodies against a myelin oligodendrocyte glycoprotein. *Amer. J. Pathol.* **130,**443–454.

Linington, C., Engelhardt, B., Kapocs, G., and Lassmann, H. (1992). Induction of persistently demyelinated lesions in the rat following the repeated adoptive transfer of encephalitogenic T cells and demyelinating antibody. *J Neuroimmunol.* **40,** 219–224.

Linington, C., and Lassmann, H. (1987). Antibody responses in chronic relapsing experimental allergic encephalomyelitis: Correlation of serum demyelinating activity with the antibody titre to the myelin/oligodendrocyte glycoprotein (MOG). *J Neuroimmunol* **17,** 61–69.

Linker, R. A., Maurer, M., Gaupp, S., Martini, R., Holtmann, B., Giess, R., Rieckmann, P., Lassmann, H., Toyka, K. V., Sendtner, M., and Gold, R. (2002). CNTF is a major protective factor in demyelinating CNS disease: A neurotrophic cytokine as modulator in neuroinflammation. *Nat Med.* **8,** 620–624.

Lipton, S. A. (1998). Neuronal injury associated with HIV-1: Approaches and treatment. *Annu Rev Pharmacol Toxicol* **38,** 159–177.

Litzenburger, T., Fässler, R., Bauer, J., Lassmann, H., Linington, C., Wekerle, H., and Iglesias, A. (1998). B lymphocytes producing demyelinating antibodies: Development and function in gene-trageted transgenic mice. *J Exp Med* **188,** 169–180.

Liu, J., Marino, M. W., Wong, G., Grail, D., Dunn, A., Bettadapura, J., Slavin, A. J., Old, L., and Bernard, C. C. (1998). TNF is a potent anti-inflammatory cytokine in autoimmune-mediated demyelination. *Nat Med.* **4,** 78–83.

Luster, A. D. (1998). Chemokines–chemotactic cytokines that mediate inflammation. *N. Engl. J. Med.* **338,** 436–445.

Maatta, J. A., Kaldman, M. D., Sakoda, S., Salmi, A. A., and Hinkkanen, A. E. (1998). Encephalitogenicity of myelin associated oligodendrocytic basic protein and 2′,3′-cyclic nucleotide 3′-phosphodieserase for BALB/c and SJL mice. *Immunology* **95,** 383–388.

Maeda, H., Okamoto, T., and Akaike, T. (1998). Human matrix metalloprotease activation by insults of bacterial infection involving proteases and free radicals. *Biol Chem.* **379,** 193–200.

Matsui, M., Weaver, J., Proudfoot, A. E. I., Wujek, J. R., Wei, T., Richter, E., Trapp, B. D., Rao, A., and Ransohoff, R. M. (2002). Treatment of experiemntal autoimmune encephalomyelitis with the chemokine receptor antagonist Met-RANTES. *J. Neuroimmunol.* **128,** 16–22.

Matsumoto, Y., and Fujiwara, M. (1986). In situ detection of class I and II major histocompatibility complex antigens in the rat central nervous system during experimental allergic encephalomyelitis. An immunohistochemical study. *J Neuroimmunol.* **12,** 265–277.

McMorris, F. A., and McKinnon, R. D. (1996). Regulation of oligodendrocyte development and CNS myelination by growth factors: Prospects for therapy of demyelinating disease. *Brain Pathol.* **6,** 313–329.

McRae, B. L., Vanderlugt, C. L., Dal-Canto, M. C., and Miller, S. D. (1995). Functional evidence for epitope spreading in the relapsing pathology of experimental autoimmune encephalomyelitis. *J Exp Med.* **182,** 75–85.

Merrill, J. E., Ignarro, L. J., Sherman, M. P., Melinek, J., and Lane, T. E. (1993). Microglial cell cytotoxicity of oligodendrocytes is mediated through nitric oxide. *J Immunol.* **151,** 2132–2141.

Miller, S. D., and Eagar, T. N. (2001). Functional role of epitope spreading in the chronic pathogenesis of autoimmune and virus-induced demyelinating diseases. *Adv Exp Med Biol.* **490,** 99–107.

Miller, S. D., Vanderlugt, C. L., Lenschow, D. J., Pope, J. G., Karandikar, N. J., Dal-Canto, M. C., and Bluestone, J. A. (1995). Blockade of CD28/B7–1 interaction prevents epitope spreading and clinical relapses of murine EAE. *Immunity.* **3,** 739–745.

Moalem, G., Gdalyahu, A., Shani, Y., Otten, U., Lazarovici, P., Cohen, I. R., and Schwartz, M. (2000). Production of neurotrophins by activated T cells: Implications for neuroprotective autoimmunity. *J Autoimmun.* **15,** 331–345.

Moalem, G., Leibowitz-Amit, R., Yoles, E., Mor, F., Cohen, I. R., and Schwartz, M. (1999). Autoimmune T cells protect neurons from secondary degeneration after central nervous system axotomy. *Nat Med.* **5,** 49–55.

Mokhtarian, F., McFarlin, D. E., and Raine, C. S. (1984). Adoptive transfer of myelin basic protein-sensitized T cells produce chronic relapsing demyelinating disease in mice. *Nature* **309,** 356–358.

Mokhtarian, F., Zhang, Z., Shi, Y., Gonzales, E., and Sobel, R. A. (1999). Molecular mimicry between a viral peptide and a myelin oligodendrocyte glycoprotein peptide induces autoimmune demyelinating disease in mice. *J Neuroimmunol.* **95,** 43–54.

Moody, D. B., and Besra, G. S. (2001). Glycolipid targets of CD1-mediated T-cell responses. *Immunology* **104,** 243–251.

Moody, D. B., Besra, G. S., Wilson, I. A., and Porcelli, S. A. (1999). The molecular basis of CD1-mediated presentation of lipid antigens. *Immunol. Reviews* **172,** 285–296.

Morris-Downes, M. M., McCormack, K., Baker, D., Sivaprasad, D., Natkunarajah, J., and Amor, S. (2002). Encephalitogenic and immunogenic potential of myelin associated glycoprotein (MAG), oligodendrocyte-specific glycoprotein (OSP) and 2′,3′-cyclic nucleotide 3′-phosphodiesterase (CNPase) in ABH and SJL mice. *J Neuroimmunol.* **122,** 20–33.

Neumann, H., Boucraut, J., Hahnel, C., Misgeld, T., and Wekerle,-H. (1996). Neuronal control of MHC class II inducibility in rat astrocytes and microglia. *Eur J Neurosci.* **8,** 2582–2590.

Neumann, H., Medana, I. M., Bauer, J., and Lassmann, H. (2002). Cytotoxic T lymphocytes in autoimmune and degenerative CNS disease. *Trends Neurosci.* **25,** 313–319.

Neumann, H., Misgeld, T., Matsumuro, K., and Wekerle, H. (1998). Neurotrophins inhibit major histocompatibility class II inducibility of microglia: Involvement of the p75 neurotrophin receptor. *Proc Natl Acad Sci US* **95,** 5779–5784.

Neumann, H., Schmidt, H., Cavalie, A., Jenne, D., and Wekerle, H. (1997). Major histocompatibility complex (MHC) class I gene expression in single neurons of the central nervous system: Differential regulation by interferon (IFN)-gamma and tumor necrosis factor (TNF)-alpha. *J Exp Med.* **185,** 305–316.

Niehaus, A., Shi, J., Grzenkowski, M., Diers-Fenger, M., Hartung, H. P,. Toyka, K., Bruck, W., and Trotter, J (2000). Patients with active relapsing-remitting multiple sclerosis synthesize antibodies recognizing oligodendrocyte progenitor cell surface protein: Implications for remyelination. *Ann Neurol.* **48,** 362–371.

Noble, P. G., Antel, J. P., and Yong, V. W. (1994). Astrocytes and catalase prevent the toxicity of catecholamines to oligodendrocytes. *Brain Res.* **633,** 83–90.

Numao, T., and Agrawal, D. K. (1992). Neuropeptides modulate human eosinophil chemotaxis. *J. Immunol.* **149,** 3309–3315.

Okuda, Y., Sakoda, S., Fujimura, H., and Yanagihara, T. (1997). Nitric oxide via an inducible isoform of nitric oxide synthase is a possible factor to eliminate inflammatory cells from the central nervous system of mice with experimental allergic encephalomyelitis. *J Neuroimmunol.* **73,** 107–116.

Oldstone, M. B., and Southern, P. J. (1993). Trafficking of activated cytotoxic T lymphocytes into the central nervous system: Use of a transgenic model. *J Neuroimmunol.* **46,** 25–31.

Olsson, T., Dahlman, I., Wallstrom, E., Weissert, R., and Piehl, F. (2000). Genetics of rat neuroinflammation. *J. Neuroimmunol.* **107,** 191–200.

Opdenakker, G., Van-Damme, J. (1994). Cytokine-regulated proteases in autoimmune diseases. *Immunol Today.* **15** 103–107.

Owens, T., Wekerle, H., and Antel, J. (2001) Genetic models for CNS inflammation. *Nature Med.* **7,** 161–166.

Paterson, P. Y. (1960). Transfer of allergic encephalomyelitis in rats by means of lymph node cells. *J. Exp. Med.* **111,** 119–135.

Pender, M. P., Nguyen, K. B., McCombe, P. A., and Kerr, J. F. (1991). Apoptosis in the nervous system in experimental allergic encephalomyelitis. *J Neurol Sci.* **104,** 81–87.

Pender, M. P and Rist, M. J. (2001). Apoptosis of inflammatory cells in immune control of the nervous system: Role of glia. *Glia.* **36,** 137–144.

Piddlesden, S. J., Storch, M., Hibbs, M., Freeman, A. M., Lassmann, H., and Morgan, B. P. (1994). Soluble recombinant complement receptor 1 inhibits inflammation and demyelination in antibody-mediated demyelinating experimental allergic encephalomyelitis. *J Immunol* **152,** 5477–5484.

Pitt, D., Werner, P., Raine, C. S. (2000). Glutamate excitotoxicity in a model of multiple sclerosis. *Nature Med* **6,** 67–70.

Prineas, J. W., and McDonald, I. W. (1997). Demyelinating diseases. *In* "Greenfield's Neuropathology" (D. I. Graham and P. L. Lantos, eds.), 6th ed., pp. 813–896. Arnold, London, Sidney, Auckland.

Probert, L., Eugster, H. P., Akassoglou, K., Bauer, J., Frei, K., Lassmann, H., and Fontana, A. (2000). TNFR1 signalling is critical for the development of demyelination and the limitation of T-cell responses during immune-mediated CNS disease. *Brain.* **123,** 2005–2019.

Raine, C. S. (1985). Experimental allergic encephalomyelitis and experimental allergic neuritis. *In* "Handbook of Clinical Neurology" (P. I. Vinken and G. W. Bruyn, eds.), Vol. 47, pp. 429–466. Elsevier, New York.

Raine, C. S., Snyder, D. H., Valsamis, M. D., and Stone, S. H. (1974). Chronic experimental allergic encephalomyelitis in inbred guinea pigs–an ultrastructural study. *Lab. Invest.* **31,** 369–380.

Ransohoff, R. M. (1999). Mechanisms of inflammation in MS tissue: Adhesion molecules and chemokines. *J Neuroimmunol* **98,** 57–68.

Remlinger, P. (1928). Les paralysies due traitment antirebique. *Annals of the Insitute Pasteur* **55** (Suppl), 35–68.

Rivers. T. M., Sprunt, D. H., and Berry, G. P. (1933). Observations on attempts to produce acute disseminated encephalomyelitis in monkeys. *J. Exp. Med.* **58,** 39–53.

Rodriguez, M., and Miller, D. J. (1994). Immune promotion of central nervous system remyelination. *Prog-Brain-Res.* **103,** 343–355.

Rosener, M. Muraro, P. A., Riethmuller, A., Kalbus, M., Sappler, G., Thompson, R. J., Lichtenfels, R., Sommer, N., McFarland, H. F., and Martin, R. (1997). 2′,3′-cyclic nucleotide 3′-phosphodiesterase: A novel candidate autoantigen in demyelinating diseases. *J Neuroimmunol* **75,** 28–34.

Ruff, M., Wahl, S. M., and Pert, C. B. (1985). Substance P receptor mediated chemotaxis of human monocytes. *Peptide* **6,** 107–111.

Ruffini, F., Furlan, R., Poliani, P. L., Brambilla, E., Marconi, P. C., Bergami, A., Desina, G., Glorioso, J. C., Comi, G., and Martino, G. (2001). Fibroblast growth factor-II gene therapy reverts the clinical course and the pathological signs of chronic experimental autoimmune encephalomyelitis in C57BL/6 mice. *Gene-Ther.* **8,** 1207–1213.

Schlüsener, H., Sobel, R. A., Linington, C., and Weiner, H. L. (1987). A monoclonal antibody against a myelin oligodendrocyte glycoprotein induces relapses and demyelination in central nervous system autoimmune disease. *J. Immunol.* **139,** 4016–4021.

Schmied, M., Breitschopf, H., Gold, R., Zischler, H., Rothe, G., Wekerle, H., and Lassmann, H. (1993). Apoptosis of T lymphocytes in experimental autoimmune encephalomyelitis: Evidence for prgrammed cell death as a mechanism to control inflammation in the brain. *Amer J Pathol* **143,** 446–452.

Schwartz, M. (2001). Harnessing the immune system for neuroprotection: Therapeutic vaccines for acute and chronic neurodegenerative disorders. *Cell Mol Neurobiol.* **21,** 617–27.

Seil, A. J., Quarles, R. H., Johnson, D., and Brady, R. O. (1981). Immunisation with purified myelin associated glycoprotein does not evoke myelination inhibiting or demyelinating antibodies. *Brain Research* **209,** 470–475.

Seil, F. J., and Agrawal, H. C. (1980). Myelin proteolipid protein does not induce demyelinating or myelin inhibiting antibodies. *Brain Research* **194,** 273–277.

Selmaj, K. W., and Raine, C. S. (1988). Tumor necrosis factor mediates myelin and oligodendrocyte damage in vitro. *Ann Neurol.* **23,** 339–346.

Serafini, B., Columba-Cabezas, S., Di Rosa F., and Aloisi, F. (2000). Intracerebral recruitment and maturation of dendritic cells in the onset and progression of experimental autoimmune encephalomyelitis. *Amer J Pathol* **157,** 1991–2002.

Shamshiev, A., Donda, A., Carena, I., Mori, L., Kappos, L., and DeLibero, G. (1999). Self glycolipids as T-cell autoantigens. *Eur. J. Immunol.* **29,** 1667–1675.

Shamshiev, A., Gober, H. J., Donda, A., Mazorra, Z., Mori, L., and DeLibero, G. (2002). Presentation of the same glycolipid by different CD1-molecules. *J. Exp. Med.* **195,** 1013–1021.

Smith, T., Groom, A., Zhu, B., and Turski, L. (2000). Autoimmune encephalomyelitis ameliorated by AMPA antagonists. *Nature Med.* **6,** 62–66.

Smith, K. J., and Lassmann, H. (2002). The role of nitric oxide in multiple sclerosis. *Lancet Neurology* **1,** 232–241.

Smith, K. J., Kapoor, R., and Felts, P. A. (1999). Demyelination: The role of reactive oxygen and nitrogen species. *Brain Pathol.* **9,** 69–92.

Smith, K. J., Kapoor, R., Hall, S. M., and Davies, M. (2001). Electrically active axons degenerate when exposed to nitric oxide. *Ann Neurol.* **49,** 470–476.

Sobel, R. A., and Colvin, R. B. (1985). The immunopathology of experiemntal allergic encephalomyelitis (EAE). III. Differential in situ expression of strain 13 Ia on endothelial and inflammatory cells of (strain 2 × strain 13) F1 guinea pigs with EAE. *J. Immunol.* **91,** 2333–2337.

Sobel, R. A., and Kuchroo, V. K. (1992). The immunopathology of acute experimental allergic encephalomyelitis induced with myelin proteolipid protein. T cell receptors in inflammatory lesions. *J. Immunol.* **149,** 1444–1451.

Springer, T. A. (1994). Traffic signals for lymphocyte recirculation and leucocyte emigration: The multistep paradigm. *Cell* **76,** 301–314.

Stefferl, A., Brehm, U., Storch, M., Lambracht-Washington, D., Bourquin, C., Wonigeit, K. Lassmann, H., and Linington, C. (1999). Myelin oligodendrocyte glycoprotein induces experimental autoimmune encephalomyelitis in the resistant Brown Norway rat: Disease susceptibility is determined by MHC and MHC-linked effects on the B-cell response. *J Immunol* **163,** 40–49.

Storch, M. K., Fischer-Colbrie, R., Smith, T., Rinner, W. A., Hickey, W. F., Cuzner, M. L., Winkler, H., and Lassmann, H. (1996). Co-localization of secretoneurin immunoreactivity and macrophage infiltration in the lesions of experiemntal autoimmune encephalomyelitis. *Neurosci.* **71,** 885–893.

Storch, M. K., Stefferl, A., Brehm, U., Weissert, R., Wallström, E., Kerschensteiner, M., Olsson, T., Linington, C., and Lassmann, H (1998). Autoimmunity to myelin oligodendrocyte glycoprotein in rats mimics the spectrum of multiple sclerosis pathology. *Brain Pathol* **8,** 681–694.

Storch, M. K., Weissert, R., Stefferl, A., Birnbacher, R., Wallstrom, E., Dahlman, I., Ostensson, C. G., Linington, C., Olsson, T and Lassmann, H. (2002). MHC gene related effects on microglia and macrophages in experiemntal autoimmune encephalomyelitis determine the extent of axonal injury. *Brain Pathol.* **12,** 287–299.

Sun, D., Qin, Y., Chluba, J.,, Epplen J. T., and Wekerle, H. (1988). Suppression of experimentally induced autoimmune encephalomyelitis by cytolytic T-T-cell interactions. *Nature* **332,** 843–845.

Sun, D., and Wekerle, H. (1986). Ia-restricted encephalitogenic T lymphocytes mediating EAE lyse autoantigen-presenting astrocytes. *Nature.* **320,** 70–72.

Sun, D., Whitaker, J. N., Huang, Z., Liu, D., Coleclough, C., Wekerle, H., and Raine, C. S. (2001). Myelin antigen specific $CD8^+$ T cells are encephalitogenic and produce severe disease in C57BL/6 mice. *J Immunol* **166,** 7579–7587.

Sundvall, M., Jirholt, J., Yang, H. T., Jansson, L., Engsröm, A., Pettersson, U., and Holmdahl, R. (1995). Identification of murine loci associated with susceptibility to chronic experimental autoimmune encephalomyelitis. *Nature Genetics* **10,** 313–317.

Swanborg, R. H. (2001). Experimental autoimmune encephalomyelitis in the rat: Lessons in T-cell immunology and autoreactivity. *Immunol. Reviews* **184,** 129–135.

Taupin, V., Renno, T., Bourbonniere, L., Peterson, A. C., Rodriguez, M., and Owens, T. (1997). Increased severity of experimental autoimmune encephalomyelitis, chronic macrophage/microglial reactivity, and demyelination in transgenic mice producing tumor necrosis factor-alpha in the central nervous system. *Eur J Immunol.* **27,** 905–913

Teesalu, T., Hinkkanen, A. E., and Vaheri, A. (2001). Coordinated induction of extracellular proteolysis systems during experimental autoimmune encephalomyelitis in mice. *Am J Pathol.* **159,** 2227–2237.

Traugott. U., Reinherz, E. L., and Raine, C. S. (1983). Multiple sclerosis: Distribution of T cell subsets within active chronic lesions. *Science* **219,** 308–310.

Tsunoda, I., Kuang, L. Q., Theil, D. J., and Fujinami, R. S. (2000). Antibody association with a novel model for primary progressive multiple sclerosis: Induction of relapsing-remitting and progressive forms of EAE in H2s mouse strains. *Brain Pathol.* **10,** 402–418.

Vanderlugt, C. L., Begolka, W. S., Neville, K. L., Katz-Levy, Y. Howard, L.,M; Eagar, T. N., Bluestone, J. A., and Miller, S. D. (1998). The functional significance of epitope spreading and its regulation by co-stimulatory molecules. *Immunol Rev.* **164,** 63–72.

Vass, K., Heininger, K., Schäfer, B., Linington, C., and Lassmann, H. (1992). Interferon-gamma potentiates antibody-mediated demyelination in vivo. *Ann. Neurol.* **32,** 189–206.

Vass, K., and Lassmann, H. (1990). Intrathecal application of interferon-gamma: Progressive appearance of MHC antigens within the rat nervous system. *Amer. J. Pathol.* **137,** 789–800.

Voskuhl, R. R. (1998). Myelin protein expression in lymphoid tissues: Implications for peripheral tolerance. *Immunol Rev.* **164,** 81–92.

Wallstrom, E., Diener, P., Ljungdahl, A., Khademi, M., Nilsson, C. G., and Olsson, T. (1996). Memantine abrogates neurological deficits, but not CNS inflammation, in Lewis rat experimental autoimmune encephalomyelitis. *J Neurol Sci.* **137,** 89–96.

Weerth, S., Berger, T., Lassmann, H., and Linington, C. (1999). Encephalitogenic and neuritogenic T cell responses ti the myelin associated glycoprotein (MAG) in the Lewis rat. *J Neuroimmunol.* **95,** 157–164.

Weissert, R., Wallstrom, E., Storch, M. K., Stefferl, A., Lorentzen, J. Lassmann, H., Linington, C., and Olsson, T. (1998). MHC haplotype-dependent regulation of MOG-induced EAE in rats. J-Clin-Invest. **102,** 1265–1273.

Wekerle, H. (1998) Immunology of multiple sclerosis. *In* "McAlpine's Multiple Sclerosis" (A. Compston, ed.), pp. 379–407. Churchill Livingstone, London.

Wekerle, H., Linington, C., Lassmann, H., and Meyermann, R. (1986). Cellular immune reactivity within the CNS. *Trends Neurosci.* **9,** 271–277.

White, C. A., McCombe, P. A., and Pender, M. P. (1998). Microglia are more susceptible than macrophages to apoptosis in the central nervous system in experimental autoimmune encephalomyelitis through a mechanism not involving Fas (CD95). *Int Immunol.* **10,** 935–941.

White, C. A., Nguyen, K. B., and Pender, M. P. (2000). B cell apoptosis in the central nervous system in experimental autoimmune encephalomyelitis: Roles of B cell CD95, CD95L and Bcl-2 expression. *J Autoimmun.* **14,** 195–204.

Willenborg, D. O., Fordham, S. A., Cowden, W. B., and Ramshaw, I. A. (1995). Cytokines and murine autoimmune encephalomyelitis: Inhibition or enhancement of disease with antibodies to select cytokines, or by delivery of exogenous cytokines using a recombinant vaccinia virus system. Scand-J-Immunol. **41,** 31–41.

Willenborg, D. O., Staykova, M. A., and Cowden, W. B. (1999). Our shifting understanding of the role of nitric oxide in autoimmune encephalomyelitis: A review. *J Neuroimmunol.* **100,** 21–35.

Wisniewski, H. M., and Bloom, B. R. (1975). Primary demyelination as a nonspecific consequence of a cell mediated immune reaction. *J. Exp. Med.* **141,** 346–459.

Wucherpfennig, K. W., and Strominger, J. L. (1995). Molecular mimicry in T cell-mediated autoimmunity: Viral peptides activate human T cell clones specific for myelin basic protein. *Cell.* **80,** 695–705.

Yednock, T. A., Cannon, C., Fritz, L. C., Sanchez-Madrid, F., and Steinman, L. (1992). Prevention of experimental autoimmune encephalomyelitis by antibodies against a4ß1 integrin. *Nature* **356,** 63–66.

Yu, M., Johnson, J. M., and Tuohy, V. K. (1996). A predictable sequential determinant spreading cascade invariably accompanies progression of experimental autoimmune encephalomyelitis: A basis for peptide-specific therapy after onset of clinical disease. *J Exp Med.* **183,** 1777–88.

Zamvil, S., Nelson, P., Trotter, J., Mitchell, D., Knobler, R., Fritz, R., and Steinman, L. (1985). T-cell clones specific for myelin basic protein induce chronic relapsing paralysis and demyelination. *Nature* **317,** 355–358.

Zettl, U. K., Mix, E., Zielasek, J., Stangel, M., Hartung, H. P., and Gold, R. (1997). Apoptosis of myelin-reactive T cells induced by reactive oxygen and nitrogen intermediates in vitro. *Cell Immunol.* **178,** 1–8.

Zhang, J., Dawson, V. L., Dawson, T. M., and Snyder, S. H. (1994). Nitric oxide activation of poly(ADP-ribose) synthetase in neurotoxicity. *Science.* **263,** 687–689.

CHAPTER

# 44

# Experimental Models of Virus-Induced Demyelination

*A. J. Bieber and M. Rodriguez*

## MEDICAL RELEVANCE OF ANIMAL MODELS OF DEMYELINATING DISEASE

Multiple sclerosis (MS) is an inflammatory demyelinating disease of the human central nervous system (CNS) and is the most common cause of acquired nontraumatic neurologic disability in young adults. The pathologic hallmark of the disease is damage to oligodendrocytes and CNS myelin, which results in demyelinated white matter lesions, followed by axonal loss and glial scarring (Lucchinetti *et al.*, 1997; Noseworthy *et al.*, 2000; Trapp *et al.*, 1998). Areas of active disease display a prominent inflammatory response with tissue infiltration by mononuclear cells, primarily T cells and macrophages. Despite decades of research, the causes of myelin damage and neurologic dysfunction in MS remain largely unknown. Chapters 29 through 33 in Section IV of these volumes provide an overview of the classification, pathology, genetics, and potential pathogenic mechanisms of multiple sclerosis.

There is no cure for MS, and attempts to develop effective therapies have met with only limited success (Noseworthy, 1998). Immunosuppression with corticosteroids is commonly used as a short-term therapy to control MS relapses. Long-term therapy generally consists of treatment with immunomodulatory drugs such as glatiramer acetate (Copolymer-1/Copaxone), interferon-β-1a (Avonex), or interferon-β-1b (Betaseron). Each of these drugs has been shown to reduce relapses of the disease, but whether they alter the long-term clinical endpoint is still being debated.

Our continued lack of understanding about the causes of MS and the mechanisms of disease progression, and the lack of truly effective therapies for the disease, underscore the need for good animal models of MS on which to conduct research. In this chapter we review two of the most widely studied animal models of virus-induced demyelinating disease: Theiler's murine encephalomyelitis virus and murine hepatitis virus. Both viruses produce acute inflammatory encephalitis that is followed by chronic CNS demyelinating disease. The clinical and pathologic correlates of virus-induced demyelination are largely immune mediated. Several pathologic mechanisms have been proposed to explain the development of myelin damage and neurologic deficits, and each of the proposed mechanisms may play a role in disease progression depending on the genetic constitution of the infected animal. The induction of demyelinating disease by virus may be directly relevant to human MS. Several viruses are known to cause demyelination in humans, and viral infection is an epidemiologic factor that is consistently associated with clinical exacerbation of MS (Sarchielli *et al.*, 1993; Sibley *et al.*, 1985). It has been suggested that viral infection may be a cause of MS, although no specific virus has been identified as a causative agent.

The clinical and pathologic presentation of virus-induced demyelination, the immune-mediated nature of the disease mechanisms, and the variability of the disease presentation depending on genetic background are all very similar to what is observed in MS. The many similarities between human MS and the demyelinating diseases that are induced by infection with TMEV and MHV make these animal models very attractive for the study of multiple sclerosis.

## THEILER'S MURINE ENCEPHALOMYELITIS VIRUS (TMEV)

Theiler's murine encephalomyelitis Virus (TMEV) belongs to the cardiovirus genus of the picornavirus family (Nitayaphan *et al.*, 1986; Pevear *et al.*, 1987). The original isolation and characterization of the virus was reported by Theiler in 1937 when the effects of TMEV infection of the CNS were observed in a mouse that spontaneously developed flaccid paralysis. The virus was subsequently transmitted to other mice by intracerebral inoculation with a suspension made from the brain and spinal cord of the infected mouse.

TMEV is a ubiquitous enteric pathogen that usually causes asymptomatic intestinal infections in mice. Occasionally, the virus will spread beyond the intestinal tract and enter the CNS, resulting in both acute and chronic CNS infections. Chronic CNS infection results in extensive demyelination with accumulating neurologic deficits and has provided a valuable experimental model for human demyelinating disease.

### Virus Biology and Life Cycle

#### *TMEV Subgroups*

Since its initial discovery, isolates of TMEV have been recovered in several laboratories. The different TMEV strains have been divided into two subgroups depending on the disease that they induce after infection of the CNS (Lorch *et al.*, 1981). The GDVII and FA strains are highly virulent with an $LD_{50}$ as low as 1 to 10 plaque forming units (PFU). CNS infection causes acute encephalitis that is characterized by the destruction of a large number of CNS neurons, especially in the cortex, hippocampus, thalamus, brain stem, and in the anterior horns of the spinal cord. The encephalitis is usually fatal, and the highly virulent strains do not result in persistent infection of the CNS.

A second TMEV subgroup is far less virulent ($LD_{50} > 10^6$ PFU) and results in a distinctly different disease presentation. This subgroup, which includes the TO4, DA, BeAn 3886, Yale, and WW strains, induces a biphasic CNS disease (Daniels *et al.*, 1952; Lipton, 1978; Wroblewska *et al.*, 1977). Following intracerebral infection, these strains replicate in neurons in the brain resulting in encephalitis similar to that observed with the GDVII strain but nonlethal. The virus is cleared from the brain by the host immune response but persists in the spinal cord, eventually resulting in the development of chronic demyelinating disease (Lehrich *et al.*, 1976; Lipton, 1975; Njenga *et al.*, 1997; Rodriguez *et al.*, 1987). The disease is characterized by viral persistence in oligodendrocytes (Rodriguez *et al.*, 1983) and macrophages (Lipton *et al.*, 1995), with chronic demyelination and progressive loss of motor function (McGavern *et al.*, 1999). The pathology is largely immune mediated with animals demonstrating a range of disease phenotypes depending on their genetic background. In the SJL strain, demyelination is evident within 30 days after infection. By 90 days, infected animals begin to develop spasticity and gait abnormalities, and weakness of the lower extremities, with paralysis eventually occurring by 6 to 9 months (Lipton and Dal Canto, 1976a).

#### *Capsid Structure*

The X-ray crystallographic structures of DA, BeAn and GDVII viruses have been determined to about 3 angstrom resolution (Grant *et al.*, 1992; Luo *et al.*, 1992, 1996; Toth *et al.*, 1993). A schematic representation of the TMEV capsid, based on the crystallograghic data, is presented in Figure 44.1. Each virus consists of a protein shell that is composed of 60

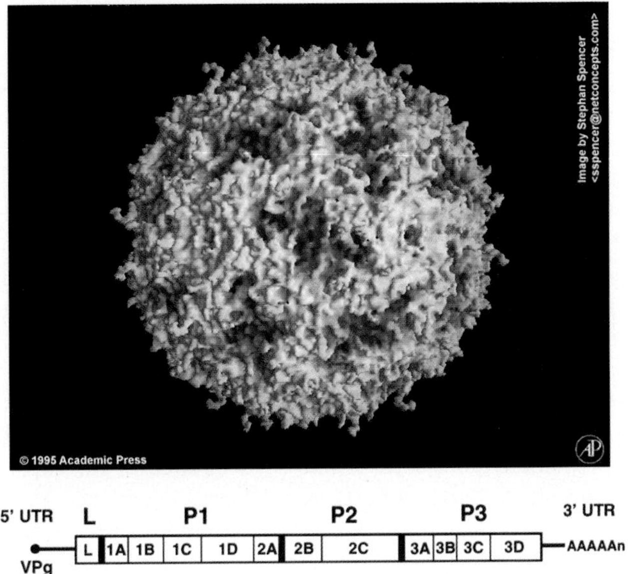


FIGURE 44.1
TMEV capsid and genome structure. The upper panel shows a schematic representation of the TMEV capsid, based on the X-ray crystallograghic data. Lower panel shows a map of the TMEV DA strain genome. The 5′ and 3′ untranslated (UTR) regions are indicated. The 5′ end of the RNA is bound by the viral VPg protein (ball) and the 3′ end is polyadenylated (AAAAAn). The open bar indicates the open reading frame from nucleotides 1066 to 7968. The heavy lines dividing the bar indicate the positions of the initial proteolytic cleavages after the leader peptide (L) and between the P1, P2, and P3 precursor peptides. The lighter lines dividing the bar indicate the arrangement of the final gene products. The identities of the final gene products are discussed in the text. The TMEV capsid structure is reproduced with permission from Webster and Granoff (1995).

protomers, arranged as 12 pentamers with icosahedral symmetry. Each protomer contains one of each of the four capsid peptides (VP1, VP2, VP3, VP4). The VP1, VP2, and VP3 capsid proteins are each composed of an eight-stranded antiparallel β-barrel. The loops that connect the strands of the β-barrel form the surface structure of the viral capsid and may play important roles as sites of binding for neutralizing antibody and in conformational determinants of virus persistence. A second surface feature, the "pit" formed at the contact region between VP1 and VP3, is the likely binding site for the cellular receptor (Zhou, *et al.*, 2000; Jnaoui, *et al.*, 2002).

### *Viral Genome*

The TMEV genome consists of a positive sense, single stranded RNA molecule. Genomes for both the GDVII and TO subgroups have been sequenced and found to be very similar, with about 90% identity at the nucleotide level and 96% at the amino acid level (Pevear *et al.*, 1988). The genome of the DA strain is 8093 nucleotides long (Ohara *et al.*, 1988) and contains a single 6903 nucleotide open reading frame that starts at nucleotide 1066 and encodes a 2301 amino acid polyprotein. The genome terminates with a poly(A) tail. The 12 mature TMEV gene products are generated from the polyprotein by post-translational proteolytic cleavage. The gene products include a leader peptide, four capsid polypeptides (VP1-4), two viral proteases, a polymerase/helicase, the RNA-dependent RNA polymerase that is involved in genome replication, and a small basic protein which becomes covalently linked to the 5′ end of viral RNAs. Two other gene products have unknown functions.

### *Virus Life Cycle*

The TMEV infection cycle is typical of the picornavirus family (Rueckert, 1996). Attachment of the virion to specific cell surface receptors serves to position the virus close to the cell membrane. Attachment also induces a conformational change in the virion that results in the loss of the VP4 capsid protein and the translocation of the RNA genome across the cell membrane and into the cytoplasm. Co-opting the translational machinery of the cell, the RNA genome directs the synthesis of a single large polyprotein. While nascent on the ribosome, the polyprotein is cleaved by virus encoded protease activity, into three large precursor proteins: P1, P2, and P3. The precursor proteins are further cleaved to produce the viral structural proteins and proteins necessary for completion of the infection cycle (Fig. 44.1).

Precursor P3 is processed to produce a viral proteinase (designated 3C), a protein involved in initiating replication of the viral genome (3B or VPg) and the viral RNA-dependent RNA polymerase (3D). The viral polymerase copies the incoming viral genome to produce a negative-strand RNA that then serves as the template for replication of the positive-strand viral genome. The newly formed positive-strand RNA molecules may be copied to form more negative-strand templates or be packaged into virions as virus assembly proceeds.

The P1 precursor protein is cleaved to produce the viral capsid proteins VP0 (1A+B), VP1 (1D), and VP3 (1C). As the concentration of capsid proteins increases in the cell, they begin to aggregate into protomers composed of one copy of each of the capsid proteins. These protomers then assemble into pentamers, and 12 pentamers assemble with a positive-stranded, VPg bound viral RNA, to produce a noninfectious provirion. The final step in maturation to infectious virus requires a maturation cleavage in which the VP0 protein is cleaved to give the final VP2 (1B) and VP4 (1A) capsid proteins that are found in the mature virus. In neonates and in some cells in culture, mature virus may accumulate to very high levels in infected cells and can often be observed as paracrystalline arrays in electron micrograghs (Fig. 44.2). Virus is generally released from the cell by infection-mediated cytolysis. The time that is required to complete the infection cycle is generally 7 to 12 hours.

### TMEV Receptor

In culture, TMEV is able to infect a wide variety of cell types from several different species. Although a unique protein receptor for the virus has not been identified, several lines of evidence suggest that cell surface carbohydrate residues may play a central role in the binding and entry of virus. Removal of sialic acid from the cell surface by treatment with sialidase significantly reduces the infectivity of BeAn virus in BHK cells (Fotiadis *et al.*, 1991). Similar decreases are observed when binding to sialic acid is blocked with wheat germ agglutinin, which binds to sialic acid on the cell surface (Fotiadis *et al.*, 1991).

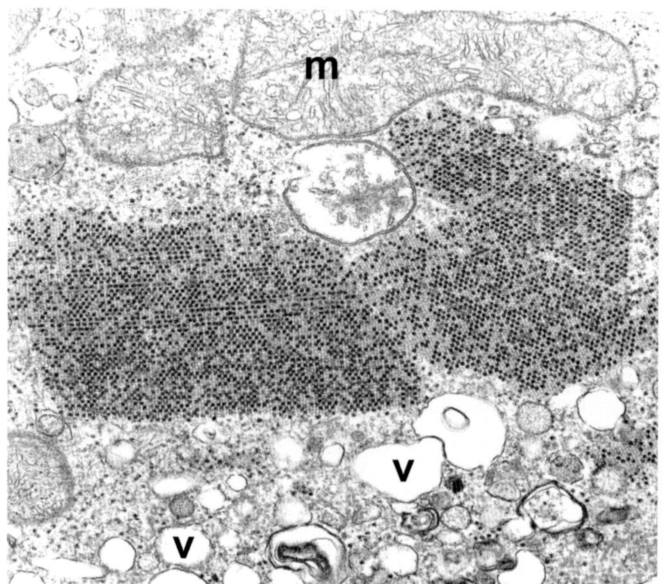


FIGURE 44.2
Crystalline virus in neonatal brain. A paracrystalline viral array in the cytoplasm of a spinal cord neuron from a neonatal SJL mouse infected with the DA strain of TMEV. An intact mitochondrion is visible (m), but the numerous cytoplasmic vacuoles (v) indicate the cytopathic effects of viral infection.

Sialyllactose comprises the terminal three sugar residues of cell surface oligosaccarides, and inclusion of sialyllactose in cell culture medium inhibits viral binding and infectivity by blocking receptor binding sites on the virus (Zhou *et al.*, 1997). Together these data demonstrate an important role for sialic acid in the recognition of the cell surface by the TO subgroup TMEV strains. Sialyloligosaccaride addition is a common post-translation modification of cell surface proteins, which is consistent with the observation that TMEV can infect a variety of cell types. Which specific sialic acid containing proteins might be required for virus binding and entry has not yet been established.

The neurovirulent strains of TMEV (GDVII and FA) do not require sialic acid for cell surface binding (Fotiadis *et al.*, 1991) but instead use cell surface heparin sulfate proteoglycan. Pretreatment of virus with heparin sulfate, treatment of host cells with heparin sulfate cleaving enzymes, or treatment with heparin sulfate specific antibodies all inhibit GDVII binding and infection (Reddi and Lipton, 2002). Proteoglycan deficient CHO cells are resistant to infection, further supporting a role for proteoglycans in GDVII binding. The interaction of proteins with heparin sulfate is usually mediated by heparin-binding domains (HBD) and a heparin-binding domain consensus sequence has been described (Cardin and Weintraub, 1989). A putative HBD is present in the amino acid sequence of the VP1 capsid protein of both the GDVII and TO subgroups. This sequence may play a role in the binding of GDVII to heparin sulfate but if so, conformational differences must exist between VP1 peptides of the TMEV subgroups because the TO subgroup viruses do not bind heparin sulfate. Proteoglycans are known to serve as co-receptors or attachment factors for a variety of different viruses. For several of these viruses, heparin sulfate acts primarily as an attachment factor and is not fully sufficient to mediate virus entry. The extent to which additional protein entry receptors are needed for GDVII infection is not yet clear (Reddi and Lipton, 2002).

## Disease Pathology

The encephalitic phase of TMEV-induced disease develops rapidly after intracerebral infection. Virus infects and replicates in neurons of the brain and spinal cord, with titers of infectious virus reaching their peak by 5 to 7 days. Immunohistochemical staining demonstrates the highest viral antigen loads in the thalamus, hypothalamus, midbrain, brain stem, and spinal cord gray matter. Neuronal infection and lysis is particularly pronounced with the GDVII subgroup viruses, and infection usually results in death soon after inoculation (Patick *et al.*, 1990).

Acute disease following infection with the TO subgroup viruses is also characterized by intense mononuclear cell infiltration in the brain and spinal cord. The combined effects of direct viral lysis of neurons and damage from infiltrating cells may result in transient flaccid paralysis within 2 weeks after infection, but in many cases the early phase of the disease is largely asymptomatic. The acute phase of the disease is followed by clearance of virus from the gray matter by the host immune response (Njenga *et al.*, 1997). Resistant strains of mice achieve virtually complete viral clearance. In susceptible strains, virus is cleared from the gray matter but persists in the white matter of the spinal cord for the lifetime of the animal.

During persistent infection, the amount of infectious virus, and the number of cells with detectable virus antigen in the spinal cord is usually quite low. This is in contrast to the high level of viral genome that is present throughout the disease (Trottier *et al.*, 2001). Infected cells most often appear in the lateral or anterior columns of the thoracic spinal cord and the presence of infected cells is often accompanied by an inflammatory parenchymal infiltrate and perivascular cuffing. The diffuse inflammatory infiltrate consists of large numbers of $CD4^+$ and $CD8^+$ T lymphocytes, activated macrophages and microglia, B cells, and reactive astrocytes (Fig. 44.3; Lindsley *et al.*, 1989). The presence of inflammatory cells correlates closely with the development of myelin damage, and electron microscopy reveals infiltrating mononuclear cells stripping myelin from axons. Macrophages containing engulfed myelin debris are numerous in demyelinating lesions. The specific roles that these different cell types play in the development of demyelination and neurologic deficits will be discussed in subsequent sections.

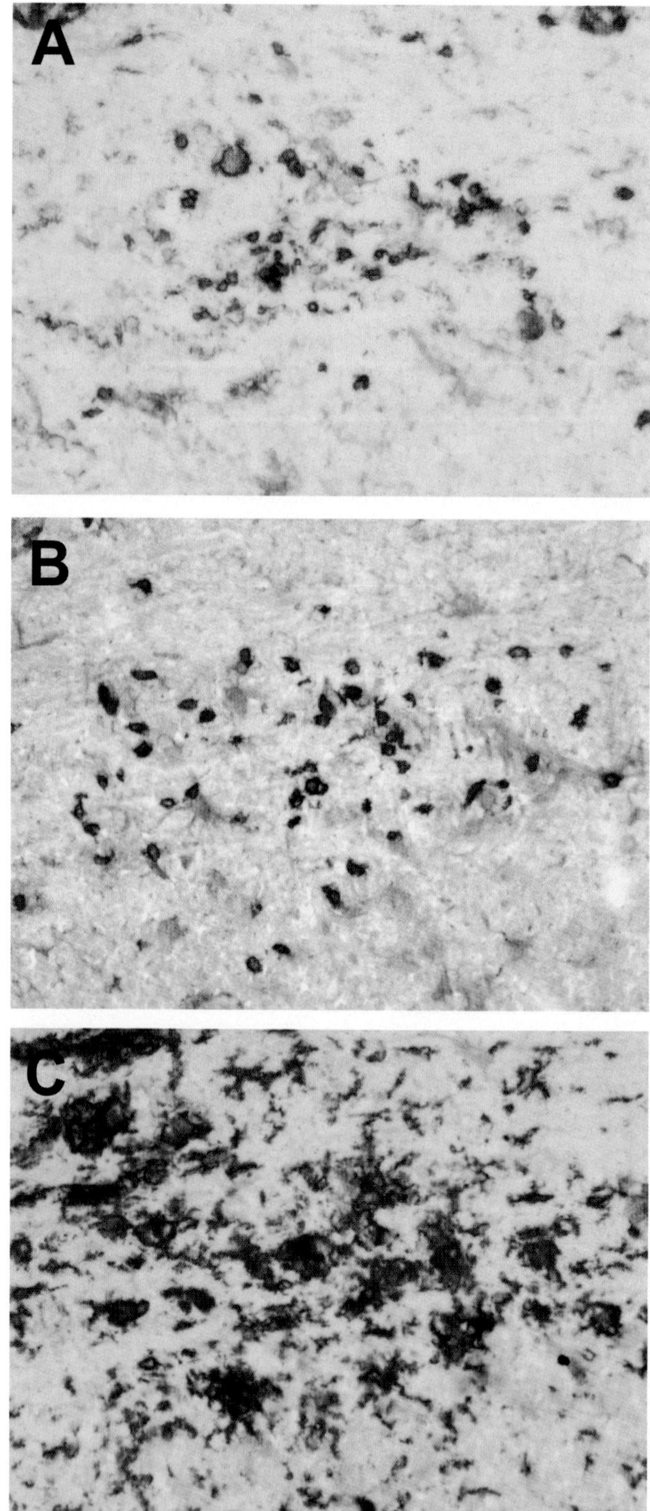


FIGURE 44.3
Immunochemical characterization of a chronic demyelinated lesion. Adjacent sections from the spinal cord of an SJL mouse, 8 months post-infection, were stained for $CD4^+$ T cells with the Ly-2 antibody (A), for $CD8^+$ T cells with the GK1.5 antibody (B) and for macrophages with the M1/70 antibody against Mac-1 (C).

Demyelination is apparent by as early as 22 days after infection and in many mouse strains, as demyelination progresses, neurologic deficits begin to appear. Demyelination pathology is illustrated in Figure 44.4. The development of neurologic deficits in

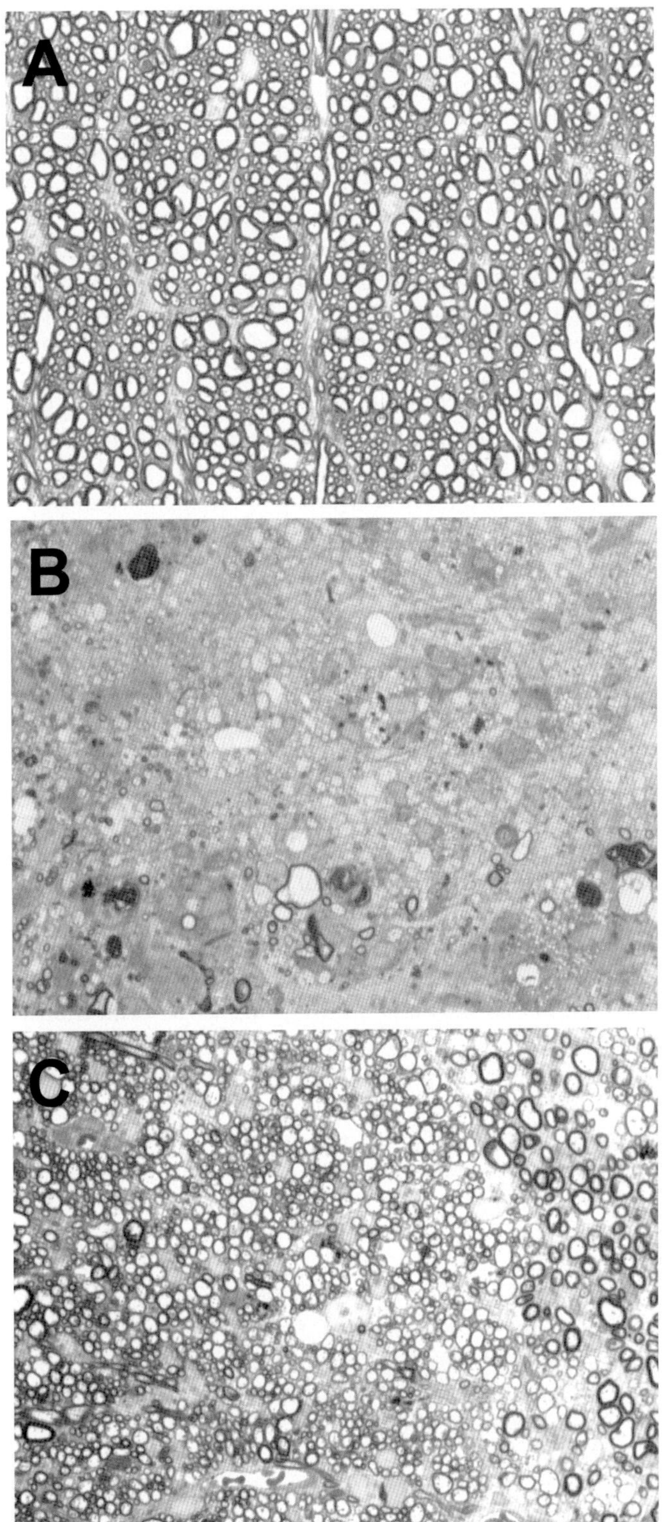


FIGURE 44.4
Demyelinated and remyelination in the TMEV-infected spinal cord. (A) Normal spinal cord white matter stained for myelin sheaths with para-phenylene-diamine. (B) A demyelinated lesion from an FVB mouse, 3 months post-infection with the DA strain of TMEV. Almost complete myelin destruction is apparent. (C) Extensive remyelination is apparent by 8 months post-infection. Schwann cell remyelination is evident as heavily stained myelin figures in the upper right corner of the panel, while the lightly staining myelin in the center of the panel is oligodendrocyte remyelination.

infected mice involves not just the disruption of neuronal function but neuronal and axonal loss as well (McGavern *et al.*, 2000). Quantitative assessment of CNS injury during TMEV-induced disease shows that significant atrophy of the lateral and anterior white matter regions of the spinal cord can be detected by 45 days post-infection. Atrophy is most pronounced in the posterior cervical and anterior thoracic regions of the spinal cord. While levels of demyelination reach a peak by 100 days post-infection, spinal cord atrophy continues to increase between 100 and 220 days. A 25% reduction was observed in the area of the anterior and lateral white matter at the C8-T11 level of the spinal cord by 195 to 229 days after infection. In this study, atrophy was specifically assessed in areas of normal appearing white matter and not in lesion areas, to avoid complications due to area changes resulting from inflammation and edema. This marked spinal cord atrophy is the result of a 30% loss of medium to large axonal fibers by 195 to 229 days post-infection. The progressive loss of axons correlates well with electrophysiologic changes in the spinal cord and with changes in motor ability. These observations demonstrate that the neurologic deficits that develop during chronic TMEV-induced demyelinating disease are primarily due to axonal damage and loss rather than to demyelination alone.

### Viral Persistence

Intracerebral inoculation with the highly virulent GDVII subgroup viruses results in fatal encephalitis, while infection with the less virulent TO viruses results in milder encephalitis, followed by clearance of virus from the brain and virus persistence in the spinal cord. There is still some debate concerning whether the difference in disease that is induced by these viruses is due simply to differences in virulence. Would the GDVII strains persist and cause demyelination if animals survived the initial encephalitis or are determinants for persistence and demyelination a specific genetic property of the TO strains? Recombinant chimeric viruses, resulting from the exchange of sequences between the GDVII and BeAn (or DA) virus genomes, have been useful in beginning to map the determinants of virus neurovirulence and persistence.

Initial studies localized the majority of neurovirulence to a segment of the GDVII genome from the middle of 1B to the middle of 2C, although additional upstream sequences had a more minor effect (Fig. 44.1; Fu *et al.*, 1990a). Infection with recombinant DA virus that contains these GDVII regions results in death at a much reduced $LD_{50}$ compared to wildtype DA virus. Subsequent studies narrowed the critical segment to a region of P1 from 1B to 1D, the capsid coding region (Zhang *et al.*, 1993). Several studies have since confirmed that major determinants of viral persistence lie in the region of the viral genome that encodes the capsid proteins and have identified regions in two of these proteins, VP1 and VP2, that appear to be necessary for persistence (Adami *et al.*, 1998; Lin *et al.*, 1998). Molecular modeling suggests that these sequences may be positioned on the surface of the virus in a manner consistent with a role in the binding of the virus to its cellular receptor (Zhou *et al.*, 1997). Differences in receptor binding between the TMEV subgroups may therefore play an important role in determining the balance between neurovirulence and the ability to produce persistent infection.

Several mutated strains of the GDVII virus have been characterized in which neurovirulence is greatly attenuated, and while these strains are viable, replicate in the brain, and may even induce encephalitis, they do not persist or induce chronic demyelinating disease (Lipton *et al.*, 1991, 1998). These experiments suggest that ability of a TMEV strain to produce persistent infection and demyelination is not solely a function of neurovirulence but may be a specific genetic property of the strain. Other investigators have reported that insertion into the GDVII backbone, of DA strain segments from across the length of the DA genome, attenuates virulence and results in virus persistence and demyelination (Fu *et al.*, 1990b; Rodriguez and Roos, 1992; see also Jakob and Roos, 1996). Further studies will be needed to determine whether there are specific genetic determinants in the TO subtype that control persistence and to map these determinants to specific viral proteins.

An additional interesting difference between the GDVII and TO subgroups involves the expression of the leader peptide region (L) of the TMEV genome at the 5′ end of the open reading frame (see Fig. 44.1). The TO strains use an alternative initiation codon to produce L*, a protein whose coding sequence is out of frame with the polyprotein reading frame. The GDVII strains do not encode the L* protein. Mutations in L* dramatically decrease virus-induced demyelination indicating that it plays a role in the development of disease (Chen *et al.*, 1995). The L* protein is essential for replication of the DA strain in a macrophage-like cell line in culture, while the GDVII strain does not replicate in these cells (Takata *et al.*, 1998). L* appears to function by preventing apoptosis of the DA-infected cells (Ghadge, *et al.*, 1998). The production of the L* protein therefore plays an essential role in the ability of TO subtype viruses to persist in specific cell types in the CNS. Analysis of the cytotoxic T lymphocyte (CTL) response in the CNS of mice infected with L* mutant virus, suggests that the inhibition of apoptosis by L* may prevent development of virus-specific cytotoxicity, permitting persistent virus infection and demyelinating disease (Lin *et al.*, 1999).

TMEV persistence in susceptible mice is associated with continuous virus replication and infectious virus and viral RNA can be isolated from the CNS for many months after initial infection. There is no single obvious cellular site of virus persistence in the spinal cord. Both viral antigen and RNA have been reported in oligodendrocytes, macrophages, and astrocytes (Aubert *et al.*, 1987; Brahic *et al.*, 1981; Lipton *et al.*, 1995; Rodriguez *et al.*, 1983). The typical observation that only very small numbers of infectious virus can be recovered from chronically infected spinal cord initially led to the notion that the virus persists at low levels in the tissue. However, recent quantitative studies on the level of viral RNA in the CNS have demonstrated the presence of large amounts of full-length viral RNA, about $10^9$ copies/spinal cord, throughout the course of the chronic disease (Trottier *et al.*, 2001). In contrast, infectious virus reaches a peak of $>10^6$ PFU/spinal cord by 15 days after intracerebral inoculation but then falls significantly to $10^2$ to $10^4$ PFU/spinal cord after 28 days. This difference between viral genome load and infectious virus may reflect the rapid neutralization of virus by virus-specific antibodies. These data indicate that active viral replication continues throughout persistent viral infection.

The identification of a primary cellular site and specific mechanism of TMEV persistence has been difficult. Based on immunostaining experiments, the predominant virus antigen burden in infected spinal cord has been reported to reside in either oligodendrocytes or macrophages (Lipton *et al.*, 1995; Rodriguez *et al.*, 1983). More recently, fractionation of macrophages and oligodendrocytes from the chronically infected CNS revealed large amounts of viral genome in both cell types (Trottier *et al.*, 2001). Restriction of virus replication has been suggested as a mechanism for virus persistence and such restriction has been reported in macrophages isolated from TMEV infected CNS (Clatch *et al.*, 1990; Levy *et al.*, 1992). However, the ratio of plus- to minus-strand TMEV RNA appears to be similar in macrophages and oligodendrocytes from infected spinal cord, suggesting that neither cell type is generally restricted for virus replication (Trottier *et al.*, 2001).

As a potential site for TMEV persistence, macrophages have been the most widely studied. As mentioned earlier, restriction of virus replication has been reported in macrophages isolated from the TMEV infected CNS, and such restriction has been suggested as a possible mechanism for persistence. Depletion of blood borne macrophages early during the course of disease (7 to 21 days post-infection) decreases the amount of viral RNA in the CNS, supporting a role for macrophages in viral persistence (Rossi *et al.*, 1997). Studies in macrophage cell lines have demonstrated a block at the point of virus assembly rather than replication and it has been demonstrated that the differentiation state of the macrophage may be critical for the ability of the cell to support persistence (Jelachich *et al.*, 1995; Shaw-Jackson and Michiels, 1997). Similar experiments, to look at potential viral persistence in the precursors of other glial types, have not yet been reported.

Other investigators have suggested a role in virus persistence for other CNS cells, such as astrocytes and vascular endothelial cells (Sapatino *et al.*, 1995; Zheng *et al.*, 2001). Whether there is a primary cellular site and a unique mechanism for TMEV persistence in the chronically infected CNS, is still an unresolved matter.

## Host Determinants of Resistance and Susceptibility

Inbred strains of mice can be either resistant or susceptible to persistent TMEV infection and demyelinating disease. Upon intracerebral infection with virus, resistant strains mount an anti-viral immune response that controls virus replication and eventually clears virus from the animal. Upon clearance, infectious virus, virus antigen, and viral RNA can no longer be detected. Susceptible strains also mount a strong immune response against virus but virus is not cleared. A persistent viral infection is established along with the development of demyelinating disease, as described earlier. Since virus clearance is mediated by the immune response, mutations that disrupt major functional elements of the immune system generally result in some level of susceptibility, even in an animal with an otherwise resistant genetic background. The effects of mutations of this type will be discussed in subsequent sections. Here we review naturally occurring genetic loci that act as modifiers of the response to TMEV infection and that have been identified using standard techniques of genetic analysis in mice.

Early studies with different strains of mice demonstrated a wide range of susceptibility to TMEV-induced disease (Lipton and Del Canto, 1979). F1 and F2 backcrossing experiments between resistant and susceptible strains revealed that several loci were important for virus clearance and that one of these loci was linked to the H-2 major histocompatibility complex on chromosome 17 (Lipton and Melvold, 1984). Further genetic analysis of this region showed that mice with certain H-2 haplotypes (H-$2^{f, p, q, r, s, v}$) are susceptible to persistent virus infection, while others (H-$2^{d,b,k}$) conferred resistance (Rodriguez and David, 1985). Resistance was a dominant effect (Patick *et al.*, 1990) and mapped to the D region of the H-2 complex, suggesting that a class-I mediated element of the immune response was essential for virus resistance (Clatch *et al.*, 1985; Rodriguez *et al.*, 1986b). Direct demonstration that an H-2 linked class-I gene was responsible for virus resistance was provided when the H-$2D^d$ class-I gene was introduced into a susceptible mouse strain and these transgenic animals were shown to be resistant (Azoulay *et al.*, 1994). A key role for class-I restricted $CD8^+$ T cells as effectors of resistance has since been confirmed with targeted mutations in CD8 and β2-microglobulin (which lacks MHC class-I function). Both of these mutations result in TMEV susceptibility in animals with otherwise resistant genetic backgrounds (Fiette *et al.*, 1993; Murray *et al.*, 1998; Pullen *et al.*, 1993; Rodriguez *et al.*, 1993). The H-$2D^b$ gene exerts its effect on the stimulation of virus-specific CTL through the presentation of an immunodominant peptide from the VP2 capsid protein: $VP2_{121-130}$ (Dethlefs *et al.*, 1997; Johnson *et al.*, 1999). There are other class-I molecules whose peptide binding sites are identical to those of the D locus and therefore have the potential to present TMEV peptide. These molecules, however, have not been shown to play a role in establishing resistance, possibly due to differential patterns of expression or to structural differences outside of the peptide binding domain that are important for antigen presentation (Altintas *et al.*, 1993; Lin *et al.*, 1997a).

Non-MHC loci also have an influence on virus resistance/susceptibility. The T-cell receptor genes lie on chromosome 6 (the *Tcrb* locus) in the mouse, and genetic mapping studies have indicated that a gene affecting resistance maps close to the *Tcrb* locus. Several commonly used strains of susceptible mice have large deletions of the Vβ T-cell receptor genes, further suggesting a link between T-cell function and virus resistance (Rodriguez *et al.*, 1992). Genetic analysis of congenic mice with specific Vβ deletions indicates that in susceptible genetic backgrounds, Vβ deletions enhance susceptibility but that have little effect on resistance. These data generally support a role for T-cell receptor genes in determining virus resistance (Rodriguez *et al.*, 1994).

Mapping experiments using the susceptible SJL strain and the resistant B10.S strain, two strains that both have the same H-$2^S$ haplotype, have identified loci on chromosomes 10 and 18 (Bihl *et al.*, 1999; Bureau *et al.*, 1993). There are two loci close to the gene for interferon-γ (Ifn-γ) on chromosome 10. While the possibility of a resistance locus at the site of the Ifn-γ gene was of obvious interest, fine mapping experiments have excluded Ifn-γ as a candidate (Bihl *et al.*, 1999). A second locus is near the gene for myelin basic protein (MBP) on chromosome 18. The exact identity of the gene involved has not yet been established but the possibility that TMEV resistance might be influenced by one of the major structural genes for myelin is intriguing. Studies on TMEV infection of MBP deficient *shiverer* mice demonstrate enhanced susceptibility in the absence of MBP, supporting the idea that MBP might play a role in determining resistance (Bihl *et al.*, 1997).

Loci that affect TMEV resistance and persistence have also been identified on chromosome 3 near the carbonic anhydrase-2 (*Car-2*) locus (Melvold *et al.*, 1990), on chromosome 11 (Aubagnac *et al.*, 1999), and on chromosome 14 (Bureau *et al.*, 1998). The identity of the genes that are involved at these loci has not yet been established. Gender has also been reported to influence the susceptibility of certain mouse strains to TMEV-induced demyelinating disease (Kappel *et al.*, 1990).

## Mechanisms of Demyelination, Axonal Damage and the Development of Neurologic Deficits

When considering TMEV-induced disease as a model for human demyelinating disease, questions regarding the mechanisms of demyelination and axonal damage are of central importance. Several different mechanisms have been proposed to explain the pathology and neurologic deficits that usually accompany persistent TMEV infection, but there is still disagreement in the field about the relative importance of the various potential mechanisms for the development of demyelination and axonal damage.

Whatever the exact mechanisms of disease resistance and susceptibility, it seems certain that a balance between persistent virus infection and immune cell activation determines whether demyelinating disease will develop in immunocompetent mice. Mice with severe combined immunodeficiency (SCID) normally die from acute encephalitis when infected with TMEV. Adoptive transfer of normal spleen cells can result in survival and the development of demyelinating disease, but the results of adoptive transfer depend critically on the number of cells transferred (Rodriguez *et al.*, 1996). Transfer of too few cells fails to ameliorate the SCID phenotype and most mice die. Transfer of too many cells results in complete virus clearance and the mice survive but do not develop disease. Only when an intermediate number of cells is transferred do the surviving mice develop persistent virus infection and demyelination. These results demonstrate the balance between immune activation and virus persistence that determines the quality and extent of demyelinating disease.

### *Mechanisms of Demyelination*

Proposed mechanisms of TMEV-induced demyelination include (1) demyelination resulting from direct virus lysis of infected oligodendrocytes or as a "dying back" response of oligodendrocytes following infection; (2) TMEV-specific, immune-mediated destruction of infected oligodendrocytes; (3) "bystander" damage to glia by toxic mediators from activated macrophages; (4) "epitope spreading," an autoimmune attack against myelin antigens resulting from the *de novo* processing and immune recognition of myelin antigens that follows the initial events of virus-induced myelin damage; and (5) "molecular mimicry," an autoimmune attack against myelin antigens based on the activity of virus-activated T cells that are cross-reactive with myelin antigens. While several distinct mechanisms of demyelination have been proposed and supported by experimental evidence, this does not preclude the likelihood that different combinations of these mechanisms may be active at various times during the course of TMEV-induced disease and in animals with varying genetic composition.

***Direct virus effects on oligodendrocytes*** While it is generally agreed that immune activation plays a major role in demyelination, several lines of evidence also support a role for direct effects of viral infection on oligodendrocytes. In cultures of mixed neonatal brain cells, TMEV infection of oligodendrocytes is primarily lytic (Graves *et al.*, 1986; Rodriguez *et al.*, 1988). Two days after infection, many cultured oligodendrocytes display cytopathic ultrastructural changes characteristic of picornavirus infection, such as numerous cytoplasmic vacuoles and disruption of the endoplasmic reticulum, with preservation of mitochondria (see Fig. 44.2). The number of oligodendrocytes in these cultures begins to diminish within 48 hours after infection and by 7 days has decreased to 50% of the value in uninfected control cultures (Rodriguez *et al.*, 1988). Since TMEV infects oligodendrocytes *in vivo* (Graves *et al.*, 1986; Ohara *et al.*, 1990; Rodriguez *et al.*, 1988) and kills these cells *in vitro*, demyelination as a direct cellular consequence of the infection of oligodendrocytes seems plausible.

A direct demonstration that infection can produce demyelination without the need for an accompanying activation of the immune response comes from studies of demyelination in nude mice which lack circulating T cells and cell mediated immunity (Roos and Wollmann, 1984; Rosenthal *et al.*, 1986). In these studies, infection of BALB/c *nu/nu* mice with the DA strain of TMEV resulted in the development of significant neurologic deficits by 2 to 3 weeks and death within 4 to 8 weeks. Demyelinated foci were observed in the spinal cord by 14 days post-infection even though inflammatory infiltrates were minimal. Electron microscopy revealed numerous infected and degenerating glial cells, some that were identified as oligodendrocytes. Damaged myelin was observed around intact axons as well as completely demyelinated axons. In general, the demyelinated lesions in these mice were small and inflammation is minimal compared to what might be expected in most susceptible strains of mice, suggesting that other mechanisms of demyelination may normally play a more prominent role. However, these observations do indicate that TMEV-induced glial damage can occur in the absence of a T-cell mediated immune response.

In immunocompetent mice, the cytoplasm of most oligodendrocytes from infected animals appears normal on electron microscopic examination (Dal Canto and Lipton, 1975; Rodriguez *et al.*, 1983), even though viral RNA and antigen have been detected in oligodendrocytes throughout the course of persistent infection (Brahic *et al.*, 1981; Rodriguez *et al.*, 1983; Trottier *et al.*, 2001). Rodriguez (Rodriguez *et al.*, 1983; Rodriguez, 1985) reported ultrastructural abnormalities of the innermost extent of the myelin sheath and has proposed a "dying back" mechanism for demyelination. In persistently infected SJL mice, the inner tongue of the myelin sheath, which is the most distal extent of the myelin lamellae, often exhibits swelling and abnormalities in the normal cytoachitecture. Abnormalities included vacuolization, degeneration of mitochondria, increased numbers of microfilaments, and the appearance of electron-dense bodies and debris. These indications of damage to the innermost layer of the myelin sheath were observed in the absence of any signs of damage to the external surface of the sheath, indicating that damage to the oligodendrocyte may occur before immune-mediated damage to the myelin surface. Immunoperoxidase studies revealed that viral antigen was present on both the inner and outer extents of the myelin lamellae, even though the ultrastructural abnormalities were restricted to the inner loops. The observed degeneration appears to begin in the inner loop of the oligodendrocyte lamellae and then proceeds proximally toward the cytoplasm with the ultimate destruction of the myelin sheath.

The "dying back" concept was initially proposed as a mechanism underlying peripheral neuropathies in which the cell body is unable to support the structure and metabolism of a distant cellular process (Spencer and Schaumburg, 1976). It seems particularly relevant that Ludwin and Johnson (1981) initially reported the "dying back" of oligodendrocytes in a very different model for CNS demyelination in which demyelination is induced by ingestion of the toxic, copper-chelating agent, cuprizone. Dying back oligodendrogliopathy may therefore represent a general mechanism for demyelination in the CNS.

***TMEV-specific immune damage*** Dying back oligodendrogliopathy could be the direct result of viral infection on the cellular physiology of oligodendrocytes. However, it has been demonstrated that the demyelination observed following persistent TMEV infection in susceptible mouse strains is, at least in part, immune mediated (Lipton and Dal Canto, 1976b). Dying back might also be the result of damage due to TMEV-specific immune reactions directed against infected oligodendrocytes.

In cultures of mixed neonatal brain cells, immunoperoxidase staining visualized with electron microscopy demonstrated large amounts of viral antigen on the oligodendrocyte cell membrane (Rodriguez *et al.*, 1988). Similarly, staining *in vivo* can detect virus antigen in persistently infected oligodendrocytes by 28 days post-infection (Rodriguez *et al.*, 1983). Antigen is present in the cell cytoplasm as well as in the myelin lamellae. Infected animals typically produce high titers of virus-specific antibody and the recognition of virus antigen on the cell surface by these immunoglobulins may result in oligodendrocyte injury through several antibody dependent mechanisms including complement activation, antibody-dependent cell-mediated cytotoxicity (ADCC), or receptor mediated phagocytosis by macrophages.

Alternatively, viral antigen might also be presented on the cell surface in the context of the MHC class I or class II proteins. MHC class I, in particular, is known to be up-regulated in oligodendrocytes following TMEV infection of the CNS (Altintas *et al.*, 1993; Lindsley *et al.*, 1992). In susceptible mouse strains, class-I MHC is up-regulated in the CNS by one day after infection and remains high in the spinal cord white matter throughout chronic infection and demyelination. A novel antigen such as viral peptide, presented on the cell surface by MHC class-I, might generate a class-I restricted cytotoxic T lymphocyte (CTL) response, which might cause primary demyelination as the result of chronic non-lethal injury to TMEV-infected oligodendrocytes. However, mice with a disrupted $\beta_2$-microglobulin ($\beta_2$-m) gene do not express significant levels of MHC class-I, do not have functional $CD8^+$ T cells, and therefore cannot mount a CTL response. When $\beta_2$-m knockout mice from a resistant haplotype are infected with TMEV, resistance is abrogated and the virus establishes persistent CNS infection. However, significant demyelination develops in these mice (Fiette *et al.*, 1993; Pullen *et al.*, 1993; Rodriguez *et al.*, 1993), demonstrating that $CD8^+$ class I-restricted cytotoxic T cells are probably not the primary mediators of CNS demyelination. In general agreement with these observations, $\beta_2$-m knockout mice from a susceptible haplotype display somewhat enhanced levels of demyelination (Begolka *et al.*, 2001). Similar results have been obtained with mice carrying a genetic deletion of the gene encoding CD8, which display little alteration in the disease phenotype in either resistant or susceptible strains (Murray *et al.*, 1998).

***Bystander damage*** In contrast to observations with MHC class-I and CD8, treatment of susceptible mice with neutralizing antibodies against MHC class-II (anti-Ia) and anti-CD4 has been shown to reduce demyelination (Gerety *et al.*, 1994; Rodriguez *et al.*, 1986a; Welsh *et al.*, 1987). These observations suggest that class-II restricted $CD4^+$ T lymphocytes might play a role in disease pathogenesis. Clatch and coworkers (1986) attempted to correlate the development of clinical disease with several pathophysiologic parameters including virus titer, titer of anti-TMEV specific antibody, delayed-type hypersensitivity (DTH), and T-cell proliferative responses. The extent of TMEV-induced demyelinating disease correlated most closely with the presence of high levels of TMEV-specific DTH.

The development of TMEV specific delayed-type hypersensitivity would require an initial presentation of virus antigen to $T_H$ cells by MHC class-II, resulting in activation and clonal expansion. Generally, the activated T cells are of the $CD4^+$ $T_H1$ subtype and are often referred to as $T_{DTH}$ cells. Upon secondary contact with antigen, $T_{DTH}$ cells secrete cytokines that recruit and activate macrophages and other nonspecific inflammatory cells. Development of the DTH response may take 48 to 72 hours and by the time the reaction is fully developed, the vast majority of the activated cells at the site of inflammation are nonspecific immune cells and macrophages which act as the primary effector cells of the DTH response. These cells release a variety of cytotoxic mediators which results in nonspecific "bystander" damage to cells in the area of the response. In the CNS of an animal with persistent TMEV infection, any cell that presents virus antigen with MHC class-II might therefore serve as a nidus for the development of a DTH response.

The concept of DTH as a mechanism of demyelination is supported by adoptive transfer experiments using the sTV1 T-cell line or using TMEV sensitized lymph node T cells. sTV1 is a DTH-mediating $CD4^+$ $T_H1$ line that is specific for the immunodominant

$VP2_{74-86}$ peptide of TMEV. Transfer of $5 \times 10^6$ peptide-stimulated sTV1 cells into SJL mice that had been infected with a suboptimal dose of virus, significantly potentiated clinical disease in the recipient mice. Animals that received cells but did not receive virus to provide secondary cellular stimulation did not develop disease. An experimental scheme using lymph node T cells from mice primed with UV-inactivated virus instead of sTV1 cells resulted in similar potentiation of disease but only when virus was present for secondary stimulation (Gerety *et al.*, 1994). Further supporting the notion of DTH mediated demyelination, induction of peripheral immune tolerance to TMEV significantly reduces the development of DTH, general inflammation, virus-specific immune responses, and demyelination, following infection with the virus (Karpus *et al.*, 1995).

***Epitope spreading*** While the precise mechanisms may not yet be clear, it is well accepted that TMEV persistence in the CNS stimulates a virus-specific immune response that initiates damage to CNS cells and myelin. Recent studies have also detected myelin-reactive T cells in chronically infected mice. The appearance of T cells that are reactive to myelin autoepitopes is presumably due to the development of an immune response to myelin antigens that are released during the initial stages of TMEV-induced demyelination. It has been proposed that these autoreactive T cells are pathogenic and that they may be a major source of pathology during the chronic stages of demyelinating disease. The generation of a myelin-specific pathologic immune response, following an initial event of virus-induced demyelination, is called "Epitope spreading" (Lehmann *et al.*, 1993; McRae *et al.*, 1995).

Earlier attempts to detect myelin reactive T cells from TMEV infected mice had been unsuccessful (Miller *et al.*, 1990). However, Miller and coworkers (1997) have now reported that 3 to 4 weeks after initiation of demyelinating disease, T-cell responses to a series of myelin autoepitopes begin to appear in an ordered progression. T-cell proliferation and DTH responses to myelin peptides were first demonstrated at about 50 days post-infection. By 164 days post-infection, reactivity was shown for multiple peptide epitopes from proteolipid protein (PLP), myelin basic protein (MBP), myelin oligodendrocyte glycoprotein (MOG), and mouse spinal cord homogenate. T-cell hybridoma clones specific for the immunodominant peptides of TMEV, and lymph node T cells from TMEV primed mice, did not show reactivity to myelin peptides. Conversely, lymph node T cells from myelin primed mice did not show reactivity to TMEV peptides. These results suggest that the reactivity to myelin epitopes was specific and not due to cross-reactivity with TMEV. Additionally, sequence comparison of the reactive myelin peptides to TMEV showed no strong homologies that might indicate a likely source of cross-reactivity.

An epitope spreading mechanism for TMEV-induced demyelinating disease would be very similar to the pathologic mechanism of EAE. Adoptive transfer of myelin reactive immune cells from animals with EAE effectively transfers the disease to naïve animals. However, attempts to transfer TMEV-induced demyelinating disease by the transfer of T cells from infected animals have been unsuccessful (Barbano *et al.*, 1984). Initial attempts to suppress TMEV-induced disease by inducing neuroantigen-specific tolerance to a heterogeneous mixture of CNS antigens were unsuccessful (Miller *et al.*, 1990). More recently, induction of myelin-specific tolerance with a fusion protein containing MBP and PLP sequences has been reported to reduce demyelination and CNS inflammation in mice with TMEV-induced demyelinating disease (Neville *et al.*, 2002).

Studies of TMEV-induced disease in CD4 knockout mice are in potential disagreement with the idea of CD4-dependent mechanisms of demyelination such as bystander damage (DTH) or epitope spreading. Murray and coworkers (1998) examined the effect of CD4 deletion in both resistant (C57BL/6) and susceptible (SJL and PLJ) genetic backgrounds. In a resistant background, the absence of CD4 resulted in the establishment of persistent viral infection in the CNS and with the development of demyelination by 90 days post-infection. In both susceptible strains, demyelination was dramatically increased.

It is not immediately obvious how best to address and reconcile the various observations described here. It might be noted, however, that CD4 plays an important role in immune control of viral infection and that TMEV titers in CD4 knockout mice were generally elevated during the disease. The development of TMEV-induced pathology likely reflects a delicate balance between viral titer and activity and a dynamic immune response to the virus. As experimental protocols alter various aspects of this balance, such as virus titer and the quality and quantity of the participating immune cells, the mechanisms of pathology may also change in ways that make the interpretation of the data less straightforward than expected. In addition to the complexity of the system, different strains of TMEV are currently being used by the most active research groups. The BeAn 8386 and Daniel's (DA) strains are both widely used and although both establish robust, persistent infections of the spinal cord, the BeAn strain is generally less virulent that the DA strain. The precise significance of the use of these two strains to the interpretation and comparison of data is not yet clear.

*Molecular mimicry* Like the epitope spreading model, molecular mimicry involves pathogenesis due to myelin reactive autoimmunity. However, in molecular mimicry, the autoimmune response results from structural homologies between TMEV and myelin proteins. Immune recognition of the virus therefore also gives rise to an anti-myelin response, and this autoimmunity is pathogenic.

While molecular mimicry is probably an important mechanism for other CNS diseases (Rouse and Deshpande, 2002; Yuki, 2001), several observations suggest that it may not play a prominent role in TMEV-induced disease. TMEV infection is followed by a rapid and robust immune response that includes the development of both TMEV-specific antibodies and T cells by 7 days post-infection. Demyelinating disease is first observed by about 21 days post-infection and does not reach a peak until 90 to 100 days. The temporal difference between the development of the TMEV-specific immune response and the appearance of demyelinating disease argues against molecular mimicry as an important component of the demyelination mechanism. Furthermore, the initial immune response to TMEV does not cross-react with several myelin antigens including MBP, PLP, and MOG (Miller *et al.*, 1997). No strong homologies have been reported between TMEV protein sequences and those of the major myelin proteins.

### *Mechanisms of Axonal Damage and the Development of Neurologic Deficits*

In the past, demyelination alone has often been considered to be sufficient for the development of axonal damage and neurologic deficits. However, both the timing and mechanisms of demyelination and axonal damage can be distinct and different in the TMEV model. Quantitative assessment of demyelination and neurologic ability in two susceptible mouse strains shows that small demyelinated lesions, accompanied by statistically significant decreases in motor ability, can occur as early as 24 days post-infection (McGavern *et al.*, 1999). However, axonal damage and neurologic deficits do not necessarily follow demyelination. Several reports have documented that deficiency of MHC class-I ($\beta_2$-microglobulin mutants) or MHC class-II ($Ab^o$ mutants) function, will abrogate resistance to TMEV-induced disease in otherwise resistant strains of mice (Fiette *et al.*, 1993; Njenga *et al.*, 1996; Pullen *et al.*, 1993; Rodriguez *et al.*, 1993). Resistant mice that are homozygous for either of these mutations develop extensive demyelination. However, class-II deficient mice develop severe neurologic deficits as indicated by significant reductions in spontaneous activity, while class-I deficient mice show no clinical signs. Electrophysiologic measurement of the conduction velocity of motor-evoked potentials shows that decreased conduction velocities accompany deficits in class-II deficient mice with chronic demyelination. Conduction velocities in class-I deficient mice are no different that those in uninfected controls (Rivera-Quinones *et al.*, 1998). These findings demonstrate that demyelination and neurologic deficits are genetically and functionally separable, and they implicate a role for MHC class-I in the development of neurologic deficits following demyelination.

A role for MHC class-I in the development of neurologic deficits implicates $CD8^+$ T cells as the pathologic effector cell for the induction of neurologic disease. Granule exocytosis (perforin release) and Fas ligand expression are two of the common cytopathic effector functions of CD8 cells, and mice deficient for perforin, Fas, and Fas ligand were tested to determine whether these molecules play a role in the development of demyelination and clinical disease (Murray *et al.*, 1998). *Lpr* (Fas mutation) and *Gld* (Fas ligand) mutant mice, on a TMEV-resistant genetic background, maintained resistance to viral persistence and demyelinating disease. Perforin-deficient mice developed persistent viral infection and chronic demyelination of spinal cord white matter. Despite demyelination and virus persistence, these mice showed only minimal neurologic deficits. These studies indicate that perforin release is the pathologic effector for the induction of neurologic disease by $CD8^+$ T cells.

The experiments described earlier for the determination of the roles played by class-I and class-II related mechanisms for the development of axonal damage were all performed in mice with the C57BL/6 or C57BL/6×129 genetic background. C57BL/6 mice mount a vigorous CTL response to TMEV. This response is predominantly directed against a single immunodominant TMEV peptide that represents amino acids 121 to 130 of the VP2 capsid protein, which is presented in the context of the H-2$D^b$ MHC class-I molecule (Borson *et al.*, 1997). At 7 days post-infection, staining of $CD8^+$ brain infiltrating lymphocytes with $D^b$:$VP2_{121-130}$ tetramers shows that 50 to 63% of the infiltrating $CD8^+$ cells are virus specific (Johnson *et al.*, 1999). Mice with a targeted disruption of the Ifn-$\gamma$ receptor gene respond to virus infection with rapidly progressing disease and severe clinical deficits. These mice also develop a class-I restricted anti-viral response that is dominanted by the $VP2_{121-130}$ epitope. In these mice, intravenous injection of the VP2 peptide one day before virus infection completely eliminates the immunodominant T-cell response (Johnson *et al.*, 2001). Elimination of the response does not cause a significant increase in viral titer. There is no change in the overall pattern of infection: by 45 days virus is primarily localized to the white matter of the spinal cord, there is no significant increase in inflammation, and demyelination is similar in extent to control animals. Elimination of the response did, however, significantly preserve motor function in infected animals. At 45 days after infection, VP2 peptide treated animals performed significantly better than control animals in tests of motor ability, although not as well as uninfected animals. These results suggest that the $CD8^+$ T cells that mediate neurologic dysfunction are most likely the TMEV-specific cells that infiltrate the CNS following infection.

In contrast to the work done in mice with the TMEV-resistant C57BL/6 genetic background, susceptible SJL mice that lack $CD8^+$ effector function ($\beta_2$-microglobulin knockouts) are not rescued from TMEV-induced neurologic deficits (Begolka *et al.*, 2001). Instead, these mice show an earlier onset of neurologic disease, with enhanced CNS demyelination and macrophage infiltration at 50 days post-infection. These results indicate that in these mice, $CD8^+$ cells are not required for the initiation or progression of demyelinating disease and may illustrate the strong influence that genetic background can have on the development of this disease.

### Remyelination Following TMEV-Induced Demyelination

Myelin repair, or remyelination, is a normal physiologic response to myelin damage. However, the ability of mice to repair the damage caused by TMEV-induced demyelinating disease is strongly dependent on the genetic constitution of the animal. $\beta_2$-microglobulin deficient mice lack MHC class-I function. On a C57BL/6×129 genetic background, these mice develop extensive demyelination following TMEV infection (Rivera-Quinones *et al.*, 1998). Despite the presence of persistent viral infection, these animals show extensive remyelination by 6 months post-infection (Miller *et al.*, 1995). This spontaneous remyelination of CNS axons involves both oligodendrocytes and Schwann cells. In contrast, MHC class-II deficient mice on the same genetic background also develop demyelinating disease but subsequent remyelination is largely absent (Njenga *et al.*, 1999). Class-II deficient mice fail to produce TMEV-specific IgG and eventually developed high viral titers. However, the animals do not die during the acute phase of the disease but survive well into the chronic demyelinating phase, even though most die by 120 days post-infection. Failure to observe remyelination may simply reflect insufficient time for myelin repair to occur before death. Significant axonal damage is also apparent in these mice and this damage may also preclude remyelination.

Like MHC class-II deficient mice, the SJL strain is susceptible to TMEV infection, develops extensive demyelinating disease, and does not repair myelin damage. In contrast to class-II deficient mice, SJL mice control viral infection effectively and can survive for over a year with persistent infection and chronic demyelinating disease. The disease in SJL mice progresses from demyelination, through mild neurologic deficits, to profound deficits and paralysis. Two general hypotheses have been proposed to explain the absence of remyelination in these mice (Miller *et al.*, 1996). First, an inhibitory local environment may be present, which prevents spontaneous repair. Local inflammation, reactive astrocytes, microglia, or damaged axons might play a role. Second, an absence of growth factors or oligodendrocyte precursor cells may prevent efficient remyelination. Which of these mechanisms is the most important remains unclear. The absence of spontaneous remyelination in SJL mice, however, has provided an excellent experimental system for the study of ways to enhance the remyelination process, and several potential therapeutic approaches have been studied and developed using this system (Asakura *et al.*, 1998; Drescher *et al.*, 1998; Njenga *et al.*, 2000; Ure and Rodriguez, 2002; Warrington *et al.*, 2000).

Whatever the mechanisms of remyelination, it seems clear that remyelination is associated with improved neurologic function. Like the SJL strain, PL/J mice develop chronic demyelinating disease but do not remyelinate. PL/J mice that are deficient for either $CD8^+$ or $CD4^+$ T cells show a significant increase in the severity of disease pathogenesis (Murray *et al.*, 1998). The disease is particularly severe in PL/J CD4 mutant mice. While early mortality is common in these animals, many survive up to 6 months post-infection, and many of the mice that survive to the chronic phase of the disease have nearly complete spontaneous remyelination. Importantly, all of the surviving mice show partial recovery of motor function that coincides with myelin repair, and the extent of recovery correlates strongly with the percentage of lesioned white matter area that has remyelinated (Murray *et al.*, 2001). These observations clearly demonstrate that functional recovery is possible despite previous demyelination and ongoing persistent virus infection, and that remyelination correlates with this recovery.

## MOUSE HEPATITIS VIRUS (MHV)

Murine hepatitis virus (MHV) is a member of the *Coronaviridae*, a family of large, enveloped, plus-strand RNA viruses. MHV is a common enteric pathogen of mice and rats that occasionally disseminates to the CNS. Like TMEV, the original isolation and characterization of one of the most commonly studied strains, MHV-JHM, occurred with the spontaneous appearance of two paralyzed mice, and the subsequent passage of the virus in mouse brain were it continued to produce paralytic disease (Cheever *et al.*, 1948; Pappenheimer, 1958). Later passages of the virus resulted primarily in encephalitic disease with accompanying demyelination. The demyelinating phase of MHV infection has been used as a model for human demyelinating disease

### Virus Biology and Life Cycle

The MHV genome is a 31 kb message-strand RNA that is capped and polyadenylated. The genomic RNA is complexed with the viral nucleocapsid phosphoprotein (N) to form a long, helical nucleocapsid. The nucleocapsid lies within a lipoprotein envelop that consists largely of intracellular host cell membrane and three viral capsid proteins: membrane protein (M), spike protein (S), and hemagglutinin-esterase protein (HE).

MHV virions bind to the plasma membrane of the host cell by the interaction of the spike proteins with the host receptor. Biliary glycoprotein 1a (Bgp1a), a member of the immunoglobulin superfamily, is a known MHV receptor (Williams *et al.*, 1991). The main determinant of cellular tropism is the ability of the spike protein to react with a suitable receptor on the cell surface and infected cell populations in the animal closely match those with demonstrated expression of the Bgp1a receptor. However, very little Bgp1a is expressed on CNS glia and neurons, and the mechanism of virus entry into these cells is still uncertain. The MHV virion also contains the HE protein. Binding of HE to 9-O-acetylated neuraminic acid residues on the plasma membrane may serve as an important pre-receptor function that facilitates viral entry.

After receptor binding, the viral envelope fuses with the plasma membrane in an S-protein mediated event. Once the RNA genome has entered the cytoplasm of the cell, it is translated into a polyprotein that is co- and post-translationally processed into multiple proteins. These proteins, which include the capsid proteins (N, M, S, and HE), the virus-specific RNA-dependent RNA polymerase, and virus encoded proteases, play various roles in the replication and development of infectious virus. The RNA-dependent RNA polymerase uses the positive-strand genomic RNA as a template to produce full-length negative-strand RNA, which in turn is used to make more positive-strand genomic RNA. Overlapping sets of 3′ co-terminal subgenomic positive-strand RNAs are also produced and translated into viral gene products. The newly synthesized genomic RNA assembles with nucleocapsid (N) protein to form the helical nucleocapsid. The S, HE, and M glycoproteins are all translated on membrane bound polysomes and are co-translationally inserted into intracellular membranes. Virions begin to form when nucleocapsids bind to intracellular membranes that contain the viral M protein and virus then buds from these specialized membranes. S and HE proteins are incorporated into the virions during budding while host proteins are excluded. After budding, mature virions accumulate in large, smooth-walled vesicles that release virus when they fuse with the plasma membrane.

### Disease Pathology

The outcome of MHV infection depends on several variables such as virus strain, virus dose and route of infection, age, and genetic composition of the host. Two different MHV strains, MHV-A59 and MHV-JHM, have been used in most studies of MHV-induced demyelination. As the name suggests, hepatitis is a common outcome of MHV infection but while infection with the MHV-A59 strain results in prominent hepatitis, MHV-JHM infected animals show little or no evidence of hepatitis. However, intracerebral or intranasal infection with either strain results in acute, sometimes fatal, encephalitis, followed by the development of chronic demyelination in animals that survive. To decrease mortality and thereby facilitate the study of MHV pathogenesis, several MHV-JHM variants have been developed that have limited neurotropism related lethality but that continue to produce an early encephalitis followed by acute primary demyelination (Erlich *et al.*, 1987; Fleming *et al.*, 1986; Haspel *et al.*, 1978).

MHV infects a variety of CNS cell types including astrocytes, oligodendrocytes, microglia and neurons. As virus replicates to high titers in the brain and spinal cord, it is controlled by the development of an anti-viral immune response that is largely restricted to the CNS. Control of infection correlates well with the appearance of an inflammatory infiltrate by 4 to 7 days post-infection. This acute inflammatory response is characterized by the influx of many types of immune effector cells including $CD4^{+}$ and $CD8^{+}$ T cells, B cells, macrophages, and natural killer cells (Williamson *et al.*, 1991). Virus neutralizing antibodies appear in the serum by 7 to 9 days post-infection but probably do not play a critical role in initial virus clearance. Infectious virus is cleared from the CNS by 10 to 14 days but complete clearance is not achieved and virus persists in the CNS. Infectious virus is rarely recovered from spinal cord tissue after the acute phase of infection. Virus antigen can be detected for several months after initial clearance and appears to persist in astrocytes and oligodendrocytes (Sun *et al.*, 1995). Viral RNA can be detected in the CNS for at least a year after infection (Lavi *et al.*, 1984).

Demyelination with axonal sparing can be detected as early as 5 days post-infection. MHV-induced demyelination is illustrated in Figure 44.5. Relatively few inflammatory cells but large numbers of debris containing macrophages characterize demyelinated lesions, and their appearance correlates well with the development of lesions (Lane *et al.*, 2000). Electron microscopy demonstrates macrophage processes extending between the

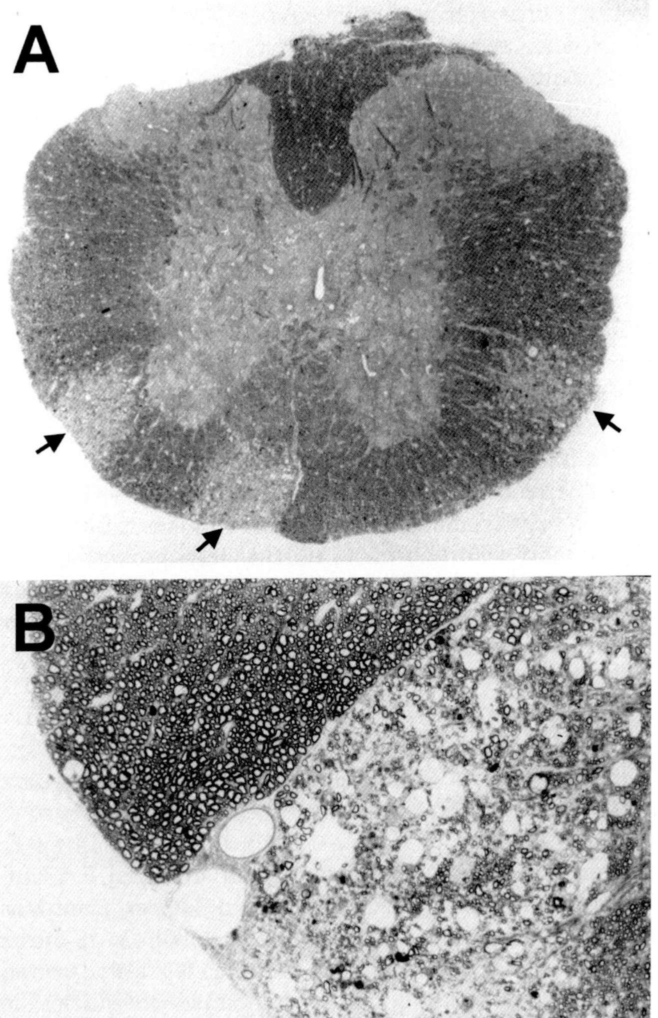


FIGURE 44.5
Pathology of the MHV-infected spinal cord. (A) A section of spinal cord tissue from an SJL mouse infected with MHV-A59 and then stained for myelin with para-phenylene-diamine shows multiple white matter lesions (arrows). (B) Normal white matter lies adjacent to a demyelinated lesion in the ventral spinal cord tracts. Myelin destruction in the lesioned area is apparent.

layers of myelin sheaths, strongly suggesting an active role for macrophages in the demyelination process (Powell and Lampert, 1975). Demyelination continues to develop until about 21 days after infection and then begins to slow. Spontaneous remyelination is common following the initial phase encephalitis and demyelination. After the initial phase of encephalitis, demyelination, and viral clearance, virus persistence results in a second phase that probably continues for the life of the animal and that is associated with the recurrent episodes of demyelination.

## Virus Resistance

Infected adult mice generate a potent immune response that clears the virus in 10 to 14 days. $CD4^+$ and $CD8^+$ T cells are the most critical elements of this response. Viral infection results in the rapid recruitment of large numbers of $CD8^+$ T cells to the CNS parenchyma, while $CD4^+$ cells are primarily localized to the perivasculature and meninges.

$CD8^+$ T cells are the primary immune effectors of virus clearance. MHC class-I tetramer staining shows that over 50% of the $CD8^+$ T cells in the CNS after infection are virus specific (Bergmann *et al.*, 1999). As virus is cleared, the total number of $CD8^+$ cells in the

CNS decreases but the percentage of cells that are virus-specific remains high. Initially the infiltrating $CD8^+$ cells display virus-specific cytolytic activity. As clearance progresses and persistence is established, these cells lose their cytolytic function while retaining their ability to secrete Ifn-$\gamma$, indicating differential regulation of $CD8^+$ effector functions as the course of infection progresses. Consistent with a role for $CD8^+$ cells in virus clearance, CD8 deficient mice show increases in viral titer, increased mortality, and an inability to efficiently clear virus after infection (Lane *et al.*, 2000; Williamson *et al.*, 1990).

$CD8^+$ cells probably use two different effector mechanisms to clear virus from different subsets of infected cells. Perforin-mediated cytolysis may play an essential role in the control of virus infection of astrocytes and microglia. Perforin deficient mice are able to clear MHV from the CNS but the clearance is delayed by several days (Lin *et al.*, 1997b), indicating that perforin-dependent CTL plays a role in viral clearance from the CNS. Histologic analysis has shown that virus-specific CTL are more efficient at the clearance of virus from astrocytes and macrophages than from oligodendrocytes (Stohlman *et al.*, 1995). Ifn-$\gamma$ is the antiviral mechanism primarily responsible for controlling the infection of oligodendrocytes (Parra *et al.*, 1999). In Ifn-$\gamma$ deficient mice, MHV infection results in increased neurologic disability and mortality that is associated with increased viral titers and delayed viral clearance. The anti-viral antibody response and the CTL response are not affected. Increases of viral antigen in Ifn-$\gamma$ deficient mice are located almost exclusively in oligodendrocytes and are accompanied by increased numbers of $CD8^+$ cells in CNS white matter. $CD8^+$ cells are therefore major participants in MHV clearance and employ at least two different effectors mechanisms to clear virus from different types of infected cells. Some studies have also suggested that the Fas-Fas ligand system may play a role (Parra *et al.*, 2000).

Although the ability to control MHV replication is predominantly controlled by $CD8^+$ cells, this response is highly dependent on the $CD4^+$ T-cell response (Stohlman *et al.*, 1998). Adoptive transfer of activated CTL into recipients that have been depleted of $CD4^+$ cells shows that although the $CD8^+$ cells can effectively traffic to sites of CNS infection in the absence of $CD4^+$ cells, once they arrive they rapidly undergo apoptosis. These observations indicate that the survival of the $CD8^+$ cells that are primarily responsible for virus clearance may depend critically on support from $CD4^+$ cells. Consistent with these observations, studies on CD4 deficient mice show increases in viral titer, increased mortality, and an inability to efficiently clear virus, a pathologic phenotype very similar to that observed for CD8 deficient mice (Lane *et al.*, 2000).

CD4 deficient mice also exhibit a significant reduction in the number of activated macrophages and microglia in the CNS of infected animals (Lane *et al.*, 2000). This may result from a decrease in the expression of the chemokine RANTES that is secreted by $CD4^+$ cells and acts to recruit infiltrating mononuclear cells to the CNS. In strong support of this idea, *in vivo* depletion of RANTES with RANTES-specific antiserum mimics the phenotype seen in CD4 deficient mice.

Despite the increases in viral titer, increased mortality, and inability to clear virus, CD4 mutant mice that survive infection show a general decrease in inflammation and demyelination. It has been proposed that these decreases may result directly from a reduction in the infiltration of macrophages that are involved in myelin destruction. However, depletion of blood-borne macrophages with toxic liposomes prior to infection has little effect on demyelination (Xue *et al.*, 1999). Large numbers of activated macrophages/microglia are still present in the CNS after liposome treatment suggesting that the activity of resident microglia may play a central role in demyelination. Macrophage depletion prior to infection does result in increased mortality, suggesting a role for macrophages in the control of viral titers prior to the development of the T-cell responses (Wijburg *et al.*, 1997; Xue *et al.*, 1999).

The role of antibody in viral clearance and the establishment of persistence has been studied in mice that lack a normal humoral immune response (Lin *et al.*, 1999). Mice homozygous for a disruption in the immunoglobulin mu gene lack B cells. In these mice, virus is cleared normally during acute infection but then virus titers increase dramatically after about 11 days post-infection, when the titer of infectious virus in wild-type animals has fallen to undetectable levels. Passive transfer of MHV immune serum following initial virus clearance prevents this secondary rise in virus titers. These data demonstrate that initial clearance of virus is largely antibody independent but that antibody may play a key role in controlling the reemergence of virus in the CNS during persistent infection.

## Mechanisms of Demyelination and Axonal Damage

The mechanisms of demyelination during MHV infection are not yet entirely clear. *A priori,* the potential mechanisms involved in MHV-induced demyelination might be similar to those involved in TMEV-induced demyelinating disease—that is, direct virus lysis of infected oligodendrocytes, virus-specific immune-mediated destruction of oligodendrocytes and myelin, macrophage-mediated "bystander" damage to oligodendrocytes and myelin, and myelin damage by "epitope spreading" or "molecular mimicry."

Several studies have shown that virus actively replicates in oligodendrocytes and that morphologic and biochemical changes accompany oligodendrocyte infection *in vivo* (Barac-Latas *et al.*, 1997; Powell *et al.*, 1975). Down-regulation of oligodendrocyte gene expression along with oligodendrocyte destruction by necrosis and apoptosis have been reported for both the early and late stages of demyelinating disease (Barac-Latas *et al.*, 1997). These types of observations have supported the suggestion that direct viral cytolysis might play a role in the development of demyelination. However, it seems clear that an immune component is essential for the full development of demyelinating disease. JHM-MHV infection of severe combined immunodeficiency (SCID) mice, which lack T lymphocytes, does not result in either demyelination or paralysis (Houtman and Fleming, 1996). Similarly, mice deficient in recombinase-activating gene (RAG) activity lack both B- and T-cell function and do not develop demyelination after MHV infection (Wu and Perlman, 1999). Infected RAG mice, whose immune system has been reconstituted by the adoptive transfer of spleen cells from genetically identical immunocompetent mice that have been immunized for MHV, developed demyelination within 7 to 9 days after transfer. Demyelination rarely occurs if donor mice have not been preimmunized against MHV, demonstrating that MHV-specific T cells are critical for the development of demyelination.

The demyelination that follows reconstitution of immune function is characterized by the extensive recruitment of activated macrophages and microglia to sites of demyelinating lesions, consistent with a potential role for these cells in the development of myelin damage. These observations are also consistent with the idea that RANTES, secreted by $CD4^+$ cells, plays a key role in the recruitment of macrophages to lesions and that activated macrophages and microglia may be primary mediators of myelin destruction (Lane *et al.*, 2000). A mechanism of $CD4^+$-dependent, nonspecific damage mediated by infiltrating macrophages bears strong resemblance to the "bystander" damage induced by the development of a DTH response in the TMEV model.

Although these data suggest a significant role for the immune system in the development of demyelination, a recent report on the infection of RAG mice with MHV-A59 demonstrated typical demyelinated lesions (Matthews *et al.*, 2002). T cells may therefore play a central role in the development of demyelination but other mechanisms may also be important, and the relative contributions of specific mechanisms may depend on variables such as virus strain and the host genetic background.

The question of axonal damage after MHV infection is separate from the question of demyelination. MHV infection is generally characterized by demyelination with axonal sparing, but axonal injury at sites of demyelination has been described (Stohlman and Weiner, 1981). In contrast to the TMEV model, where neurologic deficits tend to occur well after primary demyelination is established, most studies have shown that MHV induced paralysis and demyelination occur almost simultaneously, indicating that axonal damage occurs early in disease. In the experiments described earlier, animals that lack T cells, such as RAG and SCID mice, do not develop demyelination, but reconstitution of these animals by the adoptive transfer of spleen cells results in demyelination by 7 days post-transfer. Axonal damage appears with exactly the same pattern following MHV infection in these mice (Dandekar *et al.*, 2001). Using the appearance of nonphosphorylated neurofilament as a marker for axonal damage, the onset of axonal damage was shown to be coincident with the appearance of demyelination. Damaged axons were detected not only at sites of active demyelination but also in areas with heavy macrophage infiltration but no obvious demyelination. Axonal damage therefore occurs very early in the disease process and nonspecific inflammation may play a key role.

In the TMEV model, the secondary development of a pathogenic immune response directed against myelin antigens or "epitope spreading" has been proposed as an important mechanism for the exacerbation and maintenance of demyelination. JHM-MHV infection of either Brown Norway or Lewis rats results in a subacute demyelinating disease. Infection of Lewis rats also results in lymphocytes that proliferate in response to myelin basic protein and that produce mild encephalitis upon adoptive transfer into naïve recipients (Watanabe *et al.*, 1983). Lymphocytes from infected Brown Norway rats did not develop MBP sensitivity, demonstrating a strong host strain dependence for this response (Watanabe *et al.*, 1987). The production of pathogenic anti-myelin antibodies demonstrates potential for an epitope spreading mechanism of MHV-induced disease, but the extent to which this mechanism contributes to the development of the chronic demyelinating disease is an unresolved issue.

Antibodies, either autoreactive or anti-viral, might directly mediate demyelination by mechanisms such as antibody-dependent or complement-mediated cytotoxicity. In general, little correlation has been found between anti-MHV antibody titers and the severity of demyelination. The role of B cells and antibody has been studied directly in mice with mutations in the immunoglobulin mu gene; these mice lack B cells and make no antibody. In B-cell deficient mice, demyelination following MHV infection is significantly more severe than in controls at 30 to 60 days post-infection (Matthews *et al.*, 2002). This increase may be due to the inability of the animals to control virus after the acute phase of the disease. Animals that can produce antibody but lack antibody receptors (Fc) or components of the complement pathway are able to clear virus but still develop demyelination (Matthews *et al.*, 2002). These data indicate that antibody and antibody-dependent effector mechanisms are probably not central to the demyelination process.

Demyelination after MHV infection is clearly a complex event and probably results from some combination of direct viral destruction and immune-mediated damage. There does not, however, appear to be any single lymphocyte or monocyte function that is primarily responsible for the immune component of the damage. Both MHV-specific and nonspecific immune responses are probably involved.

## References

Adami, C., Pritchard, A. E., Knauf, T., Luo, M., and Lipton, H. L. (1998). A determinant for central nervous system persistence localized in the capsid of Theiler's murine encephalomyelitis virus by using recombinant viruses. *J. Virol.* **72,** 1662–1665.

Altintas, A., Cai, Z., Pease, L. R., and Rodriguez, M. (1993). Differential expression of H-2K and H-2D in the central nervous system of mice infected with Theiler's virus. *J. Immunol.* **151,** 2803–2812.

Asakura, K., Miller, D. J., Pease, L. R., and Rodriguez, M. (1998). Targeting of IgM kappa antibodies to oligodendrocytes promotes CNS remyelination. *J. Neurosci.* **18,** 7700–7708.

Aubagnac, S., Brahic, M., and Bureau, J. F. (1999). Viral load and a locus on chromosome 11 affect the late clinical disease caused by Theiler's virus. *J. Virol.* **73,** 7965–7971.

Aubert, C., Chamorro, M., and Brahic, M. (1987). Identification of Theiler's virus infected cells in the central nervous system of the mouse during demyelinating disease. *Microb Pathog.* **3,** 319–326.

Azoulay, A., Brahic, M., and Bureau, J. F. (1994). FVB mice transgenic for the H-2Db gene become resistant to persistent infection by Theiler's virus. *J. Virol.* **68,** 4049–4052.

Barac-Latas, V., Suchanek, G., Breitschopf, H., Stuehler, A., Wege, H., and Lassmann, H. (1997). Patterns of oligodendrocyte pathology in coronavirus-induced subacute demyelinating encephalomyelitis in the Lewis rat. *Glia* **19,** 1–12.

Barbano, R. L., and Dal Canto, M. C. (1984). Serum and cells from Theiler's virus-infected mice fail to injure myelinating cultures or to produce in vivo transfer of disease. The pathogenesis of Theiler's virus-induced demyelination appears to differ from that of EAE. *J. Neurol. Sci.* **66,** 283–293.

Begolka, W. S., Haynes, L. M., Olson, J. K., Padilla, J., Neville, K. L., Dal Canto, M., Palma, J., Kim, B. S., and Miller, S. D. (2001). CD8-deficient SJL mice display enhanced susceptibility to Theiler's virus infection and increased demyelinating pathology. *J. Neurovirol.* **7,** 409–420.

Bergmann, C. C., Altman, J. D., Hinton, D., and Stohlman, S. A. (1999). Inverted immunodominance and impaired cytolytic function of CD8$^+$ T cells during viral persistence in the central nervous system. *J. Immunol.* **163,** 3379–3387.

Bihl, F., Brahic, M., and Bureau, J. F. (1999). Two loci, *Tmevp2* and *Tmevp3*, located on the telomeric region of chromosome 10, control the persistence of Theiler's virus in the central nervous system of mice. *Genetics* **152,** 385–392.

Bihl, F., Pena-Rossi, C., Guenet, J. L., Brahic, M., and Bureau, J. F. (1997). The *shiverer* mutation affects the persistence of Theiler's virus in the central nervous system. *J. Virol.* **71,** 5025–5030.

Borson, N. D., Paul, C., Lin, X., Nevala, W. K., Strausbauch, M. A., Rodriguez, M., and Wettstein, P. J. (1997). Brain-infiltrating cytolytic T lymphocytes specific for Theiler's virus recognize H-2D$^b$ molecules complexed with a viral VP2 peptide lacking a consensus anchor residue. *J. Virol.* **71,** 5244–5250.

Brahic, M., Stroop, W. G., and Baringer, J. R. (1981). Theiler's virus persists in glial cells during demyelinating disease. *Cell* **26,** 123–128.

Bureau, J. F., Drescher, K. M., Pease, L. R., Vikoren, T., Delcroix, M., Zoecklein, L., Brahic, M., and Rodriguez, M. (1998). Chromosome 14 contains determinants that regulate susceptibility to Theiler's virus-induced demyelination in the mouse. *Genetics* **148,** 1941–1949.

Bureau, J. F., Montagutelli, X., Bihl, F., Lefebvre, S., Guenet, J. L., and Brahic, M. (1993). Mapping loci influencing the persistence of Theiler's virus in the murine central nervous system. *Nat. Genet.* **5,** 87–91.

Cardin, A. D., and Weintraub, H. J. (1989). Molecular modelling of protein-glycosaminoglycan interactions. *Arteriosclerosis* **9,** 21–32.

Cheever, F. S., Daniels, J. B., Pappenheimer, A. M., and Bailey, O. T. (1948). A murine virus (JHM) causing disseminated encephalomyelitis with extensive destruction of myelin. *J. Exp. Med.* **90,** 181–194.

Chen, H. H., Kong, W. P., Zhang, L., Ward, P. L., and Roos, R. P. (1995). A picornaviral protein synthesized out of frame with the polyprotein plays a key role in a virus-induced immune-mediated demyelinating disease. *Nat. Med.* **1,** 927–931.

Clatch, R. J., Lipton, H. L., and Miller, S. D. (1986). Characterization of Theiler's murine encephalomyelitis virus (TMEV)-specific delayed-type hypersensitivity responses in TMEV-induced demyelinating disease: Correlation with clinical signs. *J. Immunol.* **136,** 920–927.

Clatch, R. J., Melvold, R. W., Miller, S. D., and Lipton, H. L. (1985). Theiler's murine encephalomyelitis virus (TMEV)-induced demyelinating disease in mice is influenced by the H-2D region: Correlation with TEMV-specific delayed-type hypersensitivity. *J Immunol.* **135,** 1408–1414.

Clatch, R. J., Miller, S. D., Metzner, R., Dal Canto, M. C., and Lipton, H. L. (1990). Monocytes/macrophages isolated from the mouse central nervous system contain infectious Theiler's murine encephalomyelitis virus (TMEV). *Virology* **176,** 244–254.

Dal Canto, M. C., and Lipton, H. L. (1975). Primary demyelination in Theiler's virus infection. An ultrastructural study. *Lab Invest.* **33,** 626–637.

Dandekar, A. A., Wu, G. F., Pewe, L., and Perlman, S. (2001). Axonal damage is T cell mediated and occurs concomitantly with demyelination in mice infected with a neurotropic coronavirus. *J. Virol.* **75,** 6115–6120.

Daniels, J. B., Pappenheimer, A. M., and Richardson, S. (1952). Observations on Encephalitis of Mice. *J. Exp. Med.* **96,** 517.

Dethlefs, S., Escriou, N., Brahic, M., van der Werf, S., and Larsson-Sciard, E. L. (1997). Theiler's virus and Mengo virus induce cross-reactive cytotoxic T lymphocytes restricted to the same immunodominant VP2 epitope in C57BL/6 mice. *J. Virol.* **71,** 5361–5365.

Drescher, K. M., Rivera-Quinones, C., Lucchinetti, C. F., and Rodriguez, M. (1998). Failure of treatment with Linomide or oral myelin tolerization to ameliorate demyelination in a viral model of multiple sclerosis. *J. Neuroimmunol.* **88,** 111–119.

Erlich, S. S., Fleming, J. O., Stohlman, S. A., and Weiner, L. P. (1987). Experimental neuropathology of chronic demyelination induced by a JHM virus variant (DS). *Arch. Neurol.* **44,** 839–842.

Fiette, L., Aubert, C., Brahic, M., and Rossi, C. P. (1993). Theiler's virus infection of beta 2-microglobulin-deficient mice. *J. Virol.* **67,** 589–592.

Fleming, J. O., Trousdale, M. D., el-Zaatari, F. A., Stohlman, S. A., and Weiner, L. P. (1986). Pathogenicity of antigenic variants of murine coronavirus JHM selected with monoclonal antibodies. *J. Virol.* **58,** 869–875.

Fotiadis, C., Kilpatrick, D. R., and Lipton, H. L. (1991). Comparison of the binding characteristics to BHK-21 cells of viruses representing the two Theiler's virus neurovirulence groups. *Virology* **182,** 365–70.

Fu, J., Rodriguez, M., and Roos, R. P. (1990b). Strains from both Theiler's virus subgroups encode a determinant for demyelination. *J. Virol.* **64,** 6345–6348.

Fu, J. L., Stein, S., Rosenstein, L., Bodwell, T., Routbort, M., Semler, B. L., and Roos, R. P. (1990a). Neurovirulence determinants of genetically engineered Theiler viruses. *Proc. Natl. Acad. Sci. USA* **87,** 4125–4129.

Ghadge, G. D., Ma, L., Sato, S., Kim, J., and Roos, R. P. (1998). A protein critical for a Theiler's virus-induced immune system-mediated demyelinating disease has a cell type-specific antiapoptotic effect and a key role in virus persistence. *J. Virol.* **72,** 8605–8612.

Gerety, S. J., Rundell, M. K., Dal Canto, M. C., and Miller, S. D. (1994). Class II-restricted T cell responses in Theiler's murine encephalomyelitis virus-induced demyelinating disease. VI. Potentiation of demyelination with and characterization of an immunopathologic CD4$^+$ T cell line specific for an immunodominant VP2 epitope. *J. Immunol.* **152,** 919–929.

Grant, R. A., Filman, D. J., Fujinami, R. S., Icenogle, J. P., and Hogle, J. M. (1992). Three-dimensional structure of Theiler virus. *Proc. Natl. Acad. Sci. USA* **89,** 2061–2065.

Graves, M. C., Bologa, L., Siegel, L., and Londe, H. (1986). Theiler's virus in brain cell cultures: Lysis of neurons and oligodendrocytes and persistence in astrocytes and macrophages. *J. Neurosci. Res.* **15,** 491–501.

Haspel, M. V., Lampert, P. W., and Oldstone, M. B. (1978). Temperature-sensitive mutants of mouse hepatitis virus produce a high incidence of demyelination. *Proc. Natl. Acad. Sci. USA* **75,** 4033–6.

Hertzler, S., Luo, M., and Lipton, H. L. (2000). Mutation of predicted virion pit residues alters binding of Theiler's murine encephalomyelitis virus to BHK-21 cells. *J. Virol.* **74,** 1994–2004.

Houtman, J. J., and Fleming, J. O. (1996). Dissociation of demyelination and viral clearance in congenitally immunodeficient mice infected with murine coronavirus JHM. *J. Neurovirol.* **2,** 101–110.

Jakob, J., and Roos, R. P. (1996). Molecular determinants of Theiler's murine encephalomyelitis-induced disease. *J. Neurovirol.* **2,** 70–77.

Jelachich, M. L., Bandyopadhyay, P., Blum, K., and Lipton, H. L. (1995). Theiler's virus growth in murine macrophage cell lines depends on the state of differentiation. *Virology* **209,** 437–444.

Jnaoui, K., Minet, M., and Michiels, T. (2002). Mutations that affect the tropism of DA and GDVII strains of Theiler's virus *in vitro* influence sialic acid binding and pathogenicity. *J. Virol.* **76,** 8138–8147.

Johnson, A. J., Njenga, M. K., Hansen, M. J., Kuhns, S. T., Chen, L., Rodriguez, M., and Pease, L. R. (1999). Prevalent class I-restricted T-cell response to the Theiler's virus epitope $D^b$:$VP2_{121-130}$ in the absence of endogenous CD4 help, tumor necrosis factor alpha, gamma interferon, perforin, or costimulation through CD28. *J. Virol.* **73,** 3702–3708.

Johnson, A. J., Upshaw, J., Pavelko, K. D., Rodriguez, M., and Pease, L. R. (2001). Preservation of motor function by inhibition of $CD8^+$ virus peptide-specific T cells in Theiler's virus infection. *FASEB J.* **15,** 2760–2762.

Kappel, C. A., Melvold, R. W., and Kim, B. S. (1990). Influence of sex on susceptibility in the Theiler's murine encephalomyelitis virus model for multiple sclerosis. *J. Neuroimmunol.* **29,** 15–19.

Karpus, W. J., Pope, J. G., Peterson, J. D., Dal Canto, M. C., and Miller, S. D. (1995). Inhibition of Theiler's virus-mediated demyelination by peripheral immune tolerance induction. *J. Immunol.* **155,** 947–957.

Lane, T. E., Liu, M. T., Chen, B. P., Asensio, V. C., Samawi, R. M., Paoletti, A. D., Campbell, I. L., Kunkel, S. L., Fox, H. S., and Buchmeier, M. J. (2000). A central role for CD4(+) T cells and RANTES in virus-induced central nervous system inflammation and demyelination. *J. Virol.* **74,** 1415–1424.

Lavi, E., Gilden, D. H., Highkin, M. K., and Weiss, S. R. (1984). Persistence of mouse hepatitis virus A59 RNA in a slow virus demyelinating infection in mice as detected by in situ hybridization. *J. Virol.* **51,** 563–566.

Lehmann, P. V., Sercarz, E. E., Forsthuber, T., Dayan, C. M., Gammon, G. (1993). Determinant spreading and the dynamics of the autoimmune T-cell repertoire. *Immunol. Today* **14,** 203–208.

Lehrich, J. R., Arnason, B. G., and Hochberg, F. H. (1976). Demyelinative myelopathy in mice induced by the DA virus. *J. Neurol. Sci.* **29,** 149–160.

Levy, M., Aubert, C., and Brahic, M. (1992). Theiler's virus replication in brain macrophages cultured in vitro. *J. Virol.* **66,** 3188–3193.

Lin, M. T., Hinton, D. R., Marten, N. W., Bergmann, C. C., and Stohlman, S. A. (1999). Antibody prevents virus reactivation within the central nervous system. *J Immunol.* **162,** 7358–7368.

Lin, M. T., Stohlman, S. A., and Hinton, D. R. (1997b). Mouse hepatitis virus is cleared from the central nervous systems of mice lacking perforin-mediated cytolysis. *J. Virol.* **71,** 383–391.

Lin, X., Pease, L. R., and Rodriguez, M. (1997a). Differential generation of class I H-2D-versus H-2K-restricted cytotoxicity against a demyelinating virus following central nervous system infection. *Eur. J. Immunol.* **27,** 963–970.

Lin, X., Sato, S., Patick, A. K., Pease, L. R., Roos, R. P., and Rodriguez, M. (1998). Molecular characterization of a nondemyelinating variant of Daniel's strain of Theiler's virus isolated from a persistently infected glioma cell line. *J. Virol.* **72,** 1262–1269.

Lindsley, M. D., Patick, A. K., Prayoonwiwat, N., and Rodriguez, M. (1992). Coexpression of class I major histocompatibility antigen and viral RNA in central nervous system of mice infected with Theiler's virus: A model for multiple sclerosis. *Mayo Clin. Proc.* **67,** 829–838.

Lindsley, M. D., and Rodriguez, M. (1989). Characterization of the inflammatory response in the central nervous system of mice susceptible or resistant to demyelination by Theiler's virus. *J. Immunol.* **142,** 2677–2682.

Lipton, H. L. (1975). Theiler's virus infection in mice: An unusual biphasic disease process leading to demyelination. *Infect. Immun.* **11,** 1147–1155.

Lipton, H. L. (1978). Characterization of the TO strains of Theiler's mouse encephalomyelitis viruses. *Infect. Immun.* **20,** 869–872.

Lipton, H. L., Calenoff, M., Bandyopadhyay, P., Miller, S. D., Dal Canto, M. C., Gerety, S., and Jensen, K. (1991). The 5′ noncoding sequences from a less virulent Theiler's virus dramatically attenuate GDVII neurovirulence. *J. Virol.* **65,** 4370–4377.

Lipton, H. L., and Dal Canto, M. C. (1976a). Chronic neurologic disease in Theiler's virus infection of SJL/J mice. *J. Neurol. Sci.* **30,** 201–207.

Lipton, H. L., and Dal Canto, M. C. (1976b). Theiler's virus-induced demyelination: Prevention by immunosuppression. *Science* **192,** 62–64.

Lipton, H. L., and Dal Canto, M. C. (1979). Susceptibility of inbred mice to chronic central nervous system infection by Theiler's murine encephalomyelitis virus. *Infect. Immun.* **26,** 369–374.

Lipton, H. L., and Melvold, R. (1984). Genetic analysis of susceptibility to Theiler's virus-induced demyelinating disease in mice. *J. Immunol.* **132,** 1821–1825.

Lipton, H. L., Pritchard, A. E., and Calenoff, M. A. (1998). Attenuation of neurovirulence of Theiler's murine encephalomyelitis virus strain GDVII is not sufficient to establish persistence in the central nervous system. *J. Gen. Virol.* **79,** 1001–1004.

Lipton, H. L., Twaddle, G., and Jelachich, M. L. (1995). The predominant virus antigen burden is present in macrophages in Theiler's murine encephalomyelitis virus-induced demyelinating disease. *J. Virol.* **69,** 2525–2533.

Lorch, Y., Friedmann, A., Lipton, H. L., and Kotler, M. (1981). Theiler's murine encephalomyelitis virus group includes two distinct genetic subgroups that differ pathologically and biologically. *J. Virol.* **40,** 560–567.

Lucchinetti, C. F., and Rodriguez, M. (1997). The controversy surrounding the pathogenesis of the multiple sclerosis lesion. *Mayo Clin. Proc.* **72,** 665–678.

Ludwin, S. K., and Johnson, E. S. (1981). Evidence for a "dying-back" gliopathy in demyelinating disease. *Ann. Neurol.* **9,** 301–305.

Luo, M., He, C., Toth, K. S., Zhang, C. X., and Lipton, H. L. (1992). Three-dimensional structure of Theiler murine encephalomyelitis virus (BeAn strain). *Proc. Natl. Acad. Sci. USA* **89,** 2409–2413.

Luo, M., Toth, K. S., Zhou, L., Pritchard, A., and Lipton, H. L. (1996). The structure of a highly virulent Theiler's murine encephalomyelitis virus (GDVII) and implications for determinants of viral persistence. *Virology* **220,** 246–250.

Matthews, A. E., Lavi, E., Weiss, S. R., and Paterson, Y. (2002). Neither B cells nor T cells are required for CNS demyelination in mice persistently infected with MHV-A59. *J. Neurovirol.* **8,** 257–264.

McGavern, D. B., Murray, P. D., Rivera-Quinones, C., Schmelzer, J. D., Low, P. A., and Rodriguez, M. (2000). Axonal loss results in spinal cord atrophy, electrophysiological abnormalities and neurological deficits following demyelination in a chronic inflammatory model of multiple sclerosis. *Brain* **123,** 519–531.

McGavern, D. B., Zoecklein, L., Drescher, K. M., and Rodriguez, M. (1999). Quantitative assessment of neurologic deficits in a chronic progressive murine model of CNS demyelination. *Exp. Neurol.* **158,** 171–181.

McRae, B. L., Vanderlugt, C. L., Dal Canto, M. C., and Miller S. D. (1995). Functional evidence for epitope spreading in the relapsing pathology of experimental autoimmune encephalomyelitis. *J. Exp. Med.* **182,** 75–85.

Melvold, R. W., Jokinen, D. M., Miller, S. D., Dal Canto, M. C., and Lipton, H. L. (1990). Identification of a locus on mouse chromosome 3 involved in differential susceptibility to Theiler's murine encephalomyelitis virus-induced demyelinating disease. *J. Virol.* **64,** 686–690.

Miller, D. J., Asakura, K., and Rodriguez, M. (1996). Central nervous system remyelination clinical application of basic neuroscience principles. *Brain Pathol.* **6,** 331–344.

Miller, D. J., Rivera-Quinones, C., Njenga, M. K., Leibowitz, J., and Rodriguez, M. (1995). Spontaneous CNS remyelination in beta 2 microglobulin-deficient mice following virus-induced demyelination. *J. Neurosci.* **15,** 8345–8352.

Miller, S. D., Gerety, S. J., Kennedy, M. K., Peterson, J. D., Trotter, J. L., Tuohy, V. K., Waltenbaugh, C., Dal Canto, M. C., and Lipton, H. L. (1990). Class II-restricted T cell responses in Theiler's murine encephalomyelitis virus (TMEV)-induced demyelinating disease. III. Failure of neuroantigen-specific immune tolerance to affect the clinical course of demyelination. *J. Neuroimmunol.* **26,** 9–23.

Miller, S. D., Vanderlugt, C. L., Begolka, W. S., Pao, W., Yauch, R. L., Neville, K. L., Katz-Levy, Y., Carrizosa, A., and Kim, B. S. (1997). Persistent infection with Theiler's virus leads to CNS autoimmunity via epitope spreading. *Nat. Med.* **3,** 1133–1136.

Murray, P. D., McGavern, D. B., Sathornsumetee, S., and Rodriguez, M. (2001). Spontaneous remyelination following extensive demyelination is associated with improved neurological function in a viral model of multiple sclerosis. *Brain* **124,** 1403–1416.

Murray, P. D., Pavelko, K. D., Leibowitz, J., Lin, X., and Rodriguez, M. (1998). CD4(+) and CD8(+) T cells make discrete contributions to demyelination and neurologic disease in a viral model of multiple sclerosis. *J. Virol.* **72,** 7320–7329.

Neville, K. L., Padilla, J., and Miller, S. D. (2002). Myelin-specific tolerance attenuates the progression of a virus-induced demyelinating disease: Implications for the treatment of MS. *J. Neuroimmunol.* **123,** 18–29.

Nitayaphan, S., Omilianowski, D., Toth, M. M., Parks, G. D., Rueckert, R. R., Palmenberg, A. C., and Roos, R. P. (1986). Relationship of Theiler's murine encephalomyelitis viruses to the cardiovirus genus of picornaviruses. *Intervirology* **26,** 140–148.

Njenga, M. K., Asakura, K., Hunter, S. F., Wettstein, P., Pease, L. R., and Rodriguez, M. (1997). The immune system preferentially clears Theiler's virus from the gray matter of the central nervous system. *J. Virol.* **71,** 8592–8601.

Njenga, M. K., Coenen, M. J., DeCuir, N., Yeh, H. Y., and Rodriguez, M. (2000). Short-term treatment with interferon-alpha/beta promotes remyelination, whereas long-term treatment aggravates demyelination in a murine model of multiple sclerosis. *J. Neurosci. Res.* **59,** 661–670.

Njenga, M. K., Murray, P. D., McGavern, D., Lin, X., Drescher, K. M., and Rodriguez, M. (1999). Absence of spontaneous central nervous system remyelination in class II-deficient mice infected with Theiler's virus. *J. Neuropathol. Exp. Neurol.* **58,** 78–91.

Njenga, M. K., Pavelko, K. D., Baisch, J., Lin, X., David, C., Leibowitz, J., and Rodriguez, M. (1996). Theiler's virus persistence and demyelination in major histocompatibility complex class II-deficient mice. *J. Virol.* **70,** 1729–1737.

Noseworthy, J. H. (1998). Multiple sclerosis clinical trials: Old and new challenges. *Semin. Neurol.* **18,** 377–388.

Noseworthy, J. H., Lucchinetti, C., Rodriguez, M., and Weinshenker, B. G. (2000). Multiple sclerosis. *N. Engl. J. Med.* **343,** 938–952.

Ohara, Y., Konno, H., Iwasaki, Y., Yamamoto, T., Terunuma, H., and Suzuki, H. (1990). Cytotropism of Theiler's murine encephalomyelitis viruses in oligodendrocyte-enriched cultures. *Arch. Virol.* **114,** 293–298.

Ohara, Y., Stein, S., Fu, J. L., Stillman, L., Klaman, L., and Roos, R. P. (1988). Molecular cloning and sequence determination of the DA strain of Theiler's murine encephalomyelitis viruses. *Virology* **164,** 245–255.

Pappenheimer, A. M. (1958). Pathology of infection with the JHM virus. *J. Natl. Cancer Inst.* **20,** 879–891.

Parra, B., Hinton, D. R., Marten, N. W., Bergmann, C. C., Lin, M. T., Yang, C. S., and Stohlman, S. A. (1999). IFN-gamma is required for viral clearance from central nervous system oligodendroglia. *J. Immunol.* **162,** 1641–1647.

Parra, B., Lin, M. T., Stohlman, S. A., Bergmann, C. C., Atkinson, R., and Hinton, D. R. (2000). Contributions of Fas-Fas ligand interactions to the pathogenesis of mouse hepatitis virus in the central nervous system. *J. Virol.* **74,** 2447–2450.

Patick, A. K., Lindsley, M. D., and Rodriguez, M. (1990). Differential pathogenesis between mouse strains resistant and susceptible to Theiler's virus-induced demyelination. *Sem. Virol.* **1,** 281–288.

Patick, A. K., Pease, L. R., David, C. S., and Rodriguez, M. (1990). Major histocompatibility complex-conferred resistance to Theiler's virus-induced demyelinating disease is inherited as a dominant trait in B10 congenic mice. *J. Virol.* **64,** 5570–5576.

Pevear, D. C., Borkowski, J., Calenoff, M., Oh, C. K., Ostrowski, B., and Lipton, H. L. (1988). Insights into Theiler's virus neurovirulence based on a genomic comparison of the neurovirulent GDVII and less virulent BeAn strains. *Virology* **165,** 1–12.

Pevear, D. C., Calenoff, M., Rozhon, E., and Lipton, H. L. (1987). Analysis of the complete nucleotide sequence of the picornavirus Theiler's murine encephalomyelitis virus indicates that it is closely related to cardioviruses. *J. Virol.* **61,** 1507–1516.

Pevear, D. C., Luo, M., and Lipton, H. L. (1988). Three-dimensional model of the capsid proteins of two biologically different Theiler virus strains: Clustering of amino acid difference identifies possible locations of immunogenic sites on the virion. *Proc. Natl. Acad. Sci. USA* **85,** 4496–4500.

Powell, H. C., and Lampert, P. W. (1975). Oligodendrocytes and their myelin-plasma membrane connections in JHM mouse hepatitis virus encephalomyelitis. *Lab Invest.* **33**(4):440–445.

Pullen, L. C., Miller, S. D., Dal Canto, M. C., and Kim, B. S. (1993). Class I-deficient resistant mice intracerebrally inoculated with Theiler's virus show an increased T cell response to viral antigens and susceptibility to demyelination. *Eur. J. Immunol.* **23,** 2287–2293.

Reddi, H. V., and Lipton, H. L. (2002). Heparan sulfate mediates infection of high-neurovirulence Theiler's viruses. *J. Virol.* **76,** 8400–8407.

Rivera-Quinones, C., McGavern, D., Schmelzer, J. D., Hunter, S. F., Low, P. A., and Rodriguez, M. (1998). Absence of neurological deficits following extensive demyelination in a class I-deficient murine model of multiple sclerosis. *Nat. Med.* **4,** 187–193.

Rodriguez, M. (1985). Virus-induced demyelination in mice: "dying back" of oligodendrocytes. *Mayo Clin. Proc.* **60,** 433–438.

Rodriguez, M., and David, C. S. (1985). Demyelination induced by Theiler's virus: Influence of the H-2 haplotype. *J. Immunol.* **135,** 2145–2148.

Rodriguez, M., Dunkel, A. J., Thiemann, R. L., Leibowitz, J., Zijlstra, M., and Jaenisch, R. (1993). Abrogation of resistance to Theiler's virus-induced demyelination in H-$2^b$ mice deficient in beta 2-microglobulin. *J. Immunol.* **151,** 266–276.

Rodriguez, M., Lafuse, W. P., Leibowitz, J., and David, C. S. (1986a). Partial suppression of Theiler's virus-induced demyelination in vivo by administration of monoclonal antibodies to immune-response gene products (Ia antigens). *Neurology* **36,** 964–970.

Rodriguez, M., Leibowitz, J., and David, C. S. (1986b). Susceptibility to Theiler's virus-induced demyelination. Mapping of the gene within the H-2D region. *J. Exp. Med.* **163,** 620–631.

Rodriguez, M., Leibowitz, J. L., and Lampert, P. W. (1983). Persistent infection of oligodendrocytes in Theiler's virus-induced encephalomyelitis. *Ann. Neurol.* **13,** 426–433.

Rodriguez, M., Nabozny, G. H., Thiemann, R. L., and David, C. S. (1994). Influence of deletion of T cell receptor V beta genes on the Theiler's virus model of multiple sclerosis. *Autoimmunity* **19,** 221–230.

Rodriguez M, Oleszak E., and Leibowitz J. (1987). Theiler's murine encephalomyelitis: A model of demyelination and persistence of virus. *Crit Rev Immunol.* **7,** 325–365.

Rodriguez, M., Patick, A. K., Pease, L. R., and David, C. S. (1992). Role of T cell receptor V beta genes in Theiler's virus-induced demyelination of mice. *J. Immunol.* **148,** 921–927.

Rodriguez, M., Pavelko, K. D., Njenga, M. K., Logan, W. C., and Wettstein, P. J. (1996). The balance between persistent virus infection and immune cells determines demyelination. *J. Immunol.* **157,** 5699–5709.

Rodriguez, M., and Roos, R. P. (1992). Pathogenesis of early and late disease in mice infected with Theiler's virus, using intratypic recombinant GDVII/DA viruses. *J. Virol.* **66,** 217–225.

Rodriguez, M., Siegel, L. M., Hovanec-Burns, D., Bologa, L., and Graves, M. C. (1988). Theiler's virus-associated antigens on the surfaces of cultured glial cells. *Virology* **166,** 463–474.

Roos, R. P., and Wollmann, R. (1984). DA strain of Theiler's murine encephalomyelitis virus induces demyelination in nude mice. *Ann. Neurol.* **15,** 494–499.

Rosenthal, A., Fujinami, R. S., and Lampert, P. W. (1986). Mechanism of Theiler's virus-induced demyelination in nude mice. *Lab Invest.* **54,** 515–522.

Rossi, C. P., Delcroix, M., Huitinga, I., McAllister, A., van Rooijen, N., Claassen, E., and Brahic, M. (1997). Role of macrophages during Theiler's virus infection. *J. Virol.* **71,** 3336–3340.

Rouse, B. T., and Deshpande, S. (2002). Viruses and autoimmunity: An affair but not a marriage contract. *Rev. Med. Virol.* **12,** 107–113.

Rueckert, R. R. (1996). Picornaviridae: The Viruses and Their Replication. *In* "Fields Virology" (Fields, Knipe, Howley, Chanock, Melnick, Monath, Roizman, and Strauss, eds.), 3rd ed., pp. 609–654. Lippincott-Raven, Philadelphia.

Sapatino, B. V., Petrescu, A. D., Rosenbaum, B. A., Smith, R., 3rd, Piedrahita, J. A., and Welsh, C. J. Characteristics of cloned cerebrovascular endothelial cells following infection with Theiler's virus. II. Persistent infection. *J. Neuroimmunol.* **62,** 127–135.

Sarchielli, P., Trequattrini, A., Usai, F., Murasecco, D., and Gallai, V. (1993). Role of viruses in the etiopathogenesis of multiple sclerosis. *Acta Neurol. (Napoli)* **15,** 363–381.

Shaw-Jackson, C., and Michiels, T. (1997). Infection of macrophages by Theiler's murine encephalomyelitis virus is highly dependent on their activation or differentiation state. *J. Virol.* **71,** 8864–8867.

Sibley, W. A., Bamford, C. R., and Clark, K. (1985). Clinical viral infections and multiple sclerosis. *Lancet* **1,** 1313–1315.

Spencer, P. S., and Schaumburg, H. H. (1976). Central-peripheral distal axonopathy: The pathology of dying-back polyneuropathies. *Prog. Neuropathol.* **3,** 253–295.

Stohlman, S. A., and Weiner, L. P. (1981). Chronic central nervous system demyelination in mice after JHM virus infection. *Neurology* **31,** 38–44.

Stohlman, S. A., Bergmann, C. C., Lin, M. T., Cua, D. J., and Hinton, D. R. (1998). CTL effector function within the central nervous system requires $CD4^+$ T cells. *J. Immunol.* **160,** 2896–2904.

Stohlman, S. A., Bergmann, C. C., van der Veen, R. C., and Hinton, D. R. (1995). Mouse hepatitis virus-specific cytotoxic T lymphocytes protect from lethal infection without eliminating virus from the central nervous system. *J. Virol.* **69,** 684–694.

Sun, N., Grzybicki, D., Castro, R. F., Murphy, S., and Perlman, S. (1995). Activation of astrocytes in the spinal cord of mice chronically infected with a neurotropic coronavirus. *Virology* **213,** 482–493.

Takata, H., Obuchi, M., Yamamoto, J., Odagiri, T., Roos, R. P., Iizuka, H., and Ohara, Y. (1998). L* protein of the DA strain of Theiler's murine encephalomyelitis virus is important for virus growth in a murine macrophage-like cell line. *J. Virol.* **72,** 4950–4955.

Toth, K. S., Zhang, C. X., Lipton, H. L., and Luo, M. (1993). Crystallization and preliminary X-ray diffraction studies of Theiler's virus (GDVII strain). *J. Mol. Biol.* **231,** 1126–1129.

Trapp, B. D., Peterson, J., Ransohoff, R. M., Rudick, R., Mork, S., and Bo, L. (1998). Axonal transection in the lesions of multiple sclerosis. *N. Engl. J. Med.* **338,** 278–285.

Trottier, M., Kallio, P., Wang, W., and Lipton, H. L. (2001). High numbers of viral RNA copies in the central nervous system of mice during persistent infection with Theiler's virus. *J. Virol.* **75,** 7420–7428.

Ure, D. R., and Rodriguez, M. (2002). Polyreactive antibodies to glatiramer acetate promote myelin repair in murine model of demyelinating disease. *FASEB J.* **16,** 1260–1262.

Warrington, A. E., Asakura, K., Bieber, A. J., Ciric, B., Van Keulen, V., Kaveri, S. V., Kyle, R. A., Pease, L. R., and Rodriguez, M. (2000). Human monoclonal antibodies reactive to oligodendrocytes promote remyelination in a model of multiple sclerosis. *Proc. Natl. Acad. Sci. USA* **97,** 6820–6825.

Watanabe, R., Wege, H., and ter Meulen, V. (1983). Adoptive transfer of EAE-like lesions from rats with coronavirus-induced demyelinating encephalomyelitis. *Nature* **305,** 150–153.

Watanabe, R., Wege, H., and ter Meulen, V. (1987). Comparative analysis of coronavirus JHM-induced demyelinating encephalomyelitis in Lewis and Brown Norway rats. *Lab Invest.* **57,** 375–384.

Webster, R. G., and Granoff, A. (Eds.). (1995). "Encyclopedia of Virology." Academic Press, San Diego, CA.

Welsh, C. J., Tonks, P., Nash, A. A., and Blakemore, W. F. (1987). The effect of L3T4 T cell depletion on the pathogenesis of Theiler's murine encephalomyelitis virus infection in CBA mice. *J. Gen. Virol.* **68,** 1659–1667.

Wijburg, O. L., Heemskerk, M. H., Boog, C. J., and Van Rooijen, N. (1997). Role of spleen macrophages in innate and acquired immune responses against mouse hepatitis virus strain A59. *Immunology* **92,** 252–258.

Williams, R. K., Jiang, G. S., and Holmes, K. V. (1991). Receptor for mouse hepatitis virus is a member of the carcinoembryonic antigen family of glycoproteins. Proc. *Natl. Acad. Sci. USA* **88,** 5533–5536.

Williamson, J. S., and Stohlman, S. A. (1990). Effective clearance of mouse hepatitis virus from the central nervous system requires both $CD4^+$ and $CD8^+$ T cells. *J. Virol.* **64,** 4589–4592.

Williamson, J. S., Sykes, K. C., and Stohlman, S. A. (1991). Characterization of brain-infiltrating mononuclear cells during infection with mouse hepatitis virus strain JHM. *J. Neuroimmunol.* **32,** 199–207.

Wroblewska, Z., Gilden, D. H., Wellish, M., Rorke, L. B., Warren, K. G., and Wolinsky, J. S. (1977). Virus-specific intracytoplasmic inclusions in mouse brain produced by a newly isolated strain of Theiler virus. I. Virologic and morphologic studies. *Lab. Invest.* **37,** 395–602.

Wu, G. F., and Perlman, S. (1999). Macrophage infiltration, but not apoptosis, is correlated with immune-mediated demyelination following murine infection with a neurotropic coronavirus. *J. Virol.* **73,** 8771–8780.

Xue, S., Sun, N., Van Rooijen, N., and Perlman, S. (1999). Depletion of blood-borne macrophages does not reduce demyelination in mice infected with a neurotropic coronavirus. *J. Virol.* **73,** 6327–6334.

Yuki, N. (2001). Infectious origins of, and molecular mimicry in, Guillain-Barre and Fisher syndromes. *Lancet Infect. Dis.* **1,** 29–37.

Zhang, L., Senkowski, A., Shim, B., and Roos, R. P. (1993). Chimeric cDNA studies of Theiler's murine encephalomyelitis virus neurovirulence. *J. Virol.* **67,** 4404–4408.

Zheng, L., Calenoff, M. A., and Dal Canto, M. C. (2001). Astrocytes, not microglia, are the main cells responsible for viral persistence in Theiler's murine encephalomyelitis virus infection leading to demyelination. *J. Neuroimmunol.* **118,** 256–267.

Zhou, L., Lin, X., Green, T. J., Lipton, H. L., and Luo, M. (1997). Role of sialyloligosaccharide binding in Theiler's virus persistence. *J. Virol.* **71,** 9701–9712.

Zhou, L., Luo, Y., Wu, Y., Tsao, J., and Luo, M. (2000). Sialylation of the host receptor may modulate entry of demyelinating persistent Theiler's virus. *J. Virol.* **74,** 1477–1485.

CHAPTER

# 45

# Models of Krabbe Disease

*Kunihiko Suzuki*

## INTRODUCTION

The classical form of human Krabbe disease (globoid cell leukodystrophy, GLD) is caused by genetic deficiency of galactosylceramidase activity (Wenger *et al.*, 2001; also see Chapter 35, in this book). The genetic leukodystrophy in West Highland and Cairn terrier dogs had been described earlier as globoid cell leukodystrophy on the basis of the characteristic neuropathology (Fankhäuser *et al.*, 1963). As soon as the genetic enzymatic defect in the human disease was identified (Suzuki and Suzuki, 1970), the dog GLD was recognized as genetically equivalent to human disease (Suzuki *et al.*, 1970). Several years later, a spontaneous mouse mutant was discovered at the Jackson Laboratory that showed characteristic neuropathology of GLD and was named twitcher (Duchen *et al.*, 1980). Its enzymatic basis was also identified as genetic galactosylceramidase deficiency (Kobayashi *et al.*, 1980). Bridging the gap between the human and other mammalian species is a mutant that occurs in the Rhesus monkey, discovered much later (Baskin *et al.*, 1998). Galactosylceramidase cDNA was cloned, and disease-causing mutations have been identified in the mouse (Sakai *et al.*, 1996), West Highland and Cairn terriers (Victoria *et al.*, 1996), and the Rhesus monkey (Luzi *et al.*, 1997). These models have been extensively utilized for studies of the pathogenesis and treatment of GLD. They provide varying advantages and disadvantages as animal models because of their different sizes and life spans. From time to time, globoid cell leukodystrophy identified by its unique neuropathology has also been described in other mammalian species and some other strain of dogs, but these conclusions were generally sporadic and are unavailable for follow-up studies. Thus, utility of these sporadic models, even if they might be enzymatically authentic, is limited.

In addition to the naturally occurring animal models, Luzi *et al.* recently generated an experimental mouse model in which a mutation, H168C, was introduced by homologous recombination (Luzi *et al.*, 2001). A genetically distinct form of globoid cell leukodystrophy has also been experimentally generated in the mouse by inactivating one of the sphingolipid activator proteins, saposin A (Matsuda *et al.*, 2001b). This resulted in a late-onset, chronic form of GLD. All aspects of its clinical, pathological, and biochemical phenotype were consistent with impaired degradation of galactosylceramidase substrates. This model established that saposin A is indispensable for normal physiological function of galactosylceramidase *in vivo*. This chapter emphasizes the mouse models and refers to other models from time to time as appropriate. For more details on models in other species, refer to (Wenger *et al.*, 2001).

## MOUSE MODELS

### Twitcher Mutant

The twitcher mutant was originally discovered as an autosomal recessive myelin mutant in the Jackson Laboratory (Bar Harbor, Maine) in 1976. Since the first clinico-pathological documentation (Duchen *et al.*, 1980) and the identification of the genetic defect in a lysosomal hydrolase, galactosylceramidase (Kobayashi *et al.*, 1980), it has been widely used as a convenient and useful experimental tool for investigations of the pathogenesis of and therapeutic approaches to GLD. Despite the large number of known neurological mouse mutants, the twitcher remains the only naturally occurring genetically authentic mouse model of human sphingolipidoses. Although the lack of authentic models of human sphingolipidoses among small laboratory animals is no longer a problem with the advent of the homologous recombination and transgenic technology, which allows experimental generation of basically any mouse models once the gene is isolated, the twitcher mutant remains the most thoroughly characterized and most extensively utilized because of its more than 20-year history. Successful cloning of the galactosylceramidase gene (Chen *et al.*, 1993; Sakai *et al.*, 1994) has led to identification of the mutation in the twitcher mutant (Sakai *et al.*, 1996).

#### *Clinical Phenotype*

Clinical manifestations are exclusively neurological, and their onset coincides with the onset of active myelination. This is understandable because the primary substrate of the defective enzyme, galalctosylceramide, is a nearly exclusive constituent of the myelin sheath and is not even synthesized until myelin formation begins. Thus, homozygous twitcher mice are indistinguishable at birth from their unaffected littermates. Affected mice stop gaining weight and become generally less active than their littermates by 15 to 20 days. Generalized tremulousness sets in before 20 days and progressive muscle weakness and eventual paralysis develop, particularly conspicuous in the hind limbs and the neck muscles. At the terminal stage around 40 to 45 days, their body weight is about one-third of normal mice (Igisu *et al.*, 1983a). Motor functions generally deteriorate rapidly after 20 days. Genetic background appears to influence the course of the disease significantly. Currently available twitcher mice are on the genetic background of C57/BL, and their life span rarely extends beyond 45 days. However, Duchen *et al.* observed in their first description of the mutant on a different genetic background that its life span was "up to 3 months," much longer than twitcher mice on the C57/BL background (Duchen *et al.*, 1980). As in most autosomal recessive disorders, heterozygous carriers are essentially normal. However, interestingly, subtle developmental delays in neurological and neurobehavioral parameters have been described during early development in male but not in female heterozygous carriers, although they eventually caught up with wild-type littermates (Olmstead 1987).

#### *Pathology*

Neuropathology is generally well correlated with progression of the clinical manifestations and is also almost entirely limited to the nervous system. Prior to clinical onset around 15 days, no neuropathological changes are apparent on the light microscopic level, although inclusions in oligodendrocytes may be detected on the ultrastructural level as early as 5 days. Macrophages infiltrate concomitantly with myelin degeneration into the spinal cord, cerebellar white matter, and brain stem after 20 days, then into the cerebral white matter after 25 days, and into cerebellar and cerebral gray matter after 30 days. Myelin degeneration begins at 10 to 20 days after commencement of myelination in any of the given nerve fiber tracts (Taniike and Suzuki, 1994). The brain of affected mice is slightly smaller than normal at the terminal stage, but no other gross abnormalities are present. The characteristic pathology in the central nervous system is demyelination, degeneration of oligodendrocytes, reactive astrocytosis, and infiltration of macrophages that contain periodic acid-Schiff (PAS)-positive materials ("globoid cells"). The macrophages are often clustered around blood vessels. Crystalloid or slender tubular inclusions, typical in human GLD, are present most abundantly in the macrophages but also in the oligodendrocytes. These pathological features are essentially identical with those in human Krabbe disease. The cerebral cortex and other regions of gray matter are relatively unaffected pathologically, except for occasional perivascular or perineuronal microglial cells containing similar inclusions. GFAP-immunoreactive astrocytes are abundant throughout the central nervous system, including gray matter (Kobayashi *et al.*, 1986; Mikoshiba *et al.*, 1985). This increase of GFAP-immunoreactive cells is accompanied by an increase in GFAP mRNA, which is detectable as early as 10 days when demyelination is not yet obvious.

Contrary to the central nervous system, peripheral nerves are grossly abnormal. They are abnormally thick, translucent, and firm and can easily be distinguished from normal nerves by visual inspection. There is segmental demyelination with evidence of remyelination associated with infiltration of macrophages containing the typical GLD inclusions and marked endoneurial edema that widely separates individual nerve fibers (Powell *et al.*, 1983). The Schwann cells of myelinated fibers frequently contain the characteristic GLD inclusions, and the Schwann cells of unmyelinated fibers are attenuated with unusually elongated or branching processes (Duchen *et al.*, 1980; Kobayashi *et al.*, 1988). GFAP immunoreactivity increases in Schwann cells as demyelination progresses (Kobayashi *et al.*, 1986). Microglia/macrophages in both CNS and PNS react positively with anti-Mac-1 and F4/80 antibodies. Although the pathology is largely confined to the nervous system, the kidney is an exception. Abnormal inclusions are frequently present in the renal epithelial cells. This renal pathology is distinctly different from the human disease, in which the kidney is essentially normal. This difference also reflects a distinct difference in biochemical abnormalities in the kidney among the human, canine, and murine diseases (discussed later).

### *Biochemistry*

The similarities of the clinical and pathological findings of the twitcher mouse to those in human Krabbe disease strongly suggested the same biochemical basis underlying GLD in the two species. A profound deficiency in galactosylceramidase activity in the brain and liver of the twitcher mice established it as an authentic mouse model of the human disease (Kobayashi *et al.*, 1980). Clinically and pathologically normal heterozygous carrier mice showed intermediate activities. Thus, the genetic cause in the twitcher mouse is the same as that in human Krabbe disease (Suzuki and Suzuki, 1970). Enzymatic assays using tips of clipped tails of newborn mice allows identification of the genetic status and thus makes experiments before the onset of clinical symptoms feasible (Kobayashi *et al.*, 1982). These enzymatic diagnoses have been largely superceded by molecular diagnosis since the mutation underlying twitcher mouse was identified.

Twitcher mouse shares the same unusual and apparently paradoxical analytical biochemistry with the human disease. Despite the genetic defect in the lysosomal hydrolase, galactosylceramidase, its primary physiological substrate, galactosylceramide, does not accumulate abnormally in the brain. The composition of galactolipids in the brain, spinal cord, and the sciatic nerve of twitcher mice is surprisingly normal during development (Igisu *et al.*, 1983a). Galactosylceramide and sulfatide are significantly decreased in later stages in twitcher brains, but the degree of decrease is far less than that in human GLD brains. In the twitcher spinal cord, the proportions of both galactosylceramide and sulfatide in the total lipids are normal at 16 and 25 days, but at 42 days, galactosylceramide is slightly less than the control (Igisu and Suzuki, 1984a). However, the total lipid was markedly decreased in the twitcher spinal cord at this age. Therefore, there is a much greater loss of galactosylceramide and sulfatide in the spinal cord than in the brain. In contrast to the brain, there is a massive accumulation of galactosylceramide in the kidney (Ida *et al.*, 1982; Igisu and Suzuki, 1984a; Igisu *et al.*, 1983b). Both HFA- and NFA-galactosylceramides are increased even at 16 days. They increase rapidly with progression of the disease. The parallel with the human disease breaks down here in that no increase in galactosylceramide was detected in the kidneys of human GLD patients (Suzuki, 1971).

The kidney in the dog model is intermediate between the human and murine disease in that there is only a slight increase in galactosylceramide associated with occasional inclusion bodies. In addition, moderate increases of galactosylceramide occur in the liver and lung of affected mice (Igisu and Suzuki, 1984a). In contrast to galactosylceramide, another metabolically related substrate of the defective enzyme, galactosylsphingosine (psychosine), is consistently and progressively increased in CNS of twitcher mice up to 20 times normal (Igisu and Suzuki, 1984b). The degree of the psychosine accumulation generally correlates well with severity of pathology. Psychosine similarly accumulates also in human GLD brains (see Chapter 35 in this volume).

Two other minor galactolipids are also natural substrates of galactosylceramidase: monogalactosyldiglyceride and the seminolipid precursor (1-alkyl, 2-acyl, galactosylglycerol). These compounds also accumulate moderately in tissues where they are normal constituents, the seminolipid precursor almost exclusively in the testis and monogalactosyldiglyceride in the brain and kidney (Matsuda *et al.*, 2001b). Functional significance of their accumulation is not clear.

A synthetic enzyme, UDP-galactose:ceramide galactosyltransferase (CGT), catalyzes the last step of galactosylceramide synthesis. Its activity in the normal brain is known to change dramatically during CNS development in parallel to the period of active myelination (Costantino-Ceccarini and Morell, 1972). The activity is very low during the premyelination period and then increases sharply at the onset of myelination. It then declines nearly as sharply to a lower steady-state level. The activity of the enzyme in the twitcher spinal cord was normal during the early stage of myelination, but the activity decreased after 20 days (Kodama *et al.*, 1982). At 25 and 33 days, galactosyltransferase activity was drastically reduced compared to controls. Recently this study has been corroborated by quantitative estimates of CGT mRNA (Taniike *et al.*, 1998), made possible by recent cloning of the cDNA coding for rat CGT (Schulte and Stoffel, 1993; Stahl *et al.*, 1994). There was an early reduction of CGT mRNA, disproportionate to later decreases in mRNA of myelin protein genes. This pattern of decrease in enzyme activity is consistent with the morphological evidence of normal early myelination followed by destruction of myelin and oligodendrocytes after 20 days. Abnormal accumulation of a toxic metabolite, psychosine, is considered the underlying cause of this rapid degeneration of the oligodendrocytes (psychosine hypothesis) (Suzuki, 1998) (regarding detailed discussions of the psychosine hypothesis, refer to Chapter 35 in this volume).

Galactosylceramidase had for many years eluded the best efforts of several laboratories to purify. However, Wenger and colleagues recently succeeded to purify and clone the human cDNA (Chen *et al.*, 1993). Later Sakai *et al.* also cloned the cDNA independently (Sakai *et al.*, 1994). Then, the mutation underlying the twitcher mutant was identified (Sakai *et al.*, 1996). It is a nonsense mutation near the middle of the coding sequence that results in a mutation of codon 339 to a stop codon (TGG→TGA).

## Experimental Mouse Models of GLD

In addition to the naturally occurring twitcher mutant, a new experimental model of GLD due to genetic galactosylceramidase deficiency and an entirely new, genetically distinct mouse model of GLD have recently been generated. Particularly, the latter, a genetic deficiency of a sphingolipid activator protein, saposin A, introduced a new gene, defect of which can also cause impaired degradation of galactosylceramidase substrates and thus globoid cell leukodystrophy. While GLD due to saposin A deficiency is not known in humans, an equivalent human disease can be anticipated.

### *Point Mutation in Galactosylceramidase Gene*

There are several base changes in human galactosylceramidase gene, which are observed in the general population and which by themselves do not cause globoid cell leukodystrophy. They are therefore by definition polymorphisms. Some of them, however, result in galactosylceramidase protein with reduced catalytic activity, although not to the extent to cause the disease. Wenger noted that some individuals who simultaneously have three or more of these "polymorphisms" often exhibit late-onset spasticity and other white matter signs. Tested in an *in vitro* system, one of the polymorphisms, H168C, in human gene gave 80% of normal activity in COS-1 cells, but the same base change in the mouse gene gave only 10 to 20% of normal activity. Based on this observation, H168C was introduced into the mouse gene by homologous recombination technology. Mice homogygous for H168C exhibited a phenotype of GLD with slightly later onset and milder course (Luzi *et al.*, 2001). Clinical onset was about 25 to 30 days (20 days in twitcher mouse), and the average life span was about 50 days with large variations. Galactosylceramidase activities in various tissues were so low that it could not be reliably compared with that in twitcher mouse. Pathology was similar to that of the twitcher mouse. Psychosine accumulation in the brain was approximately 80% of the level observed in the twitcher mouse. Thus, although not by itself pathogenic in humans, H168C is a disease-causing mutation in the mouse. These characterizations were done relatively soon after the generation of the mutant when the genetic background was still mixed. In view of the longer-living twitcher mice with different genetic background (Duchen *et al.*, 1980), it is of interest to follow up this initial observation when the genetic background is made more homogeneous.

### *Saposin A Deficiency*

Sphingolipid activator proteins (saposins A, B, C, D) are small heat-stable glycoproteins required for *in vivo* degradation of some sphingolipids with short carbohydrate chains (Sandhoff *et al.*, 2001). They are derived from a common precursor protein (prosaposin), which is encoded by a single gene and proteolytically processed to saposins A, B, C, and D. These four saposins are all homologous to each other, having six conserved cysteines and one common glycosylation site. In spite of these structural similarities, their activator functions are relatively specific, with some overlaps, for individual sphingolipid hydrolases. Human patients with mutations in the saposin B and C domains are known and they show phenotypes of metachromatic leukodystrophy and Gaucher disease, indicating that they primarily activate arylsulfatase A and glucosylceramide *in vivo*, respectively (Christomanou *et al.*, 1986; Shapiro *et al.*, 1979). Two mutations are known in humans that result in complete inactivation of all four saposins and prosaposin (Hulková *et al.*, 2001; Schnabel *et al.*, 1992). A mouse model of human total saposin deficiency closely mimics the human disease (Fujita *et al.*, 1996). There have been circumstantial evidence that saposin A is a galactosylceramidase activator (Harzer *et al.*, 1997; Morimoto *et al.*, 1989). A saposin A-deficient mouse line has been generated experimentally by introducing an amino acid substitution (C106F) into the saposin A domain by the Cre/*lox*P system (Matsuda *et al.*, 2001b) that eliminated one of the three conserved disulfide bonds considered essential for the functional properties of saposins. In humans, an equivalent mutation in the 4th cysteine to phenylalanine in saposin C causes specific saposin C deficiency, and a mutation of the 5th cysteine to serine in saposin B causes specific saposin B deficiency (Sandhoff *et al.*, 2001). Saposin $A^{-/-}$ mice developed slowly progressive hind leg paralysis with the clinical onset around 2.5 months and survival up to 5 months. Tremors and shaking prominent in other myelin mutants were not conspicuous until the terminal stage. Both males and females of saposin A −/− are fertile, and females are able to raise pups up to three times. In every respect, pathology (firm and thick peripheral nerves, demyelination, reactive astrogliosis, and infiltration of "globoid cells" that contain the characteristic inclusion bodies) and analytical biochemistry (consequences of impaired degradation of all of the galactosylceramidase substrates in the brain, kidney, and testis) were qualitatively identical with but generally much milder than those seen in the twitcher mouse. Accumulation of psychosine in the brain was only twice normal compared to the 10- to 20-fold increase in twitcher mice. The saposin A −/− mouse clearly established that saposin A is indispensable for galactosylceramidase activation *in vivo* in the sense that normal cellular functions cannot be maintained in its absence. It should now be recognized that, in addition to galactosylceramidase deficiency, genetic saposin A deficiency can also cause chronic globoid cell leukodystrophy. Genetic saposin A deficiency should be suspected in human patients with undiagnosed late-onset chronic leukodystrophy without known enzymatic deficiencies.

## Utilities of Mouse Models

Human Krabbe disease is a rare disorder. It is always difficult to design well-controlled studies with human patients because of the relatively long life and genetic complexity. This problem is compounded when the disease is rare. Furthermore, any studies with human individuals pose serious ethical constraints. Appropriate animal models equivalent to human disease can alleviate many of these limitations of human studies. Thus, they are being utilized with increasing frequency and the GLD animal models are no exception.

### *Pathogenesis and Other Basic Studies*

Although the fundamental genetic basis of GLD is well understood and the globoid cell reaction due to impaired galactosylceramide degradation and disappearance of myelin-forming cells due to accumulation of cytotoxic psychosine appear to be the major pathogenetic mechanisms underlying the disease, many details are still uncertain. The mouse models are well suited for exploration of these questions. Some findings related to this topic are discussed in other sections of this chapter.

*Involvement of apoptotic process* While it is well accepted now that cytotoxicity of psychosine is likely to be responsible for the characteristic rapid disappearance of the oligodendrocytes, the exact mechanism is not well characterized. Involvement of the cellular apoptotic processes has been explored in this regard, and an increasing number of oligodendrocytes in twitcher mouse brains were found to be dying from apoptotic processes (Taniike and Suzuki 1995; Taniike *et al.*, 1999). This observation is consistent with an *in vitro* study, which indicated that psychosine is as potent an inducer of apoptosis as C-6 ceramide (Tohyama *et al.*, 2001).

*Involvement of immune and inflammatory processes* One of the issues related to the pathogenesis of GLD is the extent and nature of immune and inflammatory system involvement. The role of the major histocompatibility complex in the pathogenesis of twitcher mice was evaluated. With progression of demyelination, GFAP-, Mac-1- and F4/80-positive cells increased both in the twitcher CNS and PNS. Some Mac-1-positive cells also expressed the major histocompatibility complex (MHC) class II (Ia). Emergence of Ia-expressing cells was largely coincident with the onset of demyelination. Ia-immunoreactive cells gradually increased in areas of demyelination, reached a plateau between 30 to 40 days of age in the cerebrum, and then rapidly decreased despite continuous demyelination. In the spinal cord, however, Iα-immunoreactive cells did not decline even at 50 days (Ohno *et al.*, 1993). These results may indicate either a specific involvement of immunological factors in the pathogenesis of this genetic demyelinating disease or a nonspecific reaction to degenerating tissue components, such as myelin. Cross-breeding the twitcher mice with a MHC class II knockout mouse line generated a twitcher mouse line, which is also deficient with MHC class II molecules (Grusby *et al.*, 1991). In these mice, clinical symptoms and histopathology of the cerebrum and the brain stem–cerebellar region were milder than those in twitcher mice with the MHC-II positive background but there was no noticeable improvement in the pathology of the spinal cord (Matsushima *et al.*, 1994). Preliminary analysis of psychosine level also showed less accumulation than in the MHC-II-positive twitcher mice, consistent with the lesser degree of pathology in these mice. Interleukins, cytokines, and their receptors have also been examined in the twitcher mice to evaluate participation of inflammatory processes in the pathogenesis of GLD (LeVine *et al.*, 1994; LeVine and Brown 1997; Matsuda *et al.*, 2001a; Pedchenko and LeVine 1999; Podchenko *et al.*, 2000; Wu *et al.*, 2001).

*Interactions between the two lysosomal ß-galactosidases* Two ß-galactosidases are present in the lysosome. One is galactosylceramidase responsible for human Krabbe disease and several animal models. The other is acid ß-galactosidase, which primarily hydrolyzes the terminal galactose from GM1-ganglioside and its asialo-derivative, GA1, and is responsible for GM1-gangliosidosis/Morquio B disease. Cross-breeding of twitcher mice and acid ß-galactosidase knockout mice indicated that the acid ß-galactosidase gene dosage exerts unexpected and paradoxical influence on the twitcher phenotype (Tohyama *et al.*, 2000). Twitcher mice with additional complete deficiency of acid ß-galactosidase showed the mildest phenotype with the longest life span and nearly rescued CNS pathology. In contrast, twitcher mice with a single functional acid ß-galactosidase gene exhibited the most severe disease with the shortest life span. A significant proportion of these *galc −/−*, $bgal^{+/-}$ mice clinically developed additional extreme hyperreactivity and generalized seizures not seen in any other genotypes. Widespread neuronal degeneration was present in the *galc −/−*, $bgal^{+/-}$ mice, most prominently in the CA3 region of the hippocampus. The double knockout mice showed a massive accumulation of lactosylceramide in all tissues as had been expected from earlier enzymological studies (Tanaka and Suzuki, 1977). The brains inexplicably contained only a half-normal amount of galactosylceramide, which may account for the mild clinical and pathological phenotype. On the other hand, *galc −/−*, $bgal^{+/-}$ mice showed a significantly higher level of brain psychosine than other genotypes. The reduced galactosylceramide in the brain of the double knockout mice, and the significantly higher psychosine in the brain of the *galc −/−*, $bgal^{+/-}$ mice cannot readily be explained from the genotypes of these mice. These observations are contrary to the expected outcome of Mendelian autosomal recessive single gene disorders. Acid ß-galactosidase gene may function as a modifier gene for the phenotypic expression of genetic galactosylceramidase deficiency.

### *Therapeutic Trials*

***Nerve graft experiment*** The twitcher mutant has been used extensively for therapeutic trials for GLD since the identification of its underlying genetic defect as galactosylceramidase deficiency. In earlier studies, sciatic nerve of affected mice was grafted to the sciatic nerve of either normal or trembler mutant mice (Scaravilli and Jacobs, 1982; Scaravilli and Suzuki, 1983). When twitcher sciatic nerves were grafted to the sciatic nerve of normal littermates, endoneurial edema became pronounced and features of demyelination appeared 2 months after the graft operation. However, at 6 months, there were signs of improvement in pathology. Many nerve fibers were myelinated, although myelin was far thinner for the size of the axons. Galactosylceramidase activities of the grafted twitcher sciatic nerves were indistinguishable from those in the host nerves at 4, 5, and 9 months. By using trembler mice as the host, migration of host Schwann cells into the grafted twitcher nerve could be excluded as the source of the high galactosylceramidase activity in the graft.

***Bone marrow transplantation*** The bone marrow transplantation experiments prolonged life span of twitcher mice with a 36% probability of survival at 100 days in contrast to untreated mice that do not survive beyond 35 to 40 days (Hoogerbrugge *et al.*, 1988a; Yeager *et al.*, 1984). Hind limb weakness was significantly improved but tremulousness still remained. Nevertheless, body weight of the treated mice remained much below that of normal mice throughout their life span. After bone marrow transplantation, galactosylceramidase activity in the spleen and bone marrow increased to the donor level. Also the enzyme activity was significantly increased in the liver, lung and heart. In the CNS, the enzyme activity gradually increased to 15% of the control level in 100-day old treated mice (Hoogerbrugge *et al.*, 1988a). On the other hand, another group reported restoration of normal level of galactosylceramidase activity in the twitcher mouse brain by 90 days after transplantation (Ichioka *et al.*, 1987). Psychosine accumulation decreased in the CNS following bone marrow transplantation and remained stable (Hoogerbrugge *et al.*, 1988a; Ichioka *et al.*, 1987). Motor nerve conduction velocity improved in the sciatic nerve (Toyoshima *et al.*, 1986). In the late stage, morphological evidence of remyelination was present in the CNS (Suzuki *et al.*, 1988). Many nerve fibers in the cerebellum, brain stem, and spinal cord were myelinated, and myelin degeneration was rare in these regions, although thickness of the myelin sheaths was far less than expected for the size of the axons, indicating hypomyelination or remyelination. With allogeneic transplantation using C3H strain of mice [H-2K$^k$ allele of the major histocompatibility complex (MHC)] as the bone marrow donor to twitcher mice that are of C57BL strain [H-2K$^b$ allele of MHC complex], donor origin of infiltrating macrophages was demonstrated with immunocytochemical techniques (Hoogerbrugge *et al.*, 1988b; Huppes *et al.*, 1992). Other studies also showed that hematogenous cells can infiltrate into the central nervous system (Wu *et al.*, 2000a, 2000b). Remyelinating oligodendrocytes appeared normal at the light microscopic level with abundant cytoplasm. However, examination on the ultrastructural level indicated presence of GLD inclusions in their perikarya as well as in the inner or outer tongue processes (Suzuki *et al.*, 1988). Apparent recovery from demyelination in the regions where foamy cells were conspicuously present suggested that these cells were responsible for the improvement of the CNS pathology by somehow providing the normal enzyme.

***Cellular transplantation*** Transplantation of isolated and cultured glial cells has been used to remyelinate demyelinated or dysmyelinated white matter in experimental animals (Gumpel *et al.*, 1983). Transplanted glial cells migrate along the nerve fibers, blood vessels, and the subependymal region. They appear to migrate preferentially toward the site of demyelination. Intracerebrally transplanted fetal neuroglial cells were found to spread widely within the host twitcher brain (Huppes *et al.*, 1992). Intracerebal transplantation of neural stem cells is being actively pursued, and it is hoped that the results would be published in due course.

***Transgenic treatment*** Introduction of normal gene as a transgene into the genome is not and will not be in the foreseeable future a viable means for clinical treatment of genetic disease. Nevertheless, the procedure is of interest as a basic study. Matsumoto *et al.* introduced normal human galactosylceramidase cDNA as a transgene into twitcher mice under control of the promoter of a myelin-specific gene, myelin basic protein (Matsumoto *et al.*, 1997), in an attempt to influence the natural course of the disease. Expression of the transgene was unexpectedly low and could be detected only by RT-PCR. When determined at 35 days, galactosylceramidase activities in the brain and kidney showed a general trend of increasing activities from the untreated twitcher mice, twitcher mice carrying a single transgene, to twitcher mice carrying a double dose of the transgene. However, increment in the enzymatic activities in mice carrying the transgene was very minor. Nevertheless, while twitcher mice without the transgene developed the disease early, lost weight, and died by 35 $\pm$ days, those carrying one transgene developed the disease more slowly, gained weight longer, and survived generally to 50 $\pm$ days. Those with double dose of the transgene developed the disease even later, gained weight much longer, and survived up to 66 days. Pathology at 35 days suggested corresponding improvements in transgene-carrying twitcher mice. Most important, psychosine levels in the brain were reduced to nearly half of those without the transgene. This "failed" experiment with respect to "curing" the disease by introduction of the transgene nevertheless provided encouraging evidence to support the hypothesis that a relatively small increment in the enzymatic activity may be sufficient to effect "cure" of many lysosomal disorders.

***Gene therapy*** Twitcher mice are being used to explore possible avenues for gene therapy. Highly promising results have been obtained in cell culture systems (Costantino-Ceccarini *et al.*, 1999; Rafi *et al.*, 1996). The most commonly employed viral vector is the retroviruses for their well-characterized properties and the efficient and relatively nondiscriminatory capacity to infect various cellular types. If a retrovirus is appropriately modified with an inserted exogenous gene, it can infect the target cells and produce the gene product lacking in the host cell. For stable expression, the retrovirus must be integrated into the host genome, and the integration requires mitosis of the host cells. This property seriously limits the usefulness of retroviruses as the vector for gene therapy of genetic diseases of the central nervous system, in which most cells are post-mitotic. Use of either adenovirus or replication defective Herpes simplex 1 virus can overcome this disadvantage, since they do not need to be integrated into the host cell genome for its expression. Thus, the exogenous gene engineered into adenovirus or Herpes simplex 1 virus can be expressed in post-mitotic cells and actively replicating cells with similar efficiency. This ability to replicate and express its own genome independent of the host cell replication further provides an advantage in that there is much less risk of inadvertently activating oncogenes or disrupting important endogenous genes by random integration into the host genome. The disadvantage is that the introduced genes are "diluted" and eventually lost as the host cells undergo series of mitosis. More recently, adeno-associated virus (AAV) is gaining popularity as a vector for overcoming many of the shortcomings of other vectors. Some of the advantages of the AAV are (1) AAV is nonpathogenic, since the integrating DNA vector has no remaining viral genes and the co-transfected helper adenovirus is completely eliminated in time; (2) integrated gene carried by the AAV vector is stable at least in tissue culture for more than 100 passages; (3) AAV integrates itself into a small predictable region of the host genome (chromosome 19 in humans) and thus has little danger of disrupting essential host genes; (4) AAV can be introduced into most cells types; (5) the replication-defective helper adenovirus can be produced at high titers; and (6) AAV is the only known human virus that has targeting capability. AAV has also been explored as the viral vehicle for gene therapy of twitcher mice (Chen *et al.*, 1998, 1999).

***Pregnancy dramatically alleviates saposin A deficient phenotype*** During routine breeding process, it was noted that affected saposin A –/– females that were continually pregnant showed greatly improved neurological symptoms compared to affected females that do not experience pregnancy or affected males (Matsuda *et al.*, 2001a). The pathological hallmark of globoid cell leukodystrophy, demyelination with infiltration of globoid cells, largely disappeared. The immune-related gene expression (MCP-1, TNF-α) was significantly down-regulated in the brain of pregnant saposin $A^{-/-}$ mice. In addition, intense expression of estrogen receptors (ER-α and ER-β) on the globoid cells, activated astrocytes and microglia in the demyelinating area of saposin $A^{-/-}$ mice was observed. When saposin $A^{-/-}$ mice were subcutaneously implanted with time-release 17β-estradiol (E2) pellets from 30 to 90 days, the pathology was vastly improved. These findings suggest that higher level of estrogen during pregnancy is one of the important factors in the protective effect of pregnancy. While we should be cautious in extrapolating these observations in the mouse to human disease, the phenomenon is spectacularly dramatic and estrogen administration might be worth a consideration as a supplementary treatment for some chronic genetic leukodystrophies. It must be emphasized that the degree of the clinical and pathological improvement by pregnancy is much greater than those seen in any other therapeutic trials so far attempted for this disease.

***Substrate reduction*** All lysosomal diseases result from failure to degrade certain cellular constituents due to genetic defects in the degradative pathways. Radin originally proposed a concept of substrate reduction as a means to alleviate the detrimental outcome of lysosomal disease by limiting synthesis of the substrates and thus reducing burden on the degradative system (Radin, 1996, 1999; Vunnam and Radin, 1980). Radin could not test his concept because no suitable animal models were available when he proposed the idea in the 1970s. With the advent of gene targeting technology, the concept can now be tested and has in fact become fashionable. While most of the experimental tests have been done with animal models, in which glucosylceramide-based sphingolipids are stored, using inhibitors of glucosylceramide synthesis, this approach is not feasible for GLD because the disease does not involve impaired degradation of glucosylceramide-based sphingolipids. Instead, use of cycloserine, which inhibits all sphingolipid synthesis, was suggested to treat twitcher mice in 1985 (Sundaram and Lev, 1984), and recent actual trials found it to be slightly effective (Biswas and LeVine, 2002; LeVine *et al.*, 2000).

A logical weakness of all experiments with exogenous administration of inhibitors of substrate synthesis is that one can only know what the compounds do or do not do with respect to the functions tested but never know what else they might do. Thus, it is extremely difficult to prove a causal relationship between substrate inhibition and outcome on the course of the disease. A biologically "cleaner" experiment was done by cross-breeding twitcher mice with galactosylceramide synthase (UDP-galactose:ceramide galactosyltransferase, CGT) knockout mice (Ezoe *et al.*, 2000a, 2000b). The prediction that the phenotype of the doubly deficient mice should be the same as the *cgt* −/− mice, since the degrading enzyme should not be necessary if the substrate is not synthesized, proved to be only partially correct. In early stages of the disease, the doubly deficient mice (*galc* −/−, *cgt* −/−) were essentially indistinguishable from the *cgt* −/− mice. However, the doubly deficient mice had a much shorter life span than *cgt* −/− mice. Both galactosylceramide and galactosylsphingosine (psychosine) were undetectable in the brain of the *cgt* −/− and the doubly deficient mice. The characteristic twitcher pathology was never seen in the *galc* −/−, *cgt* −/− mice. However, after 43 days, neuronal pathology was observed in the brain stem and spinal cord. This late neuronal pathology has not been seen in the CGT knockout mice. These observations indicate that the functional relationship between galactosylceramidase and galactosylceramide synthase is complex.

This crossbreeding also generates hybrids with a genotype of *galc* −/−, $cgt^{+/-}$, in addition to doubly deficient mice. They are ideally suited to evaluate the potential usefulness of limiting synthesis of the substrate as a treatment of genetic disorders due to degradative enzyme defects. The rate of accretion of galactosylceramide in the brain of CGT knockout carrier mice ($cgt^{+/-}$) is approximately two-thirds of the normal rate, suggesting a gene-level compensation for the reduced gene dosage. Phenotype of twitcher mice with a single dose of normal *cgt* gene was indeed milder with statistical significance, albeit only slightly. Neuropathologists were able to distinguish blindly *galc* −/−, $cgt^{+/-}$ mice from *galc* −/−, $cgt^{+/+}$ mice. The brain psychosine level in *galc* −/−, $cgt^{+/-}$ mice was also approximately two-thirds of the *galc* −/−, $cgt^{+/+}$ mice. These observations indicate that reduction of galactosylceramide synthesis to two-thirds of the normal level results in minor but clearly detectable phenotypic improvements. This approach by itself is unlikely to be useful as the sole treatment but may be helpful as a supplement to other therapies.

## References


Baskin G. B., Ratterree M., Davison B. B., Falkenstein K. P., Clarke M. R., England J. D., Vanier M. T., Luzi P., Rafi M. A., and Wenger D. A. (1998). Genetic galactocerebrosidase deficiency (globoid cell leukodystrophy, Krabbe disease) in Rhesus monkeys (*Macaca mulatta*). *Lab. Anim. Sci.* **48,** 476–482.

Biswas S., and LeVine S. M. (2002). Substrate-reduction therapy enhances the benefits of bone marrow transplantation in young mice with globoid cell leukodystrophy. *Pediatr. Res.* **51,** 40–47.

Chen H., McCarty D. M., Bruce A. T., Suzuki K., and Suzuki K. (1998). Gene transfer and expression in oligodendrocytes under the control of myelin basic protein transcriptional control region mediated by adeno-associated virus. *Gene Therapy* **5,** 50–58.

Chen H., McCarty D. M., Bruce A. T., Suzuki K., and Suzuki K. (1999). Oligodendrocyte-specific gene expression in mouse brain: Use of a myelin-forming cell type-specific promoter in an adeno-associated virus. *J. Neurosci. Res.* **55,** 504–513.

Chen Y. Q., Rafi M. A., De Gala G., and Wenger D. A. (1993). Cloning and expression of cDNA encoding human galactocerebrosidase, the enzyme deficient in globoid cell leukodystrophy. *Hum. Mol. Genet.* **2,** 1841–1845.

Christomanou H., Aignesberger A., and Link R. P. (1986). Immunochemical characterization of two activator proteins stimulating enzymic sphingomyelin degradation in vitro: Absence of one of them in a human Gaucher disease variant. *Biol. Chem. Hoppe-Seyler* **367,** 879–890.

Costantino-Ceccarini E., Luddi A., Volterrani M., Strazza M., Rafi M. A., and Wenger D. A. (1999). Transduction of cultured oligodendrocytes from normal and twitcher mice by a retroviral vector containing human galactocerebrosidase (GALC). cDNA. *Neurochem. Res.* **24,** 287–293.

Costantino-Ceccarini E., and Morell P. (1972). Biosynthesis of brain sphingolipids and myelin accumulation in the mouse. *Lipids* **7,** 656–659.

Duchen L. W., Eicher E. M., Jacobs J. M., Scaravilli F., and Teixeira F. (1980). Hereditary leukodystrophy in the mouse – the new mutant twitcher. *Brain* **103,** 695–710.

Ezoe T., Vanier M. T., Oya Y., Popko B., Tohyama J., Matsuda J., Suzuki K., and Suzuki K. (2000a). Biochemistry and neuropathology of mice doubly deficient in synthesis and degradation of galactosylceramide. *J. Neurosci. Res.* **59,** 170–178.

Ezoe T., Vanier M. T., Oya Y., Popko B., Tohyama J., Matsuda J., Suzuki K., and Suzuki K. (2000b). Twitcher mice with only a single active galactosylceramide synthase gene exhibit clearly detectable but therapeutically minor phenotypic improvements. *J. Neurosci. Res.* **59,** 179–187.

Fankhäuser R., Luginbühl H., and Hartley W. J. (1963). Leukodystrophie vom Typus Krabbe beim Hund. *Schweiz. Arch. Tierheilkd.* **105,** 198–207.

Fujita N., Suzuki K., Vanier M. T., Popko B., Maeda N., Klein A., Henseler M., Sandhoff K., Nakayasu H., and Suzuki K. (1996). Targeted disruption of the mouse sphingolipid activator protein gene: A complex phenotype, including severe leukodystrophy and wide-spread storage of multiple sphingolipids. *Hum. Mol. Genet.* **5,** 711–725.

Grusby M. L., Johnson R. S., Papaloannou V. E., and Glimcher L. H. (1991). Depletion of CD4+ T cells in major histocompatibility compex class II-deficient mice. *Science* **253,** 670–674.

Gumpel M., Baumann N., Raoul M., and Jacque C. (1983). Survival and differentiation of oligodendrocytes from neural tissue transplanted into new-born mouse brain. *Neurosci. Lett.* **37,** 307–312.

Harzer K., Paton B. C., Christomanou H., Chatelut M., Levade T., Hiraiwa M., and O'Brien J. S. (1997). Saposins (*sap*). A and C activate the degradation of galactosylceramide in living cells. *FEBS Lett.* **417,** 270–274.

Hoogerbrugge P. M., Poorthuis B. J. H. M., Romme A. E., van de Kamp J. J. P., Wagemaker G., and van Bekkum D. W. (1988a). Effect of bone marrow transplantation on enzyme levels and clinical course in the neurologically affected twitcher mouse. *J. Clin. Invest.* **81,** 1790–1794.

Hoogerbrugge P. M., Suzuki K., Suzuki K., Poorthuis B. J. H. M., Kobayashi T., Wagemaker G., and van Bekkum D. W. (1988b). Donor derived cells in the central nervous system of twitcher mice after bone marrow transplantation. *Science* **239,** 1035–1038.

Hulková H., Cervenková M., Ledvinová J., Tochacková M., Hrebícek M., Poupetová H., Befekadu A., Berná L., Paton B. C., Harzer K., Böör A., Smíd F., and Elleder M. (2001). A novel mutation in the coding region of the prosaposin gene leads to a complete deficiency of prosaposin and saposins, and is associated with a complex sphingolipidosis dominated by lactosylceramide accumulation. *Hum. Mol. Genet.* **10,** 927–940.

Huppes W., De Groot C. J. A., Ostendorf R. H., Bauman J. G. J., Gossen J. A., Smit V., Vijg J., and Dijkstra C. D. (1992). Detection of migrated allogeneic oligodendrocytes throughout the central nervous system of the galactocerebrosidase-deficient twitcher mouse. *J Neurocytol* **21,** 129–136.

Ichioka T., Kishimoto Y., Brennan S., Santos G. W., and Yeager A. M. (1987). Hematopoietic cell transplantation in murine globoid cell leukodystrophy (the twticher mouse): Effects on levels of galactosylceramidase, psychosine, and galactocerebrosides. *Proc. Natl. Acad. Sci. USA* **84,** 4259–4263.

Ida H., Umezawa F., Kasai E., Eto Y., and Maekawa K. (1982). An accumulation of galactocerebroside in kidney from mouse globoid cell leukodystrophy (twitcher). *Biochem. Biophys. Res. Commun.* **109,** 634–638.

Igisu H., Shimomura K., Kishimoto Y., and Suzuki K. (1983a). Lipids of developing brain of twitcher mouse—An authentic murine model of human Krabbe disease. *Brain* **106,** 405–417.

Igisu H., and Suzuki K. (1984a). Glycolipids of the spinal cord, sciatic nerve and systemic organs of the twitcher mouse. *J. Neuropath. Exper. Neurol.* **43,** 22–36.

Igisu H., and Suzuki K. (1984b). Progressive accumulation of toxic metabolite in a genetic leukodystrophy. *Science* **224,** 753–755.

Igisu H., Takahashi H., Suzuki K., and Suzuki K. (1983b). Abnormal accumulation of galactosylceramide in the kidney of twitcher mouse. *Biochem. Biophys. Res. Commun.* **110,** 940–944.

Kobayashi S., Chiu F.-C., Katayama M., Sacchi R. S., Suzuki K., and Suzuki K. (1986). Expression of glial fibrillary acidic protein in the CNS and PNS of murine globoid cell leukodystrophy, the twitcher. *Am. J. Pathol.* **125,** 227–243.

Kobayashi S., Katayama M., Satoh J., Suzuki Ku., and Suzuki K. (1988). The twitcher mouse: An alteration of the unmyelinated fibers in the PNS. *Am. J. Pathol.* **131,** 308–319.

Kobayashi T., Nagara H., Suzuki K., and Suzuki K. (1982). The twitcher mouse: Determination of genetic status by galactosylceramidase assays on clipped tail. *Biochemical Medicine* **27,** 8–14.

Kobayashi T., Yamanaka T., Jacobs J. M., Teixeira F., and Suzuki K. (1980). The twitcher mouse: An enzymatically authentic model of human globoid cell leukodystrophy (Krabbe disease). *Brain Res.* **202,** 479–483.

Kodama S., Igisu H., Siegel D. A., and Suzuki K. (1982). Glycosylceramide synthesis in the developing spinal cord and kidney of the twitcher mouse, an enzymatically authentic model of human Krabbe disease. *J. Neurochem.* **39,** 1314–1318.

LeVine S. M., and Brown D. C. (1997). IL-6 and TNF$\alpha$ expression in brains of twitcher, quaking and normal mice. *J. Neuroimmunol.* **73,** 47–56.

LeVine S. M., Pedchenko T. V., Bronshteyn I. G., and Pinson D. M. (2000). L-cycloserine slows the clinical and pathological course in mice with globoid cell leukodystrophy (twitcher mice). *J. Neurosci. Res.* **60,** 231–236.

LeVine S. M., Wetzel D. L., and Eiler A. J. (1994). Neuropathology of twitcher mice: Examination by histochemistry, immunohistochemistry, lectin histochemistry and Fourier transform infrared microspectroscopy. *In. J. Develop. Neurosci.* **12,** 275–288.

Luzi P., Rafi M. A., Victoria T., Baskin G. B., and Wenger D. A. (1997). Characterization of the rhesus monkey galactocerebrosidase (GALC). cDNA and gene and identification of the mutation causing globoid cell leukodystrophy (Krabbe disease). in this primate. *Genomics* **42,** 319–324.

Luzi P., Rafi M. A., Zaka M., Curtis M., Vanier M. T., and Wenger D. A. (2001). Generation of a mouse with low galactocerebrosidase activity by gene targeting: A new model of globoid cell leukodystrophy (Krabbe disease). *Molecular Genetics and Metabolism* **73,** 211–223.

Matsuda J., Vanier M. T., Saito Y., Suzuki K., and Suzuki K. (2001a). Dramatic phenotypic improvement during pregnancy in a genetic leukodystrophy: Estrogen appears to be a critical factor. *Hum. Mol. Genet.* **10,** 2709–2715.

Matsuda J., Vanier M. T., Saito Y., Tohyama J., Suzuki K., and Suzuki K. (2001b). A mutation in the saposin A domain of the sphingolipid activator protein (prosaposin). gene causes a late-onset, slowly progressive form of globoid cell leukodystrophy in the mouse. *Hum. Mol. Genet.* **10,** 1191–1199.

Matsumoto A., Vanier M. T., Oya Y., Kelly D., Popko B., Wenger D. A., Suzuki K., and Suzuki K. (1997). Transgenic introduction of human galactosylceramidase into twitcher mouse: Significant phenotype improvement with a minimal expression. *Develop. Brain Dysfunction* **10,** 142–154.

Matsushima G. K., Taniike M., Glimcher L. H., Grusby M. J., Frelinger J. A., Suzuki K., and Ting J. P. Y. (1994). Absence of MHC class II molecules reduces CNS demyelination, microglial; macrophage infiltration, and twitching in murine globoid cell leukodystrophy. *Cell* **78,** 645–656.

Mikoshiba K., Fujishiro M., Kohsaka S., Okano H., Takamatsu K., and and Tsukada Y. (1985). Disorders in myelination in the twitcher mutant: Immunohistochemical and biochemical studies. *Neurochem. Res.* **10,** 1129–1141.

Morimoto S., Martin B. M., Yamamoto Y., Kretz K. A., O'Brien J. S., and Kishimoto Y. (1989). Saposin-A – 2nd Cerebrosidase Activator Protein. *Proc. Natl. Acad. Sci., USA* **86,** 3389–3393.

Ohno M., Komiyama A., Martin P. M., and Suzuki K. (1993). MHC class II antigen expression and T-cell infiltration in the demyelinating CNS and PNS of the twitcher mouse. *Brain Res.* **625,** 186–196.

Olmstead C. E. (1987). Neurological and neurobehavioral development of the mutant 'twitcher' mouse. *Behav. Brain Res.* **25,** 143–152.

Podchenko T. V., Broshteyn I. G., and LeVine S. M. (2000). TNF-receptor I deficiency fails to alter the clinical and pathological course in mice with globoid cell leukodystrophy (twitcher mice). but affords protection following LPS challenge. *J. Neuroimmunol.* **110,** 186–194.

Pedchenko T. V., and LeVine S. M. (1999). IL-6 deficiency causes enhanced pathology in twitcher (globoid cell leukodystrophy). mice. *Exp. Neurol.* **158,** 459–468.

Powell H. C., Knobler R. L., and Myers R. R. (1983). Peripheral neuropathy in the twitcher mutant: A new experimental model of endoneurial edema. *Lab. Invest.* **49,** 19–25.

Radin N. S. (1996). Treatment of Gaucher disease with an enzyme inhibitor. *Glycoconjugate J.* **13,** 153–157.

Radin N. S. (1999). Chemotherapy by slowing glucosphingolipid synthesis. *Biochem. Pharmacol.* **57,** 589–595.

Rafi M. A., Fugaro J., Amini S., Luzi P., De Gala G., Victoria T., Dubell C., Shahinfar M., and Wenger D. A. (1996). Retroviral vector-mediated transfer of the galactocerebrosidase (GALC). cDNA leads to overexpression and transfer of GALC activity to neighboring cells. *Biochem. Molec. Med.* **58,** 142–150.

Sakai N., Inui K., Fujii N., Fukushima H., Nishimoto J., Yanagihara I., Isegawa Y., Iwamatsu A., and Okada S. (1994). Krabbe disease: Isolation and characterization of a full-length cDNA for human galactocerebrosidase. *Biochem. Biophys. Res. Commun.* **198,** 485–491.

Sakai N., Inui K., Tatsumi N., Fukushima H., Nishigaki T., Taniike M., Nishimoto J., Tsukamoto H., Yanagihara I., Ozone K., and Okada S. (1996). Molecular cloning and expression of cDNA for murine galactocerebrosidase and mutation analysis of the twitcher mouse, a model of Krabbe disease. *J. Neurochem.* **66,** 1118–1124.

Sandhoff K., Kolter T., and Harzer K. (2001). Sphingolipid activator proteins. *In* "The Metabolic and Molecular Basis of Inherited Disease" (C. R. Scriver A. L. Beaudet, W. S. Sly, and D. Valle, eds.), pp. 3371–3388. McGraw-Hill, New York.

Scaravilli F., and Jacobs J. M. (1982). Improved myelination in nerve grafts from the leukodystrophic twitcher into trembler mice – Evidence for enzyme replacement. *Brain Res.* **237,** 163–172.

Scaravilli F., and Suzuki K. (1983). Enzyme replacement in grafted nerve of twitcher mouse. *Nature* **305,** 713–715.

Schnabel D., Schröder M., Fürst W., Klein A., Hurwitz R., Zenk T., Weber J., Harzer K., Paton B. C., Poulos A., Suzuki K., and Sandhoff K. (1992). Simultaneous deficiency of sphingolipid activator proteins 1 and 2 is caused by a mutation in the initiation codon of their common gene. *J. Biol. Chem.* **267,** 3312–3315.

Schulte S., and Stoffel W. (1993). Ceramide UDPgalactosyltransferase from myelinating rat brain: Purification, cloning, and expression. *Proc. Natl. Acad. Sci., USA* **90,** 10265–10269.

Shapiro L. J., Aleck K. A., Kaback M. M., Itabashi H., Desnick R. J., Brand N., Stevens R. L., Fluharty A. L., and Kihara H. (1979). Metachromatic leukodystrophy without arylsulfatase A deficiency. *Pediat. Res.* **13,** 1179–1181.

Stahl N., Jurevics H., Morell P., Suzuki K., and Popko B. (1994). Isolation, characterization, and expression of cDNA clones that encode rat UDP-galactose:ceramide galactosyltransferase. *J. Neurosci. Res.* **38,** 234–242.

Sundaram K. S., and Lev M. (1984). Inhibition of sphingolipid synthesis by cycloserine in vitro and in vivo. *J. Neurochem.* **42,** 577–581.

Suzuki K. (1971). Renal cerebrosides in globoid cell leukodystrophy (Krabbe disease). *Lipids* **6,** 433–436.

Suzuki K. (1998). Twenty five years of the psychosine hypothesis: A personal perspective of its history and present status. *Neurochem. Res.* **23,** 251–259.

Suzuki K., Hoogerbrugge P. M., Poorthuis B. J. H. M., Romme A. E., van de Kamp J. J. P., Wagemaker G., van Bekkum D. W., and Suzuki K. (1988). The twitcher mouse: Central nervous system pathology after bone marrow transplantation (BMT). *Lab. Invest.* **58,** 302–309.

Suzuki K., and Suzuki Y. (1970). Globoid cell leucodystrophy (Krabbe disease): Deficiency of galactocerebroside β-galactosidase. *Proc. Natl. Acad. Sci. USA* **66,** 302–309.

Suzuki Y., Austin J., Armstrong D., Suzuki K., Schlenker J., and Fletcher T. (1970). Studies in globoid leukodystrophy: Enzymatic and lipid findings in the canine form. *Exp. Neurol.* **29,** 65–75.

Tanaka H., and Suzuki K. (1977). Sustrate specificities of the two genetically distinct human brain β-galactosidases. *Brain Res.* **122,** 325–335.

Taniike M., Marcus J. R., Nishigaki T., Fujita N., Popko B., and Suzuki K. (1998). Suppressed UDP-galactose:ceramide galactosyltransferase and myelin protein mRNA in twitches mouse brain. *J. Neurosci. Res.* **51,** 536–540.

Taniike M., Mohri I., Eguchi N., Irikura D., Urade Y., Okada S., and Suzuki K. (1999). An apoptotic depletion of oligodendrocytes in the twitcher, a murine model of globoid cell leukodystrophy. *J. Neuropathol. Exp. Neurol.* **58,** 644–653.

Taniike M., and Suzuki K. (1994). Spacio-temporal progression of demyelination in twitcher mouse: With clinicopathological correlation. *Acta Neuropathol. (Berl).* **88,** 228–236.

Taniike M., and Suzuki K. (1995). Proliferative capacity of oligodendrocytes in the demyelinating twitcher spinal cord. *J Neurosci Res* **40,** 325–332.

Tohyama J., Matsuda J., and Suzuki K. (2001). Psychosine is as potent an inducer of cell death as C6-ceramide in cultured fibroblasts and in MOCH-1 cells. *Neurochem. Res.* **26,** 667–671.

Tohyama J., Vanier M. T., Suzuki K., Ezoe T., Matsuda J., and Suzuki K. (2000). Paradoxical influence of acid β-galactosidase gene dosage on phenotype of the twitcher mouse (genetic galactosylceramidase deficiency). *Hum. Mol. Genet.* **9,** 1699–1707.

Toyoshima E., Yeager A. M., Brennan S., Santos G. W., Moser H., W., and Mayer R. F. (1986). Nerve conduction studies in the twitcher mouse (murine globoid cell leukodystrophy). *J. Neurol. Sci.* **74,** 307–318

Victoria T., Rafi M. A., and Wenger D. A. (1996). Cloning of the canine GALC cDNA and identification of the mutation causing globoid cell leukodystrophy in west highland white and cairn terriers. *Genomics* **33,** 457–462.

Vunnam R. R., and Radin N. S. (1980). Analogs of ceramide that inhibit glucocerebroside synthetase in mouse brain. *Chem. Phys. Lipids* **26,** 265–278.

Wenger D. A., Suzuki K., Suzuki Y., and Suzuki K. (2001). Galactosylceramide lipidosis: Globoid cell leukodystrophy (Krabbe disease). *In* "The Metabolic and Molecular Basis of Inherited Disease" (C. R. Scriver A. L. Beaudet, W. S. Sly, and D. Valle, eds.), pp. 3669–3694. McGraw-Hill, New York.

Wu Y. P., Matsuda J., Kubota A., Suzuki K., and Suzuki K. (2000a). Infiltration of hematogenous lineage cells into the demyelinating central nervous system of twitcher mice. *J. Neuropathol. Exp. Neurol.* **59,** 628–639.

Wu Y. P., McMahon E., Kraine M. R., Tisch R., Meyers A., Frelinger J., Matsushima G. K., and Suzuki K. (2000b). Distribution and characterization of $GFP^+$ donor hematogenous cells in twitcher mice after bone marrow transplantation. *American Journal of Pathology* **156,** 1849–1854.

Wu Y. P., McMahon E. J., Matsuda J., Suzuki K., Matsushima G. K., and Suzuki K. (2001). Expression of immune-related molecules is downregulated in *Twitcher* mice following bone marrow transplantation. *J. Neuropathol. Exp. Neurol.* **60,** 1062–1074.

Yeager A. M., Brennan S., Tiffany C., Moser H. W., and Santos G. W. (1984). Prolonged survival and remyelination after hematopoietic cell transplantation in the twitcher mouse. *Science* **225,** 1053–1054.

CHAPTER

# 46

# Models of Alexander Disease

*Albee Messing and Michael Brenner*

## ALEXANDER DISEASE

Alexander disease, first described in 1949 (Alexander, 1949), is an uncommon but fatal CNS disorder usually affecting children (for a review, see chapter 36 by Messing and Goldman in this volume). In the most common form ("infantile"), children present before the age of 2 years with white matter loss especially in the frontal lobes. Seizures and spasticity that are difficult to control are prominent symptoms, as is hydrocephalus and psychomotor developmental delay. These children suffer progressive deterioration with death usually before the age of 10.

The key diagnostic feature of the neuropathology in Alexander disease is the widespread deposition of Rosenthal fibers in subpial, periventricular, and white matter astrocytes throughout the CNS. Morphologically, Rosenthal fibers consist of two components: bundles of intermediate filaments surrounding irregular deposits of dense material (Herndon *et al.*, 1970). Biochemically, Rosenthal fibers are composed of a complex ubiquitinated mixture of the intermediate filament GFAP in association with other constituents, especially the small stress proteins αB-crystallin and HSP25 (Head and Goldman, 2000; Iwaki *et al.*, 1989). Rosenthal fibers are also found sporadically in several other settings, such as some astrocytomas and chronic gliosis (their original description was in a young adult with syringomyelia; see Rosenthal, 1898), but never to the extent seen in Alexander disease.

Significant accumulations of Rosenthal fibers also occur in individuals with much later onset and different signs, which led to a broader classification of Alexander disease that now includes juvenile and adult forms. In contrast to the infantile form, where the leukodystrophy predominantly affects the frontal lobes and there is mental retardation, the older patients tend to have less cognitive impairment and the most severe pathology in the hindbrain, with corresponding prominence of bulbar signs. The extent to which infantile, juvenile, and adult forms of Alexander disease are all fundamentally the same disease is unclear (though at least some have a common genetic etiology as described later) (Russo *et al.*, 1976; see also Herndon, 1999; Li *et al.*, 2002).

Why Rosenthal fibers form, and what relation they have to the disease process, is not known. Nevertheless, the localization of Rosenthal fibers in astrocytes led to the suggestion many years ago that Alexander disease was essentially a primary disorder of astrocytes (as originally proposed by Alexander), with the drastic consequences for other cell types reflecting a secondary effect of astrocyte dysfunction (Borrett and Becker, 1985). The hydrocephalus that is often associated with infantile cases is sometimes attributed to Rosenthal fibers causing stenosis of the cerebral aqueduct (Ni *et al.*, 2002; Sherwin and Berthrong, 1970), but no direct proof of this mechanism exists and instead it could conceivably reflect primary astrocyte dysfunction.

## SPONTANEOUS ANIMAL MODELS

Based strictly on the morphological criterion of diffuse Rosenthal fiber deposition, Alexander-like diseases have been reported occasionally in dogs (Cox *et al.*, 1986; McGrath, 1980; Richardson *et al.*, 1991; Weissenböck *et al.*, 1996) and sheep (Fankhauser *et al.*, 1980), and there is an anecdotal report of a case in a captive deer. However, these cases were not extensively studied and the degree to which they truly resembled the human disease is difficult to judge. The canine cases typically presented as young adults with histories of progressive ataxia and hind-limb weakness, and on autopsy showed diffuse deposition of Rosenthal fibers in association with mild leukodystrophy. There was no frontal predominance or seizures. It is interesting that the earliest of these reports concerned two Labrador retriever littermates (McGrath, 1980), which is not the typical pattern of inheritance seen in human Alexander disease (nearly all of which have been sporadic).

## GENETIC BASIS OF ALEXANDER DISEASE

In 1998 we reported the unexpected finding that transgenic mice designed to constitutively over-express wild-type GFAP developed a lethal phenotype associated with formation of Rosenthal fibers throughout the central nervous system (Messing *et al.*, 1998). In the highest-expressing lines, GFAP levels were elevated 15- to 20-fold over controls. The mice died within a few weeks after birth with no overt symptoms other than failure to gain weight despite adequate nursing. Of particular interest was the finding that the murine Rosenthal fibers appeared indistinguishable morphologically and biochemically from human Rosenthal fibers, which led to the conclusion that formation of these complex inclusions could be initiated by a primary change in the expression of GFAP. Furthermore, given the increasing recognition of gene duplications as a mechanism in human neurological disease (Lupski *et al.*, 1991; Sistermans *et al.*, 1998), we proposed that GFAP should be evaluated as a candidate gene for Alexander disease.

Subsequent studies confirmed that GFAP indeed was the gene responsible for most cases of Alexander disease, but in the form of heterozygous missense mutations rather than gene duplications. Brenner *et al.* (2001) reported the identification of heterozygous missense mutations within the coding region of GFAP in 12 out of 13 cases of Alexander disease in whom the diagnosis had been confirmed by pathology. These mutations predicted nonconservative changes in amino acids, in each case involving an arginine (R79C, R79H, R239C, R239H, R258P, and R416W). In 7 of the original 12 cases analyzed, DNA samples were available from both parents of the affected child, and the parental samples were always normal. These findings are consistent with the hypothesis that Alexander disease usually results from dominant de novo mutations in GFAP. These results have now been confirmed in a larger group of patients, and current data show that ~95% of cases of infantile Alexander disease, and at least some of the juvenile and adult cases, are associated with mutations in GFAP (Li *et al.*, 2002). The list of known mutations has grown and now includes 20 codons, many involving amino acids other than arginine. The GFAP mutations show extensive but incomplete homologies to disease-causing mutations in other intermediate filaments, as discussed in more detail by Li *et al.* (2002). A tabulation of published GFAP mutations is being maintained at the University of Wisconsin-Madison (www.waisman.wisc.edu/alexander) and the Human Intermediate Filament Mutation Database (www.interfil.org).

## DOES ALEXANDER DISEASE REPRESENT GAIN OR LOSS OF FUNCTION IN GFAP?

The finding that most cases of Alexander disease result from heterozygous missense mutations in GFAP places it in the family of genetic disorders of intermediate filaments.

Among these disorders is the epidermolysis bullosa complex, also initially identified through analysis of mouse models that closely resembled the human phenotype and that pointed the way toward genetic analysis of the keratin genes. These other intermediate filament disorders are typically dominant, also involving heterozygous missense mutations. Such dominant effects are plausible when one considers that mature filaments are assemblies of multiple polypeptides, dysfunction of any of which might affect the whole. However, since the mouse phenocopies of the other human intermediate filament disorders are either dominant negatives or knockouts of the respective genes, the dominant mutations identified in the human patients are generally viewed as acting to induce loss of function (Fuchs and Cleveland, 1998). In contrast, GFAP filaments are present in Alexander disease patients, and GFAP null mice are fully viable and their pathology does not resemble Alexander disease (Gomi *et al.*, 1995; Liedtke *et al.*, 1996; McCall *et al.*, 1996; Pekny *et al.*, 1995). Thus the GFAP mutations in Alexander disease do not appear to be acting by reducing or eliminating normal GFAP function, but by producing a new, deleterious, activity. Further discussion on this issue and comparison with other intermediate filament diseases can be found in the review by Li *et al.* (2002). The following sections discuss the consequences of deleting or duplicating the GFAP gene in the mouse, with the goal of highlighting the strengths and limitations of these current models of Alexander disease and suggesting directions for future research.

## ASTROCYTES AND GFAP

Mature astrocytes have a complex morphology that includes extension of processes to contact multiple other cell types and structures, including formation of the glial limitans at the pial surface, glial end-feet ensheathing blood vessel walls or synapses between neurons, and contacts with axonal nodes of Ranvier. At each of these contacts, astrocytes are thought to play key roles, such as inducing the blood-brain barrier in endothelium and modulating neuronal function through regulation of the ionic or neurotransmitter content of the extracellular space. In addition, astrocytes produce numerous growth factors that act on oligodendrocytes and their precursors. Compromise of any or all of these functions could contribute to the phenotype of Alexander disease, as nothing is known about the pathogenetic mechanisms actually at work in human patients.

GFAP is the major structural protein in astrocytes, but their progenitor neural stem cells contain the nestin intermediate filament and the immediate precursors of astrocytes (as well as many mature astrocytes) express vimentin. The activation of GFAP synthesis as astrocytes mature is considered a key step in their differentiation (Dahl, 1981; Bovolenta *et al.*, 1984). Studies in cultured astrocytes and cell lines of forced over-expression of GFAP or its antisense inhibition suggested that GFAP directly controls process outgrowth (Hatten *et al.*, 1991; Rutka and Smith, 1993; Weinstein *et al.*, 1991). In response to a wide variety of insults to the CNS, astrocytes undergo the process of reactive gliosis, which consists primarily of hypertrophy accompanied by dramatic changes in gene expression (Eddleston and Mucke, 1993). Increased levels of GFAP is perhaps the most characteristic change occurring in reactive astrocytes (Amaducci *et al.*, 1981; Bignami and Dahl, 1976; Eng and Lee, 1993; Mathewson and Berry, 1985), though there is also renewed expression of vimentin (Dahl *et al.*, 1981; Pixley and de Vellis, 1984) and nestin (Clarke *et al.*, 1994; Frisén *et al.*, 1995). Nestin, vimentin, and GFAP can coassemble in the same filament (Eliasson *et al.*, 1999).

## GFAP-NULL MICE

One way to study the role of GFAP in astrocytes is to generate mice that are deficient in GFAP. Given the apparent requirement for GFAP for process formation indicated by the cell culture experiments, and the likely essential requirement for these processes in brain development and function, it was presumed that GFAP null mice would be embryonic lethals, or at least severely compromised. Consistent with this supposition, no spontaneous mutants of the murine *Gfap* gene were known. Using standard techniques of gene targeting in embryonic stem cells, four groups independently generated GFAP-null mice (Gomi *et al.*, 1995; Liedtke *et al.*, 1996; McCall *et al.*, 1996; Pekny *et al.*, 1995). The consistent result was the surprising finding that GFAP-null mice are viable, with seemingly normal life-spans, reproduction, and gross motor behavior. However, alterations in neuronal synaptic function were identified, with impaired long-term depression in the cerebellum (Shibuki *et al.*, 1996) and enhanced long-term potentiation in the hippocampus (McCall *et al.*, 1996). Ultrastructural studies in optic nerve and spinal cord suggested minor changes in astrocyte morphology, with shortening and thinning of astrocyte processes (Liedtke *et al.*, 1996; McCall *et al.*, 1996). Subsequent studies of dye-filled cells also supports this conclusion (Anderová *et al.*, 2001). Studies in cell culture suggest that GFAP-null astrocytes may alter their expression of several components of the extracellular matrix (Menet *et al.*, 2001), but whether this occurs *in vivo* is less clear (Wang *et al.*, 1997). There is some evidence for alterations in the blood brain barrier derived from cell culture models (Pekny *et al.*, 1998) and to a limited extent from studies *in vivo* (Liedtke *et al.*, 1996).

Initial injury trials with GFAP-null mice also failed to find significant effects, with the mice showing apparently normal responses to scrapie infection (Gomi *et al.*, 1995; Tatzelt *et al.*, 1996), kainic acid (Gomi *et al.*, 1995), or stab wounds (Pekny *et al.*, 1995). However, more recent studies have identified increased susceptibility to blunt head injury (Nawashiro *et al.*, 1998) or ischemia (Nawashiro *et al.*, 1998, 2000; Tanaka *et al.*, 2002), and impaired swelling following exposure to hyptonic stress *in vivo* (Anderová *et al.*, 2001), though the mechanisms are not known. When double mutant mice are made that are deficient in both GFAP and vimentin, there is reduced gliosis and increased hemorrhage following traumatic injury (Pekny *et al.*, 1999). Since there is no up-regulation of vimentin or nestin in the GFAP null mice (Gomi *et al.*, 1995; McCall *et al.*, 1996), this indicates that in the normal astrocyte either GFAP or vimentin is sufficient to maintain a subset of functions.

Two studies directly link GFAP deficiency with abnormalities of myelination. Liedtke *et al.* (1996) reported that approximately half of the GFAP-null mice in their colony developed an adult-onset degeneration of myelin, with resulting hydrocephalus. Grossly visible changes in cerebral white matter did not become apparent until mice were 18 months and older, and some white matter tracts such as optic nerve were only minimally affected, if at all. The mechanism of this myelin degeneration has not been determined, and the possible contribution of background genetics (for instance, corpus callosum defects in 129 strain mice) has not been excluded (Wahlsten, 1982). A second report from this same group determined that GFAP-null mice had increased susceptibility to experimental allergic encephalitis, with increased clinical scores and pathology (Liedtke *et al.*, 1998). However, inflammation is thought to play little role in the pathogenesis of Alexander disease (see chapter 36 by Messing and Goldman in this volume).

Overall, the relevance of GFAP-null mice to Alexander disease remains uncertain. Such mice do not develop a severe leukodystrophy and have no Rosenthal fibers, two primary characteristics of the human disease. In addition, the GFAP-null mice do not exhibit developmental delay, spasticity, seizures, ataxia, or paralysis. Nevertheless, the changes in neuronal physiology observed in GFAP-null mice (Shibuki *et al.*, 1996; McCall *et al.*, 1996), and potential effects on myelination, leaves open the possibility that at least some aspects of Alexander disease may reflect loss of function of GFAP. Furthermore, it is well known that dominant negative mutations may produce more severe phenotypes than corresponding null mutations, as recently demonstrated with keratin 10 (Reichelt *et al.*, 2001).

## GFAP TRANSGENICS

As a complementary approach to gene knockouts for studying the role of GFAP in astrocytes, we sought to force constitutive over-expression of GFAP in otherwise normal astrocytes to test whether GFAP up-regulation was sufficient to induce other aspects of reactive gliosis. Our rationale was that adding GFAP transgenes would elevate GFAP levels as a primary change in astrocytes, without the confounding effects of injuries or other treatments that are typically used to induce this response. For this purpose we used a genomic human GFAP (hGFAP) clone that we had previously isolated for transcriptional studies. The surprising result was that astrocytes in these transgenics not only became hypertrophic, but also formed Rosenthal fibers (Messing *et al.*, 1998), the first time such inclusions had been produced reliably in an *in vivo* model (Fig. 46.1). Like the Rosenthal fibers in Alexander disease, those in the mice contained GFAP and the small heat shock proteins αB-crystallin and HSP27 (the mouse homolog of HSP25), each of whose expression was also up-regulated. In addition, when astrocytes were cultured from the hGFAP transgenics in isolation from neurons, Rosenthal fibers still formed, indicating that this was a cell-autonomous phenotype (Eng *et al.*, 1998). The Rosenthal fibers in the hGFAP transgenics are distinct from the astrocytic inclusions associated with superoxide dismutase (SOD) mutations in transgenic mice (Bruijn *et al.*, 1997) and in humans with amyotrophic lateral sclerosis (Kato *et al.*, 1996), as these contain ubiquitin and SOD1 but no GFAP (Kato *et al.*, 1997).

Previously there had been considerable debate over what might precipitate formation of Rosenthal fibers, and whether the astrocyte pathology had a central role in the disease or was merely a secondary response. The hGFAP transgenic mice show that Rosenthal fibers can form as the result of a primary change in just one component, GFAP, and suggest that astrocyte dysfunction may have an active rather than passive role in the human disease.

Although the existing lines of GFAP transgenic mice are good models for studying the etiology of Rosenthal fibers, they are imperfect models of Alexander disease as they do not display several other features of the disease. Mice of the highest expressing lines did die at an early age, but without overt symptoms such as seizures. The lines now being maintained express the hGFAP transgene at lower levels, and while they also accumulate Rosenthal fibers, their only overt phenotype is a small body size compared to littermates (Messing *et al.*, manuscript in preparation). Furthermore, none of the hGFAP transgenics develop hydrocephalus or detectable white matter changes, leaving unresolved the central question of why Alexander disease in humans is often a leukodystrophy. Finally, in light of the genetic studies of human Alexander disease patients noted earlier, the GFAP-over-expressing mice do not model the true genetic lesions that have been identified in the human patients; the transgenics were made by adding copies of a wild-type human GFAP gene, whereas heterozygous missense mutations have been found in the human disease. The hGFAP transgenic mice might prove to be a model for GFAP gene duplication. It is not yet known whether such duplication might underlie any of the several Alexander disease cases for which no GFAP coding mutation has been found, or if it might be found in association with a different human disorder.

As noted earlier, the hGFAP transgenics also model the up-regulation of stress proteins found in human Alexander disease and so can serve for the further characterization of this response. In particular, αB-crystallin is a major component of the Rosenthal fibers, and one explanation for its up-regulation is that it is part of a failed protective response of the astrocyte to aberrant expression of GFAP. The αB-crystallin is thought to function as a chaperone and promotes disassembly of GFAP filaments in cell-free assays (Nicholl and Quinlan, 1994). Recent studies by Koyama and Goldman show that transfecting αB-crystallin into cultured cells counteracts the formation of aggregates produced by transfection of GFAP alone (Koyama and Goldman, 1999). These findings suggest that Alexander disease might be ameliorated were it possible to increase the level of αB-crystallin above that which normally occurs in the disease.

Johnson and colleagues recently generated a novel strain of transgenic mice that express the human placental alkaline phosphatase reporter gene under the control of a minimal antioxidant response element promoter (Johnson *et al.*, 2002). These mice thus offer an efficient means of monitoring oxidative stress, and crossing the ARE-hPAP mice with the hGFAP transgenics induces marked up-regulation of the hPAP reporter gene (Fig. 46.2). Further studies of such double transgenics will help define the relationship between oxidative stress and inclusion body formation.

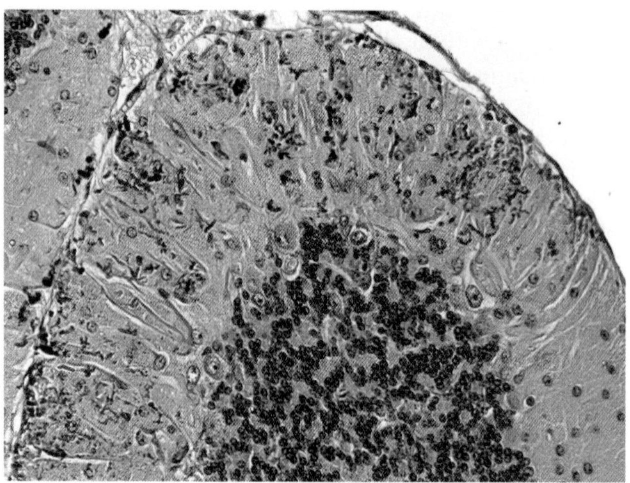

FIGURE 46.1
Rosenthal fibers in the cerebellum of an hGFAP transgenic mouse. Phloxine tartrazine stain, paraffin section.

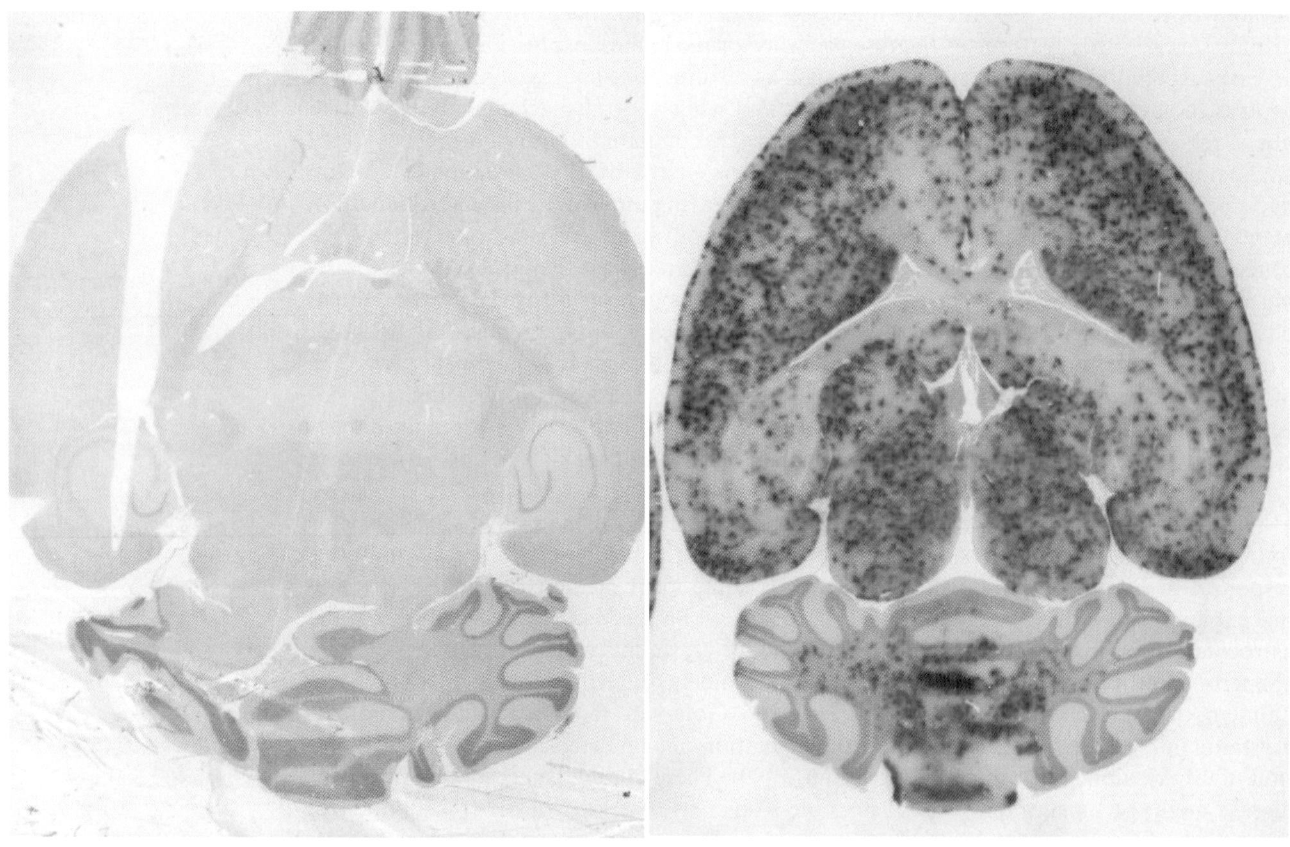


FIGURE 46.2
Extensive up-regulation of the hPAP reporter gene in ARE-hPAP/hGFAP double transgenic mice compared to single ARE-hPAP transgenic controls, tested at 3 months of age.

## NEW MOUSE MODELS

A GFAP mouse model recently produced by the Itohara laboratory (Takemura *et al.*, (2002) bears on the question of whether Rosenthal fiber formation in the hGFAP transgenics might arise from sequence incompatibility caused by the human GFAP, rather than from simple over-expression. Although there is substantial homology between human and mouse GFAP (91% identity and 95% similarity at the amino acid level) (Brenner *et al.*, 1990), it was still possible that the sequence differences could have led to the production of incompatible polypeptides with abnormalities of either assembly, disassembly, or degradation. In the Itohara mice, the entire head domain of the endogenous *Gfap* gene, where most of the species differences reside, was swapped with that of the human gene. Heterozygous mice therefore contain a normal gene copy number, carrying one allele of the normal mouse gene, and a second humanized allele with the human amino terminal end. Nevertheless, these mice developed no Rosenthal fibers or any other pathology.

As noted earlier, it is possible that the lack of leukodystrophy, seizures, and hydrocephalus in the GFAP over-expressing mice reflects a basic difference in genetic disease mechanism from that in Alexander disease. To try to develop a more accurate model, current efforts are aimed at generating mice engineered with targeted point mutations analogous to those seen in the human Alexander disease. In particular, mutations of just two amino acids (R79 and R239) account for nearly half of all reported cases, and these are the first mutations being modeled in mice. Preliminary observations indicate that such mice do indeed form Rosenthal fibers, offering formal proof that these mutations are causative for this aspect of the disease (Hagemann *et al.*, unpublished observations). It should soon be known whether these mice exhibit the full spectrum of lesions and symptoms observed in Alexander disease.

## SUMMARY

Previous transgenic results show that mice are capable of building the biochemically complex Rosenthal fibers within a short period of time *in vivo*. These transgenic lines also showed a significant phenotype, either early death or low body weight, indicating that they are sensitive to at least some forms of astrocyte dysfunction. The existing models are thus useful for examining several aspects of Alexander disease. However, since they do not display most of the common symptoms and pathology of the disorder, mice are now being produced with targeted point mutations in their endogenous *Gfap* gene. It is hoped that these will provide more complete models, leading to continued progress in unraveling the pathogenesis of Alexander disease and facilitating the development and testing of strategies for potential therapy.

### Acknowledgments

We thank our collaborators, especially James E. Goldman, who have contributed to these studies. This work was supported by grants from the National Institutes of Health (NS-22475, NS-41803).

### References

Alexander, W. S. (1949). Progressive fibrinoid degeneration of fibrillary astrocytes associated with mental retardation in a hydrocephalic infant. *Brain* **72,** 373–381.

Amaducci, L., Forno, K. I., and Eng, L. F. (1981). Glial fibrillary acidic protein in cryogenic lesions of the rat brain. *Neurosci. Lett.* **21,** 27–32.

Anderová, M., Kubinová, S., Mazel, T., Chvátal, A., Eliasson, C., Pekny, M., and Syková, E. (2001). Effect of elevated $K^+$, hypotonic stress, and cortical spreading depression on astrocyte swelling in GFAP-deficient mice. *Glia* **35,** 189–203.

Bignami, A., and Dahl, D. (1976). The astroglial response to stabbing. Immunofluorescence studies with antibodies to astrocyte-specific protein (GFA) in mammalian and submammalian species. *Neuropathol. Appl. Neurobiol.* **2,** 99–110.

Borrett, D., and Becker, L. E. (1985). Alexander's disease. A disease of astrocytes. *Brain* **108,** 367–385.

Bovolenta, P., Liem, R. K. H., and Mason, C. A. (1984). Development of cerebellar astroglia: Transitions in form and cytoskeletal content. *Dev. Biol.* **102,** 248–259.

Brenner, M., Johnson, A. B., Boespflug-Tanguy, O., Rodriguez, D., Goldman, J. E., and Messing, A. (2001). Mutations in GFAP, encoding glial fibrillary acidic protein, are associated with Alexander disease. *Nature Genet.* **27,** 117–120.

Brenner, M., Lampel, K., Nakatani, Y., Mill, J., Banner, C., Mearow, K., Dohadwala, M., Lipsky, R., and Freese, E. (1990). Characterization of human cDNA and genomic clones for glial fibrillary acidic protein. *Mol. Brain Res.* **7,** 277–286.

Bruijn, L. I., Becher, M. W., Lee, M. K., Anderson, K. L., Jenkins, N. A., Copeland, N. G., Sisodia, S. S., Rothstein, J. D., Borchelt, D. R., Price, D. L., and Cleveland, D. W. (1997). ALS-linked SOD1 mutant G85R mediates damage to astrocytes and promotes rapidly progressive disease with SOD1-containing inclusions. *Neuron* **18,** 327–338.

Clarke, S. R., Shetty, A. K., Bradley, J. L., and Turner, D. A. (1994). Reactive astrocytes express the embryonic intermediate neurofilament nestin. *NeuroReport* **5,** 1885–1888.

Cox, N. R., Kwapien, R. P., Sorjonen, D. C., and Braund, K. G. (1986). Myeloencephalopathy resembling Alexander's disease in a Scottish terrier dog. *Acta Neuropathol. (Berl.)* **71,** 163–166.

Dahl, D. (1981). The vimentin-GFA protein transition in rat neuroglia cytoskeleton occurs at the time of myelination. *J. Neurosci. Res.* **6,** 741–748.

Dahl, D., Bignami, A., Weber, K., and Osborn, M. (1981). Filament proteins in rat optic nerves undergoing Wallerian degeneration: Localization of vimentin, the fibroblastic 100-Å filament protein, in normal and reactive astrocytes. *Exp. Neurol.* **73,** 496–506.

Eddleston, M., and Mucke, L. (1993). Molecular profile of reactive astrocytes–Implications for their role in neurologic disease. *Neuroscience* **54,** 15–36.

Eliasson, C., Sahlgren, C., Berthold, C. H., Stakeberg, J., Celis, J. E., Betsholtz, C., Eriksson, J. E., and Pekny, M. (1999). Intermediate filament protein partnership in astrocytes. *J. Biol. Chem.* **274,** 23996–24006.

Eng, L. F., and Lee, Y. L. (1993). Intermediate filaments in astrocytes. *In* "Neuroglial Cells" (B. R. Ransom and H. Kettenmann, eds.). Oxford University Press, New York.

Eng, L. F., Lee, Y. L., Kwan, H., Brenner, M., and Messing, A. (1998). Astrocytes cultured from transgenic mice carrying the added human glial fibrillary acidic protein gene contain Rosenthal fibers. *J. Neurosci. Res.* **53,** 353–360.

Fankhauser, R., Fatzer, R., Bestetti, G., Deruaz, J. P., and Perentes, E. (1980). Encephalopathy with Rosenthal fibre formation in a sheep. *Acta Neuropathol. (Berl.)* **50,** 57–60.

Frisén, J., Johansson, C. B., Török, C., Risling, M., and Lendahl, U. (1995). Rapid, widespread, and longlasting induction of nestin contributes to the generation of glial scar tissue after CNS injury. *J. Cell Biol.* **131,** 453–464.

Fuchs, E., and Cleveland, D. W. (1998). A structural scaffolding of intermediate filaments in health and disease. *Science* **279,** 514–519.

Gomi, H., Yokoyama, T., Fujimoto, K., Ideka, T., Katoh, A., Itoh, T., and Itohara, S. (1995). Mice devoid of the glial fibrillary acidic protein develop normally and are susceptible to scrapie prions. *Neuron* **14,** 29–41.

Hatten, M. E., Liem, R. K. H., Shelanski, M. L., and Mason, C. A. (1991). Astroglia in CNS injury. *Glia* **4,** 233–243.

Head, M. W., and Goldman, J. E. (2000). Small heat shock proteins, the cytoskeleton, and inclusion body formation. *Neuropathology & Applied Neurobiology* **26,** 304–312.

Herndon, R. M. (1999). Is Alexander's disease a nosologic entity or a common pathologic pattern of diverse etiology? *Journal of Child Neurology* **14,** 275–276.

Herndon, R. M., Rubinstein, L. J., Freeman, J. M., and Mathieson, G. (1970). Light and electron microscopic observations on Rosenthal fibers in Alexander's disease and in multiple sclerosis. *J. Neuropathol. Exp. Neurol.* **29,** 524–551.

Iwaki, T., Kume-Iwaki, A., Liem, R. K. H., and Goldman, J. E. (1989). αB-Crystallin is expressed in non-lenticular tissues and accumulates in Alexander disease brain. *Cell* **57,** 71–78.

Johnson, D. A., Andrews, G. K., Xu, W., and Johnson, J. A. (2002). Activation of the antioxidant responsive element in primary cortical neuronal cultures derived from transgenic reporter mice. *J. Neurochem.* **81,** 1233–1241.

Kato, S., Hayashi, H., Nakashima, K., Nanba, E., Kato, M., Hirano, A., Nakano, I., Asayama, K., and Ohama, E. (1997). Pathological characterization of astrocytic hyaline inclusions in familial amyotrophic lateral sclerosis. *Am. J. Pathol* **151,** 611–620.

Kato, S., Shimoda, M., Watanabe, Y., Nakashima, K., Takahashi, K., and Ohama, E. (1996). Familial amyotrophic lateral sclerosis with a two base pair deletion in superoxide dismutase 1 gene: Multisystem degeneration with intracytoplasmic hyaline inclusions in astrocytes. *J. Neuropathol. Exp. Neurol.* **55,** 1089–1101.

Koyama, Y., and Goldman, J. E. (1999). Formation of GFAP cytoplasmic inclusions in astrocytes and their disaggregation by αB-crystallin. *Am. J. Pathol.* **154,** 1563–1572.

Li, R., Messing, A., Goldman, J. E., and Brenner, M. (2002). GFAP mutations in Alexander disease. *Int. J. Dev. Neurosci.* **20,** 259–268.

Liedtke, W., Edelmann, W., Bieri, P. L., Chiu, F. C., Cowan, N. J., Kucherlapati, R., and Raine, C. S. (1996). GFAP is necessary for the integrity of CNS white matter architecture and long-term maintenance of myelination. *Neuron* **17,** 607–615.

Liedtke, W., Edelmann, W., Chiu, F.-C., Kucherlapati, R., and Raine, C. S. (1998). Experimental autoimmune encephalomyelitis in mice lacking glial fibrillary acidic protein is characterized by a more severe clinical course and an infiltrative central nervous system lesion. *Am. J. Pathol.* **152,** 251–259.

Lupski, J. R., Montes de Oca-Luna, R., Slaugenhaupt, S., Pentao, L., Guzzetta, V., Trask, B. J., Saucedo-Cardenas, O., Barker, D. F., Killian, J. M., Garcia, C. A., Chakravarti, A., and Patel, P. I. (1991). DNA duplication associated with Charcot-Marie-Tooth disease type 1A. *Cell* **66,** 219–232.

Mathewson, A. J., and Berry, M. (1985). Observations on the astrocyte response to a cerebral stab wound in adult rats. *Brain Res.* **327,** 61–69.

McCall, M. A., Gregg, R. G., Behringer, R. R., Brenner, M., Delaney, C. L., Galbreath, E. J., Zhang, C. L., Pearce, R. A., Chiu, S. Y., and Messing, A. (1996). Targeted deletion in astrocyte intermediate filament (*Gfap*) alters neuronal physiology. *Proc. Natl. Acad. Sci. USA* **93,** 6361–6366.

McGrath, J. T. (1980). Fibrinoid leukodystrophy (Alexander's disease). *In* "Spontaneous Animal Models of Human Disease" (E. J. Andrews, B. C. Ward, and H. N. Altman, eds.), Vol. 2., pp. 147–148. Academic Press, New York.

Menet, V., Ribotta, M. G. Y., Chauvet, N., Drain, M. J., Lannoy, J., Colucci-Guyon, E., and Privat, A. (2001). Inactivation of the glial fibrillary acidic protein gene, but not that of vimentin, improves neuronal survival and neurite growth by modifying adhesion molecule expression. *J. Neurosci.* **21,** 6147–6158.

Messing, A., Head, M. W., Galles, K., Galbreath, E. J., Goldman, J. E., and Brenner, M. (1998). Fatal encephalopathy with astrocyte inclusions in GFAP transgenic mice. *Am. J. Pathol.* **152,** 391–398.

Nawashiro, H., Brenner, M., Fukui, S., Shima, K., and Hallenbeck, J. M. (2000). High susceptibility to cerebral ischemia in GFAP-null mice. *Journal of Cerebral Blood Flow & Metabolism* **20,** 1040–1044.

Nawashiro, H., Messing, A., Azzam, N., and Brenner, M. (1998). Mice lacking glial fibrillary acidic protein are hypersensitive to traumatic cerebrospinal injury. *NeuroReport* **9,** 1691–1696.

Ni, Q., Johns, G. S., Manepalli, A., Martin, D. S., and Geller, T. J. (2002). Infantile Alexander's disease: Serial neuroradiologic findings. *J. Child Neurol.* **17,** 463–466.

Nicholl, I. D., and Quinlan, R. A. (1994). Chaperone activity of α-crystallins modulates intermediate filament assembly. EMBO J. **13,** 945–953.

Pekny, M., Johansson, C. B., Eliasson, C., Stakeberg, J., Wallen, A., Perlmann, T., Lendahl, U., Betsholtz, C., Berthold, C. H., and Frisen, J. (1999). Abnormal reaction to central nervous system injury in mice lacking glial fibrillary acidic protein and vimentin. *J. Cell Biol.* **145,** 503–514.

Pekny, M., Levéen, P., Pekna, M., Eliasson, C., Berthold, C.-H., Westermark, B., and Betsholtz, C. (1995). Mice lacking glial fibrillary acidic protein display astrocytes devoid of intermediate filaments but develop and reproduce normally. *EMBO J.* **14,** 1590–1598.

Pekny, M., Stanness, K. A., Eliasson, C., Betsholtz, C., and Janigro, D. (1998). Impaired induction of blood-brain barrier properties in aortic endothelial cells by astrocytes from GFAP-deficient mice. *Glia* **22,** 390–400.

Pixley, S. K. R., and de Vellis, J. (1984). Transition between immature radial glia and mature astrocytes studied with a monoclonal antibody to vimentin. *Dev. Brain Res.* **15,** 201–209.

Reichelt, J., Bussow, H., Grund, C., and Magin, T. M. (2001). Formation of a normal epidermis supported by increased stability of keratins 5 and 14 in keratin 10 null mice. *Molecular Biology of the Cell* **12,** 1557–1568.

Richardson, J. A., Tang, K., and Burns, D. K. (1991). Myeloencephalopathy with Rosenthal fiber formation in a miniature poodle. *Vet. Pathol.* **28,** 536–538.

Rosenthal, W. (1898). Über eine eigenthümliche, mit syringomyelie complicirte geschwulst des rückenmarks. *Bietr. Pathol. Anat.* **23,** 111–143.

Russo, L. S., Jr., Aron, A., and Anderson, P. J. (1976). Alexander's disease: A report and reappraisal. *Neurology* **26,** 607–614.

Rutka, J. T., and Smith, S. L. (1993). Transfection of human astrocytoma cells with glial fibrillary acidic protein complementary DNA: Analysis of expression, proliferation, and tumorigenicity. *Cancer Res.* **53,** 3624–3631.

Sherwin, R. M., and Berthrong, M. (1970). Alexander's disease with sudanophilic leukodystrophy. *Archives of Pathology & Laboratory Medicine* **89,** 321–328.

Shibuki, K., Gomi, H., Chen, L., Bao, S. W., Kim, J. S. K., Wakatsuki, H., Fujisaki, T., Fujimoto, J., Katoh, A., Ikeda, T., Chen, C., Thompson, R. F., and Itohara, S. (1996). Deficient cerebellar long-term depression, impaired eyeblink conditioning, and normal motor coordination in GFAP mutant mice. *Neuron* **16,** 587–599.

Sistermans, E. A., Decoo, R. F. M., Dewijs, I. J., and Vanoost, B. A. (1998). Duplication of the proteolipid protein gene is the major cause of Pelizaeus-Merzbacher disease. *Neurology* **50,** 1749–1754.

Takemura, M., Nishiyama, H., and Itohara, S. (2002). Distribution of phosphorylated glial fibrillary acidic protein in the mouse central nervous system. *Genes to Cells* **7,** 295–307.

Tanaka, H., Katoh, A., Oguro, K., Shimazaki, K., Gomi, H., Itohara, S., Masuzawa, T., and Kawai, N. (2002). Disturbance of hippocampal long-term potentiation after transient ischemia in GFAP deficient mice. *J. Neurosci. Res.* **67,** 11–20.

Tatzelt, J., Maeda, N., Pekny, M., Yang, S. L., Betsholtz, C., Eliasson, C., Cayetano, J., Camerino, A. P., DeArmond, S. J., and Prusiner, S. B. (1996). Scrapie in mice deficient in apolipoprotein E or glial fibrillary acidic protein. *Neurology* **47,** 449–453.

Wahlsten, D. (1982). Deficiency of corpus callosum varies with strain and supplier of the mice. *Brain Res.* **239,** 329–347.

Wang, X., Messing, A., and David, S. (1997). Axonal and non-neuronal cell responses to spinal cord injury in mice lacking glial fibrillary acidic protein. *Exp. Neurol.* **148,** 568–576.

Weinstein, D. E., Shelanski, M. L., and Liem, R. K. H. (1991). Suppression by antisense mRNA demonstrates a requirement for the glial fibrillary acidic protein in the formation of stable astrocytic processes in response to neurons. *J. Cell Biol.* **112,** 1205–1213.

Weissenböck, H., Obermaier, G., and Dahme, E. (1996). Alexander's disease in a Bernese mountain dog. *Acta Neuropathol. (Berl.)* **91,** 200–204.

CHAPTER

# 47

# Models of Pelizeaus-Merzbacher-Disease

*Klaus-Armin Nave and Ian R. Griffiths*

## INTRODUCTION

Among inherited neurological disorders, Pelizaeus-Merzbacher disease (PMD; McKusick #312080) is a leukodystrophy well suited for modelling in rodent mutants. Myelin-deficient mice and rats with altered expression of the X chromosome-linked gene for proteolipid protein (*Plp/Dm20*) have been investigated over many years and reflect a wide spectrum of phenotypic disease expression, that is similar in many respects to human PMD (see Chapter 37) and its milder form, spastic paraplegia type 2 (SPG-2; McKusick #312920), defined by mutation of the human *PLP/DM20* gene. The virtual identity of the mouse and human myelin protein in amino acid sequence may explain, at least in part, the similarity of loss-of-function and gain-of-function effects that characterize mutant oligodendrocytes in the CNS of these species. The detailed comparison of several natural and transgenic *Plp* mutants has helped to dissect the molecular pathology of PMD at the subcellular level. Several recent reviews have covered the genetics of PMD as a human leukodystrophy (Garbern *et al.*, 1999; Hodes *et al.*, 1994; Nave and Boespflug-Tanguy, 1996; Seitelberger *et al.*, 1996; Woodward and Malcolm, 1999, 2001; Yool *et al.*, 2000) and have drawn attention to the homologous animal models (Bradl and Linington, 1996; Griffiths, 1996; Griffiths *et al.*, 1995a, 1998a; Nadon and West, 1998; Nave and Boespflug-Tanguy, 1996; Scherer, 1997; Skoff, 1995; Vela *et al.*, 1998; Werner *et al.*, 1998). Recent observations in these mice have revealed an unexpected role of PLP-expressing oligodendrocytes in maintaining the long-term integrity of myelinated CNS axons. It is hoped that animal models of PMD will aid in the development of future treatment strategies (Griffiths, 1996; Griffiths *et al.*, 1995b, 1998a).

## PROTEOLIPID PROTEIN IN MOUSE AND MAN

Proteolipid protein (PLP) is one of the major structural proteins of CNS myelin. As reviewed in more detail in Chapter 16, PLP is an integral membrane protein of 276 amino acids and a molecular weight of 30kD (Milner *et al.*, 1985; Stoffel *et al.*, 1984), comprising about 50% of total myelin protein (Lees and Brostoff, 1984). By alternative RNA splicing, a second protein isoform (termed "DM20") is generated that lacks 35 residues from an internal loop region of the polytopic membrane protein (Nave *et al.*, 1987).

Unexpectedly for a structural protein of myelin, the primary sequence of PLP and DM20 is 100% conserved between rodents (mouse, rat) and humans (Diehl *et al.*, 1986; Hudson *et al.*, 1987; Milner *et al.*, 1985; Morello *et al.* 1986), and very few amino acid differences are found in other mammalian species. This suggests that PLP engages with additional proteins, and possibly with itself, in multiple space-restricted protein interactions.

Although no *bona fide* protein structural data are available, a widely accepted model places PLP/DM20 into the family of "4-helix bundle" proteins with four transmembrane domains and intracellular protrusion of the amino- and carboxyl-termini (Popot *et al.*, 1991; Wahle and Stoffel, 1998; Weimbs and Stoffel, 1992). The identification of acylated cysteine residues has confirmed the orientation of the amino and carboxyl termini. Presumably, these acyl residues anchor the cytosolic part of the polypeptide chain close to the membrane. Posttranslational palmitylation also explains the unusual hydrophobicity of PLP and DM20 that has hampered its biochemical analysis (Laursen *et al.*, 1984; Stoffel *et al.*, 1984). Recently, PLP has been identified as a component of CHAPS-insoluble membrane lipid rafts in oligodendrocytes, and a direct binding of cholesterol to PLP has been demonstrated by UV crosslinking (Simons *et al.*, 2000). Disulfide bonds stabilize the extracellular loop regions and overall topology (Weimbs *et al.*, 1992, 1994). There is indirect evidence that PLP/DM20 assembles into an oligomeric complex prior to reaching the myelin compartment, but the stoichiometry of this hypothetical PLP oligomer is not known (Jung *et al.*, 1996; Jung and Nave, unpublished results; McLaughlin *et al.*, 2002). A functional difference between PLP and DM20 is not known. However, immunostaining of oligodendrocytes with isoform-specific antibodies has suggested that the "PLP-specific" region harbors a signal for the efficient sorting of PLP into the myelin compartment (Anderson *et al.*, 1997; McLaughlin *et al.*, 2002; Trapp *et al.*, 1997).

The rodent *Plp* gene is predominantly expressed by myelin-forming oligodendrocytes, but cells in this lineage transcribe the *Plp* gene well before myelination starts, already in a subset of bipotential neuron/glia precursor cells (Dickinson *et al.*, 1996; Goebbels, Zalc, and Nave, unpublished data; Genoud *et al.*, 2002; Spassky *et al.*, 1998; Yu *et al.*, 1994). While this has suggested a protein function in earliest oligodendrocyte differentiation, there has been little supportive evidence from the phenotypic analysis of the available *Plp* mutants.

Recent evidence suggests that a subset of CNS neurons, including brain stem motor neurons, express a previously unrecognized vesicular isoform of PLP (sr-PLP, sr-DM20 for "soma-restricted") that differs from myelin PLP by an N-terminal extension of 12 residues and its absence from myelin (Bongarzone *et al.*, 1999, 2001a, 2001b). So far, the sr-PLP encoding exon (located within the first intron) has been found only in mice. Its possible biological function remains to be determined.

Rodent Schwann cells also express the *Plp* gene at a low level, with a predominating DM20 isoform that is not found in peripheral myelin (Griffiths *et al.*, 1995a; Pucket *et al.*, 1987). The mechanism of the intracellular retention of PLP/DM20 in Schwann cells is unknown, but in PLP-overexpressing mice the protein becomes a major component of compact myelin (Anderson *et al.*, 1997). Human PLP mutations have been associated with a yet unexplained peripheral neuropathy suggesting indeed a role for PLP also in the peripheral nervous system (Garbern *et al.*, 1997; Griffiths *et al.*, 1995a; Shy *et al.*, 2003).

Mechanistically, a normal cellular function of PLP has been difficult to define, and the complex phenotype of *Plp* mutant mice was not immediately helpful. Clearly, the incorporation of PLP into compact myelin contributes to the stable association of adjacent myelin membranes that form the "intraperiod line" of compacted myelin (Boison *et al.*, 1995; Klugmann *et al.*, 1997; Rosenbluth *et al.*, 1996). As detailed later, it appears that PLP also contributes to the integrity of myelinated axons, a function that could be related to its association with membrane lipid rafts and possibly the transport of raft-associated signaling molecules.

The unknown cellular function of PLP/DM20 is likely related to that of two PLP-related tetraspan proteins, termed M6A and M6B (Kitagawa *et al.*, 1993; Werner *et al.*, 2001; Yan *et al.*, 1993). These proteolipids are expressed in both neurons and glial cells, but the mutation of either gene has no obvious developmental defect in the mouse (Werner *et al.*, unpublished results). Structurally, both M6A and M6B correspond to DM20, and additional M6B isoforms are specified by extensive alternative mRNA splicing (Werner *et al.*, 2001). PLP and M6B may have an overlapping function in developing oligodendrocytes that is only obvious in the corresponding double mutant mice (Werner *et al.*, unpublished data)

The *PLP* gene has been linked to the X chromosome in mouse and humans (Willard and Riordan, 1985) and could later be fine-mapped to human Xq22.3 (Mattei *et al.*, 1986). The X-linkage of *PLP* sparked an immediate interest in its possible role in X-linked myelin disorders, including Pelizaeus-Merzbacher disease in humans and the *jimpy* mutation of mice (for an early review see Nave and Milner, 1989).

## THE CLINICAL SPECTRUM OF PLP GENE MUTATIONS

Mouse models are most valuable if they phenocopy the human disorder both clinically and with respect to the underlying pathology. As detailed in Chapter 37, PMD was described more than 100 years ago (Merzbacher, 1910; Pelizaeus, 1885) and is clinically characterized by impaired motor development, an early onset before 1 year, and an X-linked mode of transmission. Current diagnostic criteria were defined by Boulloche and Aicardi (1986) and include electrophysiological and magnetic resonance imaging (MRI) techniques, to be applied at any time during the life of a patient. As Pelizaeus already noticed, impaired motor development presents very early, and motor handicaps are greater than the retardation of psycho-intellectual development. In the most severe type II ("connatal") form of PMD, affected males show virtually no psychomotor development and death occurs in the first decade. In the more frequent type I ("classical") form, patients reach a few motor developmental milestones up to 10 to 12 years of age, but after a plateau, have a slow deterioration (at ages 15 to 20) and death occurrs often in the fourth decade (Nave and Boespflug-Tanguy, 1996). Motor performance varies between families (i.e., *PLP* mutations) but also between affected males of the same PMD family. This suggests the existence of yet unidentified disease modifier genes that have also been noted for *Plp* mutations in different lines of inbred mice.

Histologically, the neuropathological findings in PMD are the severe hypomyelination, which is limited to the CNS, in the absence of inflammation. Islets of preserved myelin around blood vessels may result in the patchy appearence of white matter. Staining neutral lipid material in white matter areas with sudan black led to the classification of PMD as a "sudanophilic leukodystrophy." Using these neuropathological characteristics, Seitelberger *et al.* (1970) subdivided several forms of PMD, taking into account the X-linked mode of transmission, age of onset, and more recently also molecular genetics (Seitelberger *et al.*, 1996).

PMD *type I* is the slowly progressive "classical" form, described first by Pelizaeus; the more severe form *PMD type II* is "connatal" and shows rapid progression and death within 10 years of life. Clinically distinct from either form of PMD is X-linked spastic paraplegia type 2 (SPG-2) (Johnston and Mackusick, 1962) which is a milder, allelic form at the *PLP* locus (Saugier-Veber *et al.*, 1994). SPG-2 patients have progressive gait abnormalities after an almost normal motor development in the first 2 years. This makes SPG-2 a late onset disease that, nevertheless, shares clinical features with PMD (nystagmus, cerebellar ataxia, pyramidal syndrome). However, hypotonia, choreoathetosis or the bobbing movements of head and trunk, which are frequent in PMD, are rarely observed. SPG-2 patients walk unaided for many years, and most of them are able to attend school. Myelination may not be severely affected and progressive axonal involvement may be largely responsible for the clinical picture of SPG-2. Nearly the same clinical spectrum has been recognized in mouse mutants of the *Plp* gene.

## NATURAL MUTATIONS OF THE RODENT *PLP* GENE PROVIDE MODELS OF PELIZAEUS-MERZBACHER DISEASE

Spontaneous neurological mutations in the mouse that are associated with a hypomyelinated phenotype of the CNS have been known for a long time. They were studied before the molecular basis of any human leukodystrophy was known. The subgroup of X-linked recessive myelin mutants was identified by formal genetic criteria (i.e., affected males born to healthy female carriers). These mutants were allelic to each other and a mutation of the X chromosome-linked *Plp* gene has been identified in these lines. The following is a brief overview of the clinical phenotype of various *Plp* mutants, followed by a discussion of the possible disease mechanism in the natural and engineered *Plp* mutants, both of which are models for human PMD. Not covered in this chapter are *Plp* mutations in nonrodent animal species, including the *shaking pup*, a dog model (Nadon *et al.*, 1990), *paralytic tremor*, a rabbit model (Tosic *et al.*, 1994), and a congenital tremor in pig (Baumgartner and Brenig, 1996).

## The *Jimpy* Mouse

The *jimpy* mutation in the mouse (genetic symbol: $Plp^{jp}$) provided the first animal model related to PMD. This natural mutation was discovered by Phillips (1954) as a lethal X-linked trait (Sidman *et al.*, 1964) and has been maintained by the Jackson Laboratories on a CBA background (B6CBACa Aw-J/A-$Plp^{jp}$). For a long time, the genetically linked coat color gene *Tabby* (15 cM genetic distance) was the only marker of hemizygous *jimpy* males prior to the onset of symptoms, but has now been replaced by PCR-based genetic testing (Schneider *et al.*, 1995).

The clinical signs of affected males begin in the second postnatal week, coinciding with the onset of CNS myelination in wild-type mice. Ataxia, generalized body tremor that precedes locomotor activity, and seizures are similar in this and other myelin-deficient mouse mutants (Fig. 47.1). Before the fourth week of age, prolonged convulsions result in premature death (Sidman *et al.*, 1964). The final cause of the animals' death may related to the toxicity of the protein expressed in specific brain stem neurons (discussed later).

The molecular defect of *jimpy* mice is an A-to-G point mutation in the 7 exon *Plp* gene. It destroys the splice acceptor site of intron 4, thereby causing the abnormal loss of exon 5 from mature PLP and DM20 mRNA. Consequently, both PLP isoforms have truncated carboxyl-termini and lack the fourth transmembrane domain (Dautigny *et al.*, 1986; Hudson *et al.*, 1987; Macklin et al, 1987; Morello *et al.*, 1986; Nave *et al.*, 1986, 198 ).

The histological *jimpy* phenotype is the almost complete lack of myelin in the CNS, associated with the lack of mature oligodendrocytes (Hirano *et al.*, 1969; Krauss-Ruppert *et al.*, 1973; Meier and Bischoff, 1974, 1975; Meier and Bischoff, 1975) (Fig. 47.2). Increased rate of oligodendrocyte cell death (Skoff, 1982, 1995) resembles apoptosis in some but not all aspects (Knapp *et al.*, 1999a). A small percentage of *jimpy* oligodendrocytes survive and generate small patches of myelin for 1 to 2% of axons. Ultrastructurally, the intraperiod line (IPL) of myelin, normally a double-line with irregular appearance, appears fused in *jimpy* to a single electron-dense structure, indistinguishable from the major dense line (MDL). This ultrastructural abnormality suggests the lack of a "strut"-type rather than a "glue"-type molecule in compacted myelin (Duncan *et al.*, 1989; Schneider *et al.*, 1995).

Biochemical studies have failed to purifiy myelin fractions from *jimpy* mice, and the mutant PLP is nearly undetectable in total brain extracts, possibly because of instability and degradation (Benjamins *et al.*, 1994; Fannon *et al.*, 1994). As discussed further below, PLP is made in mutant oligodendrocytes but does not reach the cell surface or the myelin compartment. Peripheral myelin appears unaffected in *jimpy*, possibly reflecting the CNS-specific assembly, if not expression, of PLP/DM20.

Affected *jimpy* mice are generally smaller in size than wild-type males, and have other pathological features that are not obviously related to the primary gene defect or the lack of myelin (Gotow *et al.*, 1999; Knapp *et al.*, 1998, 1999b; Le Goascogne *et al.*, 2000; Skoff *et al.*, 1976; Vela *et al.*, 1996; Wu *et al.*, 2000). Some of these features may also be present in other mice with *Plp* point mutations, in all PLP-dependent myelin disorders, or even in unrelated dysmyelinated mice.

## The *Jimpy-msd* Mouse

The mouse mutant *msd* ($Plp^{jp\text{-}msd}$; for *myelin synthesis deficient*) was first described by Meier and MacPike (1970) and soon identified as allelic to *jimpy* (Eicher and Hoppe, 1973). The

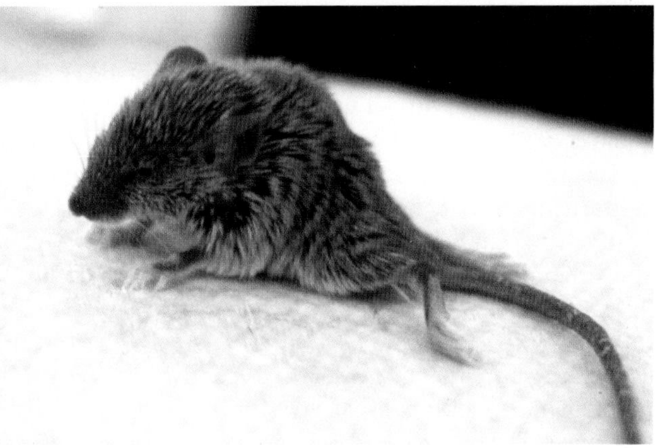

FIGURE 47.1

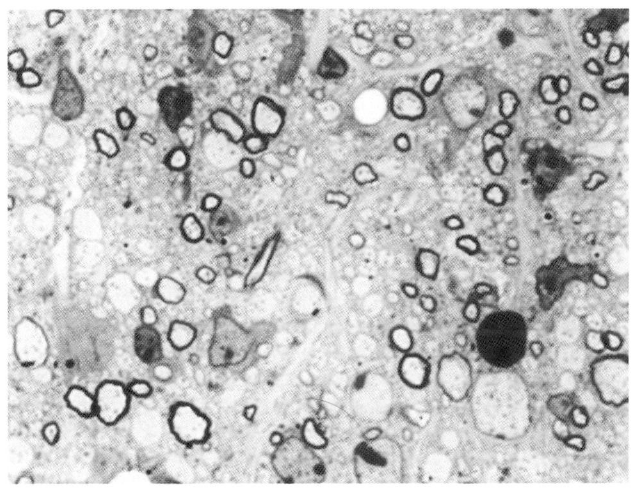

FIGURE 47.2
Light micrograph of resin section taken from the white matter of the spinal cord of a *jimpy* mouse showing many of the features associated with spontaneous *Plp* gene mutations in mice. There is an overall paucity of myelin; many axons are devoid of sheaths or associated with thin sheaths. A pyknotic nucleus is present, evidence of apoptosis, probably of an oligodendrocyte.

mouse is phenotypically, and by its reduced lifespan of 3 to 4 weeks, indistinguishable from *jimpy*, although slightly more spinal cord axons are ensheathed (Billings-Gagliardi *et al.*, 1980). Gencic *et al.* (1990) identified a point mutation in exon 7 of the *Plp* gene with a rather conservative amino acid substitution (A242V), which alters the fourth transmembrane domain of the protein. The *msd* mouse offers some experimental advantages relating to the preserved carboxylterminus of the mutant protein, to which several high-affinity antibodies are available (Gow *et al.*, 1998; Jung *et al.*, 1996; Yamamura *et al.*, 1991).

Interestingly, the same amino acid change (A242V) has been identified in one human family with connatal PMD (Komaki *et al.*, 1999), and a related human mutation (A242E) has been described by Seeman *et al.*, (2002).

## The *Jimpy-4J* Mouse

The spontaneous mutation *jimpy-4J* ($Plp^{jp\text{-}4J}$) was identified in the Jackson laboratory as a new *jimpy* allele with the most severe histological phenotype described (Billings-Gagliardi *et al.*, 1995). *Jimpy-4J* mice show the complete absence of CNS myelin, a dramatic loss of oligodendrocytes, and live for about 24 days. The mutation has been found in exon 2, predicting the substitution Ala-38-Ser in first hydrophilic loop of PLP (Pearsall *et al.*, 1997).

### The *Myelin-Deficient* Rat

The myelin-deficient *md rat* has been identified by Csiza (Csiza and Lahunta, 1979; Dentinger *et al.* 1982) and also provides a model for the connatal form of PMD associated with a lack of PLP (Koeppen *et al.*, 1987). Boison and Stoffel (1989) identified the primary defect in the rat *Plp* gene, associated with the nonconservative substitution T74P and predicting a break in the second transmembrane helix of PLP. The complete lack of mutant PLP from compact myelin results in a characteristic decrease of myelin periodicity—that is, closer apposition of myelin membranes (Duncan *et al.*, 1987)—later confirmed in *jimpy* mice (Duncan *et al.*, 1995; Schneider *et al.*, 1995), as well as subtle axonal abnormalities (Barron *et al.*, 1987; Dentinger *et al.*, 1985). Clinically, *md rats* are similar to the *Plp* mutant mice, with tremors, tonic seizures, and premature death. Recently, a longer-lived mutant substrain has been isolated in which affected males survive for about 80 days (Duncan *et al.*, 1995), suggesting the importance of yet unknown modifier genes. As larger animals, *md rats* are well suited for cell transplantation experiments (Bruestle *et al.*, 1999), for electrophysiological studies on the consequences of myelin-deficiency (Utzschneider *et al.*, 1992; Young *et al.*, 1989), and for research on the underlying cause of premature death (Miller *et al.*, 2003).

### The *Rumpshaker* Mouse

The *rumpshaker* ($Plp^{jp\text{-}rsh}$) mutation predicts the substitution Ile-186-Thr in PLP and DM20, and is associated with a relatively mild phenotype (Schneider *et al.*, 1992). The preservation of oligodendrocytes with considerably reduced cell death, when compared to *jimpy*, results in substantially improved myelination (Fig. 47.3) (Griffiths *et al.*, 1990). The optic nerve contains both amyelinated and normally myelinated axons, whereas spinal cord axons are only thinly myelinated with little growth in thickness during development (Fanarraga *et al.*, 1992). Different from *jimpy* and *jimpy-msd* mice, *rumpshaker* mutant myelin also incorporates significant amounts of proteolipids, with the DM20 isoform predominating (Fanarraga *et al.*, 1992; Karthigasan *et al.*, 1996). However, the altered ratio of PLP/DM20 is not responsible by itself for a dysmyelinated phenotype (Uschkureit *et al.*, 2001). Karthigasan *et al.* (1996) reported that the biochemical abnormalities in *rumpshaker* myelin correlate with a wider periodicity and less stable packing of the layers. *Rumpshaker* mice also demonstrated that apoptosis in other *Plp* mutants is not caused by dysmyelination per se (Schneider *et al.*, 1992), but as discussed later, rather by the toxicity of mutant PLP and DM20 isoforms when retained in the endoplasmic reticulum of oligodendrocytes (Gow and Lazzarini, 1996; Gow *et al.*, 1998).

*Rumpshaker* mice are long lived and reproduce well, although showing ataxia and mild tremor, but little seizure activity. Interestingly, the severity of their phenotype is markedly influenced by the background strain—that is, unknown modifier genes (Al-Saktawi *et al.*, 2003) (Fig. 47.4). *Rumpshaker* mice are a good animal model for SPG-2 in humans, in fact the same point mutation (I186T) was identified later in the index family of this human disease (Kobayashi *et al.*, 1994; Naidu *et al.*, 1997).

## PLP/DM20-DEPENDENT DISEASE MECHANISMS IN NATURAL AND ENGINEERED RODENT MODELS OF PMD AND SPG-2

Pelizaeus-Merzbacher disease and SPG-2 have been associated with (and are now genetically defined by) mutations of the human *PLP* locus, specifically (1) various point mutations in the coding region of the *PLP* gene and consequently the expression of mutant proteolipids, (2) with the loss of PLP function in null alleles or equivalent mutations, and (3) with the overexpression of PLP in patients that carry a gene duplication. For an updated listing of specific mutations in the *PLP* gene, see www.med.wayne.edu/Neurology/plp.html.

At the molecular level, it appears that PMD/SPG-2 is associated with three distinct pathomechanisms that act overlappingly. They have been revealed by dissecting the disease process at the cellular level in cultured cells and in corresponding mouse mutants.

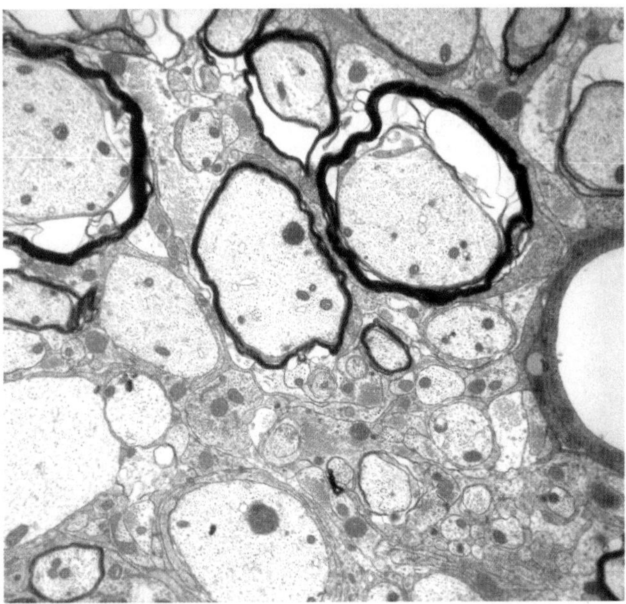

FIGURE 47.3
Electron micrograph of white matter from the spinal cord of a *rumpshaker* mouse. There is moderate dysmyelination with axons either naked or surrounded by a disproportionately thin myelin sheath. The outline of the sheaths is undulating and vacuoles are present but the majority of the myelin is compacted, although when viewed at high magnification the periodicity is reduced (not shown).

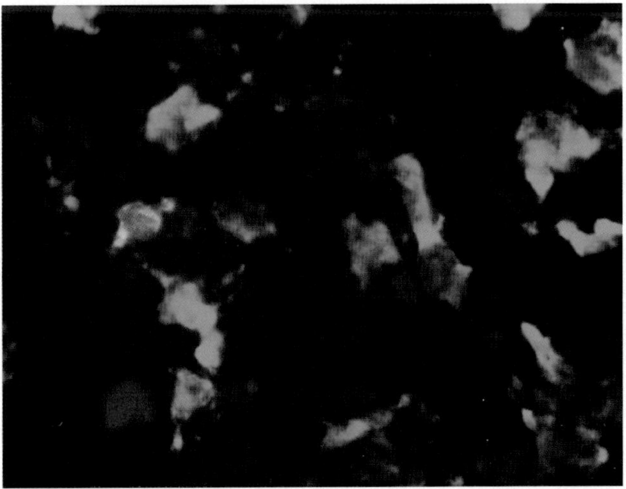

FIGURE 47.4
Area of white matter from the spinal cord of a *rumpshaker* mouse with the mutation on the C57BL/6 genetic background. When the mutation is expressed on this background the phenotype is considerably more severe than when on the C3H background (Al-Shaktawi *et al.*, 2003). The section is immunostained with the CC-1 antibody (green) to demonstrate oligodendrocytes and with the apoptotic marker, caspase-3 (red). One double labeled oligodendrocyte (orange) is undergoing apoptosis; another unidentified cell is single labeled for caspase-3 (red). Apoptotic cells are rare when the *rumpshaker* mutation is expressed on the C3H background but common when on the C57BL/6 background and also with most other spontaneous mutations of the *Plp* gene, such as *jimpy*.

## *Plp* Point Mutations and Abnormal Oligodendrocyte Death

The "classical" neurological mouse mutant *jimpy* lacks CNS myelin almost completely. The underlying histological feature is a paucity of mature oligodendrocytes and signs of abnormally increased oligodendrocyte death, such as pyknotic nuclei and TUNEL positive oligodendroglial nuclei (Skoff, 1982; Knapp *et al.*, 1986). *Jimpy* oligodendrocytes die even when maintained in cell culture and it has been impossible so far to define survival factors that prevent cell death (Bartlett *et al.*, 1998; Williams and Gard, 1997; Wolf and Holden, 1969). More recent studies suggest that abnormal cell death in *jimpy* is a combination of both apoptotic and nonapoptotic mechanisms (Cerghet *et al.*, 2001; Southwood and Gow, 2001; Thomson *et al.*, 1999). Transplantation experiments of oligodendrocytes from *jimpy* donor brains into wild-type (or *shiverer* mutant) host brains have confirmed that cell death is cell autonomous at an early window of postnatal development (Lachapelle *et al.*, 1994). It coincides with increasing expression of the mutant PLP gene, albeit the abnormal protein never accumulates to significant levels (Vermeesch *et al.*, 1990). This issue has been re-investigated at the single cell level in both *jimpy* and *jimpy-msd* mice, and also in the *md-rat*, with high-affinity PLP/DM20 antibodies, TUNEL staining, confocal immunofluorescence microscopy, in situ hybridization, and electron microscopy (Gow *et al.*, 1998; Grinspan *et al.*, 1998; Lipsitz *et al.*, 1998; Thomson *et al.*, 1999). Collectively, these studies have provided evidence that mutant oligodendrocytes mature normally up to the stage of expressing myelin proteins and other late differentiation markers, but undergo apoptosis later, presumably following a threshold expression of mutant PLP.

In normal development, oligodendrocytes are generated in excess and their final number is regulated by extrinsic signals that counteract apoptosis (Barres *et al.*, 1992; Trapp *et al.*, 1997). Theoretically, oligodendrocyte death in PLP mutants could result from disturbed glial differentiation or from the loss of a PLP/DM20 function in oligodendrocyte development. The latter seems unlikely because the complete loss of PLP in a genetic null mutant mouse does not obviously diminish oligodendrocyte survival (Stoffel *et al.*, 1984; Klugmann *et al.*, 1997; Yool *et al.*, 2001). Moreover, mutant oligodendrocytes express most of the late antigenic marker genes before they die (Gow *et al.*, 1998; Grinspan *et al.*, 1998; Pringle *et al.*, 1997). Nevertheless, Beesley *et al.* (2001) found that mutant oligodendrocytes (cultured from *md rats*) failed to express the myelin oligodendrocyte glycoprotein (MOG). Even when oligodendrocyte apoptosis was suppressed with a caspase-3 inhibitor, the expression of MOG could not be detected, suggesting a rather direct effect of mutant PLP on oligodendrocyte differentiation.

At present, oligodendrocyte death in PLP mutant mice is best explained by a "toxic" effect of aberrant *Plp* expression on oligodendrocyte survival. Using heterologous expression of *Plp* in fibroblastoid cells, Gow *et al.* (1994) observed the abnormal retention of mutant, but not wild-type, PLP and DM20 in the endoplasmic reticulum of transfected COS-7 cells. Using this cDNA expression system, a genotype-phenotype correlation between the degree of intracellular retainment of mutant proteolipid and disease severity (in PMD and the natural mouse mutants) has been established (Gow and Lazzarini, 1996). PLP and DM20 from mutant mice is indeed physically misfolded protein, as shown by the monoclonal antibody O10 that defines a conformation-sensitive epitope that is lost in PLP/DM20 isoforms derived from dysmyelinated mice (Jung *et al.*, 1996).

Expression of misfolded membrane proteins that are subsequently retained in the ER, is known to induce a cellular stress response (Ron, 2002; Sherman and Goldberg, 2001; that may lead to apoptotic cell death in vulnerable cells, such as developing oligodendrocytes. The induction of various down-stream effector genes of the ER response, including chop1, has been recently described by Gow and coworkers for *Plp*-mutant *rumpshaker* mice (Southwood *et al.*, 2002). Whether the unexpected effect of Chop1-deficiency worsening the *rumpshaker* phenotype is directly atributable to Chop1 function in stressed oligodendrocytes (Southwood *et al.*, 2002), or the effect of unknown modifier genes associated with this and other *Plp* mutations (Al-Saktawi *et al.*, 2003; Billings-Gagliardi *et al.*, 2001; Duncan *et al.*, 1995) remains to be determined.

An important physiological question is the ultimate cause of premature death of these mice after several weeks of survival. The comparison with other myelin mutants suggests that *Plp* mutants do not die as a result of dysmyelination *per se* (Billings-Gagliardi *et al.*, 1999; Wolf *et al.*, 1999). In the *md rat* it has recently been shown that the expression and toxicity of mutant PLP, detectable in a subset of glutamatergic brainstem neurons (not oligodendroglia) of the nucleus hypoglossus, perturbs the normal function of these nuclei in breathing control. Miller *et al.* (2003) found that normal ventilatory functions, following prolonged epileptic seizures and hypoxia, are not properly used for compensation. Thus, it may be a specific neuronal dysfunction and hypoxic ventilatory depression, rather than the loss of myelin, that ultimately leads to premature death.

### Transgenic *Plp* Overexpression as a Model for *PLP* Gene Duplication

The second disease mechanism underlying PMD involves the duplication of the entire X-linked *PLP/DM20* gene—that is, a mere twofold overexpression of wild-type PLP and DM20 protein. It has now been recognized that *PLP* gene duplications, rather than point mutations, underlie the majority of familial cases with PMD (Cremers, *et al.*, 1987; Ellis and Malcolm, 1994; Mimault *et al.*, 1999; Nave and Boespflug-Tanguy, 1996; Sistermans *et al.*, 1998). Turning a normal cellular gene into a lethal disease gene by two-fold overexpression is a challenge to understand at the cellular level, possibly related to overexpression of a duplicated *PMP22* gene in Charcot-Marie-Tooth disease type 1A (see Chapters 39 and 48).

Mouse models for this type of PMD have been generated inadvertantly, originally in an attempt to complement the defect of *jimpy* mice with a wild type *Plp* transgene (Kagawa *et al.*, 1994; Readhead *et al.*, 1994). An unexpected observation was a severely dysmyelinated phenotype of all those transgenic mice that overexpressed wild-type *Plp* at least two-fold (as quantified at the RNA level) (Fig. 47.5). In the study of Readhead *et al.* (1994), such mutants were homozygous or double-heterozygous for either one of two cosmid-derived full-length *Plp* transgenes (line #72 or #66). The novel phenotype was related to that of *jimpy* mice, but less severe, with later onset, and with significantly longer survival times (up to 6 months). Different from the dysmyelinated *jimpy* mouse, the histological phenotype of *Plp* overexpressors revealed a complex mixture of dys- and demyelinating features, explaining the later onset of behavioural symptoms. Abnormal oligodendrocyte death (Fig. 47.6) was less obvious in the homozygous lines #72 and #66 of Readhead *et al.* (1994), but pronounced in the shorter-lived line #4e of Kagawa *et al.* (1994), which overexpressed *Plp* at a higher level, and independently in a line of *Plp* -transgenic rats (Bradl *et al.*, 1999). The mechanisms of abnormal cell death appear different from those in *Plp*-mutant mice (Cerghet *et al.*, 2001).

A follow-up study of the PLP-transgenic rat demonstrated an intracellular accumulation of PLP together with other membrane proteins, such as MAG and MOG (but not with MBP), suggesting a rather widespread effect on the export of other myelin proteins, but also nonmyelin membrane proteins (Bauer *et al.*, 2002). ER distensions, unfolded protein response (with the induction of chaperones), and occcasional cell death was most obvious in grey matter oligodendrocytes. It is unlikely, however, that this striking cellular phenoytype is the same in human PMD, because the level of PLP overexpression is only twofold in duplication patients.

Why is PLP overexpression not tolerated? It is possible that PLP interacts stoichiometrically with cellular proteins that are required for proper PLP export. If such a stochiometry were disturbed, excess PLP may accumulate and thus mimick the retention of misfolded PLP in mutant mice. Another hypothesis has been put forward by Simons *et al.* (2002), who found that the known interaction of PLP with cholesterol in membrane lipid rafts causes PLP-overexpressing oligodendrocytes to deliver both PLP and cholesterol into the lysosomal compartment. Here, the abnormal appearance of cholesterol could conceivably alter normal lysosomal functions and thus affect general cell metabolism. Ultrastructurally, oligodendrocytes in PLP overexpressing mice contain numerous autophagic vacuoles (Readhead *et al.*, 1994) (Fig. 47.5), which is in agreement with this hypothesis. Again it is not proven that these findings can be fully extrapolated to oligodendrocytes in PMD patients with only twofold *PLP* gene dosage. Interestingly, cultured cells that are vulnerable to PLP overexpression appear less affected by overexpression of the longer srPLP isoform (Bongarzone *et al.*, 2001b).

Mice with a single copy of the *Plp* transgene (in line #66 or #72) that overexpress PLP and DM20 less than twofold at the transcriptional level (Readhead *et al.*, 1994), develop

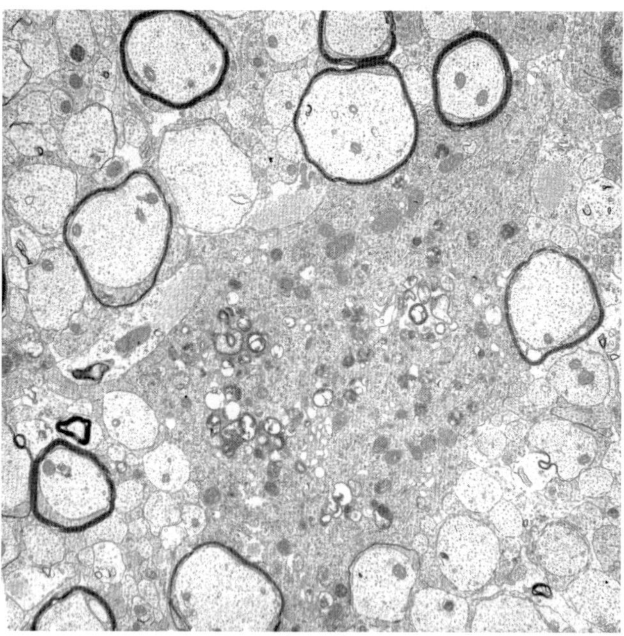

FIGURE 47.5
Electron micrograph of white matter from the spinal cord of a transgenic mouse overexpressing wild type PLP (#66, Readhead *et al.*, 1994). Dysmyelinated axons surround a central oligodendrocyte cell body in which numerous autophagic vacuoles containing membranous structures, are evident.

FIGURE 47.6
Immunostained sagittal section of cerebrum of a *Plp* overexpressing transgenic mouse showing the corpus callosum (lower aspect of figure) and the adjacent cortex (upper). The section is stained for MAG (red) which strongly labels the oligodendrocyte cell bodies. Note the paucity of myelin staining in the corpus callosum. Co-staining for caspase-3 (green) indicates several oligodendrocyes undergoing apoptosis.

normally. However, after 12 months of age, they show progressive ataxia and behavioural abnormalities. This aspect of PLP-dependent disease is caused by a (noninflammatory) demyelination with clear axonal involvement, most obvious in long tracts of the spinal cord (Anderson *et al.*, 1998). CNS demyelination has first been observed in adult mice overexpressing multiple copies of a DM20 cDNA transgene driven by a myelin-specific promoter (Mastronardi *et al.*, 1993; Simons-Johnson, et al., 1995). The mechanism underlying this late-onset neurodegeneration is unclear and its relationship to the developmental disorder in homozygous *Plp* -transgenics remains to be determined. It is likely that a similar axonal involvement contributes to the progressive nature of human PMD in patients with a *PLP* gene duplication.

## PLP/DM20-Deficient Mice: Proteolipid Function and Axonal Degeneration

Several laboratories have used gene targeting technologies and homologous recombination of in mouse embryonic stem cells to ablate the expression of PLP and DM20 (Boison and Stoffel, 1994; Klugmann *et al.*, 1997; Sporkel *et al.*, 2002; Stecca *et al.*, 2000). These mice should provide novel models of PMD, when associated with a deletion of the entire *PLP* gene (Raskind *et al.*, 1991) or an equivalent null mutation (Sistermans *et al.*, 1996), associated with a milder clinical course of disease. Moreover, null mutants should differentiate between true loss-of-function and aberrant gain-of-function effects that overlap in most mice and human patients with point mutations in this gene. Isoform-specific gene targeting should also help to understand functional differences between PLP and DM20. Surprisingly, the interpretation of all these data, when combined, is more difficult than anticipated, but the mice have clearly shown that PLP is not required for myelin formation. A toxic gain-of-function of PLP, when misfolded or overexpressed, emerges as the major cause of dysmyelination and cell death.

Stoffel and coworkers reported the first targeting of the *Plp* gene and obtained mice with a severe perturbation of *Plp* gene expression (close to a null mutation), resulting from the combination of a splice defect and anti-sense silencing by an inserted promoter sequence (Boison *et al.*, 1994). This mutation did not interfere with myelination, but the ultrastructure of CNS myelin was highly disordered. Myelin lamellae were loosely wrapped and lacked the apposition of the extracytoplasmic membrane surfaces (intraperiod line). This led to a profound reduction of conductance velocities of CNS axons (Gutierrez *et al.*, 1996), impairments in neuromotor coordination, and behavioral changes. Large diameter axons were loosely myelinated, and small axons were even unmyelinated. This led to the conclusion that adhesion properties of PLP are responsible for the tight apposition of membranes in compact myelin (Boison *et al.*, 1995). The creation of a complete PLP/DM20 null mutation in mice by Klugmann *et al.* (1997) confirmed most of these findings, but showed that the defect at the intraperiod line was highly variable, even within a single sheath with absent, condensed, and normal intraperiod lines all being observed (Klugmann *et al.*, 1997; Yool *et al.*, 2002). A tendency toward increased fixation artefacts (myelin delamination) in mutant brains was concluded and interpreted as a sign of reduced physical stability (see also Rosenbluth *et al.*, 1996). There were no motor deficits in young adult PLP-deficient mice and also the peripheral nervous system was normal, at least within the short lifespan of mice (Klugmann *et al.*, 1997), a remarkable difference from human patients with the *PLP* null mutation who develop a demyelinating peripheral neuropathy (Garbern *et al.*, 1997).

A second observation, important for the pathomechanism of PMD, was the finding that although myelin is assembled in the absence of PLP/DM20, after several months widespread axonal swellings cause neurodegeneration, predominantly of small-caliber axons (Griffiths *et al.*, 1998b) (Fig. 47.7). This fiber degeneration is probably secondary to impaired axonal transport, and is direct proof that myelinated axons require local oligodendroglial support (and that PLP/DM20 is required for this oligodendroglial function). Length-dependent axonal degenerations of the CNS have subsequently been found in both PLP-deficient mice and human patients with PMD (Garbern *et al.*, 2002). Such swellings and axonal degeneration profiles are not a feature of myelin mutants in general. They have been noted recently in the myelinated CNS of mice that carry a mutation of the oligodendrocyte-specific *Cnp1* (CNPase) gene (Lappe-Siefke *et al.*, 2003). Thus, several genes (including *Plp*) may be required by oligodendrocytes to provide axonal support, independent of myelin assembly itself. Loss of such a supportive glial function may explain the progressive axonal involvement that can be observed in several inherited and acquired myelin diseases, both in the CNS and PNS. The molecular nature of the underlying axon-glial interaction is completely unknown.

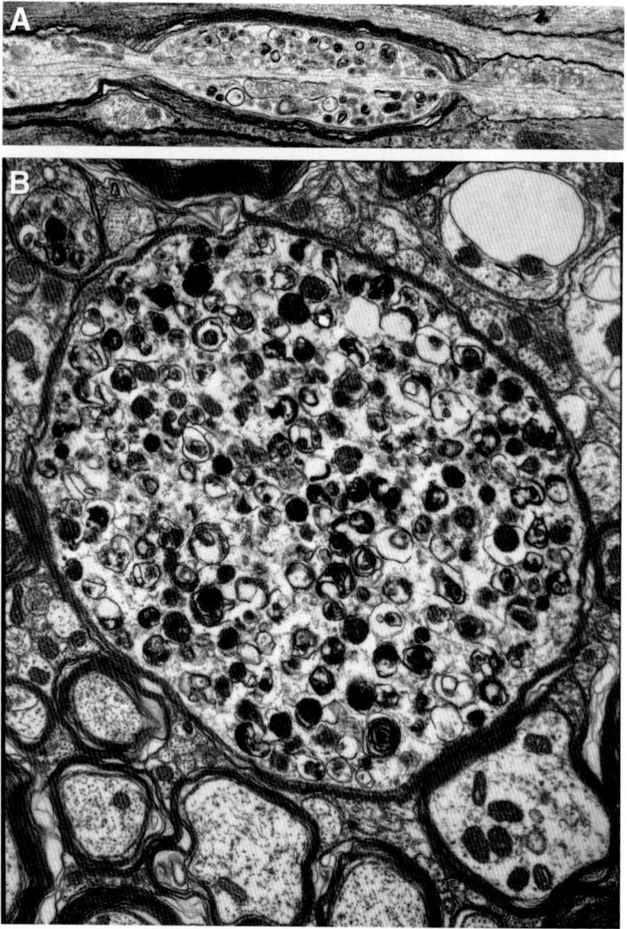


FIGURE 47.7
Electron micrograph of (A) longitudinal and (B) transverse sections of myelinated axons from a *Plp* null mouse. The axoplasm contains numerous membranous organelles, dense bodies and mitochondria. These typically accumulate initially distal to the nodal complex and are related to defects in retrograde axonal transport.

What is the molecular function and functional difference of PLP and DM20? Targeting the PLP/DM20 gene in combination with the Cre-Lox system, Stecca *et al.* (2000) have generated mice that lack alternative splicing and express, at normal levels, only the DM20 isoform. These mice showed the same phenoytype as reported for the combined PLP/DM20 null mutants, including the late onset axonal degeneration desribed by Griffiths *et al.* (1998b). This would suggest that PLP or PLP and DM20, but not DM20 alone, are required for maintaining axonal integrity. In contrast, Spörkel *et al.* (2002) who have independently created a DM20-only mouse mutant, found minimal phenotypical difference from wild-type mice, which would suggest that DM20 is sufficient for oligodendrocytes to maintain axonal integrity, and that there is little functional difference between both isoforms. This discrepancy cannot be adequately explained at the moment. However, already Griffiths *et al.* (1998b) noted that either PLP or DM20 cDNA based transgenes, when expressed in PLP/DM20 null mice, were both able to reduce the extent of axonal pathology, which agrees better with the findings of Spörkel *et al.* (2002).

The priciple cellular function of PLP and DM20 remains to be identified. It is likely that in oligodendrocytes a DM20-related proteolipid, termed M6B, serves in part a redundnant function with PLP/DM20. This is suggested because both PLP-deficient and M6B-deficient mutants are myelinated with few ultrastructural defects, whereas PLP/M6B double deficient mice have major developmental defects of CNS myelin (Werner *et al.*, in preparation).

## CONCLUSIONS

Mouse models of Pelizaeus-Merzbacher disease and SPG-2 have helped us to better understand the genetic basis and molecular pathology of the human myelin disorder and its wide clinical spectrum. This includes numerous histological, ultrastructural, and biochemical investigation of dysmyelination and demyelination in the CNS of PLP mutant mice, tracing back to the natural mutations in the 1960s and 1970s, and followed by the analysis of experimentally derived mutant lines in recent years. In conjunction with subcellular observations on mutant protein trafficking, *in vivo* and *in vitro*, a causal relationship of myelin protein misfolding, loss-of-function, abnormal gain-of-function effects, and lethal dysmyelination can be reconstructed. The greatest challenge remains in understanding the principle role that proteolipids in glia play in myelin assembly and long-term axon-glia interactions, the latter playing a major role in the progressive nature of PMD.

### References


Al-Saktawi, K., McLaughlin, M., Klugmann, M., Schneider, A., Barrie, J. A., McCulloch, M. C., Montague, P., Kirkham, D., Nave, K.-A., Griffiths, I. R., 2003, Genetic background determines phenotypic severity of the *Plp rumpshaker* mutation. *J. Neurosci. Res.* **72:**12–24.

Anderson, T. J., Montague, P., Nadon, N., Nave, K-A., Griffiths, I. R.,1997, Modification of Schwann cell phenotype with PLP transgenes: Evidence that the PLP and DM20. *J. Neurosci. Res.* **50:**13–22.

Anderson, T. J., Schneider, A., Barrie, J. A., Klugmann, M., McCulloch, M. C., Kirkham, D., Kyriakides, E., Nave, K.-A., Griffiths, I. R.,1998, Late-onset neurodegeneration in mice with increased dosage of the proteolipid protein gene. *J. Comp. Neurol.* **394:**506–519.

Barres, B. A., Hart, I. K., Coles, H. S., Burne, J. F, Voyvodic, J. T., Richardson, W. D., Raff, M. C., 1992, Cell death and control of cell survival in the oligodendrocyte lineage. *Cell* **70:**31–46.

Barron, K. D., Dentinger, M. P., Csiza, C. K., Keegan, S. M., Mankes, R., 1987, Abnormalities of central axons in a dysmyelinative rat mutant. *Exp. Mol. Pathol.* **47:**125–142.

Bartlett, W. P., Knapp, P. E., Skoff, R. P 1998, Glial conditioned medium enables jimpy oligodendrocytes to express properties of normal oligodendrocytes: Production of myelin antigens and membranes. *Glia* **1:**253–259.

Bauer, J., Bradl, M., Klein, M., Leisser, M., Deckwerth, T. L., Wekerle, H., Lassmann, H., 2002, Endoplasmic reticulum stress in PLP-overexpressing transgenic rats: Gray matter oligodendrocytes are more vulnerable than white matter oligodendrocytes. *J Neuropathol Exp Neurol.* **61:**12–22.

Baumgartner, B. G., Brenig, B., 1996, [The role of proteolipid proteins in the development of congenital tremors type AIII: A review], Dtsch. Tierarztl. *Wochenschr.* **103:**404–407.

Beesley, J. S., Lavy, L., Eraydin, N. B., Siman, R., Grinspan, J. B., 2001, Caspase-3 activation in oligodendrocytes from the myelin-deficient rat. *J Neurosci Res.* **64:**371–379.

Benjamins, J. A., Studzinski, D. M., Skoff, R. P., 1994, Analysis of myelin proteolipid protein and F0 ATPase subunit 9 in normal and jimpy CNS. *Neurochem Res.* **19:**1013–1022.

Billings-Gagliardi, S., Adcock, L. H., Wolf, M. K., 1980, Hypomyelinated mutant mice: Description of jpmsd and comparison with jp and qk on their present genetic backgrounds. *Brain Res.* **194:**325–338.

Billings-Gagliardi, S., Nunnari, J. N., Nadon, N. L., Wolf, M. K., 1999, Evidence that CNS hypomyelination does not cause death of jimpy-msd mutant mice. *Dev Neurosci.* **21:**473–82.

Billings-Gagliardi, S., Nunnari, J. J., Wolf, M. K., 2001, Rumpshaker behaves like juvenile-lethal Plp mutations when combined with shiverer in double mutant mice. *Dev Neurosci.* **23:**7–16.

Billings-Gagliardi, S., Kirschner, D. A., Nadon, N. L., DiBenedetto, L. M., Karthigasan, J., Lane, P., Pearsall, G. B., Wolf, M. K., 1995, Jimpy 4J: A new X-linked mouse mutation producing severe CNS hypomyelination. *Dev Neurosci.* **17:**300–310.

Boison, D., Stoffel, W., 1989, Myelin-deficient rat: A point mutation in exon III (A→C, Thr75→Pro) of the myelin proteolipid protein causes dysmyelination and oligodendrocyte death. *EMBO J.* **8:**3295–3302.

Boison, D., Stoffel,W., 1994, Disruption of the compacted myelin sheath of axons of the central nervous system in proteolipid protein-deficient mice. *Proc. Natl. Acad. Sci. USA* **91:**11709–11713.

Boison, D., Büssow, H., D'Urso, D., Müller, H. W., and Stoffel, W.,1995, Adhesive properties of proteolipid protein are responsible for the compaction of CNS myelin sheaths. *J. Neurosci.* **15:**5502–5513.

Bongarzone, E. R., Campagnoni, C. W., Kampf, K., Jacobs, E. C., Handley, V. W., Schonmann, V., Campagnoni, A. T., 1999, Identification of a new exon in the myelin proteolipid protein gene encoding novel protein isoforms that are restricted to the somata of oligodendrocytes and neurons. *J. Neurosci.* **19:**8349–8357.

Bongarzone, E. R., Jacobs, E., Schonmann, V., Campagnoni, A. T., 2001a, Classic and soma-restricted proteolipids are targeted to different subcellular compartments in oligodendrocytes. *J Neurosci. Res.* **65:**477–484.

Bongarzone, E. R., Jacobs, E., Schonmann, V., Kampf, K., Campagnoni, C. W., Campagnoni, A. T., 2001b, Differential sensitivity in the survival of oligodendrocyte cell lines to overexpression of myelin proteolipid protein gene products. *J Neurosci Res.* **65:**485–492.

Boulloche, J., Aicardi, J., 1986, Pelizaeus-Merzbacher disease: Clinical and nosological study. *J. Child Neurol.* **1**:233–239.

Bradl, M., Bauer, J., Inomata,T., Zielasek, J., Nave, K.-A., Toyka, K., Lassmann, H., Wekerle, H., 1999, Transgenic Lewis rats overexpressing the proteolipid protein gene: Myelin degeneration and its effect on T cell-mediated experimental autoimmune encephalomyelitis. *Acta Neuropathol.* **97**:595–606.

Bradl, M., Linington, C., 1996, Animal models of demyelination. *Brain Pathol.* **6**:303–311.

Brustle, O., Jones, K. N., Learish, R. D., Karram, K., Choudhary, K., Wiestler, O. D., Duncan, I. D., McKay, R. D., 1999, Embryonic stem cell-derived glial precursors: A source of myelinating transplants. *Science* **285,** 754–756.

Cerghet, M., Bessert, D. A., Nave, K.-A., and Skoff, R. P.,2001, Differential expression of apoptotic markers in *jimpy* and in PLP overexpressors: Evidence for different apoptotic pathways. *J. Neurocytol.* **30**:841–855.

Cremers, F. P. M., Pfeiffer, R. A., van de Pol, T. J. R., Hofker, M. H., Kruse, T. A., Wieringa, B., and Ropers, H. H.,1987, An interstitial duplication of the X chromosome in a male allows physical fine mapping of probes from the Xq13-q22 region. *Hum. Genet.* **77**:23–27.

Csiza, C. K., de Lahunta,A., 1979, Myelin deficiency (md): A neurologic mutant in the Wistar rat. *Am J Pathol.* **95**:215–223.

Dautigny, A., Mattei, M. G., Morello, D., Alliel, P. M., Pham-Dinh, D., Amar, L., Arnaud, D., Simon, D., Mattei, J. F, Guenet, J. L., *et al.*, 1986, The structural gene coding for myelin-associated proteolipid protein is mutated in jimpy mice. *Nature* **321**:867–329.

Dentinger, M. P., Barron, K. D., Csiza, C. K., 1982, Ultrastructure of the central nervous system in a myelin deficient rat. *J. Neurocytol.* **11**:671–691.

Dentinger, M. P., Barron, K. D., Csiza, C. K., 1985, Glial and axonal development in optic nerve of myelin deficient rat mutant. *Brain Res.* **344**:255–266.

Dickinson, P. J., Fanarraga, M. L., Griffiths, I. R., Barrie, J. A., Kyriakides, E., Montague, P.,1996, Oligodendrocyte progenitors in the embryonic spinal cord express DM-20. Neuropath. *Appl. Neurobiol.* **22**:188–198.

Diehl, H. J., Schaich, M., Budzinski, R. M., Stoffel, W., 1986, Individual exons encode the integral membrane domains of human myelin proteolipid protein. *Proc. Natl. Acad. Sci U S A.* **83**:9807–9811.

Duncan, I. D., Hammang, J. P., Goda, S., Quarles, R. H., 1989, Myelination in the jimpy mouse in the absence of proteolipid protein. *Glia* **2**:148–154.

Duncan, I. D., Hammang, J. P.,and Trapp, B. D., 1987, Abnormal compact myelin in the myelin-deficient rat: Absence of proteolipid protein correlates with a defect in the intraperiod line. *Proc. Natl. Acad. Sci. USA* **84**:6287–6291.

Duncan, I. D., Nadon, N. L., Hoffman, R. L., Lunn, K. F., Csiza, C., Wells, M. R., 1995, Oligodendrocyte survival and function in the long-lived strain of the myelin deficient rat. *J Neurocytol.* **24**:745–762.

Eicher, E. M., Hoppe, P. C., 1973, Use of chimeras to transmit lethal genes in the mouse and to demonstrate allelism of the two X-linked male lethal genes jp and msd. *J Exp. Zool.* **183**:181–184.

Ellis, D., Malcom S., 1994, Proteolipid protein gene dosage effect in Pelizaeus-Merzbacher disease. *Nat. Genet.* **6**: 333–334.

Fanarraga, M. L., Griffiths, I. R., McCulloch, M. C., Barrie, J. A., Kennedy, P. G. E., and Brophy, P. J., 1992, Rumpshaker: An X-linked mutation causing hypomyelination: Developmental differences in myelination and glial cells between the optic nerve and spinal cord. *Glia* **5**:161–170.

Fannon, A. M., Mastronardi, F. G., Moscarello, M. A., 1994, Isolation and identification of proteolipid proteins in jimpy mouse brain. *Neurochem Res.* **19**:1005–1012.

Filbin, M. T., Walsh, F. S., Trapp, B. D., Pizzey, J. A., and Tennekoon, G. I.,1990, Role of myelin P0 protein as a homophilic adhesion molecule. *Nature* **344**:871–872.

Garbern, J. Y., Cambi, F., Tang, X. M., Sima, A. A., Vallat, J. M., Bosch, E. P., Lewis, R., Shy, M., Sohi, J., Kraft, G., Chen, K. L., Joshi, I., Leonard, D. G., Johnson, W., Raskind, W., Dlouhy, S. R., Pratt, V., Hodes, M. E., Bird, T., and Kamholz, J., 1997, Proteolipid protein is necessary in peripheral as well as central myelin. *Neuron* **19**:205–218.

Garbern, J., Cambi, F., Shy, M., Kamholz, J., 1999, The molecular pathogenesis of Pelizaeus-Merzbacher disease. *Arch Neurol.* **56**:1210–1214.

Garbern, J. Y., Yool, D. A., Moore, G. J., Wilds, I. B., Faulk, M. W., Klugmann, M., Nave, K.-A., Sistermans, E. A., van der Knaap, M. S., Bird, T. D., Shy, M. E., Kamholz, J. A., Griffiths, I. R., 2002, Patients lacking the major CNS myelin protein, proteolipid protein 1, develop length-dependent axonal degeneration in the absence of demyelination and inflammation. *Brain* **125**:551–561.

Gencic,S., Hudson, L., 1990, Conservative amino acid substitution in the myelin proteolipid protein of jimpymsd mice. *J. Neurosci.* **10**:117–124.

Genoud, S., Lappe-Siefke, C., Goebbels, S., Radtke, F., Aguet, M., Scherer, S., Suter, U., Nave, K.-A., Mantei, N., 2002, Notch-1 control of oligodendrocyte differentiation. *J. Cell Biol.* **158,** 709–718.

Gotow, T., Leterrier, J. F., Ohsawa, Y., Watanabe, T., Isahara, K., Shibata, R., Ikenaka, K., Uchiyama, Y., 1999, Abnormal expression of neurofilament proteins in dysmyelinating axons located in the central nervous system of jimpy mutant mice. *Eur J Neurosci.* **11**:3893–3903.

Gow, A., Friedrich, V. L., Lazzarini, R. A., 1994, Many naturally occuring mutations of myelin proteolipid protein impair its intracellular transport. *J. Neurosci. Res.* **37**:574–583.

Gow, A., and Lazzarini, R. A., 1996, A cellular mechanism governing the severity of Pelizaeus-Merzbacher disease. *Nature Genetics* **13,** 422–428.

Gow, A., Southwood, C. M., Lazzarini, R. A., 1998, Disrupted proteolipid protein trafficking results in oligodendrocyte apoptosis in an animal model of Pelizaeus-Merzbacher disease. *J Cell Biol.* **140**:925–934.

Griffiths, I. R., 1996, Myelin mutants: Model systems to study normal and abnormal myelination. *BioEssays* **18:**789–797.

Griffiths, I. R., Dickinson, P., Montague, P., 1995a, Expression of the proteolipid protein gene in glial cells of the post-natal peripheral nervous system of rodents. Neuropath. *Appl. Neurobiol.* **21:**97–110.

Griffiths, I. R., Klugmann, M., Anderson, T. J., Thomson, C. E., Vouyiouklis, D. A., Nave, K.-A., 1998a, Current concepts of PLP and its role in the nervous system. *Microsc. Res. Tech.* **41:**344–358.

Griffiths, I. R., Klugmann, M., Anderson, T., Yool, D., Thomson, C.,Schwab, M. H., Schneider, A., Zimmermann, F., McCulloch, M., Nadon, N., and Nave, K.-A.,1998b, Axonal swellings and degeneration in mice lacking myelin proteolipid protein. *Science* **280:**1610–1613.

Griffiths, I. R., Schneider, A., Anderson, J., Nave, K.-A., 1995b, Transgenic and natural mouse models of proteolipid protein (PLP) related dysmyelination and demyelination. *Brain Pathol.* **5:**275–281.

Griffiths, I. R., Scott, I., McCulloch, M. C., Barrie, J. A., McPhilemy, K., Cattanach, B. M., 1990, Rumpshaker mouse: A new X-linked mutation affecting myelination: evidence for a defect in PLP expression. *J Neurocytol.* **19:**273–283.

Grinspan, J. B., Coulalaglou, M., Beesley, J. S., Carpio, D. F, Scherer, S. S., 1998, Maturation-dependent apoptotic cell death of oligodendrocytes in myelin-deficient rats. *J Neurosci Res.* **54:**623–634.

Gutierrez, R., Boison, D., Heinemann, U., Stoffel, W., 1996, Decompaction of CNS myelin leads to a reduction of the conduction velocity of action potentials in optic nerve. *Neurosci Lett.* **195:**93–96.

Hirano, A., Sax, D. S., Zimmerman, H. M., 1969, The fine structure of the cerebella of jimpy mice and their "normal" litter mates. *J. Neuropathol. Exp. Neurol.* **28:**388–400.

Hodes, M. E., Pratt, V. M., Dlouhy, S. R., 1994, Genetics of Pelizaeus-Merzbacher disease. *Dev. Neurosci.* **15:**383–394.

Hudson, L. D., Berndt, J. A., Puckett, C., Kozak, C. A., Lazzarini, R. A., 1987, Aberrant splicing of proteolipid protein mRNA in the dysmyelinating jimpy mutant mouse. *Proc. Natl. Acad. Sci. USA* **84:**1454–1458.

Hudson, L. D., Puckett, C., Berndt, J., Chan, J., Gencic, S., 1989, Mutation of the proteolipid protein gene (PLP) in a human X chromosome-linked disorder. *Proc. Natl. Acad. Sci. USA* **86:**8128–8131.

Johnston, A. W., MacKusick, V. A., 1962, A sex-linked recessive form of spastic paraplegia. *Am J. Hum. Genet.* **14:**83–94.

Jung, M., Sommer, I., Schachner, M., and Nave K-A, 1996, Monoclonal antibody O10 defines a conformationally sensitive cell-surface epitope of proteolipid protein (PLP): Evidence that PLP misfolding underlies dysmyelination in mutant mice. *J. Neurosci.* **24:**7920–7929.

Kagawa, T., Ikenaka, K., Inoue, Y., Kuriyama, S., Tsujii, T., Nakajima, J., Nakao, J., Aruga, J., Okano, H., and Mikoshiba, K., 1994, Glial cell degeneration and hypomyelination caused by overexpression of the myelin proteolipid protein gene. *Neuron* **13:**427–442.

Karthigasan, J., Evans, E. L., Vouyiouklis, D. A., Inouye, H., Borenshteyn, N., Ramamurthy, G. V., Kirschner, D. A., 1996, Effects of rumpshaker mutation on CNS myelin composition and structure. *J Neurochem.* **66:**338–345.

Kitagawa, K., Sinoway, M. P., Yang, C., Gould, R. M., Colman, D. R., 1993, A proteolipid protein gene family: Expression in sharks and rays and possible evolution from an ancestral gene encoding a pore-forming polypetide. *Neuron* **11:**433–448.

Klugmann, M., Schwab, M., Pühlhofer, A., Schneider, A., Zimmermann, F., Griffiths, I. R., Nave, K.-A., 1997, Assembly of CNS myelin in the absence of proteolipid protein. *Neuron* **18:**59–70.

Knapp, P. E., Bartlett, W. P., Williams, L. A., Yamada, M., Ikenaka, K., Skoff, R. P., 1999a, Programmed cell death without DNA fragmentation in the jimpy mouse: Secreted factors can enhance survival. *Cell Death Differ.* **6:**136–145.

Knapp, P. E., Ismaili, S., Hauser, K. F., Ghandour, M. S., 1999b, Abnormal Ca(2+) regulation in oligodendrocytes from the dysmyelinating jimpy mouse. *Brain Res* **847:**332–337.

Knapp, P. E., Maderspach, K., Hauser, K. F., 1998, Endogenous opioid system in developing normal and jimpy oligodendrocytes: Mu and kappa opioid receptors mediate differential mitogenic and growth responses. *Glia* **22:**189–201.

Knapp, P. E., Skoff, R. P., 1987, A defect in the cell cycle of neuroglia in the myelin deficient jimpy mouse. *Dev. Brain Res.* **35:**301–306.

Knapp, P. E., Skoff, R. P., Redstone, D. W., 1986, Oligodendroglial cell death in jimpy mice: An explanation for the myelin deficit. *J. Neurosci.* **6:**2813–2822.

Kobayashi, H., Hoffman, E., Marks, H., 1994, The rumpshaker mutation in spastic paraplegia. *Nat. Genet.* **7:**351–352.

Koeppen, A. H., Ronca, N. A., Greenfield, E. A., Hans, M. B., 1987, Defective biosynthesis of proteolipid protein in pelizaeus-Merzbacher disease. *Ann. Neurol.* **21:**159–170.

Komaki, H., Sasaki, M., Yamamoto, T., Iai, M., Takashima, S., 1999, Connatal Pelizaeus-Merzbacher disease associated with the jimpy(msd) mice mutation. *Pediatr Neurol.* **20:**309–311.

Kraus-Ruppert, R., Herschkowitz, N., Fürst, S., 1973, Morphological studies on neuroglial cells in the corpus callosum of the Jimpy mutant mouse. J Neuropathol Exp Neurol. **32:**197–202.

Lachapelle, F., Gumpel, M., Baumann, N., 1994, Contribution of transplantations to the understanding of the role of the PLP gene. *Neurochem. Res.* **19:**1083–1090.

Lappe-Siefke, C., Goebbels, S., Gravel, M., Nicksch, E., Lee, J., Braun, P. E., Griffiths, I. R., Nave, K.-A., 2003, Disruption of the Cnp1 gene uncouples oligodendroglial functions in axonal support and myelination. *Nat. Genet.* **33:**366– 374.

Laursen, R. A., Samiullah, M., Lees, M. B., 1984, The structure of bovine brain myelin proteolipid and its organization in myelin. *Proc Natl Acad Sci USA* **8:**2912–2916.

Lees, M,, Brostoff, S. L., 1984, Proteins of myelin. *In* "Myelin" (P. Morell, ed.), 2nd. ed., pp. 197–224. Plenum Press, New York.

Le Goascogne, C., Eychenne, B., Tonon, M. C., Lachapelle, F., Baumann, N., Robel, P., 2000, Neurosteroid progesterone is up-regulated in the brain of jimpy and shiverer mice. *Glia* **29:**14–24.

Lipsitz, D., Goetz, B. D., Duncan, I. D., 1998, Apoptotic glial cell death and kinetics in the spinal cord of the myelin-deficient rat. *J. Neurosci. Res.* **51:**497–507.

Macklin, W. B., Gardinier, M. V., King, K. D., Kampf, K., 1987, An AG-GG transition at a splice site in the myelin proteolipid protein gene in jimpy mice results in the removal of an exon. *FEBS Lett.* **223:**417–421.

Mastronardi, F. G., Ackerley, C. A., Arsenault, L., Roots, B. I., Moscarello, M. A., 1993, Demyelination in a transgenic mouse: A model for multiple sclerosis. *J Neurosci Res.* **36:**315–324.

Mattei, M. G., Alliel, P. M., Dautigny, A., Passage, E., Pham-Dinh, D., Mattei, J. F., Jolles, P., 1986, The gene encoding for the major brain proteolipid (PLP) maps on the q-22 band of the human X chromosome. *Hum. Genet.* **72:**352–353.

McLaughlin, M., Hunter, D. J. B., Thomson, C. E., Yool, D., Kirkham, D., Freer, A. A., Griffiths, I. R., 2002, Evidence for possible interactions between PLP and DM20 within the myelin sheath. *Glia* **39:**31–36.

Meier, C., Bischoff, A., 1974, Dysmyelination in "jimpy" mouse. Electron microscopic study. *J. Neuropathol. Exp. Neurol.* **33:**343–353.

Meier C, Bischoff A., 1975, Oligodendroglial cell development in jimpy mice and controls. An electron-microscopic study in the optic nerve. *J Neurol. Sci.* **26:**517–528.

Meier, C., Herschkowitz, N., Bischoff, A., 1974, Morphological and biochemical observations in the Jimpy spinal cord. *Acta Neuropathol (Berl)* **27:**349–362.

Meier, H., MacPike, A. D., 1970, A neurological mutation (msd) of the mouse causing a deficiency of myelin synthesis. *Exp Brain Res.* **10:**512–525.

Merzbacher, L., 1910, Eine eigenartige familiäre Erkrankungsform (Aplasia axialis extracorticolis congenita). *Z. Ges. Neurol. Psychiatr.* **3:**1–138.

Miller, M. J., Haxhiu, M. A., Georgiadis, P., Gudz, T. I., Kangas, C. D., Macklin, W. B., 2003, Proteolipid protein gene mutation induces altered ventilatory response to hypoxia in the myelin-deficient rat. *J Neurosci.* **23:**2265–2273.

Milner, R. J., Lai, C., Nave, K.-A., Lenoir, D., Ogata, J., Sutcliffe, J. G., 1985, Nucleotide sequences of two mRNAs for rat brain myelin proteolipid protein. *Cell* **42:**931–939.

Mimault, C., Giraud, G., Courtois, V., Cailloux, F., Boire, J. Y., Dastugue, B., Boespflug-Tanguy, O., 1999, Proteolipoprotein gene analysis in 82 patients with sporadic Pelizaeus-Merzbacher Disease: Duplications, the major cause of the disease, originate more frequently in male germ cells, but point mutations do not. The Clinical European Network on Brain Dysmyelinating Disease. *Am. J. Hum Genet.* **65:**360–369.

Morello, D., Dautigny, A., Pham-Dinh, D., Jolles, P., 1986, Myelin proteolipid protein (PLP and DM-20) transcripts are deleted in jimpy mutant mice. *EMBO J.* **5:**3489–3493.

Nadon, N. L., Arnheiter, H., Hudson, L. D., 1994, A combination of PLP and DM20 transgenes promotes partial myelination in the jimpy mouse. *J. Neurochem.* **63:**822–833.

Nadon, N. L., Duncan, I. D., Hudson, L. D., 1990, A point mutation in the proteolipid protein gene of the 'shaking pup' interrupts oligodendrocyte development. *Development* **110:**529–537.

Nadon, N. L., West, M., 1998, Myelin proteolipid protein: Function in myelin structure is distinct from its role in oligodendrocyte development. *Dev Neurosci.* **20:**533–539.

Naidu, S., Dlouhy, S. R., Geraghty, M. T., Hodes, M. E., 1997, A male child with the rumpshaker mutation, X-linked spastic paraplegia/Pelizaeus-Merzbacher disease and lysinuria. *J Inherit Metab Dis.* **20:**811–816.

Nave, K.-A., 1994, Neurological mouse mutants and genes of myelin. *J. Neurosci. Res.* **38:**607–612.

Nave, K.-A., Lai, C., Bloom, F. E., Milner, R. J., 1986, Jimpy mutant mouse: A 74-base deletion in the mRNA for myelin proteolipid protein and evidence for a primary defect in RNA splicing. *Proc. Natl. Acad. Sci. USA* **83:**9264–9268.

Nave, K.-A., Lai, C., Bloom, F. E., and Milner, R. J., 1987, Splice site selection in the proteolipid protein (PLP) gene transcript and primary structure of the DM-20 protein of central nervous system myelin. *Proc. Natl. Acad. Sci. USA* **84:**5665–5669.

Nave, K.-A., and Boespflug-Tanguy, O., 1996, Developmental defects of myelin formation: From X-linked mutations to human dysmyelinating diseases. *The Neuroscientist* **2:**33–43.

Nave, K.-A., Lai, C., Bloom, F. E., Milner, R. J., 1987, Splice site selection in the proteolipid protein (PLP) gene transcript and primary structure of the DM-20 protein of central nervous system myelin. *Proc. Natl. Acad. Sci. USA* **84:**5665–5669.

Nave, K.-A., Milner, R. J., 1989, Proteolipid proteins: Structure and genetic expression in normal and myelin-deficient mutant mice. *Crit. Rev. Neurobiol.* **5:**65–91.

Pearsall, G. B., Nadon, N. L., Wolf, M. K., Billings-Gagliardi, S., 1997, Jimpy-4J mouse has a missense mutation in exon 2 of the Plp gene. *Dev Neurosci.* **19:**337–341.

Pelizaeus, F., 1885, Über eine eigenthümliche Form spastischer Lähmung mit Cerebral erscheinungen auf hereditärer Grundlage (Multiple Sklerose). *Arch. Psychiatr.* **16:**698–710.

Phillips, R. J., 1954, *Jimpy*, a new totally sex-linked gene in the house mouse. Z. Induk. Abstamm. Vererbunsl. **86:**322

Popot, J,L., Pham-Dinh, D., Dautigny, A., 1991, Major myelin proteolipid: The 4-a-helix topology. *J. Membrane Biol.* **120:**233–246.

Pringle, N..P, Nadon, N. L., Rhode, D. M., Richardson, W. D., Duncan, I. D., 1997, Normal temporal and spatial distribution of oligodendrocyte progenitors in the myelin-deficient (md) rat. *J Neurosci Res.* **47:**264–270.

Pucket, C., Hudson, L., Ono, K., Friedrich, V., Benecke, J., Dubois-Dalcq, M., Lazzarini, R. A., 1987, Myelin specific proteolipid protein is expressed in myelinating Schwann cells but not incorporated into myelin sheaths. *J. Neurosci. Res.* **18:**511–518.

Raskind, W. H., Williams, C. A., Hudson, L. D., Bird, T. D., 1991, Complete deletion of the proteolipid protein gene (PLP) in a family with X-linked Pelizaeus-Merzbacher disease. *Am. J. Med. Genet.* **49:**1355–1360.

Readhead, C., Schneider, A., Griffiths, I., Nave, K.-A., 1994, Premature arrest of myelin formation in transgenic mice with increased proteolipoprotein gene dosage. *Neuron* **12:**583–595.

Ron, D., 2002, Translational control in the endoplasmic reticulum stress response. J Clin. Invest. **110:**1383–1388.

Rosenbluth, J., Stoffel, W., and Schiff, R., 1996, Myelin structure in proteolipid protein (PLP)-null mouse spinal cord. *J. Comp. Neurol.* **371:**336–344.

Saugier-Veber, P., Munnich, A., Bonneau, D., Rozet, J. M., Le Merrer, M., Gil, R., Boespflug-Tanguy, O., 1994, X-linked spastic paraplegia and Pelizaeus-Merzbacher disease are allelic disorders at the proteolipid protein locus. *Nat. Genet.* **6:**257–261.

Scherer, S. S., 1997, Molecular genetics of demyelination: New wrinkles on an old membrane. *Neuron* **18:**13–16.

Schneider, A., Griffiths, I. R., Readhead, C., Nave, K.-A., 1995, Dominant-negative action of the *jimpy* mutation in mice complemented with an autosomal transgene for myelin proteolipid protein. *Proc. Natl. Acad. Sci. USA* **92:**4447–4451.

Schneider, A., Montague, P., Griffiths, I., Fanarraga, M., Kennedy, P., Brophy, P., and Nave, K.-A., 1992, Uncoupling of hypomyelination and glial cell death by a mutation in the proteolipid protein gene. *Nature* **358:**758–761.

Seeman, P., Paderova, K., Benes, V. Jr, Sistermans, E. A., 2002, A severe connatal form of Pelizaeus Merzbacher disease in a Czech boy caused by a novel mutation (725C>A, Ala242Glu) at the 'jimpy(msd) codon' in the PLP gene. *Int. J. Mol. Med.* **9:**125–129.

Seitelberger, F. 1970, Pelizaeus-Merzbacher disease. *In* "Handbook of Clinical Neurology" (P. J. Vinken and G. W. Bruyn, eds.), Vol 10, pp. 150–202. North Holland, Amsterdam.

Seitelberger, F., Urbanitz, I., and Nave, K.-A. 1996, Pelizaeus-Merzbacher Disease. *In* "Handbook of Clinical Neurology" (P. J. Vinken and G. W. Bruyn, eds.), Vol. 22 (Ch. 26), pp. 559–579. Elsevier Science B. V. Amsterdam.

Sherman, M. Y., Goldberg, A. L., 2001, Cellular defenses against unfolded proteins: A cell biologist thinks about neurodegenerative diseases. *Neuron* **29:**15–32.

Shy, M. E., Hobson, G., Jain, M., Boespflug-Tanguy, O., Garbern, J., Sperle, K., Li, W., Gow, A., Rodriguez, D., Bertini, E., Mancias, P., Krajewski, K., Lewis, R., Kamholz, J., 2003, Schwann cell expression of PLP1 but not DM20 is necessary to prevent neuropathy. *Ann Neurol.* **53:**354–365.

Sidman, R. L., Dickie, M. M., Appel, S. H., 1964, Mutant mice (quaking and jimpy) with deficient myelination in the central nervous system. *Science* **144:**309–311.

Simons, M., Krämer, E. M., Macchi, P., Rathke-Hartlieb, S., Trotter, J., Nave, K.-A., Schulz, J. B., 2002, Overexpression of the myelin proteolipid protein leads to accumulation of cholesterol and proteolipid protein in endosomes/lysosomes: Implications for Pelizaeus-Merzbacher disease. *J Cell Biol.* **157:**327–336.

Simons, M., Krämer, E. M., Thiele, C., Stoffel, W., Trotter, J., 2000, Assembly of myelin by association of proteolipid protein with cholesterol- and galactosylceramide-rich membrane domains. *J Cell Biol.* **151:**143–154.

Simons-Johnson, R., Roder, J. C., Riordan, J. R., 1995, Over-expression of the DM-20 myelin proteolipid causes central nervous system demyelination in transgenic mice. *J. Neurochem.* **64:**967–976.

Sistermans, E. A., de Coo, R. F., De Wijs, I. J., Van Oost, B. A., 1998, Duplication of the proteolipid protein gene is the major cause of Pelizaeus-Merzbacher disease. *Neurology* **50:**1749–1754.

Sistermans, E. A., de Wijs, I. J., de Coo, R..F, Smit, L. M., Menko, F. H., van Oost, B. A., 1996, A (G-to-A) mutation in the initiation codon of the proteolipid protein gene causing a relatively mild form of Pelizaeus-Merzbacher disease in a Dutch family. *Hum Genet.* **97:**337–339.

Skoff, R. P., 1976, Myelin deficit in the Jimpy mouse may be due to cellular abnormalities in astroglia. *Nature* **264:**560–562.

Skoff, R. P., 1982, Increased proliferation of oligodendrocytes in the hypomyelinated mouse mutant-jimpy. *Brain Res.* **248:**19–31.

Skoff, R. P., 1995, Programmed cell death in the dysmyelinating mutants. Brain Pathol. **5:**283–288.

Snipes, G. J., Suter, U., Shooter, E., 1993, The genetics of myelin. *Curr. Op. Neurobiol.* **3:**694–702.

Southwood, C., Gow, A., 2001, Molecular pathways of oligodendrocyte apoptosis revealed by mutations in the proteolipid protein gene. *Microsc Res Tech.* **52:**700–708.

Southwood, C. M., Garbern, J., Jiang, W., Gow, A., 2002, The unfolded protein response modulates disease severity in Pelizaeus-Merzbacher disease. *Neuron* **36:**585–596.

Spassky, N., Goujet-Zalc, C., Parmantier, E., Olivier, C., Martinez, S., Ivanova, A., Ikenaka, K., Macklin, W., Cerruti, I., Zalc, B., Thomas, J. L., 1998, Multiple restricted origin of oligodendrocytes. *J. Neurosci.* **18:**8331–8343.

Sporkel, O., Uschkureit, T., Bussow, H., Stoffel, W., 2002, Oligodendrocytes expressing exclusively the DM20 isoform of the proteolipid protein gene: Myelination and development. *Glia* **37:**19–30.

Stecca, B., Southwood, C. M., Gragerov, A., Kelley, K. A., Friedrich, V. L., Gow, A., 2000, The evolution of lipophilin genes from invertebrates to tetrapods: DM-20 cannot replace proteolipid protein in CNS myelin. *J Neurosci.* **20:**4002–4010.

Stoffel, W., Hillen, H., Giersiefen, H., 1984, Structure and molecular arrangement of proteolipid protein of central nervous system myelin. *Proc. Natl. Acad. Sci. U S A.* **81:**5012–5016.

Thomson, C. E., Anderson, T. J., McCulloch, M. C., Dickinson, P. J., Vouyiouklis, D. A., Griffiths, I. R., 1999, The early phenotype associated with the jimpy mutation of the proteolipid protein gene. *J. Neurocytol.* **28:**207–221.

Tosic, M., Dolivo, M., Domanska-Janik, K., Matthieu, J. M., 1994, Paralytic tremor (pt): A new allele of the proteolipid protein gene in rabbits. *J Neurochem.* **63:**2210–2216.

Trapp, B. D., Nishiyama, A., Cheng, D., Macklin, W., 1997, Differentiation and death of premyelinating oligodendrocytes in developing rodent brain. *J Cell Biol.* **137:**459–468.

Uschkureit, T., Sporkel, O., Bussow, H., Stoffel, W., 2001, Rumpshaker-like proteolipid protein (PLP) ratio in a mouse model with unperturbed structural and functional integrity of the myelin sheath and axons in the central nervous system. *Glia* **35:**63–71.

Utzschneider, D., Black, J. A., Kocsis, J. D., 1992, Conduction properties of spinal cord axons in the myelin-deficient rat mutant. *Neuroscience* **49:**221–228.

Vela, J. M., Dalmau, I., Gonzalez, B., Castellano, B., 1996, The microglial reaction in spinal cords of jimpy mice is related to apoptotic oligodendrocytes. *Brain Res.* **712:**134–142.

Vela, J. M., Gonzalez, B., Castellano, B., 1998, Understanding glial abnormalities associated with myelin deficiency in the jimpy mutant mouse. *Brain Res. Rev.* **26:**29–42.

Vermeesch, M. K., Knapp, P. E., Skoff, R. P., Studzinski, D. M., Benjamins, J. A., 1990, Death of individual oligodendrocytes in *jimpy* brain precedes expression of proteolipid protein. *Dev. Neurosci.* **12:**303–315.

Wahle, S., Stoffel, W., 1998, Cotranslational integration of myelin proteolipid protein (PLP) into the membrane of endoplasmic reticulum: Analysis of topology by glycosylation scanning and protease domain protection assay. *Glia* **24:**226–235.

Weimbs, T., Stoffel, W., 1992, Proteolipid protein (PLP) of CNS myelin: Positions of free, disulfide-bonded, and fatty acid thioester-linked cysteine residues and implications for the membrane topology of PLP. *Biochemistry* **31:**12289–12296.

Weimbs,T., Stoffel, W., 1994, Topology of CNS myelin proteolipid protein: Evidence for the nonenzymatic glycosylation of extracytoplasmic domains in normal and diabetic animals. *Biochemistry* **33:**10408–10415.

Werner, H., Dimou, L., Klugmann, M., Pfeiffer, S., Nave, K.-A., 2001, Multiple splice isoforms of proteolipid M6B in neurons and oligodendrocytes. *Mol. Cell. Neurosci.* **18:**593–605.

Werner, H., Jung, M., Klugmann, M., Sereda, M., Griffiths, I., Nave, K.-A., 1998, Mouse models of myelin diseases. *Brain Pathol.* **8:**771–793.

Willard, H. F., Riordan, J. R., 1985, Assignment of the gene for myelin proteolipid protein to the X chromosome: Implications for X-linked myelin disorders. *Science* **230:**940–942.

Williams, W. C., Gard, A. L., 1997, In vitro death of jimpy oligodendrocytes: Correlation with onset of DM-20/PLP expression and resistance to oligodendrogliotrophic factors. *J Neurosci Res.* **50:**177–189.

Wolf, M. K., Holden, A. B., 1969, Tissue culture analysis of the inherited defect of central nervous system myelination in jimpy mice. *J Neuropathol Exp Neurol.* **28:**195–213.

Wolf, M. K., Nunnari, J. N., Billings-Gagliardi, S., 1999, Quaking*shiverer double-mutant mice survive for at least 100 days with no CNS myelin. *Dev Neurosci.* **21:**483–490.

Woodward, K., Malcolm, S., 1999, Proteolipid protein gene: Pelizaeus-Merzbacher disease in humans and neurodegeneration in mice. *Trends Genet.* **15:**125–128.

Woodward, K., Malcolm, S., 2001, CNS myelination and PLP gene dosage. Pharmacogenomics **2:**263–272.

Wu, Q., Miller, R. H., Ransohoff, R. M., Robinson, S., Bu, J., Nishiyama, A., 2000, Elevated levels of the chemokine GRO-1 correlate with elevated oligodendrocyte progenitor proliferation in the jimpy mutant. *J Neurosci.* **20:**2609–2617.

Yamamura, T., Konola, J. T., Wekerle, H., Lees, M. B., 1991, Monoclonal antibodies against myelin proteolipid protein: Identification and characterization of two major determinants. *J Neurochem.* **57:**1671–1680.

Yan, Y., Lagenaur, C., Narayanan, V., 1993, Molecular cloning of M6: Identification of a PLP/DM-20 gene family. *Neuron* **11:**423–431.

Yool, D. A., Edgar, J. M., Montague, P., Malcolm, S., 2000, The proteolipid protein gene and myelin disorders in man and animal models. *Hum. Mol. Genet.* **9:**987–992

Yool, D. A., Klugmann, M., McLaughlin, M., Vouyiouklis, D. A., Dimou, L., Barrie, J. A., McCulloch, M. C., Nave, K.-A., Griffiths, I. R., 2001, Myelin proteolipid proteins promote the interaction of oligodendrocytes and axons. *J. Neurosci. Res.* **63:**151–164.

Yool, D., Klugmann, M., Barrie, J. A., McCulloch, M. C., Nave, K.-A., Griffiths, I. R., 2002, Observations on the structure of myelin lacking the major proteolipid protein. *Neuropath. Appl. Neurobiol.* **28:**75–78.

Young, W., Rosenbluth, J., Wojak, J. C., Sakatani, K., 1989, Extracellular potassium activity and axonal conduction in spinal cord of the myelin-deficient mutant rat. *Exp. Neurol.* **106:**41–51.

Yu, W. P., Collarini, E. J., Pringle, N. P., Richardson, W. D., 1994, Embryonic expression of myelin genes: Evidence for a focal source of oligodendrocyte precursors in the ventricular zone of the neural tube. *Neuron* **12:**1353–1362.

CHAPTER

# 48

# Models of Charcot-Marie-Tooth Disease

*Lawrence Wrabetz, Maria Laura Feltri, and Ueli Suter*

## INTRODUCTION

Charcot Marie Tooth (CMT) hereditary neuropathies (including Déjérine-Sottas syndrome [DSS], congenital hypomyelinating neuropathy [CH], and hereditary neuropathy with liability to pressure palsies [HNPP]) are collectively the most common inherited neuromuscular disorder. They are inherited as dominant or recessive traits and consist of demyelinating (CMT1) or axonal (CMT2) types. Roughly one-half of CMT neuropathies are caused by a 1.4 megabase internal duplication in chromosome 17, containing *PMP22* (peripheral myelin protein 22kD gene). Another 20% are caused by specific mutations of *PMP22*, *MPZ* (myelin protein zero gene), or *CX32/GJ*β1 (Connexin 32 (Cx32) or gap junction beta 1 gene), and rarer missense, nonsense, frameshift, splice site, or other mutations in 11 additional genes. About one-third of all CMT neuropathies have yet to be associated with disease genes (see Chapter 39, "Inherited Neuropathies," and Berger *et al.*, 2002; Kleopa and Scherer, 2002; Lupski and Garcia, 2001; Wrabetz *et al.*, 2001; for recent reviews and http://molgen-www.uia.ac.be/CMTMutations for a catalog of mutations).

Even if genetically heterogeneous, the CMT phenotype is similar among the majority of patients, including progressive distal weakness and wasting in the limbs with less evident sensory loss, deformities in the feet, and reduced or absent tendon reflexes. Despite the identification of 14 disease genes, our understanding of the diverse pathogeneses of various CMT neuropathies, and how they lead to this common phenotype, is limited and has yet to reveal treatment strategies.

Disability correlates best with axonal damage in CMT neuropathies (Berciano *et al.*, 2000; Dyck *et al.*, 1989; Gabreels-Festen *et al.*, 1992; Krajewski *et al.*, 2000), even if the majority begin as demyelinating disorders. Studies of developing nerve suggest that Schwann cells and axons are reciprocally interdependent for trophic support and the determination of their respective phenotypes (see Chapters 1, 2, and 13 for details). Essentially, most if not all CMTs evolve to a disturbance of this Schwann cell/axon unit, rather than isolated damage to myelin-forming Schwann cells or axons. Therefore, to decipher the pathomechanisms of CMT neuropathy, animal models have taken center stage, as it is there that the normal three-dimensional and reciprocal relationships between Schwann cells and axons are obtained, and that chronic secondary changes may be followed.

There are four types of animal models of CMT: those resulting from naturally occurring mutations, those resulting from alterations produced through random chemical mutagenesis, those resulting from targeted mutations introduced by homologous recombination in mouse embryonic stem cells (all of these alterations reside at the endogenous gene locus), and random insertion transgenes (here extra copies of the altered gene are inserted away from the endogenous locus). Each type of model has distinct advantages, useful in order to examine the two fundamental questions raised by hereditary neuropathies: (1) How are such diverse phenotypes like CMT1, DSS, CH, and CMT2 produced from the same gene? (2) Conversely, how do mutations in these different genes, some of which are expressed specifically in Schwann cells, lead to similar axonopathy—the development of which correlates best with disability?

Here we review the animal models of CMT neuropathies, the information they have provided about natural history and pathogenesis, and treatment perspectives. See Table 48.1 for a summary list of models.

## RODENT MODELS OF CMT

### PMP22 Animal Models

#### *Introduction*

Mutations affecting the PMP22 gene (see Chapter 21, "PMP22 Gene") have been associated with various disorders of the peripheral nervous system (PNS) including CMT1A (the most common form of hereditary neuropathies), DSS, CH, and HNPP (see Chapter 39). An intrachromosomal duplication of 1.4 megabases on chromosome 17p11.2-p12, encompassing the PMP22 gene, is the most frequently encountered genetic alteration (Inoue *et al.*, 2001; Nelis *et al.*, 1996). Deletions of the same region and various frame-shift, splice site, and nonsense mutations in the PMP22 gene result in the HNPP phenotype. Some PMP22 missense mutations are associated with CMT1A, or rarely HNPP, but the majority has been linked to the more severe neuropathies of the DSS or CH type.

Various animal models for PMP22 point mutations are currently available (Tab. 48.1). Some of them have been found in normal mouse colonies and they provided the initial key to the discovery that PMP22 is a disease gene for motor and sensory neuropathies in human (Suter *et al.*, 1993). Others were isolated as part of a screen for mutagen-induced mutations (Isaacs *et al.*, 2000). Furthermore, a particular mouse line with a large in-frame deletion of PMP22 has been described (Suh *et al.*, 1997). Artificially generated transgenic lines include mice and rats overexpressing PMP22 (Huxley *et al.*, 1996; Huxley *et al.*, 1998; Magyar *et al.*, 1996; Niemann *et al.*, 2000; Norreel *et al.*, 2001; Robertson *et al.*, 2002b; Sancho *et al.*, 1999; Sancho *et al.*, 2001; Sereda *et al.*, 1996) and, although no exact human correlate has been described so far, homozygous *Pmp22*-null mice which display also a severe demyelinating neuropathy (Adlkofer *et al.*, 1995). In addition, heterozygous *Pmp22*-null (Adlkofer *et al.*, 1997a) and PMP22-antisense mRNA (Maycox *et al.*, 1997) mice have been established as models of HNPP. The generation and analysis of these animals provided the formal proof that PMP22 is the disease-causing and dosage-sensitive gene in CMT1A and HNPP (Suter and Nave, 1999). Moreover, these animals serve as models for the different forms of the disease and are valuable tools to examine disease mechanisms and potential treatment strategies.

#### *PMP22 Mutations in Natural Mouse Lines*

***Trembler mouse*** The spontaneous mouse mutant *Trembler (Tr)* was described more than 50 years ago (Falconer, 1951); soon thereafter, a second mouse line with a comparable phenotype was isolated at the Jackson Laboratory, *Trembler-J (Tr-J)* (Henry *et al.*, 1983; Henry and Sidman, 1983). Both mutants show autosomal-dominant inheritance, unsteady gait, and weakness of the hindlimbs. Furthermore, they are affected by an axial tremor and show stress-induced convulsions—hence the name "Trembler." However, no abnormalities could be detected in the central nervous system (CNS) of *Tr* animals (Braverman, 1953). Recent evidence suggests that the "trembling" behavior is caused by neuromyotonia, an increased muscle stiffness due to hyperactivity of motor units, that can also be found in other animal models of demyelinating CMT (Toyka *et al.*, 1997; Zielasek *et al.*, 2000). Interest-

TABLE 48.1 Mouse Models of CMT Neuropathies*

| CMT gene | Mouse (rat) | Mutation | Model | Reference |
|---|---|---|---|---|
| ***PMP22*** | Null(+/−). or (−/−) | neoR-ins | HNPP | (Adlkofer *et al.*, 1997a, 1995) |
| | Pmp22Antisense | $P_0$-rPmp22AS transgene | HNPP | (Maycox *et al.*, 1997) |
| | PMP22OE rat | *Pmp22*wt | CMT1A or CH | (Sereda *et al.*, 1996) |
| | PMP22OE mouse | *Pmp22*wt | CH | (Magyar *et al.*, 1996) |
| | C61, C22 | *PMP22*wt | CMT1A or CH | (Huxley *et al.*, 1996, 1998) |
| | My41 | *Pmp22*wt | CH | (Robertson *et al.*, 2002b) |
| | Conditional Pmp22 OE | Pmp22 cDNAwt | CMT1A | (Perea *et al.*, 2001) |
| | *Trembler* | G150D | DSS | (Falconer, 1951; Suter *et al.*, 1992b) |
| | *TremblerJ* | L16P | CMT1A | (Henry *et al.*, 1983; Suter *et al.*, 1992a) |
| | *TremblerNcnp* | delExonIV | CMT1A/DSS? | (Suh *et al.*, 1997) |
| | *Trembler m1H* | H12R | DSS | (Isaacs *et al.*, 2000) |
| | *Trembler m2H* | Y153X | CMT1A/DSS? | (Isaacs *et al.*, 2000) |
| ***MPZ*** | $P_0$ Null (+/−) | Tandem *Mpz*neoR-ins | CMT1B (mild) | (Martini *et al.*, 1995) |
| | $P_0$ Null (−/−) | Tandem *Mpz*neoR-ins | DSS | (Giese *et al.*, 1992) |
| | $P_0$OE | *Mpz*wt transgene | CH | (Wrabetz *et al.*, 2000; Yin *et al.*, 2000) |
| | $P_0$myc | *Mpz5'*myc transgene | CMT1B with tomacula | (Previtali *et al.*, 2000) |
| | S63del-random-ins | *Mpz*S63del transgene | CMT1B | (Wrabetz *et al.*, 2002) |
| ***GJ*β1/CX32** | Cx32 Null (y/−) | *Cx32*neoR-ins | CMT1X | (Anzini *et al.*, 1997; Scherer *et al.*, 1998) |
| | R142W-random-ins | $P_0$-*Cx32*R142W transgene | CMT1X | (Scherer *et al.*, 1999) |
| | 175fs | $P_0$-*Cx32*-175fs transgene | normal | (Abel *et al.*, 1999) |
| ***EGR2/KROX20*** | Krox20 Null (−/−) | *LacZ*/neoR-ins or Cre-ins | CH | (Topilko *et al.*, 1994; Voiculescu *et al.*, 2000) |
| | Krox20lo/lo | loxP(neoR)loxP-ins intron 1 | CH | (Nagarajan *et al.*, 2002) |
| | Krox20(floxNeo) | loxP(exon2)loxP(NeoR)loxP | ?(hypomorph) | (Taillebourg *et al.*, 2002) |
| ***PRX*** | Prx Null (−/−) | *Prx*neoR-ins | CMT4F | (Gillespie *et al.*, 2000) |
| ***KIF1B*** | KIF1B Null (+/−) | *Kif1B*neoR-ins | CMT2A | (Zhao *et al.*, 2001) |
| ***NEFL*** | L394P-random ins | MSV-*Nefl*L394P transgene | CMT2E (severe) | (Lee *et al.*, 1994) |
| ***LMNA*** | Lmna null (−/−) | *Lmna*neoR-ins | AR-CMT2 | (De Sandre-Giovannoli *et al.*, 2002; Sullivan *et al.*, 1999) |
| *???* | Clawpaw | unknown | CH with arthrogryposis | (Henry *et al.*, 1991) |

*See text or references for details of transgene structures or targeting alleles. Also see text for follow-up studies on these mice.

ingly, tremor is not uncommon in CMT patients (Cardoso and Jankovic, 1993), and severe muscle cramps have been reported as an associated feature (Hahn *et al.*, 1991).

On the molecular level, the *Tr* mutation is due to the replacement of the small, neutral amino acid glycine by the charged and bulky amino acid aspartic acid at position 150 in the last hydrophobic domain of the PMP22 protein (G150D, Suter *et al.*, 1992b). The same mutation has been found in a family diagnosed with a severe DSS neuropathy (Ionasescu *et al.*, 1997). Intracellularly, the mutation leads to a PMP22 protein trafficking defect (D'Urso *et al.*, 1998; Naef *et al.*, 1997). Furthermore, a particular propensity for aggregation of the Tr protein has been reported, which may contribute to the cellular basis of the phenotype (Tobler *et al.*, 2002). Adult *Tr* mutants show severe hypomyelination of peripheral nerves (Ayers and Anderson, 1973, 1975, 1976; Henry *et al.*, 1983; Low, 1976a, 1976b, 1977), increased Schwann cell number and Schwann cell proliferation (Perkins *et al.*, 1981; Sancho *et al.*, 2001), and reduced NCV (Low and McLeod, 1975). During development (Fig. 48.1), the onset of myelination is delayed (Henry *et al.*, 1983). Furthermore, structural abnormalities in myelin of heterozygous *Tr* mice have been described (Kirschner and Sidman, 1976). Homozygous *Tr* mice have a normal life span, although they lack myelinated fibers almost completely (Henry and Sidman, 1988).

Hypomyelination in *Tr* is associated with a general downregulation of myelin protein components, including PMP22 (Adlkofer *et al.*, 1997b; Bascles *et al.*, 1992; Costaglioli *et al.*, 2001; Garbay *et al.*, 1995; Garbay and Bonnet, 1992; Maier *et al.*, 2002a; Vallat *et al.*,

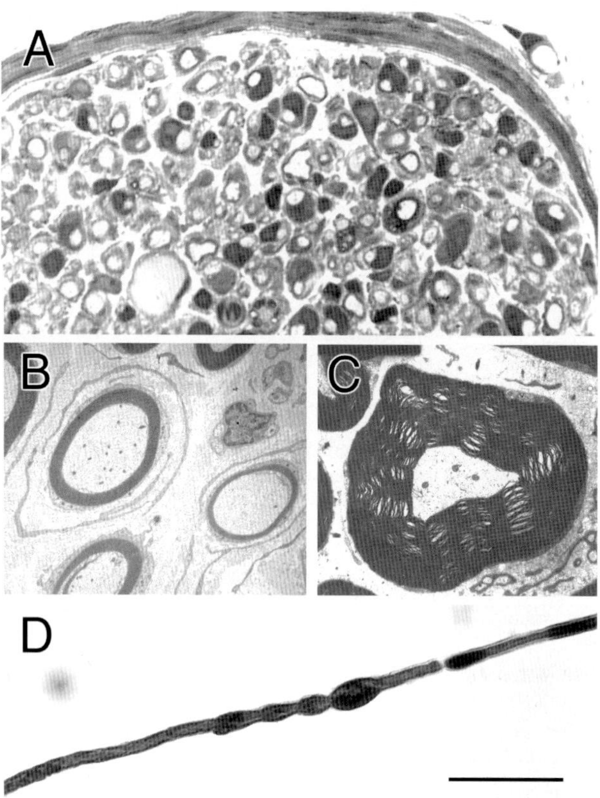


FIGURE 48.1
Specific pathological alterations of CMT1A due to *PMP22*$^{G150D}$, CMT1A with duplication, and HNPP are reproduced in *Trembler* mouse (A), the Pmp22 overexpressing rat (B), and heterozygous *Pmp22*-null mouse (C and D), respectively. (A) Severe hypomyelination is revealed in a semithin section of P18 *Trembler* peripheral nerve. (B). Typical onion bulbs are detected in peripheral nerve of a 2-month-old rat. (C). An electron micrograph and (D) teased fiber preparation of the quadriceps nerve of adult heterozygous *Pmp22*-null mice show tomacula. Bar (in D) = 12 μm (A), 4 μm (B), 5 μm (C), and 75 μm (D).

1999) and mislocalization of MAG (Vallat *et al.*, 1999). In addition, the lipid metabolism of myelinated peripheral nerves is strongly altered (Boiron-Sargueil *et al.*, 1995; Garbay *et al.*, 1998; Garbay and Cassagne, 1994; Heape *et al.*, 1995; Heape *et al.*, 1996; Salles *et al.*, 2002; Sargueil *et al.*, 1999). Grafting experiments have demonstrated that the myelination defect in *Tr* is largely Schwann cell-autonomous (Aguayo *et al.*, 1977), consistent with the high expression of PMP22 in normal myelinating Schwann cells. Nevertheless, there is also a strong effect of the mutant *Tr* Schwann cells on the axon (Maier *et al.*, 2002b). This includes decreased axonal caliber, increased neurofilament density, and decreased slow axonal transport (de Waegh and Brady, 1990; de Waegh and Brady, 1991; de Waegh *et al.*, 1992). In addition, the microtubule cytoskeleton and its associated proteins are altered in composition and phosphorylation (Kirkpatrick and Brady, 1994). Interestingly, xenograft experiments of nerve biopsies from a patient carrying a PMP22 point mutation into nude mice have yielded similar results (Chance and Dyck, 1998; Sahenk *et al.*, 1998), suggesting only a minor role (if any) of neuronally expressed PMP22 in the disease process (De Leon *et al.*, 1994; Parmantier *et al.*, 1997).

The *Tr* mouse has also been used to show that compact myelin is not required for the initial clustering of voltage-gated sodium channels, ankyrinG 480/270 kDa and cell adhesion molecules leading to the formation of the node of Ranvier in peripheral nerves (Lambert *et al.*, 1997). However, the juxtaparanodal potassium channels Kv1.1 and Kv1.2 are redistributed in *Tr* nerves (Wang *et al.*, 1995). The influence of demyelination and dysmyelination on axonal proteins in CMT1A models has not been investigated in detail, although it certainly contributes to the phenotype (Neuberg *et al.*, 1999).

***Trembler-J mouse*** A missense mutation exchanging a proline residue for a leucine at position 16 in the first hydrophobic domain of PMP22 has been found in *Tr-J* mice (L16P, Suter *et al.*, 1992a). The same mutation has also been described in a family with severe Charcot-Marie-Tooth disease type 1 (Valentijn *et al.*, 1992). The Tr-J protein appears to reach the intermediate compartment between the endoplasmic reticulum and the Golgi apparatus but cannot be transported further (D'Urso *et al.*, 1998; Tobler *et al.*, 1999). The mutant protein forms multimers with wild-type PMP22 protein, accumulates partially in aggresomes, and is degraded via the lysosomal and proteasomal pathways (Notterpek *et al.*, 1997; Ryan *et al.*, 2002; Tobler *et al.*, 2002). Furthermore, the Tr-J protein shows a prolonged interaction with the chaperone calnexin and sequesters calnexin into myelin-like intracellular figures (Dickson *et al.*, 2002). Thus, the cellular basis for the resulting disease may involve the loss of this folding partner for other proteins. The pathology in adult heterozygous *Tr-J* mice is qualitatively similar but less pronounced than in *Tr* (Henry *et al.*, 1983). Thinly myelinated axons, Schwann cell onion bulb formations, abnormalities in myelin compaction, and signs of altered axon-glia interactions are the main features (Heath *et al.*, 1991; Notterpek *et al.*, 1997; Robertson *et al.*, 1997). Whereas the levels of protein components of compact myelin, including PMP22, $P_0$ and MBP, are decreased, MAG protein, thought to mediate Schwann cell/axon interactions, shows only altered glycosylation (Bartoszewics *et al.*, 1996; Inuzuka *et al.*, 1985; Notterpek *et al.*, 1997).

***Trembler-Ncnp mouse*** A third spontaneous PMP22 mouse mutant named *Tr-Ncnp* (Sakai *et al.*, 1999; Suh *et al.*, 1997) is associated with an in-frame deletion of exon IV (Suter *et al.*, 1994). Thus, the resulting PMP22 protein lacks the second and part of the third hydrophobic domain (Taylor *et al.*, 2000). *Tr-Ncnp* differs from *Tr* and *Tr-J* in that giant vacuoles are present in the sciatic nerve of homozygous animals resembling swollen endoplasmic reticulum of Schwann cells. Furthermore, significant cell death was found in the nerves of these animals, a feature that is also present in other PMP22 mutants (Sancho *et al.*, 2001).

### *Artificial PMP22 Mutants*

***Mutagen-induced PMP22 mutants*** A large scale *N*-ethyl-*N*-nitrosurea (ENU) mutagenesis project in the mouse has yielded two new mouse lines with PMP22 point mutations (Isaacs *et al.*, 2000). The first mutation replaces a histidine at position 12 by an arginine residue (H12R). A mutation at the same position (H12Q) is associated with DSS in humans (Valentijn *et al.*, 1995). As expected, the phenotype of this mouse is pronounced with severe tremor and paucity of myelination—only occasional thin myelin sheaths are found. The second mutant line carries a nonsense mutation at position 153 (Y153X) with no human genetic correlate. These mice are less affected clinically but have also strongly hypomyelinated peripheral nerves.

### *Models with Increased PMP22 Gene Dosage*

***PMP22 trangenic mouse*** Different strategies have been employed to generate animal models for CMT1A associated with increased PMP22 gene dosage. Transgenic mice and rats have been generated and analyzed that carry varying numbers of extra copies of the mouse PMP22 gene. Mice with 16 or 30 additional copies display a severe congenital hypomyelinating neuropathy with an almost complete lack of myelinated large caliber axons, associated with pronounced slowing of nerve conduction velocity (NCV) (Magyar *et al.*, 1996). Affected nerves contain an increased number of Schwann cells that are aligned along axons. Cellular onion bulbs are rare but empty basal laminae, probably remnants of degenerated supernumerary Schwann cells and their processes, are common. The mutant Schwann cells are in a promyelination-like state since they express the early Schwann cell markers $p75^{NTR}$, N-CAM and L1. Thus, mutant Schwann cells are unable to differentiate toward the myelinating phenotype.

Increased Schwann cell proliferation and Schwann cell death were also found in postnatal development of PMP22 mutant nerves (Sancho *et al.*, 2001). The degree of cell death correlated with increased proliferation (as in homozygous *Pmp22*-null and *Tr* mice), implicating general mechanisms that normally regulate Schwann cell number in developing nerve. Thus, a primary influence of PMP22 on proliferation and cell death, as suggested by cell culture experiments, seems unlikely in postnatal development. Interestingly, if postnatal rat Schwann cells are tranduced with a viral construct to overexpress PMP22, and allowed to myelinate dorsal root ganglia (DRG) axons in culture, initial myelin spiraling and myelin compaction are normal (D'Urso *et al.*, 1997), whereas animal models suggest that PMP22 overexpression can alter or even prevent normal myelination. Thus, expression of PMP22 in embryonic Schwann cells may be critical (Hagedorn *et al.*, 1999; Paratore *et al.*, 2002), although differences in the levels of overexpression *in vitro* and *in vivo* can not be excluded as an explanation for these observations.

Further analysis revealed that the mutant mice are also affected by a distally accentuated axonopathy (Sancho *et al.*, 1999). Such axonal loss, most probably due to altered Schwann cell-axon interactions, has also been observed in homozygous *Pmp22*-null and heterozygous *Mpz*-null mice (Frei *et al.*, 1999). Degenerating axons seem to be preferentially associated with demyelinating or dysmyelinating Schwann cells. Thus, these animals provide a valuable model in which to identify the responsible signals.

A pronounced muscular phenotype is also observed, most likely as a secondary effect (Maier *et al.*, 2002b). Single atrophied, triangle-shaped muscle fibers and massive loss of muscle fibers leading to fascicular muscle atrophy are seen. In atrophied muscles, ultraterminal sprouting and elongated endplates with abnormal morphology as well as polyinnervation of the neuromuscular junction are frequent. It will be an important issue to characterize the nature of this muscular atrophy and the precise process of denervation and reinvervation at the cellular and molecular level.

***PMP22 transgenic rat*** The same PMP22 transgene described earlier was used to generate PMP22 overexpressor rats (Niemann *et al.*, 2000; Sereda *et al.*, 1996). A single line with three transgenic *Pmp22* copies was derived. The animals develop gait abnormalities caused by a peripheral hypomyelination, Schwann cell hypertrophy, and muscle weakness. In particular, these mutant rats are the only CMT1A model with abundant onion bulb formation (Fig. 48.1), suggesting active demyelination in peripheral nerves, similar to nerves of patients. Intracellular myelin-like figures that might be related to the structures described by Dickson *et al.* (2002) in PMP22-transfected cells (discussed earlier), and in *Tr-J*, and *Tr* nerves (Adlkofer *et al.*, 1997b), are also present (Niemann *et al.*, 2000).

Myelin abnormalities are more pronounced in ventral than in dorsal roots, as has been noted in other animal models for CMT and CH (Martini, 1997; Wrabetz *et al.*, 2000). If the PMP22 gene dosage is doubled in homozygous transgenic rats, no myelin is formed. PMP22 appears to be blocked in a late Golgi compartment, while the program of myelin gene expression is not affected (Niemann *et al.*, 2000). Similar to CMT1A patients the visible, electrophysiological, and pathological phenotypes in heterozygous and homozygous PMP22-transgenic rats are highly variable from animal to animal and correlate with variability in PMP22 mRNA overexpression. The molecular basis for this observation remains unclear, but the data are consistent with the results obtained from PMP22 transgenic mice that carry different copy numbers of a yeast artificial chromosome (YAC) containing the human PMP22 gene (Huxley *et al.*, 1996). In these mice, varying levels of PMP22 expression correlate with the degree of demyelination and reduced NCV (Huxley *et al.*, 1998; Norreel *et al.*, 2001).

As measured by its nuclear localization, cyclin D1 is active as Schwann cells proliferate after nerve injury, but not during development (Atanasoski *et al.*, 2001). What about in CMT1A? Analysis in PMP22-transgenic rats revealed that proliferating Schwann cells associated with demyelinated axons show nuclear cyclin D1 expression (Atanasoski *et al.*, 2002). Thus, these demyelinated axons produce signals in Schwann cells more like those of nerve injury than development.

***Conditional PMP22 overexpressing mouse*** Perea and colleagues have recently generated a mouse model with conditional PMP22 overexpression (Perea *et al.*, 2001; Robertson *et al.*, 2002a). They used a tetracyline-regulatable system to demonstrate that PMP22 overexpression rapidly induces demyelination even in adult mice that have developed with normal PMP22 expression. This experiment shows conclusively that adult, fully differentiated Schwann cells are vulnerable to PMP22 overexpression. Conversely, adult animals that developed with PMP22 overexpression showed rapid, partial remyelination when PMP22 expression was normalized. These results are encouraging from a disease point of view, since they suggest that mutant Schwann cells may not be irreversibly damaged in adult CMT1A patient and might be able to remyelinate if PMP22 overexpression can be corrected. Due to technical limitations of the experimental system, however, it was not possible to examine whether remyelination was specific to Schwann cells with normalized PMP22 expression and whether this effect would also lead to an amelioration of the axonopathy, muscle atrophy, and clinical behavior of the mice.

***Mice with decreased PMP22 gene dosage*** Mice with genetic disruption of the PMP22 gene are viable but develop walking difficulties due to progressive weakness of the hind limbs (Adlkofer *et al.*, 1995). Onset of myelination is slightly delayed indicating a crucial role of PMP22 in the initial steps of myelination, a conclusion that is supported by the morphological analysis of PMP22 transgenic and *Tr-J* mice (Robertson *et al.*, 1999). Myelination is altered by the characteristic formation of mainly paranodal, but also internodal tomacula. Furthermore, the myelin structure appears to be more sensitive to myelin splitting artefacts. Hypermyelination structures (tomacula) are unstable and degenerate with age. Demyelination and remyelination, indicated by thinly myelinated axons and Schwann cell onion bulbs, and associated with very slow NCV, are the predominant feature in older animals although some tomacula can still be found (Adlkofer *et al.*, 1995; Sancho *et al.*, 1999). Homozygous *Pmp22* null mice also develop a distal axonopathy with definitive signs of active axonal degeneration seen in older animals (Sancho *et al.*, 1999). As a consequence of the neural phenotype, a muscular atrophy arises as indicated by extensive type grouping of muscle fibers. No obvious pathological alterations have been detected in other tissues that normally express PMP22 although major functions of PMP22 in regulating cell death (Wilson *et al.*, 2002) and as a component of tight junctions have been described (Notterpek *et al.*, 2001). Whether this is due to more subtle effects yet to be discovered or possible compensatory effects by other members of the PMP22/EMP/MP20 family remains to be determined.

Heterozygous "knock-out" PMP22 (+/0) mice are an animal model for HNPP and show the characteristic tomacula as observed in human nerves (Adlkofer *et al.*, 1997a, and Fig. 48.1). These structures develop already in young PMP22 (+/0) mice. With age, some electrophysiological abnormalities can be detected accompanied by a significant number of abnormally swollen and degenerating tomacula. Thinly myelinated axons and Schwann cell onion bulbs appear, indicating ongoing demyelination and remyelination. Such findings have also been reproduced in another transgenic HNPP model using the $P_0$ promoter to drive rat antisense PMP22 mRNA expression (Maycox *et al.*, 1997). Similar to the observed progressive degenerative events in the mouse model, some aging HNPP patients develop a chronic form of neuropathy with similarities to CMT1 (Windebank, 1993). Whether the intrinsic instability of tomaculous myelin is also involved in the transient symptoms experienced by HNPP patients after nerve trauma remains to be determined.

Finally, available PMP22 alleles were exploited in cross-breeding experiments to generate more information about the genetic mechanism of missense mutants of PMP22 (Adlkofer *et al.*, 1997b). These studies revealed that the *Tr* allele is able to act as a true gain-of-function mutation on a null background (*Tr/0*) as well as in homozygous *Tr* animals (*Tr/Tr*). That is, the $PMP22^{Tr}$ is able to produce dose-dependent, toxic gain of function in Schwann cells, independent of any effect on wild-type PMP22 (see Chapter 39 for pathogenetic details).

## $P_0$ Animal Models

### *Introduction*

$P_0$ glycoprotein is the most abundant protein in peripheral nerve myelin (Greenfield *et al.*, 1973, see Chapter 20, "The P0 Protein Gene," for details). It is a single pass transmembrane protein with an immunoglobulin(Ig)-like fold, predicting a role in adhesion (Lemke and Axel, 1985). Aggregation assays of transfected cells showed that the extracellular domain of $P_0$ can mediate homophilic intermolecular interactions (D'Urso *et al.*, 1990; Filbin *et al.*, 1990; Schneider-Schaulies *et al.*, 1990). Crystallographic analysis of the extracellular domain suggests that four $P_0$ molecules form a tetramer in cis that interacts homophilically in trans with tetramers in apposing myelin lamellae (Shapiro *et al.*, 1996) to form the intraperiod line. In fact, complete disruption of $P_0$ expression in homozygous *Mpz*-null mice leads to uncompaction of the myelin sheath, including disruption of the intraperiod line (Giese *et al.*, 1992). *MPZ* in human maps to chromosome 1 and is mutated in CMT1B. CMT1B cases tend to manifest a more severe phenotype than the median CMT1; more rapidly progressive, with more profoundly slowed NCV (Bird, 1999). Pathological features include hypomyelination, onion bulbs, rarely tomacula, and loss of large fibers.

Thus far, more than 80 mutations have been identified in *MPZ*. They account for 4 to 14% of CMT not due to chromosome 17 duplication in various series (see Table 39.2 in Chapter 39). Missense, nonsense, and frameshift mutations have been reported (reviewed in Nelis *et al.*, 1999), but no deletion or duplication of the gene. The mutations are distributed primarily in the extracellular domain, but also within the transmembrane and intracellular domains. Mutations in *MPZ* generate perhaps the widest diversity of CMT phenotypes—ranging from mild CMT1B, typical CMT1, or HNPP-like, to the more severe DSS and CH or even CMT2—as well as pathologies—including demyelination, dysmyelination, florid tomacula, myelin outfolding, or axonal loss with clusters of regenerating axons. Commonly, specific mutations reproducibly generate certain phenotypes. For example, mutations S44F, T124M, D61G, and Y119C usually cause CMT2-like neuropathy (Marrosu *et al.*, 1998; Senderek *et al.*, 2000). How these mutations in a myelin protein influence primarly axons is an interesting question. Such diverse phenotypes suggest mutation-specific cellular pathomechanisms that can be readily investigated in animal models.

### *Loss-of-Function Models of MPZ-Related Neuropathies*

Most MPZ mutations produce neuropathy in heterozygotes. Thus, one possible explanation for diverse phenotypes is variable loss of function. At least one *MPZ* mutation, V102FS, probably represents a complete null allele (Pareyson *et al.*, 1999; Warner *et al.*, 1996), as virtual translation predicts a protein of only 78 aminoacids that contains no transmembrane domain. However, in an extended family, a phenotype in heterozygous parents and grandparents was recognized only after homozygous children presented with DSS. The children showed delayed motor milestones, severe weakness, and very slow NCV of less than 4m/s. Nerve biopsies showed markedly reduced numbers of myelinated fibers, thin myelin sheaths, and numerous basal lamina onion bulbs. Heterozygous relatives, instead, were asymptomatic with only mildly slowed NCV (median motor 40 to 48m/s) (Sghirlanzoni *et al.*, 1992).

These two situations are well modelled by heterozygous *Mpz*-null and homozygous *Mpz*-null mice, respectively. Heterozygous-null mice develop a late-onset neuropathy, with thin myelin sheaths and progressive demyelination and subtle onion bulb formation (Fig. 48.2) starting at 4 months of age (Martini *et al.*, 1995). In contrast, homozygous-null mice show severe hypomyelination, with poorly compacted myelin sheaths, and some axons surrounded by reduced or absent wraps of Schwann cell membrane, redundant basal lamina, and with age the formation of rudimentary onion bulbs (Giese *et al.*, 1992; Martini *et al.*, 1995). Consistent with this, NCV are only mildly decreased in heterozygous-null mice, but are severely reduced in homozygous-null mice, with low amplitude compound motor action potentials (CMAP) (Zielasek *et al.*, 1996). Therefore, the majority of *MPZ*-related neuropathies probably fall in an interval between loss of function of one (mild CMT1B) and two (DSS-like) alleles. This is consistent with dominant-negative gain of abnormal function (Martini, 1997); that is, the mutant allele loses adhesive function and provokes varying loss of function in the partner wild-type allele. A series of experiments *in vitro* and *in vivo* (discussed later) provide further support for this hypothesis.

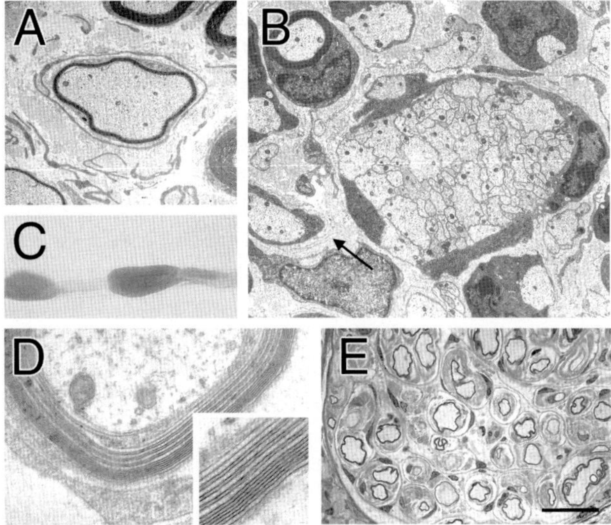


FIGURE 48.2
Different pathogenetic mechanisms in transgenic mice reproduce diverse pathological alterations as described in *MPZ*-related neuropathies. (A) A quadriceps nerve from a 13-month-old heterozygous *Mpz*-null mouse contains a typical onion bulb with supernumerary Schwann cell processes encircling a thin myelin sheath. (B) A low-power electron micrograph of $P_0$ overexpressor sciatic nerve at P28 shows paucity of myelin, with many Schwann cells arrested at the promyelin stage, occasional bundles of unsorted naked axons and redundant basal lamina (arrow). $P_0$myc mice manifest both tomacula, seen in a teased fiber (C) and uncompaction, as represented in a micrograph (D). Finally, semithin section analysis of $P_0$S63del sciatic nerves at 18 months old reveals florid onion bulbs (E). Bar (in E) = 4μm (A), 1.5μm (B), 20μm (C), 1.5μm (D), and 25μm (E).

Since progression of disability in CMT neuropathy correlates with axonal damage, a model of the more severe DSS neuropathy might manifest axonal changes. That CMAP amplitudes were reduced to less than 25% of normal in homozygous-null mice was also suggestive (Martini *et al.*, 1995; Zielasek *et al.*, 1996). Martini and colleagues confirmed this anatomically, as homozygous-null mice develop a distal axonopathy with loss of distal axons and sensory Merkel cells, and angulated fibers in muscle suggesting denervation (Frei *et al.*, 1999).

Interestingly, an inflammatory infiltration consisting of T lymphocytes and macrophages was also detected in nerves of heterozygous *Mpz*-null mice (Martini *et al.*, 1995; Shy *et al.*, 1997). Increasing infiltration paralleled progressive demyelination. Indeed, by crossing these mice with mice deficient in T lymphocytes (*Rag1*-null or *T cell receptor* α-null) or in macrophage activation (*Osteopetrosis*/macrophage colony stimulating factor-deficient), demyelination was ameliorated (Carenini *et al.*, 2001; Schmid *et al.*, 2000). Moreover, reconstitution of the immune system by transplant of wild-type bone marrow into *Mpz*(+/−)/*Rag1*(−/−) mice reproduced the worse demyelinating phenotype of native *Mpz*(+/−) mice (Maurer *et al.*, 2001). Taken together with the T lymphocyte and macrophage infiltration also described in *Cx32* deficient mice (Kobsar *et al.*, 2002), these data suggest that immune response may generally modulate the phenotype of hereditary neuropathies. Therefore, immunomodulation therapy in CMT patients may be worth exploring. In addition, by reconstituting specific elements (e.g., subsets of antigen-specific T cells) of the immune system in *Mpz*(+/−)/*Rag1*(−/−) mice, it may be possible to more specifically target immunotherapy (Maurer *et al.*, 2001, 2002).

### *Gain-of-Function Models of* MPZ*-Related Neuropathies*

Given that complete haploinsufficience of $P_0$ in human and mouse produces only mild neuropathy, many *MPZ*-related neuropathies probably include an additional gain of abnormal function mechanism—either a dominant-negative effect, most likely originating in the myelin sheath, or a "toxic" effect of the mutant protein initiating from any intracellular location during the synthesis and trafficking of $P_0$. But how can such gain of function mechanisms be correlated with the diverse *MPZ*-related phenotypes?

Evidence from human nerves, *in vitro* experiments, and transgenic mice support the notion of gain of function. Specific myelin packing defects affecting the intraperiod line have been detected in CMT1B nerves associated with several extracellular domain mutations (S63del, R98H, R98C, Kirschner *et al.*, 1996), suggesting that the mutant proteins are expressed and inserted in the myelin sheath. When coexpressed with wild-type $P_0$, either $P_0$ truncated in the cytoplasmic domain or $P_0$ unable to form a disulfide bond in the extracellular domain impaired the adhesion normally mediated by wild-type $P_0$ between transfected CHO cells, demonstrating a dominant-negative gain of function (Wong and Filbin, 1996; Zhang and Filbin, 1998).

In contrast to PMP22, there are no naturally occuring mouse mutants with *Mpz* point mutations. To test for diverse gain of function mechanisms, various *MPZ* mutations were engineered in the *Mpz* gene, which was then inserted as a random transgene, in addition to the two endogenous *Mpz* alleles, in mice. In this way loss of mutant $P_0$ function in these mice should be invisible.

As a control, it has been shown that additional copies of wild-type *Mpz* as a randomly inserted transgene produce $P_0$ overexpression ($P_0$OE) and dose-dependent congenital hypomyelinating neuropathy (CHN) in mice (Wrabetz *et al.*, 2000). In $P_0$OE nerves, many myelin-forming Schwann cells had appropriately ensheathed single axons, but the membrane spiraling around the axon (inner mesaxon) was arrested after 1 to 2 turns (Fig. 48.2) by adhesion and reduced space between the first two wraps, associated with premature arrival of $P_0$ (Yin *et al.*, 2000). This represents a gain of normal function, in that it is homophilic adhesion located in the forming myelin sheath, but at the wrong time. This study also determined that less than 50% overexpression of $P_0$ permitted normal myelination.

Also, random insertion of a transgene encoding $P_0$ with a myc epitope tag at the mature amino terminus ($P_0$myc) produced a severe demyelinating neuropathy, even when overexpressed at only 50% relative to endogenous $P_0$ (Previtali *et al.*, 2000). $P_0$myc mice had nerve morphology reminiscent of two subgroups of CMT1B neuropathies, both including amino acid substitutions predicted by the crystal structure of the $P_0$ extracellular domain to be near the amino terminus. Pathological features included tomacula and redundant myelin loops, and uncompaction of the myelin sheath (Fig. 48.2)—neither were seen with $P_0$ wild-type overexpression. $P_0$myc was located by immunoelectronmicroscopy in the myelin sheath, in areas of uncompacted myelin. Moreover, the intraperiod line (where opposing $P_0$ECD interact in trans to compact myelin) was widened, suggesting a steric, dominant-negative, gain of function mechanism.

Finally, mice that contain the CMT1B allele *Mpz*S63del (deletion of serine 63) as a random insertion transgene develop adult-onset, hypertrophic, demyelinating neuropathy, with motor NCV reduced to 24 m/sec (Wrabetz *et al.*, 2002, and manuscript in preparation). Numerous, large onion bulbs were observed, perhaps the most florid described in an animal model of CMT neuropathy (Fig. 48.2). Of note, onion bulbs were never observed in $P_0$ overexpressor or $P_0$myc mice. Even when the total *Mpz* dosage was reduced to normal by crossing the *Mpz*S63del transgene into the *Mpz*(+/−) background, neuropathy remained, confirming that it was specified by the S63del mutation. This shows that a gain of abnormal function not related to overexpression is sufficient to produce a CMT1B neuropathy in mice.

Surprisingly, further analysis showed that the $P_0$S63del mutant protein is retained in the endoplasmic reticulum, is subsequently partially degraded, and does not arrive to the myelin sheath (Wrabetz *et al.*, 2002, and manuscript in preparation). Thus, the $P_0$S63del mouse provides another good model (in addition to *Trembler* and *TremblerJ*) in which to ask how mutant myelin proteins can provoke demyelination from an intracellular location away from myelin.

Taken together, these gain of function *Mpz* models strongly suggest that *MPZ* mutations act through various pathogenetic mechanisms, some mutation specific, that originate from various intracellular locations in Schwann cells, in order to produce the remarkably diverse *MPZ*-related phenotypes.

## Cx32 Animal Models

*CX32* mutations were first described in X-linked CMT disease (CMT1X) by Bergoffen and colleagues (1993) based on genetic mapping experiments and the discovery of high-level Cx32 expression by myelinating Schwann cells. CMT1X accounts for 7 to 16% of all forms of CMT (Table 39.2, Chapter 39) and is particularly characterized by prominent axonal loss and regenerative clusters, in addition to the classically observed variable demyelination and remyelination (Hahn *et al.*, 1990). This specific feature has led to the diagnosis of axonal CMT (CMT2) in some patients (Scherer and Fischbeck, 1999).

In peripheral nerves, Cx32 is found in uncompacted domains along the myelin internode—the paranodes and Schmidt-Lanterman incisures (Scherer *et al.*, 1995a). The incisures traverse the compact myelin sheath as a conical spiral and generate a cytoplasmic connection between the outer, perinuclear and the inner, periaxonal Schwann cell cytoplasm. It is thought that supply and retrieval of biosynthetic components and ions take place at the myelin-cytoplasmic channel interface as well as between outer, abaxonal and inner, adaxonal Schwann cell cytoplasm. Functional, reflexive gap junction channels have been described in incisures suggesting the formation of a more direct radial pathway across the myelin sheath (Balice-Gordon *et al.*, 1998). However, the rate of (injected) dye diffusion across the sheath was not disturbed in *Cx32*-null mice suggesting that other gap junction proteins might be expressed and functional in the myelin sheath of peripheral nerves. Indeed, mouse Cx29 (putative human orthologue: Cx31.3) has been detected in the innermost aspects of the myelin sheath, the paranode, the juxtaparanode, the inner mesaxon and the Schmidt-Lanterman incisures in adult sciatic nerves (Altevogt *et al.*, 2002). Whether this protein is required for efficient transport through incisures or myelin integrity awaits the corresponding mouse mutant or the discovery of *Cx31.3* mutations in human pedigrees.

Some *CX32* mutations seem to result in null alleles (Fischbeck *et al.*, 1999; Scherer *et al.*, 1999, see Chapter 39); and thus, *Cx32*-null mice have been analyzed as potential models of CMT1X (Anzini *et al.*, 1997; Nelles *et al.*, 1996; Scherer *et al.*, 1998). This analysis revealed near normal NCV, but with aging, *Cx32*-null mice developed a late-onset, progressive peripheral neuropathy with characteristics similar to CMT1X. Cellular onion bulbs as signs of demyelination and remyelination were present and teased nerve fiber analysis revealed segmental demyelination. As observed in other CMT1 models, the motor nerves were more affected than sensory branches. Conspicuously abnormal, enlarged periaxonal collars (Figure 48.3) and cytoplasmic thickenings of other noncompacted compartments, such as Schmidt-Lanterman incisures and paranodal loops, were frequently seen. Disorganization of the inner Schwann cell compartment in *Cx32*-deficient mice may reflect the consequence of disturbed communication between the outer and inner cytoplasmic aspects of myelinating Schwann cells. Furthermore, regenerative clusters indicative of axonal degeneration are present. Heterozygous female animals show segmental loss of Cx32 expression and less signs of demyelination than age-matched homozygous mice, consistent with the finding that the X-linked *Cx32* gene is randomly inactivated. As first observed in *Mpz*-deficient mice, macrophages modulate the demyelinating phenotype of *Cx32*-null mice (Kobsar *et al.*, 2002; Maurer *et al.*, 2002).

Gene-expression profiling of *Cx32*-null mice revealed marked upregulation of the cytoskeletal protein glial fibrillary acidic protein (GFAP) of yet unknown significance (Nicholson *et al.*, 2001). Altered molecular architecture of peripheral nerves in *Cx32*-null mice has been reported, but the localization of the axonal proteins Caspr and Kv1.1 and 1.2 appears not to be disrupted (Arroyo *et al.*, 1999; Neuberg *et al.*, 1999).

Although *Cx32*-deficient mice reflect the CMT1X phenotype quite accurately, there seem to be considerable differences among species in the role of Cx32 outside of the PNS. Some *CX32* mutations also produce CNS symptoms (Kleopa *et al.*, 2002; Paulson *et al.*, 2002), but no other consistent phenotype has been described. In the *Cx32*-null mouse, however, disrupted metabolic cooperativity among hepatocytes results in reduced glucose release upon stimulation of the sympathetic nerves in the liver (Nelles *et al.*, 1996).

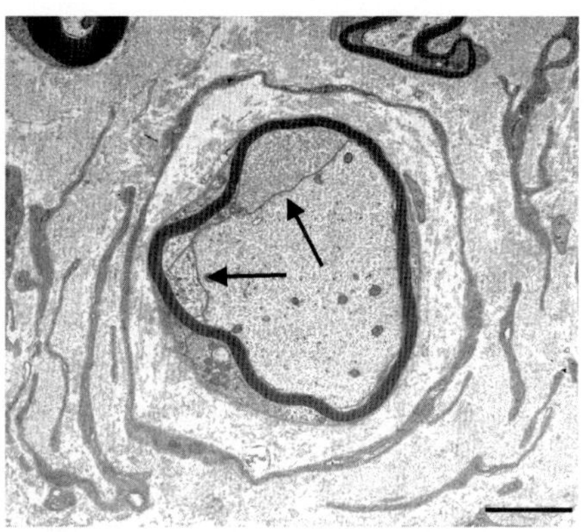

FIGURE 48.3
Alterations at the axoglial junction of CMT1X are reproduced in *Cx32*-null mice. Note the enlarged periaxonal collar typical of CMT1X fibers (arrows). Bar = 2 μm.

Furthermore, adult *Cx32*-deficient mice are more susceptible to chemically induced tumors and display more spontaneous liver tumors than age-matched wild-type mice (Temme *et al.*, 1997; and for discussion see Willecke *et al.*, 1999).

Potential gain-of-function disease mechanisms of several *CX32* mutations have been tested by expressing (under the control of the $P_0$ promoter) the mutant allele in myelinating Schwann cells of transgenic mice. This analysis revealed that a frame-shifting mutation at codon 175 (175fs) was only expressed at the mRNA level, apparently without other effects, consistent with a loss-of-function mechanism (Abel *et al.*, 1999). In contrast, in R142W transgenic mice, the mutant Cx32 accumulated in the perinuclear cytoplasm without reaching the Schmidt-Lanterman incisures or the paranodes (Scherer *et al.*, 1999). In addition, endogenous Cx32 expression was reduced and wild-type Cx32 was retained intracellularly, suggesting a "dominant-negative" effect of the mutated protein (Fischbeck *et al.*, 1999). Similar to mice completely deficient in Cx32, R142W-mutant mice developed a late-onset demyelinating neuropathy. It should be noted, however, that a direct "dominant-negative" effect between mutant and wild-type Cx32 is unlikely to occur in CMT1X patients since there is only one allele expressed per Schwann cell. Nevertheless, the mutated protein may interact with other connexins and generate an adverse effect. In other myelinopathies, aberrant trafficking of other myelin proteins like proteolipid protein (PLP) (Gow *et al.*, 1998), PMP22 (discussed earlier) and P0 (discussed earlier) has been described and may contribute to the pathogenesis (Southwood *et al.*, 2002). Thus, intracellular accumulation and sequestration of chaperones by mutated proteins (Dickson *et al.*, 2002) might be a common denominator in the pathophysiology of diseases affecting myelinating cells.

## EGR2/Krox20 Animal Models

Altered dosage of various myelin genes (including *PMP22*, *MPZ* in the PNS, and *PLP* in the CNS) perturbs normal myelination. So it is not surprising that mutations in a transcription factor, encoded by *EGR2*, are associated with CMT. *EGR2* is a member of the early growth response gene family and encodes the zinc-finger transcription factor Krox20. As predicted by segment-specific expression of Krox20 in developing hindbrain, *Krox20*-null mice had defective formation of rhombomeres 3 and 5 (Schneider-Maunoury *et al.*, 1993; Swiatek and Gridley, 1993). Unexpectedly, *Krox20* null mice also manifested dysmyelination in peripheral nerve (Topilko *et al.*, 1994).

Most *Krox20*-null mice die shortly after birth, before significant peripheral myelination has begun. However, a few homozygous-null mice can survive for as much as 2 weeks after birth (Schneider-Maunoury *et al.*, 1993; Topilko *et al.*, 1994), in a strain-dependent fashion (L. Wrabetz, personal observation). In outlier *Krox20*-null mice, myelination is blocked at an early stage, in which Schwann cells begin to wrap axons, express early markers such as myelin associated glycoprotein (MAG), but do not induce the expression of other myelin genes, including *Mpz* and *Mbp* (myelin basic protein gene) (Topilko *et al.*, 1994). This observation has been further confirmed in mice homozygous for the hypomorphic *Krox20lo* gene, a "knock-down" allele created by inserting a neoR gene into the *Egr2* intron. Homozygotes routinely survive for 3 to 4 weeks after birth, but still manage essentially no peripheral nerve myelination (Nagarajan *et al.*, 2002, and J. Svaren personal communication).

Krox20 is thought to link axonal signals to induction of myelin gene expression and myelination by Schwann cells (Murphy *et al.*, 1996). Indeed, adenoviral overexpression of Krox20 in cultured Schwann cells markedly activates expression of the program of myelin-related genes, including *Pmp22* and *Mpz* within 24 hours (Nagarajan *et al.*, 2001). Like other EGR family members, Krox20 also contains a conserved R1 repressor domain, bound by the NAB corepressor proteins, that serves to modulate transcriptional activation of Krox20 target genes (Svaren *et al.*, 1998). Six of seven *EGR2* mutations are dominant, associated with CMT1, DSS and CH, and fall in the highly conserved zinc finger DNA binding domains, supporting that Krox20 transcriptional function is important for myelination, whereas one recessive mutation (I268N), causing CH, falls in the R1 domain preventing interactions with NAB corepressors and superactivating a synthetic Krox20 target promoter by 15-fold *in vitro* (Warner *et al.*, 1998, 1999, and see Chapter 39).

Heterozygous *Krox20*-null mice show normal myelination (Topilko *et al.*, 1994), whereas dominant *EGR2* mutations manifest in heterozygotes, suggesting that these mutations act at least in part though gain of function. In keeping with this idea, the S382R/D383Y mutant inhibits the activation of endogenous myelin genes by wild-type Krox20 in cotransduced Schwann cells (Nagarajan *et al.*, 2001). Therefore, to study the pathomechanisms of these mutations *in vivo*, it will be necessary to engineer mice with authentic mutations introduced by homologous recombination in ES cells.

The recessive I268N mutation is associated with CH in the homozygous state and therefore could be modelled by homozygous *Krox20* null mouse. However, unlike the mouse, I268N produces no evidence of brain stem or bone abnormalities in patients, thus it is unlikely to represent a null allele. Instead, I268N may be released from NAB regulation, and derepress a Krox20 target gene (15-fold), such that Warner *et al.* (1998) proposed a gene dosage neuropathy. *PMP22* and *MPZ* would be good candidate targets, as significant overexpression of either produces a CH-like neuropathy in mice (discussed earlier).

## Periaxin-Null Mice Model CMT4F

The autosomal recessive demyelinating neuropathies (CMT4) are less common than CMT1 and tend to be more severe (Chapter 39). Out of eight CMT4 loci, five disease genes have been identified (CMT4A:*GDAP1*, CMT4B1:*MTMR2*, CMT4B2:*MTMR13/SBF2*, CMT4D:*NDRG1*, and CMT4F:*PRX*), and most mutations are thought to produce loss of function.

Periaxin is a PDZ domain protein that was identified as a Schwann cell-specific cytoskeletal protein (Gillespie *et al.*, 1994). Periaxin expression is polarized during development first to the inner cytoplasmic domain of the Schwann cell, facing the axon, and then in mature nerves to the outer cytoplasmic domain, away from the axon (Scherer *et al.*, 1995b). Here it interacts via dystrophin related protein -2 (DRP-2) with the dystroglycan complex, which in turn links laminin-2 in the basal lamina to the actin cytoskeleton in the cytoplasm (Sherman *et al.*, 2001). Furthermore, this complex may also activate signal transduction from laminin to the Schwann cell (Wrabetz and Feltri, 2001).

Homozygous or compound heterozygous nonsense and frameshift mutations in *PRX* have been associated with CMT4F or DSS, as well as milder CMT1-like phenotypes (Boerkoel *et al.*, 2001; Guilbot *et al.*, 2001; Takashima *et al.*, 2002); all are predicted to produce loss of function, confirmed thus far in one patient whose sural nerve biopsy contained no periaxin (Guilbot *et al.*, 2001; Takashima *et al.*, 2002). Therefore, the *Prx*-null mouse is a potential animal model of CMT4F due to *PRX* mutations.

Prx-null mice develop a phenotype with peculiar characteristics remarkably similar to those of CMT4F patients (Gillespie *et al.*, 2000). *Prx*-null mice form normal myelin, but the myelin sheath is unstable and after 6 weeks of age mice develop myelin infolding/thickening, followed by hypomyelination, segmental demyelination with onion bulbs, and tomacula around "compressed" axons by 6 to 8 months of age. Interestingly, these mice have a more prominent sensory neuropathy relative to motor involvement, in contrast to other myelin mutant mice. Allodynia, hyperalgesia, and neuropathic pain (Gillespie *et al.*, 2000) were documented by reduced conduction velocity of afferent myelinated fibers in the saphenous nerve after von Frey filament stimulation and increased withdrawal response to mechanical and thermal stimulation. Similarly, CMT4F patients develop a severe neuropathy, with both motor involvement as well as pronounced sensory abnormalities and neuropathic pain, and morphologically, loss of myelinated fibers, onion bulbs, myelin out- and infolding and axonal compression (see Figure 6 in Guilbot *et al.*, 2001; Takashima *et al.*, 2002).

## CMT2 Animal Models

### *Introduction*

In CMT2 hereditary neuropathies, axons are primarily and more severely affected. CMT1 and 2 are distinguished by clinical, electrophysiological, and histological characteristics; in particular, by the NCV in the forearm (below 38m/sec in CMT1 and above 38m/sec in CMT2). At least 13 genetic loci have been described, and disease genes have been identified in three autosomal dominant forms, *KIF1B* for CMT2A, *RAB7* for CMT2B, and *NEFL* for CMT2E, and in one autosomal recessive form, *LMNA* for autosomal recessive (AR)-CMT2A. In addition, certain *MPZ* mutations are associated with a CMT2-like phenotype, and *GJ*β1 mutations produce a CMT1X phenotype with axonal characteristics that in part overlap CMT2 (see Chapter 39 for further discussion). Animal models have been described for *KIF1B*, *NEFL*, and *LMNA*.

### *Kif1B-Null Mice Model CMT2A*

*Kif1B* is a member of the kinesin gene superfamily, and produces two alternatively spliced variants, termed α and β, that encode a common N-terminal ATPase motor domain fused to one of two divergent C-terminal cargo domains. A loss of function Q98L mutation in the ATP binding site in the motor domain causes CMT2A (Zhao *et al.*, 2001). Homozygous *Kif1b*-null mice die from apnea due to loss of CNS neurons. Heterozygous-null mice develop a late-onset, axonal neuropathy confirming that haploinsufficiency can explain neuropathy in CMT2A. Neuropathy was characterized by impaired motor (rotarod performance) but not sensory (hotplate test) capacity, with reduced CMAP and preserved NCV; no nerve histology was described (Zhao *et al.*, 2001). Kinesin 1Bα carries mitochondria, and via PDZ-containing linker proteins such as PSD-95 and synaptic scaffolding molecule-90, interacts with potassium channels, NMDA receptor subunits, and neuronal nitric oxide synathase; whereas Kinesin 1Bß carries synaptic vesicle precursor proteins—heterozygous-null mice showed decreased axonal transport of the latter (Zhao *et al.*, 2001). It remains to be determined which cargo is important to the pathogenesis of CMT2A (Mok *et al.*, 2002), but in any case this provides a potentially satisfying explanation for length-dependent axonal damage typical of CMT2; the distal part of longer axons should require more efficient axonal transport.

### *Do Nefl-Null Mice Model CMT2E?*

Neurofilaments are the major intermediate filaments of neurons and axons and are assembled by copolymerization of heavy, medium, and low molecular weight monomers, NF-H, M, and L. Neurofilaments are an important component of axonal cytoskeleton and determinant of axonal caliber. Decreased neurofilament phosphorylation and spacing, axonal caliber, and slow axonal transport were detected in dysmyelinated axons of *Trembler* or *MAG*-null mice (de Waegh *et al.*, 1992; Yin *et al.*, 1998). In demyelinating neuropathies, these effects are non-cell autonomous, as they are detected in wild-type mouse axons regenerated through sural nerve xenografts from patients with CMT (Sahenk, 1999; Sahenk *et al.*, 1999).

It is perhaps not surprising, therefore, that *NEFL*, encoding the NF-L subunit, could be a CMT2 disease gene. Multiple *NEFL* mutations have been identified in CMT2E, most missense, and several segregating faithfully with axonal neuropathy in multigeneration families (De Jonghe *et al.*, 2001; Jordanova *et al.*, 2003; Mersiyanova *et al.*, 2000; Yoshihara *et al.*, 2002). The genetic mechanism is likely to be gain of abnormal function, as CMT2E segregates as a dominant trait, most mutations are missense, and two CMT2E mutant NF-L subunits disrupt assembly and axonal transport of neurofilaments in transfected DRG neurons (Brownlees *et al.*, 2002; Perez-Olle *et al.*, 2002).

Mouse models relevant to *Nefl* support this idea, as heterozygous *Nefl*-null mice manifest reduced axonal caliber, but do not develop a CMT2-like phenotype (Zhu *et al.*, 1997). In contrast, the expression of an NF-L missense mutant (L394P) in transgenic mice, predicted to alter the coil 2B domain and disrupt neurofilament assembly, causes a very severe neuronopathy/neuropathy with abnormal gait and weakness (Lee *et al.*, 1994). Finally, a series of transgenic studies of neurodegenerative diseases such as Amyotrophic Lateral Sclerosis have revealed that gain of function mechanisms are far more important than loss of function mechanisms in neurofilament-related pathological processes (reviewed in Julien *et al.*, 1998). Thus, valid animal models of CMT2E will probably be produced only via introduction of missense *NEFL* mutations by homologous recombination in ES cells.

It is worth emphasizing that disability in CMT neuropathies correlates with axonal damage (see the introduction). Both primary demyelinating and axonal neuropathies produce similar neurofilament alterations, with consequential effects on axonal caliber, nerve conduction velocity, and axonal transport that could account for length-dependent axonal damage. Thus, this point of convergence in the pathogenesis of some axonal and demyelinating neuropathies is a valid therapeutic target.

#### *Lmna–Null Mice Model AR-CMT2A Neuropathy*

Lamin A/C isoforms, encoded by *LMNA*, are widely expressed nuclear envelope proteins. Mutations in *LMNA* have been associated with various diseases, including limb-girdle and Emery-Dreifuss muscular dystrophies, dilated cardiomyopathy 1A, partial lipodystrophy, and mandibuloacral dysplasia (reviewed in Moir and Spann, 2001). Recently, a homozygous R298C mutation was reported in three families with AR-CMT2A (Chaouch *et al.*, 2003; De Sandre-Giovannoli *et al.*, 2002). R298C probably produces lamin A/C loss of function in nerve, as reevaluation of the homozygous *Lmna*-null mouse (Sullivan *et al.*, 1999) revealed a peripheral neuropathy, with abnormally stiff gait, weak grip, and loss of myelinated fibers and more amyelinated axons of increased caliber (De Sandre-Giovannoli *et al.*, 2002). Further characterization will determine whether this fully models the human neuropathy characterized by weakness and atrophy of both distal and proximal muscles, distal loss of sensation, normal motor NCV and reduced or absent sensory nerve action potentials, and histology showing profound loss of large myelinated fibers, regenerating clusters of axons, and the absence of onion bulbs (Chaouch *et al.*, 2003; De Sandre-Giovannoli *et al.*, 2002). Most of the other *LMNA* mutations produce diverse diseases in heterozygosity, suggesting varying gain of function effects.

## MODELS OF SYNDROMIC NEUROPATHIES WITH CMT-LIKE FEATURES

Several syndromes include neuropathies with CMT-like features (see Chapter 39 by Wrabetz, *et al.*, for discussion of syndromic neuropathies). The presence or absence of neuropathy in mouse models with diverse mutations in the corresponding genes may provide clues as to how the original mutations in human cause neuropathy.

### Desert Hedgehog-Null Mice

*Desert Hedgehog*, together with *Sonic Hedgehog* and *Indian Hedgehog* are homologous to the Drosophila Hedgehog segment polarity gene and belong to a family of signaling molecules crucially important for early development (reviewed in Ingham and McMahon,

2001). Desert Hedgehog is secreted by Schwann cells in the endoneurium, from where it acts on perineurial cells through the Patched receptor, to regulate perineurial formation (Parmantier *et al.*, 1999). Umehara *et al.* (2000) described a family with members homozygous for *DHH*-null mutations, who develop gonadal dysgenesis and a minifascicular neuropathy remarkably similar to that of *Dhh*-null mice. Numerous minifascicles subdivide the endoneurium, each containing several Schwann cell-axon units surrounded by perineurial-like cells. Further analysis in *Dhh*-null mice revealed that the formation of epineurium and perineurium nerve sheaths is defective. Perineurial tight junctions are abnormal, resulting in increased permeability of the perineurial blood/nerve barrier. Abnormalities in the endoneurial environment may cause secondary degeneration of nerve fibers, as patients show a mild reduction in the density of myelinated fibers (Umehara *et al.*, 2000).

### PLP-Null Mice

In contrast, the peripheral neuropathy associated with some other human syndromic myelinopathies is not reproduced in animal models. For example, *PLP* produces two alternatively spliced transcripts that encode PLP and DM20, together the major component of CNS myelin. PLP contains a specific 35 amino acid domain not found in DM20. *PLP* is also expressed by myelin-forming Schwann cells in peripheral nerve, albeit at low levels. Mutations in PLP/DM-20 cause Pelizeaus-Merzbacher disease, an X-linked leukodystrophy (see Chapter 37 for details). Patients with mutations that eliminate the expression of both PLP and DM20 also develop a peripheral neuropathy (Garbern *et al.*, 1997; Shy *et al.*, 2003). Of note, mutations predicted to eliminate PLP, but maintain expression of DM20, cause neuropathy, whereas mutations that preserve the PLP-specific domain do not (Shy *et al.*, 2003). This suggests that the PLP-specific domain is required for peripheral nerve function. However, even though *Plp* produces similar isoforms in mouse, *Plp/DM20*-null mice do not develop a peripheral neuropathy (Griffiths *et al.*, 1998; Klugmann *et al.*, 1997). Perhaps other lipophilin family members, such as M6B (Werner *et al.*, 2001), may compensate for the absence of PLP in mouse, but not human, nerve.

### Heterozygous *Sox10*-Null Mice and Myelinopathy

Sox10 is a transcription factor required for normal development of several neural crest derivatives. *Sox10* is expressed at all stages of Schwann cell lineage (Kuhlbrodt *et al.*, 1998), during which it cooperates with other transcription factors, such as Oct6, Pax3, and Egr2, and ultimately activates myelin-specific genes as Schwann cells terminally differentiate (Kuhlbrodt *et al.*, 1998; Peirano *et al.*, 2000). Homozygous *Sox10*-null mice do not develop peripheral glia, including Schwann cells (Britsch *et al.*, 2001). In addition, Sox10 is required for normal differentiation of oligodendrocytes (Stolt *et al.*, 2002).

Heterozygous mutations in *SOX10* in humans give rise to Waardenburg-Shah (WS4) syndrome, which presents with intestinal aganglionosis (Hirschprung disease), depigmentation, and deafness (Waardenburg syndrome) (Pingault *et al.*, 1998). Absence of several neural crest derivatives, such as enteric ganglion cells and melanocytes, account for the phenotype, but these patients do not develop myelin-related diseases. Instead, several WS patients with putative dominant-negative mutations (DNA binding domain retained; activation domain altered) in *SOX10* had peripheral and sometimes central dysmyelination similar to Pelizeus-Merzbacher disease and CMT1 or CH (Inoue *et al.*, 2002; 1999; Pingault *et al.*, 2001).

One hypothesis is that Waardenburg/Hirschprung symptoms derive from haploinsufficiency, whereas the myelinopathies derive from a dominant-negative gain of function for mutated *SOX10*. In mouse, a spontaneous mutation in *Sox10* causes a similar syndrome called Dominant Megacolon (*dom*). Heterozygous *Sox10*-null mice manifest pigmentation and megacolon defects, confirming that these symptoms in *dom* mice and Waardenburg/Hirschprung patients represent haploinsufficiency; no peripheral nerve defects have been reported in heterozygous *Sox10*-null mice (Britsch *et al.*, 2001). As for many CMT neuropathies, transgenic mice with myelinopathy-specific *Sox10* mutations will probably be required to test the dominant-negative hypothesis.

## ANIMAL MODELS WITH PATHOLOGICAL SIMILARITY TO HEREDITARY NEUROPATHIES

Several animal models phenocopy human neuropathies, but result from genetic alterations not yet described in humans, or are not even associated with a disease gene yet. An example of the former, *Mpz* overexpression in mice phenocopies CH, with many Schwann cells unable to sort axons, arrested in the promyelin stage, or associated with a thin myelin sheath. These nerves also contain increased endoneurial collagen, and redundant Schwann cell basal lamina, without evidence of myelin destruction or Schwann cell onion bulbs (Fig. 48.2). Finally, the myelination defect improves somewhat with time. All of these features compare well with CH in human (Phillips *et al.*, 1999). However, no corresponding human case of *MPZ* duplication has been documented, although the pathogenesis of *EGR2* mutant I268N may include myelin gene overexpression (see the earlier discussion and Wrabetz *et al.*, 2000).

A fascinating example of a genetically unidentified model is *Claw Paw (clp)*, a spontaneous autosomal recessive mutant that arose in the C57BL/6J-obese strain and has CH with abnormal posture of the forelimbs (sometimes called arthrogryposis, but in *clp/clp* mice it does not initially represent fixed joint contractures, as they retain the full range of passive motion). Nerve histology showed diffuse hypomyelination, with Schwann cells temporarily blocked at the promyelinating stage, followed by improvement and progressive myelination of a subset of axons after the first 2 to 4 weeks of life (Henry *et al.*, 1991). In the adult, *clp/clp* is one of the few myelin mutants that shows equal or worse dysmyelination in the dorsal as compared to ventral roots. The pathological effect of *clp* is at least in part Schwann cell autonomous, where it functions downstream of or in parallel with the Pou3f1/Oct6/SCIP transcription factor (Darbas *et al.*, 2002). Also, *clp* maps to mouse chromosome 7 (Henry *et al.*, 1991) and has been localized to an interval of less than 1 megabase (J. Bermingham and D. Meijer, personal communication). Screening of candidate genes is underway, and may produce a disease gene for CH in human.

## GENERALIZATIONS FROM ANIMAL MODELS

What generalizations emerge from the animal models of CMT? First, dys- or demyelinating animals phenocopy corresponding human CMT neuropathies reasonably well (models of axonal neuropathies are too few and too sparsely characterized to form generalizations). Specific morphological alterations are produced in myelin (e.g., tomacula in heterozygous PMP22 null or myelin infolding in homozygous periaxin-null mice) that produce electrophysiological and behavioural alterations consistent with clinical characteristics of associated CMT neuropathies. Moreover, the onset and progression are consistent with, but also flesh out, the partial data set deduced from clinical studies. So for example, we have learned that tomacula form and then degenerate to produce a more general demyelinating neuropathy in HNPP model mice.

Second, CMT animal models have proven genetic cause and revealed cell biological pathogenesis. For example, it is clear that PMP22 overexpression or haploinsufficience are the relevant causes of CMT1A and HNPP related to chromosome 17 duplication or deletion, respectively. Also some missense mutants of PMP22 or P0 produce a toxic gain of abnormal function related to retention at various points in the biosynthetic pathway, suggesting an important role for altered protein quality control in CMT neuropathies.

Third, the analysis of CMT models is beginning to uncover common consequences that may serve as general therapeutic targets. So the immune response to myelin damage is present in CMT1X and CMT1B models and modulates the phenotype. Also, as in human, probably all demyelinating mouse models develop secondary axonal damage. However, it must be noted that axonal damage is underwhelming in these mice as compared to humans, perhaps because mice have shorter nerves and life spans (see Martini, 1997, 2000, and 2001 for further discussion). As mouse models of axonal CMT2 neuropathies are analyzed further, it will be important to compare axonal damage in them to the corresponding human CMT2.

Finally, studies of animal models have also indicated potential difficulties for the treatment of CMT neuropathies. Thus, where pathogenesis includes loss of function, replacement therapy will require precise control. Dosage of most myelin related genes is tightly regulated. For example, over- or underexpression of *PMP22* or *MPZ* by only about 50% itself produces neuropathy—a real challenge for the gene therapy vectors currently in use. Second, the cell-autonomous pathogenesis, even for alterations of the same gene, is many times mutation specific. Thus, an important challenge is to identify further common consequences that could represent therapeutic targets for all CMT neuropathies.

## CONCLUSIONS

Animals models relevant to 8 of 14 CMT genes have been characterized. The majority are behaviorally, electrophysiologically, and pathologically similar to the corresponding human diseases. These models have produced new information about the normal function of CMT genes, as well as the natural history of CMT neuropathies, and emphasize that the pathogenesis usually begins cell-autonomously and is often mutation specific, even for diverse alterations of the same gene. However, corollary immune responses and initial axonal damage may be common features of CMT neuropathies that are reproduced in animal models of CMT and represent promising targets for the development of new therapies.

### Acknowledgments

L. W. and M. L. F. have been supported by the National Institutes of Health (NS41319 and NS45630); Telethon, Italy; Great Britain Multiple Sclerosis Society; and the European Community. U. S. has been supported by the Swiss National Science Foundation, the Swiss Muscle Disease Foundation, the National Center of Competence in Research "Neural Plasticity and Repair," and the Swiss Bundesamt for Science related to the Commission of the European Communities, specific Research, Technological Development and Demonstration program "Quality of Life and Management of Living Resources," QLK6-CT-2000-00179. We thank our many colleagues whose work has contributed to this area. We also thank Rudolf Martini, Igor Kobsar, and Michael Sereda for the gift of micrographs.

### References

Abel, A., Bone, L. J., Messing, A., Scherer, S. S., and Fischbeck, K. H. (1999). Studies in transgenic mice indicate a loss of connexin32 function in X-linked Charcot-Marie-Tooth disease. *J Neuropathol Exp Neurol*, **58,** 702–710.

Adlkofer, K., Frei, R., Neuberg, D. H., Zielasek, J., Toyka, K. V., and Suter, U. (1997a). Heterozygous peripheral myelin protein 22-deficient mice are affected by a progressive demyelinating tomaculous neuropathy. *J Neurosci*, **17,** 4662–4671.

Adlkofer, K., Martini, R., Aguzzi, A., Zielasek, J., Toyka, K. V., and Suter, U. (1995). Hypermyelination and demyelinating peripheral neuropathy in Pmp22-deficient mice. *Nat Genet*, **11,** 274–280.

Adlkofer, K., Naef, R., and Suter, U. (1997b). Analysis of compound heterozygous mice reveals that the Trembler mutation can behave as a gain-of-function allele. *J Neurosci Res*, **49,** 671–680.

Aguayo, A. J., Attiwell, M., Trecarten, J., Perkins, S., and Bray, G. M. (1977). Abnormal myelination in transplanted Trembler mouse Schwann cells. *Nature*, **265,** 73–75.

Altevogt, B. M., Kleopa, K. A., Postma, F. R., Scherer, S. S., and Paul, D. L. (2002). Connexin29 is uniquely distributed within myelinating glial cells of the central and peripheral nervous systems. *J Neurosci*, **22,** 6458–6470.

Anzini, P., Neuberg, D. H., Schachner, M., Nelles, E., Willecke, K., Zielasek, J., Toyka, K. V., Suter, U., and Martini, R. (1997). Structural abnormalities and deficient maintenance of peripheral nerve myelin in mice lacking the gap junction protein connexin 32. *J Neurosci*, **17,** 4545–4551.

Arroyo, E. J., Xu, Y. T., Zhou, L., Messing, A., Peles, E., Chiu, S. Y., and Scherer, S. S. (1999). Myelinating Schwann cells determine the internodal localization of Kv1.1, Kv1.2, Kvbeta2, and Caspr. *J Neurocytol*, **28,** 333–347.

Atanasoski, S., Scherer, S. S., Nave, K. A., and Suter, U. (2002). Proliferation of Schwann cells and regulation of cyclin D1 expression in an animal model of Charcot-Marie-Tooth disease type 1A. *J Neurosci Res*, **67,** 443–449.

Atanasoski, S., Shumas, S., Dickson, C., Scherer, S. S., and Suter, U. (2001). Differential cyclin D1 requirements of proliferating Schwann cells during development and after injury. *Mol Cell Neurosci*, **18,** 581–592.

Ayers, M. M., and Anderson, R. M. (1973). Onion bulb neuropathy in the Trembler mouse: A model of hypertrophic interstitial neuropathy (Dejerine-Sottas). in man. *Acta Neuropathol*, **25,** 54–70.

Ayers, M. M., and Anderson, R. M. (1975). Development of onion bulb neuropathy in the Trembler mouse. Comparison with normal nerve maturation. *Acta Neuropathol*, **32,** 43–59.

Ayers, M. M., and Anderson, R. M. (1976). Development of onion bulb neuropathy in the Trembler mouse. Morphometric study. *Acta Neuropathol*, **36,** 137–152.

Balice-Gordon, R. J., Bone, L. J., and Scherer, S. S. (1998). Functional gap junctions in the schwann cell myelin sheath. *J Cell Biol*, **142,** 1095–1104.

Bartoszewics, Z. P., Lauter, C. J., and Quarles, R. H. (1996). The myelin-associated glycoprotein of the peripheral nervous system in trembler mutants contains increased α2–3 sialic acid and galactose. *J Neurosci Res*, **43,** 587–593.

Bascles, L., Bonnet, J., and Garbay, B. (1992). Expression of the PMP-22 gene in Trembler mutant mice: Comparison with the other myelin protein genes. *Dev Neurosci*, **14,** 336–341.

Berciano, J., Garcia, A., Calleja, J., and Combarros, O. (2000). Clinico-electrophysiological correlation of extensor digitorum brevis muscle atrophy in children with charcot-marie-tooth disease 1A duplication. *Neuromuscul Disord*, **10,** 419–424.

Berger, P., Young, P., and Suter, U. (2002). Molecular cell biology of Charcot-Marie-Tooth disease. *Neurogenetics*, **4,** 1–15.

Bergoffen, J., Scherer, S. S., Wang, S., Scott, M. O., Bone, L. J., Paul, D. L., Chen, K., Lensch, M. W., Chance, P. F., and Fischbeck, K. H. (1993). Connexin mutations in X-linked Charcot-Marie-Tooth disease. *Science*, **262,** 2039–2042.

Bird, T. D. (1999). Historical perspective of defining Charcot-Marie-Tooth type 1B. *Ann N Y Acad Sci*, **883,** 6–13.

Boerkoel, C. F., Takashima, H., Stankiewicz, P., Garcia, C. A., Leber, S. M., Rhee-Morris, L., and Lupski, J. R. (2001). Periaxin mutations cause recessive Dejerine-Sottas neuropathy. *Am J Hum Genet*, **68,** 325–333.

Boiron-Sargueil, F., Heape, A., Garbay, B., and Cassagne, C. (1995). Cerebroside formation in the peripheral nervous system of normal and Trembler mice. *Neurosci Lett*, **186,** 21–24.

Braverman, I. M. (1953). Neurological actions caused by the mutant gene "Trembler" in the house mouse (Mus musculus L.): An investigation. *J Neuropathol Exp Neurol*, **12,** 64–72.

Britsch, S., Goerich, D. E., Riethmacher, D., Peirano, R. I., Rossner, M., Nave, K. A., Birchmeier, C., and Wegner, M. (2001). The transcription factor Sox10 is a key regulator of peripheral glial development. *Genes Dev*, **15,** 66–78.

Brownlees, J., Ackerley, S., Grierson, A. J., Jacobsen, N. J., Shea, K., Anderton, B. H., Leigh, P. N., Shaw, C. E., and Miller, C. C. (2002). Charcot-Marie-Tooth disease neurofilament mutations disrupt neurofilament assembly and axonal transport. *Hum Mol Genet*, **11,** 2837–2844.

Cardoso, F. E., and Jankovic, J. (1993). Hereditary motor-sensory neuropathy and movement disorders. *Muscle Nerve*, **16,** 904–910.

Carenini, S., Maurer, M., Werner, A., Blazyca, H., Toyka, K. V., Schmid, C. D., Raivich, G., and Martini, R. (2001). The role of macrophages in demyelinating peripheral nervous system of mice heterozygously deficient in P0. *J Cell Biol*, **152,** 301–308.

Chance, P. F., and Dyck, P. J. (1998). Hereditary neuropathy with liability to pressure palsies: A patient's point mutation in a mouse model. *Neurology*, **51,** 664–665.

Chaouch, M., Allal, Y., De Sandre-Giovannoli, A., Vallat, J. M., Amer-el-Khedoud, A., Kassouri, N., Chaouch, A., Sindou, P., Hammadouche, T., Tazir, M., Levy, N., and Grid, D. (2003). The phenotypic manifestations of autosomal recessive axonalCharcot-Marie-Tooth due to a mutation in Lamin A/C gene. *Neuromuscul Disord*, **13,** 60–67.

Costaglioli, P., Come, C., Knoll-Gellida, A., Salles, J., Cassagne, C., and Garbay, B. (2001). The homeotic protein dlk is expressed during peripheral nerve development. *FEBS Lett*, **509,** 413–416.

D'Urso, D., Brophy, P. J., Staugaitis, S. M., Gillespie, C. S., Frey, A. B., Stempak, J. G., and Colman, D. R. (1990). Protein zero of peripheral nerve myelin: Biosynthesis, membrane insertion, and evidence for homotypic interaction. *Neuron*, **4,** 449–460.

D'Urso, D., Prior, R., Greiner-Petter, R., Gabreels-Festen, A. A., and Muller, H. W. (1998). Overloaded endoplasmic reticulum-Golgi compartments, a possible pathomechanism of peripheral neuropathies caused by mutations of the peripheral myelin protein PMP22. *J Neurosci*, **18,** 731–740.

D'Urso, D., Schmalenbach, C., Zoidl, G., Prior, R., and Muller, H. W. (1997). Studies on the effects of altered PMP22 expression during myelination in vitro. *J Neurosci Res*, **48,** 31–42.

Darbas, A., Jaegle, M., Walbeehm, E., Grosveld F, E., and Meijer, D. (2002). Schwann cell autonomy of the claw paw gene. *Glia*, **38,** S68.

De Jonghe, P., Mersivanova, I., Nelis, E., Del Favero, J., Martin, J. J., Van Broeckhoven, C., Evgrafov, O., and Timmerman, V. (2001). Further evidence that neurofilament light chain gene mutations can cause Charcot-Marie-Tooth disease type 2E. *Ann Neurol*, **49,** 245–249.

De Leon, M., Nahin, R. L., Mendoza, M. E., and Ruda, M. A. (1994). SR13/PMP-22 expression in rat nervous system, in PC12 cells, and C6 glial cell lines. *J Neurosci Res*, **38,** 167–181.

De Sandre-Giovannoli, A., Chaouch, M., Kozlov, S., Vallat, J. M., Tazir, M., Kassouri, N., Szepetowski, P., Hammadouche, T., Vandenberghe, A., Stewart, C. L., Grid, D., and Levy, N. (2002). Homozygous defects in LMNA, encoding lamin A/C nuclear-envelope proteins, cause autosomal recessive axonal neuropathy in human (Charcot-Marie-Tooth disorder type 2)., and mouse. *Am J Hum Genet*, **70,** 726–736.

de Waegh, S., and Brady, S. T. (1990). Altered slow axonal transport and regeneration in a myelin-deficient mutant mouse: The trembler as an in vivo model for Schwann cell-axon interactions. *J Neurosci*, **10,** 1855–1865.

de Waegh, S. M., and Brady, S. T. (1991). Local control of axonal properties by Schwann cells: Neurofilaments and axonal transport in homologous and heterologous nerve grafts. *J Neurosci Res*, **30,** 201–212.

de Waegh, S. M., Lee, V. M., and Brady, S. T. (1992). Local modulation of neurofilament phosphorylation, axonal caliber, and slow axonal transport by myelinating Schwann cells. *Cell*, **68,** 451–463.

Dickson, K. M., Bergeron, J. J., Shames, I., Colby, J., Nguyen, D. T., Chevet, E., Thomas, D. Y., and Snipes, G. J. (2002). Association of calnexin with mutant peripheral myelin protein-22 ex vivo: A basis for "gain-of-function" ER diseases. *Proc Natl Acad Sci U S A*, **99,** 9852–9857.

Dyck, P. J., Karnes, J. L., and Lambert, E. H. (1989). Longitudinal study of neuropathic deficits and nerve conduction abnormalities in hereditary motor and sensory neuropathy type 1. *Neurology*, **39,** 1302–1308.

Falconer, D. S. (1951). Two new mutants, "Trembler" and "Reeler" with neurological actions in the house mouse. *Genetics*, **50,** 192–201.

Filbin, M., Walsh, F., Trapp, B., Pizzey, J., and Tennekoon, G. (1990). Role of myelin Po protein as a homophilic adhesion molecule. *Nature*, **344,** 871–872.

Fischbeck, K. H., Abel, A., Lin, G. S., and Scherer, S. S. (1999). X-linked Charcot-Marie-Tooth disease and connexin32. *Ann N Y Acad Sci*, **883,** 36–41.

Frei, R., Motzing, S., Kinkelin, I., Schachner, M., Koltzenburg, M., and Martini, R. (1999). Loss of distal axons and sensory Merkel cells and features indicative of muscle denervation in hindlimbs of P0-deficient mice. *J Neurosci*, **19,** 6058–6067.

Gabreels-Festen, A. A., Joosten, E. M., Gabreels, F. J., Jennekens, F. G., and Janssen-van Kempen, T. W. (1992). Early morphological features in dominantly inherited demyelinating motor and sensory neuropathy (HMSN type I). *J Neurol Sci*, **107,** 145–154.

Garbay, B., Boiron-Sargueil, F., and Cassagne, C. (1995). Expression of the exon 1A-containing PMP22 transcript is altered in the trembler mouse. *Neurosci Lett*, **198,** 157–160.

Garbay, B., Boiron-Sargueil, F., Shy, M., Chbihi, T., Jiang, H., Kamholz, J., and Cassagne, C. (1998). Regulation of oleoyl-CoA synthesis in the peripheral nervous system: Demonstration of a link with myelin synthesis. *J Neurochem*, **71,** 1719–1726.

Garbay, B., and Bonnet, J. (1992). P0 protein in normal, trembler heterozygous/homozygous mice during active PNS myelination. *Neuroreport*, **3,** 594–596.

Garbay, B., and Cassagne, C. (1994). Expression of the ceramide galactosyltransferase gene during myelination of the mouse nervous system. Comparison with the genes encoding myelin basic proteins, choline kinase and CTP:phosphocholine cytidyltransferase. *Dev Brain Res*, **83,** 119–124.

Garbern, J. Y., Cambi, F., Tang, X. M., Sima, A. A., Vallat, J. M., Bosch, E. P., Lewis, R., Shy, M., Sohi, J., Kraft, G., Chen, K. L., Joshi, I., Leonard, D. G., Johnson, W., Raskind, W., Dlouhy, S. R., Pratt, V., Hodes, M. E., Bird, T., and Kamholz, J. (1997). Proteolipid protein is necessary in peripheral as well as central myelin. *Neuron*, **19,** 205–218.

Giese, K. P., Martini, R., Lemke, G., Soriano, P., and Schachner, M. (1992). Mouse P0 gene disruption leads to hypomyelination, abnormal expression of recognition molecules, and degeneration of myelin and axons. *Cell*, **71,** 565–576.

Gillespie, C. S., Sherman, D. L., Blair, G. E., and Brophy, P. J. (1994). Periaxin, a novel protein of myelinating Schwann cells with a possible role in axonal ensheathment. *Neuron*, **12,** 497–508.

Gillespie, C. S., Sherman, D. L., Fleetwood-Walker, S. M., Cottrell, D. F., Tait, S., Garry, E. M., Wallace, V. C., Ure, J., Griffiths, I. R., Smith, A., and Brophy, P. J. (2000). Peripheral demyelination and neuropathic pain behavior in periaxin-deficient mice. *Neuron*, **26,** 523–531.

Gow, A., Southwood, C. M., and Lazzarini, R. A. (1998). Disrupted proteolipid protein trafficking results in oligodendrocyte apoptosis in an animal model of Pelizaeus-Merzbacher disease. *J Cell Biol*, **140,** 925–934.

Greenfield, S., Brostoff, S., Eylar, E. H., and Morell, P. (1973). Protein composition of myelin of the peripheral nervous system. *J. Neurochem*, **20,** 1207–1216.

Griffiths, I., Klugmann, M., Anderson, T., Yool, D., Thomson, C., Schwab, M. H., Schneider, A., Zimmermann, F., McCulloch, M., Nadon, N., and Nave, K. A. (1998). Axonal swellings and degeneration in mice lacking the major proteolipid of myelin. *Science*, **280,** 1610–1613.

Guilbot, A., Williams, A., Ravise, N., Verny, C., Brice, A., Sherman, D. L., Brophy, P. J., LeGuern, E., Delague, V., Bareil, C., Megarbane, A., and Claustres, M. (2001). A mutation in periaxin is responsible for CMT4F, an autosomal recessive form of Charcot-Marie-Tooth disease. *Hum Mol Genet*, **10,** 415–421.

Hagedorn, L., Suter, U., and Sommer, L. (1999). P0 and PMP22 mark a multipotent neural crest-derived cell type that displays community effects in response to TGF-beta family factors. *Development*, **126,** 3781–3794.

Hahn, A. F., Parkes, A. W., Bolton, C. F., and Stewart, S. A. (1991). Neuromyotonia in hereditary motor neuropathy. *J Neurol Neurosurg Psychiatry*, **54,** 230–235.

Heape, A. M., Bessoule, J. J., Boiron-Sargueil, F., and Cassagne, C. (1996). Pathways of incorporation of fatty acid into glycerolipids of the murine peripheral nervous system in vivo: Alterations in the dysmyelinating mutant trembler mouse. *Neurochem Int*, **29,** 607–622.

Heape, A. M., Bessoule, J.-J., Boiron-Sargueil, F., Garbay, B., and Cassagne, C. (1995). Sphingolipid metabolic disorders in Trembler mouse peripheral nerves in vivo result from an abnormal substrate supply. *J Neurochem*, **65,** 1665–1673.

Heath, J. W., Inuzuka, T., Quarles, R. H., and Trapp, B. D. (1991). Distribution of P0 protein and the myelin-associated glycoprotein in peripheral nerves from Trembler mice. *J Neurocytol*, **20,** 439–449.

Henry, E. W., Cowen, J. S., and Sidman, R. L. (1983). Comparison of trembler and trembler-J phenotypes: Varying severity of peripheral hypomyelination. *J Neuropathol Exp Neurol*, **42,** 688–706.

Henry, E. W., Eicher, E. M., and Sidman, R. L. (1991). The mouse mutation claw paw: Forelimb deformity and delayed myelination throughout the peripheral nervous system. *J Hered*, **82,** 287–294.

Henry, E. W., and Sidman, R. L. (1983). The murine mutation trembler-J: Proof of semi-dominant expression by the use of the linked vestigial tail marker. *J Neurogen*, **1,** 39–52.

Henry, E. W., and Sidman, R. L. (1988). Long lives for homozygous trembler mutant mice despite virtual absence of peripheral myelin. *Science*, **241,** 344–346.

Huxley, C., Passage, E., Manson, A., Putzu, G., Figarella-Branger, D., Pellissier, J. F., and Fontes, M. (1996). Construction of a mouse model of Charcot-Marie-Tooth disease type 1A by pronuclear injection of human YAC DNA. *Hum Mol Genet*, **5,** 563–569.

Huxley, C., Passage, E., Robertson, A. M., Youl, B., Huston, S., Manson, A., Saberan-Djoniedi, D., Figarella-Branger, D., Pellissier, J. F., Thomas, P. K., and Fontes, M. (1998). Correlation between varying levels of PMP22 expression and the degree of demyelination and reduction in nerve conduction velocity in transgenic mice. *Hum Mol Genet*, **7,** 449–458.

Ingham, P. W., and McMahon, A. P. (2001). Hedgehog signaling in animal development: Paradigms and principles. *Genes Dev*, **15,** 3059–3087.

Inoue, K., Dewar, K., Katsanis, N., Reiter, L. T., Lander, E. S., Devon, K. L., Wyman, D. W., Lupski, J. R., and Birren, B. (2001). The 1.4-Mb CMT1A duplication/HNPP deletion genomic region reveals unique genome architectural features and provides insights into the recent evolution of new genes. *Genome Res*, **11,** 1018–1033.

Inoue, K., Shilo, K., Boerkoel, C. F., Crowe, C., Sawady, J., Lupski, J. R., and Agamanolis, D. P. (2002). Congenital hypomyelinating neuropathy, central dysmyelination, and Waardenburg-Hirschsprung disease: Phenotypes linked by SOX10 mutation. *Ann Neurol*, **52,** 836–842.

Inoue, K., Tanabe, Y., and Lupski, J. R. (1999). Myelin deficiencies in both the central and the peripheral nervous systems associated with a SOX10 mutation. *Ann Neurol*, **46,** 313–318.

Inuzuka, T., Quarles, R. H., Heath, J., and Trapp, B. D. (1985). Myelin-associated glycoprotein and other proteins in Trembler mice. *J Neurochem*, **44,** 793–797.

Ionasescu, V. V., Searby, C. C., Ionasescu, R., Chatkupt, S., Patel, N., and Koenigsberger, R. (1997). Dejerine-Sottas neuropathy in mother and son with same point mutation of PMP22 gene. *Muscle Nerve*, **20,** 97–99.

Isaacs, A. M., Davies, K. E., Hunter, A. J., Nolan, P. M., Vizor, L., Peters, J., Gale, D. G., Kelsell, D. P., Latham, I. D., Chase, J. M., Fisher, E. M., Bouzyk, M. M., Potter, A., Masih, M., Walsh, F. S., Sims, M. A., Doncaster, K. E., Parsons, C. A., Martin, J., Brown, S. D., Rastan, S., Spurr, N. K., and Gray, I. C. (2000). Identification of two new Pmp22 mouse mutants using large-scale mutagenesis and a novel rapid mapping strategy. *Hum Mol Genet*, **9,** 1865–1871.

Jordanova, A., De Jonghe, P., Boerkoel, C. F., Takashima, H., De Vriendt, E., Ceuterick, C., Martin, J. J., Butler, I. J., Mancias, P., Papasozomenos, S. C., Terespolsky, D., Potocki, L., Brown, C. W., Shy, M., Rita, D. A., Tournev, I., Kremensky, I., Lupski, J. R., and Timmerman, V. (2003). Mutations in the neurofilament light chain gene (NEFL). cause early onset severe Charcot-Marie-Tooth disease. *Brain*, **126,** 590–597.

Julien, J. P., Couillard-Despres, S., and Meier, J. (1998). Transgenic mice in the study of ALS: The role of neurofilaments. *Brain Pathol*, **8,** 759–769.

Kirkpatrick, L. L., and Brady, S. T. (1994). Modulation of the axonal microtubule cytoskeleton by myelinating Schwann cells. *J Neurosci*, **14,** 7440–7450.

Kirschner, D. A., and Sidman, R. L. (1976). X-ray diffraction study of myelin structure in immature and mutant mice. *Biochim Biophys Acta*, **448,** 73–87.

Kirschner, D. A., Szumowski, K., Gabreel-Festen, A. A. W. M., J. E., H., and P. A., B. (1996). Inherited demyelinating peripheral neuropathies: Relating myelin packing abnormalities to Po molecular defects. *J. Neurosci. Res.*, **46,** 502–508.

Kleopa, K. A., and Scherer, S. S. (2002). Inherited neuropathies. *Neurol Clin*, **20,** 679–709.

Kleopa, K. A., Yum, S. W., and Scherer, S. S. (2002). Cellular mechanisms of connexin32 mutations associated with CNS manifestations. *J Neurosci Res*, **68,** 522–534.

Klugmann, M., Schwab, M. H., Puhlhofer, A., Schneider, A., Zimmermann, F., Griffiths, I. R., and Nave, K. A. (1997). Assembly of CNS myelin in the absence of proteolipid protein. *Neuron*, **18,** 59–70.

Kobsar, I., Maurer, M., Ott, T., and Martini, R. (2002). Macrophage-related demyelination in peripheral nerves of mice deficient in the gap junction protein connexin 32. *Neurosci Lett*, **320,** 17–20.

Krajewski, K. M., Lewis, R. A., Fuerst, D. R., Turansky, C., Hinderer, S. R., Garbern, J., Kamholz, J., and Shy, M. E. (2000). Neurological dysfunction and axonal degeneration in Charcot-Marie-Tooth disease type 1A. *Brain*, **123,** 1516–1527.

Kuhlbrodt, K., Herbarth, B., Sock, E., Hermans-Borgmeyer, I., and Wegner, M. (1998). Sox10, a novel transcriptional modulator in glial cells. *J Neurosci*, **18,** 237–250.

Lambert, S., Davis, J. Q., and Bennett, V. (1997). Morphogenesis of the node of Ranvier: Co-clusters of ankyrin and ankyrin-binding integral proteins define early developmental intermediates. *J Neurosci*, **17,** 7025–7036.

Lee, M. K., Marszalek, J. R., and Cleveland, D. W. (1994). A mutant neurofilament subunit causes massive, selective motor neuron death: Implications for the pathogenesis of human motor neuron disease. *Neuron*, **13,** 975–988.

Lemke, G., and Axel, R. (1985). Isolation and sequence of a cDNA encoding the major structural protein of peripheral nerve myelin. *Cell*, **40,** 501–508.

Low, P. A. (1976a). Hereditary hypertrophic neuropathy in the trembler mouse: Part 1: Histopathological studies: Light microscopy. *J Neurol Sci*, **30,** 327–341.

Low, P. A. (1976b). Hereditary hypertrophic neuropathy in the trembler mouse: Part 2: Histopathological studies: Electron microscopy. *J Neurol Sci*, **30,** 343–368.

Low, P. A. (1977). The evolution of 'onion bulbs' in the hereditary hypertrophic neuropathy of the Trembler mouse. *Neuropath Appl Neurobiol*, **3,** 81–92.

Low, P. A., and McLeod, J. G. (1975). Hereditary demyelinating neuropathy in the trembler mouse. *J Neurol Sci*, **26,** 565–575.

Lupski, J., and Garcia, C. (2001). Charcot-Marie-Tooth peripheral neuropathies and related disorders. *In* "The Metabolic & Molecular Bases of Inherited Disease" (C. R. Scriver, A. L. Beaudet, W. S. Sly, D. Valle, B. Childs, K. W. Kinzler, and B. Vogelstein, eds.), Vol. 3, pp. 5759–5788. McGraw-Hill, New York.

Magyar, J. P., Martini, R., Ruelicke, T., Aguzzi, A., Adlkofer, K., Dembic, Z., Zielasek, J., Toyka, K. V., and Suter, U. (1996). Impaired differentiation of Schwann cells in transgenic mice with increased PMP22 gene dosage. *J Neurosci*, **16,** 5351–5360.

Maier, M., Berger, P., Nave, K. A., and Suter, U. (2002a). Identification of the regulatory region of the peripheral myelin protein 22 (PMP22). gene that directs temporal and spatial expression in development and regeneration of peripheral nerves. *Mol Cell Neurosci*, **20,** 93–109.

Maier, M., Berger, P., and Suter, U. (2002b). Understanding Schwann cell-neurone interactions: The key to Charcot-Marie-Tooth disease? *J Anat*, **200,** 357–366.

Marrosu, M. G., Vaccargiu, S., Marrosu, G., Vannelli, A., Cianchetti, C., and Muntoni, F. (1998). Charcot-Marie-Tooth disease type 2 associated with mutation of the myelin protein zero gene. *Neurology*, **50,** 1397–1401.

Martini, R. (1997). Animal models for inherited peripheral neuropathies. *J Anat*, **191,** 321–336.

Martini, R. (2000). Animal models for inherited peripheral neuropathies: Chances to find treatment strategies? *J Neurosci Res*, **61,** 244–250.

Martini, R. (2001). The effect of myelinating Schwann cells on axons. *Muscle Nerve*, **24,** 456–466.

Martini, R., Zielasek, J., Toyka, K. V., Giese, K. P., and Schachner, M. (1995). Protein zero (P0)-deficient mice show myelin degeneration in peripheral nerves characteristic of inherited human neuropathies. *Nat. Genet.*, **11,** 281–286.

Maurer, M., Kobsar, I., Berghoff, M., Schmid, C. D., Carenini, S., and Martini, R. (2002). Role of immune cells in animal models for inherited neuropathies: Facts and visions. *J Anat*, **200,** 405–414.

Maurer, M., Schmid, C. D., Bootz, F., Zielasek, J., Toyka, K. V., Oehen, S., and Martini, R. (2001). Bone marrow transfer from wild-type mice reverts the beneficial effect of genetically mediated immune deficiency in myelin mutants. *Mol Cell Neurosci*, **17,** 1094–1101.

Maycox, P. R., Ortuno, D., Burrola, P., Kuhn, R., Bieri, P. L., Arrezo, J. C., and Lemke, G. (1997). A transgenic mouse model for human hereditary neuropathy with liability to pressure palsies. *Mol Cell Neurosci*, **8,** 405–416.

Mersiyanova, I. V., Perepelov, A. V., Polyakov, A. V., Sitnikov, V. F., Dadali, E. L., Oparin, R. B., Petrin, A. N., and Evgrafov, O. V. (2000). A new variant of Charcot-Marie-Tooth disease type 2 is probably the result of a mutation in the neurofilament-light gene. *Am J Hum Genet*, **67,** 37–46.

Moir, R. D., and Spann, T. P. (2001). The structure and function of nuclear lamins: Implications for disease. *Cell Mol Life Sci*, **58,** 1748–1757.

Mok, H., Shin, H., Kim, S., Lee, J. R., Yoon, J., and Kim, E. (2002). Association of the kinesin superfamily motor protein KIF1Balpha with postsynaptic density-95 (PSD-95), synapse-associated protein-97, and synaptic scaffolding molecule PSD-95/discs large/zona occludens-1 proteins. *J Neurosci*, **22,** 5253–5258.

Murphy, P., Topilko, P., Schneider-Maunoury, S., Seitanidou, T., Baron-Van Evercooren, A., and Charnay, P. (1996). The regulation of Krox-20 expression reveals important steps in the control of peripheral glial cell development. *Development*, **122,** 2847–2857.

Naef, R., Adlkofer, K., Lescher, B., and Suter, U. (1997). Aberrant protein trafficking in Trembler suggests a disease mechanism for hereditary human peripheral neuropathies. *Mol Cell Neurosci*, **9,** 13–25.

Nagarajan, R., Le, N., Mahoney, H., Araki, T., and Milbrandt, J. (2002). Deciphering peripheral nerve myelination by using Schwann cell expression profiling. *Proc Natl Acad Sci U S A*, **99,** 8998–9003.

Nagarajan, R., Svaren, J., Le, N., Araki, T., Watson, M., and Milbrandt, J. (2001). EGR2 mutations in inherited neuropathies dominant-negatively inhibit myelin gene expression. *Neuron*, **30,** 355–368.

Nelis, E., Haites, N., and Van Broeckhoven, C. (1999). Mutations in the peripheral myelin genes and associated genes in inherited peripheral neuropathies. *Hum Mutat*, **13,** 11–28.

Nelis, E., Van Broeckhoven, C., De Jonghe, P., Lofgren, A., Vandenberghe, A., Latour, P., Le Guern, E., Brice, A., Mostacciuolo, M. L., Schiavon, F., Palau, F., Bort, S., Upadhyaya, M., Rocchi, M., Archidiacono, N., Mandich, P., Bellone, E., Silander, K., Savontaus, M. L., Navon, R., Goldberg-Stern, H., Estivill, X., Volpini, V., Friedl, W., Gal, A., *et al.* (1996). Estimation of the mutation frequencies in Charcot-Marie-Tooth disease type 1 and hereditary neuropathy with liability to pressure palsies: A European collaborative study. *Eur J Hum Genet*, **4,** 25–33.

Nelles, E., Butzler, C., Jung, D., Temme, A., Gabriel, H. D., Dahl, U., Traub, O., Stumpel, F., Jungermann, K., Zielasek, J., Toyka, K. V., Dermietzel, R., and Willecke, K. (1996). Defective propagation of signals generated by sympathetic nerve stimulation in the liver of connexin32-deficient mice. *Proc Natl Acad Sci U S A*, **93,** 9565–9570.

Neuberg, D. H., Sancho, S., and Suter, U. (1999). Altered molecular architecture of peripheral nerves in mice lacking the peripheral myelin protein 22 or connexin32. *J Neurosci Res*, **58,** 612–623.

Nicholson, S. M., Gomes, D., de Nechaud, B., and Bruzzone, R. (2001). Altered gene expression in Schwann cells of connexin32 knockout animals. *J Neurosci Res*, **66,** 23–36.

Niemann, S., Sereda, M. W., Suter, U., Griffiths, I. R., and Nave, K. A. (2000). Uncoupling of myelin assembly and schwann cell differentiation by transgenic overexpression of peripheral myelin protein 22. *J Neurosci*, **20,** 4120–4128.

Norreel, J. C., Jamon, M., Riviere, G., Passage, E., Fontes, M., and Clarac, F. (2001). Behavioural profiling of a murine Charcot-Marie-Tooth disease type 1A model. *Eur J Neurosci*, **13,** 1625–1634.

Notterpek, L., Roux, K. J., Amici, S. A., Yazdanpour, A., Rahner, C., and Fletcher, B. S. (2001). Peripheral myelin protein 22 is a constituent of intercellular junctions in epithelia. *Proc Natl Acad Sci U S A*, **98,** 14404–14409.

Notterpek, L., Shooter, E. M., and Snipes, G. J. (1997). Upregulation of the endosomal-lysosomal pathway in the trembler-J neuropathy. *J Neurosci*, **17,** 4190–4200.

Paratore, P., Hagedorn, L., Floris, J., Hari, L., Kleber, M., Suter, U., and Sommer, L. (2002). Cell-intrinsic and cell-extrinsic cues regulating lineage decisions in multipotent neural crest-derived progenitor cells. *Int J Dev Biol 46: 193–200 (2002)*, **46,** 193–200.

Pareyson, D., Menichella, D., Botti, S., Sghirlanzoni, A., Fallica, E., Mora, M., Ciano, C., Shy, M. E., and Taroni, F. (1999). Heterozygous null mutation in the P0 gene associated with mild Charcot-Marie-Tooth disease. *Ann N Y Acad Sci*, **883,** 477–480.

Parmantier, E., Braun, C., Thomas, J. L., Peyron, F., Martinez, S., and Zalc, B. (1997). PMP-22 expression in the central nervous system of the embryonic mouse defines potential transverse segments and longitudinal columns. *J Comp Neurol*, **378,** 159–172.

Parmantier, E., Lynn, B., Lawson, D., Turmaine, M., Namini, S. S., Chakrabarti, L., McMahon, A. P., Jessen, K. R., and Mirsky, R. (1999). Schwann cell-derived Desert hedgehog controls the development of peripheral nerve sheaths. *Neuron*, **23,** 713–724.

Paulson, H. L., Garbern, J. Y., Hoban, T. F., Krajewski, K. M., Lewis, R. A., Fischbeck, K. H., Grossman, R. I., Lenkinski, R., Kamholz, J. A., and Shy, M. E. (2002). Transient central nervous system white matter abnormality in X-linked Charcot-Marie-Tooth disease. *Ann Neurol*, **52,** 429–434.

Peirano, R. I., Goerich, D. E., Riethmacher, D., and Wegner, M. (2000). Protein zero gene expression is regulated by the glial transcription factor Sox10. *Mol Cell Biol*, **20,** 3198–3209.

Perea, J., Robertson, A., Tolmachova, T., Muddle, J., King, R. H., Ponsford, S., Thomas, P. K., and Huxley, C. (2001). Induced myelination and demyelination in a conditional mouse model of Charcot-Marie-Tooth disease type 1A. *Hum Mol Genet*, **10,** 1007–1018.

Perez-Olle, R., Leung, C. L., and Liem, R. K. (2002). Effects of Charcot-Marie-Tooth-linked mutations of the neurofilament light subunit on intermediate filament formation. *J Cell Sci*, **115,** 4937–4946.

Perkins, C. S., Aguayo, A. J., and Bray, G. M. (1981). Schwann cell multiplication in Trembler mice. *Neuropathol Appl Neurobiol*, **7,** 115–126.

Phillips, J. P., Warner, L. E., Lupski, J. R., and Garg, B. P. (1999). Congenital hypomyelinating neuropathy: Two patients with long-term follow-up. *Pediatr. Neurol.*, **20,** 226–232.

Pingault, V., Bondurand, N., Kuhlbrodt, K., Goerich, D. E., Prehu, M. O., Puliti, A., Herbarth, B., Hermans-Borgmeyer, I., Legius, E., Matthijs, G., Amiel, J., Lyonnet, S., Ceccherini, I., Romeo, G., Smith, J. C., Read, A. P., Wegner, M., and Goossens, M. (1998). SOX10 mutations in patients with Waardenburg-Hirschsprung disease. *Nat Genet*, **18,** 171–173.

Pingault, V., Bondurand, N., Le Caignec, C., Tardieu, S., Lemort, N., Dubourg, O., Le Guern, E., Goossens, M., and Boespflug-Tanguy, O. (2001). The SOX10 transcription factor: Evaluation as a candidate gene for central and peripheral hereditary myelin disorders. *J Neurol*, **248,** 496–499.

Previtali, S. C., Quattrini, A., Fasolini, M., Panzeri, M. C., Villa, A., Filbin, M. T., Li, W., Chiu, S. Y., Messing, A., Wrabetz, L., and Feltri, M. L. (2000). Epitope-tagged P(0). glycoprotein causes charcot-marie-tooth-like neuropathy in transgenic mice. *J. Cell Biol.*, **151,** 1035–1046.

Robertson, A., Perea, J., Tolmachova, T., Thomas, P. K., and Huxley, C. (2002a). Effects of mouse strain, position of integration and tetracycline analogue on the tetracycline conditional system in transgenic mice. *Gene*, **282,** 65–74.

Robertson, A. M., Huxley, C., King, R. H., and Thomas, P. K. (1999). Development of early postnatal peripheral nerve abnormalities in Trembler-J and PMP22 transgenic mice. *J Anat*, **195,** 331–339.

Robertson, A. M., King, R. H., Muddle, J. R., and Thomas, P. K. (1997). Abnormal Schwann cell/axon interactions in the Trembler-J mouse. *J Anat*, **190,** 423–432.

Robertson, A. M., Perea, J., McGuigan, A., King, R. H., Muddle, J. R., Gabreels-Festen, A. A., Thomas, P. K., and Huxley, C. (2002b). Comparison of a new pmp22 transgenic mouse line with other mouse models and human patients with CMT1A. *J Anat*, **200,** 377–390.

Ryan, M. C., Shooter, E. M., and Notterpek, L. (2002). Aggresome formation in neuropathy models based on peripheral myelin protein 22 mutations. *Neurobiol Dis*, **10,** 109–118.

Sahenk, Z. (1999). Abnormal Schwann cell-axon interactions in CMT neuropathies. The effects of mutant Schwann cells on the axonal cytoskeleton and regeneration-associated myelination. *Ann N Y Acad Sci*, **883,** 415–426.

Sahenk, Z., Chen, L., and Freimer, M. (1998). A novel PMP22 point mutation causing HNPP phenotype: Studies on nerve xenografts. *Neurology*, **51,** 702–707.

Sahenk, Z., Chen, L., and Mendell, J. R. (1999). Effects of PMP22 duplication and deletions on the axonal cytoskeleton. *Ann Neurol*, **45,** 16–24.

Sakai, Y., Nakabayashi, O., Kikuchi, T., and Wada, K. (1999). Identification of break points in mutated PMP22 gene in a new Trembler (Tr-Ncnp). mouse. *Neuroscience*, **88,** 989–991.

Salles, J., Sargueil, F., Knoll-Gellida, A., Witters, L. A., Shy, M., Jiang, H., Cassagne, C., and Garbay, B. (2002). Fatty acid synthase expression during peripheral nervous system myelination. *Brain Res Mol Brain Res*, **101,** 52–58.

Sancho, S., Magyar, J. P., Aguzzi, A., and Suter, U. (1999). Distal axonopathy in peripheral nerves of PMP22-mutant mice. *Brain*, **122,** 1563–1577.

Sancho, S., Young, P., and Suter, U. (2001). Regulation of Schwann cell proliferation and apoptosis in PMP22-deficient mice and mouse models of Charcot-Marie-Tooth disease type 1A. *Brain*, **124,** 2177–2187.

Sargueil, F., Knoll, A., Salles, J., Garbay, B., and Cassagne, C. (1999). High metabolism and subsequent elongation of 3-hydroxyeicosanoyl-CoA in very-long-chain fatty acid deficient PNS of Trembler mice. *Neurosci Lett*, **273,** 29–32.

Scherer, S. S., Bone, L. J., Deschenes, S. M., Abel, A., Balice-Gordon, R. J., and Fischbeck, K. H. (1999). The role of the gap junction protein connexin32 in the pathogenesis of X-linked Charcot-Marie-Tooth disease. *Novartis Found Symp*, **219,** 175–185.

Scherer, S. S., Deschenes, S. M., Xu, Y. T., Grinspan, J. B., Fischbeck, K. H., and Paul, D. L. (1995a). Connexin32 is a myelin-related protein in the PNS and CNS. *J Neurosci*, **15,** 8281–8294.

Scherer, S. S., and Fischbeck, K. H. (1999). Is CMTX an axonopathy? *Neurology*, **52,** 432–433.

Scherer, S. S., Xu, Y. T., Bannerman, P. G., Sherman, D. L., and Brophy, P. J. (1995b). Periaxin expression in myelinating Schwann cells: Modulation by axon-glial interactions and polarized localization during development. *Development*, **121,** 4265–4273.

Scherer, S. S., Xu, Y. T., Nelles, E., Fischbeck, K., Willecke, K., and Bone, L. J. (1998). Connexin32-null mice develop demyelinating peripheral neuropathy. *Glia*, **24,** 8–20.

Schmid, C. D., Stienekemeier, M., Oehen, S., Bootz, F., Zielasek, J., Gold, R., Toyka, K. V., Schachner, M., and Martini, R. (2000). Immune deficiency in mouse models for inherited peripheral neuropathies leads to improved myelin maintenance. *J Neurosci*, **20,** 729–735.

Schneider-Maunoury, S., Topilko, P., Seitandou, T., Levi, G., Cohen-Tannoudji, M., Pournin, S., Babinet, C., and Charnay, P. (1993). Disruption of Krox-20 results in alteration of rhombomeres 3 and 5 in the developing hindbrain. *Cell*, **75,** 1199–1214.

Schneider-Schaulies, J., Brunn, A. V., and Schachner, M. (1990). Recombinant peripheral myelin protein Po confers both adhesion and neurite outgrowth-promoting properties. *J. Neuroscience Research*, **27,** 286–297.

Senderek, J., Hermanns, B., Lehmann, U., Bergmann, C., Marx, G., Kabus, C., Timmerman, V., Stoltenburg-Didinger, G., and Schroder, J. M. (2000). Charcot-Marie-Tooth neuropathy type 2 and P0 point mutations: Two novel amino acid substitutions (Asp61Gly; Tyr119Cys)., and a possible "hotspot" on Thr124Met. *Brain Pathol*, **10,** 235–248.

Sereda, M., Griffiths, I., Puhlhofer, A., Stewart, H., Rossner, M. J., Zimmerman, F., Magyar, J. P., Schneider, A., Hund, E., Meinck, H. M., Suter, U., and Nave, K. A. (1996). A transgenic rat model of Charcot-Marie-Tooth disease. *Neuron*, **16,** 1049–1060.

Sghirlanzoni, A., Pareyson, D., Balestrini, M. R., Bellone, E., Berta, E., Ciano, C., Mandich, P., and Marazzi, R. (1992). HMSN III phenotype due to homozygous expression of a dominant HMSN II gene. *Neurology*, **42,** 2201–2204.

Shapiro, L., Doyle, J. P., Hensley, P., Colman, D. R., and Hendrickson, W. A. (1996). Crystal structure of the extracellular domain from P0, the major structural protein of peripheral nerve myelin. *Neuron*, **17,** 435–449.

Sherman, D. L., Fabrizi, C., Gillespie, C. S., and Brophy, P. J. (2001). Specific disruption of a schwann cell dystrophin-related protein complex in a demyelinating neuropathy. *Neuron*, **30,** 677–687.

Shy, M. E., Arroyo, E., Sladky, J., Menichella, D., Jiang, H., Xu, W., Kamholz, J., and Scherer, S. S. (1997). Heterozygous P0 knockout mice develop a peripheral neuropathy that resembles chronic inflammatory demyelinating polyneuropathy (CIDP). *J Neuropathol Exp Neurol*, **56,** 811–821.

Shy, M. E., Hobson, G., Jain, M., Boespflug-Tanguy, O., Garbern, J., Sperle, K., Li, W., Gow, A., Rodriguez, D., Bertini, E., Mancias, P., Krajewski, K., Lewis, R., and Kamholz, J. (2003). Schwann cell expression of PLP1 but not DM20 is necessary to prevent neuropathy. *Ann Neurol*, **53,** 354–365.

Southwood, C. M., Garbern, J., Jiang, W., and Gow, A. (2002). The unfolded protein response modulates disease severity in Pelizaeus-Merzbacher disease. *Neuron*, **36,** 585–596.

Stolt, C. C., Rehberg, S., Ader, M., Lommes, P., Riethmacher, D., Schachner, M., Bartsch, U., and Wegner, M. (2002). Terminal differentiation of myelin-forming oligodendrocytes depends on the transcription factor Sox10. *Genes Dev*, **16,** 165–170.

Suh, J. G., Ichihara, N., Saigoh, K., Nakabayashi, O., Yamanishi, T., Tanaka, K., Wada, K., and Kikuchi, T. (1997). An in-frame deletion in peripheral myelin protein-22 gene causes hypomyelination and cell death of the Schwann cells in the new Trembler mutant mice. *Neuroscience*, **79,** 735–744.

Sullivan, T., Escalante-Alcalde, D., Bhatt, H., Anver, M., Bhat, N., Nagashima, K., Stewart, C. L., and Burke, B. (1999). Loss of A-type lamin expression compromises nuclear envelope integrity leading to muscular dystrophy. *J Cell Biol*, **147,** 913–920.

Suter, U., Moskow, J. J., Welcher, A. A., Snipes, G. J., Kosaras, B., Sidman, R. L., Buchberg, A. M., and Shooter, E. M. (1992a). A leucine-to-proline mutation in the putative first transmembrane domain of the 22-kDa peripheral myelin protein in the trembler-J mouse. *Proc Natl Acad Sci U S A*, **89,** 4382–4386.

Suter, U., and Nave, K. A. (1999). Transgenic mouse models of CMT1A and HNPP. *Ann N Y Acad Sci*, **883,** 247–253.

Suter, U., Snipes, G. J., Schoener-Scott, R., Welcher, A. A., Pareek, S., Lupski, J. R., Murphy, R. A., Shooter, E. M., and Patel, P. I. (1994). Regulation of tissue-specific expression of alternative peripheral myelin protein-22 (*PMP22*). gene transcripts by two promoters. *J Biol Chem*, **269,** 25795–25808.

Suter, U., Welcher, A. A., Ozcelik, T., Snipes, G. J., Kosaras, B., Francke, U., Billings-Gagliardi, S., Sidman, R. L., and Shooter, E. M. (1992b). Trembler mouse carries a point mutation in a myelin gene. *Nature*, **356,** 241–244.

Suter, U., Welcher, A. A., and Snipes, G. J. (1993). Progress in the molecular understanding of hereditary peripheral neuropathies reveals new insights into the biology of the peripheral nervous system. *Trends Neurosci*, **16,** 50–56.

Svaren, J., Sevetson, B. R., Golda, T., Stanton, J. J., Swirnoff, A. H., and Milbrandt, J. (1998). Novel mutants of NAB corepressors enhance activation by Egr transactivators. *Embo J*, **17,** 6010–6019.

Swiatek, P. J., and Gridley, T. (1993). Perinatal lethality and defects in hindbrain development in mice homozygous for a targeted mutation of the zinc finger gene Krox20. *Genes Dev*, **7,** 2071–2084.

Taillebourg, E., Buart, S., and Charnay, P. (2002). Conditional, floxed allele of the Krox20 gene. *Genesis*, **32,** 112–113.

Takashima, H., Boerkoel, C. F., De Jonghe, P., Ceuterick, C., Martin, J. J., Voit, T., Schroder, J. M., Williams, A., Brophy, P. J., Timmerman, V., and Lupski, J. R. (2002). Periaxin mutations cause a broad spectrum of demyelinating neuropathies. *Ann Neurol*, **51,** 709–715.

Taylor, V., Zgraggen, C., Naef, R., and Suter, U. (2000). Membrane topology of peripheral myelin protein 22. *J Neurosci Res*, **62,** 15–27.

Temme, A., Buchmann, A., Gabriel, H. D., Nelles, E., Schwarz, M., and Willecke, K. (1997). High incidence of spontaneous and chemically induced liver tumors in mice deficient for connexin32. *Curr Biol*, **7,** 713–716.

Tobler, A. R., Liu, N., Mueller, L., and Shooter, E. M. (2002). Differential aggregation of the Trembler and Trembler J mutants of peripheral myelin protein 22. *Proc Natl Acad Sci U S A*, **99,** 483–488.

Tobler, A. R., Notterpek, L., Naef, R., Taylor, V., Suter, U., and Shooter, E. M. (1999). Transport of Trembler-J mutant peripheral myelin protein 22 is blocked in the intermediate compartment and affects the transport of the wild-type protein by direct interaction. *J Neurosci*, **19,** 2027–2036.

Topilko, P., Schneider-Maunoury, S., Levi, G., Baron-Van Evercooren, A., Chennoufi, A. B., Seitanidou, T., Babinet, C., and Charnay, P. (1994). Krox-20 controls myelination in the peripheral nervous system. *Nature*, **371,** 796–799.

Toyka, K. V., Zielasek, J., Ricker, K., Adlkofer, K., and Suter, U. (1997). Hereditary neuromyotonia: A mouse model associated with deficiency or increased gene dosage of the PMP22 gene. *J Neurol Neurosurg Psychiatry*, **63,** 812–813.

Umehara, F., Tate, G., Itoh, K., Yamaguchi, N., Douchi, T., Mitsuya, T., and Osame, M. (2000). A novel mutation of desert hedgehog in a patient with 46,XY partial gonadal dysgenesis accompanied by minifascicular neuropathy. *Am J Hum Genet*, **67,** 1302–1305.

Valentijn, L. J., Baas, F., Wolterman, R. A., Hoogendijk, J. E., van den Bosch, N. H., Zorn, I., Gabreels-Festen, A. W., de Visser, M., and Bolhuis, P. A. (1992). Identical point mutations of PMP-22 in Trembler-J mouse and Charcot-Marie-Tooth disease type 1A. *Nat Genet*, **2,** 288–291.

Valentijn, L. J., Ouvrier, R. A., van den Bosch, N. H., Bolhuis, P. A., Baas, F., and Nicholson, G. A. (1995). Dejerine-Sottas neuropathy is associated with a de novo PMP22 mutation. *Hum Mutat*, **5,** 76–80.

Vallat, J. M., Sindou, P., Garbay, B., Preux, P. M., Anani, T., Richard, L., and Diot, M. (1999). Expression of myelin proteins in the adult heterozygous Trembler mouse. *Acta Neuropathol (Berl)*, **98,** 281–287.

Voiculescu, O., Charnay, P., and Schneider-Maunoury, S. (2000). Expression pattern of a Krox-20/Cre knock-in allele in the developing hindbrain, bones, and peripheral nervous system. *Genesis*, **26,** 123–126.

Wang, H., Allen, M. L., Grigg, J. J., Noebels, J. L., and Tempel, B. L. (1995). Hypomyelination alters K+ channel expression in mouse mutants shiverer and Trembler. *Neuron*, **15,** 1337–1347.

Warner, L. E., Hilz, M. J., Appel, S. T., Killian, J. M., Kolodny, E. H., Karpati, G., Carpenter, S., Watters, G. V., Wheeler, C., Witt, D., Bodell, A., Nelis, E., Broeckhoven, C. V., and Lupski, J. R. (1996). Clinical phenotypes of different MPZ (Po) mutations may include Charcot-Marie-Tooth type 1b, Dejerine-Sottas, and Congenital Hypomyelination. *Neuron*, **17,** 451–460.

Warner, L. E., Mancias, P., Butler, I. J., McDonald, C. M., Keppen, L., Koob, K. G., and Lupski, J. R. (1998). Mutations in the early growth response 2 (EGR2) gene are associated with hereditary myelinopathies. *Nat Genet*, **18,** 382–384.

Warner, L. E., Svaren, J., Milbrandt, J., and Lupski, J. R. (1999). Functional consequences of mutations in the early growth response 2 gene (EGR2). correlate with severity of human myelinopathies. *Hum Mol Genet*, **8,** 1245–1251.

Werner, H., Dimou, L., Klugmann, M., Pfeiffer, S., and Nave, K. A. (2001). Multiple splice isoforms of proteolipid M6B in neurons and oligodendrocytes. *Mol Cell Neurosci*, **18,** 593–605.

Willecke, K., Temme, A., Teubner, B., and Ott, T. (1999). Characterization of targeted connexin32-deficient mice: A model for the human Charcot-Marie-Tooth (X-type). inherited disease. *Ann N Y Acad Sci*, **883,** 302–309.

Wilson, H. L., Wilson, S. A., Surprenant, A., and North, R. A. (2002). Epithelial membrane proteins induce membrane blebbing and interact with the P2X7 receptor C-terminus. *J Biol Chem*, in press.

Windebank, A. J. (1993). Inherited recurrent neuropathy. *In* "Peripheral Neuropathy" (P. J. Dyck, P. K. Thomas, J. W. Griffin, P. A. Low, and J. F. Poduslo, eds.), pp. 1094–1136. WB Saunders, Philadelphia.

Wong, M. H., and Filbin, M. T. (1996). Dominant-negative effect on adhesion by myelin Po protein truncated in its cytoplasmic domain. *J. Cell Biol.*, **134,** 1531–1541.

Wrabetz, L., D'Antonio, M., Dati, G., Fratta, P., Previtali, S., Imperiale, D., Zielasek, J., Toyka, K., Messing, A., Feltri, M.-L., and Quattrini, A. (2002). Transgenic mice expressing the CMT1B mutant *Mpz*(delser63). develop demyelinating neuropathy. *2002 Abstract Viewer/Itinerary Planner. Washington, DC: Society for Neuroscience*, **(Online),** Program No. 523.527.

Wrabetz, L., and Feltri, M. L. (2001). Do Schwann cells stop, DR(o)P2, and roll? *Neuron*, **30,** 642–644.

Wrabetz, L., Feltri, M. L., Hanemann, C. O., and Müller, H. W. (2001). The molecular genetics of hereditary demyelinating neuropathies. *In* "Glial Cell Development: Basic Principles and Clinical Relevance" (K. R. Jessen, and W. R. Richardson, eds.), pp. 327–351. Oxford University Press, Oxford.

Wrabetz, L., Feltri, M. L., Quattrini, A., Imperiale, D., Previtali, S., D'Antonio, M., Martini, R., Yin, X., Trapp, B. D., Zhou, L., Chiu, S. Y., and Messing, A. (2000). P(0) glycoprotein overexpression causes congenital hypomyelination of peripheral nerves. *J Cell Biol*, **148,** 1021–1034.

Yin, X., Crawford, T. O., Griffin, J. W., Tu, P., Lee, V. M., Li, C., Roder, J., and Trapp, B. D. (1998). Myelin-associated glycoprotein is a myelin signal that modulates the caliber of myelinated axons. *J Neurosci*, **18,** 1953–1962.

Yin, X., Kidd, G. J., Wrabetz, L., Feltri, M. L., Messing, A., and Trapp, B. D. (2000). Schwann cell myelination requires timely and precise targeting of P(0). protein. *J Cell Biol*, **148,** 1009–1020.

Yoshihara, T., Yamamoto, M., Hattori, N., Misu, K., Mori, K., Koike, H., and Sobue, G. (2002). Identification of novel sequence variants in the neurofilament-light gene in a Japanese population: Analysis of Charcot-Marie-Tooth disease patients and normal individuals. *J Peripher Nerv Syst*, **7,** 221–224.

Zhang, K., and Filbin, M. T. (1998). Myelin Po protein mutated at Cys21 has a dominant-negative effect on adhesion of wild type Po. *J. Neurosci Res.*, **53,** 1–6.

Zhao, C., Takita, J., Tanaka, Y., Setou, M., Nakagawa, T., Takeda, S., Yang, H. W., Terada, S., Nakata, T., Takei, Y., Saito, M., Tsuji, S., Hayashi, Y., and Hirokawa, N. (2001). Charcot-Marie-Tooth disease type 2A caused by mutation in a microtubule motor KIF1Bbeta. *Cell*, **105,** 587–597.

Zhu, Q., Couillard-Despres, S., and Julien, J. P. (1997). Delayed maturation of regenerating myelinated axons in mice lacking neurofilaments. *Exp Neurol*, **148,** 299–316.

Zielasek, J., Martini, R., Suter, U., and Toyka, K. V. (2000). Neuromyotonia in mice with hereditary myelinopathies. *Muscle Nerve*, **23,** 696–701.

Zielasek, J., Martini, R., and Toyka, K. V. (1996). Functional Abnormalities in P-0-Deficient Mice Resemble Human Hereditary Neuropathies Linked to P-0 Gene Mutations. *Muscle & Nerve*, **19,** 946–952.

# Index